Handbook of
Mental Health and Aging

Handbook of
Mental Health and Aging

Second Edition _____

Editors

James E. Birren
Borun Center for
Gerontological Research
University of California,
Los Angeles
Los Angeles, California

R. Bruce Sloane
Department of Psychiatry
University of Southern California
Medical Center
Los Angeles, California

Gene D. Cohen
National Institute on Aging
Bethesda, Maryland

Associate Editors

Nancy R. Hooyman
School of Social Work
University of Washington
Seattle, Washington

Barry D. Lebowitz
National Institute
of Mental Health
Rockville, Maryland

May Wykle
Gerontological Nursing
FPB School of Nursing
Cleveland, Ohio

Editorial Coordinator

Donna E. Deutchman
Borun Center for
Gerontological Research
University of California,
Los Angeles
Los Angeles, California

Academic Press, Inc.
Harcourt Brace Jovanovich, Publishers

San Diego   New York   Boston
London   Sydney   Tokyo   Toronto

Front Cover Photograph: Sculpture of *Old Woman and Young Man* by Gustav Vigeland, Vigeland Sculpture Park, Oslo, Norway.

This book is printed on acid-free paper. ∞

Academic Press, Inc.
1250 Sixth Avenue
San Diego, California 92101

United Kingdom Edition published by
Academic Press Limited
24–28 Oval Road, London NW1 7DX

Library of Congress Cataloging-in-Publication Data

Handbook of mental health and aging / edited by James E. Birren, R. Bruce Sloane, Gene D. Cohen. -- 2nd ed.
   p. cm.
  Includes bibliographical references and index
  ISBN 0-12-101277-8
   1. Geriatric psychiatry--Handbooks, manuals, etc. 2. Aged--Mental health--Handbooks, manuals, etc. 3. Aged--Psychology--Handbooks, manuals, etc. I. Birren, James E. II. Sloane, R. Bruce, date.
III. Cohen, Gene D.
   [DNLM: 1. Aging. 2. Mental Disorders--in old age. WT 150 H2355]
RC451.4.A5H38 1991
618.97'689--dc20
DNLM/DLC
for Library of Congress   91-41083
                                            CIP

PRINTED IN THE UNITED STATES OF AMERICA
92 93 94 95 96 97   HA   9 8 7 6 5 4 3 2 1

Contents

Contributors xv
Preface xix

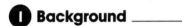 **Background**

1. Concepts and Issues in Mental Health and Aging

Barry D. Lebowitz and George Niederehe

I. Introduction 3
II. A Decade of Research Progress 5
III. A Bio-Psycho-Social Perspective 6
IV. Concepts of Mental Health and Mental Illness 7
V. Intellectual Underpinnings 10
VI. Future Research Issues 13
VII. Service System Policy Dilemmas for the 1990s 16
VIII. Education and the Need for Trained Personnel 20
IX. Conclusion 22
References 23

2. The Epidemiology of Selected Mental Disorders in Later Life

James C. Anthony and Ahmed Aboraya

I. Introduction 28
II. Dementia Syndromes 32
III. Depressive Disorders 41
IV. Panic Disorder 48
V. Phobic Disorders 51
VI. Obsessive-Compulsive Disorders 54
VII. Syndromes of Dependence and Abuse Involving Alcohol and Other Drugs 57
VIII. Summary and Future Directions 63
References 66

3. Culture and Mental Health in Later Life

David Gutmann

I. Introduction: A Field without a Literature   75
II. Fieldwork and the Limitations of Academic Geropsychology   76
III. Culture   78
IV. Deculturation and the Elders   88
References   96

4. Gender and Ethnicity Patterns

E. Percil Stanford and Barbara C. Du Bois

I. Introduction   99
II. Demographic Considerations   100
III. Definitions and Conceptual Underpinnings   102
IV. The Role of Stress, Social Supports, and Coping in Mental Health   105
V. Prevalence of Mental Health Disorders   106
VI. Approaches to Community Mental Health   112
VII. Recommendations for the Future   114
VIII. Summary   114
References   115

5. Adult Life Crises

Morton A. Lieberman and Harvey Peskin

I. Defining Adult Life Crises   120
II. A First Look: Salience of Life Events on Mental Health Consequences   122
III. Adult Life Crises and Psychiatric Disorders   124
IV. Life Crises and Adaptation   128
V. Adult Crisis as Transformative   131
VI. Dynamic Theories of Adult Crises: A Child-Centered versus Adult-Centered View   133
VII. A Cautionary Note   138
VIII. Clinical Aspects of Crisis   138
IX. A Summing Up   140
References   141

ⓘ Neuroscience and Aging

6. Structural Changes in the Aging Brain

Arnold B. Scheibel

I. Introduction   147
II. Historical Evolution of Ideas   148

III. Gross Changes   149
IV. Microscopic Changes   151
V. Changes in the Vascular System   163
VI. Structural Change and Behavioral Change: An Overview   167
References   169

7. Neurochemical Changes with Aging: Predisposition towards Age-Related Mental Disorders
David G. Morgan

I. General Anatomical Changes in the Brain with Normal Aging   175
II. Aging Changes in Synaptic Neurochemistry   178
III. Usual Aging in the Dopamine System, Schizophrenia, and Parkinson's Disease   184
IV. The Interaction of Aging with the Pathological Features of Alzheimer's Disease   187
V. Summary and Conclusions   193
References   194

8. Cerebral Metabolism in Aging and Dementia
Cheryl L. Grady and Stanley I. Rapoport

I. Introduction   201
II. Cerebral Metabolism and Aging   204
III. Dementia of the Alzheimer Type   209
IV. Other Dementias   219
V. Future Directions   221
VI. Summary and Conclusions   222
References   223

9. The Outcomes of Psychiatric Disorder in the Elderly: Relevance to Quality of Life
Barry Gurland and Sidney Katz

I. Centrality of the Quality of Life   230
II. Domains   232
III. Interactions among Domains   238
IV. Needed Developments   242
V. Prospect   245
References   246

III Behavioral Sciences and Aging

10. Aging and the Senses
Frank Schieber

I. Vision 252
II. Hearing 265
III. Taste 278
IV. Olfaction 285
V. Cutaneous Sensitivity 288
VI. Future Considerations 293
References 295

11. Memory, Learning, and Attention
Judith A. Sugar and Joan M. McDowd

I. Introduction 307
II. Memory and Learning 308
III. Attention and Aging 319
IV. Mental Health Issues 326
V. Future Research Directions 330
References 331

12. Intellectual Functioning in Relation to Mental Health
Walter R. Cunningham and Kirsten L. Haman

I. Studies of Structure 340
II. Change in Level 341
III. Extraneous Influences on Intellectual Performance in the Elderly 343
IV. Developing New Tests for the Elderly? 351
References 352

13. Emotion and Personality
Hans Thomae

I. Stability and Change of Emotional and Behavioral Dispositions 356
II. Cognition: Emotion Interactions and Research on Personality and Aging 360
III. Conclusions 371
References 371

Ⅳ Psychopathology of Later Life _____

14. Mood Disorders and Suicide

Harold G. Koenig and Dan G. Blazer

    I. Introduction   380
   II. Classification and Clinical Presentation   380
  III. Epidemiology   383
  IV. Prognosis and Course   384
   V. Differential Diagnosis   386
  VI. Laboratory Evaluation   390
 VII. Management   391
VIII. Suicide   397
     References   400

15. Anxiety and Its Disorders in Old Age

Javaid I. Sheikh

    I. Introduction   410
   II. Epidemiologic Studies   411
  III. Classification and Phenomenology of Anxiety Disorders   413
  IV. Models of Anxiety and Phobias   416
   V. Evaluation of Anxiety   418
  VI. Mixed Anxiety–Depression Syndromes   419
 VII. Anxiety and Medical Illness   420
VIII. Psychological Treatments   422
  IX. Pharmacological Treatments   423
   X. Knowledge Gaps and Future Directions   425
  XI. Conclusion   426
     References   427

16. Personality Disorders in Old Age

Joel Sadavoy and Barry Fogel

    I. Background   433
   II. Classification of Personality Disorders   435
  III. Stability of Personality   435
  IV. Epidemiology of Personality Disorder in Old Age   437
   V. Evolution of Personality Disorder Symptoms with Age   439
  VI. Symptom Expression in the Elderly   441
 VII. Residual and Emergent Personality Disorders   445
VIII. Special Considerations   447

IX. Research Directions   454
       References   457

17. Schizophrenia and Psychotic States

Peter V. Rabins

   I. Schizophrenia   464
  II. Late-Life-Onset Schizophrenia   466
 III. Chronic Schizophrenia with Early-Life Onset   469
 IV. Other Conditions   470
    References   473

18. Alzheimer's Disease and Other Dementing Disorders

Murray A. Raskind and Elaine R. Peskind

    I. Dementia   478
   II. Alzheimer's Disease   478
  III. Dementia in Parkinson's Disease and the Spectrum of Lewy Body
      Diseases   487
  IV. Multi-Infarct Dementia   490
   V. Pick's Disease   492
  VI. Normal-Pressure Hydrocephalus   493
 VII. Metabolic Dementing Disorders   494
VIII. Infectious Dementing Disorders   494
  IX. Alcoholic Dementia   496
   X. Treatment of Secondary Behavioral Problems in Dementia   497
  XI. Dementia and Depression   499
 XII. The Relationship of Depression in Parkinson's Disease to Dementia in
      Parkinson's Disease   501
XIII. Delirium   502
XIV. Conclusion   503
    References   503

19. Alcohol and Substance-Use Disorders in the Elderly

Roland M. Atkinson, Linda Ganzini, and Michael J. Bernstein

   I. Introduction   516
  II. Epidemiology   516
 III. Principles of Assessment and Management   521
 IV. Alcohol-Use Disorders   522
  V. Prescription Psychoactive Drug-Use Disorders   529
 VI. Other Substances   536

VII. Looking Ahead   543
References   545

20. Sleep Disorders and Aging

Carolyn C. Hoch, Daniel J. Buysse, Timothy H. Monk, and Charles F. Reynolds III

I. Introduction   557
II. Sleep and Aging   558
III. Sleep Disturbances   562
IV. Clinical and Laboratory Assessment   573
V. Pharmacologic Treatment Approaches   574
VI. Nonpharmacologic Treatment Approaches   576
VII. Conclusions   576
References   577

21. Aging in Persons with Developmental Disabilities

Marsha Mailick Seltzer

I. Introduction   583
II. Population Characteristics and Demographic Trends   585
III. Age-Related Changes   587
IV. Formal and Informal Supports   590
V. Summary   594
VI. The Need for Future Research: The Mental Health of Older Persons
with Developmental Disabilities   595
References   596

Ⓥ Assessment, Treatment, and Prevention _____

22. Neuropsychiatric Assessment

Eric D. Caine and Hillel T. Grossman

I. Introduction   603
II. Framework for Assessment   605
III. Data Acquisition   608
IV. Differential Diagnosis   625
V. Conclusion of Assessment   636
References   637

23. Neuropsychological Assessment

Asenath La Rue, Janet Yang, and Sheryl Osato

I. Introduction   643
II. Trends in Research and Practice   644

III. Diagnostic Applications 649
IV. Treatment Planning and Evaluation 660
V. Summary and Conclusions 662
   References 663

24. Functional Assessment in Geriatric Mental Health

Bryan J. Kemp and Judith Mitchell

I. The Conceptual Basis of Functional Assessment 672
II. The Effect of Mental Illness on Function 679
III. Functional Assessment Principles 681
IV. Survey of Functional Assessment Instruments 684
V. Discussion and Summary 693
   References 694

25. Behavioral and Psychotherapeutic Interventions

Nancy A. Newton and Lawrence W. Lazarus

I. Introduction 699
II. Establishing the Therapeutic Relationship 700
III. Individual Psychotherapy: Psychodynamic Approaches 702
IV. Individual Psychotherapy: Behavioral Interventions 705
V. Individual Psychotherapy: Empirical Investigations 709
VI. Group Psychotherapy 710
VII. Marital Therapy 712
VIII. Multigenerational Family Therapy 712
IX. Conclusions 714
   References 715

26. Psychopharmacologic Treatment

Carl Salzman and Joyce Nevis-Olesen

I. Overview 722
II. Factors Complicating Prescription of Psychotropic Drugs 723
III. Age-Related Changes in Pharmacologic Drug Effect 729
IV. Psychotropic Treatment of Behavior Disorders, Agitation, and Psychosis 732
V. Treatment of Depression 738
VI. Treatment of Mania 744
VIII. Treatment of Anxiety 745
VIII. Treatment of Sleep Disorders 750
IX. Treatment of Memory Loss and Cognitive Dysfunction 752

X. Summary and Conclusions   755
References   756

27. Environmental Interventions for Cognitively Impaired Older Persons

Victor Regnier and Jon Pynoos

I. Introduction   764
II. Twelve Environment–Behavior Principles   766
III. Application of These Principles to Institutional Environments   769
IV. Home Settings: Strategies for Environmental Management   782
V. Future Directions   789
References   790

28. Community and Home Care for Mentally Ill Older Adults

Linda K. George

I. Need for Mental Health Services: Heterogeneity of the Mentally Ill   794
II. Community-Based Mental Health Services   796
III. Mental Health Service Use   799
IV. Home Care of Mentally Ill Older Adults   804
V. The Interface between Community Care and Home Care   806
VI. Conclusions and Recommendations   809
References   810

29. Mental Health and Aging: Hospital Care—A Nursing Perspective

May H. Wykle, Mary E. Segall, and Stephanie Nagley

I. Background   816
II. Admission of the Geriatric Mental Health Patient   817
III. Specific Behavior Problems in the Older Adult   818
IV. Formal Assessment   825
V. Mental Health Interventions for Hospitalized Aged Persons   826
VI. Summary and Future Research Needs   829
References   829

30. Nursing Home Care

Benjamin Liptzin

I. Background   833
II. Epidemiology of Mental Disorders in Nursing Homes   834

III. Public Policy Issues   848
References   849

31. Forensic and Ethical Issues
Spencer Eth and Gregory B. Leong

I. Competency   854
II. Confidentiality   866
III. Boundary Issues   867
IV. Conclusion   868
References   868

32. Economic Issues and Geriatric Mental Health Care
Gary L. Gottlieb

I. Introduction   873
II. Economic and Health Policy Issues   874
III. The Medicare System   876
IV. Medicaid   883
V. Private Insurance and Out-of-Pocket Expenditures   884
VI. Innovative Delivery Models: Cost Containment and Improved
Access   885
VII. Conclusion   888
References   889

Ⅵ The Future

33. The Future of Mental Health and Aging
Gene D. Cohen

I. Historic Moment in the Field of Mental Health and Aging   894
II. Concepts Shaping the Direction of the Field   895
III. Research on Aging—Relevance to All Age Groups   898
IV. The Significance of Time and the Capacity to Change with
Aging   899
V. Epidemiological Trends in Mental Health and Aging   901
VI. The Mental Health–Physical Health Interface in Later Life   906
VII. Public Policy and Social Values—Lessons from Anthropology   909
VIII. Selected Summary of Mental Health and Aging Trends toward the
Future   910
IX. Conclusion   911
References   912

Author Index   915
Subject Index   981

Contributors

Numbers in parentheses indicate the pages on which the authors' contributions begin.

Ahmed Aboraya (27), Fellow, Psychiatric Epidemiology and Aging, The Johns Hopkins University, Baltimore, Maryland 21205

James C. Anthony (27), Department of Mental Hygiene, The Johns Hopkins University, Baltimore, Maryland 21205

Roland M. Atkinson (515), Veterans Affairs Medical Center, Portland, Oregon 97201, and Department of Psychiatry, School of Medicine, Oregon Health Sciences University, Portland, Oregon 97201

Michael J. Bernstein (515), Veterans Affairs Medical Center, Portland, Oregon 97201, and Department of Psychiatry, School of Medicine, Oregon Health Sciences University, Portland, Oregon 97201

Dan G. Blazer (379), Department of Psychiatry, Duke University Medical Center, Durham, North Carolina 27705

Daniel J. Buysse (557), Fleet Evaluation Center, Pittsburgh, Pennsylvania 15213

Eric D. Caine (603), UR-NIMH Clinical Research Center for the Study of Psychopathology of the Elderly, Department of Psychiatry, University of Rochester School of Medicine and Dentistry, Rochester, New York 14642

Gene D. Cohen (893), National Institute on Aging, Bethesda, Maryland 20892

Walter R. Cunningham (339), Department of Psychology, University of Florida, Gainesville, Florida 32611

Barbara C. Du Bois (99), University Center on Aging, College of Health and Human Services, San Diego State University, San Diego, California 92182

Spencer Eth (853), Department of Psychiatry and Biobehavioral Sciences, School of Medicine, University of California, Los Angeles, California 90024, and Psychiatry Service, West Los Angeles Veterans Affairs Medical Center, Los Angeles, California 90073

Barry Fogel (433), Center for Gerontology and Health Care Research, Brown University, Providence, Rhode Island 02912

Linda Ganzini (515), Veterans Affairs Medical Center, Portland, Oregon 97201, and Department of Psychiatry, School of Medicine, Oregon Health Sciences University, Portland, Oregon 97201

Linda K. George (793), Department of Psychiatry and Center for the Study of Aging, Duke University Medical Center, Durham, North Carolina 27710

Gary L. Gottlieb (873), Department of Geriatric Psychiatry, Hospital of the University of Pennsylvania, Leonard Davis Institute of Health Economics, Philadelphia, Pennsylvania 19104

Cheryl L. Grady (201), Laboratory of Neurosciences, National Institute on Aging, Bethesda, Maryland 20892

Hillel T. Grossman (603), UR-NIMH Clinical Research Center for the Study of Psychopathology of the Elderly, Department of Psychiatry, University of Rochester School of Medicine and Dentistry, Rochester, New York 14642

Barry Gurland (229), Center for Geriatrics and Gerontology, Columbia University Faculty of Medicine, New York State Office of Mental Health, New York, New York 10032

David Gutmann (75), Institute of Psychiatry, Northwestern University, Chicago, Illinois 60611

Kirsten L. Haman (339), Department of Psychology, University of Florida, Gainesville, Florida 32611

Carolyn C. Hoch (557), Fleet Evaluation Center, Pittsburgh, Pennsylvania 15213

Sidney Katz (229), Columbia University Faculty of Medicine, New York State Office of Mental Health, New York, New York 10032

Bryan J. Kemp (671), Clinical Gerontology Service, Rancho Los Amigos Medical Center, Downey, California 90242, and Rehabilitation Research and Training Center on Aging, Departments of Psychiatry and Family Medicine and Gerontology, University of Southern California, Los Angeles, California 90007

Harold G. Koenig (379), Department of Psychiatry, Duke University Medical Center, Durham, North Carolina 27705

Asenath La Rue (643), Department of Psychiatry and Behavioral Sciences, University of California, Los Angeles, California 90024

Lawrence W. Lazarus (699), Rush Medical School, Chicago, Illinois 60612

Barry D. Lebowitz (3), National Institute of Mental Health, Rockville, Maryland 20857

Gregory B. Leong (853), Department of Psychiatry and Biobehavioral Sciences, School of Medicine, University of California, Los Angeles, and Psychiatry Service, West Los Angeles Veterans Affairs Medical Center, Los Angeles, California 90073

Morton A. Lieberman (119), Center for Social Sciences, University of California, San Francisco, San Francisco, California 94143

Benjamin Liptzin (833), Tufts University School of Medicine, Boston, Massachusetts, and Baystate Medical Center, Springfield, Massachusetts 01199

Joan M. McDowd (307), Department of Psychology, University of Southern California, Los Angeles, California 90089

Judith Mitchell (671), Rehabilitation Research and Training Center on Aging, School of Family Medicine, University of Southern California, Los Angeles, California 90007

Timothy H. Monk (557), Fleet Evaluation Center, Pittsburgh, Pennsylvania 15213

David G. Morgan (175), Division of Neurogerontology and Department of Biological Sciences, University of Southern California, Los Angeles, California 90089

Stephanie Nagley (815), Frances Payne Bolton School of Nursing, Case Western Reserve University, Cleveland, Ohio 44106

Joyce Nevis-Olesen (721), Harvard Medical School—Affiliated Teaching Hospitals, Boston, Massachusetts 02115

Nancy A. Newton (699), Chicago School of Professional Psychology, Chicago, Illinois 60605

George Niederehe (3), National Institute of Mental Health, Rockville, Maryland 20857

Sheryl Osato (643), Geropsychiatry Service, West Los Angeles VA Medical Center, Brentwood Division, Los Angeles, California 90024

Harvey Peskin (119), San Francisco State University, San Francisco, California 94143

Elaine R. Peskind (477), Department of Psychiatry and Behavioral Sciences, University of Washington, School of Medicine, Seattle, Washington 98195

Jon Pynoos (763), Andrus Gerontology Center, University of Southern California, Los Angeles, California 90089

Peter V. Rabins (463), Department of Psychiatry and Behavioral Sciences, Johns Hopkins School of Medicine, Baltimore, Maryland 21205

Stanley I. Rapoport (201), Laboratory of Neurosciences, National Institute on Aging, Bethesda, Maryland 20892

Murray A. Raskind (477), Department of Psychiatry and Behavioral Sciences, University of Washington, School of Medicine, Seattle, Washington 98195

Victor Regnier (763), Departments of Architecture and Gerontology, University of Southern California, Los Angeles, California 90089

Charles F. Reynolds III (557), Fleet Evaluation Center, Pittsburgh, Pennsylvania 15213

Joel Sadavoy (433), Department of Psychiatry, University of Toronto, Baycrest Centre for Geriatric Care, Toronto, Ontario M6A 2E1, Canada

Carl Salzman (721), Department of Psychopharmacology, Harvard Medical School, Massachusetts Mental Health Center, Boston, Massachusetts 02115

Arnold B. Scheibel (147), Departments of Anatomy and Cell Biology, Psychiatry, and Brain Research Institute, University of California, Los Angeles, Medical Center, Los Angeles, California 90024

Frank Schieber (251), Department of Psychology, Oakland University, Rochester, Michigan 48309

Mary E. Segall (815), Frances Payne Bolton School of Nursing, Case Western Reserve University, Cleveland, Ohio 44106

Marsha Mailick Seltzer (583), University of Wisconsin, Madison, and Waisman Center, Madison, Wisconsin 53705

Javaid I. Sheikh (409), Department of Psychiatry and Behavioral Sciences, Stanford University School of Medicine, Stanford, California 94305

E. Percil Stanford (99), University Center on Aging, College of Health and Human Services, San Diego State University, San Diego, California 92182

Judith A. Sugar (307), Department of Psychology, Colorado State University, Fort Collins, Colorado 80523

Hans Thomae (355), Department of Psychology, Langemarck 387, University of Bonn, 5300 Bonn 3, Germany

May H. Wykle (815), Frances Payne Bolton School of Nursing, Case Western Reserve University, Cleveland, Ohio 44106

Janet Yang (643), Department of Psychiatry and Behavioral Sciences, University of California, Los Angeles, Los Angeles, California 90024

Preface

The first edition of the *Handbook of Mental Health and Aging* was published in 1980. Supported by the National Institute of Mental Health, the first edition aimed to survey a subject matter that was predicted to grow in significance. That prediction has proved to be correct; the subject matter has grown enormously since the first edition. A dramatic increase in the population of older persons has focused international attention on the well-being of older persons—their mental and physical health. Advances in medicine and increases in longevity have presented new concerns in the area of mental health and aging, for example, how to treat the new and burgeoning population of persons with developmental disabilities who are surviving into late life. Increasing life expectancy and trends towards earlier retirement have meant that many people can expect to survive almost two decades past retirement. Maintaining mental health and productivity during this period is of critical importance.

In the scientific and professional communities there has been a marked increase in research and an exponential growth in published literature. This is not evidence that the mental health of older persons has improved, only that we are better equipped to study its many aspects. This top-down view of the subject matter suggests that improvements can follow if training of qualified personnel also becomes a higher priority in our professions and sciences. However, the number of personnel devoted to study and service in mental health and aging remains very small. While devoted primarily to the understanding of phenomena of mental health and aging, we hope that this volume will contribute to an improvement in the mental life of older adults and in the quality of life for the growing millions of older persons.

The purpose of this *Handbook* is to provide authoritative reviews and reference sources to the scientific and professional literature on mental health and aging. It is intended to be a definitive reference work for professional personnel, researchers, and advanced students. The chapters describe the changes in mental well-being that can occur with advancing age as a result of many influences: biological, social, and behavioral.

Mental health of the older population is a function of many aspects of modern society: family life, caregivers, community and institutional care, ethnic and sociocultural differences, and urbanization, among many other influences. The subject matter appears as broad as the content of life itself; in fact, one might argue that mental health is about the content and processes of life. If so, then the agenda for services, training, research, and scholarship must be broad. In turn, the content of this volume is necessarily broad but also reports in depth on the many facets of human life in the later adult years.

There is "regional intellectual" prosperity shown in the growth of many new specialty journals. Since the first edition, an International Psychogeriatric Association has been founded that organizes international meetings and publishes a journal, *International Psychogeriatrics*. The American Psychological Association in the past decade began the publication of *Psychology and Aging,* and many other new relevant journals are appearing. Examples include the *International Journal of Geriatric Psychiatry* and *Alzheimer's Disease and Associated Disorders*. This activity is healthy and promotes an air of optimism about the future of the subject matter.

This *Handbook* assumes the task of keeping an integrated view of mental health. As we learn more about difficult phenomena of aging (e.g., Alzheimer's Disease, behavioral genetics, and memory), there is a tendency to split the subject matter into subspecialities that have less intercommunication. This volume is intended to provide a place where all of the pieces are fitted together, however provisionally. The editors have encouraged efforts to consolidate information about mental health and aging during a time of furious expansion of knowledge about brain, behavior, and well-being. They are grateful to the many excellent authors for meeting this challenge.

We hope that this book will provide the background and motivation to stimulate future research, scholarship, and services in this important area of human concern.

We are grateful to the Anna and Harry Borun Foundation for support of the senior editor. We also gratefully acknowledge the work of Lisa Dieckmann, who undertook the painstaking task of indexing this volume. Finally, we acknowledge the unfailing efforts of Alieh Mehri Eslami and Emily Zoller; without their administrative expertise the present volume would not have been possible.

Background

۲

1

Concepts and Issues in Mental Health and Aging _____

Barry D. Lebowitz and George Niederehe

    I. Introduction
   II. A Decade of Research Progress
  III. A Bio-Psycho-Social Perspective
  IV. Concepts of Mental Health and Mental Illness
      A. Norms and Abnormality
      B. Controllability and the Labeling of Abnormality as a Disease
      C. Positive Mental Health
    V. Intellectual Underpinnings
      A. Major Themes
      B. Time Dimensions
      C. Negative Age Stereotypes
   VI. Future Research Issues
      A. Likely Trends
      B. Research Needs and Key Issues
  VII. Service System Policy Dilemmas for the 1990s
      A. Mental Health Service Use
      B. Primary Care and Mental Health
      C. Family Support and the Caregiver at Risk
      D. Long-Term Care
      E. Disability
      F. Too Old, Too Sick
 VIII. Education and the Need for Trained Personnel
   IX. Conclusion
      References

I. Introduction _____

In the ten years that have followed upon publication of the first edition of this *Handbook,* the field of mental health and aging has undergone steady evolution, not the least of which

Handbook of Mental Health and Aging, Second Edition
Copyright © 1992 by Academic Press, Inc. All rights of reproduction in any form reserved.

has stemmed from the continuing demographic growth and transformation in characteristics of the generation of individuals now elderly. In terms of research, very significant advances have been made in our capacity to characterize, understand, and treat mental disorders among the aged. Changes in the mental health service system to improve care for the elderly population have not, however, tended to keep pace with this overall record of scientific progress.

In this chapter, our primary purpose is to provide an overview of the current status of the field. As such, we break no new ground; rather, we synthesize and appraise an accumulation of knowledge and experience from the recent decade of work in mental health and aging. We also review a number of fundamental concepts, note various areas of progress, and highlight particular issues of special or continuing importance for the field. In doing so, we acknowledge the significant contribution of Birren and Renner (1980) in the first edition of this *Handbook.* In many ways this chapter constitutes an update of that earlier chapter, and the reader is referred to that document for its exposition of the historical and conceptual background of the field.

Our scope in this chapter is broad rather than deep, and selective rather than encyclopedic. We have attempted to address only a limited number of concerns for which sufficient information has accumulated over the past decade to allow either a more precise delineation of research questions or further specification of conclusions. Though our selection of topics may thus represent a blueprint for consideration and potential action, as with any blueprint, the outcomes to be anticipated from implementation remain highly tentative and subject to influence from a variety of forces.

The mental disorders of late life are widespread and serious and have pervasive effects on older persons and those who are close to them. In later chapters in this *Handbook,* the full scope of these disorders will be presented. It is clear from examining the data in these chapters on the prevalence and distribution of the mental disorders that much remains to be learned about risk factors, predictors of treatment response, and the general burdens of disability and dysfunction in the present cohorts of older persons as well as those to come in the future. Nonetheless, these data also belie most of the typical cliches about mental disorders in the elderly. Old age is not inevitably a period of successive losses—a view that has led many to assume, falsely, that mental illness occurs with a disproportionately high prevalence among the elderly. Nor is aging so characterized by a process of natural selection or survival of the fittest that one can assume that mental illness is uncommonly rare among the surviving elderly. Differences among age groups in prevalence rates appear more likely to be reflective of cohort differences than they are of aging effects.

As will be addressed at greater depth in later chapters, however, accurate recognition of the pervasiveness of late-life mental disorders needs to be matched with a corresponding sense of their treatability, rather than viewed with therapeutic pessimism. Though research is always needed to further specify the nature, applicability, and limitations of treatment, over the past decade we have witnessed the emergence of a broad array of efficacious pharmacologic, somatic, and psychotherapeutic strategies for treatment of late-life mental disorders and management of associated symptoms. This broad therapeutic armamentarium, now accessible to clinicians in a variety of settings and systems, represents one of the great stories of success and accomplishment in the field, and the systematic and cumulative body of knowledge underlying it deserves widespread recognition and application.

II. A Decade of Research Progress

The broad topic of mental health and aging extends to almost all areas of contemporary research in the biological, clinical, behavioral, and psychosocial areas. This wide domain is currently experiencing an excitement and a burst of scientific creativity not previously seen; it promises to advance markedly our understanding of the field.

The past decade has seen mental health issues brought to the forefront of gerontological and geriatric discussion and, conversely, has seen aging issues being examined by those in the mental health field. These developments are made all the more striking when viewed in the context of the tremendous gains in a number of areas of basic science such as fundamental neuroscience, mechanisms of cognitive and intellectual function, and social network theory.

Research progress in the last decade has been substantial. Using the latest approaches and conceptualizations in basic neurobiology, scientists have identified the processes by which nerve cells change to create pathology. In addition, using high-powered imaging techniques, investigators have developed methods for directly studying the brain and for linking functional abnormalities with structural lesions. Progress in understanding the nature and progression of Alzheimer's disease has been particularly notable.

Research in epidemiology has highlighted the growing significance of age of onset. Clinical research has identified features of depression and schizophrenia that can be used to distinguish late-onset disease from that exhibited by patients who developed these diseases earlier in life.

The approaches of psychoneuroimmunology have been used to demonstrate the mutual reinforcement of psychosocial and neurobiological factors in morbidity and mortality. This research has been instrumental in allowing us to move beyond the individual patient and to highlight the consequences of long-term caregiving for the spouses and other family members of patients with Alzheimer's disease and other chronic conditions.

Well-controlled clinical trials of pharmacologic, psychotherapeutic, and combined treatments that have been launched in the last decade have resulted in the establishment of validated treatment protocols in a number of major disorders. Longitudinal methods have made possible increased attention to issues of clinical course and outcome of disease and have demonstrated the need for continuation and maintenance treatment following the acute treatment phase. Long-term symptom management has emerged as a major focus of concern and, along with this, issues around appropriate systems of care and the need for changes in the methods of payment and reimbursement have emerged as primary.

Thus, developments in basic science and clinical investigation are providing a firm base for treatment and prevention of the major mental disorders among the aged. Directions for future research are clearly established. This rich body of scientific achievement has developed a significant momentum with an ever-increasing pace of achievement and development.

At the same time, important developments in methodology have provided the impetus for creative and sophisticated theory building. These developments have made it possible to make more precise characterizations and examine increasingly complex models of the phenomena of interest in this field. In doing so, the artificial distinctions between disciplines have been pushed aside, and attention to the mutual reinforcement of biological, clinical, behavioral, and psychosocial factors in mental health and mental illness has become a central part of the methodology of choice in complex, multidisciplinary studies.

III. A Bio-Psycho-Social Perspective

Mental disorders including the dementias, particularly in the elderly, are bio-psycho-social phenomena (Kahn, 1971; Wang & Busse, 1971), and their understanding requires the integration of biological, psychological, social, and environmental perspectives and factors. Furthermore, aging-related developments in each of these spheres influence outcomes. However, aging also seems to reduce the degree of differentiation that can actually be observed among these subsystems of influences. Many prior discussions of this topic have indicated the importance of differentiating biological, psychological, and social processes of aging.

The individual's state of physical health and other biological factors are generally more telling influences on mental health than is the person's chronological age. Both in clinical treatment and research, patterns of mental illness in the aged must be referenced against the individual's physical health, consumption of medications, the possibility of undetected underlying diseases, and the like. Conditions such as arthritis, hypertension, and cardiovascular disease particularly influence the degree of mental and functional disability.

Among psychological factors, prior personality is thought to have a major effect on both vulnerability to mental disorder and on the *choice* of symptoms displayed when psychologically distressed, suggesting the importance of the study of lives in improving understanding of late-life mental disorders. On one hand, much research indicates remarkable stability in personality over time, suggesting that factors such as long-term neuroticism merit greater attention as psychological factors implicated in late-life disorders (Costa, 1985). On the other hand, disordered behavior in the aged may represent exacerbations or the going astray of psychological changes that develop as part of normal aging. For example, hypochondriasis may be the manifestation of too great a swing toward the *body monitoring* that quite generally increases in later life, beginning in middle age (Neugarten, 1970). Other psychiatric disorders can equally be viewed as elaborations on other psychological shifts that are quite universal with age, such as change in time perspectives, increased interiority or introspection, personalization of death, or efforts at achieving ego integrity rather than despair in the face of increasing physical limitations. In addition, individuals' perceptions of control over their situations (whether objective or not) are very predictive of their situational adjustment (Rodin & Langer, 1980).

Objective situational factors also become increasingly powerful influences with age, particularly with decline in the individual's physical and cognitive abilities for coping with the ever-present demands of their *environmental press*. This has been described as the principal of *environmental docility* (Lawton & Nahemow, 1973), and is particularly important in considering the functional adjustment of those elderly persons with physical and cognitive disabilities, such as those residing in nursing homes. Family elements of the social environment are especially salient in mental health. For example, marital status has major effects—not well understood—on the prevalence of mental disorders.

IV. Concepts of Mental Health and Mental Illness _____

Like aging, mental health is a multifaceted concept that refers more clearly to a field of research and clinical activity than to a unitary theoretical entity. Though any number of definitions may be (and have been) offered, we prefer an operational approach and opt to emphasize here simply that most attempts to define the concept combine in complex fashion several elements: statistical normality, relationship of individual functioning to group or species norms, controllability or treatability of disordered states, and ideals of positive functioning. The conceptual background for mental health constructs within gerontology has been discussed extensively by Birren and Renner (1980). Conventional operational definitions of mentally disordered states are provided by such current diagnostic systems as the revised third edition of the *Diagnostic and Statistical Manual of Mental Disorders* (DSM-III-R; American Psychiatric Association, 1987) or the International Classification of Diseases (ICD-9) of the World Health Organization, as well as by observer rating and self-report measures of various symptoms and traits commonly used in the mental health research field. Operational definitions of positive mental health are less well established.

Mental health phenomena emerge from the interplay of multiple contributing subsystems, and require multisystemic thinking to be understood. Some theorists hold, furthermore, that problems build to become major mental disorders only over a lengthy time course and following a process in which interpersonal problems are transmitted between generations within families (e.g., Bowen, 1978) or as the individual passes through various developmental life stages.

A. Norms and Abnormality

Although varying contributory factors may be emphasized in terms of etiology, in general we identify mental disorder initially in behavioral terms, e.g., an individual behaves deviantly, acting, thinking, or communicating in ways that break the norms of socially acceptable behavior, or living in styles that are maladjusted relative to expectations in his or her community or culture. The normality component within mental health, which can be understood only by contrast with the corresponding concept of mental disorder, implies an underlying statistical dimension along which atypical behavior is differentiated in its frequency from that which is commonplace. Normality in terms of biological functioning is determined largely in terms of what is biologically typical of the species, or within typical physiological limits (Birren & Renner, 1980). The normality of social behavior tends to be defined in terms of not only frequency but also conformity with customs and norms. Based on the assumption that most people abide by the norms, behavior that is conventional is apt to be statistically normal as well.

The link between abnormal behavior and norms is thus close and inherent. Our everyday understanding of behavior is rooted in norms (rules for behavior that are accepted by members of a society via convention). In our modern Western culture, a behavioral pattern is typically explained as acceptably rational in one of two primary ways, both traceable to underlying cultural concepts deeply embedded in our language—either by pointing out that the behavior is conventional (most people typically do the same under similar circumstances) or, if it departs from normative expectations, by proffering other evidence suggesting that the individual had a specific goal-directed intent or motive (Peters, 1958). Psychoanalytic theorists such as Freud expanded the consideration of goal-directed behavior by introducing the concept of unconscious as well as conscious motives. Unconventional behavior is most likely to be judged abnormal or deviant from a mental health–method illness perspective when (1) it deviates from norms that describe aspects of social behavior or biological functioning that are very highly valued and desirable; (2) the degree of deviation or norm-breaking is great; and (3) the deviation does not seem linked to socially acceptable goals.

Both in psychiatry and in behavioral and biological sciences, distinctions are made between several differing ways of failing to satisfy norms. Forms of behavior that are deficient relative to standards regarding expected levels of performance may be termed deficits or *negative symptoms*. These differ greatly in meaning from so-called dysfunctions or *positive symptoms*, the presence of alternative behaviors that are inconsistent with or actively contravene norms. Still other patterns develop from the interplay of positive symptoms and deficits (e.g., positive symptoms often represent secondary attempts to cope with or compensate for primary deficits).

Broader issues about the age stratification and organization of norms within society may make recognition of deviant behavior by the elderly more difficult than that of younger adults. Some have argued that the disengagement (or disenfranchisement) of the aged from former social roles leaves this age group relatively roleless, with a lack of social norms to define the boundaries of appropriate behavior (Kuypers & Bengtson, 1973; Rosow, 1985). Against such a backdrop of role loss and status changes, it may be difficult to ascertain problem conditions that manifest themselves in deviant behavior.

In recent years, conventional diagnostic standards in psychiatry (such as DSM-III-R) have increasingly emphasized the degree of interference with the individual's normal roles as a criterion for judging symptomatic conditions as mental disorders. This convention can be problematic in the absence of work and occupational features in the individual's life, as is typical of most older adults. In this context, judgments of symptomatic interference are commonly reduced to whether the person can carry out the most basic everyday functions, or the so-called activities of daily living (ADLs). Other more subtle disruptions may be more difficult to define clearly in the aged, retired individual (Linn, 1988).

B. Controllability and the Labeling of Abnormality as a Disease

All societies develop and institutionalize both legal–political and extralegal means of counteracting and controlling deviant behavior, mimimizing its potentially disruptive impact on the social order and maintaining established norms for acceptable behavior (Parsons, 1964). Our modern society understands forms of deviant behavior that appear both unmotivated and outside the legal–political sphere mainly according to a metaphor of disease or illness, and considers their control a responsibility of the health profession, broadly speaking.[1] Most health professionals thus tend to be concerned primarily with problematic aspects of mental health, and to label the conditions dealt with as diseases, disorders, or at least *syndromes*. For practical purposes, this labeling can be seen as synonymous with identifying the labeled problems as within the profession's purview.

Experience in other fields suggests that as knowledge of the mental health issues of aging expands, more disease states will be identified. Since human conditions tend to be defined as diseases when professional means are available to treat or otherwise deal with them effectively, as knowledge of various problem areas grows and avenues for potential intervention increase, so does the likelihood that these problems will be labeled diseases (Englehardt, 1979). Conversely, normal aging tends to be treated as a residual category of change processes that are not amenable to professional treatment or control.

C. Positive Mental Health

Mental health is a broader notion than simply the absence of mental disorder. It implies in addition that the individual functions in desirably positive ways, manifesting some aspects of the ideal of health (even though complete attainment of the ideal may be atypical in a statistical sense). A subjective sense of well-being (as defined by such related notions as happiness, good morale, and life satisfaction) is one of the prominent features. Other aspects of positive mental health include positive self-attitudes, growth and self-actualization, integration of the personality, autonomy, reality perception, and environmental mastery (Jahoda, 1958). Since each of these criteria can be viewed on a continuum, an individual's overall mental health should not be considered only as the absence of the abnormal, but must also be treated as a matter of degree or trend toward the ideal.

At the clinical level, we need a balanced consideration of patients' strengths as well as weaknesses or symptoms. For example, when doing neuropsychological or mental status assessments, clinicians must not attend only to the evidence of cognitive deterioration, assuming this to be inevitable with age, but also must identify the aspects of the person's functioning that imply his or her potential for productive intellectual activity. More generally, whereas there has too often been a prevailing assumption of inevitable disease and deterioration with age, increasingly clinicians and researchers are recognizing the importance of attending to perspectives that emphasize the older person's continuing psychological growth and maturity and potential for positive mental health (Cohen, this volume; Gutmann, 1982).

---

[1] It has not always been so. For example, in earlier eras when the church was the prevailing social institution, abnormal behavior was typically viewed according to a metaphor of sinfulness and handled by ecclesiastical personnel (Szasz, 1970).

V. Intellectual Underpinnings

A. Major Themes

Five themes combine to create a unique characterization of the subject matter of mental health and aging. These are

The gerontological revolution, brought about by improvement in public health and life style, and resulting in increases in active life expectancy and reductions in age-specific mortality. These, in turn, result in large numbers of healthy people staying well throughout most of their lives until risk factors accumulate to the point of disease and disability. Late-life diseases—with the prototype being Alzheimer's disease, but also including late-onset forms of anxiety and affective disorders, psychotic disorders, and perhaps personality disorders—constitute the general framework of concern with this question (Manton, 1990; Myers, 1990).

The geriatric revolution, brought about by the same dynamic that produced the gerontological revolution, but applied in this instance to persons with chronic disease or disability developed at birth or during early adulthood. The extension of life for those with Down's syndrome and other developmental disabilities and of those with schizophrenia are the prime examples of this phenomenon (Kramer, 1980).

Senescence or normal processes of development and change in biological, psychological, cognitive, and behavioral systems. These provide an important backdrop for recognizing and understanding pathology in late life. Age-related changes have been documented in nervous system structure and function, vision, hearing, gastrointestinal function, the musculoskeletal system, and many others (Schneider & Rowe, 1990; Birren & Schaie, 1990).

Comorbidity of physical illness and mental disorder is also common—significantly more so in geriatrics than in the adult population where disorders are much more likely to be seen alone. For example, depression is a common feature of stroke and Parkinson's disease, and anxiety is frequently seen accompanying gastrointestinal, cardiovascular, and pulmonary disease. Many commonly used medications affect mood or cognition. Since many medical illnesses can present with psychiatric, cognitive, emotional, and behavioral components, and since many age-related changes also influence these same issues, the tasks of diagnosis, treatment selection and response, and outcome are all especially complex and difficult in clinical approaches to the geriatric patient (Cohen, 1988).

Each of these features combines with the well-established *heterogeneity* of the population (by age, gender, race, ethnicity, etc.) to complete the overall background prospective on the area of aging and mental health.

These five characteristics combine to influence the presentation, course, response to treatment, and outcome of major mental disorders and combine as well to influence psychological development and the promotion of positive mental health.

B. Time Dimensions

Analytically, it is important to distinguish three uses of *age* or time dimensions with specific reference to mental disorders in the aged. We will speak, therefore, of *age of the patient, age of onset,* and *age of the disorder.* As indicated by Schaie's (1965) analysis of analogous constructs in developmental research, these notions are so inherently linked (or confounded) that it is not possible to treat all three simultaneously as independent variables. By determining or fixing any two of the three, the third is already determined.

Most obvious, perhaps, is the age of the patient, a notion that in the elderly implies certain probable maturational features in terms of both biological senescence and experiential stage of life. The comorbidity theme mentioned above is linked with age of the patient. For example, the aged show frequent comorbidity of Alzheimer's disease and depression and anxiety, and many medical illnesses present with anxietylike, dementialike, and depressionlike symptoms.

Furthermore, the dynamics of symptomatic presentation and course of disorders may differ in the elderly. For example, though mental health personnel tend to understand the basic processes and principles of depression similarly in younger and older adults, certain symptom patterns do appear to become more common with age. The elderly depressed individual may more likely complain of physical problems, but be less apt to acknowledge mood changes.

The young-old versus old-old distinction (Neugarten, 1974) is also crucial to determining mental health priorities among the aged. Numerous factors in combination appear to indicate that the physical changes and diseases of aging take their toll on mental functioning predominantly after age 75, so that disabilities are highly clustered in increasingly older age groups.

Among the most important, but frequently forgotten, distinctions among mental disorders within the elderly population, is that between those developing for the first time in late life (which thus are appropriately termed geriatric in origin) and those that developed for the first time earlier in life and have endured or reemerged. A critical intellectual question is whether age of onset has major clinical significance. For example, is depression first appearing in late life the same disorder as the depression that appears earlier? Is the clinical presentation the same? Should treatment strategies by similar? These questions also have important implications for our understanding of the brain and of basic brain–behavioral relationships.

There appear to be numerous differences between the patients showing early- or late-onset forms of various disorders (particularly in coping resources and prognosis for recovery). Age of onset has been highlighted as significant in certain disorders (depression and schizophrenia), but has been downplayed in others (Alzheimer's disease and related dementias). The course of illness is highly variable in older persons with early-onset disease: the positive symptoms of schizophrenia become less prominent, while the negative symptoms become more prominent; suicide becomes a greater and more direct risk. Symptomatology may reach high levels while rates of diagnosed disease have low prevalence, as in depression.

In terms of the third concept, age or chronicity of the disorder, the applicability to the aged cannot be denied of the ubiquitous behavioral principle that *past is prologue* (Busse & Pfeiffer, 1977), or that the best predictor of future behavior is past behavior. Accordingly, for those individuals for whom mental problems have been a long-standing or recurrent matter across the life cycle, the chronicity of the problems often assumes greater importance than the age of the patient. The difficulty of treating these problems needs to be clearly conceptualized as a function of the tendency forged by repetition to perseverate in long-standing behavior patterns rather than as a property of chronological age or life stage as such. An interesting question among those with chronic mental illnesses, however, is whether aging is associated with symptomatic *burnout* or remission in some disorders (Miller & Cohen, 1987).

A final time-dimensional notion to be considered here is that of age cohorts.[2] There are major difficulties in concluding from the available information on mental disorders what aspects are aging-related versus what are historically specific to the generations now old, and those now younger. This is particularly true in terms of patterns of help-seeking and service use. It has long been anticipated that, as the cohort of those in the late stages of life becomes increasingly well-educated and affluent, becomes a group who has been informed about and has held lifelong acceptance of a positive belief system about mental health, use of mental health services by the aged may increase dramatically. For example, whereas the median education of the aged in 1952 was only 8.2 years, by 1990 it has been expected to be about 12 years. Similarly, many believe that the rates of various mental disorders may characterize different generations in fairly stable ways; thus, the pattern that currently younger generations show higher rates of depression may presage high rates in the future when these generations reach their old age.

C. Negative Age Stereotypes

Though considerable enlightenment and improvement in attitudes have occurred in recent years, the mental health of the aged remains an area rife with negative stereotypes about the aging process. The necessity of resisting and counteracting these misconceptions and the resulting age discriminations is likely to continue to be a motive force shaping many efforts within the geriatric mental health field.

Even the field of gerontology is not exempt from the influence of such myths and misconceptions. Any piece of research rests upon assumptions and implicit definitions about growing old. As already mentioned, research in the mental health and aging area has tended to reflect predominantly negative expectations about the aging process—a decremental or catastrophic model of aging that assumes decline is inevitable.

At the same time, misconceptions may also color researchers' views of the social contexts in which older adults actually live, and to which their problems may be erroneously attributed. For example, one viewpoint has been that many of the mental health problems of the aged stem simply from the neglect of older persons by younger generations. While, as in all myths, there are elements of truth to this viewpoint, the weight of the evidence available fails to document such neglect or to support it as a major explanation for mental disorders in the aged. In particular, the notion that younger family members abandon their mentally impaired older relatives or "dump" them readily into nursing homes, though repeatedly debunked, has proven to be a hydra-headed myth that is very difficult to dispel (Shanas, 1979).

---

[2]Conceptually, though not always empirically, differentiable within this category are the notions of generation effects versus historical period effects (Bengtson, Cutler, Mangen, & Marshall, 1985; Maddox & Campbell, 1985).

VI. Future Research Issues _____

Research in mental health and aging in the next decade probably will, and should, expand on major trends that have developed over recent years. At the same time, we anticipate and wish to encourage increasing research attention to certain key issues and to gaps in the knowledge base that have gone relatively unnoticed among recent efforts. We turn now to a brief consideration of the elements we would place high on the future research agenda for the field. While we suspect that the field's progress will depend strongly on the degree of scientific advance that is achieved in these areas, we acknowledge both that the list is far from exhaustive and that the difficulties to be addressed in some areas may mean that progress will be slow to develop, even given a substantial infusion of research resources. Following consideration of these research issues, we take up in the next section a series of service system dilemmas that will also benefit from research attention, but for which the ultimate resolution will have to be reached at a public policy level.

A. Likely Trends

Undoubtedly, research advances in mental health and aging will continue to capitalize on new developments in neurosciences, computer technology, and other basic scientific and technological fields. The fact that scientific knowledge about fundamental mechanisms in geriatric mental health has expanded dramatically over recent years should mean that increasing attention will be paid to practical applications of this knowledge base in the years ahead. An example of this trend can be seen in the field of aging and sleep research, where increasing scientific understanding of the salience of such phenomena as sleep apnea and myoclonus among aging-related sleep changes has fostered exploration of selective treatment approaches to these aspects of disturbed sleep (Vitiello & Prinz, 1988). Linkages of sleep disorders to mental health issues such as disturbed sleep in dementia syndromes and depressive disorders are also being investigated (Reynolds *et al.,* 1988).

Though some have felt that recent emphasis on neuroscientific advances has detracted from commensurate attention to the context of mental illness, creating a danger of neglect of social and cultural factors, in fact a number of such issues are coming increasingly to the fore and are likely to be the subject of considerable research attention in future years. In epidemiological work on Alzheimer's disease, for instance, cognitive performance differences due to differing education, ethnicity, and socioeconomic status have become a prime focus (Katzman *et al.,* 1988; Valle, 1989). Research on ethnic minority and gender influences on mental health in the aged should be emphasized more generally (Harper, 1990; Jackson, Newton, Ostfeld, Savage, & Schneider, 1988).

The role in late-life mental illness played by a number of *social pathologies,* such as loneliness, social isolation (Murphy, 1982), bereavement and widowhood (Gallagher, Breckinridge, Thompson, & Dessonville, 1982), and rolelessness, is receiving continued attention. More research is needed as well regarding life stresses and quality-of-life issues, particularly since bioethical issues pertaining to the use of medical and other technological interventions are likely to dominate discussions of the final stages of life over the next decade.

Though a substantial body of studies has now looked at the mental health implications of caregiving (Light & Lebowitz, 1989), the future research agenda will likely give broader attention to the *natural ecology* of mental disorders in the aged, including family influences on their mental health. The manner in which families respond to a psychiatrically disturbed family member is critical to the patient's emotional state and experience of mental disorder, including patients with dementing conditions (Fruge & Niederehe, 1985; Lebowitz, 1985; Niederehe & Fruge, 1984; Zarit, Orr, & Zarit, 1985). At the very least, the family context can offer the patient tremendous reassurance or can add immensely to his or her emotional distress. In some cases, family conflicts may figure importantly in the genesis of the disorder itself.

B. Research Needs and Key Issues

As suggested by our above discussion of the bio-psycho-social perspective, we see a particular need for research that integrates biological with psychological and social variables affecting the mental health of the aged. Several other issues or themes mentioned above also deserve major research attention though, since already covered, they will not be further discussed here. These include the clinical significance of age of onset in various disorders, and the issues of comorbidity that touch on all late-life disorders.

At the same time, research efforts must be expanded to better address certain disorders which to date have not received adequate attention. Among such understudied topics, information is clearly needed in much greater depth regarding anxiety disorders in the aged (Salzman & Lebowitz, 1991), behavioral disturbances among the cognitively impaired (Cohen-Mansfield, 1986; Merriam, Aronson, Gaston, Weh, & Katz, 1988; Swearer, Drachman, O'Donnell, & Mitchell, 1988; Teri, Larson, & Reifler, 1988), mania, and personality disorders in late life. The newly defined construct of age-associated memory impairment (AAMI; Crook, 1986) addresses both the keen popular concerns and substantive clinical questions relating to subsyndromal cognitive decrements in many elderly persons. Though the construct has been criticized by some on conceptual and methodological grounds (Rosen, in press), since it has generated considerable research activity, the current lack of relevant empirical information in this area may soon be lessened considerably. Similar efforts at conceptualization and focused research are needed regarding the subsyndromal depression (dysphoria, demoralization) that numerous observers have noted to be an extremely common problem in the elderly population (Blazer, Hughes, & George, 1987; Blazer & Williams, 1980; Gurland, 1976). Likewise, more research should be directed at improving understanding of cognitive dysfunction, sometimes transient, in nondementing mental disorders in this age group, sometimes referred to as pseudodementia (Caine, 1981; Emery, 1988; Reifler, 1982; Wells, 1979), particularly in light of recent findings that white-matter brain lesions appear with unusual frequency in elderly depressed patients (Coffey, Figiel, Djang, Saunders, & Weiner, 1989; Zubenko *et al.*, 1990).

A welcome trend over the past decade has been the development and refinement of improved research instruments for assessing mental symptoms, psychiatric syndromes, treatment outcomes, and other relevant variables among the elderly. Although many examples could be cited of new or modified measures now available that are attuned to, and validated to take into account, the special conditions, settings, and response requirements of elderly individuals, perhaps several illustrative examples will suffice to make the point. Included among useful measures developed during the past decade are the Geriatric Depression Scale (Yesavage *et al.*, 1983), discrete research scales to disaggregate various components of caregiving situations (Pearlin, Mullan, Semple, & Skaff, 1990), various scales for differentially quantifying both objective cognitive dysfunctions and subjective memory complaints (Poon *et al.*, 1985), and emerging computerized assessment batteries for a wide range of neuropsychological functions (Ferris, Flicker, & Reisberg, 1988; Larrabee & Crook, 1988). Increasing standardization of procedures for assessment of dementia patients, such as has been occurring under the Consortium to Establish a Registry for Alzheimer's Disease (CERAD; Morris, Mohs, Rogers, Fillenbaum, & Heyman, 1988) also promises to enhance diagnostic assessment capabilities in that particular area. Further work was accomplished with the Multiphasic Environmental Assessment Procedure (Moos, Gauvain, Lemke, Max, & Mehren, 1979), which provides a template for assessing relevant features of sheltered long-term care settings. Although the greater availability of age-appropriate instruments constitutes a definitely improved methodological capability within the field, much additional work is needed to establish the *age invariance* or stability of factor structures across age groups for general-purpose instruments that are used with multiple age cohorts. Although the subject of attention by some mental health researchers (McGarvey, Gallagher, Thompson, & Zelinski, 1982; Foelker, Shewchuk, & Niederehe, 1987), to a large degree this methodological issue remains yet to be faced in the area of geriatric mental health assessments. For more detailed consideration of available instruments in the above-mentioned and other areas of assessment, the reader is referred to the volume edited by Raskin and Niederehe (1988).

The previously mentioned considerations about negative age stereotypes suggest the need for a new emphasis on the treatability of mental disorders among the aged, and for increased efforts at mental health promotion in this age group. Both clinical intervention and service delivery research need to be expanded. Many questions about the natural history of late-life mental disorders, and intervention and prevention efforts to serve the elderly population, still require a great deal of empirical investigation. For example, does psychotherapy need to be conducted differently with aged patients? Research on acute treatment of depression in older patients has shown that treatment response to both psychotherapy (Thompson & Gallagher, 1984) and medications (Rockwell, Lamb, & Zisook, 1988) is substantial, though naturalistic followup has shown high rates of relapse and recurrence. Research to establish protocols for continuation and maintenance treatment is now underway.

Somatic treatment issues are confounded by age-related changes in pharmacokinetics and by the vulnerability of older persons to anticholinergic and cardiovascular side-effects of many commonly used medications. Researchers must continue investigating how psychopharmacological treatments are best managed to achieve desired treatment effects yet minimize potential adverse effects, such as the risk of developing tardive dyskinesia (Jeste & Wyatt, 1987; Schooler, 1988).

One of the greatest needs is for more research that follows patients over considerably longer periods than has typically been the case, to clarify the natural course of various mental disorders in the later stages of the life cycle and the life *trajectories* followed by patients with chronic or recurrent disorders as they age.

Whereas longitudinal studies highlight aging-related changes, also needed are cohort-based analyses of the predictable characteristics and mental health needs that can be expected of the future aged (Gatz & Smyer, 1990). Many mental health patterns may remain quite stable for each generation over time, yet be historically specific to that age cohort. The characteristics of the oldest generation may then be gradually transformed over time as today's elderly die and are replaced by others growing old—a transformation resulting from age differences among cohorts rather than from the aging process. Analyses of the future aged, based on what is already known about patterns of mental health and illness and utilization of mental health services in today's younger generations, can assist in long-range planning for the kind of mental health system that is most likely to be called for when these generations reach their old age. For example, will narcissistic disorders become more common when the "me" generation reaches old age? Various observers have noted that the increasing educational attainment, affluence, and exposure to psychological concepts (psychological mindedness) that will characterize tomorrow's aged presage likely tendencies in the future aged toward greater self-diagnosis of problems as psychological in nature, greater self-advocacy for appropriate treatment, and reduced compliance with professional attitudes of therapeutic pessimism regarding the aged, and perhaps greater reliance on self-help organizations (e.g., Kahn, 1975).

VII. Service System Policy Dilemmas for the 1990s _____

Some of the problems faced by the elderly needing mental health services stem from the fragmented system of services that has grown up in patchwork fashion, owing to the politics of establishing benefits for the aged and reaching typical political compromises. Services for older persons with mental disorders remain fragmentary, nonpredictable, and subject to wide local variation. Clearly, innovative program directors and clinicians have developed important and effective approaches, and determined individuals have been able to organize useful service resources to meet their needs. Nonetheless, these accomplishments have too often been achieved in spite of current systems and regulations and not because of them. This problem persists in spite of numerous studies, commissions, and recommendations for action, and therefore remains an important priority concern for policy and program development. As well, over the last two decades, mental health care for the aged has become largely institutionalized in long-term care facilities (in line with the deinstitutionalization movement from state mental hospitals), and increasingly privatized (Gatz & Smyer, 1990; Kahn, 1975). We must conclude that in spite of the few dramatic positive examples, the mental health system as a whole is not prepared to fully address the broad set of treatment needs of older persons with mental disorders.

The sections below outline a series of selective issues that we view as key to addressing improved care for the aged within the mental health service system in the years ahead.

A. Mental Health Service Use

The availability and accessibility of community-based mental health services for the elderly have been issues of major concern for over a decade (Lebowitz, 1988). The disparity between the need for service and the small caseload of elderly patients generally documented in community mental health centers (CMHCs) has become even more notable as research in geriatrics has expanded and as the broad range of serious disorders and mental health problems experienced by older persons has been identified.

A combination of factors is thought to account for the low utilization of CMHC services by elderly patients, including health care system variables. CMHC programs are not widely accessible and, even where available, tend to be isolated from the mainstream of community health and social services to the elderly. Mental health service programs have typically not engaged in aggressive outreach and case finding but instead have been content to rely on referrals and self-identification of potential patients or clients. Furthermore, reimbursement for treatment of mental disorder under Medicare is substantially different from and less complete than reimbursement for physical disorder. The recognition of mental disorder in nursing homes is restricted by regulations that limit the number of residents with a primary psychiatric diagnosis, thereby limiting a potentially important site for development of CMHC services.

Elderly individuals for whom psychological treatment would be beneficial are apt to encounter ageist attitudes that may impede their access to appropriate services, partly because few mental health professionals have been trained to work with older persons. Despite much evidence to the contrary, many professionals continue to harbor a therapeutic nihilism or pessimism about the elderly's ability to change or make progress, or avoid professional involvement with the aged and their problems. Unfamiliarity with state-of-the-art research and practice has led many clinicians to conclude that no effective treatments or preventive interventions are available for use with older persons. Older persons have been seen as noncompliant, uninteresting, and generally inappropriate for treatment by many mental health professionals, who would rather deal with younger persons who are considered attractive, verbal, intelligent, and sophisticated.

At the same time, members of the older generation in a pattern of mutual avoidance (Kahn, 1975) cling to negative attitudes learned earlier in life about the mental health profession and decline to view their problems as psychological in nature. The stigma of mental illness is especially strong in the current cohort of elderly people, who tend to associate mental disorder with personal failure, spiritual deficiency, or some other stereotypic view. Thus, the need for mental health treatment is not accurately or appropriately recognized (or is denied) by patients, members of their families, and even the primary care physicians who provide most of the care to the elderly.

Despite these formidable obstacles, it is becoming clear that some CMHCs have developed services for the elderly that have had higher utilization than is the norm for CMHCs in general. The success of these programs is very strongly related to two factors: the existence of an aging-services unit within the CMHC staffed by professionals with specialized training in geriatrics, and coordinated relationships between the CMHC and its local community counterpart for aging services, usually known as the area agency on aging (Lebowitz, Light, & Bailey, 1987; Light, Lebowitz, & Bailey, 1986).

B. Primary Care and Mental Health

Use of prescription medications by the elderly is very high, and multiple medication use is common. According to the 1980 National Ambulatory Medical Care Survey, almost 70% of physician visits by patients older than 75 result in at least one prescribed medication, and 44% of these patients receive multiple medications (National Center for Health Statistics, 1983). Furthermore, about 10% of physician visits by persons older than 65 result in a psychotropic drug prescription—a figure relatively consistent across all older age groups. Most prescriptions are for anxiolytics, sedatives, and hypnotics (64%), with the remainder being for antidepressants (24%) and antipsychotic and antimanic agents (12%). For persons of all ages, multiple psychotropic drugs are prescribed in 10% of visits, and multiple prescriptions that include one psychotropic agent are given in another roughly similar proportion of cases.

Approximately 95% of visits resulting in psychotropic drug prescription are made to nonpsychiatrist physicians. Compliance with physician-prescribed therapeutic regimens is generally thought to be as high as 80% in geriatric patients, though this is not exclusive to psychotropic drugs (German and Burton, 1989). Noncompliance tends to be limited to underuse, with few studies reporting overuse or abuse. While reflecting the prevalence of psychiatric symptomatology in elderly persons seen in general medical practice, the frequency of psychotropic drug use requires continuing investigation of the efficacy and safety of these treatments both in themselves and as applied in primary care settings. More generally, issues of polypharmacy, drug misuse, and the potential of these factors for producing iatrogenic dysfunction in the elderly must be a continuing focus for future research and service planning (Niederehe & Fruge, 1985).

In addition, a majority of nursing home patients are prescribed psychotropic medication (50–60%) over the course of a year—a significant portion of these (approximately 20%) without recording of an appropriate diagnosis. An estimated 25% of nursing home patients receive antipsychotic medication: 7%, antidepressants; 7%, anxiolytics; and 7%, sedative–hypnotics (Beardsley, Larson, Burns, Thompson, & Kamerow, 1989).

The existence of this *de facto* system of mental health care needs to be acknowledged and programmatic initiatives need to be developed to assure that optimal care is provided in such settings.

C. Family Support and the Caregiver at Risk

The family is a major source in the care of older patients; most patients have family members who are willing to assist in care regardless of the substantial financial and emotional burden this entails. The family is now seen as central to the support of the geriatric patient and as a key component in the planning of a long-term continuum of care that could include community-based services such as activity centers, day care, congregate meals, assisted housing, and respite care, as well as institutional services in the hospital or nursing-home setting.

Providing this care is not without cost, however. In particular, those who are caring for the most impaired older persons (those with Alzheimer's disease, for example) report very high rates of guilt, demoralization, and depression associated with the great burden of care

(Brody, 1989). Caregivers in these situations also show significant suppression of a number of immune system parameters, thus making them more susceptible to illness and death from infections, influenza, etc. (Kiecolt-Glaser & Glaser, 1989). Clearly, addressing the needs of the family along with those of the patient will remain an important concern for program and policy development.

D. Long-Term Care

As a broader range of community-based services has become available and the so-called continuum-of-care has become more highly elaborated, a paradox has also become apparent. This paradox, stated at its simplest, is that *as the range of community-based services has grown, the need for long-term institutional care has also expanded.* Community services have not substituted for institutional care and, in fact, it has become apparent that community services do not serve as alternatives for institutional care (Callahan, 1989). There has been a clear displacement of services (e.g., nursing homes and not psychiatric hospitals have emerged as the most frequent site for care of the elderly mentally ill), but there has been no reduction in the demand for institutional care.

Indeed, one could argue that systems of care, rationally designed and widely accessible, have as their major result an increase in the life expectancy of those who receive service. In this framework, mortality varies as a function of the availability of services, where, simply put, people die when there are no appropriate services available to them. These services do not cure disease or reverse disability, however. Therefore, one can expect that functional disability and debilitation will continue until such time as institutional placement becomes appropriate. But more people will survive to that point.

Therefore, while services can delay institutionalization or divert placement on a single-case basis at one time, it is clear that looking at populations from a longitudinal perspective leads to the paradoxical conclusion of a positive relationship between services and institutionalization.

E. Disability

Disability, age, and diagnosis provide contradictory bases for policy development and service eligibility. Public discussion of appropriate treatment for major disorders has been informed by conceptualization of a metric of function, namely, the ability to accomplish various ADLs; a number of well-validated instruments for functional assessment have been developed and effectively used in both individual treatment planning and in overall health policy and planning (Kane & Kane, 1981). For example, ADLs have been used as the basis for eligibility in a number of state and federal proposals for legislation in the area of long-term care. At the same time, however, both age and the diagnostic pathway by which a patient reaches a certain level of ADL function can determine not only treatment setting and modality but also eligibility and exclusion. In the area of mental retardation and developmental disabilities, for example, many patients and their families have been denied continued participation in community programs because the individual has grown too old for continued eligibility. Portions of the recently enacted nursing home reforms in the 1987 Omnibus Budget Reconciliation Act (OBRA '87, Public Law 100-203) exclude from admission those potential patients who otherwise meet ADL criteria for nursing homes if the source of their disability is a major mental disorder.

The implications of these disparities in different areas of policy development are yet to be fully determined, but they do represent a clear signal that age and diagnosis, and not strictly ADLs, are the important determinants of disability and treatment availability in at least that group of patients with mental disorder.

F. Too Old, Too Sick

Community services for the mentally ill have traditionally focused upon providing appropriate living and vocational skills to adult chronic patients. These services, such as those generally referred to as community support programs, are meant to maintain the adult chronic patient in the community and to prevent long-term hospitalization in inpatient mental health facilities. The services are heavily psychosocial and rehabilitative in terms of living skills and have a strong vocational component. This mix of services is clearly oriented to the adults with serious and persistent mental disorders—usually schizophrenia—but who are otherwise free of disease or disability from sources other than the mental illness. Most older patients, with their multitude of coexisting mental and physical conditions and without need for vocational training, would be clearly inappropriate for participation in this type of service.

At the same time, it appears that community services for older persons are equally incapable of dealing with potential clients with mental disorder. The ability to accommodate the special needs of those with mental disorder in day care, nutrition services, congregate housing, and other similar settings seems to decrease with the severity of the disability and the intensity of the supervision required. Mild confusion and disorientation are generally not problematic, but more serious difficulties and behavioral disturbances such as assaultive or aggressive behavior are grounds for ineligibility or elimination from many programs. Thus a new challenge has emerged. Where the issue for program development was formerly how (or whether) to integrate those with mental disorder in institutional long-term care, the question is now how (or whether) to integrate those with mental disorder in community long-term care services. Few models exist to guide program development in this area of emerging importance.

Thus, those most in need of services in the community become the least likely to get them; in the proverbial sense, they have fallen through the crack between programs. This is not to say that there are no elegant and effective models of community programs for older persons with mental illness. There are many. Yet a consistent and coherent nationwide approach to these issues does not exist.

VIII. Education and the Need for Trained Personnel _____

Opportunities for education in gerontology and geriatrics are increasing at a significant rate. In medicine, geriatric subspecialization has been gaining acceptance; added qualifications through fellowship training or examination have been adopted for internal medicine, family practice, and psychiatry. Significant curriculum-development efforts have been carried out in all mental health disciplines, and the number of texts, monographs, and specialized journals in gerontology and geriatrics has multiplied significantly. Psychology internships may be expanded and restructured to strengthen clinical specialization in particular areas, such as work with the elderly.

The number of postgraduate specialty training programs focused on services for the elderly has increased substantially in the past decade in all the mental health disciplines, so that there are now over 50 such programs. It is clear that these programs have had a substantial impact on the availability and accessibility of mental health services to older persons.

Estimates of numbers of personnel needed for the mental health disciplines are based upon the perspective that (1) almost all clinicians in practice can provide service to geriatric patients; (2) some of these clinicians will choose to concentrate their practice in the area of geriatrics; and (3) a small group of academic geriatric specialists will assume leadership positions in education and research at universities, schools of medicine, and at major teaching hospitals.

Projections of need for trained specialists in geriatric mental health have been developed by the Committee on Personnel for Health Needs of the Elderly (1988). Using estimates of need for treatment as revealed in epidemiological studies and medical care utilization surveys, the Committee determined the need for academic geriatric psychiatrists to provide leadership in education, training, and research at 400 to 500. Similar estimates were made by the Committee for many other health professions. Of particular interest are the estimates for academics needed in the other core disciplines in the geriatric mental health field: psychology (900); social work (800); and psychiatric nursing (500).

In light of these estimates, the Committee identified three types of training needs:

1. geriatrics should be part of the training of all clinicians, with appropriate didactic and clinical experience in the undergraduate professional curriculum as well as in postgraduate training and as part of continuing education;
2. increased educational experiences for special competency should be available; and
3. advanced training, through special postgraduate fellowships should be available for those seeking academic careers.

The quality of clinical training in geriatrics is an area that has received insufficient attention. In the absence of external standards usable for evaluation, practitioners can designate any content, curriculum, or experience as specialized training simply by naming it as such. Specialization, indeed, could be established simply by assertion—for example, by an advertisement claiming specialization. That is not to say that curriculum standards do not exist—indeed, one can argue that consensus has developed around courses, content, and settings appropriate for geriatric training. Most clinicians trained in gerontology and geriatrics can be expected to have mastered a core didactic subject matter that could be applied with effectiveness in the clinical setting, given appropriate clinical training experiences and supervision. Then, too, external criteria of clinical preparedness are beginning to be applied, particularly in geriatric psychiatry where added qualifications examinations will require fellowship training in a program that has been accredited by a national review body. Similar structures for review, evaluation, and accreditation exist in psychology, social work, psychiatric nursing, and family and marital therapy, albeit currently directed toward generalist rather than specialty levels of training.

In the face of this gain and record of success, however, the prospects for long-range stability in funding are highly uncertain in light of regularly declining appropriations and the absence of clear statutory mandates through targeted legislative development. Consequently, the personnel question remains a critical one for policy development and action.

IX. Conclusion

The population of the United States, and of the entire world, is growing older (we have gained nearly 30 years of life expectancy in this century). The elderly population is itself growing older (with the greatest proportionate increase projected in those age 85 and older). With those older than age 65 already including one in every eight Americans, reduced birthrates and lowered mortality rates in adulthood lead to projections that the elderly will come to constitute nearly one in five within the American population in the first quarter of the 21st century. Such unprecedented growth in the proportion of older people has led to unprecedented challenge to established systems of service delivery and medical care. Free-standing systems of social services for the elderly have been established; large citizen-based groups have developed with the goal of articulating the interests of older persons; scientific societies and subsocieties have proliferated, along with scientific meetings, journals, and presentations; subspecialization in geriatrics has been established in internal medicine, family practice, and psychiatry; and legislation addressing some particular aspect of health care, income maintenance, or social services for the elderly constitute a major concern of federal, state, and local governments.

The 1990s have been designated the Decade of the Brain by President George Bush following a Joint Resolution of the Congress. The Decade of the Brain calls for enhanced efforts in the basic and clinical neurosciences to aid in overcoming severe brain disorders, among which the mental disorders are paramount. The diseases of brain and behavior, of which the geriatric mental disorders are prime examples, are central to the scientific agenda of the Decade of the Brain.

Developments in basic science and clinical investigation are providing a firm base for treatment and prevention as well as for educational programs and for further research. Investigators are using the best of contemporary approaches to address questions on the onset, course, and outcome of disease, on the interaction of disease with normal age-associated changes in adult development, on the impact of comorbidity of acute or chronic conditions, and on the significance of age of onset of disorder. This rich body of science has developed a significant momentum with an ever-accelerating pace of achievement.

As the field has expanded, the continued growth of the investments in research has become increasingly apparent. Individual research projects, principally supported by the federal agencies, compose the main source of research support for investigators in the field. Mental health researchers are provided support from a number of sources, both public and private (such as foundations, the pharmaceutical industry, and institutional endowments). Funding for all these programs must be assured, and long-term growth and stability must be attained so that a productive framework for the support of research can be maintained.

At the same time, attention must be paid to the need to build the base for this research effort through the support of research centers, training programs, data banks, cell and tissue depositories, animal resources, and the like. Though not the most glamorous aspects of research, these provide the foundation upon which the research enterprise is built. Thus, a two-pronged strategy for the continued support of research must be developed so that projects and research resources can be supported as appropriate.

Issues identified in this chapter, and in the remainder of this volume, represent the main areas of concern in mental health and aging. Each is a piece of the overall picture, and even a brief overview shows the interlocking nature of the concerns. Over the past decade there has been substantial development in each of these areas. At the same time, the concerns and need for improvement have become equally apparent. Fulfillment of the promise in these areas will require the sustained efforts of many individual investigators, educators, and clinicians, whose work already demonstrates the potential that policy development can try to capture and formalize so that new levels in the state of the art can be achieved. These achievements, in turn, can be realized only if shaped by the leadership of forward-looking and innovative policy-makers at all levels of government and non-governmental bodies. The challenge is enormous, but the rewards in development of successful approaches to the needs of sick old people and those who care for and about them are well worth the efforts of all of us.

References

Advisory Panel on Alzheimer's Disease. (1989). *Report of the Advisory Panel on Alzheimer's Disease, 1988–1989*. DHHS Pub. No. (ADM) 89-1644. Washington, DC: U.S. Government Printing Office.

American Psychiatric Association (1987). *DSM-III-R: Diagnostic and Statistical Manual of Mental Disorders* (3rd rev. ed.). Washington, DC: American Psychiatric Association.

Beardsley, R. S., Larson, D. B., Burns, B. J., Thompson, J. W., & Kamerow, D. B. (1989). Prescribing of psychotropics in nursing home patients. *Journal of the American Geriatrics Society, 37,* 327–330.

Bengtson, V. L., Cutler, N. E., Mangen, D. J., Marshall, V. W. (1985). Generations, cohorts, and relations between age groups. In R. H. Binstock & E. Shanas (Eds.), *Handbook of Aging and the Social Sciences* (2nd ed.), (pp. 304–338). New York: Van Nostrand Reinhold.

Birren, J. E., & Renner, V. J. (1980). Concepts and issues of mental health and aging. In J. E. Birren & R. B. Sloane (Eds.), *Handbook of Mental Health and Aging* (pp. 3–33). Englewood Cliffs, NJ: Prentice-Hall.

Birren, J. E., Schaie, K. W. (Eds.). (1990). *Handbook of the Psychology of Aging* (3rd ed.). San Diego: Academic Press.

Blazer, D., Hughes, D. C., & George, L. K. (1987). The epidemiology of depression in an elderly community population. *The Gerontologist, 27,* 281–287.

Blazer, D., & Williams, C. D. (1980). Epidemiology of dysphoria and depression in an elderly community population. *American Journal of Psychiatry, 137,* 439–444.

Bowen, M. (1978). *Family Therapy in Clinical Practice*. New York: Jason Aronson.

Brody, E. M. (1989). The family at risk. In E. Light & B. D. Lebowitz (Eds.), *Alzheimer's Disease Treatment and Family Stress: Directions for Research* (pp. 2–49). Washington, DC: U.S. Government Printing Office.

Busse, E. W. & Pfeiffer, E. (1977). Functional psychiatric disorders in old age. In E. W. Busse & E. Pfeiffer (Eds.), *Behavior and Adaptation in Late Life* (2nd ed.) (pp. 158–211). Boston: Little, Brown.

Caine, E. D. (1981). Pseudodementia: Current concepts and future directions. *Archives of General psychiatry, 38,* 1359–1364.

Callahan, J. J. (1989). Play it again Sam—There is no impact. *The Gerontologist, 29,* 5–6.

Coffey, C. E., Figiel, G. S., Djang, W. T., Saunders, W. B., & Weiner, R. D. (1989). White matter hyperintensity of magnetic resonance imaging: Clinical and neuroanatomic correlates in the depressed elderly. *Journal of Neuropsychiatry, 1,* 135–144.

Cohen, G. D. (1988). *The Brain and Human Aging.* New York: Springer.

Cohen-Mansfield, J. (1986). Agitated behaviors in the elderly: II. Preliminary results in the cognitively deteriorated. *Journal of the American Geriatrics Society, 34,* 722–727.

Committee on Personnel for Health Needs of the Elderly Through the Year 2020 (1988). Report. Washington, DC: U.S. Government Printing Office.

Costa, P. T., Jr. (1985). Longitudinal stability of personality and its relation to health perceptions. In C. M. Gaitz, G. Niederehe & N. L. Wilson (Eds.), *Aging 2000: Our Health Care Destiny, Volume II: Psychosocial and Policy Issues* (pp. 75–84). New York: Springer-Verlag.

Crook, T., Bartus, R., Ferris, S., Whitehouse, P., Cohen, G., & Gershon, S. (1986). Age-associated memory impairment: Proposed diagnostic criteria and measures of clinical change—Report of a National Institute of Mental Health work group. *Developmental Neuropsychology, 2,* 261–276.

Emery, V. O. B. (1988). *Pseudodementia: A theoretical and empirical discussion.* Western Reserve Geriatric Education Center Interdisciplinary Monograph Series, No. 4. Cleveland, OH: Case Western Reserve University School of Medicine.

Englehardt, H. T., Jr. (1979). Is aging a disease? In R. Beatch (Ed.), *Life Span: Values and life-expanding technologies* pp. 184–194). San Francisco: Harper & Row.

Ferris, S. H., Flicker, C., & Reisberg, B. (1988). NYU computerized test battery for assessing cognition in aging and dementia. *Psychopharmacology Bulletin, 24,* 699–702.

Foelker, G. A., Jr., Shewchuk, R. M., & Niederehe, G. (1987). Confirmatory factor analysis of the short-form Beck Depression Inventory in elderly community samples. *Journal of Clinical Psychology, 43,* 111–118.

Fruge, E., & Niederehe, G. (1985). Family dimensions of health care for the aged. In S. Henao & N. P. Grose (Eds.), *Principles of family systems in family medicine* (pp. 165–191). New York: Brunner/Mazel.

Gallagher, D., Breckenridge, J. N., Thompson, L. W., & Dessonville, C. (1982). Similarities and differences between normal grief and depression in older adults. *Essence, 5,* 127–140.

Gatz, M., & Smyer, M. A. (1990, August). *The mental health system and the older adult in the 1990s.* Invited address at 98th Annual Convention of the American Psychological Association, Boston.

German, P. S., & Burton, L. C. (1989). Medication and the elderly: Issues of prescription and use. *Journal of Aging and Health, 1,* 4–34.

Gurland, B. (1976). The comparative frequency of depression in various adult age groups. *Journal of Gerontology, 31,* 283–292.

Gutmann, D. (1982). Training in the clinical psychology of aging: Observations and recommendations. In J. Santos & G. R. VandenBos (Eds.), *Psychology and the older adult: Challenges for training in the 1980s* (pp. 97–107). Washington, DC: American Psychological Association.

Harper, M. S. (Ed.). (1990). *Minority Aging: Essential Curricula Content for Selected Health and Allied Health Professions.* DHHS Pub. No. HRS (P-DV-90-4). Washington, DC: U.S. Government Printing Office.

Jackson, J. S., Newton, P., Ostfeld, A., Savage, D., & Schneider, E. L. (Eds.) (1988). *The Black American elderly: Research on physical and psychosocial health.* New York: Springer.

Jahoda, M. (1958). *Current Concepts of Positive Mental Health.* New York: Basic Books.

Jeste, D. V., & Wyatt, R. J. (1987). Aging and tardive dyskinesia. In N. E. Miller & G. D. Cohen (Eds.), *Schizophrenia and aging* (pp. 275–286). New York: Guilford Press.

Kahn, R. L. (1971). Psychological aspects of aging. In I. Rossman (Ed.), *Clinical geriatrics* (pp. 107–113). Philadelphia: J. B. Lippincott.

Kahn, R. L. (1975). The mental health system and the future aged. *The Gerontologist, 15,* 24–31.

Kane, R. H., & Kane, R. L. (1981). *Assessing the elderly: A practical guide to measurement.* Lexington, MA: D. C. Heath.

Katzman, R., Zhang, M., Qu, Q.-Y., Wang, Z., Liu, W. T., Yu, E. Wong, S.-C., Salmon, D. P., & Grant, I. (1988). A Chinese version of the Mini-Mental State Examination: Impact of illiteracy in a Shanghai dementia survey. *Journal of Clinical Epidemiology, 41,* 971–978.

Kiecolt-Glaser, J., & Glaser, R. (1989). Caregiving, mental health, and immune functioning. In E. Light & B. D. Lebowitz (Eds.), *Alzheimer's disease treatment and family stress: Directions for research* (pp. 245–266). Washington, DC: U.S. Government Printing Office.

Kramer, M. (1980). The rising pandemic of mental disorders and associated chronic diseases and disabilities. *Acta Psychiatrica Scandinavica, 62(Suppl. 285),* 382–397.

Kuypers, J. A., & Bengtson, V. L. (1973). Social breakdown and competence: A model of normal aging. *Human Development, 16,* 181–201.

Larrabee, G. J., & Crook, T. (1988). A computerized everyday memory battery for assessing treatment effects. *Psychopharmacology Bulletin, 24,* 695–697.

Lawton, M. P., & Nahemow, L. (1973). Ecology and the aging process. In C. Eisdorfer & M. P. Lawton (Eds.), *psychology of adult development and aging* (pp. 619–674). Washington, DC: American Psychological Association.

Lebowitz, B. D. (1985). Family caregiving in old age. *Hospital and Community Psychiatry, 36,* 457–458.

Lebowitz, B. D. (1988). Mental health services. In G. L. Maddox (Ed.), *Encyclopedia of Aging* (pp. 440–442). New York: Springer.

Lebowitz, B. D., Light, E., & Bailey, F. (1987). Mental health center services for the elderly: The impact of coordination with Area Agencies on Aging. *The Gerontologist, 27,* 699–702.

Light, E., & Lebowitz, B. D. (Eds.). (1989). *Alzheimer's disease treatment and family stress: Directions for research.* DHHS Publ. No. (ADM)89-1569. Washington, DC: U.S. Government Printing Office.

Light, E., Lebowitz, B. D., & Bailey, F. (1986). CMHCs and elderly services: An analysis of direct and indirect services and service delivery sites. *Community Mental Health Journal, 22,* 294–302.

Linn, M. W. (1988). A critical review of scales used to evaluate social and interpersonal adjustment in the community. *Psychopharmacology Bulletin, 24,* 615–621.

Maddox, G. L., & Campbell, R. T. (1985). Scope, concepts, and methods in the study of aging. In R. H. Binstock & E. Shanas (Eds.), *Handbook of aging and the social sciences* (2nd ed.) (pp. 3–31). New York: Van Nostrand Reinhold.

Manton, K. G. (1990). Mortality and morbidity. In R. H. Binstock & L. K. George (Eds.), *Handbook of aging and the social sciences* (3rd ed.) (pp. 59–90). San Diego: Academic Press.

McGarvey, B., Gallagher, D., Thompson, L. W., & Zelinski, E. (1982). Reliability and factor structure of the Zung self-rating depression scale in three age groups. *Essence, 5,* 141–151.

Merriam, A. E., Aronson, M. K., Gaston, P., Wey, S.-L., & Katz, I. (1988). The psychiatric symptoms of Alzheimer's disease. *Journal of the American Geriatrics Society, 36,* 7–12.

Miller, N. E., & Cohen, G. D. (Eds.). (1987). *Schizophrenia and aging.* New York: Guilford Press.

Moos, R. H., Gauvain, M., Lemke, S., Max, W., & Mehren, B. (1979). Assessing the social environments of sheltered care settings. *The Gerontologist, 19,* 74–82.

Morris, J. C., Mohs, R. C., Rogers, H., Fillenbaum, G., & Heyman, A. (1988). Consortium to Establish a Registry for Alzheimer's Disease (CERAD) clinical and neuropsychological assessment of Alzheimer's disease. *Psychopharmacology Bulletin, 24,* 641–652.

Murphy, E. (1982). Social origins of depression in old age. *British Journal of Psychiatry, 141,* 135–142.

Myers, G. C. (1990). Demography of aging. In R. H. Binstock & L. K. George (Eds.), *Handbook of aging and the social sciences* (3rd ed.) (pp. 19–44). San Diego, CA: Academic Press.

National Center for Health Statistics (1983, June). Utilization of psychotropic drugs in office-based ambulatory care: National Ambulatory Medical Care Survey, 1980 and 1981 (by Koch H). *Advanced data from vital and health statistics, No. 90.* DHHS Pub. No. (PHS) 83-n250. Hyattsville, MD: Public Health Service.

Neugarten, B. L. (1970). Dynamics of transition of middle age to old age: Adaptation and the life cycle. *Journal of Geriatric Psychiatry, 4,* 71–87.

Neugarten, B. L. (1974). Age groups in American society and the rise of the young-old. *Annals of Political and Social Sciences Sept.,* 187–198.

Niederehe, G., & Fruge, E. (1984). Dementia and family dynamics: Clinical research issues. *Journal of Geriatric Psychiatry, 17,* 21–56.

Parsons, T. (1964). Definitions of health and illness in the light of American values and social structure. In T. Parsons (Ed.), *Social structure and personality* (pp. 257–291). London: The Free Press.

Pearlin, L. I., Mullan, J. T., Semple, S. J., & Skaff, M. M. (1990). Caregiving and the stress process: An overview of concepts and their measures. *The Gerontologist, 30,* 583–594.

Peters, R. S. (1958). *The Concept of Motivation*. London: Routledge & Kegan Paul.

Poon, L. W., Crook, T., Davis, K. L., Eisdorfer, C., Gurland, B. J., Kazniak, A. W., & Thompson, L. W. (Eds.). (1986). *Handbook for clinical memory assessment of older adults*. Washington, DC: American Psychological Association.

Raskin, A., & Niederehe, G. (Eds.). (1988). *Assessment in diagnosis and treatment of geropsychiatric patients*. Special Issue of *Psychopharmacology Bulletin* (Vol. 24, Whole No. 4). DHHS Pub. No. (ADM)88-173. Rockville, MD: Alcohol, Drug Abuse, and Mental Health Administration.

Reifler, B. V. (1982). Arguments for abandoning the term pseudodementia. *Journal of the American Geriatrics Society, 30*, 665–668.

Reynolds, C. F., Kupfer, D. J., Houck, P. R., Hoch, C. C., Stack, J. A., Berman, S. R., & Zimmer, B. (1988). Reliable discrimination of elderly depressed and demented patients by EEG sleep data. *Archives of General Psychiatry, 45*, 258–264.

Rockwell, E., Lam, R. W., & Zisook, S. (1988). Antidepressant drug studies in the elderly. *Psychiatric Clinics of North America, 11*, 215–233.

Rodin, J., & Langer, E. (1980). Aging labels: The decline of control and the fall of self-esteem. *Journal of Social Issues, 36*, 12–29.

Rosen, T. J. (in press). Age-associated memory impairment: A critique. *European Journal of Cognitive Psychology*.

Rosow, I. (1985). Status and role change through the life cycle. In R. H. Binstock & E. Shanas (Eds.), *Handbook of aging and the social sciences* (2nd ed.) (pp. 62–93). New York: Van Nostrand Reinhold.

Salzman, C., & Lebowitz, B. D. (Eds.). (1991). *Anxiety in the elderly*. New York: Springer.

Schaie, K. W. (1965). A general model for the study of developmental problems. *Psychological Bulletin, 64*, 72–107.

Schneider, E. L., & Rowe, J. W. (Eds.). (1990). *Handbook of the Biology of Aging* (3rd ed.). San Diego, CA: Academic Press.

Schooler, N. (1988). Evaluation of drug-related movement disorders in the aged. *Psychopharmacology Bulletin, 24*, 603–607.

Shanas, E. (1979). Social myth as hypothesis: The case of the family relations of old people. *The Gerontologist, 19*, 3–9.

Swearer, J. M., Drachman, D. A., O'Donnell, B. F., & Mitchell, A. L. (1988). Troublesome and disruptive behaviors in dementia: Relationships to diagnosis and disease severity. *Journal of the American Geriatrics Society, 36*, 784–790.

Szasz, T. S. (1970). *The manufacture of madness*. New York: Delta.

Teri, L., Larson, E. B., & Reifler, B. V. (1988). Behavioral disturbance in dementia of the Alzheimer's type. *Journal of the American Geriatrics Society, 36*, 1–6.

Thompson, L. W., & Gallagher, D. (1984). Efficacy of psychotherapy in the treatment of late-life depression. *Advances in Behavioral Research and Therapy, 6*, 127–139.

Valle, R. (1989). Cultural and ethnic issues in Alzheimer's disease family research. In E. Light & B. D. Lebowitz (Eds.), *Alzheimer's disease treatment and family stress: Directions for research*. DHHS Publ. No. (ADM)89-1569 (pp. 122–154). Washington, DC: U.S. Government Printing Office.

Vitiello, M. V., & Prinz, P. N. (1988). Aging and sleep disorders. In R. Williams, I. Karacan, & C. Moore (Eds.), *Sleep disorders: Diagnosis and treatment* (pp. 293–312). New York: John Wiley & Sons.

Wang, H.-S., & Busse, E. W. (1971). Dementia in old age. In C. E. Wells (Ed.), *Dementia* (pp. 152–162). Philadelphia, PA: F. A. Davis.

Wells, C. E. (1979). Pseudodementia. *American Journal of Psychiatry, 136*, 895–900.

Yesavage, J. A., Brink, T. L., Rose, T. L., Lum, O., Huang, V., Adey, M. B., & Leirer, V. O. (1983). Development and validation of a geriatric depression screening scale: A preliminary report. *Journal of Psychiatric Research, 39*, 37–49.

Zarit, S. H., Orr, N. K., & Zarit, J. M. (1985). *The hidden victims of Alzheimer's disease: Families under stress*. New York: New York University Press.

Zubenko, G. S., Sullivan, P., Nelson, J. P., Belle, S. H., Huff, F. J., & Wolf, G. L. (1990). Brain imaging abnormalities in mental disorders of late life. *Archives of Neurology, 47*, 1107–1111.

2

The Epidemiology of Selected Mental Disorders in Later Life ___

James C. Anthony and Ahmed Aboraya

I. Introduction
    A. Epidemiology as a Basic Science of Causes and Prevention
    B. The Scope, Purposes, and Organization of the Chapter
II. Dementia Syndromes
    A. The Estimated Prevalence of the Dementias
    B. The Estimated Risk of Dementia and Cognitive Impairment in Later Life
    C. Suspected Risk Factors for the Dementias in Later Life
III. Depressive Disorders
    A. The Estimated Prevalence of Depression
    B. The Estimated Risk of Depression
    C. Sex and Gender, Age and Aging as Risk Factors for Depression
    D. Other Suspected Risk Factors for Depression in Later Life
IV. Panic Disorder
    A. The Estimated Prevalence of Panic Disorder
    B. The Estimated Risk of Panic Disorder
    C. Suspected Risk Factors for Panic Disorder in Later Life
V. Phobic Disorders
    A. The Estimated Prevalence of Phobic Disorders
    B. The Estimated Risk of Phobic Disorders
    C. Suspected Risk Factors for Phobic Disorders
VI. Obsessive-Compulsive Disorders
    A. The Estimated Prevalence of Obsessive-Compulsive Disorder
    B. The Estimated Risk of Obsessive-Compulsive Disorder
    C. Suspected Risk Factors for Obsessive-Compulsive Disorders in Later Life
VII. Syndromes of Dependence and Abuse Involving Alcohol and Other Drugs
    A. The Estimated Prevalence of Alcohol and Drug Abuse–Dependence
    B. The Estimated Risk of Alcohol and Drug Abuse–Dependence
    C. Suspected Risk Factors for Alcohol and Drug Abuse–Dependence in Later Life
VIII. Summary and Future Directions
    References

I. Introduction ───

A. Epidemiology as a Basic Science of Causes and Prevention

All over the world, more and more people are living longer. Large numbers have reached the seventh and eighth decades of human life, and many now survive past age 80 (Macfadyen, 1990). These later years of life are a time of great satisfaction, well-being, and success for a surprising majority (Rowe & Kahn, 1987). Nonetheless, with increasing age, far too many people fall victim to dementia, depression, and other disturbances of mind and behavior.

Epidemiology is one important way to learn about conditions and processes that can influence the occurrence and duration of these mental and behavioral disturbances in the later years of human life. Epidemiology is distinctive because in a special sense it calls for close attention to both the sick and the well. Its concern is not only the cases of mental disorders that arise and come to clinical attention, but also the total population experience out of which these cases have surfaced, including the experience of untreated cases and non-cases. This distinction is especially important in later life, when a greater proportion of mental disorder cases remain untreated (Hagnell, 1966; Gruenberg, 1980; George, Blazer, Winfield-Laird, Leaf, & Fischbach, 1988).

In many respects, epidemiology is a basic science in the search for causes of mental disorders, and also in the search for practical methods to prevent and control these disorders. Epidemiologic reasoning and analysis are crucial stages of inquiry as the germ of each idea about mental disorder causation or prevention moves toward acceptance as a well-established scientific fact (Morris, 1975; Gruenberg, 1980; Turner, 1987; Anthony, 1990).

The need for epidemiologic reasoning appears early when suspected clinicopathologic associations are probed for causal implications. Studying patients, clinical scientists often find ostensible abnormalities that might be markers or traces of important causal disease processes. In the scientific workup of these clues, two linked questions to be asked are "Abnormal? Compared to what?" A thoroughgoing attempt to answer these questions demands a reach beyond the case material readily available to clinical scientists, a reach toward the population experience out of which the cases surfaced. However difficult, this reach is essential to answer key questions in the estimation and evaluation of causal associations, if such findings are to be taken seriously when forging chains of causal inference concerning disease.

The special capacities and strengths of epidemiology show most clearly in research problems of this type, in which the readily available case material is not enough to delve into a suspected association of causal significance or a promising preventive intervention. These strengths and capacities are not always so obvious in epidemiologic evidence from cross-sectional field surveys of community populations. Evidence from these field surveys allows us to describe the magnitude of a health problem in terms of its prevalence, and can help us form hypotheses. These surveys rarely are designed to test etiologic theory.

Epidemiologic field surveys are limited in part because they can estimate the *prevalence* of mental and behavioral disturbances, but they typically cannot speak to issues of *incidence* or *risk*. Prevalence is defined in a way that mixes the forces affecting incidence and risk together with the separate and separable forces influencing duration of mental and behavior disturbances (see Kramer, Von Korff, & Kessler, 1980). As a result, when a survey shows that depression is more prevalent among women as compared to men, by itself this association does not reveal that being a woman is a risk factor for depression. The association can emerge when depression in women lasts longer than depression in men, even when the two sexes bear equal risk of depression (see Murphy, Olivier, Monson, Sobol, & Leighton, 1988). Mortimer (1988) has drawn attention to this problem in relation to cross-national comparison of dementia prevalence values.

Mental disorder risk factors are conditions and processes that clearly are associated with the *risk* of developing a disturbance in mental life or behavior, and also are judged to have causal significance just short of what is needed to regard them as causes (Kleinbaum, Kupper, & Morgenstern, 1982). In making this point, Lilienfeld drew attention to origins of the risk factor concept in cardiovascular disease epidemiology. Age was discovered to be associated with risk of developing cardiovascular disease, and in many respects the association met accepted criteria for causal significance. However, the distinctive causal processes linking age to disease were a matter of speculation, and no experimental intervention to change age was possible. Hence age became known as a cardiovascular disease risk factor, a variable having values that signaled different levels of risk, and which was *judged* to have some causal significance (A. Lilienfeld, personal communication, 1982).

In contrast with the usual field-survey method, the modern epidemiologic case-control strategy and its extensions via case-base and case-cohort sampling have been designed specifically to probe hypotheses about risk factors and other suspected causal associations by reaching for information about the population from which the cases have surfaced. The inquiry often begins with a search for individual risk-associated variables, and later moves toward more rigorous evaluation of consistently observed associations, for example, by means of multiple regression modeling (Schlesselman, 1982; Miettinen, 1985; Prentice, 1986; Anthony, 1988). When possible, prospective or longitudinal studies and the epidemiologic field experiment can augment the inquiry, particularly in the instance of prevention research designed to test causal hypotheses at the same time preventive strategies are being evaluated (Lilienfeld, 1976; Kellam, Anthony, Brown, & Dolan, 1989; Anthony, 1990).

B. The Scope, Purposes, and Organization of the Chapter

This chapter concerns the epidemiology of mental disorders in later life, i.e., after age 60 or 65. Its focus is on two distinct topics for epidemiologic research: first, the estimation of age-related prevalence and risk for a selection of specific mental disorders; and second, an overview of the evidence on risk factors for these mental disorders in later life, as observed by means of epidemiologic research. Suggestions for future research directions also are offered. Other chapters discuss separate important epidemiologic topics such as prevention of mental disorders in later life, and use of mental health services by the elderly, as well as categories of mental disorders that are not addressed here.

One of our purposes in this chapter is to draw attention to underlying substantive theory associated with the *null* hypothesis in risk factor studies of mental disorders in later life. To some extent, reports on these studies have stressed an alternative hypothesis without drawing attention to the substantive implications of the null. In so doing, an impression may be left that the null is substantively empty: all is random, and what we have observed can be explained by chance alone (Oakes, 1990).

From our perspective on risk factor research concerning mental disorders in later life, we find that the operative theory associated with the null often seems to be one of so-called normal aging or inevitable senescence in the human species at this stage in evolu-tionary process. For example, in theory, the neurobiologic differences identified by Alz-heimer in studies of dementia and clarified in later research (e.g., Blessed, Tomlinson, & Roth, 1968; Roth, 1986) might be viewed as a manifestation of senescence in which specific extrinsic influences are unnecessary to account for degeneration of cortical and subcortical neurons (e.g., see Miller, 1977). These changes might be identified with later damage from a gene or genes that bestowed advantage to the species earlier in life (Williams, 1957; Sluss, Gruenberg, & Kramer, 1981), possibly a species-wide breakdown in the process of somatic repair that otherwise would check progressive accumulation of randomly occurring damage (Kirkwood, 1981). The risk factor research challenges the senescence theory to the extent that it yields consistent evidence of specific extrinsic influences that are associated with earlier onset or greater incidence of mental disorders in the population. While senescence theory might prove to be little more than a straw man, it generally has defied rejection in epidemiologic analysis, as we shall see. We are left with all the more reason to take note of any disconfirming instances where it regularly is found that any specific exposure or other specific extrinsic influence has mattered (Oakes, 1990).

It appears that some 30 years ago Karl Jaspers (1963) already had drawn a conclusion about the senescence theory in respect to most mental disorders in later life: "The psychoses that can actually be attributed to aging get fewer in number. Perhaps senile dementia is the only disease of age (p. 687)." Surely, in some degree, Jaspers was influenced by the work of Sir Martin Roth, whose studies have challenged the idea that "all mental maladies of old age derive from cerebral degenerative disease (p. 206)" (Roth, 1980), either of the senile or arteriosclerotic type (Roth, 1955). In this challenge, Roth and his collaborators made prime contributions to psychopathology by showing a relative heterogeneity between categories of mental disorders seen after age 60, and homogeneity within these categories. Going far beyond differences and similarities of clinical picture observed cross-sectionally in patients, the assembled evidence now ranges to prognostic characteristics for external validation: case fatality rates; percentage dis-charged (alive) within 6 to 24 months of admission for inpatient care; length of inpatient stay (Roth, 1955, 1972, 1976; Blessed & Wilson, 1982); and also to pathologic features such as a postmortem count of amyloid plaques (Blessed, Tomlinson, & Roth, 1968), change in neurotransmitters and other neurochemical lesions (Mountjoy, 1986; Roth, 1986), systolic blood pressure readings made before death (St. Clair & Whalley, 1983), and regional cerebral brain flow and brain electrical activity (John, Prichep, Fridman, & Easton, 1988).

While there are several vantages from which to attack the validity of specific diagnostic categories and classifications advanced in psychiatric studies (e.g., see Roth, 1984), it is difficult to ignore them in research on mental health and mental morbidity in later life.

There is an enduring need to weigh the value of diagnostic categories, but the ultimate valuation in epidemiologic risk factor research is pragmatic with respect to scientific goals. We must ask whether these categories help in testing theories about the conditions under which mental and behavioral disturbances occur or in learning how to prevent occurrence of these disturbances. At present, the answer to this question seems affirmative, to the extent that the categories mark off useful etiologic classes within which there is a relative homogeneity of causal conditions.

Considering theory in epidemiologic research as it relates to diagnostic categories and classifications, it is important to note that the newer rubrics do not use age as a defining feature. Thus, when we speak of mental disorders in later life, this refers to the timing of their occurrence, and not to any particular form or content.

Commenting on this change in the diagnostic rubrics, Jablensky recently noted that Jaspers' ideas about mental disorders and aging have been played out in the international consensus process leading to the newest International Classification of Diseases (ICD), Tenth Revision (World Health Organization, 1990): "Mental disorders occurring in the elderly are no longer considered to belong in a separate category of morbidity (p. 683)" (Jablensky, 1990). These developments also converge with Roth's position that in old age the variety of mental disorders generally are the same as can be seen at earlier ages, but under different conditions (Roth, 1976).

Consistent with these developments, there have been changes in the original categories proposed by Roth more than 30 years ago when he was working to challenge the generalized theory of cerebral degeneration. For the most part, Roth's category of *senile psychosis* has been replaced by categories such as *primary degenerative dementia* and *senile dementia—Alzheimer's type* (SDAT); *arteriosclerotic psychosis* by *multi-infarct dementia* or less specific *vascular dementia; acute confusion* by *delirium* and other so-called organic syndromes of relatively short duration but important health impact; and *paraphrenia* has been replaced by *schizophrenia* and other differentiated categories of schizophrenia-like or paranoid psychoses. *Affective psychosis* has been split apart into several categories under general headings such as *affective disorders,* which admit the possibility of psychotic features in the context of depressed mood or mania (e.g., in major depression or in bipolar disorder).

The present chapter has been organized in relation to the more recent DSM-III rubrics, but to some extent we have reached for evidence gathered in relation to older categories of similar form and content, also summarized elsewhere (e.g., Kay & Bergmann, 1980; Gurland & Cross, 1982; Henderson & Kay, 1984). Most recent epidemiologic evidence pertains to the dementias and to depressive disorders; this accounts for a relative emphasis on these conditions. We have also touched upon alcohol and other drug abuse and dependence in later life, as well as the DSM-III anxiety disorders group: panic disorder, phobic disorders, and obsessive-compulsive disorder. Unfortunately, delirium, intoxication, and related acute confusional states, the schizophrenias, and the personality disorders of later life generally have been neglected in recent epidemiologic studies. The present chapter, with a focus on recent research, mirrors this neglect.

Finally, we should mention the analysis of mortality rates, which nearly always has been a mainstay of epidemiologic research. This has not been true in respect to the epidemiology of mental disorders, primarily for two reasons. First, mental disorders are conditions encountered during life. Often, they leave behind no more than a rapidly decaying trace after a death typically due to other causes (Gruenberg, 1980). Second, even when terminal disease processes are biological substrates for mental disorders, as in the dementia associated with Alzheimer's disease, there is a documented problem of suspected variability in routine diagnostic practices and death certification (e.g., Jorm, Henderson, & Jacomb, 1989). This problem now undermines confidence about the vital statistics data pertinent to mental disorders.

II. Dementia Syndromes

A pithy definition for the dementia syndrome is "global deterioration of intellectual functions in clear consciousness (p. 228)." This definition declares dementia to be a disorder of cognition, and its individual words and phrases serve to set dementia apart from the other primary disorders of cognition: mental retardation, delirium, and intoxication states, as well as focal cognitive deficit states such as the amnestic syndrome (Folstein, Anthony, Parhad, Duffy, & Gruenberg, 1985).

Recent diagnostic criteria embellish this definition and call for attention to the specific known or suspected causes of dementia. A dementia syndrome can be due to proximal head trauma, repeated blows to the head (as in professional boxing), communicating hydrocephalus, mutations in mitochondrial DNA (e.g., in MERRF, myclonic epilepsy with ragged red fibers), trisomies associated with Down's syndrome, and other genetic diseases (e.g., Huntington's disease), vascular disease (as in multi-infarct dementia), mood disorders (dementia syndrome of depression), avitaminoses (e.g., nicotinamide deficiency), infections (as in neurosyphilis, Kuru, dementia attributed to human immunodeficiency virus (HIV) infection and acquired immunodeficiency syndrome (AIDS), and brain tumors, as well as other causes mentioned elsewhere (McKhann *et al.*, 1984; Marsden, 1984; Kiloh, 1986; American Psychiatric Association, 1987; World Health Organization, 1990).

Typically, dementias said to be caused by Alzheimer's disease are diagnosed only after the known or suspected causes have been ruled out on the basis of laboratory tests, history, or clinical inference. During life, and even when causes of death are certified, clinical diagnoses of dementia due to Alzheimer's disease must be relied upon, with no expert search for neuropathological changes in specific cortical regions (e.g., plaques or tangles in frontal, temporal regions, cingulate gyrus, and hippocampus) or in subcortical regions (e.g., neuronal fallout in the nucleus basalis of Meynert) (Marsden, 1984; Roth, 1986). As a result, death certificates have uncertain value in the epidemiologic study of Alzheimer's disease and dementia (Jorm *et al.*, 1989).

The neurobiologic changes identified by Alzheimer are suspected to account for some 50–60% of recognized dementia cases after age 60, and possibly as much as 20% more in accompaniment with vascular disease or some other cause (Marsden, 1984; Henderson, 1986; Kohlmeyer, 1986). Evans *et al.* (1989) have reported corresponding values of 84% and 7% for East Boston community residents age 65 and older. Nonetheless, in some community surveys, multi-infarct dementia has been found to be more common than Alzheimer's dementia (AD), most notably in Japan and China (e.g., Shibayama, Kasahara, & Kobiyashi, 1986; Li, Shen, Chen, Zhao, & Li, 1989), but not exclusively (e.g., Folstein *et al.*, 1985; Rorsman, Hagnell, & Lanke, 1986). While this appearance of international disparities should prompt substantive epidemiologic reasoning, differences in method have not been ruled out. Moreover, given a focus on prevailing cases rather than incident cases in virtually all of these studies, the observed variation can be attributable to differing case fatality rates for dementia across various study areas, or even to inadvertent under-representation of multi-infarct dementias in the case material (Jorm, Korten, & Henderson, 1987; Mortimer, 1988).

A. The Estimated Prevalence of the Dementias

The world literature on the epidemiology of dementia syndromes now includes more than 50 prevalence surveys, most with a concentration of survey respondents aged 60–79 years. Survey-based estimates for prevalence of moderate and severe dementia in elderly populations generally have ranged upward from about 1%, centering close to 5%, and with almost all values falling between 2 and 14%. Prevalence estimates for Alzheimer's dementia typically have been about one half the overall dementia prevalence value.

To illustrate, Folstein *et al.* (1985) surveyed 923 elderly subjects, selected in 1981 to be representative of adult household residents in eastern Baltimore, aged 65 years and older. The survey was distinctive in its use of standardized dementia case definitions and a three-stage survey design for screening, medical–psychiatric examination, and differential diagnosis of identified dementia syndromes. The resulting prevalence estimate for *definite dementia syndrome* was 6.1% (± 2.3%), subdivided as 2.0% for Alzheimer's dementia, 2.8% for multi-infarct (vascular) dementia, and 1.3% for other dementias, primarily mixed AD and multi-infarct dementia.

By comparison, a more recent, carefully executed community survey in East Boston found an Alzheimer's dementia prevalence of 12.3%, once other causes of dementia syndromes had been ruled out (Evans *et al.*, 1989). A survey estimate of this size could mean that the elderly residents of East Boston have become affected at an exceptionally high rate, or that dementia cases remain in the East Boston community for a longer period, or even that prevalence values from other surveys were underestimates, perhaps due to less sensitive and accurate case detection methods. Additional studies are needed to resolve these issues, but it is known that prevalence values substantially higher than 12% can be obtained when dementia syndromes from all causes are counted, when the computation includes mild dementia as well as more severely affected cases, and when other features of the survey method are favorable (Gurland, Dean, Cross, & Golden, 1980; Henderson & Huppert, 1984; Kay *et al.*, 1985; Jorm *et al.*, 1987).

B. The Estimated Risk of Dementia and Severe Cognitive Impairment in Later Life

Two remarkable sets of estimates for the incidence of dementia have come from the Lundby studies based at the University of Lund in Sweden and from the Olmsted County medical record–linkage studies at the Mayo Clinic in Rochester, Minnesota. The Lundby studies began in 1947 with a mental morbidity prevalence survey of 2,550 community residents, inhabitants of all ages living within a circumscribed area some distance from the university (Essen-Moller, 1956). These inhabitants were resurveyed after 10 years (Hagnell, 1966) and 25 years (Hagnell et al., 1983; Rorsman et al., 1986), in order to reconstruct the population's experience of psychiatric disturbances during the interim. The prospective data for 1947 to 1957 showed the incidence of senile dementia after age 60 to be .67% per year for men, .84% per year for women (presumed Alzheimer type, all grades of impairment). Corresponding values for multi-infarct dementia were 1.1% and .67% per year for men and women, respectively. Somewhat lower estimates were obtained from the 1957 to 1972 followup data, each set of estimates showing a pattern of age-related increases generally congruent with patterns of age-specific prevalence (Rorsman et al., 1986).

The Olmsted County studies have been based upon surveillance of the health of approximately 55,000 community residents via record linkage between medical facilities, nursing homes, state medical institutions, and private practitioners. During the period 1960 to 1964, a total of 165 dementia cases aged 60 and older were identified, yielding the following age-specific incidence estimates: .13% per year for the ages 60–69, .74% per year for the ages 70–79, and 2.18% per year for the ages 80 and older. Corresponding values for Alzheimer's dementia were .1% per year for 60- to 69-year-olds, .53% per year for 70- to 79-year-olds, and 1.43% per year for those 80 and older (Schoenberg, Kokmen, & Okazaki, 1987). In general, Alzheimer's dementia estimates subsequently reported for 1965 to 1969 and for 1970 to 1974 were slightly lower than those reported for 1960 to 1964. Despite congruence with trend data from the Lundby study, the investigators did not believe the apparent decline merited discussion (Kokmen, Chandra, & Schoenberg, 1988).

The National Institute of Mental Health Epidemiologic Catchment Area (ECA) was a five-site collaborative study of mental disorders in community populations within the United States, completed between 1980 and 1985. The ECA samples were drawn as probability samples to represent adult household and institutionalized populations in each community. Participants included more than 20,000 sampled respondents who agreed to complete the baseline interview and a followup interview one year later. To assess the occurrence of psychiatric disorders, trained lay interviewers administered the Diagnostic Interview Schedule (DIS), a highly standardized assessment for selected mental disorders as defined in the Diagnostic and Statistical Manual, Third Edition (DSM-III) (APA, 1980). After data gathering, a computer program was used to sort respondents' mental and behavioral disturbances into categories, using the DSM-III criteria. ECA estimates for the prevalence of specific mental disorders in the community have been made by using computerized diagnoses from the baseline interviews with these respondents (Regier et al., 1988). ECA estimates for the incidence of specific mental disorders have been made by comparing computerized diagnoses from the followup interviews at four sites with diagnoses made at baseline (Eaton et al., 1989).

The ECA Program produced data on incidence and prevalence of operationally defined impairment in cognitive functioning, but not on dementia syndromes per se. Early validation data led the ECA Program Steering Committee to measure cognitive functioning with the Mini-Mental State Examination (MMSE), a brief test to grade cognitive mental status, interpreting a score in the range from 0 to 17 (many errors) as an operational measure for a construct of *severe cognitive impairment* from all causes (Folstein, Folstein, & McHugh, 1975; Anthony, LeResche, Niaz, Von Korff, & Folstein, 1982; Folstein *et al.*, 1985; George, Landerman, Blazer, & Anthony, 1991). As it turned out, elderly community subjects with scores in the 0–17 range were more likely than not to qualify as cases of dementia or to have other psychiatric disorders with impaired cognitive functioning as a central feature. Some 95% of elderly community residents scored in the 18–30 range, most in the 26–30 range (0–4 errors) where the probability of independently diagnosed dementia has been found to be under 5%.

Using this operational measure, the ECA investigators have estimated the prevalence of severe cognitive impairment from all causes to be 4.9% (± 0.4%) for community residents aged 65 years and older. Prevalence was estimated as 2.9% for persons 65–69 years old, 6.8% for those 75–84 years old, and 15.8% for those who had survived past their 85th birthdays (Regier *et al.*, 1988).

Published ECA estimates for the risk of developing severe cognitive impairment have been based upon an observed difference in performance on the MMSE from baseline to followup administration about one year later at four ECA sites. These ECA risk estimates show the probability of scoring in the low range at followup, among persons who scored above that range at baseline. For all persons aged 65 years and older, this probability was estimated to be 4.64% (Eaton *et al.*, 1989), a value not too distant from the prevalence value of 4.9%, but substantially larger than estimates for annual incidence of dementia reported for Lundby and Olmsted County.

Figure 1a (for males) and Figure 1b (for females) each display two sets of age-specific estimates for risk of severe cognitive impairment among community residents who were between the ages of 18 and 90 at baseline. In this figure and subsequently, the broad sweep of risk in relation to age is conveyed by a solid line of smoothed estimates for individuals of each stated age, where the smoothing of possible discontinuities from age to age has been accomplished by means of a multiple logistic regression model (Eaton *et al.*, 1989). We have used a different procedure, the generalized additive model (GAM) of Hastie and Tibshirani (1990), to explore age-related risks in more detail and to probe for possible discontinuities in risk across the age strata. This procedure involved iterative fitting of the logistic regression model to the previously analyzed data. However, in order to produce a risk estimate for any given age, the GAM smoothing routine borrowed heavily from neighboring age strata and borrowed little or nothing from individuals considerably younger or older (as in estimation procedures based on moving averages). In the figures, our risk estimates from the more exploratory but probative GAM procedure are represented as boxes.

Despite encumbrances in the ECA approach to definition and measurement of cognitive impairment, as well as some uncertainty about error in measurement of age, the age-specific risk estimates shown in Figures 1a and 1b are generally understandable in relation to known causes of impairment in cognitive functioning across age strata. For both men and women, there was a sharp upturn in the risk estimates for the older age strata, following the pattern observed for age-specific incidence of the dementias. At the same time, it must be acknowledged that the magnitudes of these ECA risk estimates

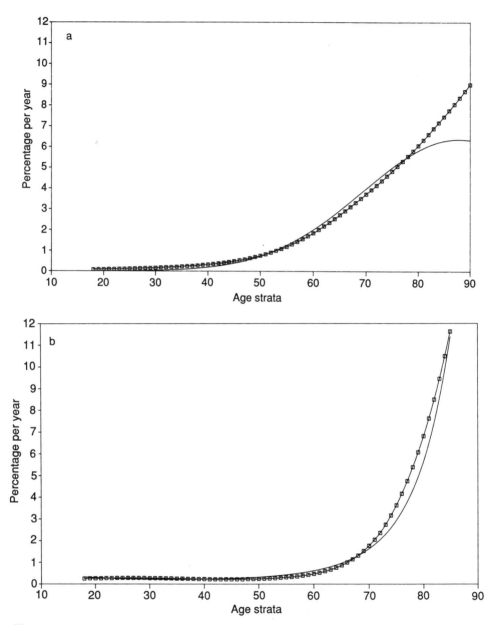

Figure 1 (a) Estimated annual incidence (percent per year) of DIS/DSM-III Severe Cognitive Impairment (MMSE) by age, for males. (Estimates from the generalized additive model have been plotted as boxes, estimates from the original multiple regression model as a solid line.) (b) Estimated annual incidence (percent per year) of DIS/DSM-III Severe Cognitive Impairment (MMSE) by age, for females. (Estimates from the generalized additive model have been plotted as boxes, estimates from the original multiple regression model as a solid line.)

could be overstated to the extent that the baseline method failed to detect mildly affected dementia cases who deteriorated further and were detectable at followup. These estimates also might exceed dementia incidence values because severe cognitive impairment is defined to encompass many other conditions (e.g., delirium and intoxication; see George *et al.*, 1991).

To the extent that pre-senile dementia was a potent, separate determinant of severe cognitive impairment, one might expect some evidence of an early peak in the risk curves for men and women in their 50s and early 60s, followed by a sharp increase in the later years. In the middle-age strata, the level of risk for men was found to be higher than that observed for women, in part reflecting sex differences in alcohol consumption and consequences of alcohol intoxication observed at followup but not at baseline. Further, if there had been an early peak associated with pre-senile dementia, it must have been swamped by other determinants of severe cognitive impairment during those years. Nonetheless, at age 85, the sex differences were less pronounced, with evidence of a slight female excess (10% per year for women age 85 versus 8% per year for men at that age).

The more probative GAM procedure pointed toward increasing risk of cognitive impairment with age for both men and women; after age 85, there was an appearance of greater risk for women versus men. For men, this finding was at odds with results from the usual logistic regression procedure, which showed some evidence of plateau in risk after age 80 (solid line in Figure 1). On one hand, the discrepancy of results is disappointing because of age-related plateau in risks for one sex but not the other prompts consideration of important questions. For example, the interaction challenges the simplest models of senescence as a satisfactory explanation for the occurrence of cognitive difficulty in late life—it begs for attention as to how it is that risk for long-surviving men might plateau, while risk for long-surviving women reaches higher levels in successive age strata. On the other hand, it is important to note that others have observed a decline in incidence of the dementias after age 85 (e.g., Hagnell *et al.*, 1983) and in prevalence of mild dementia as well (e.g., Essen-Moller, 1956; Nielsen, 1962). Further, in two of three autopsy series, the prevalence of Alzheimer-type histologic changes has reached plateau levels in very late life (Evans, 1988; Miller, Hicks, D'Amato, & Landis, 1984). The accumulated evidence concerning these plateaus raises possibilities such as selective mortality of high-risk individuals (Mortimer, 1988), and should temper any premature judgment that Alzheimer's dementia is an inevitable consequence of aging.

C. Suspected Risk Factors for the Dementias in Later Life

The known causes of the dementia syndrome often are other diseases or their biologic substrates, standing as intermediaries between the time of gametogenesis and the occurrence of dementia (e.g., vascular disease or mood disorders, the trisomies underlying Down's syndrome, and HIV infection). Even though some of these intermediary conditions are rare, their contribution to public health burden in the form of dementia is yet another reason to speed toward discovery of what causes these intermediate conditions, the nature of causal linkage to dementia, beneficial treatments, and effective preventive measures. Evans (1988) has discussed these issues with respect to multi-infarct dementia, and vascular dementias in general.

For the most part, epidemiologic research on suspected risk factors for Alzheimer's dementia has been a search for specific extrinsic influences that might challenge a presumptive senescence theory, or alternately, a search for equally challenging evidence of familial aggregation and inheritance. Evans (1988) has pointed out three lines of evidence against simple senescence and against simple genetic theories: (1) observed discordance in studies of identical twins presumed monozygous; (2) epidemiologic evidence of temporal variation in risk, as reported by Hagnell *et al.* (1983) and Rorsman *et al.,* (1986) for the Lundby research group; and (3) epidemiologic evidence of cross-national and regional variation in occurrence of Alzheimer's dementia, including one study suggesting that New York dementia prevalence was greater than dementia prevalence in London (Copeland *et al.,* 1987). From this foundation, he offered a model of gene–environment interaction involving an extrinsic factor to which a great majority of the population might be exposed, capable of producing Alzheimer's-type brain changes and associated dementia in all subjects surviving into the later years of life, given sufficient exposure. A separate causal component showing familial aggregation might be a genetically determined special susceptibility to the exposure, which could lead to an earlier age at onset of Alzheimer dementia (Evans, 1988).

There are several plausible risk factors for Alzheimer's dementia that entail sustained exposures at the high prevalence levels required by Evans' model. For example, a very large proportion of the population is exposed in childhood to the varicella-zoster (V-Z) virus, a DNA-virus of the herpesvirus group shown to be responsible both for chickenpox and, after a period of latency and then reactivation, for herpes zoster (shingles). In both chickenpox and herpes zoster, there is a continuum of responses involving nerve cells, with encephalitis and other central nervous system complications at one extreme. Moreover, the long period of latency following V-Z virus infection in childhood might meet Evans' requirement for sufficient exposure over time. Nonetheless, it should be emphasized that this is a matter of speculation; there now is no definitive evidence implicating V-Z virus or other herpesviruses as being of etiologic importance in relation to Alzheimer's dementia.

Henderson (1988) has provided an overview of more than 20 plausible risk factors for Alzheimer's dementia, including many for which there is meager evidence or none at all. For this chapter, our intent is more limited. We sought regularities in the epidemiologic evidence on AD risk factors, as observed in published case-control comparisons (Soininen & Heinonen, 1982; Heyman *et al.,* 1984; Mortimer, French, Hutton, & Schuman, 1985; French *et al.,* 1985; Amaducci *et al.,* 1986; Chandra, Philipose, Bell, Lazaroff, & Schoenberg, 1987; Shalat, Seltzer, Pidcock, & Baker, 1987; Broe *et al.,* 1990). For the most part, these were clinic-based studies, and the cases were patients referred to specialists in neurology or psychiatry and diagnosed as having a probable or definite late-life dementia for which there was no known cause. A methodologically notable exception was the case-control study conducted by Broe *et al.* (1990), organized around surveillance for new occurrence of dementia in a predesignated general practice study base, with sampling of matched non-cases from within that base. Two of the studies had both hospital controls (with other medical conditions) and population controls. All studies gathered data on suspected risk factors from knowledgeable informants by reasonably standardized interview methods, sometimes augmented by the medical record. To date, only one study has reported results from multiple regression modeling (Soininen & Heinonen, 1982).

Figure 2 is a summary of evidence from these epidemiologic studies, concerning seven suspected risk factors for which there were at least four relative risk estimates and necessary data to derive test-based 95% confidence intervals (Miettinen, 1985). Here, *relative risk* is meant to convey the risk of dementia in Alzheimer's disease among persons *exposed to* or with a specific characteristic (e.g., head injury), divided by the risk of AD

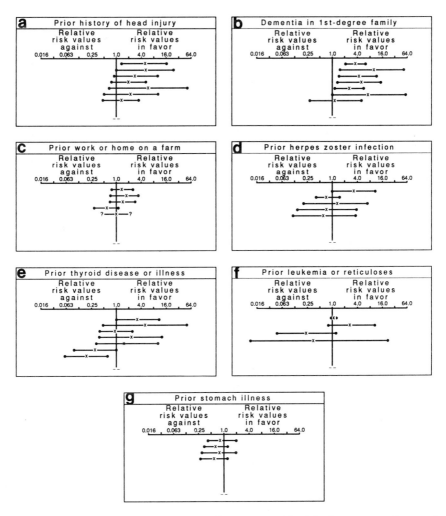

Figure 2 Summary of relative risk estimates from seven epidemiologic case-control comparisons of suspected risk factors for dementia associated with Alzheimer's disease. (The point estimates for relative risk from each case-control comparison are marked with an X, and the test-based 95% confidence intervals are drawn as line segments.)

among those without the characteristic. It follows that relative risk values of 1.0 indicate no difference in risk; those exceeding 1.0 indicate greater risk among the exposed; those under 1.0 indicate greater risk among the nonexposed (see Lilienfeld, 1976; Breslow & Day, 1980; Schlesselman, 1982; or Anthony, 1988).

Several regularities appear in these data. As shown in Figure 2a, seven of seven case-control comparisons gave relative risk estimates in excess of 1.0 (marked by an X), signaling increased risk of AD among persons with head injury, typically defined to include loss of consciousness but no cognitive impairment of note after the immediate period of post-trauma recovery. Also shown in Figure 2a, the 95% confidence intervals for most studies trapped the relative risk value corresponding to no association (RR=1.0), but the balance of support weighed in favor of head injury as a risk factor for AD. The first-published case-control report was an inverse association involving head injury (Soininen and Heinonen, 1982), but data needed to estimate relative risk for the matched pairs under study were not available. Despite the exception, the epidemiologic evidence generally converged with theory, clinical studies, and one twin study according to which head injury caused or has hastened onset of AD (Corsellis, Bruton, & Freeman-Browne, 1973; Evans, 1988; Gedye, Beattie, Tuokko, Horton, & Korsarek, 1989), perhaps by damage to the brain's reserve capacity or to other compensatory and protective mechanisms (see Roth, 1986; Carlsson, 1986). Because it poses a strong challenge to the prevailing senescence theory, this potential clue about AD etiology deserves additional scrutiny to rule out sources of spurious association (see Henderson, 1986; Sackett, 1979).

In general, the recent case-control studies also have pointed toward increased risk of dementia in Alzheimer's disease for individuals who have had first-degree relatives with a dementia (Figure 2b). Here, most of the estimated associations were of moderate strength (RR > 2.0), and had 95% lower limits above 1.0. While the epidemiologic evidence was in accord with many prior clinical studies and family-genetic investigations (summarized by Kay, 1986; Martin, Gerteis, & Gabrielli, 1988), it did not speak to specific genetic models or linkages (e.g., see Breitner, Folstein, & Murphy, 1986; St. George-Hyslop et al., 1987). Moreover, these epidemiologic studies have not yet settled an enduring controversy about differential importance of familial Alzheimer's disease in early-onset versus late-onset cases (see Gruenberg, 1977; Henderson, 1988; Evans, 1988).

A history of living or working on a farm has some plausibility as a risk factor for Alzheimer's disease because of differential exposures (e.g., to livestock and their infections) (Henderson, 1986, 1988). Nonetheless, the available epidemiologic evidence indicates that working or living on a farm had no more than a weak association with occurrence of AD, if any (Figure 2c).

Apropos the discussion of V-Z virus, the evidence on herpes zoster also has been mixed, the balance of available estimates suggesting no strong association with risk of AD (Figure 2d). However, because a history of herpes zoster might not serve well to index activity of the V-Z virus, serologic probes may be needed to yield more definitive evidence on this possible risk factor.

In respect to thyroid disease and thyroid gland dysfunction, the mixed evidence from case-control comparisons is counterbalanced by a backdrop of relevant theory and clinical observation (e.g., Whybrow, Prange, & Treadway, 1969). Four of seven current estimates favored a positive association (RR > 1.0), two showed inverse associations (RR < 1.0), and one comparison showed no association (RR=1.0) (Figure 2e).

The current evidence on prior leukemia or reticuloses is quite evenly balanced, with two estimates showing inverse associations, two showing positive associations, and none reliably different from the null relative risk (RR=1.0) (Figure 2f). In contrast, a history of stomach problems has had a consistently inverse association with occurrence of AD in the reported comparisons (Figure 2g). Nonetheless, the estimated degree of association conveyed by these estimates is not strong (RR < 0.50), and the link to associated theory is not clear.

III. Depressive Disorders

The recent epidemiologic evidence on depressive disorders in later life mainly concerns major depression, and several studies have considered dysthymia (depressive neurosis), as defined in DSM-III (APA, 1980). Major depression involves at least one persistent and prominent episode of depressed mood or anhedonia, with at least four allied symptoms each lasting for two weeks or more during the episode. Psychotic features can be present, but according to DSM-III rules, the diagnosis of major depression should not be made when the episode of depression can be understood in the context of pre-existing or concurrent severe mental disorders such as an intoxication or organic affective syndrome, schizophrenia, or paranoid disorder, or in relation to simple bereavement. By comparison, dysthymic disorder also involves a persistent and prominent depression, but the required duration is two years or more, the number of allied symptoms is three, and no psychotic features can be present. DSM-III also included diagnostic categories for other mood disturbances, such as bipolar disorder, atypical depression, organic affective syndromes, and adjustment disorder with depression. These categories have not figured prominently in epidemiologic research on mental disorders occurring in later life, in part due to apparently low prevalence and incidence (e.g., see George *et al.*, 1988; Regier *et al.*, 1988; Weissman, Bruce, Leaf, Florio, & Holzer, 1991).

A. The Estimated Prevalence of Depression

Almost all epidemiologic evidence shows that depression in older adults is too common to be ignored. For example, we have estimated that slightly more than 5% of adults aged 65 years and older have currently active mood disorders, based on analysis of data from standardized examinations conducted by psychiatrists in the eastern Baltimore community survey (Folstein *et al.*, 1985; Anthony *et al.*, 1985). Applying DSM-III diagnostic criteria, the psychiatrists found an estimated 2.9% of the elderly community population to have an active organic affective syndrome; 0.8% with active major affective disorders such as major depression; and 2.0% with other active depressions such as dysthymic disorder and adjustment disorder with depressed mood. Grouping active major depression and manic episodes with dysthymic disorder into a single DSM-III *affective disorders* category, George *et al.* (1988) analyzed DIS data from four ECA sites and found fairly consistent prevalence estimates for elderly adults (age 65+), ranging from 1.5% (in St. Louis) to 2.9% (in New Haven)—but the DIS method did not attempt to assess DSM-III organic affective syndromes nor adjustment disorder with depressed mood.

At one extreme, community surveys using symptom scales have tended to produce substantially higher estimates of depression prevalence in the later years of life, such as the prevalence value of 34% reported by Turner and Noh (1988). At the other extreme, when only affective psychoses were counted, or when DSM-III criteria for major depression have been applied to elderly community residents, as a rule the survey-based estimates generally have been in the .5%–2.0% range (e.g., Nielsen, 1962; Kay, Beamish, & Roth, 1964; Perrson, 1980; Blazer & Williams, 1980; Weissman *et al.*, 1985; Copeland *et al.*, 1987; Weissman *et al.*, 1991). Exceptions to this rule are noteworthy, as in community survey data from Hobart (Tasmania) showing DSM-III Major Depression prevalence of 6.3% for 70 to 79 year olds and 15.5% for those age 80 and older (Kay *et al.*, 1985), and survey data from Ahtari (Finland), where prevalence of DSM-III dysthymic disorder was 20.6% for adults aged 60 and older (Kivela & Pahkala, 1989). As elucidated by others (e.g., Gurland, Dean, Cross, & Golden, 1980; Kay *et al.*, 1985), the magnitude of these depression-prevalence estimates cannot be understood without taking survey methods into account, especially diagnostic criteria, thresholds, and case ascertainment methods.

Epidemiologic evidence tends to challenge once-prevailing views that depressive illnesses are more common past age 60 or 65, as compared with earlier adult years, and that these illnesses become more common in successive age strata. In their analysis of ECA data on DIS/DSM-III affective disorders, George *et al.* (1988) found generally declining prevalence values past age 55 at three of four ECA sites. The most dramatic decline was observed at the St. Louis site where 6.2% of adults aged 55–64 years had DIS/DSM-III affective disorders, as compared to 2.0% of those aged 65–74 years, .6% of those aged 75–84 years, and .7% of those aged 85 years and older. A tendency toward increasing prevalence was observed only at the central North Carolina ECA site, in the Durham-Piedmont area, where 4.0% of 55- to 64-year-olds, 1.7% of 65- to 74-year-olds, 2.7% of 75- to 84-year-olds, and 3.7% of older adults (85+) were found to have DIS/DSM-III affective disorders.

Feinson (1989) recently summarized evidence from 25 reports on community surveys of depression conducted between 1969 and the present, with a range of methods extending from depression symptom scales to diagnostic instruments like the DIS. She found only two surveys showing increased depression prevalence in older adults as compared to younger adults; the others showed no differences or a tendency for depression prevalence to be greater in younger age strata.

B. The Estimated Risk of Depression

Based on DIS data from the ECA incidence study, estimated risk of developing DSM-III Major Depression for the first time was 1.59% per year for all adults, 1.25% per year for adults age 65 years and older. For older men (65+), estimated risk was 0.9% per year (±

0.7%). For older women (65+), estimated risk was about 50% greater, 1.48% per year (±0.6%) (Eaton et al., 1989).

Among men, estimated risk ranged between .5 and 1.5% per year in successive strata from age 18 to age 90, and there was a very weak tendency for risk to be lower in older strata (Figure 3a). We have been able to suppress the DSM-III exclusion of major depressive episodes occurring in the context of bereavement after death of a loved one. In so doing, we found slight increases in the risk estimates for virtually all age strata, especially for men who survived past age 60 (Figure 3b). In the ninth decade of life, there was a doubling of risk estimates for major depression when we counted episodes associated with grieving, to an extent that estimated risk values for men in their 80s equaled or exceeded values for those in their 20s (Figure 3b).

Among women, risk estimates from the Generalized Additive Model (GAM) ranged from a low of about .5% per year in the oldest age strata to peak values of about 3% per year for women in their mid-20s and 4–5% per year for women in their mid-40s. In the seventh decade, there was a tertiary peak at about 2% per year (Figure 3c).

Grief-associated episodes of the DSM-III major depression syndrome had some impact on risk estimates for women age 25 to 45, but mattered little in older age strata (Figure 3d). It is likely that deaths to loved ones (especially spouses) more often are experienced as off-time events for younger women, possibly accounting for this pattern of depression risk. As suggested by Bebbington (1987), it also is likely that younger women who lose their spouses have greater hardship in respect to child-rearing and finances.

There was a considerable drop in estimated risk from the peaks to the troughs in Figure 3c. This magnitude of difference from age strata some 10 years apart might be within the range of sampling variability. However, the fairly large numbers of women in each stratum, year by year, made for reasonably precise age-specific risk estimates until the age group 85 to 90 was reached, where the number of respondents was much smaller. Despite these smaller numbers in the oldest old age strata, it is of note that the risk of DIS/DSM-III Major Depression showed age-specific declines in the 8th and 9th decades of life for women. These trends in prospectively obtained risk estimates for major depression differ from recently published hazard rate estimates derived from retrospective age of onset data gathered for ECA baseline interviews (Burke, Burke, Regier, & Rae, 1990). Methods differences most likely account for this variation in that the retrospective age of onset data rely somewhat more heavily upon accuracy of recall over long spans of developmental time (Parker, 1987).

In Hagnell's 1957 to 1972 followup data for women in Lundby, the only non-zero risk values for *severe* depression were found in three age strata: 20–29, 60–69, and 70–79, with the larger values being in later life. For men, severe depression occurred from age 20 through age 59. When severe cases were combined with moderate and mild cases, the data on males showed a peak value for 20 to 29 year olds, followed by gradually declining values until a fairly sharp drop at age 70–79. For women, this aggregation of depression levels produced a sharply rising value from 10 to 19 to 20 to 29, and thereafter relative stability at comparable levels for all 10-year age strata from 20 to 29 through 60 to 69, with a somewhat smaller risk estimate for the 70- to 79-year-olds (Hagnell, Lanke, Rorsman, & Ojesjo, 1982). Thus, the Swedish estimates were not entirely inconsistent

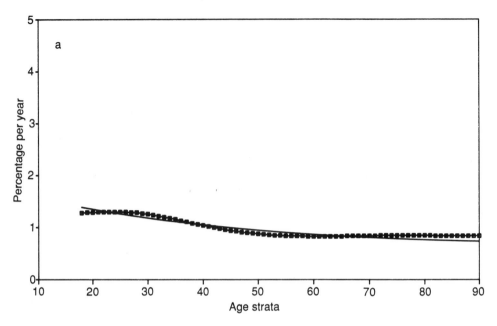

Figure 3a Estimated annual incidence (percent per year) of DIS/DSM-III Major Depression by age, for males. (Estimates from the generalized additive model have been plotted as boxes, estimates from the original multiple regression model as a solid line.)

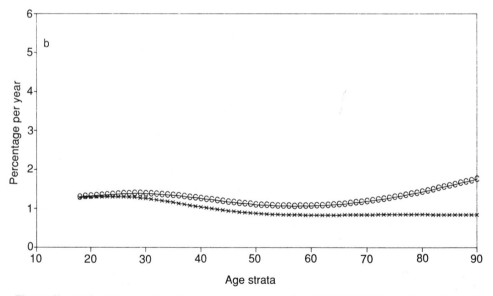

Figure 3b Estimated annual incidence (percent per year) for DIS/DSM-III Major Depression, with and without exclusion of grief-related episodes, by age for males. (Generalized additive model estimates for major depression excluding grief-related episodes have been plotted as Xs, generalized additive model estimates for major depressive episodes including grief-related episodes as Os.)

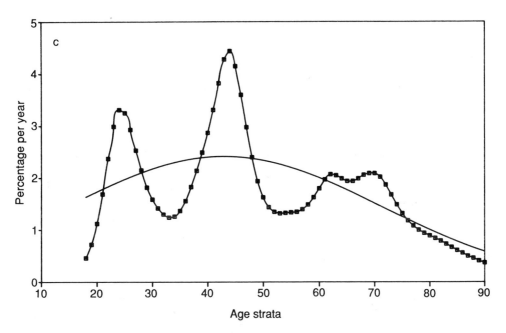

Figure 3c Estimated annual incidence (percent per year) of DIS/DSM-III Major Depression by age, for females. (Estimates from the generalized additive model have been plotted as boxes, estimates from the original multiple regression model as a solid line.)

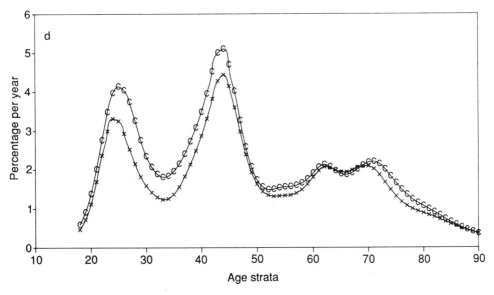

Figure 3d Estimated annual incidence (percent per year) for DIS/DSM-III Major Depression, with and without exclusion of grief-related episodes, by age for females. (Generalized additive model estimates for major depression excluding grief-related episodes have been plotted as Xs, generalized additive model estimates for major depressive episodes including grief-related episodes as Os.)

with those reported here, though they were based upon different sampling schemes, diagnostic classifications and definitions, and methods of measurement. Moreover, the numbers of cases and respondents in the Swedish study were considerably smaller than those studied for ECA incidence estimates.

C. Sex and Gender, Age and Aging as Risk Factors for Depression

The depressions occurring in later life have not been a frequent subject of epidemiologic case-control studies, or of large-scale prospective risk-factor studies. For this reason, it has not been possible to summarize regularities in the evidence on suspected risk factors as was done for dementia in Alzheimer's disease. Nonetheless, a review of published studies allows some generalizations about sex and gender, age and aging, as well as several other suspected risk factors.

1. Male–Female Differences

Notwithstanding several contradictory results (see Murphy *et al.*, 1988; Romanoski *et al.*, submitted), the balance of clinical and epidemiologic evidence has implied that women are at least 1.5 times more likely than men to develop major depression and other depressive disorders (Weissman & Klerman, 1985; Bebbington, 1988), with the possible exception of organic affective syndromes. The ECA major depression risk estimates have rekindled interest in whether there is a reversal of the male:female ratio in risk of depression after the seventh decade of life, a question also raised in a number of clinical studies and community prevalence surveys (e.g., Gurland *et al.*, 1980; Copeland *et al.*, 1987; Conwell, Nelson, Kim, & Mazure, 1989).

2. Age and Aging

There is a common idea that depression risk increases with age, consonant with views on age and depression prevalence, and also with rates of first admissions for depressive psychoses (Bebbington, 1987). Current risk estimates based on prospective study of community samples are opposite, as are rates of first admissions for nonpsychotic depression (Bebbington, 1987). Concerning women, Hagnell's Swedish data and the American ECA data suggest that risk declines after age 69. Concerning men, there is evidence of declining risk (Hagnell *et al.*, 1982) or no difference with age in the later years (Figure 3a).

   Pearlson and Rabins (1988) have noted that the concept of late-onset depression in women is linked to the concept of involutional melancholia, implicitly caused by age-related menopausal changes. This causal linkage retains an enduring plausibility, though the available evidence is mixed, at best (Weissman, 1979). As an illustration, the GAM risk estimates for major depression showed sharp declines across the age strata from 45 years to 50 years, and stayed at relatively low levels during the early and mid-50s (Figure 3c). For most women, these are the ages when menstruation ceases.

   In the context of studying age in association with risk of depression, it is of interest to note an accumulating body of evidence from the United States, Sweden, and elsewhere concerning possible cohort differences in risks of depressive disorders or illnesses, a possibility first noted almost 20 years ago (Schwab, Holzer, & Warheit, 1973). Hagnell's Swedish data from Lundby constitute the most persuasive evidence that birth cohorts born after World War II have experienced increased risk of depressive illnesses (Hagnell *et al.*, 1982). This evidence is corroborated by American estimates obtained retrospectively in the ECA baseline interviews and elsewhere (Rice *et al.*, 1984; Weissman *et al.*, 1984; Klerman *et al.*, 1985; Klerman, 1986; Wickramaratne, Weissman, Leaf, & Holford, 1989; Weissman, Bruce, Leaf, Florio, & Holzer, 1991), but not entirely by trend data from Stirling County, Nova Scotia (Murphy, Sobol, Neff, Olivier, & Leighton, 1984).

Although the reported cohort differences in depression risk can be understood as methodologic artifacts (see Anthony, 1987; Hasin & Link, 1988), major cohort effects might be occurring. If so, it would be a mistake to draw firm conclusions about age and depression prevalence without taking these effects into account. Relatively greater depression prevalence among younger adults, due to cohort or period effects, might mask what otherwise would be an age-related increase in prevalence of depression.

D. Other Suspected Risk Factors for Depression in Later Life

1. Age-Related Pathologies

To some degree, ideas about age and depression have been shaped by decades-old observations that mood disturbances can arise in the course of separable age-related diseases, including the cerebral degenerative pathologies cited by Roth (1980) and discussed in this chapter under the heading of dementia risk factors. Lehmann (1982) has cited examples of age-related diseases causing depression from within broad categories of neoplasms, cardiovascular disease, metabolic disorders, and the degenerative diseases. Studies restricted to clinical samples can offer persuasive arguments that depression syndromes arise as part of separable disease processes occurring in the later years of life (e.g., Robinson *et al.*, 1984; Holland *et al.*, 1986). In this tradition, Cadoret and Widmer (1988) have used a prospective study design to examine temporal sequencing, finding that severe illness predicted depression symptoms among elderly men, not elderly women. In the tradition of community surveys, Kivela and Pahkala (1989) found both major depression and dysthymic disorder to be associated with the presence of clinician-rated health problems, but did not clarify the temporal sequence giving rise to the association.

2. Age-Related Biologic Changes

Bebbington (1987, 1988) has drawn attention to the possibility that age exerts a releasing effect on severe affective disorders, and has speculated about possible mediation through biological mechanisms. Lipton (1976) reviewed several age-related biologic changes that might be plausible mediators: depletion of relevant biogenic amines via increased monoamine oxidase (MAO) activity, linkages between functioning of the gonads and MAO, and change in thyroid function. More recent evidence implicates other aspects of the hypothalamic–pituitary–adrenal axis, serotonin receptor activity, and deficits in central norepinephrine function (Doyle, George, Ravindran, & Philpott, 1985; Schneider, Severson,

Sloan, & Frederickson, 1988). Meyers and Alexopoulos (1988) have speculated that late-onset depression in some instances might represent acceleration of a normally distributed rate of brain aging, e.g., as manifest in premature depletion of biogenic amines. Considering morphologic and structural brain changes, Pearlson and Rabins (1988) have discussed nonspecific brain atrophy as a factor that possibly unmasks a predisposition to depression.

Emerging evidence on these matters of brain structure and function will require epidemiologic reasoning of a type previously used to examine the co-occurrence of functional disorders with cerebral disease and central nervous system insults like head injury. Key issues in this reasoning involve whether the degree of co-occurrence is beyond fortuitous coincidence, and whether clinic-attending patients with non-specific brain atrophy are a biased sampling of cases in which depressions are over-represented (Roth, 1955).

3. Family and the Risk of Affective Disorders

There is some evidence that family history is associated with occurrence of depressive disorders in the later years of adulthood, but to a lesser extent than in earlier life (e.g., Mendlewicz, 1988; Conwell *et al.*, 1989). Levels of these associations in late-life depression might be biased to a greater extent than in studies of earlier-onset depressions, for example, through variation in recall of family history by affected probands (Sackett, 1979).

4. Demographic and Social Role Characteristics

We recently have completed new analyses of ECA prospective data on major depression occurring for the first time after age 40. These multiple logistic regression analyses have shown patterns of association between risk of depression in middle to later adulthood and the following demographic and social role characteristics: being separated or divorced; being unemployed; having failed to complete 12 years of schooling; and being White–Not Hispanic (Royall & Anthony, submitted manuscript). Similar relationships emerged when analyses were restricted to adults older than 59. For almost all of these demographic and social role characteristics, there is supportive evidence from prevalence surveys and other sources (e.g., Weissman *et al.*, 1991; Bebbington, 1987, 1988; Kivela & Pahkala, 1989), but support from other prospective studies and from case-control studies is lacking. Thus, further inquiry is essential before firm conclusions can be drawn about these suspected sociodemographic risk factors for depression in later life.

IV. Panic Disorder

Panic disorder, one of several DSM-III anxiety disorders, involves recurrent, unexplained attacks of apprehension or fear, with at least four allied symptoms (e.g., palpitations, dizziness, trembling or shaking, feelings of unreality). As such, in DSM-III, panic disorder is distinguished from agoraphobia, major depression, and other DSM-III mental disorder categories, though panic attacks may occur in the context of these other disorders (APA, 1980).

A. The Estimated Prevalence of Panic Disorder

According to ECA results, an estimated 0.5% (± 0.1%) of adults have active panic disorder, with at least one panic attack in the recent past. The prevalence estimate was 0.1% (± 0.1%) for those aged 65 and older, with little evidence of variation across sites. No active cases were found among older men, and the prevalence value for older women was .2% (± .1%) (George et al., 1988; Regier et al., 1988).

B. The Estimated Risk of Panic Disorder

Considering all adults, the estimated risk of developing panic disorder for the first time was 0.56% per year, with peak values occurring between age 30 and age 64. The male peak was close to 0.5% per year, and was observed in the late 30s. By comparison, the female peak was slightly greater than 1.0% per year, and was observed in the early 40s. All incident cases past age 60 were women, and for women age 65 and older the estimated risk of panic disorder was 0.07% (± 0.05%) per year (Eaton et al., 1989).

According to these risk estimates, panic disorder has been a fairly infrequent occurrence in later life, but there are important associations between age and risk of panic disorder. The usual logistic regression model showed peak values occurring between age 35 and 45 for both men and women, but the GAM procedure pointed toward two peaks, one occurring in the late 20s and the other occurring in the mid-50s (Figures 4a and 4b). The GAM risk curves are consistent with results from a recently published multiple-regression analysis of risk factors for panic disorder (Keyl & Eaton, 1990).

C. Suspected Risk Factors for Panic Disorder in Later Life

Though scanty, available evidence suggests that age, being female, marital status, and social class merit continuing attention in risk-factor models for occurrence of panic disorder in later years of life (Eaton, Dryman, & Weissman, 1991). Nonetheless, this conclusion rests solely upon the observation that age did not modify observed associations in multiple regression analyses focused upon risk of panic disorder in adulthood generally (Keyl and Eaton, 1990). Clearly, more study is needed.

In the absence of firm evidence, we offer a speculation that panic disorder occurring after age 50 often will coincide with cardiovascular disease, or with fear of incipient heart attack. If this is so, it might be worthwhile to draw a distinction between panic attacks involving cardiovascular complaints and those restricted to psychosensory and psychologic complaints, as practiced elsewhere (Keyl & Eaton, 1990). It follows that the DSM-III rule to exclude panic disorder *due to physical disorder* may prove difficult to implement in both clinical practice and epidemiologic studies.

It also is quite plausible that serious life events, or more specifically, an enduring severe danger of such events, merit consideration in risk-factor models for panic disorder in late life, as observed in other age groups (e.g., Finlay-Jones, 1981). These conditions

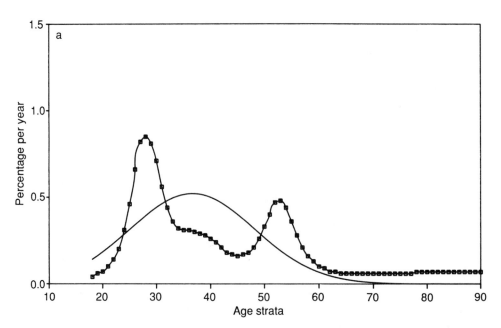

Figure 4a Estimated annual incidence (percent per year) of DIS/DSM-III Panic Disorder by age, for males. (Estimates from the generalized additive model have been plotted as boxes, estimates from the original multiple regression model as a solid line.)

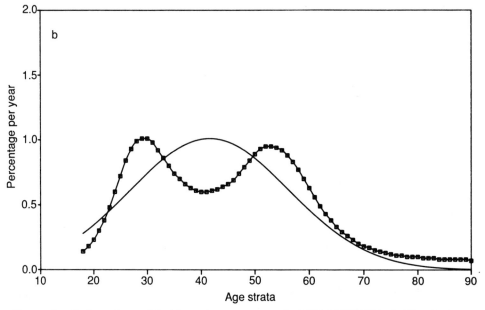

Figure 4b Estimated annual incidence (percent per year) of DIS/DSM-III Panic Disorder by age, for females. (Estimates from the generalized additive model have been plotted as boxes, estimates from the original multiple regression model as a solid line.)

have been accorded causal importance in clinical reports about anxiety syndromes in old age, which will be mentioned in relation to risk factors for phobic disorders.

Finally, the relatively low risk of panic disorder in late life might be linked to age-associated declines in brain concentrations of the monoamine neurotransmitters. This linkage would be consistent with one of the hypothesized neurobiologic mechanisms for panic attacks, involving monoamine-containing neurons in the locus ceruleus and other brain regions (see Gelder, 1986).

V. Phobic Disorders

The phobic disorders include agoraphobia, social phobia, and simple phobia. By DSM-III rules, these anxiety disorders involve more enduring and unreasonable fear than panic disorder, often in response to specific phobic stimuli. For simple phobia, the stimuli typically are readily identified objects or settings such as spiders, dogs, closets, and high places. By comparison, social phobia is activated in specific contexts, such as speaking in public or meeting new people. Agoraphobia, arguably the most severe form of phobia, is defined in relation to marked fear and avoidance of "being alone or in public places from which escape might be difficult or help not available in case of sudden incapacitation, e.g., crowds, tunnels, bridges, public transportation (p. 227)" (APA, 1980). Recent latent structure analyses of epidemiologic data suggest a value in distinguishing two subtypes of agoraphobia. *Classic* agoraphobia primarily involves fear and avoidance of going out (of the home) alone, of being alone, and of crowds, but not so frequently fear of public transportation, tunnels, or bridges. *Situational* agoraphobia more often involves fear and avoidance of public transportation, tunnels, or bridges, but not going out alone or being alone (Eaton & Keyl, 1990).

A. The Estimated Prevalence of Phobic Disorders

Based on ECA surveys, an estimated 6.2% (± 0.2%) of adults have a phobic disorder with phobic anxiety in the prior month. For older adults (age 65+), the estimate was 4.8% (± 0.3%). Estimated prevalence for older women was found to be substantially higher than for older men (6.1% versus 2.9%) (Regier et al., 1988).

Within the ECA Program, there was a remarkable site-to-site variation in the prevalence of phobic disorders. Lower values were observed at the St. Louis (MO) and Los Angeles (CA) sites, higher values at the Baltimore (MD) site and the Durham-Piedmont site in central North Carolina. To illustrate, for elders living in St. Louis, the prevalence of recently active simple phobia was 1.7%, as compared to 10.0% and 9.7% for those in Baltimore and central North Carolina, respectively. Similar differences were found for agoraphobia (.6% versus 5.0% and 5.2%) and for social phobia as well (.2% versus 1.6% and 1.4%) (George et al., 1988).

For adults age 65 and over, simple phobia was the most common, with prevalence values ranging from 1.7% at the St. Louis site to 9.7% in central North Carolina and 10.0% in Baltimore. Agoraphobia was next most common in later life, with a prevalence value of .6% in St. Louis, 5.0% in Baltimore, and 5.2% in central North Carolina. Social phobia was observed less frequently: .2% in St. Louis, 1.4% in central North Carolina, and 1.6% in Baltimore (George *et al.,* 1988).

B. The Estimated Risk of Phobic Disorders

ECA estimates show that risk of developing DSM-III Phobic Disorder for the first time was 3.98% (0.30%) per year for adults of all ages. Estimated risk for adults aged 65 years and older was at a comparable level, 4.29% (± 0.58%) (Eaton *et al.,* 1989). Phobia risk values of this magnitude were unexpected, and lower prevalence values in later life had led many to draw premature conclusions about lower risk. Although present space does not allow discussion of the underlying substantive and methodologic issues, interested readers can refer to source material on these topics (e.g., Eaton *et al.,* 1985, 1989; Eaton, Dryman, & Weissman, 1991).

ECA risk estimates for cognitive impairment, major depression, and panic disorder showed considerable nonlinearity in relation to age. This was not found for phobic disorders, where the risk estimates varied little or not at all from one age stratum to the next (Figures 5a and 5b). The curves in Figure 5b show some age-related declining risk after the middle years, but this has been found to be more artifact than real (Eaton *et al.,* 1989). Thus, these estimates run counter to the once-prevailing view that older adults are not at risk of anxiety disorders. Moreover, if middle age is a peak period for risk of anxiety disorders (e.g., Shepherd & Gruenberg, 1957), then the peak must be induced by disorders other than the phobias (e.g., by panic disorder).

Eaton & Keyl (1990) have reported on ECA analyses in which it was found that risk of classic agoraphobia was extremely low for adults age 65 years and older, as compared to younger adults. In contrast, the older adults were found to have slightly greater risk of situational agoraphobia, as compared to younger adults. Risk estimates for the other specific phobic disorders are not yet available.

C. Suspected Risk Factors for Phobic Disorders

The epidemiologic findings on phobia risk in later life substantiate earlier discussions by Roth (1959) and other clinicians who have observed patients with adult-onset of phobic anxiety, sometimes occurring in the midst or aftermath of serious life events. Along these lines, Marks (1987) has discussed space phobias that have begun or become worse after a fall, and has related them to fears of falling in old age, when there may be poorer agility, greater risk of fractures, loss of righting reflexes as a result of neuronal fallout, and focal neurological damage, as well as greater risk of a serious fracture.

To our knowledge, being female is the only suspected risk factor to be implicated consistently in epidemiologic studies on phobic disorders in late life (Eaton, Dryman, & Weissman, 1991; Eaton & Keyl, 1990). In order to understand the observed variation in prevalence of phobic disorders across ECA sites, it will be necessary to study ethnic and sociocultural differences in more detail than present data allow (Brown, Eaton, & Suss-

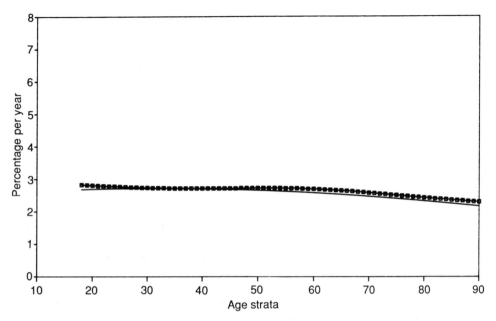

Figure 5a Estimated annual incidence (percent per year) of DIS/DSM-III Phobic Disorder by age, for males. (Estimates from the generalized additive model have been plotted as boxes, estimates from the original multiple regression model as a solid line.)

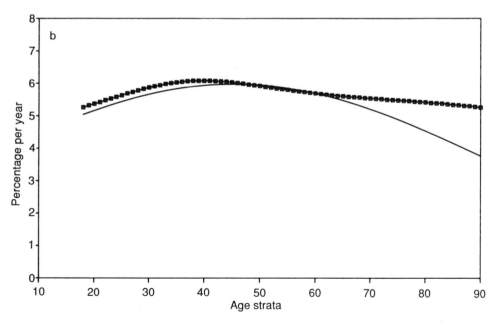

Figure 5b Estimated annual incidence (percent per year) of DIS/DSM-III Phobic Disorder by age, for females. (Estimates from the generalized additive model have been plotted as boxes, estimates from the original multiple regression model as a solid line.)

man, 1990). Other observed associations that should be examined in future research involve the extent to which a history of panic attacks is essential to the development of agoraphobia or other subtypes of phobic disorders in late life, and whether pre-existing mental disorders increase risk of phobic disorders in late life, as appears to be the case in earlier years of adulthood (Eaton & Keyl, 1990).

VI. Obsessive-Compulsive Disorders

Notwithstanding some controversy (e.g., Roth, 1984), obsessive-compulsive disorder was grouped with panic disorder and the phobias within the DSM-III category for Anxiety Disorders. DSM-III criteria for obsessive-compulsive disorder (OCD) call for presence of either an obsession or a compulsion that is a significant source of distress or impaired functioning. DSM-III defines obsessions as recurrent and persistent ego-dystonic ideas, thoughts, images, or impulses that are experienced as senseless or repugnant. Compulsions are defined as "repetitive and seemingly purposeful behaviors that are performed according to certain rules or in a stereotyped fashion (p. 235)," intended to produce or prevent some future event or situation, and performed with a sense of compulsion. According to DSM-III rules, OCD is not to be diagnosed if it can be attributed to some other mental disorder (APA, 1980).

A. The Estimated Prevalence of Obsessive-Compulsive Disorder

According to ECA estimates based on DSM-III diagnostic criteria and the DIS method, the prevalence of recently active obsessive-compulsive disorder was just under one percent (0.85%) among adults aged 65 years and older. By comparison, prevalence estimates were 2.23% for 18- to 29-year-olds, 2.06% for 30- to 44-year-olds, and 1.01% for 45- to 64-year-olds (Karno & Golding, 1991). Corresponding estimates for elderly community residents at four ECA sites ranged from .7% (in New Haven) to 1.4% (in Central North Carolina) (George et al., 1988).

B. The Estimated Risk of Obsessive-Compulsive Disorder

Based on DIS data from the ECA incidence study, estimated risk of developing DSM-III Obsessive-Compulsive Disorder for the first time was .69% per year for all adults, not too different from the value of .64% per year observed for adults aged 65 years and older (Eaton et al., 1989). For older men (65+), estimated risk was .12% per year (± 0.09%). For older women (65+), estimated risk was about eight times greater, 1.00% per year (± 0.29%) (Eaton et al., 1989).

Among men, the highest estimates were observed for the youngest adults, where the risk of developing obsessive-compulsive disorder was just above 0.5% per year. There was some tendency for the risk values to decline across age strata, leading to values just under .12% per year for men in their ninth decade (Figure 6a).

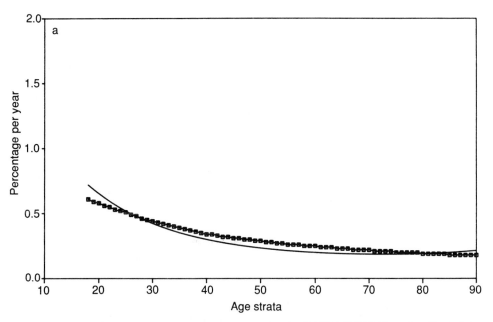

Figure 6a Estimated annual incidence (percent per year) of DIS/DSM-III Obsessive-Compulsive Disorder by age, for males. (Estimates from the generalized additive model have been plotted as boxes, estimates from the original multiple regression model as a solid line.)

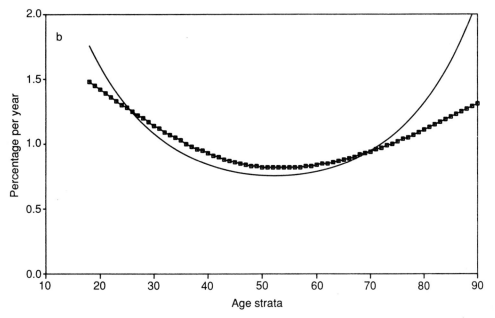

Figure 6b Estimated annual incidence (percent per year) of DIS/DSM-III Obsessive-Compulsive Disorder by age, for females. (Estimates from the generalized additive model have been plotted as boxes, estimates from the original multiple regression model as a solid line.)

Among women, the risk estimates followed a U-shaped curve. The GAM estimates were about 1.5% per year for the youngest adult women, with a drop to about .7% per year in the middle years of adulthood, and then a climb to the 1.0–1.25% per year range between the ages of 75 and 90 (Figure 6b). Previously published risk estimates based on the usual logistic regression model also followed a U-shaped curve, but with somewhat higher values for the youngest women and the oldest old women (Eaton *et al.*, 1989).

A possibility of increased OCD risk among women in very late life also emerged in survival analyses of retrospective age of onset data obtained in ECA baseline interviews (Burke *et al.*, 1990). Thus, the prospective risk estimates and those based on retrospection appear to contradict a prior impression that obsessive-compulsive disorder (OCD) is "a disorder with early age of onset (p. 209)" (Karno & Golding, 1991).

If the up-turning OCD risk curve in later years can be substantiated in future studies, it might prove useful to probe its linkage with aging processes such as age-related declines in brain concentrations of serotonin and norepinephrine. These are biogenic amines previously implicated in neurobiologic speculations and research probing the etiology and pathology of OCD (Insel *et al.*, 1985; Hollander, Fay, & Leibowitz, 1988). In addition, occurrence of OCD has been linked to neurological illnesses, some of which become more common with age (Grimshaw, 1964). Finally, obsession-like and compulsion-like behavior can emerge in response to perceived or real declines in cognitive functioning (Evans, 1990). Even among individuals without OCD, both younger and older, concerns about forgetfulness can lead to distressing behavior such as returning over and over to check whether the stove has been turned off or whether the door was locked; there can be concerned rumination about whether tasks such as these have been forgotten. Whereas these behaviors might come to qualify as obsessional or compulsive traits or behavior patterns, it also is conceivable that the DIS/DSM-III method involves a mislabeling of these behaviors as if they were evidence of primary mental disorders.

If our speculations about cognition and OCD are correct, the apparently greater and increasing risk of OCD among older women as compared to older men might follow from the role of women as the primary or sole homemakers responsible for tasks that can be dangerous if left untended. In addition, or perhaps separately, the sex differences in pattern and level of risk might be due to an apparently greater risk of cognitive difficulty among women in their 80s and 90s, as compared to men who have survived to corresponding ages (Figure 1b).

C. Suspected Risk Factors for Obsessive-Compulsive Disorders in Later Life

1. Male–Female Differences

A large number of clinical studies have pointed toward a preponderance of women among patients being treated for OCD, and greater prevalence of OCD was found among women in the ECA surveys. However, when multiple regression methods were used to control for social and economic factors, it was concluded that the apparent male–female difference in prevalence should be attributed to these factors (Karno, Golding, Sorenson, & Burnam, 1988). Without intending to gainsay these results from analyses of prevalence data, we believe that the apparent sex differences in ECA risk estimates for older adults merit further study.

2. Education

Some clinical researchers have been impressed by an unexpected high educational achievement among patients with OCD, but analyses of ECA lifetime prevalence data have raised a possibility that individuals who started high school but did not graduate are just as likely to have developed OCD as college graduates (perhaps more so); for high school graduates, the OCD lifetime prevalence estimate was lower than for either of these groups (Karno & Golding, 1991). Future studies are needed to clarify this possibly important risk factor relationship, and to determine whether a similar relationship holds for older adults.

3. Variation across ECA Sites

Regier *et al.* (1988), as well as Karno and Golding (1991), have reported OCD estimates for all adults that give an impression of greater prevalence in the eastern Baltimore community and in the Durham-Piedmont community of central North Carolina, as compared to the other three ECA sites. In prevalence estimates for older adults (age 65+), George *et al.* (1988) also found higher values at the North Carolina site. Although this variation across ECA sites might be within the bounds of sampling variability, the possibility of site-specific differences based on factors such as physical geography and culture should not be dismissed before additional study, particularly in view of similar patterns observed for phobic disorders.

VII. Syndromes of Dependence and Abuse Involving Alcohol and Other Drugs _____

Within DSM-III, the broad class of Substance Use Disorders encompasses syndromes of psychoactive drug dependence and also syndromes of psychoactive drug abuse. To some degree, the case criteria for these syndromes depend upon the drug involved (e.g., alcohol versus cocaine). Nonetheless, for alcohol and many other drugs, DSM-III defined the dependence syndrome by requiring presence of (1) either a pattern of pathological use or evidence of impaired social or occupational functioning due to drug use, and (2) either evidence of tolerance after sustained use or a withdrawal syndrome when sustained use is disrupted by abstinence or by pharmacologic antagonism. By comparison, the abuse syndrome generally was defined by presence of both pathological drug use and impaired social or occupational functioning due to drug use, and the abuse episode must last for at least one month (APA, 1980; Anthony & Helzer, 1991). In the ICD-10 and DSM-IIIR, psychoactive drug dependence and abuse are defined somewhat differently, but at present there are no published reports of epidemiologic data based on these newer criteria (APA, 1987; WHO, 1990).

Consistent with prior reports concerning the epidemiology of DSM-III substance use disorders, this chapter combines DSM-III alcohol abuse and alcohol dependence under a single heading of alcohol abuse–dependence, implying presence of either abuse or dependence, or both. Likewise, abuse and dependence involving barbiturates, tranquilizers, marijuana, cocaine, and other internationally regulated substances have been grouped together and labeled drug abuse–dependence—neither alcohol nor tobacco nor caffeine is considered under the heading of drug abuse–dependence (Helzer *et al.*, 1991; Anthony and Helzer, 1991).

A. The Estimated Prevalence of Alcohol and Other Drug Abuse–Dependence

To a large extent, the occurrence and epidemiologic distribution of dependence and abuse syndromes involving alcohol and other psychoactive drugs are dependent upon patterns of exposure to these drugs and their consumption. As in Frost's early formulation of epidemiologic theory for infectious diseases, the epidemiology of these conditions is influenced not only by what determines exposure and effective contact with the human organism, but also by what determines response once exposure and effective contact have occurred (Anthony & Helzer, 1991; Anthony, 1990). For the most part, this important distinction has not been given attention in epidemiologic studies of the alcohol and drug syndromes that appear in later life. As a result, the epidemiologic evidence presented here typically involves study of abuse–dependence in relation to all other persons, with no discrimination of drinkers or drug users who have not developed abuse–dependence syndromes.

An estimated 2.8% ($\pm$ 0.2%) of adults qualify as currently active cases of alcohol abuse–dependence, according to DIS/DSM-III diagnoses made for the ECA surveys. Strong associations were found to exist between prevalence of alcohol abuse–dependence, sex, and age. By way of illustration, prevalence was estimated as 6.0% for men age 18–29, 6.2% for 30 to 44 year olds, 4.0% for 45 to 64 year olds, and 1.8% for those 65 and older. Corresponding values for women were 2.3%, 1.1%, .3%, and .3% (Regier *et al.*, 1988). Site-specific prevalence estimates for the elderly, reported by George *et al.* (1988), have revealed important variations deserving continued study. At the Baltimore and St. Louis sites, active alcohol abuse–dependence was found in about 1.5% of those age 65 and over, versus prevalence values of .4% in central North Carolina and 0.8% in New Haven. This observed variation might be due to variability in alcohol beverage consumption across these regions, but final interpretation is made difficult by complicated patterns of urban-rural differences within population subgroups at several sites (Helzer *et al.*, 1991; Blazer, George, Woodbury, Manton, & Jordan, 1984).

Holzer *et al.* (1984), analyzing data on elderly respondents at the first three ECA sites (New Haven, Baltimore, St. Louis), found that virtually all recently active cases of alcohol abuse–dependence were in the younger-old strata from age 60 to age 79. No recently active cases of alcohol abuse–dependence were found among 989 women aged 75 and older, and none among 87 men aged 85 and older.

While there can be no escape from the possibility that the DIS method failed to diagnose alcohol abuse–dependence properly, it is of interest to note generally comparable prevalence values and age-associated trends in other surveys. For example, in the

Baltimore survey with standardized examinations by psychiatrists, cases were identified according to DSM-III criteria, but potentially more sensitive probing and cross-examination methods were used (Anthony *et al.*, 1985). The prevalence estimate for DSM-III alcohol abuse–dependence, based on psychiatric examination of community residents aged 65 and over, was 1.6%—a value not too distant from the contemporaneous DIS/DSM-III estimate of 1.4% in Baltimore.

Setting aside the DIS method, use of DSM-III criteria for the ECA surveys might have led to under-identification of alcohol dependence or abuse in later life. However, Weissman *et al.* (1980) reported on a New Haven field survey that used different criteria (i.e., Research Diagnostic Criteria, RDC) and methods (i.e., Schedule for Affective Disorders and Schizophrenia, SADS), and found evidence of probable or definite active alcoholism among 1.6% of 66- to 75-year-olds, but no active cases were found after age 75. Of course, it is a truism that different prevalence rates can be obtained by relaxing diagnostic criteria or by studying drinking patterns only (Blazer and Pennybacker, 1984), and different age-associated trends can emerge as well. For example, drawing from a national sample survey conducted in 1979 for the National Institute on Alcohol Abuse and Alcoholism in the United States, Gomberg (1982) reported an age-associated decline in prevalence of heavy drinking among older women, from 1.0% for women age 61–70 to .0% for women age 71 and over, but an age-associated increase in prevalence of heavy drinking among older men, from 8% for the 61–70 year olds to 13% for those past 70. However, the same investigation found age-associated decline in prevalence of recent drinking problems. The prevalence estimate for showing loss of control over drinking in the prior year or at least two other symptoms of alcohol dependence was 6.0% for men age 61–70, only 2.0% for those past 70. Corresponding values for recent adverse social consequences attributed to drinking were 5% and 4%. Neither loss of control, nor two dependence symptoms, nor adverse drinking consequences were found among women past age 60 (Clark & Midanik, 1982). Thus, at least for the oldest men, there was greater prevalence of recent heavy drinking, but fewer of the drinkers reported alcohol problems.

Recently published community surveys of drinking and drinking problems around the world generally mirror the patterns of age-associated decline in prevalence observed in United States populations. Sometimes, higher or lower prevalence of drinking problems in later life has been found. For example, in Smart and Liban's Canadian community survey, almost 11% of adults aged 60 and older had one or more problems of alcohol dependence (Smart & Liban, 1981). At the other extreme, Kua (1990) surveyed a random sample of 612 elderly Chinese and found that 3.2% drank four or more times each week, but only four subjects had symptoms of alcohol abuse or dependence (e.g., alcohol-related gastritis).

Substantially higher prevalence values also can be obtained by considering formerly active alcohol abuse–dependence, in addition to currently or recently active alcoholism. To illustrate, the DIS/DSM-III method has been used to survey community residents in metropolitan Taipei City and two townships on Taiwan, in Edmonton (Canada), in Puerto Rico, and in South Korea. There now is no published report on prevalence of active alcohol syndromes from this cross-national study. However, the estimated proportion of men aged 65 and older with a history of past or current abuse–dependence (*lifetime prevalence*) was just under 20% in Canada, and close to six percent in Taiwan, as compared to values of 7%, 17%, and 20% for men aged 60 and older in New Haven, St. Louis, and Baltimore, respectively. Further, there were age-associated declines at each of these sites after peak values occurring between ages 25 and 44 (Holzer *et al.*, 1984; Helzer *et al.*, 1991). The work in South Korea and Puerto Rico did not include older community residents, but these surveys showed unanticipated age-associated increases in lifetime prevalence from age 18–24 to 25–44 to 45–64 (Helzer *et al.*, 1990). Treacherous conceptual and methodologic difficulties must be faced in the interpretation and comparison of lifetime prevalence estimates (see Kramer, Von Korff, & Kessler, 1980; Holzer *et al.*, 1984; Helzer *et al.*, 1990). Nonetheless, these epidemiologic findings are clues about possibly important age, cohort, and cross-national differences that should be investigated in future inquiries, both methodologic and substantive. The importance of variation in drinking practices by age, period, and cohort has been underscored by recent analyses of both cross-sectional and longitudinal data from several countries (e.g., Holzer *et al.*, 1984; Makkai & McAllister, 1990; Adams, Garry, Rhyne, Hunt, & Goodwin, 1990).

Whereas older adults clearly face many hazards associated with medicine use (e.g., see Henderson & Kay, 1984), the present evidence indicates exceptionally low prevalence of abuse–dependence syndromes associated with self-administered psychoactive medicines such as tranquilizers and sleeping preparations. The DIS/DSM-III method at five ECA sites revealed no cases of currently active drug abuse–dependence among 5,702 household residents aged 65 and older, even when deliberate misuse of prescribed medicines was taken into account (Regier *et al.*, 1988). In the Baltimore survey based on more thorough examinations, the psychiatrists found very few active cases among elderly subjects, yielding an estimated prevalence of .2% by psychiatrists. By comparison, DIS/DSM-III active drug abuse–dependence affected 1.3% (± .1%) of adults of all ages (Regier *et al.*, 1988), and 3.5% of the 18–24 year olds. In large part, the age-associated decline in prevalence of drug abuse–dependence followed age-associated declines in the proportion reporting a history of ever having taken a medicine or other drug without medical authorization or more than was prescribed (Anthony & Helzer, 1991).

It would seem that to obtain higher prevalence values for active drug abuse–dependence it might be necessary to relax substantially the diagnostic criteria for these syndromes, perhaps to the extent that instances of prescriber error and oversedation by nursing staff are included. Alternately, there might be defects in current field survey methods to detect drug abuse–dependence in later life, analogous to those discussed in relation to alcohol drinking practices and problems (e.g., Gomberg, 1982; Blazer & Pennybacker, 1984; Werch, 1989).

B. The Risk of Alcohol and Other Drug Abuse–Dependence

According to ECA estimates, the estimated risk of developing alcohol abuse–dependence for the first time in adulthood varied roughly in parallel with age relationships observed for the prevalence of these syndromes. For all adults, the estimated risk was 1.79% (± .22%) per year, with peak values among the youngest adults, both male and female. Estimated risk for adults age 65 and older was 1.2% (± .68%) per year for males, .27% (± 0.16%) for females (Eaton *et al.*, 1989).

Shown in Figure 7a, the alcohol abuse–dependence risk curves dropped sharply from

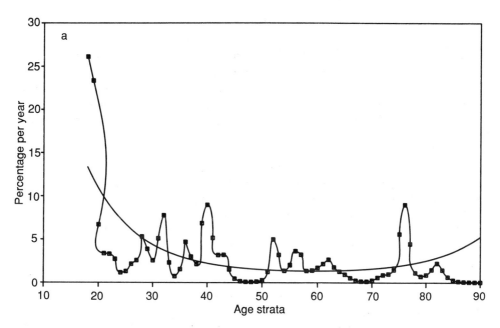

Figure 7a Estimated annual incidence (percent per year) of DIS/DSM-III Alcohol Abuse-Dependence Disorders by age, for males. (Estimates from the generalized additive model have been plotted as boxes, estimates from the original multiple regression model as a solid line.)

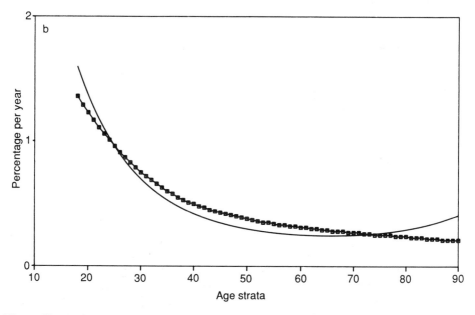

Figure 7b Estimated annual incidence (percent per year) of DIS/DSM-III Alcohol Abuse-Dependence Disorders by age, for females. (Estimates from the generalized additive model have been plotted as boxes, estimates from the original multiple regression model as a solid line.)

high values in the late teens. The GAM procedure hinted toward subsequent peak values in the early 30s and at age 40, with later peaks in the mid-50s, and again after age 70. The broad sweep of estimates from the usual logistic regression model also showed an upturn past age 70. The GAM estimates made this upturn more clear: it was due to several new cases occurring in the mid-70s and just past age 80; there were no new cases among males after age 85.

By comparison with the alcohol abuse–dependence risk curves for males, those for women were of substantially lower magnitude, though the broad sweep of the age-specific risk values was not too different (Figure 7b). However, for the women, the GAM estimates contradicted an apparent upturn in risk past age 70.

It is of note that the male age-specific annual incidence estimates for DSM-III alcohol abuse–dependence syndromes in the Swedish Lundby study also followed a pattern similar to the broad sweep of the ECA risk curve for males, though the Swedish data were based on substantially smaller numbers of cases. Among adult males, peak values were observed in the teen years, with subsequent declines until age 60, when the annual incidence rate increased slightly for the age strata 60–69 and 70–79. Moreover, there were no new cases past age 80 (Ojesjo, Hagnell, & Lanke, 1982).

Based on ECA estimates, the risk of developing drug abuse–dependence for the first time during adulthood was 1.09% (± .17%) per year for both sexes, 1.66% (± .36%) per year for men, and .66% (± .16%) per year for women. Consistent with the age-specific prevalence estimates, no incident cases were observed in age strata beyond the middle years of adulthood, although many of the respondents were in middle age and later life. Due to space limitations, the risk values for drug abuse–dependence are not shown in a figure here; interested readers are referred to the prior report by Eaton *et al.* (1989).

C. Suspected Risk Factors for Alcohol and Drug Abuse–Dependence in Later Life

Owing to the observed low prevalence and risk values, the published literature offers little more than suggestions about risk factors for alcohol and drug abuse–dependency syndromes in later life, derived primarily from clinical experience with treated patients. On this basis, following Rosin and Glatt, Blazer and Pennybacker (1984) have mentioned the possibility that onset of alcoholism in later life is *reactive* to life experiences such as bereavement, retirement, loneliness, infirmity, or marital stress. They also noted that personality factors might play a smaller role in late-onset alcoholism.

Some very careful analyses of prospective Lundby data on DSM-III alcohol abuse and dependence have shown that risk of these alcohol syndromes between the ages of 25 and 59 was strongly associated with a number of plausible risk factors, including family history of alcoholism (estimated RR = 7.4), marital crisis (estimated RR = 22.1), and a socially disintegrated environment characterized by hostility, poverty, and loose or weak social ties (estimated RR = 19.3). However, there were too few incident cases past age 60 to provide for study of risk factors for later-onset alcoholism. Whether the epidemiologic evidence on risk factors for alcohol or drug abuse–dependence syndromes in the later years will conform to patterns observed for younger age strata remains a topic for future study, which should tease apart important period and cohort effects manifest since the ending of Prohibition in the U.S. and since World War II.

VIII. Summary and Future Directions

If each era of epidemiologic research has a character, the last four decades of work are marked by an increased awareness that prevalence surveys can tell us much about the numbers and proportions who have fallen victim to mental and behavioral disturbances, but they yield far too little information about important conditions and processes that influence occurrence of these disturbances in human populations. We now can read literally hundreds of papers based on field surveys that have looked for the dementias and the depressions occurring in later life. On this basis, we know how dreadfully often older people are afflicted with these conditions in later life, we have found that these disorders are quite likely to be unrecognized and untreated by local health authorities, and we know something of how to study these conditions in the field. Beyond this, we have produced no real breakthrough discoveries, either in etiology, or in the planning or evaluation of services.

To some extent, it has been a low yield from epidemiologic field surveys that has slowed progress in development of new knowledge about the occurrence and distribution of the schizophrenias, affective psychoses, delirium, and other mental disorders in later life that have been neglected in this chapter's coverage. A repetitious experience of finding few cases in community samples, coupled with especially difficult measurement problems, has set back epidemiologic research on these disorders, despite their clear importance in relation to the public health and impact on the lives of affected cases and their families.

Against this dismal backdrop, it is encouraging to see a shift toward prospective and longitudinal studies of samples defined and selected epidemiologically, and toward the epidemiologic case-control strategy and its variants. In the case of dementias with unknown cause, there is good reason to be enthusiastic about an increasing number of clinic-based, case-control studies with either hospital or population controls, properly selected. Until more compelling theory is stated, we will need more of these studies. Like a fleet of fishing boats, they can spread out and try many hypotheses at once, without the person-years of effort and expense spent on each longitudinal study, which necessarily must have a sharper focus. In view of the age-associated risks of dementia in later life, and the growing numbers of people surviving to face those risks, we should mount a mammoth fishing expedition with many nets and lines in the water. Problems of multiple significance tests, spurious association, confounding variables, and Berkson's bias can be worked out in a later sequence of replications and targetted prospective studies that pursue important, specific leads.

To be sure, there are ways to improve a new generation of epidemiologic research on the dementias. Case-control studies can be designed with a clearer view of the underlying substantive null hypothesis and its alternatives. More attention can be paid to standardized assessment of suspected risk factors, complementing retrospective reports from readily available informants with biologic probes (e.g., for antigen response) and with other augmented efforts to evaluate pertinent exposures earlier in the lifespan of the cases (e.g., via retrieval of personal records from schools, hospitals, and places of employment). Better statistical theory and method can be called into play. Multisite collaborative studies and planning for future meta-analyses are other areas needing developmental work.

At the present stage of work on the dementias, the observed and replicated association involving history of head injury now should be a focus in the planning of prospective studies. These might be nonconcurrent in design, using records of head injuries occurring in times past—for example, as recorded in modern shock–trauma networks. However, once brain imaging can provide a clear scan of Alzheimer's-type lesions known or judged to pre-date the trauma, it would be foolish to postpone the design of large-sample, concurrent prospective investigations of head-injured patients stratified by type and magnitude of the lesions, as well as by family history of dementia subtype.

For many of the suspected dementia risk factors, long noticed or newly discovered, it now has become possible to take advantage of current and emerging prospective studies of cancer, cardiovascular disease, and other chronic diseases occurring in the later years of life. For example, recently initiated prospective studies originating with a focus on cardiovascular disease and stroke are being supplemented to probe dementia risk factors at the same time, to the extent that the risk-factor profiles can be made to overlap.

In respect to the affective and anxiety disorders, the schizophrenias, and other less frequent disturbances occurring later in life, we need to take pages from the book of the dementia epidemiologists. More epidemiologic case-control studies of these conditions are needed, starting with clinic-based samples, and followed by more probing inquiries. Just as ongoing studies of other diseases are being tapped for study of the dementias, these studies can be harnessed for prospective study of less frequent disturbances of mind and behavior. To some extent, this already is being accomplished in contexts such as the National Institute on Aging's multisite collaborative epidemiologic studies of elderly populations (EPES). Other opportunities exist, but have not been harnessed. To the extent that these investigations already are measuring age-associated changes in immune response, endocrine systems, neurotransmitters, and brain electrical activity, they will offer unprecedented opportunities for coordinated epidemiologic study of mental disorders occurring in later life.

The recent research on alcohol and drug abuse–dependence in later life signals a need for continued emphasis on conceptual and methodologic development, if not a revised nosology. Contrary to the impressions of many clinicians, the available epidemiologic evidence on risk of these syndromes suggests surprising low values. While the problem might stem from too-heavy reliance upon self-report measures and recall (Werch, 1989), and there is a possibility that the wrong behaviors are being assessed (Blankfield & Maritz, 1990), it is conceivable that the clinicians serving older alcohol- and drug-dependent patients are seeing a somewhat different phenomenon, one that could merit redefinition with more specificity to older populations (Blazer & Pennybacker, 1984).

A similar critique is possible in relation to the depressions and the anxiety disorders, particularly in view of suggestions that the observed epidemiologic prevalence estimates are too low (see Blazer & Williams, 1980; Feinson, 1989). And dementia is not immune to a similar line of attack: for example, Evans (1988) has suggested reconsideration of whether dementia in Alzheimer's disease should be conceptualized as disease; Jorm

(1986) has raised interest in subtypes defined by presenting features of information processing.

It is not too late to conduct the clinical and epidemiologic investigations required to address these issues. For example, recent analyses of field survey data have demonstrated an exploration of the latent structure of complaints, symptoms, and signs used to define the DSM-III mental disorder categories. Eaton and Keyl have presented results on situational and classic agoraphobia as well as subtypes of panic disorder (Eaton & Keyl, 1990; Keyl & Eaton, 1990), Blazer *et al.* (1984) on alcohol abuse and dependence, Gurland *et al.* (1980) on dementia and depression. We now need a coordinated effort through which the field survey findings of this type will be evaluated in the context of clinical practice and research. After all, if we are to come to grips with the problems of mental disorders in later life, it is essential to build deliberate bridges between laboratory research on these conditions, epidemiologic research, and both clinical research and practice (see Anthony, 1988). For the past several decades, epidemiologists have tried to take the clinical concepts and methods into the context of field studies, and they will continue to do so. The bridges can be strengthened further when clinicians and laboratory scientists try the epidemiology-forged concepts and methods in their work as well.

Finally, we wish to direct attention to a basic epidemiologic principle that will prove to have an increasing importance in the remaining years of this century and well into the next century: namely, that rarely occurring events might not appear until after a large accumulation in person-years of experience. This principle now serves as a foundation stone in the modern development of medicinals within the context of the pharmaceutical industry and drug regulation decisions, and helps explain why postmarketing surveillance for adverse drug reactions has become an important tool for new drug development. Rare but extremely important adverse reactions may not be apparent in the earlier stages of drug development, when relatively limited numbers of patients are exposed to a new medicine. As rare events, these adversities begin to emerge only with the dramatic increase in person-years of population experience that effective marketing can bring.

To this point, there has been little opportunity for rigorous, scientific study of the population's experience in health and disease past the 8th decade of life. This aspect of our history as a species is changing, and there is a rapid and growing accumulation of person-years of experience during a period of life that now is mainly uncharted. As these person-years of experience continue to accumulate, we should expect to find some unexpected events, perhaps in the form of new diseases that now pass without clinical recognition, perhaps in the form of new types or clusters of disturbed mental life and behavior. To the extent that we look only for mental disorders as they now are codified in the diagnostic and statistical manuals of our time, we will miss these events as they emerge. To bring them into view, we must gaze with informed but open minds toward and beyond the new horizons in the later years of life.

Acknowledgments

The Epidemiologic Catchment Area Program was a multisite collaborative study of psychiatric disorders, carried out in five United States metropolitan areas by University-based research teams in collaboration with staff of the Division of Biometry and Epidemiology

(DBE) of the National Institute of Mental Health (NIMH). During the period of data collection, the ECA Program was supported by cooperative agreements. The NIMH Principal Collaborators were Darrel A. Regier, Ben Z. Locke, William W. Eaton, and Jack Burke; NIMH Project Officers were Carl A. Taube and William Huber. The Principal Investigators and Co-Pls from the five sites were Yale University, MH34224—Jerome K. Myers, Myrna M. Weissman, and Gary L. Tischler; The Johns Hopkins University, MH33870—Morton Kramer, Ernest Gruenberg, and Sam Shapiro; Washington University, St. Louis, MH33883—Lee N. Robins and John Helzer; Duke University, MH35386—Dan Blazer and Linda George; University of California, Los Angeles, MH35865—Marvin Karno, Richard L. Hough, Javier I. Escobar, M. Audrey Burnam, and Dianne Timbers. Preparation of this paper was supported by ADAMHA and NIA Research and Training Grants MH41908, MH14592, AG00161, DA04823. Appreciation is extended to Ms. Denise Spriggs and Ms. Jean Lavelle for their bibliographic and manuscript-processing assistance.

References

Adams, W. L., Garry, P. J., Rhyne, R., Hunt, W. C. & Goodwin, J. S. (1990). Alcohol intake in the healthy elderly: Changes with age in a cross-sectional and longitudinal study. *Journal of the American Geriatrics Society, 38*, 211–216.

Amaducci, L. A., Fratiglioni, L., Rocca, W. A., Fieschi, C., Livrea, P., Pedone, D., Bracco, L., Lippi, A., Gandolfo, C. (1986). Risk factors for clinically diagnosed Alzheimer's disease: A case-control study of an Italian population. *Neurology, 36*, 922–931.

American Psychiatric Association (1980). *Diagnostic and statistical manual of mental disorders* (3rd ed.). Washington, DC: American Psychiatric Association.

American Psychiatric Association (1987). *Diagnostic and statistical manual of mental disorders* (3rd rev. ed.) (*DSM-III-R*). Washington, DC: American Psychiatric Association.

Anthony, J. C., LeResche, L. R., Niaz, U., Von Korff, M. R., & Folstein, M. F. (1982). Limits of the "Mini-Mental State" as a screening test for dementia and delirium among hospital patients. *Psychological Medicine, 12*, 397–408.

Anthony, J. C., Folstein, M. F., Romanoski, A., Von Korff, M. R., Nestadt, G., Chahal, R., Merchant, A., Brown, C. H., Shapiro, S., Kramer, M., & Gruenberg, E. M. (1985). Comparison of the lay Diagnostic Interview Schedule and a standardized psychiatric diagnosis: Experience in eastern Baltimore. *Archives of General Psychiatry, 42*, 667–675.

Anthony, J. C. (1987). A potential artifact in determining rates of depression (Letter). *Archives of General Psychiatry, 44*, 759–760.

Anthony, J. C. (1988). The epidemiologic case-control strategy, with applications in psychiatric research. In A. S. Henderson & G. D. Burrows (Eds.), *Handbook of social psychiatry* (pp. 152–172). Amsterdam: Elsevier Science Publishers.

Anthony, J. C. (1990). Prevention research in the context of epidemiology, with a discussion of public health models. In P. Muehrer (Ed.), *Conceptual research models for preventing mental disorders* (pp. 1–32). Washington: National Institute of Mental Health.

Anthony, J. C., & Helzer, J. E. (1991). Syndromes of drug abuse and dependence. In L. N. Robins & D. A. Regier (Eds.), *Psychiatric Disorders in America* (pp. 116–154). New York: The Free Press.

Avison, W. R., & Turner, R. J. (1988). Stressful life events and depressive symptoms: Disaggregating the effects of acute stressors and chronic strains. *Journal of Health and Social Behavior, 29*, 253–264.

Bebbington, P. E. (1987). Marital status and depression: A study of English national admission statistics. *Acta Psychiatrica Scandinavica, 75*, 640–650.

Bebbington, P.E. (1988). The social epidemiology of clinical depression. In A. S. Henderson & G. D. Burrows (Eds.), *Handbook of social psychiatry* (pp. 87–102). Amsterdam: Elsevier Science Publishers.

Berry, J. M., Storandt, M., & Coyne, A. (1984). Age and sex differences in somatic complaints associated with depression. *Journal of Gerontology, 39,* 465–467.

Blankfield, A., & Maritz, J. S. (1990). Female alcoholics. III. Some clinical associations of the Michigan Alcoholism Screening Test and diagnostic implications. *Acta Psychiatrica Scandinavica, 81(5),* 483–487.

Blazer, D., & Williams, C. D. (1980). Epidemiology of dysphoria and depression in an elderly population. *American Journal of Psychiatry, 137,* 439–444.

Blazer, D. G., George, L. K., Woodbury, M. A., Manton, K. G., & Jordan, B. K. (1984). The elderly alcoholic: A profile. In G. L. Maddox, L. N. Robins, & N. Rosenberg (Eds.), *Nature and extent of alcohol problems among the elderly* (NIAAA research Monograph No. 14) (pp. 275–297). Rockville, MD: National Institute of Alcohol Abuse and Alcoholism.

Blazer, D. G., & Pennybacker, M. (1984). Epidemiology of alcoholism in the elderly. In J. T. Hartford & T. Samorajski (Eds.), *Alcoholism in the elderly: Medical, social, and biomedical issues (Aging Vol. 25)* (pp. 25–33). New York: Raven Press.

Blessed, G., Tomlinson, B. E., & Roth, M. (1968). The association between quantitative measures of dementia and of senile change in the cerebral grey matter of elderly subjects. *British Journal of Psychiatry, 114,* 797–811.

Blessed, G., & Wilson, I. D. (1982). The contemporary natural history of mental disorder in old age. *British Journal of Psychiatry, 141,* 59–67.

Breitner, J. C. S., Folstein, M. F., & Murphy, E. A. (1986). Familial aggregation in Alzheimer's dementia. I. A model for the age-dependent expression of the autosomal dominant gene. *Journal of Psychiatric Research, 20,* 31–43.

Breslau, N., & Davis, G. C. (1986). Chronic stress and major depression. *Acta Psychiatrica Scandinavica, 43,* 309–314.

Breslow, N. E., & Day, N. E. (1980). *Statistical methods in cancer research: Vol. 1. The analysis of case-control studies* (32nd ed). Lyon, France: International Agency for Research on Cancer.

Broe, G. A., Henderson, A. S., Creasey, H., McCusker, E. Korten, A. E., Jorm, A. F., Longley, W., & Anthony, J. C. (1990). A case-control study of Alzheimer's disease in Australia. *Neurology, 20,* 31–43.

Brown, D. R., Eaton, W. W., & Sussman, L. (1990). Racial differences in the prevalence of phobic disorders. *Journal of Nervous and Mental Disease, 178,* 434–441.

Burke, K. C., Burke, J. D., Regier, D. A., & Rae, D. S. (1990). Age at onset of selected mental disorders in five community populations. *Archives of General Psychiatry, 47,* 511–518.

Cadoret, R. J., & Widmer, R. B. (1988). The development of depressive symptoms in elderly following onset of severe physical illness. *Journal of Family Practice, 1,* 71–76.

Carlsson, A. (1986). Neurotransmitters in old age and dementia. In H. Hafner, G. Moschel, & N. Satorius (Eds.), *Mental health in the elderly: A review of the present state of research* (pp. 29–34). New York: Springer-Verlag.

Chandra, V., Philipose, V., Bell, P. A., Lazaroff, A., & Schoenberg, B. S. (1987). Case-control study of late-onset "probable Alzheimer's disease". *Neurology, 37,* 1295–1300.

Clark, W. B., & Midanik, L. (1982). Alcohol use and alcohol problems among U.S. adults: Results of the 1979 national survey. In National Institute on Alcohol Abuse and Alcoholism (Ed.), *Alcohol consumption and related problems (Alcohol and health monograph No. 1)* (pp. 3–52). Washington, DC: U.S. Department of Health and Human Services.

Conwell, Y., Nelson, J. C., Kim, K. M., & Mazure, C. M. (1989). Depression in late life: Age of onset as marker of a subtype. *Journal of Affective Disorders, 17,* 189–195.

Copeland, J. R. M., Gurland, B. J., Dewey, M. E., Kelleher, M. J., Smith, A. M. R., & Davidson, I. A. (1987). Is there more dementia, depression, and neurosis in New York? A comparative study of the elderly in New York and London using the computer diagnosis AGECAT. *British Journal of Psychiatry, 151,* 466–473.

Corsellis, J. A. N., Bruton, C. J., & Freeman-Browne, D. (1973). The aftermath of boxing. *Psychological Medicine, 3,* 270–303.

Doyle, M. C., George, A. J., Ravindran, A. V., & Philpott, R. (1985). Platelet alpha$_2$-adrenoreceptor binding in elderly depressed patients. *American Journal of Psychiatry, 142,* 1489–1490.

Eaton, W. W., Weissman, M. M., Anthony, J. C., Robins, L. N., Blazer, D. G., Karno, M. (1985). Problems in the definition and measurement of prevalence and incidence of psychiatric disorders. In W. W. Eaton & L.

G. Kessler (Eds.), *Epidemiologic field methods in psychiatry: The NIMH Epidemiologic Catchment Area Program* (pp. 311–326). San Francisco: Academic Press.

Eaton, W. W., Dryman, A., & Weissman, M. M. (1991). Panic and phobia. In L. N. Robins & D. A. Regier (Eds.), *Psychiatric disorders in America* (pp. 155–179). New York: Free Press.

Eaton, W. W., & Keyl, P. M. (1990). Risk factors for the onset of DIS/DSM-III Agoraphobia in a prospective, population-based study. *Archives of General Psychiatry, 47,* 819–824.

Eaton, W. W., Kramer, M., Anthony, J. C., Dryman, A., Shapiro, S., & Locke, B. Z. (1989). The incidence of specific DIS/DSM-III mental disorders: Data from the NIMH Epidemiologic Catchment Area Program. *Acta Psychiatrica Scandinavica, 79,* 163–178.

Essen-Moller, E. (1956). Individual traits and morbidity in a Swedish rural population. *Acta Psychiatrica Scandinavica, Supple. 100,* 5–160.

Evans, D. A., Funkenstein, H. H., Albert, M. S., Scherr, P. A., Cook, N. R., Chown, M. J., Hubert, L. E., Hennekens, C. H, & Taylor, J. D. (1989). Prevalence of Alzheimer's disease in a community population of older persons: Higher than previously reported. *Journal of the American Medical Association, 262,* 2551–2556.

Evans, J. G. (1988). The epidemiology of the dementias of the elderly. In J. A. Brody & G. L. Maddox (Eds.), *Epidemiology and aging* (pp. 36–53). New York: Springer.

Evans, J. G. (1990). How are the elderly different. In R. L. Kane, J. G. Evans, & D. Macfadyen (Eds), *Improving the health of older people: A world view* (pp. 50–68). Oxford: WHO/Oxford University Press.

Feinson, M. C. (1989). Are psychological disorders most prevalent among older adults? Examining the evidence. *Social Science and Medicine, 29,* 1175–1181.

Finlay-Jones, R. (1981). The diagnosis of a case by a global rating method. In J. K. Wing, P. Bebbington, & L. N. Robins (Eds.), *What is a case? The problem of definition in psychiatric community surveys* (pp. 70–75). London: Grant McIntyre.

Folstein, M. F., Anthony, J. C., Parhad, I., Duffy, B., & Gruenberg, E. M. (1985). The meaning of cognitive impairment in the elderly. *Journal of the American Geriatrics Society, 33,* 228–235.

Folstein, M. F., Folstein, S. E., & McHugh, P. R. (1975). "Mini-Mental State": A practical method for grading the cognitive state of patients for the clinician. *Journal of Psychiatric Research, 12,* 189–198.

French, L. R., Schuman, L. M., Mortimer, J. A., Hutton, J. T., Boatman, R. A., & Christians, B. (1985). A case-control study of dementia of the Alzheimer type. *American Journal of Epidemiology, 121(3),* 414–421.

Gedye, A., Beattie, B. L., Tuokko, H., Horton, A., & Korsarek, E. (1989). Severe head injury hastens age of onset of Alzheimer's disease. *Journal of the American Geriatrics Society, 37,* 970–973.

Gelder, M. G. (1986). Panic attacks: New approaches to an old problem. *British Journal of Psychiatry, 149,* 346–352.

George, L. K., Blazer, D. G., Winfield-Laird, I., Leaf, P. J., & Fischbach, R. L. (1988). Psychiatric disorders and mental health service use in later life: Evidence from the Epidemiologic Catchment Area Program. In J. Brody & G. L. Maddox (Eds.), *Epidemiology and Aging* (pp. 189–219). New York: Springer.

George, L. K., Landerman, R., Blazer, D., & Anthony, J. C. (1991). Cognitive impairment. In L. N. Robins & D. A. Regier (Eds.), *Psychiatric disorders in America* (pp. 291–327). New York: The Free Press.

Gomberg, E. S. L. (1982). Alcohol use and problems among the elderly (Alcohol and health monograph No. 4). In National Institute on Alcohol Abuse and Alcoholism (Ed.), *Special population issues* (pp. 263–290). Washington, DC: U.S. Department of Health and Human Services/Government Printing Office.

Grimshaw, L. (1964). Obsessional disorder and neurological illness. *Journal of Neurology, Neurosurgery, and Psychiatry, 27,* 229-231.

Gruenberg, E. M. (1977). The failures of success. *Milbank Memorial Fund Quarterly. Health and Society, 55(1),* 3–24.

Gruenberg, E. M. (1980). Mental disorders. In J. M. Last (Ed.), *Maxcy-Rosenau public health and preventive medicine* (11th ed., pp. 1303–1358). New York: Appleton-Century-Crofts.

Gurland, B., Dean, L., Cross, P., & Golden, R. (1980). The epidemiology of depression and dementia in the elderly: The use of multiple indicators of these conditions. In J. O. Cole & J. Barrett (Eds.), *Psychopathology in the aged* (pp. 37–62). New York: Raven Press.

Gurland, B. J. & Cross, P. S. (1982). Epidemiology of psychopathology in old age: Some implications for clinical services. *Psychiatric Clinics of North America, 5,* 11–26.

Hagnell, O. (1966). *A Prospective Study of the Incidence of Mental Disorder.* Norstedts, Sweden: Svenska Bokforlaget.

Hagnell, O., Lanke, J., Rorsman, B., & Ohman, R. (1986). Predictors of alcoholism in the Lundby Study. III. Social risk factors for alcoholism. *European Archives of Psychiatry and Neurological Sciences, 235,* 197– 199.

Hagnell, O., Lanke, J., Rorsman, B., Ohman, R., & Ojesjo, L. (1983). Current trends in the incidence of senile and multi-infarct dementia. *Archiv Fur Psychiatrie Und Nervenkrankheiten, 233,* 423–438.

Hagnell, O., Lanke, J., Rorsman, B., & Ojesjo, L. (1982). Are we entering an age of melancholy? Depressive illnesses in a prospective epidemiological study over 25 years: The Lundby Study, Sweden. *Psychological Medicine, 12,* 279–289.

Hagnell, O. (1986). The 25-year follow-up of the Lundby Study: Incidence and risk of alcoholism, depression, and disorders of the senium. In J. E. Barrett & R. M. Rose (Eds.), *Mental disorders in the community* (pp. 89–110). New York: The Guilford Press.

Hallstrom, T. (1987a). Major depression, parental mental disorder, and early family relationships. *Acta Psychiatrica Scandinavica, 75,* 259–263.

Hallstrom, T. (1987b). The relationships of childhood socio-demographic factors and early parental loss to major depression in adult life. *Acta Psychiatrica Scandinavica, 75,* 212–216.

Hasin, D., & Link, B. (1988). Age and recognition of depression: Implications for a cohort effect in major depression. *Psychological Medicine, 18,* 683–688.

Hastie, T., & Tibshirani, R. J. (1990). *Generalized additive models* (*Monograph on statistics and applied probability series #43*). London: Rutledge, Chapman, & Hall.

Helzer, J. E. (1987). Epidemiology of alcoholism. *Journal of Consulting and Clinical Psychology, 55,* 284– 292.

Helzer, J. E., Burnam, A., & McEvoy, L. T. (1991). Alcohol abuse and dependence. In L. N. Robins & D. A. Regier (Eds.), *Psychiatric disorders in America* (pp. 81–116). New York: The Free Press.

Helzer, J. E., Canino, G. J., Yeh, E. K., Bland, R. C., Lee, C. K., Hwu, H. G., & Newmans, S. (1990). Alcoholism—North America and Asia. *Archives of General Psychiatry, 47(4),* 313–319.

Henderson, A. S. (1986). The epidemiology of Alzheimer's disease. *British Medical Bulletin, 42,* 3–10.

Henderson, A. S. (1988). The risk factors for Alzheimer's disease: A review and a hypothesis. *Acta Psychiatrica Scandinavica, 78,* 257–275.

Henderson, A. S., & Huppert, F. A. (1984). The problem of mild dementia. *Psychological Medicine, 14,* 5–11.

Henderson, A. S., & Kay, D. W. K. (1984). The epidemiology of mental disorders. In D. W. K. Kay & G. D. Burrows (Eds.), *Handbook of studies on psychiatry and old age* (pp. 53–88). Amsterdam: Elsevier.

Heyman, A., Wilkinson, W. E., Stafford, J. A., Helms, M. J., Sigmon, A. H., & Weinberger, T. (1984). Alzheimer's disease: A study of epidemiological aspects. *Annals of Neurology, 15,* 335–341.

Holland, J. C., Korzun, A. H., Tross, S., Siberfarb, P., Perry, M., Cornis, R., & Oster, M. (1986). Comparative psychological disturbance in patients with pancreatic and gastric cancer. *American Journal of Psychiatry, 143,* 982–986.

Hollander, E., Fay, M., & Leibowitz, M. R. (1988). Clonidine and clomipramine in obsessive-compulsive disorder. *American Journal of Psychiatry, 145,* 388–389.

Holzer, C. E. III., Robins, L. N., Myers, J. K., Weissman, M. M., Tischler, G. L., Leaf, P. J., Anthony, J. C., & Bednarski, P. (1984). Antecedents and correlates of alcohol abuse and dependence in the elderly. In G. L. Maddox, L. N. Robins, & N. Rosenberg (Eds.), *Nature and Extent of Alcohol Problems among the Elderly, NIAAA Research Monograph 14* (pp. 217–244). Rockville, MD: National Institute on Alcohol Abuse and Alcoholism.

Insel, T. R., Mueller, E. A., Alterman, I., Linnoila, M., & Murphy, D. L. (1985). Obsessive-compulsive disorder and serotonin: Is there a connection? *Biological Psychiatry, 20,* 1174–1188.

Jablensky, A. (1990). Diagnosis and classification of dementias in the elderly with special reference to the tenth revision of the international classification of diseases (ICD-10) (Appendix). In R. L. Kane, J. G. Evans & D. Macfadyen (Eds.), *Improving the health of older people: A world view* (pp. 683–693). Oxford: WHO/Oxford University Press.

Jaspers, K. (1963). *General psychopathology* (7th ed). Chicago: University of Chicago Press.

John, E. R., Prichep, L. S., Fridman, J., & Easton, P. (1988). Neurometrics: Computer-assisted differential diagnosis of brain dysfunctions. *Science, 239(4836),* 162–169.

Jorm, A. F., Henderson, A. S., & Jacomb, P. A. (1989). Regional differences in mortality from dementia in Australia: An analysis of death certificate data. *Acta Psychiatrica Scandinavica, 79*(2), 179–185.

Jorm, A. F., Korten, A. E., & Henderson, A. S. (1987). The prevalence of dementia: A quantitative integration of the literature. *Acta Psychiatrica Scandinavica, 76*, 465–479.

Karno, M., & Golding, J. M. (1991). Obsessive compulsive disorder. In L. N. Robins & D. A. Regier (Eds.), *Psychiatric disorders in America* (pp. 204–219). New York: The Free Press.

Karno, M., Golding, J. M., Sorenson, S. B., & Burnam, A. (1988). The epidemiology of obsessive-compulsive disorder in five U.S. communities. *Archives of General Psychiatry, 45*, 1094–1099.

Kay, D. W. K. (1986). The genetics of Alzheimer's disease. *British Medical Bulletin, 42*(1), 19–23.

Kay, D. W. K., Beamish, P., & Roth, M. (1964). Old age mental disorders in Newcastle-upon-Tyne. I. A study of prevalence. *British Journal of Psychiatry, 110*, 146–158.

Kay, D. W. K., & Bergmann, K. (1980). Epidemiology of mental disorders among the aged in the community. In J. E. Birren & R. B. Sloane (Eds.), *Handbook of mental health and aging* (pp. 34–56). Englewood Cliffs, NJ: Prentice-Hall.

Kay, D. W. K., Henderson, A. S., Scott, R., Wilson, J., Rickwood, D., & Grayson, D. A. (1985). Dementia and depression among the elderly living in the Hobart community: The effect of diagnostic criteria on the prevalence rates. *Psychological Medicine, 15*, 771–788.

Kellam, S. G., Anthony, J. C., Brown, C. H., & Dolan, L. (1989). Prevention research and early risk behaviors in cross-cultural studies. In M. H. Schmidt & H. Remschmidt (Eds.), *Needs and prospects of child and adolescent psychiatry* (pp. 241–254). Toronto: Hans Huber Verlag.

Keyl, P. M., & Eaton, W. W. (1990). Risk factors for the onset of panic disorder and other panic attacks in a prospective, population-based study. *American Journal of Epidemiology, 131*, 301–311.

Kiloh, L. G. (1986). The secondary dementias of middle and later life. *British Medical Bulletin, 42*(1), 106–110.

Kirkwood, T. B. L. (1981). Repair and its evolution: survival versus reproduction. In C. R. Townsend & P. Calow (Eds.), *Physiological ecology: An evolutionary approach to resource use* (pp. 165–189). Sunderland, MA: Sinauer Associates.

Kivela, S. L., & Pahkala, K. (1989). Dysthymic disorder in the aged in the community. *Social Psychiatry and Psychiatric Epidemiology, 24*(2), 77–83.

Kleinbaum, D. G., Kupper, L. L., & Morgenstern, H. (1982). *Epidemiologic research: Principles and quantitative research.* Belmont, California: Lifetime Learning Publications.

Klerman, G. L., Lavori, P. W., Rice, J., Reich, T., Endicott, J., Adreason, N. C., Keller, M. B., & Hirschfield, M. A. (1985). Birth cohort trends in rates of major depressive disorder among relatives of patients with affective disorder. *Archives of General Psychiatry, 42*, 689–693.

Klerman, G. L. (1986). Evidence of increase in rates of depression in North American and Western Europe in recent decades. In H. Hippius, G. L. Klerman, & N. Mattusek (Eds.), *New results in depression research* (pp. 7–15). Berlin: Springer-Verlag.

Kohlmeyer, K. (1986). Morphology of the brain in normal aging and in processes of dementia: Neuropathology and CT-findings. In H. Hafner, G. Moschel, & N. Satorius (Eds.), *Mental health in the elderly: A review of the present state of research* (pp. 117–126). New York: Springer-Verlag.

Kokmen, E., Chandra, V., & Schoenberg, B. S. (1988). Trends in incidence of dementing illness in Rochester, Minnesota, in three quinquennial periods, 1960–1974. *Neurology, 38*, 975–980.

Kramer, M., Von Korff, M. R., & Kessler, L. G. (1980). The lifetime prevalence of mental disorders: Estimation, uses, and limitations. *Psychological Medicine, 10*, 429–435.

Kua, E. H. (1990). Drinking habits of elderly Chinese. *British Journal of Addiction, 85*, 571–573.

Lehmann, H. E. (1982). Affective disorders in the aged. *Psychiatric Clinics of North America, 5*(1), 27–44.

Li, G., Shen, Y. C., Chen, C. H., Zhao, Y. W., & Li, S. R. (1989). An epidemiological survey of age-related dementia in an urban area of Bejing. *Acta Psychiatrica Scandinavica, 79*, 557–563.

Lilienfeld, A. M. (1976). *Foundations of epidemiology.* New York: Oxford University Press.

Lipton, M. A. (1976). Age differentiation in depression: Biochemical aspects. *Journal of Gerontology, 31*, 293–299.

Macfadyen, D. (1990). International demographic trends. In R. L. Kane, J. G. Evans, & D. Macfadyen (Eds.), *Improving the health of older people: A world view* (pp. 19–29). Oxford: WHO/Oxford University Press.

Makkai, T., & McAllister, I. (1990). Alcohol consumption across the life-cycle in Australia, 1985–1988. *Drug and Alcohol Dependence, 25*, 305–313.

Marks, I. M. (1987). *Fears, phobias, and rituals*. New York: Oxford University Press.

Marsden, C. D. (1984). Neurological causes of dementia other than Alzheimer's disease. In D. W. K. Kay & G. D. Burrows (Eds.), *Handbook of studies on psychiatry and old age* (pp. 145–167). Amsterdam: Elsevier.

Martin, R. L., Gerteis, G., & Gabrielli, W. F. (1988). A family-genetic study of dementia of Alzheimer type. *Archives of General Psychiatry, 45*, 894–900.

McKhann, G., Drachman, D., Folstein, M. F., Katzman, R., Price, D., & Stadlan, E. M. (1984). Clinical diagnosis of Alzheimer's disease: Report of the NINCDS-ADRDA work group under the auspices of Department of Health and Human Services Task Force on Alzheimer's Disease. *Neurology, 34*, 939–944.

Mendlewicz, J. (1988). Population and family studies in depression and mania. *British Journal of Psychiatry, 153(suppl.3)*, 16–25.

Meyers, B. S., & Alexopoulos, G. S. (1988). Age of onset and studies of late-life depression. *International Journal of Geriatric Psychiatry, 3*, 219–228.

Miettinen, O. S. (1985). *Theoretical epidemiology: Principles of occurrence research in medicine*. New York: John Wiley and Sons.

Miller, E. (1977). *Abnormal Aging: The psychology of senile and presenile dementia*. New York: John Wiley and Sons.

Miller, F. D., Hicks, S. P., D'Amato, C. J., & Landis, R. (1984). A descriptive study of neuritic plaques and neurofibrillary tangles in an autopsy population. *American Journal of Epidemiology, 120*, 331–341.

Morris, J. N. (1975). *Uses of epidemiology*. London: Churchill Livingstone.

Mortimer, J. A., French, L. R., Hutton, J. T., & Schuman, L. M. (1985). Head injury as a risk factor for Alzheimer's disease. *Neurology, 35*, 264–267.

Mortimer, J. A. (1988). Epidemiology of dementia: International comparisons. In J. A. Brody & G. L. Maddox (Eds.), *Epidemiology and aging* (pp. 150–164). New York: Springer.

Mountjoy, C. Q. (1986). Correlations between neuropathological and neurochemical changes. *British Medical Bulletin, 42(1)*, 81–85.

Murphy, J. M., Olivier, D. C., Monson, R. P., Sobol, A. M., & Leighton, A. H. (1988). Incidence of depression and anxiety. The Stirling County Study. *American Journal of Public Health, 78*, 534–540.

Murphy, J. M., Sobol, A. M., Neff, R. K., Olivier, D. C., & Leighton, A. M. (1984). Stability of prevalence: Depression and anxiety disorders. *Archives of General Psychiatry, 41*, 990–997.

Nielsen, J. (1962). Geronto-psychiatric period-prevalence investigation in a geographically delimited population. *Acta Psychiatrica Scandinavica, 38*, 307–330.

Oakes, M. (1990). *Statistical inference*. Chestnut Hill, MA: Epidemiology Resources, Inc.

Ojesjo, L., Hagnell, O., & Lanke, J. (1982). Incidence of alcoholism among men in the Lundby Community Cohort—Sweden, 1957–1972. *Journal of Studies on Alcohol, 43*, 1190–1198.

Osuntokun, B. S. (1986). The value of collaborative research in aging. In H. Hafner, G. Moschel, & N. Sartorius (Eds.), *Mental health in the elderly: A review of the present state of research* (pp. 162–165). New York: Springer-Verlag.

Parker, G. (1987). Are the lifetime prevalence estimates in the ECA study accurate? *Psychological Medicine, 17*, 275–282.

Pearlson, G., & Rabins, P. (1988). The late-onset psychoses. *Psychiatric Clinics of North America, 11*, 15–32.

Perrson, G. (1980). Prevalence of mental disorders in a 70-year-old urban population. *Acta Psychiatrica Scandinavica, 62*, 119–139.

Prentice, R. L. (1986). On the design of synthetic case-control studies. *Biometrics, 42*, 301–310.

Regier, D. A., Boyd, J. H., Burke, J. D., Locke, B. Z., Rae, D. S., Myers, J. K., Kramer, M., & Robins, L. N., George L. K., Karno, M., & Locke, B. Z. (1988). One-month prevalence of mental disorders in the U.S.: Based on five epidemiologic catchment area sites. *Archives of General Psychiatry, 45*, 977–986.

Rice, J., Reich, T., Andreasen, N. C., Lavori, P. W., Endicott, J., Clayton, P. J., Keller, M. B., Hirschfield, R. M. A., & Klerman, G. L. (1984). Sex-related differences in depression: Familial evidence. *Journal of Affective Disorders, 77*, 199–210.

Robinson, R. G., Kubos, K. L., Starr, L. B., Rao, K., & Price, T. R. (1984). Mood disorders in stroke patients. *Brain, 107*, 81–93.

Rorsman, B., Hagnell, O., & Lanke, J. (1986). Prevalence and incidence of senile and multi-infarct dementia in the Lundby Study: A comparison between the time periods 1947–1957 and 1957–1972. *Neuropsychobiology, 15*, 122–129.

Roth, M. (1955). The natural history of mental disorder in old age. *Journal of Mental Science, 101*, 281–301.

Roth, M. (1959). The phobic-anxiety-depersonalization syndrome. *Proceedings of the Royal Society of Medicine, 52,* 587–595.

Roth, M. (1972). Recent progress in the psychiatry of old age and its bearing on certain problems of psychiatry in earlier life. *Biological Psychiatry, 5*(2), 103–125.

Roth, M. (1976). The psychiatric disorders of later life. *Psychiatric Annals, 6,* 417–445.

Roth, M. (1980). Senile dementia and its borderlands. In J. O. Cole & J. E. Barrett (Eds.), *Psychopathology in the aged* (pp. 205–232). New York: Raven Press.

Roth, M. (1984). Agoraphobia, panic disorder, and generalized anxiety disorder: Some implications of recent advances. *Psychiatric Developments, 2,* 31–52.

Roth, M. (1986). The association of clinical and neurological findings and its bearings on the classification and aetiology of Alzheimer's disease. *British Medical Bulletin, 42*(1), 42–50.

Rowe, J. W., & Kahn, R. L. (1987). Human aging: Usual and successful. *Science, 237*(4811), 143–149.

Sackett, D. L. (1979). Bias in analytic research (with comment by M. P. Vessey and discussion). *Journal of Chronic Diseases, 32,* 51–63.

Sayetta, R. B. (1986). Rates of senile dementia—Alzheimer's type in the Baltimore longitudinal study. *Journal of Chronic Diseases, 39,* 271–286.

Schlesselman, J. J. (1982). *Case-Control Studies: Design, conduct, analysis.* New York: Oxford University Press.

Royall, D., & Anthony, J.C. (submitted). Risk factors for major depression in middle age and in later life. The Johns Hopkins University (unpublished manuscript).

Schneider, L. S., Severson, J. A., Sloane, R. B., & Fredrickson, E. (1988). Decreased platelet ^{3}H-imipramine binding in elderly outpatients with primary depression compared to secondary depression. *Journal of Affective Disorders, 15,* 195–200.

Schoenberg, B., Kokmen, E., & Okazaki, H. (1987). Alzheimer's disease and other dementing illnesses in a defined United States population: Incidence rates and clinical features. *Annals of Neurology, 22,* 724–729.

Schwab, J. J., Holzer, C. E., & Warheit, G. J. (1973). Depressive symptomatology and age. *Psychosomatics, 14,* 135–141.

Shalat, S. L., Seltzer, B., Pidcock, C., & Baker, E. L. (1987). Risk factors for Alzheimer's disease: A case-control study. *Neurology, 37,* 1630–1633.

Shepherd, M., & Gruenberg, E. M. (1957). The age of neuroses. *Milbank Memorial Fund Quarterly. Health and Society, 35,* 258–265.

Shibayama, H., Kasahara, Y., & Kobayashi, H. (1986). Prevalence of dementia in a Japanese elderly population. *Acta Psychiatrica Scandinavica, 74,* 144–151.

Sluss, T. K., Gruenberg, E. M., & Kramer, M. (1981). The use of longitudinal studies in the investigation of risk factors of senile dementia—Alzheimer type. In J. Mortimer & L. Schuman (Eds.), *The epidemiology of dementia* (pp. 132–154). New York: Oxford University Press.

Smart, R. G., & Liban, C. B. (1981). Predictors of problem drinking among the elderly, middle-aged, and youthful drinkers. *Journal of Psychoactive Drugs, 13,* 153–163.

Soininen, H., & Heinonen, O.P. (1982). Clinical and etiological aspects of senile dementia. *European Neurology, 21,* 401–410.

St. Clair, D., & Whalley, L. J. (1983). Hypertension, multiinfarct dementia and Alzheimer's disease. *British Journal of Psychiatry, 143,* 274–276.

St. George-Hyslop, Tanzi, R. E., Polinsky, R. J., Haines, J. L., Nee, L., Watkins, P. C., Myers, R. H., Feldman, R. G., Pollen, D., Drachman, D., Growdon, J., Bruni, A. J., Fonein, J. F., Salmon, D., Frommeti, P., Anaducci, L., Sorbi, S., Piacentini, S., Stewart, G. D., Hobbs, W. J., Conneally, P. M., & Gusella, J. F. (1987). The genetic defect causing familial Alzheimer's disease maps on chromosome 21. *Science, 235,* 885–890.

Turner, R. J. (1987). In pursuit of socially malleable contingencies in mental health: An epidemiological perspective. In J. A. Steinberg & M. M. Silverman (Eds.), *Preventing mental disorders: A research perspective* (pp. 160–171). Washington, DC: National Institute of Mental Health/U.S. Government Printing Office.

Turner, R. J., & Noh, S. (1988). Physical disability and depression: A longitudinal analysis. *Journal of Health and Social Behavior, 29,* 23–27.

Weissman, M. M. (1979). The myth of involutional melancholia. *Journal of the American Medical Association,* *242,* 742–744.

Weissman, M. M., Wickramaratne, P. J., Merikangas, K. R., Leckman, J. F., Prusoff, B. A., Caruso, K. A., Kidd, K. K., & Gammon, G. D. (1984). Onset of major depression in early adulthood: Increased familial loading and specificity. *Archives of General Psychiatry, 41,* 1136–1143.

Weissman, M. M., Bruce, M. L., Leaf, P. J., Florio, L. P., & Holzer, C. E. (1991). Affective disorders. In L. N. Robins & D. A. Regier (Eds.), *Psychiatric disorders in America* (pp. 53–80). New York: The Free Press.

Weissman, M. M., & Klerman, G. L. (1985). Gender and depression. *Trends in Neuroscience, 8,* 416–420.

Weissman, M. M., Myers, J. K., & Harding, P. S. (1980). Prevalence and psychiatric heterogenity of alcoholism in a United States urban community. *Journal of Studies on Alcohol, 41,* 672–681.

Weissman, M. M., Myers, J. K., Tischler, G. L., Holzer, C. E., Leaf, P. J., Orvaschel, H., & Brody, J. A. (1985). Psychiatric disorders (DSM-III) and cognitive impairment among the elderly in a U.S. urban community. *Acta Psychiatrica Scandinavica, 71,* 366–379.

Werch, C. E. (1989). Quantity-frequency and diary measures of alcohol consumption for elderly drinkers. *International Journal of the Addictions, 24(9),* 859–865.

Whybrow, P. C., Prange, A. J., & Treadway, C. R. (1969). Mental changes accompanying thyroid gland dysfunction. *Archives of General Psychiatry, 20,* 48–53.

Wickramaratne, P. J., Weissman, M. M., Leaf, P. J., & Holford, T. R. (1989). Age, period, and cohort effects on the risk of major depression: Results from five United States communities. *Journal of Clinical Epidemiology, 42,* 333–343.

Williams, G. C. (1957). Pleiotropy, natural selection, and the evolution of senescence. *Evolution, 11,* 396–411.

World Health Organization (1990). *Chapter V: Mental and behavioural disorders (including disorders of psychological development). Diagnostic criteria for research. (February 1990 draft for field trials).* (Document no. MNH/MEP/89.2, Rev. 1.) Geneva, Switzerland: WHO.

Culture and Mental Health in Later Life Revisited

David Gutmann

I. Introduction: A Field without a Literature
II. Fieldwork and the Limitations of Academic Geropsychology
III. Culture
   A. The Need for a Psychosocial Definition
   B. In Relation to Social and Psychic Structures
   C. The Stimulus Barrier
   D. Narcissism
   E. The Cultural Uses of Splitting and Projection
   F. Inner Controls
   G. Self-Continuity
   H. The Components of Culture
   I. Elders: The Wardens of Culture
   J. Elder Passivity and Elder Power
   K. Mental Health and the Traditional Elder
IV. Deculturation and the Elders
   A. Economic Power and Elder Power
   B. Deculturation and the Druze
   C. Deculturation and the High Culture
   D. The Aging Strangers
   E. Some Geropsychological Consequences
   F. Deculturation and Geriatric Psychopathology
References

I. Introduction: A Field without a Literature

In 1980, writing the chapter on Culture, Mental Health, and Aging (Gutmann, 1980) for the first edition of this series, I found very little literature addressed to the title topic;

clearly, the psychological status of elders under varying cultural conditions was not then a hot subject in gerontology. Ten years later, a definitive literature on the geropsychology of culture–personality relations is still not much in evidence.

But the beginning of a beginning has been made: in the interim, the cultural if not the psychological aspect has in fact received some coverage. In large part stimulated by the recently formed Association for Anthropology and Gerontology, a long overdue ethnogerontology literature is now showing up: *Culture* and particularly *cohort* have become buzz-words in gerontology. Predictably, these ethnographic reports do not address the question of mental health; instead, they quite properly report on matters that interest anthropologists more than they do psychologists: The social roles of elders; the rituals through which they enter and exit from age-graded statuses; the characteristics of their social relationships, both formal and informal; the quality of elder-care in various societies, etc. While carefully wrought descriptions of this sort are immensely useful in breaking down culture-bound stereotypes about the aging process, and in establishing social gerontology as a natural science, such accounts—which record the normative consequences of social adaptation—cannot tell us much about psychological contributions either to adaptation or to psychopathology. In short, an anthropologist can tell us interesting things about the cultural antecedents of a psychiatric patient, but he cannot, on that basis alone, make the clinical diagnosis. By the same token, social status does not reliably predict mental health or illness; madness occurs in the best of families (and, as the playwright Philip Barry reminds us, especially the best).

Indeed, the elevated status of the aged can even put them at risk. Thus, Opler (1959) found that young Tonga (Africa) tribesmen revere their elders, but also believe that they achieve longevity through human sacrifice. Vampirelike, they presumably steal the life-force of their youthful victims, and so are blamed for the death of young people. In my own field work among the Highland Maya (1968), I observed that elders were treated with great deference, but respect was mingled with fear, because these same elders were suspected of demonic practices. Village lore had it that the *Naguales* (the animal familiars) of elderly Highland Maya men would meet on mountain tops, and these covens would decide the fate of individual villagers. Accordingly, deaths caused by epidemics were sometimes blamed on the *Naguales* of powerful old men; and these unfortunates were occasionally shot from ambush by vengeful survivors. However we choose to define this construct, the mental health of Highland Maya elders did not reflect their position in society. Summing up his essential posture, an aged informant told me, "I keep quiet" ("Quedo callado").

Clearly then, ethnographic accounts bearing on the social status and roles of human elders can give us—at the most—very imprecise and even misleading information about their psychological status.

II. Fieldwork and the Limitations of Academic Geropsychology ____

But neither do we get much help from psychology. A minority of ethnopsychologists do report on the feelings, attitudes, self-conceptions and mental symptoms of elders in various societies; but while they claim to study aging psychology, their work, like that of the ethnogerontologists, does not really tell us much about the mental health of elders, or its mediation by culture. My major objection is that only a few of the relevant studies utilize the depth-psychological instruments that were specifically crafted to probe the unconscious dynamisms underlying mental health, or psychopathology. Instead, the usual study is based on *standard* instruments—often standardly administered pencil and paper tests—which purport to measure the life satisfaction, stress, mental symptoms, etc., of elders in various societies. But standardization is a subjective rather than an objective condition; it is not reached *via* precoded instruments, or standard instructions given by examiners whose behavior is invariant from subject to subject. Such procedures give the illusion of standardization; they reassure investigators as to their "scientific" credentials; but they do not reassure unsophisticated, often preliterate subjects, who routinely suspect that the foreign investigator is a witch, or a government spy. Indeed, these essentially bureaucratic research procedures fuel such suspicions. Despite its cross-cultural pretensions, academic geropsychology—with a few notable exceptions (Cohler & Lieberman, 1979; LeVine, 1978a, 1978b; Shanan, 1985)—remains steadfastly culture-bound.

Psychologists could break out of that constraint by adopting less concretely behavioral guidelines for our field methods. The standard condition that we should aim for with naive or preliterate subjects is best covered by the term rapport—that special state wherein the subject *wants* to explore matters that are of importance to him, and of scientific interest to the investigator. Rapport is in all cases achieved by nonstandard, *ad hoc* methods, by procedures that are responsive to the fears and special concerns of the particular respondent. But when the real goal is methodological purity rather than illumination, we get instead expressions of test anxiety, social desirability, and the naive subject's fear of a foreign investigator.[1] What we do *not* get is an accurate reading of the subject's psychological strengths, vulnerabilities and pathologies.

---

[1] I have carried out comparative research on the personality dynamics of older people in a variety of preliterate cultures. Early on, I found that pre-coded, self-report interview schedules did not generate useful data bearing on the covert aspects of personality, those that were likely to change with age, or in the transition to a postparental stage of life. Before administering any instruments, I found that I had to first *legitimize* myself in the eyes of informants, by allowing them to interview me about my purposes and sponsorship. Without this *invited interview*, subjects tended to mistrust the foreign investigator, believing me to be a spy, a government agent, a limb of the devil, rather than a scientist. Lacking the invited interview, subjects would give evasive and guardedly plausible answers, designed to confound the malign stranger, rather than assist the scientist. In general, I have found that the degree of personal disclosure is a direct function of the degree of investigator–subject *rapport*.

Thus, a Navajo father, whose retarded daughter suffered from epileptiform disease gave me, in the course of one relatively brief interview, four different accounts of her trouble. At first, thinking that I was a public health service doctor, he described her disease as a congenital disorder, exacerbated by early measles. Then, after I revealed some knowledge of the Navajo medicine culture, he spoke to me as Navajo to anthropologist: "There was a witch, some man way out there who envied our wealth in sheep and turquoise jewelry. Out of envy he did this." But when I addressed him as a clinical psychologist, suggesting that there must have been some intense and complex personal relationship between the subjects' family and the witch, the informant's wife chimed in. The sorcerer was actually her father, a powerful medicine man who had "gone to the bad side." He had become a sorcerer, she said, in order to satisfy the insatiable demands of his young second wife for goods and wealth. In order to enter the society of witches, her father had to violate the firmest Navajo taboos against harming a blood relative; but it was her hated step-mother who had put him up to it. Quite suddenly, we were far away from the culture of the medical clinic or the medicine culture of the Navajo; by now, we were *jointly* exploring the universal *human* context, of generic family dynamics: Oedipal rivalry, the daughter's hatred for the young step-

III. Culture

A. The Need for a Psychosocial Definition

In sum, the developing science of comparative geropsychology is in part retarded by the methodological orthodoxies of academic psychology, but most stringently by the conceptual biases of the cultural anthropologists. The latter group *own* the definitions of culture that are applied to culture–personality studies, but these have the unfortunate result of bending both domains—psychology *and* culture—out of shape. Thus, despite substantial disagreements among cultural anthropologists, the majority join in treating culture as an independent variable, and in asserting that all expressive behavior is socially patterned. The proponents of this externalized view—many psychologists among them—hold that nurture in the form of cultural indoctrination is supreme, and that there are no *natural,* organismic sources of coherent, organized behavior. In effect, the culture-centric view establishes, at the very heart of the social sciences, a mind–body dichotomy: the body, its imperatives, rhythms, and appetites, is only a source of anarchy, not order; and in later life, of debility and decay.

These definitions, of culture as dominant, serve the academic imperialism of anthropologists, but they retard our understanding of psychological adaptation or breakdown at any age. Such a view of personality as the dependent, unmediated product of culture is particularly misleading in gerontology, and does violence to the observed facts. It does not, for example, help us to understand—without forcing the data into a procrustean bed—the finding (see Gutmann, 1987) of universal, culture-free personality change in later life.

At worst, such externalized understandings of human psychology lead to a simpleminded *Lumpen*-Marxism: Motives, attitudes and their attendant behaviors are ascribed to economic conditions, to *social class,* or to *"the later stages of capitalism."* More commonly, given the exaggerated scientism of American social scientists, the search for quantifiable dependent (psychological) and independent (cultural) variables does violence to the natural systems being studied. *Culture* and *personality* are not easily assimilated to glib independent–dependent variable sequences or designs.

Christine Fry (1985) is one of the few ethnogerontologists who resists the conceptual colonialism of her discipline: She proposes a partnership, an implicit equality between culture and those aspects of personality that mature in encultured frameworks. Thus Professor Fry:

> Individuals are not the passive recipients of knowledge, rules and standards from enculturators who are older, bigger, stronger, or more important than they are. Knowledge, rules, and standards are not learned to be blindly followed in motivating action or determin-

---

mother who had replaced her deceased blood mother in the father's bed. This family drama could not have been predicted from the accounts that I had initially elicited, in the guise of Anglo clinician or Anglo ethnographer. These introductory versions were plausible resistances against the *real* story, and were designed to obfuscate and lead me away from the emotionally charged *stepmother* tale. After experiencing a number of revelations like this one, in a variety of field settings, I stopped using standard interview schedules and procedures; and I came to mistrust any study that reported findings based exclusively on such methods and data.

ing responses. . . . Culture is a model each individual has formed of what others know, believe, and mean. . . . People use their models to generate the actions they think will lead others to *validate a certain identity*. People conform to rules to demonstrate to themselves and to others that they are a particular kind of person (p. 217). (Italics mine).

Fry speaks out of the psychoethological position first enunciated by Erik Erikson (1959). In his view, the universal or structural aspects of culture have co-evolved with the *deep structures* of the mind—the ego executive capacities that, while they develop under conditions of sociality, also function so as to maintain the nurturing conditions that sponsored them. Thus, culture and individual personality are equal partners, metaphors of each other, entwined in a dialectic exchange. Culture is not individual personality writ large, nor is personality only a print-out of local norms, cohort influences, and belief systems: It is not culture writ small. Clearly, investigations devoted to the linkage between culture and elderly mental health should attend to those aspects of culture that extend and sponsor psychological capacities, particularly those that underwrite a culturally regulated social life.

In the balance of this essay I will put forward some conceptions of culture that take into account its functions *vis-à-vis* the social collectivity as well as its functions *vis-à-vis* individual personality. This discussion will focus on two related phenomena: the special role that older individuals play in maintaining the ritual aspects of culture; and the special bonus of mental health that elders may receive in exchange for this service. I will also discuss the pathogenic consequences for elders when, under conditions of deculturation, they lose their special, privileged relationship to culture.

B. In Relation to Social and Psychic Structure

While culture requires the human mind as a precondition for its continuity, it is also a *social* reality, existing apart from particular brains. Like language, it outlasts its founders, it is transmitted in recognizable form from generation to generation, and it is based in those parts of the mental apparatus that (like the deep structures of linguistics) are common to all socialized adults. Possessing in these senses an objective reality, culture is a guarantor of individual as well as social *continuity*. Social scientists emphasize mainly the part played by culture in bringing about the continuity of trustworthy communities rather than trustworthy individuals. Culture is invoked by them as the proper context for understanding social conformity, social continuity, and social change in any organized, corporate body. In their designs, individuals are only the *genes* of culture. Thus, cultural anthropologists generally use individuals as informants not on their own lives, but on the beliefs and customs of their local culture. In their view culture is mapped into the *tabula rasa* of the individual gene through formal and informal learning; and while psychological conflict may trouble the mind, it originates externally in discrepant social norms, rather than in necessary conflict between competing needs or appetites. But a truly psychological conception treats culture not as prior to the psyche, but as the counterpart and sponsor, on the collective scale, of the mental processes that guarantee the individual's delay, rationality, and control.

C. The Stimulus Barrier

The psychosocial role of culture is clarified when we consider an overriding need of the human psyche: to establish autonomy from stimulus overload, the blur and buzz of immediate experience. The mental apparatus has preformed deep structures to match that need: inbuilt potentials to abstract, to symbolize, to *name*. The ego generalizes: it abstracts *categories* out of the regularities that it discovers in the wash of events, it *names* these categories, and it endows them with the tonus of reality. Having constructed these constancies, these *objects,* the psyche has established the structural base of its autonomy, its freedom from the tyranny of the immediate. Rather than endure the shock of unbuffered experience, the ego can fix attention on its own constructions *about* reality; in so doing, it gains the capacity for delay of impulse and gratification that is fundamental to rationality and mastery.

Redfield (1947) held that any proper culture is a coherent system of *shared understandings* as to what is good and bad, possible and impossible, thinkable and unthinkable. So construed, culture facilitates the psyche's *conquest of experience:* it restricts in advance the range of permissible mental and physical activity, and it provides already established *names*—as well as the precedents that names imply—to neutralize the individual encounter with the new and the strange. *Via* language, culture speeds the process of bringing order, predictability, and significance to new experience.

D. Narcissism

But culture is the counterpart and reciprocal of the irrational as well as the rational, order-seeking side of the psyche; more than a collection of shared and shareable understandings, culture is reciprocal to the narcissistic tendencies studied by psychoanalysts such as Kohut (1978) and Kernberg (1975). By restoring the individual's conviction of centrality, and by supplying emergency rations of self-esteem, narcissism buffers the vulnerable individual against the "slings and arrows of outrageous fortune." Thus, narcissism fosters the illusion of security, either by elevating the self, or by endowing those parts of the world related to the self with unordinary stature, power, and grace.

In particular, culture sponsors a central aspect of narcissism: the plasticity of this powerful tendency. Narcissism can lead to an excessive glorification of the isolate individual self, or it can lead to the idealization of the social objects that condense out of collective experience. Under the sway of culture, the balance tilts toward society: the narcissistic investment is shifted away from the self, away from personal grandiosity, toward idealization of the cultural icons and institutions.

The great power that culture wields in this regard derives from its ubiquitous relationship to the founding myth, the legend that is graven in the annals of all vital societies. The cultural mystery is typically a drama of redemption. It tells how a special people, in dire straits, were rescued by the intervention of unordinary beings—whether gods (Yahweh at the Red Sea Crossing) or mortal though legendary heroes (George Washington, at Valley Forge). The founding myth is the power-shed of the encultured society: it lends significance to shared values, for these express the nature of the gods; and it lends dignity to conforming behavior, for such discipline is required by the gods and pleases them.

In effect, the myth is a narcissistic dream on the collective scale: the people's vulnerability countered by the *Deus ex machina,* the omnipotent, rescuing deity or hero. Thus, culture meets the human need to create illusory security by encumbering parts of the world with more than ordinary stature or power; in short, culture offers *objects of veneration.* These attract individual narcissism, and bind it to the communal service. Culture's great achievement is to transform potentially asocial narcissism into prosocial idealization of venerated gods, the traditions that reflect their nature, and the institutions that, through ritual, uphold these founding traditions. Culture is not—as some anthropologists would hold—the sum of distinctive group habits (in that limited sense, baboon bands could be said to have culture); culture is the system of idealized objects, including the institutions that service and defend them. Culture is what you will die for, or send your sons to die for.

E. The Cultural Uses of Splitting and Projection

But power–particularly the *tabu* power of the gods that causes them to be venerated—is always ambivalent, double-edged: like fire, it can warm your house, or burn it down. Likewise, the empowered, venerated gods, because they are vessels of power, may destroy their followers. Children deal with this dilemma, the essential unreliability of powerful providers, via the psychic mechanisms of *splitting* and *projection.* Malign aspects of the parent, those that detract from the ideal image, are deleted, and projected on some alternate—a stepparent, a strict teacher, or the "Bogey-Man." As a consequence, parts of the child's world may become frightening, but the Good Parent, the reassuring rescuer, is preserved. Culture uses these primitive defenses, whose first goal is to protect the immature self, for its own higher purpose: the protection of the idealized constructs, and by extension, the social order.

Thus, as they impanel demonic representations of bad power, cultures provide a *projective ecology* to accommodate the dark side of ambivalence. The world fills with devils, witches, or traitors, but the venerated objects remain uncorrupted. In adult life, splitting and projection can fuel individual paranoia, but culture is the talisman that converts these defenses to prosocial uses: the preservation of the collective icons. Culture uses evil, the names of the Devil, to protect the good.

F. Inner Controls

Erik Erikson once pointed out (personal communication, 1961) that deprivation *per se* is not psychologically destructive; it is only deprivation without *meaning* that is psychologically destructive. In this succinct thought, the great psychologist summed up the essential contribution of culture to the integrity of the psyche, and to its vital system of inner controls. By satisfying the hunger for the ideal, culture supplies encultured individuals with the sense of *meaning* that makes possible—even palatable—the conformities, disciplines, and sacrifices that are required by decent social life and by adequate parenting. A viable society requires predictable, *seemly* behavior; in the encultured society, such conformity is not a mark of shameful passivity. Instead, it becomes an aspect of ritual, a link to the founding mystery. To conform, to act in a seemly way is to garner—better, to recapture—for the self, some of the ideal qualities that have been conceded to the cultural icons. Thus *laundered* or neutralized, narcissism reverts to the self, in the form of self-esteem rather than megalomania. In effect, culture functions as the immune system of the social body: by providing individuals with meaning in exchange for their controlled, conforming behavior, it protects the social order against anarchy and unbridled asocial narcissism.

G. Self-Continuity

Strong cultures provide the ecology not only for inner controls, but also for a secure sense of selfhood. In particular, culture provides the conditions for an automatic sense of rootedness and inclusion. As Sigmund Freud (1922) pointed out in *Group Psychology and the Analysis of the Ego*, individuals who idealize the same leader automatically come together as a group. Each follower discovers in the other believers a piece of himself—the identification that is held in common. As a consequence, he endows his fellow believers with some portion of self-love, thereby forming a group. But culture, to bring about social bonding, goes beyond the *Führer Prinzip:* even in the absence of a charismatic leader, culture-mates recognize in each other a portion of themselves—the shared identification with the cultural icons, and the values that these represent. Encultured individuals *know* each other without prior acquaintance, through self-examination, through knowing themselves. Culture performs the great work of transforming potential strangers into familiars, and asocial narcissism into social bonds. The encultured individual has an automatic sense of recognition and inclusion, of being folded into a larger social body composed of those others who are, in important ways, extensions of self. The tie to leaders, those who best exemplify the virtues of ancestors and sponsoring gods, gives to the encultured individual the sense of being in touch with the redeeming powers who once rescued his people and who will now succor him; he discovers an echo of the founding mystery at the very core of self. A strong culture at the social level provokes a strong sense of identity at the individual level.

H. The Components of Culture

Summing up, the particular aspects of culture that co-act with individual needs for community, security and self-continuity are these:

A founding myth: The legend of special beginnings of a special people, favored by special gods.
Traditions: Formats for collective ritual, belief, and social action that reflect the ways of the founders, and partake of their sacred nature.
Institutions: Organized bodies, persisting across generations, that represent, guard, and enact the cultural myths and traditions. In general, religious institutions are wardens of the founding myth, while secular institutions are wardens of tradition.
Rituals: Patterns of stylized action choreographed by religious institutions to be metaphors, enact-

ments of the founding myth. Ritual practices provide encultured individuals with some sense of participation in the mystery, and its powers.

Age grade systems: Status *elevators* that reliably move accredited individuals, in their seniority, to the seats of institutional power, and to the gates of the mystery.

Strong cultures, no matter what their value content, meet these criteria. When culture is in these terms strong, then its adherents will be encultured, the culture will be a daily reality in the life of the people, and its values will be securely lodged in the mental life of the typical citizen. These internal certainties will constrain individual behavior, and lead to the perpetuation of culture by the next generation. When culture is in this sense perceivable, rooted, and transmissible, then the society is in a condition of culturation: whatever its ethnicity, whatever its particular values, whatever its economics, whatever its terrain, then there are predictable consequences, arising from the condition of culturation alone, for the collective and individual life. Whether pacific or war-like, the culturated society will almost certainly maintain strong families, trustworthy parents, emotionally sturdy children, and—however much it may trouble the peace of other societies—a relatively orderly, usually productive civil life. Finally, the vulnerable pre- or post-productive members of a culturated society—children, the infirm, and the old—are likely to be protected rather than grossly exploited by the strong.

I. Elders: The Wardens of Culture

Thus, the aged are major beneficiaries of a culturated society; but those who review the status and functions of the elders across cultures will find that the elders are also the most vital supporters of a strong culture, particularly in its mythic or *numinous* aspects.

The elder's special relation to culture helps us to understand male gerontocracy, another unique feature of human social organization. Among the subhuman primates, aging males drop out of the dominance hierarchy when they can no longer, by sheer muscular strength, maintain their rank and their unchallenged access to females. It is only when we cross the ape–human boundary that we encounter the institution of male gerontocracy. The ethnographic literature makes it clear that such governance is almost universally the rule in the folk, tradition-directed, encultured society. specifically, Leo Simmons' (1945) review of ethnographic studies of aging shows that older men were chiefs in 56 of the sample societies, that they could choose to hold office in eight more, and that in no case were they deposed on account of age. Humans then are the only primate species in which the older male, despite his loss of physical strength, his warrior's edge, can find alternate sources of spiritual strength to sustain and even increase his status. The special strength, even *charisma,* of the older traditional male comes not from his physical dominance, but from a resource that hairier apes do not have: his special, privileged access to *culture,* and to the power inherent in the cultural myths.

Older traditionals, because of their special access to the gods, to the myth-embracing past, and to the spiritualized ancestors, become the living exemplars of the founding legend. It is they, the elders, who bypass the time gap between then and now, bringing the two into conjunction. *Via* the elders, the mythic past and the mundane present are interpenetrated, and the climate of mythic origins is brought forward, into the here and now. Through the rituals managed by the older men, the power-shed of the past is tapped, and the *mana* that once rescued a desperate people reenters the world to heal the ill, to bring reviving rain down to a wasted land, or to move puny boys into strong manhood.

A substantial number of ethnographers report (and their accounts accord with my observations of the Navajo, Highland Maya, and Druze) that when society maintains a traditional consensus, older men lead the congregation. Thus, the correlational study by Timothy Sheehan (1976) of the relationship between societal type and senior prestige reveals that, for a sample of 47 preliterate groups, a settled, non-nomadic, relatively isolated and traditional society provides the best communal ecology for the aged and cultural life. There is folklore to be guarded and handed down by seniors, there is religious thought, cosmic ceremony and *rites de passage* through which they gain special access to the empowering gods.

Individual ethnographic accounts from a broad range of traditional societies bear out Sheehan's generalizations. Thus, from the Orient, Kalab (1990) reports on the ascension of Khmer elders, as they acquire new learning, to high rank in the Buddhist religion. Cowgill (1972) found that Thai elders withdraw gracefully from formal roles in society, but show marked increase in religious observance.

Shelton (1972) observed that Igbo (Africa) elders were thought to be exemplars of the life force, and were "most like a spirit." According to Biesele and Howell (1981), the title *big* is respectfully added to Kalahari Bushman seniors. Fuller (1972) who worked among the African Bantu, discovered their elders to be wardens of the land. They come to personify their clan lineage, and they are regarded as the living link to the ancestors. Similarly in Samoa, Holmes (1972) observed that older men have special access to the spirit world.

In the course of my own field work among the Druze, I found that Middle Easterners are no exception to the general rule. At around age 55, postparental Druze men, those who have lived an exemplary life and raised exemplary children, are invited to join the ranks of the *Aqil,* the accredited elders who guard the secret religion that defines their sect.

Coming full circle, back to our continent, we find that older American Indians "return to the blanket" and take up the traditional religion, even in the face of rapid modernization and deculturation. Thus, Fowler (1990) notes that Arapaho elders will maintain high social standing, despite loss of economic security, so long as they can enhance their ritual role in the native religion. Amoss and Harrell (1981) assert that, paradoxically, the prestige of the Indian elder in North America has risen, owing to a modern development: The return to nativistic roots on the part of young, relatively deculturated Indians. The revival of interest in tradition and ritual has brought with it a special advantage to those remaining elders who still remember—or can claim to remember—the old ways.

Summing up, we find a general rule that drives gerontocracy, across cultures: Older persons are less apt to control resources that have to do with pragmatic, economic production, but by the same token, their grip over the ritual sources of sacred power increases with age. In effect, young men kill with edged weapons, but older men can kill with a curse. Thus Lucien Levy-Bruhl (1928) observed that, in the preliterate folk society, the old man is possessed by an essence so pervasive that his body parts and even his excrement can be the residence of *tabu* power.

Claude Lévi-Strauss (1983) says it best: For him, the old are to the young as culture is to nature. He thereby implies an intrinsic connection between the elder and the human construction of society, which is *culture*. Society is a *natural* event. Individuals who find each other to be similar in important (usually physical) respects are automatically drawn together to from social *groups*. But society in its natural state, based on mechanical solidarity, is *raw*, either anarchic or subject to the harsh rule of the strongest, most ferocious leaders. It is only under the sway of culture that living becomes orderly and predictably calm. The young and especially untutored children are naturally social, but without being cultured. Their groups are like the packs of animals, predatory and unruly. It is the aged who represent the specifically human creation of culture. They know its ways, they have lived under its discipline, and they had daily knowledge of the ancestors. They have become part of the mystique from which the society derives its traditions, its rituals and its enduring strength. In traditional societies, the aged are seen to be iso-morphic with culture; they are its human face.

J. Elder Passivity and Elder Power

The older traditional's special access to spiritual power rests on a number of bases, including the endowment of wisdom, which is most evident under the redundant, rela-tively predictable circumstances of the small, isolated society. In addition, those hardy individuals who survive to old age under the stringent circumstances of the preliterate society are quite naturally regarded as special, unordinary. They have a special edge, which—since it does not come from their depleted bodies—must be the gift of the favoring gods. Their wrinkles do not betoken weakness, but duelling scars from god.

   Wisdom and longevity should bring prestige in any social setting; but I have speculated elsewhere (Gutmann, 1987) that the aged are additionally favored, under traditional culture, by qualities that can lead to their stigmatization, and social disadvantage under modern conditions. For example, as noted by Simone de Beauvoir (1972), the aged are always in danger of becoming the *stranger*, the *other*. The stranger is eerie, not quite human, even revolting, but also strong. And in the traditional assemblage, the aging strangers are told off to deal with the ultimate aliens, the gods. There, instead of revul-sion, the aspect of strength is underlined, and amplified, *via* the vivid contact with the gods. The passivity that surfaces in men's later years (see Gutmann, 1987) can also lead to stigma and shame in our society, but under the conditions of traditional culture, the same dangerous quality fits the older male for his special, power-giving relationship to the gods. In the encultured traditional society, the pacified older man acts as the intermediary between the society and its nurturing but also potentially dangerous, easily offended gods. There, accumulating the gods' *tabu* power for social purposes is not a task for Promethean young men. The necessary passivity is alien to them; their boldness would insult the gods, and—like Oedipus—bring disaster on the community and on themselves. To avoid this fate, the power brokers who man the sacred perimeter of the community must, in their own nature, be metaphors of the benign power that they would attract. Accordingly, in the traditional and religious community, it is the postparental older men, cleansed of sex and aggression, humble in bearing, who can beseech the nurturing influences of the gods, without offending the divinity. What we activist Americans might think of as shameful passivity becomes, under encultured conditions, the essential requirement for the strong traditional elder. Older men discover in the supernaturals the strength that they no longer find within themselves; they use prayer, *au fond* a passive-dependent modality, to beseech, for themselves and for the people, their fire from the gods.

K. Mental Health and the Traditional Elder

The older traditional not only revivifies himself through ritual, but he is also the power broker for society, the splice between the folk and its gods. The *mana* imported by the elder power-bringer revives not only him, but also the natural environment and social organs of his community. He becomes, for his people, the prime source of luck, of success in battle, of ripe crops, of fat herds, of healthy children.

Returning to the subject of this chapter, mental health and the elder, our model allows us to make a prediction for which confirmatory data does not yet exist: namely, that under conditions of gerontocracy and strong culture, even economic hardship will not detract from the psychological resilience of traditional elders.[2] This prediction takes into account the traditional elder's special relationship to cultural institutions, particularly those that convert narcissism to social bonds, that support inner controls, and that counteract existential terror. Thus, through his or her special linkage to the gods, the older traditional makes the sense of divinity manifest to the community as a whole. Through their social contact and personal identifications with the elder, individuals of all ages can feel themselves to be connected to, included in, the vital center. Thus enabled, they can discover echoes of that vital center within themselves. Via the intercessions of the traditional elder, the encultured person of any age receives the sense of grace that is vital to their self-esteem and the sense of significance that underpins their self-control. By the same token, given their special relation to the sacred aspect of culture, the older traditionals inherit important (though not always sufficient) prerequisites of their own psychological health: social status; respect, often verging on fear and awe; the assurance of social security from obligated kinfolk; and the sense of connection to a benevolent, supernatural order.

I am not suggesting a comprehensive theory of mental health or pathogenesis in later life; this discussion is limited to specific features of the mental life that normally become critical in the later years: inner controls, narcissistic fixations, self-continuity. I will briefly consider the influence of a strong culture in preventing those narcissistic disorders that result from weakened controls, impulse disorders, and disruptions in the experience of self.

Developmental as well as sociocultural forces act to bring about salutary transformations of narcissism. Particularly during the years of active parenthood, idealization of the

---

[2]As noted earlier, there are few reliable references in the cross-cultural literature to elderly mental health. The majority of these report on mental status issues, such as the presence or absence of dementia in particular groups. Most observers, such as Shelton among the Ibo (1965), Fuller (1972) among the Bantu, or Syryani *et al.* (1988) among the traditional Balinese, report the low incidence, even the complete absence, of dementing conditions. However, these findings might be an artifact of poor medical care in the traditional sector, rather than evidence of a social climate supportive of elderly mental health.

self and its goals is, if things go as they should, supplanted by the condition of *generativity* (Erikson, 1963): parental narcissism is conceded to the now-idealized child. The child should live forever, should not experience grief or want, should inherit the promise of the future, etc. This generational transfer of narcissism is vital to the child's development during its years of early vulnerability, before it has formed its own capacities, or found its own allies. But as children grow up, and as the sense of *parental emergency* (Gutmann, 1987) phases out, they do not need, nor do they justify, donations of parental narcissism. They have their own supplies; and, having revealed their own limitations, they are no longer creatures of infinite promise. As a consequence, in the postparental years, as in the preparental years, narcissism may again be retained for the self, in its unbuffered— hence pathogenic—form. Hypochondria, egocentricity, fussily obsessive rituals, hypersensitivity to minor slights, and depression in reaction to major insults can result, particularly for those older individuals with life-long narcissistic character disorders. But in the postparental years, a strong culture can provide, despite the emptied nest, new catalysts for healthy, phase-specific transformations of narcissism. In their seniority, traditional elders do not—as claimed by Cummings and Henry (1961)—disengage from social interaction into self-absorption (actually, disengagement is much more likely to occur under conditions of modernity and secularization). Instead, the traditional elder typically becomes the *warden* of the cultural myths and becomes merged, identified with the representations of that mystery: the cultural objects of veneration. In short, through the intervention of culture, traditional elders can shift self-concern away from themselves to transcendent icons, thereby converting pathogenic narcissism into idealism. Thus, instead of fussing over his private obsessions, the older traditional can choreograph the details of shared ritual: the ballet of seemly behavior that ties the people to their gods. His own fate becomes incidental; what counts is not the persistence of the individual self, but of the people and the ways in which they serve their god.

In sum, a strong culture, by buffering and neutralizing narcissism, deflects one of the leading *specific* threats to mental health in later life. By the same token, as elders themselves approach the iconic status, their sense of personal significance, the *meaning* of their service to the venerated objects, increases. In their adult years their self-control was validated by the imperatives of parenthood; in their postparental years, their self-control finds new justification, and now derives from their own venerated status, and from their special closeness to the gods. The vital sense of self-continuity is normally at risk in later life, eroded by critical changes in the inner and outer *ecologies of the self*. Most geropsychologists (see Atchley, 1989) hold that self-continuity later in life is threatened by expectable changes in familiar social domains: retirement, losses of spouse, kin, friends, etc. However, our studies of late-onset psychopathology at Northwestern Medical School have shown that *tectonic* inner shocks, having to do with important shifts in basic appetites, sexual identifications, and associated fantasies can also bring about profound revisions in the experience of self. Intrapsychic changes powerful enough to alter self-continuity can result from developmental transitions of the postparental period, and also from the weakening of inner controls. Despite their different origins, all such eruptive changes have similar effects: the older individual may feel that an alien, uninvited presence has taken over some part of the personal space, leaving him estranged from himself. In short, the integrity of the self is intimately linked to the integrity of inner controls; and, as we have already observed, these require endowments of cultural meaning to compensate for the deprivation inherent in such controls. In later life particularly, inner controls are threatened by the narcissistic wish for omniconsumption and omnigratification; strong cultures provide the intrapsychic controls with new anchors against the regressive pull. Culture functions as the immune system of society, and it also braces the psychological immune system of the traditional elder.

IV. Deculturation and the Elders

Culture has both structural and content features. The structural aspect, quite independent of particular contents, has to do with what can be called the *density* and *interiority* of a cultural regime—the degree to which it is a constant *presence* in the life of encultured individuals. The usual assumption in geropsychology is that the mental health of elders in a given society varies according to changes in the *content* features of culture: the mental health of older Americans is presumably at risk because they live in a society that values youth, etc. But the argument of this essay is that *deculturation*—the weakening or loss of culture—has the most profound consequences for the mental condition of the elderly. As long as culture is intact in the structural sense then variations in value consensus will have little effect on their psychic constitution. Thus, as we have seen in Iran, a holy Imam in his ninth decade, allied to the icons of Islam, could send revolutionary youth frenzied into the streets. Khomeini's special charisma for Iranian youth did not have to do with the fact that he was a revolutionary—these are common in the Middle East—but that he personified for them the timeless purity of Islam: through him, the Prophet was reborn.

As the Iranian example shows, traditional cultures can be very durable; many influences must combine to set in train the processes of social entropy that lead ultimately to deculturation, and the psychic deracination of the elders. These influences cannot be glibly summarized under the heading of either modernization or urbanization. While these processes can be part of a common sequence, modernization and urbanization often work independent of each other.

Briefly, modernity refers to influences that, while they usually originate in cities, are not exclusive to them: literacy, electrification, advanced modes of technology and manufacture, as well as *rationalized* uses of labor. Urbanization refers to the forms of association that typically occur in the city—with or without electricity or trams—but rarely in the village: the mingling of foreigners, the mixing of social classes and their contrasting ways, the open clash of philosophies—the city as market place of lifeways, ideas, and goods.

Stable, insular, usually rural societies are the best setting for strong cultures. So long as traditional beliefs and values can flourish in their own niche, uncontested by alternate world views (particularly those emanating from more developed societies), they avoid the fate of being relativized and called into question. An inevitable consequence of modernity is loss of physical distance between hitherto isolate societies; and when a modernizing society moves out of its isolation—or is moved out of it, by conquest or colonization—the people are automatically brought into contact with contrasting, even conflicting conceptions as to what is good and bad, possible and impossible, holy and impure. Despite this disorienting and relativizing contact, the emerging society may retain much of the ideological content of its culture; but the structural relationship between the people and their special beliefs must change as a result. The shock is most severe when the emerging society makes contact with the beliefs and practices of a technologically advanced society, one whose engineering and medical skills bring about immediate, tangible "miracles," wonders that cannot be matched by prayer and ritual. Thus, in the course of my own fieldwork I saw how the power of the Navajo medicine man was broken, not by white missionaries, but by Anglo medical interns working out of the Public Health Service hospitals scattered across the reservation. Despite his awesome dignity, despite being crusted with silver and turquoise, the medicine man's prayers cannot save a child with intestinal infections. The singer will chant powerfully for nine nights, while the feverish child dehydrates and dies. As concerned parents, the Navajo have learned that a callow white intern, who commands penicillin, can save the child that the magnificent medicine man will lose. Accordingly, at-risk children survive, but the mythic basis of Navajo culture is at the same time called into question, and Navajo lifeways lose their power to provide individuals with sacred sentiments, self-esteem, and discipline. Under such conditions, the cultural conceptions may still be widely distributed, familiar to most affiliates of the society; but now they are known to be no more than symbols, rather than substance. They are no longer the basic, power-compelling axioms of the universe. And as the sacred ideas become relativized, as symbol is split from substance, the elders who represent and expound these ideas are likewise split from their special powers. The elder loses the special cachet of "wise man" or "wise woman."

A. Economic Power and Elder Power

The economic changes that come with modernity are mainly important insofar as they degrade traditional ideas of sacred power, and the access to such power. *Wealth* in the folk mind is important only insofar as it links up with traditional ideas about *tabu* power, to the degree that it represents favor from the gods (or the power of witchcraft used in the service of envy-driven acquisition). As *objective* economics intrudes into the folk world, the traditional conception of sacred power loses its commanding position within a special preserve, while the *modern* forms of power take on some of the vibrancy that the traditional forms have lost. Power becomes secularized, represented by cash, by machines, by the products of machines, and even by beverage alcohol. In effect, under the new economics, the distinction between totemic and secular power phases out, and the power boundary is reset, no longer dividing the sacred from the ordinary world, but instead standing between the underdeveloped community and the modern or Western world. The effect on elders is profound: the aged are the monitors and heroes of the old power frontier that faces gods and demons; it is the young who cross the new frontier between societies to bring back alien power, in the form of cash, weapons, and technology, for themselves and their community. This is a role for the Promethean young and not for the cautious elders. If anything, the role of the elders on the new frontier is a reactionary and even destructive one. They tend to distrust the new, deritualized sources of power; and they impede development, the flow of modern forms of power, from the developed world into the still relatively powerless, emerging community.

The sons of the old traditionals are also caught up in the economics of modernity in ways that endow them not only with the new *financial* coinage of power, but also with the *mana* that their fathers are losing. The modernizing society typically provides a labor pool for the developed world; and the young men, instead of staying home to work their father's fields, leave the traditional village to find wage employment in the plantations, mines, mills, and armies of the more developed sectors. There, the young discover an economic base of power to which they have privileged access, resources not under the control of their fathers. They no longer have to ask him for the bride price that will accelerate their change from boys into men. The confirmatory power now comes from outside the community, rather than from within it. Thus, Rowe (1961) finds that Indian village gerontocracy has eroded as a direct result of changing employment. The young men find wage work in the cities and return home impatient with tradition, with the rule of the father, and with the slow-paced village life. And the wealth that they bring back undercuts the traditional association between affluence and advanced age, further corroding the status of the aged. Press and McKool (1972) find that when they shift from agricultural to wage work, young village Maya can buy their own land long before their father is ready to surrender the family holdings in their favor. In his dotage, the father now comes to live in the son's house, rather than granting the son's family a place in the patriarchal compound. The once mighty leading men, the *principles,* are degraded, and aging fathers who hold on to their land, refusing to recognize this shift in power, are sometimes murdered by their own sons. West and south of the Yucatan, among the Zapotec Indians, Adams (1972) found that the elder man's importance declines in step with the weakening of the *cargo* system, the age-graded order of responsibilities for church and ritual.

A number of African studies bear out the Mexican reports. Thus, Cattell (1989) notes that, in Western Kenya, elder knowledge is exclusively *local* in its scope. Modernization brings about the *delocalization* of knowledge, and the aged lose their special edge, their reputation for wisdom. For similar reasons, social change toward modernity induces doubt of their elders among young men of the Ethiopian Sidamo (Hamer, 1972). Fuller (1972) tells us that nowadays young Bantu find brides and "become men" without economic assistance from their fathers, or even in defiance of them. In his needful old age, his sons feel little obligation toward their father.

B. Deculturation and the Druze

Such observations, in settings as diverse as village India and rural Mexico, are confirmed by mine among the Druze sect of the Golan Heights. There, I learned that the various consequences of modernization are synergistic, mutually supporting. While carrying out a longitudinal study of aging psychology among the Golan Druze, I noted the ways in which economic, cognitive, and ritual changes bear on the fortunes of the elders in a traditional, classically gerontocratic village. Clearly, in the Druze community, the generational transfer of sacred power does at least begin in the pocketbook. During these years of Israeli hegemony, the young Golan Druze, who used to work their fathers' land while waiting to inherit, now find wage work in the *kibbutzim* and industries across the Jordan, in the Jewish sector. Again, they become less dependent for resource on their fathers' whim or generosity, and their exposure to modern people who do not respect or fear their fathers gives them further reason to doubt their hitherto-unquestioned power. Furthermore, affluence and modernization mean machinery. In Majd-Al-Shams, the donkey has largely been replaced by the tractor, and while the old men might understand donkeys, it is the young men, with their trade school and Syrian Army experience, who understand tractors. They can command the exotic power of the machine and make it available for the general purposes of the Druze. They play the interceding role in regard to machine power, that of harnessing it for their underpowered community, that their fathers play in regard to the powers of Allah. As a consequence, there is notably less deference toward the aged on the part of the Golan young, who begin to resemble the young men of the less-traditional (Israeli or Galilean Druze) sectors of their society. A generation gap has opened, such that their manner toward older traditional relatives begins to be patronizing, and even insulting.

It is evident then, that as the traditional young discover an economic base outside of their village and family, they acquire more than bank accounts: they begin to inherit the *mana* that was once exclusive to their fathers and grandfathers. As the society opens up to alien influences, new images and new myths, based on the power of aliens and of contemporary heroes who stole alien power, (and got away with it), fill the cultural space. The young can interpret and fit into these myths, for they have been to the place of the aliens; they have endured strange power, and they have—like Prometheus—captured some small part of it in the form of wages, technical knowledge, and even weapons. The young begin to take on some of the glamour of those who have danced before the gods and have survived the awesome contact with strange power.

Inevitably, as the young take on the bridgehead functions *vis-à-vis* alien power that the aged once performed, the prestige of the young is elevated, and the prestige of the traditional aged declines. Tectonic changes of this sort can take place in the cultural structure, long before there is any evident change in its *official* values: The disrespectful modernized young of the Golan are still very aware of the Druze norm of cowed respect for the old. The cultural contents still persist, and are given fine lip service, but the *density* and *interiority* of the venerated ideas and objects are reduced, as is their power over behavior and the mental life. Now there is crime, neighbor against neighbor, in the Golan villages.

C. Deculturation and the High Culture

As we have seen, modernization, whether it takes place in the village or in the city, undercuts the elders' monopoly on *tabu* power by creating alternate power bases, rooted in the new economies and the miraculous products of technology to which the young have privileged access. The contragerontic influences of the city act to degrade the sources of *tabu* power by attacking the symbolic bases—the specific icons and totems—on which gerontocracy is based. Furthermore, while modernization and urbanization can proceed independently, in the growing city these tendencies are most likely to potentiate, to amplify each other's deculturating effects. In the city, the traditional culture is not only weakened by the fallout from contrasting values and lifeways; it is also actively opposed by the society of critical elites that forms naturally on the nutriments provided by the liberal city. The high culture of creative literature, experimental theater, academic criticism and free inquiry, etc., gains its particular morale and vitality precisely by attacking, even symbolically murdering, the traditional, myth-centered culture. Thus, the high culture makes its agenda out of questioning certainties, of exploding hallowed myths, of ridiculing conformity, and exposing the frailties, physical and moral, of commonly revered figures: George Washington had wooden teeth; Thomas Jefferson kept slaves; Abe Lincoln was a manic-depressive, etc. The activists of high culture kill off the traditional culture for the same reasons that young men attack gerontocracy: in order to remove the dead hand of the past, the established precedents that block curiosity, creativity, and the experimentation with new, undreamed-of pleasures. Unfortunately, while the high culture makes the urban scene more vivid and amusing, it has no capacity whatever to support the more prosaic, undramatic civil life, the quotidian decencies that underwrite social security, domestic security, and sturdy children.

D. The Aging Strangers

Furthermore, in U.S. urban settings, we threaten the integrity of the founding culture in particularly American ways. Thus, the American impulse toward equality, which first struggles against the restrictions on ordinary civil rights, ends by politicizing the chronic complaint against existential restrictions. Individual Americans were long ago granted the right to choose their own leaders, careers, and political parties; but in recent times the principle of equality attacks a core cultural assumption, of commonly held, unquestioned values. Until recently, these were regarded as objective: fixed social realities to be internalized by the individual, but to be created and maintained apart from that same individual, by idealized cultural institutions and their leaders. But in recent times, the high culture has succeeded in democratizing the process of value formation to the point where it has been taken out of the institutional province and given over to the private individual. Moving thus, from the social to the personal sphere, values lose their shared and objective character, to become private and subjective. In effect, we have democratized and relativized the process of value formation to the point where each citizen is conceded the right to decide personally the standards against which he should be measured.

Outside of a courtroom, the assertion "I'm just doing my own thing," is coming to be the ultimate justification for any action short of murder. In our obsessive pursuit of equality we have succeeded in subjectivizing values to the point where weakened culture no longer coheres shared ideals. Thus, in the city the common culture is weakened by a dual assault: from the high culture; and, paradoxically, from the operation of a principle—equality—that is fundamental to our common culture. But whatever the causes of the decay, a depleted common culture loses the power to convert strangers into familiars, and narcissistic potentials into enduring social bonds. The consequent deculturation soon leads to social crisis.

The attack by the high culture on sacrosanct myths is particularly damaging to the elders. So long as the founding legends go unchallenged, their special tie to the mystery gives elders the charisma of the awesome rather than the repulsive stranger; and the culture's all-including *we* overrides the alienating effects of age, cohort, and cosmetic differences between the young and the old. Again, the encultured know themselves and their fellows through their association with transcending, idealized collectivities. But, much like the processes of aging, deculturation undercuts the institutions that direct the transformations of narcissism, from its raw asocial to its sculpted, prosocial state. Under the conditions of deculturation, narcissistic preference dictates the lines of affiliation. Decultured persons only extend the tonus of familiarity and we-ness to those who resemble them in the most concrete, immediately sensible respects: those who share the same skin color, the same body conformation, the same genitalia, the same sexual appetites, and the same age group. With deculturation, the principles of association are no longer based on shared standards but become instead the politics of narcissism: racist, sexist, homoerotic, and ageist. When the deculturating society fragments along the natural cleavage lines of race, gender, dominant erotic appetite, and generation, then the *stranger* potential of the aged is underscored rather than overridden. A strong culture underwrites the strong face of aging; but deculturation brings forth its weak face. The decultured society is automatically *gerophobic*.

Under conditions of deculturation, the gender and age distinctions that divide the larger society penetrate to the heart of the modern family. To the degree that family solidarity still persists across the generations in urban societies, it is mainly between the grandmothers, daughters, and granddaughters of the female line, more and more excluding of men. And by the same token, the mistrust between generations that is often a feature of the general social life under deculturation has invaded the heart of the family itself. The family, whether nuclear or extended, is usually the one enclave in which generational distinctions are overlooked, in favor of some higher principle of kinship solidarity. But the generation gap that is strikingly absent in the traditional village family bisects the heart of the nuclear and modified extended family in the city. The urban aged begin to know alienation even within their own primary groups.

E. Some Geropsychological Consequences

The fate of elders and children is everywhere linked, such that the condition of one group, whether good or bad, predicts directly the condition of the other. Encultured societies extend protection, automatically, to preproductive children, and to postproductive elders. But as the society decultures, as it loses idealized icons, the individual self becomes its own venerated object, and narcissism—as we have seen—becomes increasingly the coinage of social relationships. Under these conditions the pre- and postproductive cohorts are at risk, on the grounds that children and elders both require inordinate amounts of unreciprocated care. Thus, while child abuse is a major topic of contemporary congresses on family dynamics, papers on elder abuse now dominate the proceedings of the Gerontological Society.

I have argued that the encultured society provides a facilitating developmental milieu, one in which the nascent potentials of later life are shaped, to become the special capacities of the traditional elder. thus, entropic deculturation not only deprives the aged of congenial, development-sponsoring social circumstances; it also depletes their intrapsychic domain. As a consequence, important developmental transitions of later life—particularly, the transformations of narcissism into idealization—are less likely to come about. These failures of later-life development are likely to leave decultured elders vulnerable not only to the narcissism of the young, but also to their own. Aged Druze, who have converted narcissism into worship of Allah, can look with equanimity on the prospect of their death, saying to me only, "This is Allah's will; to complain about my sickness or death would be to dispute his will." These aged Druze, because they feel identified with their changeless god, are able to accommodate, without much sense of shock or insult, catastrophic change, including the final transition into death.

However, the changes affecting the density and interiority of culture that arrive with modernity seem to release a more narcissistic, greedy nature, even in ostensibly traditional elders. This effect was revealed through a study on the *oral* Dimension of Aging Personality (Gutmann, 1971) carried out among traditional Navajo and Druze. Having found strong correlations between passive-dependency and the degree of specifically oral concerns in Druze and Navajo subjects, I went on to examine the effects of age, culture and modernity, as these affected the orality variable. Two statistically significant main effects were found. Orality increased with age, and with urban-proximal residence, regardless of age. Culture *per se* has *no* effect on orality: It climbs at the same rate with age among Navajo and Druze. Thus, as predicted, narcissistic self-concerns—as measured by the orality (or "feed me!") variable—goes up with age. But while oral narcissism is not affected by differences in the value consensus between two very different cultures, it is strongly affected by the structural aspects of culture, as these weaken along the folk-urban axis of two traditional societies.

Again, the value content of Druze and Navajo culture does not change significantly in the transition from isolate-traditional to near-urban–traditional settings; the real change is in the structural features of culture, and these do affect the management—if not the intensity—of individual oral appetites. The personality differences between the rural isolate and urban-proximal traditionals are not trivial: the high-orality, urbanized Navajo express their greater passive-dependency through alcoholism, psychosomatic illness, and even criminality.

F. Deculturation and Geriatric Psychopathology

The linkage discovered among the Navajo, between senescent orality and pathogenesis, gives clues to the fate of the decultured, openly narcissistic elder, who is in the peak period for physical, cognitive, cosmetic, social and existential losses. If the intense focus on self continues, the result is an increasing sense of vulnerability: the normal losses and changes of aging become insults, outrages, and terrors. Depression and hypochondriasis, as well as delusional attempts to deny depletion and imperfection, can be the too-frequent result. In our clinical studies of late-onset disorders at Northwestern University Medical School (see Gutmann, 1988), we note that many emotional disorders of later life represent frantic attempts to overcome the sense of insult and depression on the part of older individuals who have not relinquished their conviction of centrality and perfection. In them, psychiatric breakdown occurs when the need to deny loss and insult, or to project onto others the responsibility for imperfection, is so strong that reality is abandoned in favor of the defense. Thus, *denial* of loss and threat, sometimes taking the form of manic psychosis, is one major defense of the older patient. A paranoid state, in which the sense of blemish or the responsibility for the blemish, is projected onto others, is an alternate but equally strong possibility. Severe depression and even lethal illness can result when these primitive defenses fail. In a real sense, later-life psychosis represents a hectic attempt to supply, for the self, the donations of self esteem that are routinely donated to elders by an encultured society.

In sum, deculturation and the weakening of the extended family have major effects that particularly disadvantage older individuals. Wrenched away from culture, they lose their special developmental milieux, they lose their special bases for self-esteem, and they are transformed from *elders* into *the aging.* Losing their traditional character as hero, they take on their modern character, as victim. The weak face of aging appears; and this debility can be expressed in the form of individual psychopathology.

A *caveat* is in order: lacking reliable comparative mental health data from traditional societies, we cannot confidently assert that geriatric psychopathology increases under conditions of modernity, secularization, or deculturation. It may be, though it is not likely, that the rates of elderly depression and psychosis in more folk-like societies match those of the "first" world. But if this were the case, then ethnographers who study the condition of traditional elders in naturalistic ways would report at least anecdotal evidence of such trouble. Usually living among their subjects, not buffered from them by standard instruments, these qualitative investigators develop the heightened sensitivities, the early warning systems, that would pick up the signs of emotional distress among their elderly informants. But, as we have seen, these dedicated ethnogerontologists are much more apt to report the high status, the powers, and the seeming contentment of traditional elders. Save for the Highland Maya of Chiapas, whose elders had high status and were hated for it, I came back from the field with similar impressions and with interview data to back them up. Accordingly, until we get trustworthy reports to the contrary, I will stick with this possibly shaky assumption: Modernity, *if* it leads to deculturation, is not good for elderly mental health. In addition, I have tried to show that the pathogenic causes lie not in changing cultural content, or *cohort influences,* but in a much more ominous development: the degradation of culture itself.

Organized gerontology avoids this grim truth. For one thing, our sterile methods, driven by the narcissistic need for invulnerability rather than revelation, are themselves a symptom of deculturation. Additionally, while dimly recognizing the trouble, we try to confine it to the aged: *They* will suffer the consequences of deculturation; it is our job as gerontologists to study them while it happens. But just as the study of aging does not stop gerontologists from getting old, the study of elder abuse will not protect us from the general decay of decency in our society. It is a common tragedy; and by not acknowledging it we accelerate the process of social entropy.

But we should remember that our elders, though they have lost their traditional link to culture in its external institutional form, still preserve culture in its internalized form:

During a time of rapid deculturation, the elders are still the most encultured minority among us. Contrary to the impression propagated by mass media and congresses of gerontology, the great majority of our elderly—even when enfeebled—are *not* candidates for long-term care. Quite the contrary: as inheritors of the now deconstructed American culture that suckled their characters, they still live by the *ethos* of rugged independence and self-sufficiency. They avoid long-term care up to the last moment of possibility. Our elders do have their psychic vulnerabilities and pathologies, and some of these are based on their unrelinquished pride; but they are still the wardens of what was once our common culture. Instead of devoting the bulk of our energy and concern to the elderly candidates for long-term care, we should think about the proper therapy for the silent majority, of stubbornly autonomous, still encultured elders. Perhaps the best therapy for these counter-dependant cohorts is to let *them* help us. They can counsel us concerning the maintenance of culture, and the proper steps towards its restoration.

References

Adams, F. (1972). The role of old people in Santo Tomas Mazaltepec. In D. Cowgill & L. Holmes. (Eds.), *Aging and Modernization* (pp. 103–126). New York: Appleton-Century-Crofts.

Amoss, P. T., & Harrell, S. (Eds.). (1981). Introduction. In *Other ways of growing old: An anthropological perspective* (pp. 1–24). Stanford: Stanford University Press.

Atchley, R. C. (1989). A continuity theory of normal aging. *The Gerontologist, 29*, 183–190.

Biesele, M., & Howell, N. (1981). "The old people give you life": Aging among !Kung hunter-gatherers. In P. T. Amoss & S. Harrell (Eds.), *Other ways of growing old*, Anthropological Perspectives. Stanford: Stanford University Press.

Cattell, M. (1989). Knowledge and social change in Samia, Western Kenya. *Journal of Cross-Cultural Gerontology, 4*, 225–244.

Cohler, B. J., & Lieberman, M. A. (1979). Personality change across the second half of life: Findings from a study of Irish, Italian, and Polish-American men and women. In D. E. Gelfand & A. J. Kutzik (Eds.), *Ethnicity and Aging* (pp. 227–245). New York: Springer.

Cowgill, D. (1968). The social life of the aging in Thailand. *The Gerontologist, 8*, 159–163.

Cowgill, D. (1972). *Aging and modernization*. New York: Appleton-Century-Crofts.

Cummings, E., & Henry, W. (1961). *Growing old: The process of disengagement*. New York: Basic Books.

de Beauvoir, S. (1972). *The coming of age*. New York: Putnam.

Erikson, E. (1963). *Childhood and society* (2nd ed.). New York: Norton.

Erikson, E. (1959). Identity and the life cycle. *Psychological Issues, 1*, (Monograph I). New York: International University Press.

Fowler, L. (1990). Colonial context and age group relations among plains Indians. *Journal of Cross-Cultural Gerontology, 5*, 149–168.

Freud, S. (1922). *Group psychology of the ego* (No. 6). London: International Psychoanalytic Library.

Fry, C. (1985). Culture, behavior and aging in the comparative perspective. In J. Birren & K. Schaie (Eds.). *Handbook of the psychology of aging* (2nd ed., pp. 216–244). New York: Van Nostrand Reinhold.

Fuller, C. (1972). Aging among the Southern African Bantu. In D. Cowgill & L. Holmes (Eds.), *Aging and modernization* (pp. 51–72). New York: Appleton-Century-Crofts.

Gutmann, D. (1968). Aging among the Highland Maya: A comparative study. *Journal of Personality and Social Psychology, 7*, 28–35.

Gutmann, D. (1971). Navajo dependency and illness. In E. Palmore (Ed.), *Prediction of life span* (pp. 181–198). Lexington, MA: D. C. Heath.

Gutmann, D. (1980). Observations on culture and mental health in later life. In J. Birren & R. Bruce Sloan (Eds.), *Handbook of Mental Health and Aging* (pp. 429–447). Englewood Cliffs, NJ: Prentice-Hall.

Gutmann, D. (1987). *Reclaimed powers: Toward a new psychology of men and women in later life*. New York: Basic Books.

Gutmann, D. (1988). Late-onset pathogenesis: Dynamic models. *Topics in Geriatric Rehabilitation, 3,* 1–8.

Hamer, J. (1972). Aging in a gerontocratic society: The Sidamo of Southwest Ethiopia. In D. Cowgill & L. Holmes (Eds.), *Aging and modernization* (pp. 15–30). New York: Appleton-Century-Crofts.

Holmes, L. (1972). The role and status of the aged in a changing Samoa. In D. Cowgill & L. Holmes (Eds.), *Aging and Modernization* (pp. 73–90). New York: Appleton-Century-Crofts.

Kalab, M. (1990). Buddhism and emotional support for elderly people. *Journal of Cross-Cultural Gerontology, 5,* 7–19.

Kernberg, O. (1975). *Borderline conditions and pathological narcissism.* New York: Jason Aronson.

Kohut, H. (1978). *The restoration of the self.* New York: International University Press.

LeVine, R. (1978a). Adulthood and aging in cross-cultural perspective. *Items, 31/32,* 1–5.

LeVine, R. (1978b). Comparative notes on the life course. In T. K. Hareven (Ed.), *Transitions: The family and the life course in historical perspective* (pp. 287–297). New York: Academic Press.

Lévi-Strauss, C. (1983). *The raw and the cooked.* Chicago: University of Chicago Press.

Levy-Bruhl, L. (1928). *The "soul" of the primitive.* London: Allen and Unwin.

Opler, M. E. (1959). *Culture and mental health: Cross-cultural studies.* New York: Macmillan.

Press, I., & McKool, M. (1972). Social structure and status of the aged: Toward some valid cross-cultural generalizations. *Aging and Human Development, 3,* 297–306.

Redfield, R. (1947). the folk society. *American Journal of Sociology, 2,* 293–308.

Rowe, W. (1961). The middle and later years in Indian society. In R. Kleemeier (Ed.), *Aging and leisure* (pp. 104–112). New York: Oxford University Press.

Shanan, J. (1985). Personality types and culture in late adulthood. In J. Meacham (Ed.), *Contributions to human development (Vol. 12,* pp. 1–144). Basel: S. Karger.

Sheehan, T. (1976). Senior esteem as a factor of socio-economic complexity. *Gerontologist, 16,* 433–440.

Shelton, A. (1965). Ibo aging and eldership: Notes for gerontologists and others. *Gerontologist, 5,* 20–23.

Shelton, A. (1972). The aged and eldership among the Igbo. In D. Cowgill (Ed.), *Aging and modernization* (pp. 31–50). New York: Appleton-Century-Crofts.

Simmons, L. (1945). *The role of the aged in primitive society.* New Haven: Yale University Press.

Syryani, L., Kamar, T., Andjana, A., Thong, D., Manik, I. Putra, D., Widjaja, W., Tama, D., & Jensen, G. (1988). The physical and mental health of elderly in a Balinese village. *Journal of Cross-Cultural Gerontology, 3,* 105–120.

4

Gender and Ethnicity Patterns ___

E. Percil Stanford and Barbara C. Du Bois

I. Introduction
II. Demographic Considerations
III. Definitions and Conceptual Underpinnings
    A. Aging
    B. Gender
    C. Ethnicity
IV. The Role of Stress, Social Supports, and Coping in Mental Health
    A. Psychosocial Stress
    B. Social Support Resources
    C. Coping and Adaptation
V. Prevalence of Mental Health Disorders
    A. African-American Elderly
    B. Hispanic Elderly
    C. American Indian Elderly
    D. Asian-Pacific Island Elderly
VI. Approaches to Community Mental Health
    A. Cultural Sensitivity and the Mental Health Care System
    B. Eliminating Barriers to the Mental Health System
VII. Recommendations for the Future
VIII. Summary
    References

I. Introduction ___

Aging research and program development should incorporate more systematic methods to better understand the role of gender and ethnicity in the mental health status of older individuals. Current information and programmatic models are predicated on what are presumed to be the needs of the average older male; however, the majority of older individuals are female, especially after the age of 80. In addition, little attention has been given to ethnicity and its bearing on the mental health status of older people. The lower life expectancies of minorities in the United States provide ample evidence of the role of ethnicity in morbidity and mortality. There is evidence that mental health status is affected by ethnicity, gender, and age; however, there is a paucity of systematic information that clearly delineates age and sex differentials in mental health by ethnic groups. Although greater attention should be directed toward understanding these influences on mental health, researchers and professionals in the field are limited by the absence of these data.

The ideas and issues presented in this chapter are intended to challenge practitioners, researchers, and academicians to further consider the impact of older persons' gender and ethnicity on their mental health and well-being. This chapter provides background for (1) demographic considerations; (2) definitions of aging, gender, and ethnicity; (3) the role of stress, social supports, and coping in mental health; (4) the prevalence of mental health disorders by ethnic group and, where possible, by age and gender; (5) approaches to community mental health; and (6) implications for the fields of mental health and aging now and in the future.

There are incremental changes in mental health status with advancing age. Emotional and mental disorders occur with higher frequency. Although evidence suggests that many of these changes may have a genetic basis, some factors appear to promote mental disorders in susceptible populations. Risk factors that are among the primary antecedents to mental disorders are gender, advancing older age, ethnicity, socioeconomic and environmental factors, health behavioral and health care utilization patterns, psychosocial stress and coping resources, and factors related to culture change, such as acculturation, modernization, and migration.

There is a popular notion that loss accounts for the apparent increase of psychopathology in the aged. Loss may be construed as loss of loved ones, loss of social role, loss of occupation through retirement, and loss of socioeconomic status. Although loss may be associated with changes in mental health status, there is increasing evidence that well-being is positively associated with aging (Markides, 1986); thus, there is an apparent reversal of this notion from a negative to a more positive formulation. With advances in medical treatment and lifestyle changes, significantly more elderly are living to older age. The presence of Medicare and various aging network services provide a larger economic safety net for many elderly.

II. Demographic Considerations

As shown in Table I, there are large differences in total population and cohort size between ethnic minority groups and whites. Significant increases occurred between 1980 and 1990 in the population older than 65 for Hispanics (55%), African-Americans (25%), and whites (23%). Funding for programs and services for minorities tends to target younger more than older age groups (U.S. Department of Health and Human Services, 1985); however, with such significant increases in the age group older than 65 and among minority populations, funding priorities need to be re-examined. Table II provides an overview of population projections of those 45 and older by sex, age, and ethnicity for the years 1990, 2000, and 2010. The distribution of total females is between 2 and 4% higher

Table I

Population Distribution and Projections of Ethnic Minority Groups
in the United States 1980–1990[a]

Ethnic group	Total number 1980	65 and older 1980	Percentage of group	Projected 65 and older 1990	Percentage increase 1980 to 1990
White	188,340,790	22,944,033	12.2	28,300,000	23.3
African-American	26,488,218	2,085,826	7.9	2,600,000	24.7
American Indian	1,418,195	74,788	5.3	80,000	6.5
Asian and Pacific islanders	3,500,636	211,834	6.0	222,000	4.8
Spanish origin	14,605,883	708,785	4.8	1,100,000	55.2
Total	**232,935,527**	**25,950,478**	Percentage of total population **11.1**	**32,302,000**	

[a]Adapted from Markides & Mindel (1987) and Taeuber (1990).

than that of total males, with largest differences occurring among *blacks* and *other races*. The largest percentage change in population size will occur among minorities, with largest increases occurring by 1990 (blacks, 16%; other races, 67%; whites, 8%), followed by less robust but still significant change for the years 2000 (blacks, 13%; other races, 35%; whites, 5%) and 2010 (blacks, 11%; other races, 27%; whites, 3%). Such population projections are critical in guiding mental health care planners and providers.

Migration patterns also have an important impact on the demographic structure of older age groups. Much of the increase in population size of other races, indicated by Table II, is attributable to Hispanic and Asian immigrants. Uhlenberg (1977) indicated that the number of white foreign-born persons older than 60 has dropped from one third of the population in 1900 to about 6% in 1980. The aged population will become more diverse as cohorts of more recent immigrants reach older ages. The Hispanic population is the best example of a group whose numbers continue to surge and who will need more mental health services. By the year 2005, the number of Hispanic persons age 65 and older will have increased fourfold from the proportion found in 1985 (U.S. Bureau of the Census, 1986). Taeuber (1990) reaffirmed that racial and ethnic diversity will intensify.

Survivorship is highly selective with regard to socioeconomic status, genetics, and environmental factors; however, females across all ethnic groups live longer than males for a variety of reasons. Lifestyle factors interacting with genetic predispositions probably account for the higher mortality rates among men from major chronic diseases, especially coronary heart disease. Socioeconomic and environmental factors may severely affect an individual's ability to seek health care and alternative sources of support, thus rendering

Table II

Projection of the Total Population by Age, Sex, and Race: 1990 to 2010[a]

Age, sex, and race	Population (1000)			Percentage distribution			Percentage change		
	1990	2000	2010	1990	2000	2010	1990	2000	2010
	250,410	**268,266**	**282,575**	**100.0**	**100.0**	**100.0**	**9.9**	**7.1**	**5.3**
45–54 years	25,487	37,223	43,207	10.2	13.9	15.3	12.0	46.0	16.1
55–64 years	21,364	24,158	35,430	8.5	9.0	12.5	−1.8	13.1	46.7
65–74 years	18,373	18,243	21,039	7.3	6.8	7.4	17.4	−.7	15.3
75+ years	13,187	16,639	18,323	5.3	6.2	6.5	31.2	26.2	10.1
Male, total	**122,243**	**131,191**	**138,333**	**100.0**	**100.0**	**100.0**	**10.2**	**7.3**	**5.4**
Female, total	**128,167**	**137,076**	**144,241**	**100.0**	**100.0**	**100.0**	**9.7**	**7.0**	**5.2**
White, total	**210,616**	**221,514**	**228,978**	**100.0**	**100.0**	**100.0**	**7.7**	**5.2**	**3.4**
45+ years									
Male	103,184	108,774	112,610	49.0	49.1	49.2	8.0	5.4	3.5
Female	107,432	112,739	116,368	51.0	50.8	50.8	7.4	4.9	3.2
Black, total	**31,148**	**35,129**	**38,833**	**100.0**	**100.0**	**100.0**	**15.8**	**12.8**	**10.6**
45+ years									
Male	14,835	16,787	18,602	47.6	47.8	47.9	16.2	13.2	10.8
Female	16,313	18,342	20,231	52.4	52.2	52.1	15.4	12.4	10.3
Other races, total	**8,646**	**11,624**	**14,764**	**100.0**	**100.0**	**100.0**	**67.2**	**34.5**	**27.0**
45+ years									
Male	4,224	5,629	7,122	48.9	48.4	48.2	66.5	33.3	26.5
Female	4,422	5,995	7,642	51.1	51.6	51.8	67.8	35.6	27.5

[a]Adapted from U.S. Department of Commerce, Statistical Abstract of the U.S. 1990, p. 16.

an individual more susceptible to end-stage diseases. Additionally the stress of poverty may predispose certain genetically susceptible individuals to higher rates of disease.

Environment may be an important factor for understanding diversity among ethnic groups because it helps to explain differences in lifestyle between urban–rural populations and those from broadly different geographic regions. The 1980 census showed that the majority of blacks continue to reside in rural areas of the South (U.S. Bureau of the Census, 1980). This contrasts sharply with the larger urban residences of blacks in other parts of the country. Trends that account for this may in part be socioeconomic (i.e., higher rate of affordable housing in inner cities) as well as cultural (i.e., residence near members of your own ethnic group).

III. Definitions and Conceptual Underpinnings ⎯⎯⎯⎯⎯⎯⎯⎯⎯⎯

The following definitions of *aging, gender,* and *ethnicity* will be adopted for the purposes of the present chapter.

A. Aging

Aging refers

> to the regular changes that occur in mature, genetically representative organisms living under representative environmental conditions as they advance in chronological age. (Birren & Renner, 1977, p. 4)

B. Gender

In 1980, women represented 54.7% of the U.S. population 40 years of age and older, and 59% of those 60 and older (U.S. Bureau of the Census, 1980). A white female can expect to live approximately eight years longer than her male counterpart, and a nonwhite female is expected to live nine years longer than her male peer. Among those aged 65 to 69, there are approximately 127 females to every 100 males, but by age 85 and older, there are roughly 220 women to every 100 men. Given the demographic profile of the elderly in the United States and the significantly higher number of women than men living to older age, it is reasonable to give more attention to planning mental health care services for older women.

One of the striking differences between aged men and women, regardless of ethnicity, is that slightly more than three fourths of all men 65 and over are married, while slightly over one third of the women 65 and over are married; thus, there are many widows among older women. Men are likely to remarry at a higher rate than their female counterparts and are also likely to marry younger, rather than same age or older, women (Markson, 1983).

Minority status and ethnicity are associated with the potential of becoming a widow, and of widowhood's having an impact on living arrangements. Pelham and Clark (1987) indicated that widows from both white and African-American groups tend to live alone, while widows from Hispanic and Asian groups tend to live with others. Because of these circumstances, it is likely that the latter have more ongoing support than the former (Dowd & Bengston, 1978; Pelham & Clark, 1987).

The interaction of gender and marital status is an important consideration in understanding the health conditions of all groups of elders (Gove, 1973). For example, in comparison to widows, widowers experience more negative health problems, are more socially isolated, have fewer emotional ties with families, and are less likely to have a confidant (Strain & Chappell, 1982). With advancing age and an increase in functional limitations, the differences between widows and widowers become less obvious (Martin-Matthews, 1987).

The average older woman is often pictured as living alone, in poverty or with low income, in substandard housing, with very little medical care and few opportunities for gainful employment. This scenario creates a very bleak picture for older women in our society. The reality is that some women face these circumstances regardless of ethnic background. On the other hand, women from minority groups generally do not have optimal income or living arrangements, but they may have socially beneficial and supportive relationships with family and friends.

C. Ethnicity

Gordon (1978) described ethnicity from a functional perspective, categorizing groups of persons within the natural boundaries of the United States. These groupings are distinguished by race, religion, national origin, or some combination of the above.

> Race refers to differential concentrations of gene frequencies responsible for traits, which are confined to physical manifestations, such as skin color or hair form. It has no causative connection with cultural patterns and institutions. (Gordon, 1978, p. 111)

The concept of ethnic group can be used to refer to those persons who have common racial and cultural backgrounds. Ethnic identity preserves cultural uniqueness, but ethnicity may also be used to prevent access to the larger society. An ethnic group may become a minority group when, according to an early definition by Wirth,

> a group of people who, because of their physical or cultural characteristics, are singled out from others in the society in which they live for differential and unequal treatment, and who therefore regard themselves as objects of collective discrimination. (Wirth, 1945, p. 346)

In spite of the powerful assimilative forces in the larger society, ethnicity and ethnic group identity persist. Greeley (1974) used the concept of ethno-genesis to explain the tenacious quality of ethnicity in multicultural settings. The very forces that shape loss of ethnic identity may well act to preserve certain characteristics of ethnicity as groups adapt to a complex society. To better understand social stratification in a complex society, social scientists recommend that ethnicity be considered in relation to specific demographic characteristics, such as sex, age, social class, and socioeconomic status. The bulk of research on minorities tends to focus on the most deprived members and fails to distinguish ethnic and cultural factors from the effects of social class and racial discrimination (Markides, 1982). Within ethnic minority groups, wide variability is a function of social class, socioeconomic status, and effects of discrimination. Cool (1986) suggests that the concept of ethnic group encompasses socially significant characteristics of an aggregate of people within a larger context. The members themselves define the social significance of ethnic group characteristics, and this process is undertaken within a framework of alternative cultural modalities. Research among specific groups may demonstrate variable ethnic-adaptive patterns. Elderly Jewish populations have been shown to make aging a part of life's career; hence, Jewish ethnicity provides a powerful source of reinforcement and support for successful aging (Myerhoff, 1978). Valle (1988–1989) discusses ethnicity in terms of group identification based upon a common cultural heritage. Customs are followed, beliefs are held, and a predominant language is used. Valle further states the importance of linking *ethnicity* to *minority* when discussing American Indians, African-Americans, Asian–Pacific Islanders, and Hispanics. The rationale for doing so is that these groups are minorities from the standpoint of their social, political, and economic status.

The idea that all ethnic minority older people can be treated without attention to cultural background began to disappear in the 1950s when it became evident that the *melting-pot* theory was no longer relevant (Gelfand, 1979). Sopolopski (1985) aptly pointed out that ethnicity and ethnic-related patterns are so diverse that more individuals are increasingly moving back to their ethnicity as a point of reference.

IV. The Role of Stress, Social Supports, and Coping in Mental Health

A. Psychosocial Stress

The psychosocial stress process involves cognitive appraisal of the particular stressor or problem, assessment of internal and external resources for mediating the problem (e.g., internal locus of control, personality styles, social support solicitation, social network interaction), and coping and adaptation (Moos, 1979). What constitutes a stressor may be different from one individual to another because it requires a unique appraisal of potential threat. There are, however, different kinds of stressors. Some may be short lived, while others may be indicative of a more serious problem.

The common notion underlying studies of psychopathology in ethnic minority populations has focused on the effects of lower social class on mental disorders (Dohrenwend & Dohrenwend, 1969; Fried, 1975; Kessler, 1979). Lower socioeconomic status is associated with greater levels of stress and fewer coping resources in general. Combining lower social class, higher levels of stress, and older age result in greater risk for mental disorder for most ethnic minority elderly (Kessler & Cleary, 1980; Markides, 1986).

The predominant mechanisms by which this occurs are through discrimination and exclusion, immigration, and the stress of acculturation (Markides, 1986). The cumulative net savings for older age are a function of lifetime earning potential. When this economic potential is restricted, regardless of the specific mechanism, more ethnic minority elders will experience the hardship of reduced or limited income at a time when they may need it the most. Thus, the economic stress associated with ethnic identity and discrimination in general may well be precursors to mental health outcomes in older age. As noted by Markides (1986) from several studies of mental hospital admissions, foreign-born patients are significantly over-represented as patients. Although the stress of migration and adaptation may provide an important mechanism for the development of mental disorder, there are many conditioning factors that may serve to mitigate the stress of acculturation in the migrant community, such as size of the community, similarity of culture between the place of origin and the new location, and length of stay.

B. Social Support Resources

Lin (1986) conceptualized social support as having two components: the social component concerns the individuals' linkages with their social environment, while the support environment concerns the instrumental and expressive activities of support. In the latter, there are differences in perceived and actual access to support resources. Thus, social support is construed as "the perceived or actual instrumental and/or expressive provisions supplied by the community, social networks, and confiding partners" (Lin, 1986, p. 18). Social support theory proposes that social support mediates the negative effects of stress, thereby reducing susceptibility to stress-related disease. If certain types of stressors predispose to mental health outcomes, then social support can influence mental health (Cohen & Syme, 1985).

There may be commonalities across ethnic groups regarding the function of social support systems; however, differences in the type, structure, quality, and availability of social supports cannot be overemphasized (Kobata, Lockery, & Moriwaki, 1980). Kobata and colleagues indicated that the family, church, and community have been primary focal points of support for ethnic minority groups. The family represents a primary support group taking responsibility for the physical, emotional, psychological, economic, and social welfare of its members. The role of the family and extended family continues to be of primary importance in transmitting cultural values, beliefs, customs, and practices. Examples of the family support system are the important emphasis placed on filial piety among Asians; the idealized role given to the extended family among Mexican-Americans, in which relatives play an important role; the extended or augmented families in black communities that provide support; and the kinship systems that continue to function among Native Americans. These examples also represent ways in which ethnic identity is maintained through the operation of the family support system. The church, as well as community organizations, serves as reinforcement to group identity through shared values, beliefs, and activities.

C. Coping and Adaptation

The process of coping results from variable patterns of behavior that promote differential adaptation (Moos, 1979). Coping may be represented as specific behaviors, such as affect regulation or emotional outburst. Coping may be the specific act of soliciting more instrumental aid and assistance to assist with adaptation. Adaptation, the sum result of the psychosocial stress process, results in different types of outcomes, which may be positive, negative, or moderately effective. Poor adaptation may result in higher morbidity, while successful adaptation may promote an inoculation effect.

The process of acculturation may show different patterns of immigrant cultural adaptation related to health outcomes. Immigrant families from Southeast Asia must deal with more egalitarian roles for men and women, and between older and younger generations. The traditional authority of the elders may be diminished as younger wage earners provide financial security for the family. This may create family discord and result in higher rate of mental disorder (Yee, 1990).

V. Prevalence of Mental Health Disorders _____

Two specific types of mental health research have been conducted regarding ethnic minority populations: (1) clinic or institution-based research, and (2) community or epidemiological surveys. Results from clinic–institution-based research may provide evidence of certain behavioral, demographic, or cultural patterns that are indicative of mental health status; however, the primary weakness in such studies is the self-selection of the patient to the institutional setting. Do the rates of mental impairment truly represent community rates? The second line of inquiry is the community or epidemiological surveys to ascertain representative rates of mental disorder. Community studies may also not report accurate prevalence rates if appropriate sampling designs are not used. The epidemiological catchment area (ECA) studies have been conducted in five primary sites in the United States (Baltimore, New Haven, Piedmont in North Carolina, St. Louis, and Los Angeles). With regard to the aged and minority groups, the surveys were conducted in settings where there was ethnic and socioeconomic diversity. Appropriate sampling frames were implemented to obtain a representative sample of subjects from each ECA site. Assessment of mental health status represented a significant component to the ECA studies and the first attempt to determine prevalence rates of cognitive impairment in older age groups.

A. African-American Elderly

Racism has been called the number one mental health problem among African-Americans by the American Psychiatric Association (Butler & Lewis, 1973). Race alone has confounded acceptance of African-Americans in society and has damaged self-dignity and respect. Age compounds the handicaps already experienced by many. A comparative study of psychological distress among older blacks and whites (Ulbrich & Warheit, 1989) showed that blacks scored significantly higher in distress with the death of a relative or friend, financial concerns, and activities of daily living. These distress scores were mitigated by significantly higher rates of social support utilization and social network interaction with relatives and friends than in the white cohort. There were no rates established for black females.

The National Health and Nutritional Examination Surveys (NHANES) indicated that the adjusted prevalence of depression in the black population was 23% (Eaton & Kessler, 1981). The Center for Epidemiological Studies in Depression (CES-D) Scale has been used to make nonclinical diagnoses of possible and probable depression, using cutpoints of 16 or greater. In comparative studies between blacks and whites and after controlling for the effects of income, there were no significant differences in depression scores between the two groups (Comstock & Helsing, 1976). In a related study examining the tails of the distribution of CES-D scores, results showed that a higher proportion of blacks were more severely depressed than whites, even after controlling for demographic and economic effects (Eaton & Kessler, 1981). Although these results are somewhat equivocal, the evidence suggests that after controlling for economic effects, blacks are no more likely to experience depression than are whites. In a recent community study of depression among black elderly, the rate of depression was 15.6%, comparable to rates established in other community studies of African Americans (Du Bois *et al.*, 1991). Depression rates of older individuals were highest among those having poor financial resources, reduced social network contact, and inadequate caregiver support. Although black females had higher rates of depression than did males, gender differences were not so important for mental health outcomes as social support resources.

The ECA studies evaluated levels of cognitive impairment in cross-cultural samples from East Baltimore and St. Louis (Fillenbaum, Hughes, Heyman, George, & Blazer, 1988). Using the Mini-Mental State Examination (MMSE), which consists of 35 scorable items and comparing black and white MMSE scores, preliminary evaluations showed that 56% of black subjects age 60 and older showed mild to severe impairment, while 24% of white subjects showed impairment. Although being female was associated with higher rates of cognitive impairment, the differences were of little statistical importance. Further analyses showed that performance on the MMSE was sensitive to education, age, race, and ability to perform instrumental activities of daily living. Thus, results strongly suggested that adjustments for education, age, and race should be considered to assess the prevalence of cognitive impairment in cross-cultural settings.

Anxiety disorders are among the most common of psychiatric impairments in the general population. Results from the ECA studies in Baltimore and St. Louis (Brown, Eaton, & Sussman, 1990; Eaton, Regier, Locke, & Taupe, 1981) showed a significantly higher prevalence of phobic disorder in black females than in males or any other population cohort. Upon reaching the age of 65, phobic disorders declined significantly. Highest rates occurred among females between the ages of 45 and 64, those previously married, those with fewer than eight years of education, and with low occupational prestige.

Comparisons of life satisfaction between whites and blacks have shown that blacks have significantly higher levels of general life satisfaction after age 65 in addition to greater happiness, although the latter was a nonsignificant trend (Ortega, Crutchfield, & Rushing, 1983). The relatively high participation in black churches by the elderly is considered the primary reason for these life-satisfaction differentials. In a related study (Ward & Kilburn, 1983), good health, children, and higher education accounted for a significant amount of variance in life satisfaction among black elderly. There were no gender differences in life satisfaction in either study.

B. Hispanic Elderly

Although data on the mental health status of Hispanics are not extensive (Jones, Grey, & Parson, 1983), the ECA data from Los Angeles have provided the most complete epidemiological profile of psychiatric impairment to date. Among Hispanic women older than 40, the six-month prevalence rates of the most common disorders are phobia (13.4/100 or 13.4 cases per 100 people, adjusted for age and sex), major depression (4.4/100), cognitive impairment (3/100), panic disorder (3/100), alcohol abuse–dependence (2/100), and obsessive-compulsive disorder (1/100) (Burnam et al., 1987). Prevalence rates for Hispanic men over age 40 indicate that alcohol abuse–dependence is the predominant psychiatric disorder (6.2/100), followed by phobia (3/100), cognitive impairment (2/100), major depression (1.2/100), and drug abuse–dependence (.5/100). Examining significant differences between Hispanic and non-Hispanic white women of comparable age, more Hispanic women suffer from major depression, abuse alcohol, suffer phobic and panic disorders, and show higher levels of cognitive impairment. The particularly high rate of phobia may be due to greater levels of social and economic stress. In contrast to white males older than 40, Hispanic males have higher rates of alcohol abuse, phobia, and cognitive impairment. Rates of cognitive impairment for males and females should be used with caution. The MMSE used by the ECA studies has come under increasing scrutiny owing to the culture bias of the instrument (Bird, Canino, Stipec, & Shrout, 1987). Having low or no education may produce false-positives.

The Los Angeles ECA study (Karno *et al.*, 1987) determined lifetime prevalence rates expressed as percentages, which showed that the predominant impairments for Hispanic females older than 40 were the affective disorders of dysthymia (9.4%) and major depressive episodes (6.5%), and the anxiety–somatoform disorders of phobia (20.7%) and panic disorder (3.4%). Lifetime prevalence rates for males older than 40 were highest for alcohol abuse (28.5%), followed by phobia (7.2%), major depressive disorder (3.4%), and dysthymia (3.1%).

An epidemiological study of health status and health care needs of elderly Hispanics was conducted in Los Angeles (Lopez-Aqueres, Kemp, Plopper, Staples, & Brummel-Smith, 1984). Employing the use of the Comprehensive Assessment and Referral evaluation (CARE), the study determined that 14% of older subjects were affected by cognitive impairment, 31% by depression–demoralization, 28% by financial hardship, 17% by problems with ambulation, and 25% by activity limitation. Nineteen percent needed assistance or used social services (22%). In comparison to men, women composed the largest group of those affected by cognitive impairment (17 versus 10%), depression (37 versus 22%), problems with ambulation (22 versus 11%), activity limitations (27 versus 22%), and need for assistance (24 versus 13%). A related study of dysphoria and depression from the Hispanic CARE project showed that 27% were found to have depression or dysphoria, 5% were rated dysphoric, 1% had major depressive disorder, 4% were dysphoric with dementia, 3% had major depression with dementia, 8% were dysphoric with medical disability, and 7% had major depression with disability (Kemp, Staples, & Lopez-Aqueres, 1987). For all depressed subjects, 71% were elderly females, and 29% were males. The largest proportion of depressed elderly were in the 60–64 age cohort (35%). Significantly, the highest number of depressed individuals spoke no English (70%) or were widowed (45%). Depression was also related to fewer than 5 years of education (66%) and yearly income below $6,000 (69%). A community study of depression among Mexican-American adults 45 and older in San Diego, reported depression rates of 26% (Morton, Schoenrock, Stanford, Peddecord, & Molgaard, 1989). Hispanic women had significantly higher rates of depression than did men.

Hispanic mental health data support the notion that problems due to acculturation and poor socioeconomic status account for a significant proportion of the most common psychiatric impairments (Burnam *et al.*, 1987; Golding & Burnam, 1990). Hispanic elderly at greatest risk for mental impairments tend to suffer from higher levels of social and economic deprivation than those less at risk (Cooper, Kendell, & Gurland, 1972). In one study of native-born versus immigrant Mexican-Americans, native-born Mexican-Americans who are highly acculturated to American cultural values and behaviors exhibit significantly higher levels of impairment than those who are Mexican-American immigrants and less acculturated by virtue of their immigrant status (Burnam *et al.*, 1987). Disparity between cultural beliefs and practice appears to be a significant risk factor for acculturation stress.

Accumulating evidence on the protective effects of the Hispanic family and kin network support the hypothesis that social support resources tend to mitigate the more negative effects of acculturation or socioeconomic stress (Kall, 1989). Further evidence of the role of the family–kin support system in relation to the health of the elderly is provided by community health care utilization data (Hough *et al.*, 1987; Wells, Hough, Golding, Burnam & Karno, 1987). Hispanic elderly underutilize health and mental health care services even though they may be less ambulatory and exhibit higher levels of impairment than their white counterparts. In those situations in which these individuals receive higher levels of informal support, their need for community care options tends to lesson (Greene & Monahan, 1984).

Although researchers have suggested that Mexican-Americans have at least as many episodes of mental illness as whites (Roberts, 1980; Markides, 1980; Vega, Warheit, Buhl-Auth, & Meinhardt, 1984), the rates of underutilization of mental health care services do not support this proposition. Barriers to mental health care utilization that impede access have been the absence of bilingual, bicultural services. Such culturally appropriate services go far toward making mental health care services more available to Hispanic patients (Reeves, 1986).

C. American Indian Elderly

Elderly American Indians come from a diversity of backgrounds within the American Indian community, yet all share a similar experience that would appear to strongly predispose them to mental disorders. The emotional impact of the disruption of the American Indian way of life is difficult to quantify, although speculation is that the psychological effect on the American Indian elder has been significant.

The disruption of their cultural value systems when Europeans arrived led to tremendous conflict, personal disorganization, and an increase in mental, emotional, and social problems (Markides, 1986). The leading mental health problem of Native Americans is alcoholism. Few efforts have been directed toward exploring personality disorders and the mental health status of American Indians, much less examining the rates among the older age groups by gender and age differences. A study of Indian Health Service utilization data (Rhoades, Marshall, Attneave, Bjork, & Baiser, 1980) showed that visits for all mental disorders was lowest among those 65 and older, while the diagnosis of organic brain syndrome was highest among this cohort. There was a sharp reduction in service utilization among those suffering from depression, anxiety, and alcoholism. The higher mortality rate of alcoholics would suppress health care utilization rates.

In terms of the stress of acculturation, those who maintain tribal identity have fewer problems in general. This same pattern would likely be present with mental health disorders. There is significant agreement that the elder American Indian may be the most significantly deprived individual in the country, but there is a paucity of information regarding how this deprivation translates into mental disorders. A study of mental health scores and life satisfaction among the elderly was conducted among five ethnic groups (blacks, Hispanics, Jews, Indians, and whites) (Johnson *et al.*, 1988). Using the Older American Resources Survey (OARS) multidimensional functional assessment questionnaire and the Life Satisfaction Index-Z Scale (LSI-Z), results showed that American

Indians had median mental health scores comparable to whites and blacks, better scores than Hispanics, but worse scores than Jewish subjects. Although they scored in the lower ranks of life satisfaction along with Hispanics and Jews and lower than whites and blacks, median life satisfaction scores for older American Indians showed scores well above the median cutpoint of the scale. The results of both analyses are somewhat equivocal, however, because the effects for income were not controlled. In a related study of mental health and life satisfaction among elderly Indians (Johnson *et al.*, 1986), results showed a relatively high level of life satisfaction (64%) among American Indians. There is a positive association between life satisfaction and mental health in older American Indians.

D. Asian–Pacific Island Elderly

Preliminary results from the Los Angeles ECA study reported prevalence rates for mental health status for Japanese, Filipino, and Chinese-American elderly (Yamamoto *et al.*, 1985). The Diagnostic Interview Schedules II and III and the Folstein MMSE were used. Lifetime prevalence data indicated that 28–36% of Japanese elderly had symptoms indicative of organic brain syndrome; 60%, somatization disorder; 27–39% dysthymic disorder; 1–5% manic disorder episodes; 3–16% depressive disorder; 2–10% schizophrenic disorder; 9% panic disorder; 36% antisocial personality; 9% anorexia nervosa; and 1% alcohol abuse–dependence. Females had higher prevalence rates than males for dysthymic disorder, somatization disorder, and schizophrenic disorder, while males had higher prevalence of antisocial personality disorder and alcohol abuse–dependence. Organic brain syndrome showed generally comparable rates between males and females. Preliminary data were reported on a small sample of elderly Filipinos and indicated that 13% had symptoms for psychosexual dysfunction and 9%, major depressive disorder. Alcohol abuse, obsessive-compulsive disorder, agoraphobia, somatization disorder, and pathological gambling had low prevalence (2%). Data on Chinese elderly indicated that psychosexual dysfunction and organic brain syndrome were the predominant mental health disorders (50% and 45%), followed by tobacco dependence, alcohol abuse–dependence, and agoraphobia (5%). Results by gender were not reported for either group.

Depressive scores were reported for Chinese, Korean, Japanese, and Filipino elderly in Seattle (Kuo, 1984). Using the CES-D scale, mean rates showed that Asian-Americans across all age groups score as high as whites. Unique ethnic differences in acculturation stress showed that Koreans, the most recent migrants, had higher overall depression scores than any other Asian group. For all Asian groups, marriage, higher income, being age 60 or older, and being male were related to lower depression scores in general. Women across all Asian–Pacific Island groups tend to be at greater risk for depression, especially Filipino and Korean women; however, these risks are mitigated somewhat by reaching the age of 60, when the beneficial effects of elder status are attained (Kuo, 1984). Korean women, however, remain the exception. Asian-Americans tend to rely on natural support groups in their communities and may not avail themselves of public mental health services (Kitano, 1982; Yip, 1990); thus, underutilization of the mental health system is not attributable to a lower rate of mental disorder, which these data support.

Although mental health information on Asian–Pacific Island elderly is scarce, available data indicate that the majority suffer from problems that are largely so-cioeconomic in nature, thus supporting the acculturation stress hypothesis. The effects of lower income, limited access to transportation, medical care, housing, and employment all affect the well-being of these elderly (Lee, 1987). With the additional problems of minority status, discrimination, cultural dissimilarity, and linguistic barriers, these elderly remain an at-risk group.

Asian-American elders are not unlike other ethnic minority elders. The elderly, in general, are expected to show greater levels of mental disorder. The stress of accultura-tion, lower socioeconomic status, and fewer social resources are presumed to predispose Asian–Pacific Island elderly to higher rates of mental disorder (Kessler & Cleary, 1980). However, demographic data provide evidence among these elderly of differential patterns of adaptation and coping that are a function of length of residency in the United States, historical events that lead up to migration, and degree of familiarity with the larger culture. In point of fact, recent Southeast Asian refugees show significantly higher rates of psychiatric and social impairments from war trauma than those migrants who arrived earlier. These impairments severely affect their ability to adjust to their new homeland (Mollica, Wyshak, & Lavelle, 1987). The Hmong are a particularly at-risk group, having very limited exposure to modern lifestyles in Asia, and thus were less prepared for the migration experience than were their Cambodian, Vietnamese, or Lao counterparts (West-ermeyer, 1988; Westermeyer, Vang, & Neider, 1983).

Historical antecedents may account for the differences in the ways the elderly adapt to life in the United States. The discriminatory treatment of Chinese immigrants in the 19th century accounts for a higher proportion of males to females today (Butler & Lewis, 1973). Chinese male immigrants were prohibited from bringing wives from China or intermarrying. This produced an imbalance in the sex ratio, which is still in evidence among older Chinese Americans. A similar sex-ratio difference exists among aged Filipi-no males, although the historical circumstances are somewhat different. The ratio of males to females among the Japanese-American community is more equitable, because family members were allowed to accompany them during early migration periods.

VI. Approaches to Community Mental Health

The continuum of mental health model, proposed by Goldsmith (1984), is a community-based approach for the delivery of mental health services to the population. The approach emphasizes coordination of mental health services in the community and linkage of clients with appropriate services. The continuum of mental health model includes a range of care options from long-term institutional care to community-based services for those with chronic disabilities, intensive and accessible services to the mentally impaired, and tar-geted prevention services to those at high risk for mental illness.

Ethnic minority elders need community-based resources in order to successfully adjust to increasing physical deterioration. The minority elderly run the risk of becoming iso-lated within their own communities. They commonly do not venture outside their commu-nities for health or mental health treatment; thus, the community mental health framework is the most appropriate model for individuals from diverse ethnic backgrounds.

A. Cultural Sensitivity and the Mental Health Care System

A low priority is given to minority patients entering the mental health care system (Kobata, Lockery, & Moriwaki, 1980). There is even less emphasis placed upon the cultural context of mental health problems of the minority elder patient. There is little known regarding culturally acceptable parameters for defining mental health, psychological adjustment, self-esteem, or happiness for minority elderly. Cultural norms for acceptable behavior by ethnic group are not incorporated into the diagnostic or treatment regimens used in the mental health system (Kobata *et al.*, 1980). To provide optimal service, mental health professionals should be acquainted with the ethnic backgrounds of patients and trained to be culturally sensitive. This is all the more important for future mental health planning because a significant proportion of patients will be represented by ethnic minorities. In addition, adequate cross-cultural data bases need to be compiled for research and the design of feasible community mental health programs.

A major deterrent to effective treatment of individuals from different cultures is the lack of understanding on the part of the mental health care professional regarding the appropriate point of intervention in the patient's life. Treating the *family* as the patient rather than the symptomatic *individual* is commonly practiced in less industrialized countries (Kleinman, 1980). This practice results in the patient's remaining a part of the family system and promotes a wider social reinforcement for recovery. Because the family shares the burden of the diagnosis, there is less stigma attached to the patient from the labeling of the disorder. The family also knows that ill health is a transitory condition in most cases; thus, everyone including the patient has an expectation of recovery. Including family members in the treatment regimen of the patient enhances opportunities for compliance and recovery.

B. Eliminating Barriers to the Mental Health System

The utilization of mental health services by minority elderly is affected by language barriers, limited access to information regarding available services, transportation, cultural dissimilarity, and reduced social and economic resources. The impact of mental illness on refugee families appears to be significantly more severe, owing to these barriers. Support is often minimal, especially with groups such as the Lao and Cambodians (Yip, 1990). Many of these individuals do not understand the need for services or the necessity to comply with a treatment regimen.

Much of the current literature in gerontology has focused on what has been called successful aging, adaptation to aging, or positive adjustment to aging (Markides, 1986). Too little emphasis has been placed on the prevention of mental health problems as individuals approach older age. There is currently little information on the relationships between stressors and the development of stress-related disease and mental disorders among minority populations (Cuellar & Roberts, 1984).

Awareness of mental health status and prevention are not the sole responsibility of the patient. An institutional responsibility is also required for effective treatment. Williams (1980) suggested that multiple strategies be implemented to ensure that the customs, attitudes, and expectations of ethnic minorities are integrated into mental health planning programs. Individuals who are both bilingual and bicultural should be involved in identifying these gaps in service delivery to the communities.

VII. Recommendations for the Future

The data on gender, ethnicity, and aging attest to the fact that greater emphasis should be assigned to ethnic minority women by academicians, researchers, policy makers, and planners for the mental health care system. The special circumstances surrounding the mental health status of ethnic minority elderly women should receive higher priority for future research (Bastida, 1990). For the 1990s, research on gender and ethnic issues should be directed toward closing loopholes left by a decade or more of exploratory investigations.

Clinicians and mental health professionals should bring their knowledge to bear upon ways in which gender and ethnic minority issues will continue to be addressed. Currently, there is enough bicultural experience to begin formally organizing information toward the treatment and prevention of specific mental health problems of ethnic minorities in general, and minority women in particular (Kalish & Moriwaki, 1973).

VIII. Summary

An emerging pattern among ethnic minority populations has shown that the mental impairments associated with aging are amplified by problems related to ethnicity and gender. The effects of poor socioeconomic status produce an increased susceptibility to mental disorders in an already vulnerable group of people. To assist research in aging and efforts toward program development, studies must incorporate greater specification of age, sex, and ethnic cohorts as they relate to the mental health status of the elderly.

Future demographic trends are currently projected for the minority elderly. Ethnic minority elderly will represent a rapidly increasing segment of the total elderly population. Additionally, more women than men across all ethnic groups will live to older age.

When comparing and contrasting mental impairments of African-American, Hispanic, American Indian, and Asian–Pacific Island elderly, the overriding impact of poor social and economic resources is substantial on the mental health status of both males and females; however, females tend to have higher rates of impairment in the areas of affective disorders and anxiety–somatoform disorders, while males tend to have higher rates of substance abuse–dependence.

Approaches to community mental health highlight the importance of cultural sensitivity and cross-cultural training of mental health professionals, attempts to eliminate the barriers to greater utilization of the mental health care system by ethnic minority elderly, and developing institutional arrangements to enhance services to elderly minority females.

References

Bastida, E. (1990). *Older Hispanics: A state-of-the-art review*. Bethesda, MD: National Institute on Aging.

Bird, H. R., Canino, G., Stipec, M. R., & Shrout, P. (1987). Use of mini-mental state examination in a probability sample of a Hispanic population. *The Journal of Nervous and Mental Disease, 175*, 731–737.

Birren, J. E., & Renner, V. J. (1977). Research on the psychology of aging: Principles and experimentation. In J. Birren & K. W. Schaie (Eds.), *Handbook of the psychology of aging* (pp. 3–38). New York: Van Nostrand Reinhold.

Brown, D. R., Eaton, W. W., & Sussman, L. (1990). Racial differences in prevalence of phobic disorders. *The Journal of Nervous and Mental Disease, 178*, 434–441.

Burnam, M. A., Hough, R. L., Escobar, J. I., Karno, M., Timbers, D. M., Telles, C. A., & Locke, B. Z. (1987). Six-month prevalence of specific psychiatric disorders among Mexican Americans and non-Hispanic whites in Los Angeles. *Archives of General Psychiatry, 44*, 687–694.

Burnam, M. A., Hough, R. L., Karno, M., Escobar, J. I., & Telles, C. A. (1987). Acculturation and lifetime prevalence of psychiatric disorders among Mexican Americans in Los Angeles. *Journal of Health and Social Behavior, 28*, 89–102.

Butler, R. N., & Lewis, M. I. (1973). *Aging and mental health positive psychosocial approaches* (2nd ed.). St. Louis, MO: C. V. Mosby.

Cohen, S., & Syme, S. (1985). *Social support and health*. San Diego, CA: Academic Press.

Comstock, G. W., & Helsing, K. J. (1976). Symptoms of depression in two communities. *Psychological Medicine, 6*, 551–563.

Cool, L. (1986). Ethnicity: Its significance and measurement. In C. L. Fry and J. Keith (Eds.), *Methods for old age* (pp. 263–280). South Hadley, MA: Bergin and Garvey.

Cooper, J. E., Kendell, R. E., & Gurland, B. J. (1972). *Psychiatric diagnosis in New York and London: A comparative study of mental hospital admissions*. London: Oxford University Press.

Cuellar, I. & Roberts, R. (1984). Psychological disorders among Chicanos. In J. L. Martinez and R. Mendoza (Eds.), *Chicano psychology* (2nd ed., pp. 133–161). New York: Academic Press.

Dohrenwend, B. P., & Dohrenwend, B. S. (1969). *Social status and psychological disorders*. New York: Wiley.

Dowd, J., & Bengtson, V. L. (1978). Aging in minority populations: An examination of the double jeopardy hypothesis. *Journal of Gerontology, 33*, 427–436.

Du Bois, B. C., Stanford, E. P., Goodman, J. D., Morton, D. J., Happersett, C., & Molgaard, C. (1991). Depression, social support, and socioeconomic resources among older African Americans. *Journal of Aging and Health* (submitted).

Eaton, W. W., & Kessler, L. G. (1981). Rates of symptoms of depression in a national sample. *American Journal of Epidemiology, 114*, 528–538.

Eaton, W. W., Regier, D. A., Locke, B. Z., & Taube, C. A. (1981). The epidemiological catchment area program of the National Institute of Mental Health. *Public Health Report, 96*, 319–325.

Fillenbaum, G. G., Hughes, D. C., Heyman, A., George, L. K., & Blazer, D. G. (1988). Relationship of health and demographic characteristics to mini-mental state examination score among community residents. *Psychological Medicine, 18*, 719–726.

Gelfand, D. E. (1979–1980). Ethnicity, aging, and mental health. *International Journal of Aging and Human Development, 10*, 289–298.

Golding, J. M., & Burnam, M. A. (1990). Immigration, stress, and depressive symptoms in a Mexican-American community. *The Journal of Nervous and Mental Disease, 178*, 161–171.

Goldsmith, J. M. (1984). *Final report of the governor's select commission on the future of the state–local mental health system*. Albany, NY: New York State Office of Mental Health.

Gordon, M. M. (1978). *Human nature, class, and ethnicity*. New York: Oxford University Press.

Gove, W. (1973). Sex, marital status, and mortality. *American Journal of Sociology, 79*, 45–46.

Greeley, A. (1974). *Ethnicity in the United States*. New York: Wiley and Sons.

Greene, V. L., & Monahan, D. J. (1984). Comparative utilization of community-based long-term care services by Hispanic and Anglo elderly in a case management system. *Journal of Gerontology, 39*, 730–735.

Hough, R. L., Landsverk, J. A., Karno, M., Burnam, A., Timbers, D., Escobar, J. I., & Regier, D. A. (1987). Utilization of health and mental health services by Los Angeles Mexican Americans and non-Hispanic whites. *Archives of General Psychiatry, 44*, 702–709.

Johnson, F. L., Foxall, M. J., Kelleher, E., Kentopp, E., Mannlein, E. A., & Cook, E. (1988). Comparison of mental health life satisfaction of five elderly ethnic groups. *Western Journal of Nursing, 10,* 613–628.

Johnson, F. L., Foxall, M. J., Kelleher, E., Kentopp, E., Mannlein, E. A., & Cook, E. (1986). Life satisfaction of the elderly American Indian. *International Journal of Nursing Studies, 23,* 265–273.

Jones, B. E., Grey, B. A., & Parson, E. B. (1983). Manic-depressive illness among poor urban Hispanics. *American Journal of Psychiatry, 140,* 1208–1210.

Kall, B. L. (1989). Drugs, gender, and ethnicity: Is the older minority woman at risk? *The Journal of Drug Issues, 19,* 171–189.

Kalish, R. A., & Moriwaki, S. (1973). The world of the elderly Asian American. *Journal of Social Issues, 29,* 187–209.

Karno, M., Hough, R. L., Burnam, M. A., Escobar, J. I., Timbers, D. M., Santana, F., & Boyd, J. H. (1987). Lifetime prevalence of specific psychiatric disorders among Mexican Americans and non-Hispanic Whites in Los Angeles. *Archives of General Psychiatry, 44,* 695–701.

Kemp, B. J., Staples, F., & Lopez-Aqueres, W. (1987). Epidemiology of depression and dysphoria in an elderly Hispanic population. *Journal of American Geriatric Society, 35,* 920–926.

Kessler, R. C. (1979). Stress, social status, and psychological distress. *Journal of Health and Social Behavior, 20,* 100–108.

Kessler, R. C., & Cleary, P. D. (1980). Social class and psychological distress. *American Sociological Review, 45,* 463–478.

Kitano, H. H. (1982). Mental health in the Japanese-American community. In E. E. Jones and S. J. Korchin (Eds.), *Minority mental health* (pp. 149–164). New York: Praeger.

Kleinman, A. (1980). *Patients and healers in the context of culture: An exploration of the borderland between anthropology, medicine, and psychiatry.* Los Angeles: University of California Press.

Kobata, F. S., Lockery, S. A., & Moriwaki, S. Y. (1980). Minority issues in mental health and aging. In J. E. Birren and R. B. Sloan (Eds.), *Handbook of mental health and aging* (pp. 448–466). New York: Prentice-Hall.

Kuo, W. H. (1984). Prevalence of depression among Asian Americans. *The Journal of Nervous and Mental Disease, 172,* 449–457.

Lee, J. (1987). Asian American elderly: A neglected minority group. *Journal of Gerontological Social Work, 9,* 103–116.

Lin, N. (1986). Conceptualizing social support. In N. Lin, A. Dean & W. Ensel (Eds.), *Social Support, Life Events, and Depression* (pp. 17–30). San Diego: Academic Press.

Lopez-Aqueres, W., Kemp, B., Plopper, M., Staples, F., & Brummel-Smith, K. (1984). Health needs of the Hispanic elderly. *Journal of the American Geriatrics Society, 32,* 191–198.

Markides, K. S. (1980). Correlates of life satisfaction among older Mexican Americans and Anglos. *Journal of Minority Aging, 5,* 183–190.

Markides, K. S. (1982). Ethnicity and aging: A comment. *The Gerontologist, 22,* 467–470.

Markides, K. S. (1986). Minority status: Aging and mental health. *International Journal of Aging and Human Development, 23,* 285–300.

Markides, K. S., & Mindel, C. H. (1987). *Aging and Ethnicity.* Volume 163, Sage Library of Social Research, Newbury Park, California.

Markson, E. W. (Ed.). (1983). *Older women: Issues and prospects.* Lexington, MA: Lexington Books.

Martin-Matthews, A. (1987). Widowhood as an expectable life event. In V. W. Marshall (Ed.), *Aging in Canada: Social perspectives* (2nd ed, pp. 343–366). Markham, Ontario, Canada: Fitzhenry & Whiteside.

Mollica, R. F., Wyshak, G., & Lavelle, J. (1987). The psychosocial impact of war trauma and torture on Southeast Asian refugees. *American Journal of Psychiatry, 144,* 1567–1572.

Moos, R. (1979). Social-ecological perspectives on health. In G. C. Stone, F. Cohen, & N. Adler (Eds.), *Health psychology handbook.* San Francisco: Jossey-Bass.

Morton, D. J., Schoenrock, S. A., Stanford, E. P., Peddecord, K. M., & Molgaard, C. A. (1989). Use of the CES-D among a community sample of older Mexican-Americans. *Journal of Cross Cultural Gerontology, 4,* 289–306.

Myerhoff, B. (1978). *Number Our Days.* New York: Dutton.

Ortega, S. T., Crutchfield, R. D., & Rushing, W. A. (1983). Race differences in elderly personal well-being. *Research on Aging, 5,* 101–118.

Pelham, A. O., & Clark, W. F. (1987). Widowhood among low-income racial and ethnic groups in California. In H. Lopata (Ed.), *Widows in North America* (pp. 191–222). Durham, NC: Duke University Press.

Reeves, K. (1986). Hispanic utilization of an ethnic mental health clinic. *Journal of Psychosocial Nursing, 24,* 23–26.

Rhoades, E., Marshall, M., Attneave, C., Bjork, J., & Beiser, M. (1980). Impact of mental disorders upon elderly American Indians as reflected in visits to ambulatory care facilities. *Journal of the American Geriatrics Society, 28,* 33–39.

Roberts, R. E. (1980). Prevalence of psychological distress among Mexican-Americans. *Journal of Health and Social Behavior, 25,* 134–145.

Sokolovsky, J. (1985). Ethnicity, culture and aging: Do differences really make a difference? *The Journal of Applied Gerontology, 4,* 6–17.

Strain, L. A., & Chappell, N. L. (1982). Confidants: Do they make a difference in quality of life? *Research on Aging, 4,* 479–502.

Taeuber, C. (1990). Diversity: The dramatic reality. In S. A. Bass, E. A. Kutza, & F. M. Torres-Gil (Eds.), *Diversity in aging* (pp. 1–45). Glenview, IL: Scott, Foresman.

Uhlenberg, P. (1977). Changing structure of the older population of the USA during the twentieth century. *The Gerontologist, 17,* 197–202.

Ulbrich, R. M., & Warheit, G. J. (1989). Social support, stress, and psychological distress among older black and white adults. *Journal of Aging and Health, 1,* 286–305.

U.S. Bureau of the Census (1986). Projections of the Hispanic population: 1983 to 2080. G. Spencer, *Current population reports* (Series P-25, No. 995). Washington, DC: U.S. Government Printing Office.

U.S. Bureau of the Census (1980). *General social and economic characteristics* PC80-1-C1, U.S. Summary, Washington, DC: Government Printing Office, December 1983, Table 120.

U.S. Bureau of Commerce (1990). *Statistical abstracts of the U.S.,* 16.

U.S. Department of Health and Human Services, Health Resources and Services Administration (1985). *Health status of minorities and low income groups.* Washington, DC: U.S. Government Printing Office.

Valle, R. (1988–1989). Outreach to ethnic minorities with Alzheimer's disease: The challenge to the community. *Health Matrix, 6,* p. 14.

Vega, W., Warheit, G., Buhl-Auth, J., & Meinhardt, K. (1984). The prevalence of depressive symptoms among Mexican Americans and Anglos. *American Journal of Epidemiology, 120,* 592–607.

Ward, R. A., & Kilburn, H. (1983). Community access and satisfaction: Racial differences in later life. *International Journal of Aging and Human Development, 16,* 209–219.

Wells, K. B., Hough, R. L., Golding, J. M., Burnam, M. A., & Karno, M. (1987). Which Mexican-Americans underutilize health services? *American Journal of Psychiatry, 144,* 918–922.

Westermeyer, J. (1988). DSM-III psychiatric disorders among Hmong refugees in the United States: A point prevalence study. *American Journal of Psychiatry, 145,* 197–202.

Westermeyer, J., Vang, T. F., & Neider, J. (1983). Migration and mental health among Hmong refugees. *The Journal of Nervous and Mental Disease, 171,* 92–96.

Williams, D. A. (1980). Considerations for comprehensive health planning for elderly minority populations. In E. P. Stanford (Ed.), *Minority aging: Policy issues for the 80s.* San Diego, CA: University Center on Aging, College of Health and Human Services, San Diego State University.

Wirth, L. (1945). The problems of minority groups. In R. Linton (Ed.), *The science of man in the world crisis.* New York: Columbia University Press.

Yamamoto, J., Machizawa, S., Araki, F., Reece, S., Steinberg, A., Leung, J., & Cater, R. (1985). Mental health of elderly Asian Americans in Los Angeles. *The American Journal of Social Psychiatry, 1,* 37–46.

Yee, B. W. K. (1990). Gender and family issues in minority groups. *Generations, 14,* (3), 39–42.

Yip, B. (1990). Impact of mental illness on support networks from a community based, multi-service organization perspective: The union of Pan Asian communities. In E. P. Stanford, S. A. Lockery, & S. A. Schoenrock (Eds.), *Ethnicity and aging: Mental health issues* (pp. 33–39). San Diego, CA: University Center on Aging, College of Health and Human Services, San Diego State University.

5

Adult Life Crises

Morton A. Lieberman and Harvey Peskin

   I. Defining Adult Life Crises
  II. A First Look: Salience of Life Events on Mental Health Consequences
 III. Adult Life Crises and Psychiatric Disorders
     A. Methodological Considerations
     B. Stress and Anxiety Disorders
     C. Stress and Schizophrenia
     D. Depressive Illnesses
  IV. Life Crises and Adaptation
     A. Spousal Loss
   V. Adult Crises as Transformative
  VI. Dynamic Theories of Adult Crises: A Child-Centered versus Adult-Centered View
     A. Self-Discovery as the Province of the Later Adult Crisis
     B. The Gender Crisis at Midlife
     C. Relational Investment as a Consequence of Adult Crises
 VII. A Cautionary Note
VIII. Clinical Aspects of Crisis
  IX. A Summing up
     References

The chapter's goals are to examine the empirical and conceptual work that addresses the central question of the effects of adult life crises on the level of mental health functioning of adults. The area does not represent a coherent intellectual discipline but rather is a theme constructed from a vast and diverse aggregate of empirical studies and conceptual perspectives that threads through a host of academic disciplines: epidemiology, sociology and psychology, psychiatry, psychoanalysis, and adult development.

    Our chapter addresses the central question from several interrelated approaches. We start with the issue of defining adult life crises, and then move to comparing various types or categories of crises. Are some more salient in their impact on mental health? The main body of the chapter is organized around an examination of the consequences for adults of life crises looked at from three perspectives commonly used to index consequences— the development of psychopathology, adaptive outcomes and perspectives on transformation or change. We end our chapter with an examination of the field for clinical practice.

I. Defining Adult Life Crises

How do we determine what external life events or inner manifestations are appropriately designated adult life crises? By definition, life crises are normatively defined by each society. Crises otherwise ignored by society are relegated to, and become the province of, certain institutions that deal with the marginal, the ill, and the disabled. Thus psychiatry and its allied professions have become the repository for those individuals whose disrupted emotional lives receive no other succorance or aid. One approach, then, for defining the current arena of adult life crises is to examine the array of institutions that society has made available to ameliorate the psychological consequences of life stresses. If, for example, psychiatry has historically functioned to contain the most ill people, community-based psychological resources, such as self-help groups and adult education have become newly available to minimize or master such consequences, by supporting adults who are confronting issues beyond the individual's capacity to solve. A catalog of self-help groups (Gartner & Riessman, 1977; Lieberman & Borman, 1979) might provide a ready picture of what contemporary American culture recognizes as adult life crises. This definition of adult crises based on community response has changed historically and of course does not produce a fixed and eternal list.

The usual academic definition of adult life crises involves discrete changes in life events that are consensually recognized as entailing some degree of distress, challenge, and/or hazard by the individual and members of his or her social group. The common-sense meaning is contained in the list of major life events, both normative (marriage, birth of a child, retirement) and those nonscheduled but all too common life events such as divorce and widowhood. Interest for many investigators is in the particular event (widowhood, retirement, marriage, divorce, and so forth), a class of events (losses), or on the accumulation of life events (life stress). Numerous modifiers may also be invoked to explain the linkages between life crises and responses. Often the major point of departure is not the event, but the modifier.

A phenomenological perspective has guided the life-events research of several investigators. Although they begin with real external events that have an objective definition in time and place, interest is in the processing of these events rather than the events themselves (e.g., Lazarus & Folkman, 1984).

Life-crisis research is also represented by a distinct developmental position. The work of Buhler (1935), Jung (1933), Erikson (1982), Levinson, Darrow, Klein, Levinson, and Mckee (1978), Gutmann (1987), and Gould (1978) articulate a broad formulation of crisis as engendering major transformations. Adult life crises are seen as representing or inaugurating distinct psychological stages, which require energy and effort for salutary change.

Although *developmentalists* link crises to external events, these events are not at the forefront of their theory.

Although there is considerable correspondence between these methods of defining crises, distinct differences do exist. For example, we are not aware of self-help groups that deal with job promotion. Yet social scientists have made us well aware of its power to create distress as well as pleasure. Conversely, the stress of caregiving for aging parents by adult children has been newly legitimized by the community, as evidenced by the proliferation of self-help groups and adult education. Historically, this was not defined as a crisis, but was part of the family life cycle, rather than an abrupt entrance into a new role. The profound changes in our social structure within the memory of most of us have propelled *parent caring* into the nomenclature of adult life crisis. Noticing the adult's predicament of simultaneously caring for children and parents (the so-called sandwich generation) has also become a sign of wider community commitment to social and economic justice. Such societal recognition moves the problem from an individual focus to a social issue involving both the person and society's structures.

Mental health consequences are usually indexed by one of two general approaches: (1) the assessment of illness by classifying people into standard psychopathological categories, or (2) the effects on adaptation measured by assessing a variety of indications, such as depression, as symptom rather than as illness. Other common indicators include anxiety, social functioning, self-esteem, and role performance. Both approaches are embedded in a homeostatic framework that assumes that the organism perturbed by life crises seeks to rectify disequilibrium by returning to prior levels of adaptation. In contrast, investigators interested in transformations look at the development of new qualities, new characteristics, and enhanced functioning as a consequence of life crises. They emphasize changes in personality, in world view, in perspective, and in self-image. Obviously, this represents a distinctly separate tradition from *caseness* and adaptation for understanding human behavior. Table I provides, in telegraphic fashion, the categories of consequences, various perspectives on adult life crises, and the mediators examined for linking life event to consequence.

The chapter's intention is to ask how well these various perspectives on crises and consequences have served the field. Do they provide an adequate explanation of the development of psychopathology in adult lives? Do they help organize and provide an understanding of the course of adult development? Are they able to provide conceptual answers to the trite but true observation that twenty-year-olds are different from thirty-year-olds, and both are different from those older than sixty? And finally, how well do these various perspectives and the empirical information they have generated serve the clinician? Do they aid in diagnosis? In treatment? Do they have a practical fallout for altering and channeling how clinicians think about the adults they see in their practices? These are the questions we optimistically set for ourselves as we developed the material for this chapter.

The chapter is organized as a sequence of topics each portraying an essential relationship between life crises and consequences. As we move from an examination of the life-crises effects on psychopathology, on adaptation and on transformations, the links between event and outcome will increase in complexity by the addition of modifiers and concepts describing consequences.

Table I

Linking Life Event to Consequence

Life crises	Consequences

Specific Events
  Modifiers
    Negative
    Loss
    Controllability
    Predictability
    Normative
    Expectable Life Cycle
    Role Exit
    Role Entrance
    Timing (off/on)
    Historical Changes in Timing
    Multiple Time Tables
Accumulation of events "life-stress"
Phenomenology or subjective meaning of life events
Life-cycle stages: Events as inner manifestations
Events as anticipations
	1. Development of psychopathology; cases of mental illness
	2. Effects on external adaptation—depressive symptoms, anxiety, social functioning, self-esteem, performance
	3. Transformations of personality, world view, perspectives, self-image

II. A First Look: Salience of Life Events on Mental Health Consequences

Figures 1–3 list the events of the adult life cycle that have commonly been examined for their impact on lives.[1] Many involve role exits; some, role entrances. Most represent losses; fewer, gains. More events seem negative than positive. Some of the events would be classified as controllable; most would not. Four measures of consequences, subsequent to the occurrence of the event, are portrayed. The impact of events on mental illness is indexed by depressive symptoms; transforming qualities by self-(image) changes. The other two are phenomenological measures—events as life changing; and preoccupation, the degree to which the event is active in the psyche of the person months or years after.

Events differ in their impact on people. Some are associated with increases in depression for nearly all, while others affect a much smaller number of people. The salience of any particular life event is to a large extent dependent on how the consequences are assessed. Our response to the question of what life events have an impact is answerable only in context; i.e., according to whether the question addresses mental health consequences or, on the other hand, the transforming characteristics of an event, such as changes in the self-image. There is no single perspective that could answer the question of

[1]The data are drawn from a panel study of a random sample of 2300 subject's age 18–65 at Time 1 and followed again five years later. Event cited occurred between the two measurement times; the consequent measures are T_2 scores (Pearlin & Lieberman, 1979).

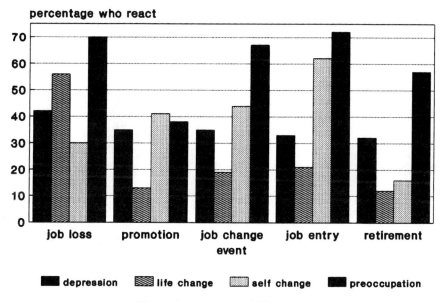

Figure 1   Occupational life events.

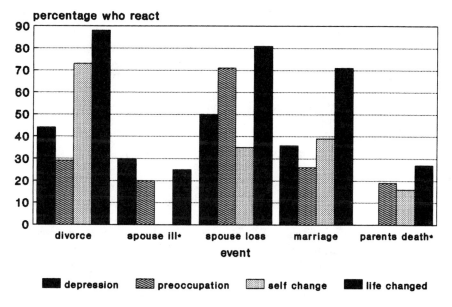

Figure 2   Marital life events. *information not available.

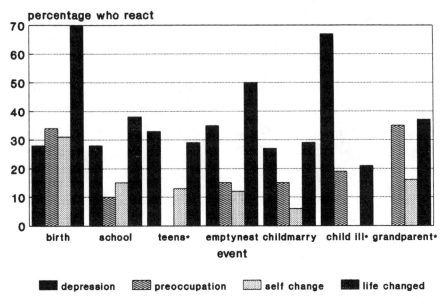

Figure 3   Family life events. *information not available.

what are the salient and significant transitional crises of the adult life cycle. Context includes, of course, not only consequences, but predisposing factors such as social class, gender, and stage of life.

An analysis of the data displayed in Figures 1–3 (not graphed) based upon decade of life (20s through the 70s), found relatively little systematic influence of chronological age on the reactions to life events. Of course, the frequency of occurrence of different life events is age-linked. In general, with increasing age, subjects perceive relatively lower amounts of change in the self-image.

These findings from a large random sample serve to underscore the complexity of the chapter's topic. The various conceptual frames used to understand the role that adult life crises play in the lives of adults are reflected in the remainder of our chapter.

III. Adult Life Crises and Psychiatric Disorders

This section reviews what is known about the causal role of adult life crises on the onset, timing, and course of mental disorders. Much of this review is garnered from empirical knowledge that has evolved from *life stress* studies, a more inclusive framework that subsumes *adult life crises*. It examines how such knowledge has been generated and the attendant methodological problems. Three classes of mental disorders have received the most attention in illuminating the linkage between life crises and psychiatric illness—the anxiety, depressive, and schizophrenic disorders.

There are at least three working models linking stress or crises to mental disorders. The *innocent-victim* model sees the prospective patient as exposed by chance to environmental events or circumstances that lead to the psychiatric disorder. The *vulnerability* model sees chance exposures to a stressor as triggering illness onset, but adds that the toll is greater for those made vulnerable by social deficits (social roles, social position), and for those with fewer social resources, particularly the availability of significant others for support. The *interactive* model suggests that because of preexisting psychological deficiencies in coping and interpersonal skills, people who become clinically ill either are unable to avoid the occurrence of undesirable life events or actively provoke them.

There are two different life-events literatures, one grounded in epidemiology and the other in case-control clinical studies. In the former, investigators ordinarily focus on the association between recent life events and some measure of mental distress in a general population. Psychopathology is usually defined by measures of psychological distress, e.g., a symptom checklist. (Not all epidemiologically based studies, however, rely on this. For example, the work of Brown and Harris [1978] utilized a well-validated case-finding procedure in an epidemiological framework.) In contrast, most case-controlled, clinical studies begin with a sample of carefully diagnosed psychiatric patients and compare them to a sample drawn from the general population or from other psychopathology samples. This research tradition ordinarily relies on small samples whose members have been victimized by one particular life crisis.

A. Methodological Considerations

Three major strategies have been used to investigate the linkage between life events and psychiatric illness: to study those who have a particular disorder in order to assess frequency of stressors; to study those who have experienced an event (for example, a natural disaster) in order to assess who and how many become ill; or to follow a randomly selected community cohort over time to see who experiences stressors and who becomes ill. Most studies of stress and psychiatric disorder have used the first strategy, that of studying life events experienced and reported by different patient groups. This form of evidence, however, is the least contributory to a statement about causal linkages to the development of illness (Rabkin, 1980).

Each of the three approaches presents characteristic methods problems. Much of the epidemiological-based research linking life events to mental disorders fails to establish clinical diagnosis of illness, relying rather on global ratings or counting of psychological symptoms. On the other hand, many of the case-controlled studies that have developed sophisticated differential diagnoses rely on retrospective design. Such designs produce frequent errors of recall and retrospective falsification of pre–morbid life events. In both strategies, the problem in documenting the impact of more common stressor events is that prior emotional difficulties can bring about some events, such as divorce or job loss, thus leading to ambiguity in the causal meaning of association of life events and disorder. Indeed, a substantial percentage of the events in standard life-event inventories have been judged to be symptoms of emotional disorder (Dohrenwend, Dohrenwend, Dodson, & Strout, 1984). In general, case-control studies can at best show what proportion of those in a given illness or control group experience particular life events, providing a measure of association but no direct insight into etiology. In contrast, the rarer prospective studies indicate what proportion of those who experience the life event become ill.

B. Stress and Anxiety Disorders

Studies of phobic disorders, the main anxiety disorder examined, (Rabkin, 1980) can be grouped into two types: those in which the investigator assumes that each illness has a precipitant and the task is to identify it; and those that ask whether or not illness onset is preceded by an identifiable stressor. Studies of the first type usually consist of event frequencies preceding illness onset. In such studies, the absence of control groups together with lack of precision in definition of both stress and diagnosis render findings virtually uninterpretable. Both types are open to the criticism that the question itself is of doubtful validity since nearly any illness or behavioral change will be identified with a precipitant if the patient is asked to produce one (Sim & Houghton, 1966).

Despite both clinical and lay expectations that phobic disorders are triggered if not caused by a particular stressor, investigators have not found a strong association. In a well-controlled study, Clarke and Kreetmann (1977) compared 30 agoraphobic housewives and 30 controls. The authors conclude that the data showed no evidence that a specific stimulus commonly initiated the phobia. Other studies report that about two thirds of phobics reported a precipitating stressor, although the researchers themselves did not always agree with the patient's assessment (Roberts, 1964; Shafar, 1976).

C. Stress and Schizophrenia

Clinicians regard the presence of a particular event or experience directly before onset of a schizophrenic episode as either an etiological or a precipitating factor. Such an event is commonly believed to contribute to the cause or timing of schizophrenia and to influence prognosis. However, a prodromal phase of variable length preceding the acute psychosis (that manifests itself in behavioral changes such as impaired routine daily functioning, social withdrawal, diminished effectiveness at work, irritability, markedly eccentric behavior, and personality changes) makes it difficult to establish the impact of life events on the outbreak of psychotic functioning.

Investigators then have been cautious in attributing an etiological role to stressful events; rather they emphasize stressor influence on the timing of the illness episode. The focus, therefore, is on the precipitating role of events in already vulnerable people. Researchers look at whether schizophrenics, compared either to normals or to those with other psychiatric conditions report events that are more severe, more frequent, of a singular nature, or of a specific type. Overall there is little evidence that events reported by schizophrenics are more frequent than those reported by other diagnostic groups preceding illness onset. One study that evaluated magnitude of stress associated with events found that events reported by schizophrenics were less *objectively* hazardous or troublesome than those reported by depressives (Beck & Worthen, 1972). Those who become schizophrenic are believed to be exceptionally sensitive to perceived or actual threats to self-esteem, and psychotic episodes may follow situations not ordinarily regarded as objectively stressful or hazardous (Lehmann, 1975).

The studies of Brown, Harris, and Peto, (1973), Jacobs and Meyers (1976) and Serban (1975) do not point to any decisive agreement on the degree of influence of life crises in precipitating illness onset. Brown, Harris, and Peto (1973) regard life events as significant precipitants that influence the timing, if not the probability of illness. They find that more life events are reported by schizophrenics than by normals in the three weeks immediately preceding illness, both in comparison to normals in the same period and in comparison with their own reports for earlier periods. Jacobs and Meyers (1976) are more cautious in attributing a significant role for recent life events, and Serban (1974) is least convinced about their influence. In a recent review of evidence concerning schizophrenia, Kandler (1988) cites five recent studies based on methods of blind diagnosis, control groups, personal interviews, and operationalized diagnostic criteria, which provide robust methodological studies to assess this question. The role of life crises was not paramount.

Rabkin's (1980) summary succinctly characterizes studies of schizophrenia:

Cumulatively, such results demonstrate that life events may contribute incrementally to an already inflated stress level and so might influence the timing if not the probability of illness onset. Overall, the research evidence indicates that a weaker relationship between life events and schizophrenia onset exists than the clinical literature suggests, although methodological limitations preclude firm conclusions at this time (p. 424).

D. Depressive Illnesses

The major depressive illnesses have traditionally been the one class of psychiatric disturbances most closely linked to adult life crises. Historically, psychiatry has made a major diagnostic distinction between reactive and endogenous depressive disorders based on external stressors as precipitants in the former. Such a distinction has not held up in most empirical studies. For example, Paykel (1979) found that life events accounted for less than three percent of the variance in illness subtypes. Overall, it has been concluded that depressive subtypes are not differentiated by frequency of stressful precipitants in the classification systems so far examined in the literature.

The cumulative evidence does suggest that depressed patients do report more events in the period preceding the start of an illness episode. When compared to normal controls, there is a significant increase in life events. Studies such as those by Brown and his colleagues (1973) found that the three-week period directly preceding illness was a critical juncture, distinguishing depressed patients from controls. Overall, although such differences are neither large nor consistently reported, most of the evidence suggests that there is an association between increased frequency of life events and onset of depressive illness in comparison both to other patient groups and to the general population.

Measurement strategies that obtain contextually specific information about events (Brown & Harris, 1978) promise to clarify the role of life crises in the development of depressive disorders. Thoits (1983) has concluded that the features of crises documented as most important for the development of psychopathology are undesirability, magnitude, and time clustering.

Despite the consensus in the field, the magnitude of the relationship between adult life crises and the onset of illness is small, and at best accounts for 10% of the variance. Most people do not become mentally ill even when terrible things happen to them. Studies of various specific stressors, particularly role exits, do not support the contribution of life events as crucial in the development of major depressive disorders. Such precipitating *stress* is not necessary or sufficient to account for depressive onset. Although a certain amount of specificity has been verified, the evidence for high levels of specificity with particular types of adult life crises and the onset of depressive illness is not strong.

Generally, the very modest relationships and their inconsistent showings are probably in part a product of the methodological problems outlined previously in this section, such as diagnostic heterogeneity, sampling biases, and numerous ambiguities in conceptualizing and studying the nature of the crises. More complex models, such as developed by Dohrenwend and Dohrenwend (1978), as well as contextual studies like those of Brown and his colleagues, are necessary to trace the contribution of adult life crises and the development of major depressive disorders. Clearly some form of relationship exists, but the level of linkage at this juncture probably makes the accumulated research findings less than relevant to the working clinician.

Dynamically oriented clinicians have addressed the relationship between adult life crises and the development of psychopathology through studies of late-onset psychiatric illness. They attempt to trace the complex chain of both inner and outer factors of individual lives in order to explain why seemingly stable individuals without a history of gross mental disorders are rendered ill in late life by stresses that more obviously burdened people might shrug off (Gutmann, Griffin, & Graves, 1982). Collectively, clinicians working in this tradition have developed intriguing and complex hypotheses to account for the above-mentioned observations. At this juncture, however, accumulated empirical research is too sparse and too diffuse to permit a meaningful evaluation of the contribution of this perspective for adult life crises and mental illness.

IV. Life Crises and Adaptation

Adaptational studies range from clinical case exemplars to well-specified epidemiological surveys. Some researchers use a *cumulative life-stress* framework; others look at *specific* crises.

The literature on cumulative life events is vast and diversified, and numerous review articles and monographs are available. Overall, the message that may be garnered is that there is ample evidence of a small but consistent relationship between the accumulation of life events and negative consequences.

Investigations of *specific* adult life crises—both normative life transitions and eruptive, unanticipated events—also make up a variegated field. Countless research articles, reviews, and monographs exist on the specific adult crises of marriage, divorce, widowhood, remarriage, and remaining single. The same is true for family events, e.g., the birth of a child, the exit of children from the home, the marriage of a child, and grandparenthood. In the occupational area, numerous studies of the effects of unemployment, retirement, demotions, promotions, and entrance into the job world are available. Empirical investigations of any single life crisis usually demonstrate a wide range of effects. Although studies of retirement have generally not shown high rates of negative consequences, some studies of specific occupation and condition of retirement demonstrate negative impact. Simple generalizations about the impact of adult life crises then are not possible. Often the event modifiers (see list, Table I) have more impact on consequences than does the simple occurrence of the events. It is certainly beyond the scope of this chapter or the capacity of the authors to master or systematize this diversified body of accumulated knowledge.

A. Spousal Loss

We have chosen one life crisis to illustrate the issues confronting investigators who study adult life crises from an adaptational perspective. Moreover, the loss of a spouse exemplifies the conceptual and methodological promise and problems inherent in the study of adult life crises. Spousal-loss research is of interest to the mental health disciplines, sociology, and epidemiology. The history of such research also demonstrates changing methods and respecifications of the relevant questions and the conceptual frames to explicate this singular adult life crisis.

In the language of the modifiers of life crises, spousal bereavement represents a negative event. It is both a role exit and a loss that is not controllable, yet is, especially for women, part of the expectable life cycle. Studies of spousal bereavement are imbedded in a homeostatic model. Loss is seen as creating a disturbance, while the mourning processes serve as the mechanism that returns the organism to prior levels of adaptation. The factors affecting the successful working through of grief and mourning emphasize individual differences in prior losses, the relationship with the deceased spouse, and current or past *other* psychological problems. It has been shown that timing (in the sense of on-time or off-time) influences the consequence of widowhood or widowerhood. Available evidence also suggests that the consequences of this life event have changed dramatically over large periods of historical time. In these senses, then, the loss of a spouse is an ideal surrogate for many other adult life crises.

Classical spousal-loss research (Bowlby, 1980; Osterweis, Solomon, & Green, 1984; Raphael, 1983) lays emphasis on the loss consequences for psychological health through a focus on the vicissitudes of mourning and grief. Much of the early work in the classical view was based on small, opportunistic samples, skewed to the mentally distressed who sought help. The early interest was in determining processes that led to restoring the person to previous levels of functioning. Particularly important in Freud's (1917) thinking was an emphasis on reattachment; mourning was a gradual surrender of psychological attachment to the deceased in order to liberate the bereaved for new attachments. Freud believed that relinquishment of the love object involves an internal struggle between intense yearning for the lost loved one and the reality of the loved one's absence. It was Freud who advanced the idea that many psychiatric illnesses are expressions of pathological mourning. Such pathology includes not only excessive grief but also failure to grieve and suppression or denial of emotional feelings. Conversely, psychological health after spousal loss is said to depend on capacity to grieve as reflected in depressive reactions.

Studies (Clayton, Halikas, & Maurice, 1972; Vachon, 1976) have raised questions about the model of adaptation outlined by Freud and other dynamic theories that imply that absence of grieving is linked to negative outcomes, signified by a delay, suppression, or denial of effect. (See Osterweis, *et al.*, 1984 and C. B. Wortman & Silver, 1987 for excellent reviews of the empirical literature). Many widows and widowers, however, who show no evidence of grieving, have been found to be well adapted subsequent to the loss of their spouse. Little evidence is available to document the hypothesis that manifestly undistressed or undepressed widows and widowers are at high risk for subsequent maladaptation because of not managing the process of grieving. Lieberman (1991) classified the recently widowed into four patterns of grieving by assessing grief appraisals soon after the death of their husband (T_1) and again one year later (T_2). Thirty-seven percent showed no grief at T_1 or T_2, 37% showed chronic grief (high at T_1 and T_2), 17% were characterized as recovered at T_2, and 9% as delayed grievers (low at T_1 and high at T_2). The best adapted (social functioning and mental health measures) widows at T_2 were the nongrievers; next were those that appeared to resolve their grief over the year; worst off were the chronic grievers. A simple loss model to explain reactions and adaptation to spousal loss is neither theoretically robust nor empirically supported. Studies need to focus on the range of social and psychological issues engendered by widowhood and widowerhood.

Beyond grieving and loss of the partner, the spousally bereaved are faced with a set of challenges and alternative paths. It disrupts plans, hopes, and dreams for the future (Silver & Wortman, 1980). The loss also challenges individuals' beliefs and assumptions about their world. Social supports and social network must be renegotiated (Lieberman, Heller, and Mullan, 1990). The spousally bereaved must reexamine their self-images which have been embedded in long-term relationships, and move to selves based on *I* rather than *we*. Many of the spousally bereaved are faced with inner psychological tasks that can be described by the label existential dilemmas—confrontations of their regrets not only in regard to the deficits of their past marital relationships but also to undeveloped aspects of their own lives. Such confrontations lead some from a sense of aloneness to the *closeness* of their own death, and then to seeking new meanings in life (Yalom & Lieberman, 1991). Such challenges can be a source of distress for many; for others, however, it can provide a sense of accomplishment.

Studies on the transforming characteristics of spousal bereavement are not numerous, yet their findings are evocative. They depart from the predominantly homeostatic model specifying restoration to initial (pre-loss) levels. Yalom & Lieberman (1991) found that 27% of the spousally bereaved showed clear-cut evidence of growth. Growth was defined in terms of new behaviors, new ways of doing things, restructuring of the self in relationship to behaviors, and so forth. The study also demonstrated that a particular process, namely involvement in existential exploration, was significantly related to growth. The growth of new behaviors and the exploration of existential issues were not related to the typical measures of recovery, such as depression levels, social functioning, and grief resolution.

Lieberman (1992) replicated the growth findings in a panel study of nonclinical widows followed for seven years. Fifty-three percent of the widows showed some evidence of growth, i.e., new patterns of behavior and/or ways of thinking.

As attention turned toward other types of samples and different researchable hypotheses about spousal loss, evidence began to accumulate that (1) grief reactions to spousal loss are not universal; (2) adaptation is not highly predictable, in a normative sample, from the dynamics of mourning; (3) classical risk factors (other losses and an ambivalent relationship to the deceased) do not account for most of the variations in successful–unsuccessful adaptation. Increasingly, concern has been with the modifiers rather than affective reactions to spousal bereavement. Attention has moved from an internal dynamic to external conditions such as social supports, social contexts, and cognitive characteristics such as coping strategies and adaptive skills. For example, akin to the findings repeatedly shown for almost all crises or stress studies, modest relationships between social supports and success of adaptation have been repeatedly reported. The magnitude of the relationship clearly requires consideration of other explanatory factors to understand the complex processes of adaptation in reaction to spousal loss. Although such newer studies represent a shift in both method and paradigm, most still share a common homeostatic framework for indexing consequences, that of restoring the widow–widower to their initial adaptive levels.

Clearly, loss of a spouse in mid and late life is a complex event that can lead not only to adaptive failures and illness, but also to enhanced functioning. The narrow confines of a homeostatic framework for understanding the impact of adult crises need expansion. This perspective on spousal loss provides a useful bridge to the chapter's next section; the transforming potential of adult life crises described by a number of classic views on the meaning of adult life crises from a developmental perspective. The next section provides an exploration of adult crises theories that have enhanced functioning as their central tenet.

V. Adult Crisis as Transformative

Crisis as a catalyst for development has become a virtual cornerstone of adult lifespan study. Concepts relating crisis to favorable outcomes rather than to arrest and deficit have more and more illuminated the growing discipline of late-life personality development. Rather than a forewarning of developmental regression and adaptive losses, crisis from this perspective has come to convey a vigorous personal unfolding that carries the individual across a threshold to new experience, meanings, and inner psychological states. Adult crises are seen as essentially transformative, where the self is released to realize its potential for new differentiations, structures, and organizations. In this sense, crisis creates new forms by discarding, amending, or reconfiguring old ones, and thus belongs within a sequence of alternating order and change. Within this perspective, the study of adult crisis, then, is virtually the study of lifespan development itself.

While our previous sections considered crisis as strain and loss induced by external and cumulative stressors, crisis as transformation is greater than the sum of losses (empty nest, divorce, widowhood, parental death) and gains (marriage, parenthood, job promotion). A transformative process means rather a new gestalt of self-recognition in which a triggering loss (or gain) may induce a new recognition of hidden capacities and a wider grasp of human experiencing. Thus, the envy of youth in middle age may mobilize untapped resources of caring (Kernberg, 1980); the keener awareness of death in middle age may permit a more equanimous attitude toward one's mortality, a lessening of strivings for perfection, and a new realization of creative potential (Jaques, 1965); the death of a loved parent may help free the survivor to become more his or her own person (Pollock, 1961). In transformative crisis, then, the past is not surmounted by the present but integrated with it.

Crises that result in such positive changes may depend crucially on a facilitating environment that allows for transformative outcomes. Such allowance calls especially for an appreciation of the experimental and provisional nature of human behavior at such vulnerable times, as Erikson (1963) understood in designating adolescence as a moratorium. Without such ameliorative attention to crisis, the potential gains that might be liberated by confronting obvious loss in such real-life events as widowhood (as in our example in the preceding section) may be drained off into unavailing guilt or depression.

Strong emotionality may be neither sufficient nor perhaps even necessary for such transformative outcomes. Against the tumult of transformative crisis in Jung's (1933) stage model and the findings of Levinson *et al.* (1978) in which adults come painfully to question essential aspects of their lives, there is the more continuous and quieter change of Erikson's (1963) epigenetic scheme. In this scheme, each adult developmental step— from intimacy to generativity to integrity—builds on, rather than deconstructs, the relational competencies of the prior stage.

Theorists' choice of event and timing that crystallize such crisis reflects their conceptual opinions of the essential lines of adult development. Birth and death for *event,* and midlife for *timing,* occupy the lead positions in most formulations of transformative crisis. Regarding birth, the beginning and/or end of parenting are deemed transformative turning points in the theories of Erikson (1963, 1982) and Gutmann (1987). They differ, however, in the literalness of definition: Gutmann means parenting exclusively, so that a childless woman may be liable to a depressive reaction for missing this life stage (Gutmann, Griffin, & Grunes, 1982), whereas Erikson views parenting as one of several alternative ways of acquitting a sense of generativity. Moreover, in Gutmann's social–anthropological framework, parents discharge an essential tribal and species responsibility, which will earn them the right to develop their inner selves. For Erikson, to parent is to transform the sense of *intimacy* with a partner into intergenerational *generativity,* preparatory to a full sense of relational *integrity* with culture and civilization. Although there has been more consensus than critical debate among lifespan theorists, one might discern in Gutmann's and Erikson's positions the arguable issue of whether adult transformations normatively bend the adult toward increasing self-centeredness (narcissism, disengagement) or toward a broader relational investment in the world.

Regarding awareness of mortality, adults' transformative potentials are illuminated in the midlife light and again, in the late-life shadow of one's own approaching death. Contrasting outcomes of confronting one's mortality at mid-life and late life are seen in the new creative powers at midlife in Jaques' formulation versus a critical life-review of the self in Butler's (1963) view of late aging.

Notwithstanding the diversity of adult models, midlife is a critical passage for most theorists (Jung, Gutmann, Levinson, Jaques, Gould), perhaps because it approximates the powerful confluence of the on-time end of active parenting and the awareness of death.

VI. Dynamic Theories of Adult Crises: A Child-Centered versus Adult-Centered View

An adult-centered concept makes crisis accessible to, and consonant with the self's emerging purposes and capacities, whereas a child-centered concept presumes crisis to be dissonant and divisive to the self. The traditional child-centered view that treats adult stability as unconditionally favorable to personality adjustment has been opposed by an adult-centered position that links such stability to the failure of development. Virtually all lifespan viewpoints suggest that major personal struggle precedes true psychological coherence and, with it, the sense of becoming more *oneself.* This is especially so in the culminating *midlife crisis,* the conceptual centerpiece for such theorists as Jung, Levinson, Gutmann, Neugarten, and Jaques.

Adult crisis in child- and adult-oriented theory has received quite different attributions for personality development. In the adult-centered view, periods of adult crises and transitions are times of natural growth and therapeutic efficacy. In the child-centered view, adult crisis is the echo of delayed stress or trauma that presupposes regressive retreats from developmental paths to initial points of vulnerability. The revival of long-suspended stress might be triggered in later adulthood by the phasing out of life-course regimens that had kept such stress at bay—notably the ending of child rearing or retirement.

An adult-centered view is most persuasive when adults are given repeated opportunities to demonstrate their changing perspectives and uses of the past. We are cautioned, then, against taking as fixed those life-history narratives, such as obtained by Levinson, which draw from only one adult era. His midlife informants have provided just one version of their lives, including the reconstruction of prior crisis periods, that best suits their sense of consistency about who they have presently become. Longitudinal research is obviously the design of choice to demonstrate the fluidity of lives between, say, the disparate crises of midlife and old age.

Reformulating crisis in adult-centered terms leads to fresh ways of thinking about the organization of the past. If adulthood has a momentum of its own, it cannot then be a permanent vantage point for an unchanging reconstruction of childhood; if adulthood too, like youth and adolescence, is formative, then adult retrospection cannot be a motionless and transparent medium, but a richly opaque one into the past. As an expression of its own design and purpose, adulthood may then be said to cast its own view on the early past, as well as be cast by that early past. Perhaps just as children mirror and animate their changing sense of themselves in the endless possible designs of their futures, so might adults rewrite or *re-emplot* the narrative of their pasts as an expression of the new or renewed self-understandings that successful crisis resolution brings.

Not only might changing self-perceptions of one's personal history illuminate the present, but they might also actively promote certain courses of action. In the adult-centered view, adulthood not only throws its own shadow, but also draws a map of itself across the past to chart the destination of, and give direction to current life tasks. One's *same* early past may be remapped and redirected again and again as such life tasks change. This mapping metaphor emphasizes understudied aspects of adult crisis, namely access to the past as source of new motivation and resources, in short, uses of the past. Moreover, ameliorating an adult issue may open up new avenues to the unsolved crises of the past and with it, new perceptions there of unseen potentials. This is the situation in which a current life crisis is resolved in a manner that illuminates alternate ways of approaching earlier conflict or draws isolated parts of the self into present functioning. That such opportunities to renegotiate early conflict may appear over the adult lifespan presupposes a more varied and interesting terrain for adulthood than the notion of adulthood as a smooth plateau, favored by the traditional, child-oriented psychodynamic schools.

Revisions and uses of the past in an adult-centered view have guided longitudinal studies by Peskin (1987), Peskin and Livson (1981), Peskin and Gigy (1977), and Gigy (1982). An illustrative study by Peskin and Gigy demonstrates the impact of new parenting on such revisions. Women who became mothers over this period were more likely to rate their current year as more satisfying than before, but their early childhood years as more stressful than before, compared to women who had remained childless. The parenthood *imperative,* we inferred, not only enhanced the mothers' present quality of life, but with this enhanced well-being, promoted a revision of the past that allowed for the acknowledgement of early-life stresses.

Underlying the debate between child- and adult-centered positions on the nature of lifespan crisis is the question of whether adulthood itself is truly a time of progressive psychological development or progressive loss. The child-oriented position answers in the negative, mostly by implication from its basic premise that childhood prefigures adulthood, so that the agents of change are always behind the adult, never ahead, and still further behind with aging. Cautioning against the unrewarding project of treating the older patient, Freud (1898) was unabashedly ageist by present-day standards in holding to these child-centered presuppositions.

No less than Freud's, Jung's thinking about later-life development and later-life psychotherapy was dictated by unconditional, if quite opposite, premises about the nature of development. Jung's focus was on exploring the self which, far from being hidden in one's personal history, did not reach its ascendancy until middle age and could not be resolutely explored until then. Just as the second half of life could not be governed by the principles of the first, Jung would not trust the discovery of the self to early adulthood. The meaning of one's individual life was hardly to be found in the pre-midlife occupation with the tangible and the attainable, nor, of course, in their infantile roots. It was rather to be found in relinquishing the egoistic power of the achievement motive.

Jung appealed to vague maturational necessity to account for stage change, dismissing external or internal stressors. Even nearness of death was discounted as pivotal, notwithstanding its obvious suggestion in Jung's (1933) famous image of the rising and setting sun upon which he otherwise drew to capture the maturational inevitability of the midlife reversal of life's purpose.

Jung's depiction of the transformative crisis between life's first and second half remains the essential core of several contemporary lifespan theories. Levinson's *seasons,* Gould's

(1978) rich adult-history narratives, and Gutmann's *parental imperative,* however, have appreciably dignified the periods and crises of pre-midlife to which Jung gave short shrift. Recent thinkers have also elucidated a sophisticated and tangible social causality for the midlife crisis. The cycle of parenting and intergenerational reordering has especially helped to demystify Jung's singular reliance on an obscure *maturational* process. Moreover, the recognition of an historical causality as well for the midlife crisis necessarily disputes its timeless universality. The midlife crisis, even in its seeming physical signs of bodily and sexual decline, may be more a creation of the small modern family, with its early dethronement of the adults from the once ceaseless parental role in the large family (Demos, 1986).

We have chosen three specific areas of *transformation* for more detailed examination.

A. Self-Discovery as the Province of Later Adult Crisis

Minimizing early self-experience seems an occupational hazard for theorists who, like Jung, detach their model of the adult lifespan from early development. This disinterest has been supported by a few reviewers (e.g., Cohler & Galatzer-Levy, 1990) who argue that extant longitudinal studies confirm the unpredictability and discontinuity, rather than the stability of personality parameters between youth to adulthood. Stability of personality, however, is the dominant view among personality theorists (Block, 1971; Costa & Mc-Crae, 1987). Even investigators who have studied broad adult adaptational patterns rather than single traits (e.g., Peskin, 1987) find predictability and continuity between behavior in youth and later psychological health.

The discounting of early self-experience may be part of a larger presumption that a later adult era comes closer than the prior era to one's personal authenticity and true self. This linear notion overlooks the likelihood that in earlier stages an individual may have boldly wrestled with personal truths that were compromised in later life. An adult crisis may be initiated by the opportunity or necessity for the older adult to meet and confront the disavowed ideals (not merely ambitions, as in Levinson's young-adult Dream) of his or her youth. Even one's own adolescent or young-adult offspring, in the service of self-discovery beyond the family orbit, might launch a parent's self-confrontation. Similarly, Erikson's underpinning of the adult self in the identity crisis of adolescence brings into question the notion that the self's true development only comes in later adulthood. The otherwise meager conceptual interest by adult theorists of self-discovery in childhood, youth, and early adulthood leaves fallow important empirical questions on how the early life course might shape later adult crises.

B. The Gender Crisis at Midlife

The Jungian core in much contemporary theory of adult crisis is contained in Jung's well-known proposal that the inner resources that become newly available at midlife contain the opposite gender qualities of the first half of life: the male's *unused supply* of femininity and the female's unused masculinity. This reversal of gender qualities occupies a central position in the formulations of midlife crisis of Gutmann, Levinson and Gould: men and women are released from both the constraint and stability of their gendered roles once they have acquitted the gendered responsibilities of parenting, family survival, and social empowerment.

The accessibility of such unused gender traits after midlife is illustrated by some longitudinal findings from the Intergenerational Studies of the Institute of Human Development. Peskin and Livson (1981) and Peskin (1987) found that adaptation between pre- and post-midlife depends partly on the reversal of gendered traits from adolescence. Psychologically healthy men in their early 40s draw on behaviors from adolescence that reflected the classic, outer-directed portrait of the established, instrumental male. It is the image of the male who prizes masculinity, power, sociability, conventional values, and wariness of imagination and fantasy. Psychologically healthy men in their early 50s, however, show a dramatic reversal of these adolescent traits: their adolescent years were concerned not with willpower and masculinity but rather with inner psychological states invested in fantasy and unconventional thinking. Healthy women in their early 50s who are in the empty nest and beyond the parental imperative, show a corresponding reversal of gendered adolescent traits: they draw on adolescent behaviors of low responsibility, low nurturance, and low guilt. By contrast, healthy women who are still actively parenting at this age organize their past around high responsibility, nurturance, and guilt.

Explanations of the gender crisis at midlife do not address the relational implications of the gender reversal. Where does this gender change leave the long-term relationship between a man and a woman? Is the relationship after midlife likely to be as polarized between the sexes as in the first half of life, only now with the man and woman at new opposite poles? Or, on the other hand, does the manifest reversal build on the core gender, so that a new mutuality, rather than a renewed antithesis between the sexes evolves at mid-life? Clearly, the relational possibilities of the gender crisis raise evocative and under-studied questions.

C. Relational Investment as a Consequence of Adult Crises

The Jungian-based ethos of Levinson and Gutmann tends to situate the full expression of the self outside the interpersonal sphere of mutual responsibilities, such as family build-ing. For them, the surest flowering of selfhood comes in later adulthood when tribal *emergencies* have been outlived and personal autonomy reclaimed; here, then, socializa-tion and selfhood are adversaries. For Erikson, they are psychosocial allies at best, perhaps codependents at worse (when the adult loses himself in the community), but always partners in the actualization of *life tasks*.

Erikson's ego-relational formulation is a major exception to the general trend of adult theories to be rooted in the inner sense of self at the price of underestimating the impor-tance of human interdependency in late life, especially in the areas of intimacy, empathy, and responsibility. Indeed, most theorists view interdependency in middle and late life as diminishing, whether from a Jungian base of increased introversion or a Freudian one of strengthened (or threatened) narcissism. They presume that the later-life change from active to passive mastery of the environment—a hallmark of interiority—spells a withdrawal and disengagement from experiencing the outer world (Neugarten, 1968; Cumming & Henry, 1961). Erikson, in contrast, views an invested life in a relational order as the *sine qua non* of mature resolution of the adult crises, including the most interior and culminating crisis of integrity versus despair when the aging adult apprehends internally whether he has over his lifetime "taken care of things and people." This relational quality of interiority is, of course, also captured in Butler's life-review.

Differentiating interiority from disengagement after midlife requires a level of observation beyond simple assessment of discrete traits and behaviors. For example, capacity for fantasy or unconventional thinking can reasonably support the contrary positions of interiority or disengagement as being normative to males' mid and late life, unless the wider context of an adult's personal and relational adaptation is taken into account. For the normative potential of an era is represented by personality functioning under the most salutary psychosocial conditions. Our longitudinal findings (Peskin & Livson, 1981) and Peskin (1987), discussed above, support the normative midlife turn to interiority, since those who have shown essential inward dispositions in their youth are the most high functioning, psychologically healthy and least detached older males in the sample. Our results suggest that such inward dispositions, incipient in adolescence, "come of age" in the interiority of a healthfully relational second half of life.

The role of relational investment and interdependency in precipitating and resolving adult crisis is arguably a fruitful area for investigation. Our own contribution is to suggest that there is a cumulative adult crisis in middle and late life whose purpose (unlike the prototypical midlife crisis of new interiority and new gendered dispositions) is to reconfirm the older developmental achievements of the first half of life, especially the sense of one's autonomous identity. The need for such reconfirmation arises because the more complex relational world of the older adult taxes and challenges personal autonomy more heavily than had been the case in the simpler individualistic and achievement-oriented ambiance of the first half of life.

The lives of middle-aged and older individuals are embedded in extensive social networks of generational and intergenerational role responsibilities, commitments, and entitlements. Accordingly, their earlier personal autonomy must be confirmed and established again in relationship rather than in separation (as in the adolescent prototype of family leave-taking and psychic distancing). Crisis resolution in late life then involves sustaining personal autonomy by realigning primary relationships rather than detaching from them. Such new alignments might assume the appearance of solitude and separation, as in a mother's refusal to reparent her adult daughter by being a caretaker to her grandchildren (Cohler & Grunebaum, 1981). But these relational changes, once the passing of the parental imperative has relieved them of obligatory bonding, may actually represent parents' autonomous attempts to redefine, rather than relinquish their relationships with adult children. By this view, a mother becomes freer to spend more time with an adult daughter with whom she prefers to visit than with another adult offspring who needs her more. This transformation might be called a related autonomy, whereby a higher level of autonomy becomes congruent with a higher level of relatedness.

By now, the reader is aware that we wish to make a place for an important kind of adult crisis that is not as easily discernible among the more bounded life transitions (instigated by role entrances, exits, and anticipations), wherein old traits recede and new traits ascend. Our perspective raises the issue of how the older adult also sustains, rather than jettisons, the self-identity of early life in the face of the relatively complex relational world of later life. Stated in this manner, transformative crises should include not only cycles of trait recession–ascendance or reversals, but also the reconciliation and new integration of apparently contradictory personality forces. In this light, we have indicated that interiority and autonomy in later life may undergo a transformation into the parodox-ical achievements of *relational interiority* and *relational autonomy*. Again, as a concep-tual alternative to the midlife male's feminine *reversal*, one might speak of a *relational masculinity* that integrates the *separated* masculinity of early life with the strengthened affiliative motive of the later years.

VII. A Cautionary Note

Postulating adult life crises as transformative offers a rich conceptual step to the eventual systematization of adult development. We believe, however, that a number of conceptual and methodological concerns demand attention. Although transformative concepts are evocative and challenging, they are often underspecified, limiting the ability of others to replicate.

We found the common assumption of universality disturbing. We believe that adult life crises are products of a particular social context, and the attribution of universality may hinder more than help scholarship. Similarly, we question another major assumption that an individual's failure to address a particular crisis, defined of course from the point of view of the investigator, leads to untoward psychological outcomes. Too often in these theories, change is equated with the good, the true, and the beautiful; stability of psycho-logical processes with the bad, the imperfect, or the pathological. Moreover, most of the transformation theories are often ambiguous concerning what is transformed: Does one look at rate of transformation? Type of transformation? Quality of transformation?

Most of the reviewed theoretical positions are based upon the study of elites. More serious, they often do not represent longitudinal samples. The problems of equating cross-sectional designs to repeated followups are by now well enough known in the adult-development field that no explanation is required here. Obviously at issue is that in order for adult-crisis transformation theories to move beyond mere tautologies, lives must be examined before, during, and after the event. There must be a mechanism for defining who is in a crisis and who is not now in crisis nor has ever been. Only then and with more specification of consequences would it become possible to appreciate the true utility of such concepts for the study of the adult life cycle. Currently we believe that, across studies, no cumulative evidence is available to render a reasonable opinion about both the promise and limitations of this perspective.

VIII. Clinical Aspects of Crisis

What utility can the working clinician find in what we have said, given the diversity of views and the disparity of empirical findings that compose the complex and unbounded field of adult crisis? Certainly, the documentation is weak that adult life crises, either singly or in combination, are intrinsically linked to the development of mental disorders. The timing of such disorders, particularly those representing depressive illness, finds somewhat more support in the empirical literature, although this finding is by no means accepted by all investigators. What stands out is that the linkage between adult crises, whether externally defined or representing perspectives on meaning, requires a complex chain of psychological and social modifers between the event and the consequence. A person's place in society, historical time, and idiosyncratic perceptions have enormous influence on the linkage between crises and their consequences. Broadening the perspective and viewing crisis, not only as a source of potential distress for human adaptation but also as a signal for potential development, brings us finally to the clinical arena. Here, the perspectives of distress and development seem unlikely allies. Yet they too are interdependent, with development drawing energy for transforming hardly manageable crises into self-controlled and self-constructed transitions.

This final section of our paper presents a clinical perspective for thinking about adult crisis, both in evaluating those who come for help and in developing strategies for intervention. Our view is frankly psychodynamic, but not as usually rendered in an exclusive child-oriented view. Rather, we briefly describe and illustrate a framework which includes the adult-oriented position that locates the crucial causes of psychopathology and the pathways to therapeutic change in later life.

The workable resolution of adult crisis, including its integration into further personality development, must ultimately draw on both the child- and adult-oriented viewpoints. In the psychotherapy of adult crisis, where strong emotional upheaval seems unbidden and disorganizing, child-centered formulations complement adult-centered ones focused on active mastery of conflict. This integrative view stands as the cornerstone of Erikson's epigenetic model of development where early crises "pre-face" current issues (child-centered), while current issues reciprocally "re-face" early ones (adult-centered). Early life crises, then, must be resolved in terms of current issues. New resolutions are not foreclosed by how the adult "did" earlier phases, but how he or she "re-faces" them again in later opportunities along the life span. Erikson's (1976) cogent example, drawn from the Bergmann film *Wild Strawberries,* aptly captures this dual perspective. The film portrays an aging, emotionally deadened professor who is taken through a peripatetic life review by his estranged son that ultimately allows him to re-face—to re-surface and to re-build—his relationships to his offspring and to the rejected figures of his past.

Gutmann, et al. (1982) discuss late-life psychopathologies in a manner that similarly integrates both viewpoints for diagnosis and treatment planning. The male's normal midlife transition to post-parental passivity becomes particularly crisis-ridden for men whose early-life fears of femininity have unduly kept them in an inflexible, hyper-masculine adjustment during young adulthood. In a treatment context, it would be reasonable to suppose that the early-life conflict becomes more current and accessible under the maturational press of the midlife crisis than in the prior periods of the aggressive pursuit of normal male adult tasks pertaining to occupation, breadwinning, and parenting. This position, of course, is directly contrary to holding that stable periods are preferred for childhood conflict resolution.

Consider briefly the situation of a newly retired, near 65-year-old man whose mounting depression and anxiety since his retirement as a corporation executive is naturally attributed to role loss. Returning to being a performing artist, a career path not taken since college, initially excites him and calms his anguish, but eventually the full brunt of the stress returns, and the role loss becomes the major understanding for it. In psychotherapy, he allows himself to confront the question of whether the career path not taken as an adolescent, because of his father's refusal to allow it, still remains an active, current conflict. He considers the possibility that his re-entry into the jazz field provokes anxiety not only because of his untried abilities after many years (anticipatory risk). He also discovers that he has compounded the difficulty with the stern judgement, taken over from his late father's early disapproval, that he could never supplement his retirement income by this new career. He realizes that he is at the dangerous point of acceding once again, this time internally, to his father's authority. Clearly, the early-life conflict has become current and resolvable as a consequence of the retirement crisis.

Again, consider the situation of a 50-year-old woman who comes for help to grieve the recent death of her father. Her efforts to do so seem destined to be short-lived by the very difficulty to mourn, which brought her to the treatment initially. The therapist's reminder of this initial difficulty encourages her to remain in therapy and, beyond that, leads her to re-face an earlier personal loss that she had never mourned, perhaps because it had gone quite entirely unacknowledged by significant others: that of having to relinquish, due to back surgery in preadolescence, her love of skating and the dream of a career as an ice-skater. The loss had insinuated itself into a lifestyle resigned to withdrawal from animated activity, including play and protest. This vignette suggests again the integrated, reciprocal viewpoint of adult and child crisis: the *pre-facing* of the difficulty to mourn her father's death once she had failed to recognize her own preadolescent grief, and the *re-facing* of the unresolved grief of the surgery once the need to grieve for her father's death received the kind of serious attention by the therapist that her family had earlier withdrawn from her surgery. This case vignette also recalls our opening discussion on the relational nature of adult crisis and its amelioration. And so, we come to the close of this chapter where we began: the recognition of crisis by significant others alters the crisis from being felt as unmasterable, socially isolating, and demeaningly immature.

IX. A Summing up

Although we have criticized both the concepts and studies linking adult life crises to the development of psychopathology and other types of maladaptive responses, the chapter's message should not be taken to signify that such crises are innocuous in the lives of adults. Studies that have unambiguously demonstrated that adult life crises threaten stability and portend a threat to mental health encompass frameworks based on the complexity of adult lives. It is in the study of the complex internal and external mediators between the occurrence of event and its consequences that the oft-tenuous associations found between events and consequences can be strengthened and clarified. Furthermore, concepts and measures must be increasingly developed and used that permit evaluation of adult life crises both as potentially harmful to adaptation and as productive for change or growth.

Recent research in specifying vulnerability, based on both person and social-surround characteristics is critical for increased precision in identifying the role of adult life crises in the development and course of psychopathology. Unfortunately, such specifications of vulnerability do not as yet represent a useful, conceptual, or empirical consensus.

The optimistic expectations of adult developmentalists that the sequence of adult life crises could be relied on to organize the life cycle has not been fulfilled. Simple models linking crises to consequences woefully underreflect the complexity of the processes. More sophisticated frameworks that reflect characteristics of the persons and their social surrounds are required before the optimism of several decades ago can be realized.

We also believe that more attention should be addressed to the role of social structure in defining and providing mechanisms for help as people face adult crises. It is, of course, not only the care and concern of significant others that can help transform intense adult crises into developmental advances. Recent changes in the structure of lifespan crisis itself may also have helped ease the adult's sudden plunge into the new roles of normative crisis. Such changing models of life crisis have often been directed to maintaining dependable social supports in a manner that mitigates the abruptness of these developmental shifts. Cohabitation arrangements outside of formal marriage are a prominent example because they do not typically demand the abrupt changeover of important family relationships to an exclusive relational focus on a single partner. Such arrangements allow for much more experimental leverage in accommodating relational and autonomous needs, rather than enforcing by formal marriage an often premature relinquishment of essential social attachments, especially for younger adults.

The move toward pluralistic rather than monolithic arrangements of other key lifespan junctures—from paternity work-leaves to the plethora of retirement options—will continue to set the stage for a less procrustean fit of the adult to his or her *life task*. Not only will such wider choice cushion the developmental fall of the more vulnerable who reel at the accelerated pace of adult crisis, but such choice will also release new existential possibilities for the less vulnerable. Perhaps for all adults, such restructuring of adult crisis will make of these difficult passages an effort not only to survive, but also to prosper.

References

Beck, J., & Worthen, K. (1972). Precipitating stress, crisis theory, and hospitalization in schizophrenia and depression. *Archives of General Psychiatry, 26,* 123–129.

Block, J. (1971). *Lives through time.* Berkeley: Bancroft Books.

Bowlby, J. (1980). *Attachment and loss (Vol. 3). Loss: Sadness and depression.* London: Hogarth Press.

Brown, G. W. (1974). Meaning, measurement, and stress of life events. In B. S. Dohrenwend, B. P. Dohrenwend (Eds.), *Stressful life events: Their nature and effects* (pp. 217–244). New York: Wiley.

Brown, G. W., & Harris, T. (1978). *Social origins of depression.* London: Tavistock.

Brown, G. W., Harris, T., & Peto, J. (1973). Life events and psychiatric disorders: Part II. Nature of causal link. *Psychological Medicine, 3,* 159–176.

Buhler, C. (1935). The curve of life as studied in biographies. *Journal of Applied Psychology, 19,* 405–409 (138).

Butler, R. (1963). The life review: An interpretation of reminiscence in the aged. *Psychiatry, 26,* 65–76.

Clayton, P. J., Halikas, J. A., & Maurice, W. I. (1972). The depression of widowhood. *British Journal of Psychiatry, 120,* 71–78.

Cohler, B., & Galatzer-Levy, R. (1990). Self, meaning, and morale across the second half of life. In R. Nemiroff & C. Colarusso (Eds.), *New dimensions in adult development* (pp. 214–263). New York: Basic Books.

Cohler, B., & Grunebaum, H. (1981). *Mothers, granddaughters, and daughters: Personality and child care in three-generation families.* New York: Wiley-Interscience.

Costa, P., & McCrae, R. (1987). The case for personality stability. In G. Maddow & E. Busse (Eds.), *Aging: The universal human experience* (pp. 418–431). New York: Springer.

Cumming, E., & Henry, W. (1961). *Growing old: The process of disengagement.* New York: Basic Books.

Demos, J. (1986). *Past, present, and personal: The family and the life course in American history.* New York: Oxford University Press.

Dohrenwend, B. S., & Dohrenwend, B. P. (1978). Some issues in research on stressful life events. *Journal of Nervous and Mental Disease, 166,* 7–15.

Dohrenwend, B. S., Dohrenwend, B. P., Dodson, M., & Strout, P. E. (1984). Symptoms, hassles, social supports, and life events: Problem of confounding measures. *Journal of Abnormal Psychology, 93,* 222–230.

Erikson, E. (1963). *Childhood and society.* New York: Norton.

Erikson, E. (1976). Reflections on Dr. Borg's life cycle. *Daedelus, 105*(2), 1–28.

Erikson, E. (1982). *The life cycle completed.* New York: Norton.

Freud, S. (1898). Sexuality in the aetiology of the neuroses. In J. Strachey (Ed.), *The standard edition of the complete psychological works of Sigmund Freud (Vol. 3)* (pp. 261–285). London: Hogarth Press.

Freud, S. (1917). Mourning and melancholia. In J. Strachey (Ed.), *The standard edition of the complete psychological works of Sigmund Freud (Vol. 14)* (pp. 237–258). London: Hogarth Press.

Gartner, A., & Riessman, F. (1977). *Self-help in the human services.* San Francisco: Jossey-Bass.

Gigy, L. (1982). Women's adjustment to retirement: Use of the personal past. (Unpublished doctoral dissertation, University of California, San Francisco).

Gould, R. (1978). *Transformations: Growth and change in adult life.* New York: Simon and Schuster.

Gutmann, D. (1987). *Reclaimed powers: Towards a psychology of men and women in later life.* New York: Basic Books.

Gutmann, D., Griffin, B., & Grunes, J. (1982). Developmental contributions to the late-onset affective disorders. In P. Baltes & O. Brim (Eds.), *Life-span development and behavior* (pp. 244–263). New York: Academic Press.

Jacobs, S., & Myers, J. (1976). Recent life events and acute schizophrenic psychosis: A controlled study. *Journal of Nervous and Mental Disease, 162,* 75–87.

Jaques, E. (1965). Death and the mid-life crisis. *International Journal of Psychoanalysis, 46,* 502–514.

Jung, C. (1933). *Modern man in search of a soul.* New York: Harcourt, Brace, & World.

Kandler, K. S. (1988). The genetics of schizophrenia and related disorders. In D. L. Donner, E. S. Gershon, & J. E. Barrett (Eds.), *Relatives at risk for mental disorder.* New York: Raven Press.

Kernberg, O. (1980). Normal narcissism in middle age. In O. Kernberg (Ed.), *Internal world and external reality: Object relations theory applied* (pp. 121–134). New York: Jason Aronson.

Lazarus, R. S., & Folkman, S. (1984). *Stress, appraisal and coping.* New York: Springer.

Lehmann, H. (1975). Schizophrenia: Clinical features. (1975). In A. Freedman, H. Kaplan, & G. Sadock (Eds.), *Comprehensive textbook of psychiatry II* (Vol. 1, 2nd ed.). Baltimore, MD: Williams & Wilkins.

Levinson, D., Darrow, G., Klein, E., Levinson, M., & McKee, B. (1978). *The seasons of a man's life.* New York: Knopf.

Lieberman, M. A. (1991). Patterns of grieving and long-term adaptation. (Unpublished manuscript.)

Lieberman, M. A. (1992). A re-examination of adult life crises: Spousal loss in mid and late life. In G. H. Pollock (Ed.), *The course of life.* New York: International Universities Press.

Lieberman, M. A., and Borman, L. (1979). *Self-help groups for coping with crises: Origins, members, processes and impact.* San Francisco: Jossey-Bass.

Lieberman, M. A., Heller, K., & Mullan, J. (1990). Predicting effects of social network and social supports on adaptation. (Unpublished manuscript.)

Neugarten, B. (1968). Adult personality: Toward a psychology of the life cycle. In B. Neugarten (Ed.), *Middle age and aging* (pp. 137–147). Chicago: The University of Chicago Press.

Osterweis, M., Solomon, F., & Green, M. (1984). (Eds.), *Bereavement: Reactions, consequences, and care.* Washington, DC: National Academy Press.

Paykel, E. S. (1979). Causal relations between clinical depression and life events. In J. E. Barrett, R. M. Rose, & G. L. Klerman (Eds.), *Stress and mental disorder.* New York: Raven Press.

Pearlin, L. I., and Lieberman, M. A. (1979). Social sources of emotional and distress. *Research in Community and Mental Health, 1,* 217–248.

Peskin, H. (1987). Uses of the past in the adult lifespan. In G. Maddox & E. Busse (Eds.), *Aging: The universal human experience* (pp. 432–440). New York: Springer.

Peskin, H., & Gigy, L. (1977). Time perspective in adult transitions. In symposium, *Transitions and the adult life course.* Gerontological Society of America, San Francisco.

Peskin, H., & Livson, N. (1981). Uses of the past in adult psychological health. In D. Eichorn, J. Clausen, N. Haan, M. Honzik, & P. Mussen (Eds.), *Present and past in middle life.* New York: Academic Press.

Pollock, G. (1961). Mourning and adaptation. *International Journal of Psychoanalysis, 42,* 341–361.

Rabkin, J. G. (1980). Stressful life events and schizophrenia: A review of the research literature. *Psychological Bulletin, 87,* No. 2, 408–425.

Raphael, B. (1983). *The anatomy of bereavement.* New York: Basic Books.

Roberts, A. H. (1964). Housebound housewife: A follow-up study of a phobic anxiety state. *British Journal of Psychiatry, 110,* 191–197.

Serban, G. (1974). Relationship between pre- and post-morbid psychological stress on schizophrenics. *Psychological Reports, 35,* 507–517.

Serban, G. (1975). Stress in normals and schizophrenics. *British Journal of Psychiatry, 126,* 394–407.

Shafar, S. (1976). Aspects of phobic illness: A study of 90 research cases. *British Journal of Medical Psychology, 49* (3), 221–236.

Silver, R. L., & Wortman, C. B. (1980). Coping with undesirable life events. In J. Garber, & M. E. P. Seligman, (Eds.), *Human helplessness: Theory and applications* (pp. 279–375). New York: Academic Press.

Sim, M., & Houghton, H. (1966). Phobic anxiety and its treatment. *Journal of Nervous and Mental Disease, 143,* 484–491.

Thoits, P. A. (1983). Dimensions of life events that influence psychological distress: An evaluation and synthesis of the literature. In H. B. Kaplan (Ed.), *Psychosocial stress: Trends in theory and research* (pp. 33–103). New York: Academic Press.

Vachon, M. L. S. (1976). Grief and bereavement following the death of a spouse. *Canadian Psychiatric Journal, 21:* 35–44.

Wortman, C. B., & Silver, R. L. (1987). Coping with irrevocable loss. In G. L. Vanden Bos & B. K. Bryant (Eds.), *Cataclysms, crises, and catastrophes: Psychology in action* (pp. 189–233). Washington, DC: American Psychiatric Association.

Yalom, I., and Lieberman, M. A. (1991). Spousal bereavement and heightened existential awareness. *Psychiatry* (in press).

Neuroscience and Aging

6

Structural Changes in the Aging Brain

Arnold B. Scheibel

I. Introduction
II. Historical Evolution of Ideas
III. Gross Changes
IV. Microscopic Changes
   A. The Problem of Neuron Loss
   B. Changes in Neuronal Structure and Organization
   C. Dendrite Systems
V. Changes in the Vascular System
VI. Structural Change and Behavioral Change: An Overview
   References

I. Introduction

Therefore my age is as a lusty winter, Frosty but kindly
William Shakespeare, As You Like It, Act 2

The phenomenon of aging should be considered a part of a continuous developmental sequence commencing with embryogenesis and proceeding through a number of maturational phases during the lifespan of the organism. In many respects, brain tissue may be the most revealing mirror for this process since the neuron is essentially nonreplaceable. For those neurons that persist throughout the massive replicative phases of early and mid-pregnancy and the almost equally dramatic pruning phenomena of the late gestational and perinatal periods, the maturative, adult, and aging periods represent a continuous time for evolutionary adaptation and physical self-maintenance. The structural picture that nerve cells show at each phase of this continuum can be taken in a sense as index, both of the particular phase of the individual's lifespan, and the relative state of health or dysfunction at the time.

Cutler (1982) has emphasized the correlation between the longevity of an individual and its dependence for its evolutionary success on 'learned behavior' as opposed to 'instinctive behavior' (p. 2). The increasing lifespan, which has characterized recent human history, may reflect both the progressive increment in our learned behavior and the increasing challenge the nonreplicating neuronal population must face as a result of this increased longevity. This latter factor may be in part responsible for the still-blurred interface between normal healthy aging and the various manifestations of age-related disease. We may safely state at the outset that a broad range of age-related alterations occur in the structural matrix, from brain to brain, just as there is marked variation in the degree of cognitive, motor and psychosocial intactness among the aged. Indeed, one can plot a spectrum of psychopathology and histopathology ranging from those individuals demented and dying of Alzheimer's presenile dementia during their late 40s and 50s, to those who may be approaching their hundredth year while still alert, active, and reasonably productive. Our major goal will be to describe the structural characteristics of healthy aged brain tissue and to contrast this with the manifestations of pathological aging. Even now, this represents a problematic area, and a short review of the historical aspects of this problem emphasizes its inherent ambiguities.

II. Historical Evolution of Ideas

Remarkably little notice can be found in the anatomical or medical literature concerning age or dementia-related structural change in the brain until the observations of the English pathologist, Baillie. In 1795 he noted that the brains of very old patients were sometimes considerably firmer than those of younger individuals, and in some of these, the ventricles were enlarged and "full of water" (Baillie, 1977). The first clear-cut description of brain atrophy is probably attributable to Wilks (1864), who remarked on this change in senile dementia as well as in central nervous system (CNS) syphilis and chronic alcoholism. His description of the hemispheres is remarkably modern. "Instead of the sulci meeting, they are widely separated and their intervals filled with serum and which, on being removed with the pia mater, the full depth of the sulci can be seen" (Wilks, p. 383). Clouston (1911) remarked on the progression from focal softening to atrophy of parts or all of the hemispheres (Clouston, p. 649) while Alzheimer (1907), in his famous description of the brain of a demented 51-year-old woman from a Frankfurt "insane asylum," noted widespread atrophy and arteriosclerotic changes in the larger cerebral vessels. In addition, he described unusual, thickened intraneuronal fibrillar tangles, which seemed to persist after neuronal death, and finally, large numbers of miliary foci made up of a peculiar substance that could often be recognized without staining. Simchowitz (1910) further enlarged the picture with his discussions of granulovacuolar degeneration. The overall picture of age- and dementia-related structural changes was therefore essentially in place by the beginning of the second decade of the twentieth century. Despite the rising tide of relevant literature, especially during the past 30 years, it is remarkable how little more has been added, even with the use of increasingly powerful technological tools.

III. Gross Changes

The process of aging exerts its effects on all organs of the body, and the brain is no exception. Some degree of loss of substance seems to be the most obvious characteristic of the normal aging process, but the degree of alteration varies enormously among subjects. The unique combination of genetic and epigenetic factors each individual represents is powerfully reflected in brain structure and function. Indeed, the brain of a vigorous 80-year-old patient may show fewer changes than that of an individual 20 years his junior. This spectrum of age-related patterns is further enhanced by the range of dementing illnesses to which the individual is increasingly vulnerable as the course of life progresses. In this section we will review some of these alterations, with one caveat. Excluding overt progressive pathological processes such as Alzheimer's disease and multi-infarct dementia, we remain uncertain as to the relative contributions of the intrinsic biologic aging process, and that provided by the cognitive, motor, and psychological *slowing,* which most of us seem to consider an inevitable part of growing old. Abundant experimental evidence (Diamond, Johnson & Ingham, 1975, Diamond, 1988; Greenough, Juraska & Volkmar, 1979) suggests that the old dictum, "Use it or lose it," may be just as applicable to brain tissue as it is to muscle tissue. For that reason, the following descriptions of brain specimens can be taken at face value, but with the realization that they have not been correlated with the histories and lifestyles of the individuals who originally used them.

In general, the brain decreases in size as a function of age, while the leptomeninges become thickened, opaque, and increasingly adherent. As the cerebral convolutions tend to narrow and the sulci to widen, an excess of cerebrospinal fluid collects between the leptomeninges and the cortical surface. The pattern of gyral atrophy (Figure 1), noted most usually in the frontal and temporal regions, varies widely, and in some cases may escape detection by the naked eye. Except in the case of the *old* old (i.e., beyond age 75), most brain shrinkage appears due to loss of mass in the white matter. The ventricular system is often (although not always) enlarged to visual examination. Brain weight, while not considered, in and of itself, a reliable measure of age-related change, does tend to decline after the fourth decade. If the average weight of the male brain is 1399.8 g at age 20, it is 1360.8 g between the ages of 41 and 50; 1,337.6 g between 51 and 60; 1306.4 g between 61 and 70; 1265.9 g between 71 and 80; and 11790.9 g beyond the age of 80 (Greenfield, 1967). It is calculated that the *free space* between brain and skull approximately doubles between the ages of 20 and 70. These changes are all intensified in the presence of the dementias, the specific pattern again depending on the disease and the time of onset. Gyral atrophy and ventricular widening often appear greater in the presenile form of Alzheimer's disease than in the senile variant. Narrowing of the convolutions and widening of the sulci may be generalized or primarily obvious over one or more of the major lobes, e.g., (pre) frontal and temporo-parietal. White matter pathology, primarily softening or infarction, may be seen in Alzheimer's disease (Englund, Brun, & Persson, 1987), although not so frequently or intensively as that described in the Binswanger type of vascular dementia (Olszewski, 1962).

The development of noninvasive imaging techniques over the past 15 years has

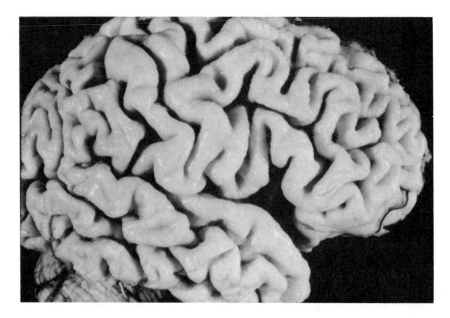

Figure 1   Cerebral hemisphere from an 85-year-old individual with symptoms of moderate dementia. Note generalized marked gyral atrophy and increased width of sulci.

contributed significant information on the processes of brain maturation and aging and also on the structural concomitants of the developing dementias. A number of studies of normally aging individuals employed computed tomography (CT) to determine brain morphometrics (Gyldensted, 1977; Brinkman, Sarwar, Leven & Morris, 1981; Schwartz *et al.,* 1985). Although several different techniques of measurement were used, all reported varying amounts of age-related loss of grey and/or white matter and progressive dilation of cerebrospinal fluid spaces. The total volume of grey matter was correlated negatively with age, while the volume of cerebrospinal fluid showed an age-positive correlation. "The volume of the lateral and third ventricles was elevated in the elderly, and volumes of the thalamus and lenticular nuclei were reduced" (Schwartz *et al.,* 1985; p. 146). Several reports refer specifically to cortical atrophy in the left temporal region, particularly in those presumably normal elderly showing benign senescent forgetfulness. However, conflicting data have been reported on the relationship between ventricular size and increasing cognitive impairment. Problems in establishing the position of the brain–ventricular borders with some degree of rigor are presumed to be largely responsible for the discrepancies in results. With improved methodology it now appears that there is some degree of ventricular enlargement with normal aging and an additional enhancement in size, proportional to the degree of cognitive deficit. However, correlative measures between ventricular enlargement and cognitive levels remain relatively weak (George *et al.,* 1983). The ventricular:brain ratio has proven a more reliable yardstick for correlation with neuropsychologic performance. Correlation coefficients of 0.725 or better are reported by Eslinger, Damasio, Graff-Radford,, & Damasio (1984).

A rapidly developing body of literature documents the robust correlation between the dementias and CT scans. Creasey, Schwartz, Fredericksen, Hoxby, and Rapoport (1986) found significantly larger degrees of brain atrophy and ventricular dilation in patients with senile dementia, Alzheimer type (DAT) compared to age-matched, nondemented controls. Male patients with mild dementia showed larger mean third-ventricle volumes, while those with more severe dementia showed increased volume of lateral and third ventricles, and reduced amounts of grey matter. "Statistically significant and appropriate correlations between several dementia scales and CT measures in the DAT patients indicated that brain atrophy and ventricular dilation were related to the severity of the dementia" (Creasey *et al.*, 1986; p. 1563). These results agree with studies such as those of Gado *et al.* (1982) who found that volumetric indices of ventricular and sulcal size as determined by pixel counts for demented subjects were very significantly greater than those for age-matched controls ($p < 0.0001$). In contrast, Bigler, Hubler, Cullum, and Turkheimer (1985) found no significant difference between ventricular size and performance on Wechsler Adult Intelligence (WAIS) or Wechsler Memory Scales (WMS). However, the index of cerebral atrophy was found to correlate negatively with various performance measures of the WAIS and WMS.

The clash of data revealed by these studies undoubtedly attests not only to the considerable variation in the ways in which gross brain structure reflects those processes related to aging and senescence, but also to problems inherent in quantification of CT and magnetic resonance imaging (MRI) scans. However, the unique capability of the MRI to explore tissue resonance phenomena after radio excitation (relaxation time, T_1, T_2) has added another type of insight to studies of this kind, i.e., white matter abnormalities. As an example, Henderson *et al.* (1988) describe "confluent perifocal periventricular white matter hyper-intensity on T_2 weighted images in 75% (15 of 20) of elderly demented patients (137). Other types of dementia-related white matter lesions can now be described in multi-infarct dementia, Binswanger's disease and Jacob-Creutzfeld disease using similar techniques (Brun, 1988). Although the resolution capacity of such methods is unlikely to increase indefinitely, it seems clear that they have already added powerful tools to the qualitative and quantitative description of the processes of brain aging. While beyond the scope of this chapter (see chapter by Grady and Rapoport, this volume) it should be added that positron emission tomography (PET) has already revealed impressive dementia-related alterations in metabolic patterns throughout the cerebral cortex and particularly in frontal, parietal, and temporal association cortices, with little or no changes in primary sensory and motor areas, basal ganglia, and cerebellum (Kuhl, 1986; Haxby & Rapoport, 1988). Thus the way has been opened to follow the development and progression of age- and dementia-related processes in specific brain structures.

IV. Microscopic Changes

The literature that addresses the problem of age- and dementia-related histological change in the central nervous system is both rapidly growing and tenaciously enigmatic. There are many reasons for the problematic nature of these data. A host of technological factors must be considered including problems in obtaining specimens, intervals between death and tissue fixation, the selection of methods for tissue preparation, modes of study, both qualitative and quantitative, and techniques for assessing and reporting the data. There are inherent limitations in the stop-frame method of investigation to which we are limited by the methods of histology and pathology. These provide us with one *look* at the specimen, frozen in time, and without relationship to the earlier or later characteristic of the same brain. This, in turn, introduces the single overarching problem of any type of analysis of human brain material, the enormous interindividual variation. Each brain is obviously the product of its own unique genomic pattern. However, we now realize that the genes paint with broad strokes and that epigenetic factors, the idiosyncratic input stimuli and life experiences of each individual, sculpt the final product (Diamond, Johnson, & Ingham, 1975; Diamond, Johnson, & Gold, 1977; Greenough, *et al.* 1979). Patterns of aging are as variable as personality, and the challenge and stress of 50 years of life for one individual may exceed that of 80 years for another. Accordingly, descriptions of age-related histological changes in the brain must be considered approximations, those alterations most likely to be found under the *bell-shaped curve* at any one epoch, but with the understanding that these are at best models that may bear little relevance to the individual *normally aging* subject with whom we are concerned.

In addition to these considerations, the entire range of age-related dementias add further variables to the picture. Although Alzheimer's disease and multi-infarct dementia cannot be considered part of normal aging, they share—in greatly augmented form— many of the structural and perhaps chemical characteristics of normal aging. Some believe that we are dealing with a spectrum of phenomena and that senile dementias such as Alzheimer's disease represent an intensification, or better, a caricature of the normal aging process. For others, it is a discrete syndrome or group of syndromes that develop, preferentially, within the matrix of an aging nervous system. We will discuss those histological manifestations most often found in brain tissue of the healthy aged human subject, with the already mentioned caveats, and then contrast them with the much more robust alterations usually seen in the most frequent age-related dementia, Alzheimer's disease.

A. The Problem of Neuron Loss

One of the most popular bromides about aging is that we lose 100,000 nerve cells each day. It is not clear how this sobering figure was arrived at, but it is safe to say that the problem of age-related neuron loss has been of formal interest for almost 100 years. The pioneering study of Hodge (1894) set the stage for such concerns by demonstrating age-related nerve cell loss in both humans and honey bees. More than a half century later, the much-quoted but inadequately controlled work of Brody (1955, 1970) appeared to provide strong support for this idea by reporting decreases in neuron density in the superior temporal gyrus of 50 to 60% between the age of 18 and 95. The superior frontal gyrus showed a 50% density decrease over an almost equivalent interval, while primary sensory and motor cortical strips showed apparent losses of approximately one half as much. All cortical layers seemed to participate in this loss, with the greatest declines in layers II and IV.

The general concept of age-related loss of neurons in human brain tissue has been supported by many (but not all) studies (Shefer, 1973; Mouritzen Dam, 1979; Miller,

Alston, Mountjoy, & Corsellis, 1984). With this has come the concomitant realization that patterns of loss are both lamina-specific and region-specific. In addition, it is increasingly clear as Coleman and Flood (1987) have pointed out, that *two-point studies* may be insufficiently sensitive to pick up maturation and age-related changes that are not monotonic. Furthermore, it seems very likely that the increasingly robust decrements in cell number occurring in the eighth and ninth decades of life may still pale before the massive elimination of neurons effected during the late prenatal and perinatal periods. A still unanswered question is the degree to which old-age–related inactivity and terminal physical disease may contribute to the picture of neuronal pathology and loss noted in neurohistological brain specimens from other patients. It is interesting to note in passing that careful multiepoch studies of aging rat cortex, reveal "significant decrease in the density of neurons between 41 and 108 days of age, followed by stability in number until 904 days of age" (Diamond, 1988; p. 47).

Another variable in the pattern of age-related cell loss in the human cerebrum is cell size. Using automated cell-counting methods, Terry, DeTeresa, and Hansen (1987) described a selective decrease in density of large neurons and an apparent increase in the density of small cells. They attributed this phenomenon to shrinkage of the large neurons, an interpretation that has problematic aspects because of the possibility of mistaking neuroglia for small nerve cells. Although Terry and colleagues were aware of this possibility and resorted to on-line editing of the computer-operated system, age-related increase in astroglia plus decreasing cortical volume (Hubbard & Anderson, 1981) undoubtedly provide reason for residual concern about these results.

Data derived from analysis of limbic system structures generally echo the theme of moderate but consistent age-related loss of cells. Hippocampal pyramidal cells are lost at a rate of somewhere between 4 and 10% per decade (Mouritzen Dam, 1979; Anderson, Hubbard, Coghill, & Sliders, 1983; Miller *et al.*, 1984). Disappearance of dentate granule cells seems to occur primarily in the *older old*. Mouritzen Dam (1979) reported losses of 15% when comparing a younger (21–56 years) with an older (68–91 years) group. Cell loss also occurs in the amygdala, but curiously enough, only in the phylogenetically *older* (cortico-medial) portions (Beal & Martin, 1986).

A much more varied picture is presented by subcortical structures. Cerebellar Purkinje cells show modest progressive loss in both cerebellar hemispheres (Hall, Miller, & Corsellis, 1975) and vermis (Torvik, Torp, & Linboe, 1986). Data relating to the far more numerous granule cells seem inconclusive thus far, although structural changes, if not loss, of granule cell axons (parallel fibers) may occur. The picture remains equally confusing with regard to the basal ganglia, but there is consensus that most brain stem and cranial nerve nuclei (with a few notable exceptions) remain essentially intact.

Of particular interest are those subcortical nuclei associated with the production and distribution of acetylcholine and the catecholamines. The nucleus basalis of Meynert of the basal forebrain complex is recognized as one of the primary sources of cholinergic innervation of the forebrain. In view of the postulated relationship of this neurotransmitter with a number of very significant cognitive activities including memory, it is interesting to note the clash of data on this subject. Marked neuronal loss has been reported by Mann, Yates, and Marcyniuk (1984) and by the McGeer group (McGeer, McGeer, Suzuki, Dolman, & Nagai, 1984) while Chui, Bondareff, Zarow, and Slazer (1984) and Whitehouse, *et al.* (1983) noticed no decrement in cell numbers. The reasons behind these conflicting reports are difficult to understand. However, it should be noted that the first two reports that found cell loss included data from children, while the others used only material from adults over 25 years of age. As Coleman and Flood (1987) have pointed out in their detailed review, this might indicate that a significant portion of whatever neuron loss occurs here, may in fact occur early in life, with relatively more stable numbers being maintained from adulthood into old age. There is more consensus on the age-related loss of pigmented neurons in the catecholaminergic locus ceruleus, subceruleus, and the noradrenergic cell group (A2) of the vagal motor nuclear complex (Mann, Yates, and Hawkes, 1983; Vijayashankar & Brody, 1979; Tomlinson, Irving, & Blessed, 1981; Mann *et al.* 1984). Pigmented neurons are also apparently lost in the substantia nigra, although the temporal patterns and amounts of loss are less clear (McGeer, McGeer, & Suzuki, 1977; Mann *et al.,* 1984).

The actual significance of numerical measures of cell loss has been called into question by Bondareff (1987). For example, there appears to be a disproportionately small loss of norepinephrine (NE) in anterior cingulate cortex (2%) relative to neuronal loss (27%) in the locus ceruleus (Bondareff, Mountjoy, Roth, Rossor, & Iversen, unpublished data, quoted by Bondareff, 1987) in Alzheimer patients beyond 79 years of age at death. On the other hand, a more proportionate relationship exists between cortical neurotransmitter loss and parent neuronal loss, i.e., cortical NE loss, 65%; loss of locus coruleus neurons, 48%, in Alzheimer patients dying before the age of 79. Bondareff (1987) postulates that decreased levels of cortical neurotransmitter may reflect down-regulation of enzyme synthesis in surviving neurons of origin in younger Alzheimer patients, whereas in the older patient group, the surviving neurons may be capable of working at a higher level of efficiency, compensating for decreased levels of cortical NE. This interpretation is attractive in view of the generally more malignant nature of earlier appearing (presenile) Alzheimer syndromes, which almost invariably involve greater brain tissue destruction, increased levels of senile plaques and tangles (see next section) and shortened life expectancy.

B. Changes in Neuronal Structure and Organization

A significant number of presumably age-related alterations in the morphology of neurons has been described during the past century. The possibility that cell bodies may change in size (e.g., the decrease in size or shrinkage of large pyramidal cells), has already been alluded to in the previous section. Of even greater interest is the probability that discrete populations of neurons may undergo selective alterations of intrasomal and dendritic structure resulting in atrophy and loss. A noteworthy example of this process occurs in the case of the giant pyramidal cells of Betz, and will be discussed in detail later.

The most prominent and widespread age-related changes of a structural nature are undoubtedly the development of intrasomal inclusions. Accumulations of lipochrome bodies or lipofuscins (Borst, 1922) are found in the vast majority of nerve cell bodies by the seventh or eighth decade of life, and there is reason to believe that they begin to appear much earlier. Knowledge of their origin and pathogenesis and their impact upon cell function remain unsatisfactory. In terms of their staining reactions, it seems clear that they are acid fast periodic acid–Schiff (PAS)-positive, and oil-red-O positive. They are believed to represent pigmented cellular waste products (Figure 2), the accumulated residues of incompletely degraded membrane fragments from lysosomes and perhaps mitochondria (Minckler, 1968). They are not believed to be toxic in and of themselves, but like most of the other cellular inclusions we will discuss, may prove ultimately injurious to the cell by occupying intrasomal space needed for the protein-synthesizing machinery (i.e., the endoplasmic reticulum and Golgi bodies) of the cell. Some support for this emerges from the study of Hydén and Lindstrom (1950), who showed that ribonuclease is inactive in areas of cytoplasm containing the yellow pigment and that an inverse relationship exists between the amount of yellow pigment and ribonucleic acid content of the cell. However, lipofuscin pigments may appear as early as the sixth postnatal year in the inferior olive, a nucleus now recognized to maintain its full complement of neurons throughout life (Vijayashankar & Body, 1977).

Granulovacuolar degeneration is largely confined to the large pyramids of the hippocampal formation and subiculum. It is characterized by the presence of 1 μ argyrophilic core granules contained in vacuoles of 3 to 5 μ in diameter. The vacuole is membrane-bound and the core is electron dense. The structures tend to congregate near the apical end of the neuron and gradually displace intracytoplasmic RNA. The regional predilection

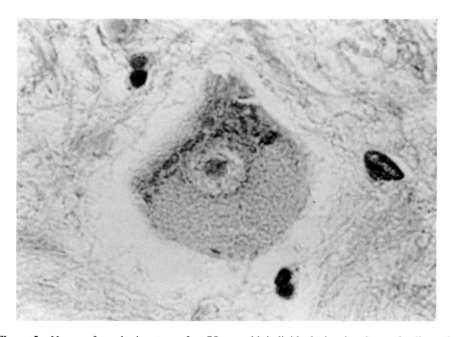

Figure 2 Neuron from brain stem of a 75-year-old individual showing heavy loading with lipofuscin granules. Note that the protein-synthesizing organelles of the cytoplasm such as the endoplasmic reticulum are compressed into a small fraction of the cell body volume. Cresyl violet stain. Original magnification ×980.

(subiculum and field H. of the cornu Ammonis) suggests to some that a common neuro-transmitter substrate, possibly acetylcholine, may be involved (Ball, 1983). Mention may also be made of the Hirano body, an eosinophilic rod type of inclusion, 15–30 μ in length, sometimes seen in hippocampal pyramids. The nature and pathogenesis of this structure remain uncertain (Brun, 1983).

The presence of skein-like tangles of fibers within nerve cell bodies was first described by Alois Alzheimer (1907) in the brain of a demented 51-year-old woman. These neu-rofibrillary tangles (Figure 3) have become one of the hallmarks of Alzheimer's disease and undoubtedly represent the single most destructive intracellular inclusion. They are of more than passing interest to any student of the normally healthy aging brain because of their presence in small numbers in the healthy aged individual. They were initially identified in reduced silver stains but can readily be identified by their green birefringence in polarized light after staining with Congo red. In this attribute they resemble amyloid-containing senile plaques, although the similarity is believed more likely due to certain physical (a β-pleated sheet secondary structure) rather than to chemical similarities.

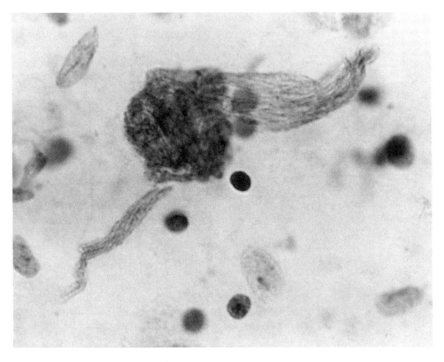

Figure 3   Neurofibrillary tangles in a pyramidal cell of the hippocampal cortex of a patient with senile dementia of Alzheimer. Tangles in the cell body tend to be arranged in swirls or packets, while those in the apical and basal dendrites are arranged in linear ensembles. These structures are immunohistochemically stained by antibody to paired helical filaments (donated by Dr. D.J. Selkoe) and counterstained with cresyl violet. Final print magnification ×990. (Courtesy of Dr. Taihung Duong).

Tangles are found primarily in cortical pyramidal cells and are especially noticeable in hippocampal pyramidal cells of Sommer's sector and in association areas (frontal and temporal) of the neocortex. They have also been described in the amygdala, basal forebrain, and in catecholaminergic nuclei of the brain stem.

At the ultrastructural level, they are composed of paired helical filaments (PHF). Each filament of a pair is 10–12 nM in diameter and wound around the adjacent fiber of the pair in a left-handed helical configuration with a half periodicity of 80 nM (Kidd, 1963; Terry, Gonatas, & Weiss, 1964). The PHF is totally unlike either neurofilaments or microtubules, and there is no major immunocytochemical cross-reaction with these normal elements of the neuronal endoskeleton. However, some studies indicate that certain polyclonal and monoclonal antibodies to neurofilaments may stain tangles *in situ*, the reason for which is not yet clear (Miller, Haugh, Kahn, & Anderton, 1986). The source and pathogenesis of PHFs are unknown, but some investigators have suggested that posttranslational modifications occurring within the affected neurons may lead to their development (Iqbal & Wisniewski, 1983). Ihara and Kondo (1989) have recently reported that PHFs are composed entirely of ubiquitin in conjugated form and tau protein. The remarkable stability of the tangles in both fresh and frozen tissue, their insolubility under physiological conditions, and their resistance to proteolytic digestion and even to mild acids and alkalis provide some hint to their capacity for producing permanent damage once they are laid in the cell.

The senile plaque, the other major hallmark of Alzheimer's disease, is, like the neurofibrillary tangle, also invariably present in brain tissue of the normally aging individual, but again, in very much reduced numbers. Although described previously, the relationship of the plaque to human dementias was first documented by Alzheimer (1907) and Simchowitz (1910). Plaques are essentially foci of neuropil destruction surrounding, in most cases, a central core of amyloid (Figure 4). *Primitive* plaques consist primarily of degenerating neuronal and glial processes surrounding a fine feltwork of amyloid fibers. *Classic* plaques are presumably more completely developed and consist of a central amyloid core surrounded by neuroglia and fragmented masses of neuronal processes. In some cases, the amyloid plaque appears to stand alone. They are easily made visible in light microscope preparations through a number of stains including hematoxylin and eosin, PAS, Congo red, thioflavin S, reduced silver, etc. Electron microscopy indicates that the amyloid fibers are made up of paired helical filaments, although appreciably smaller and somewhat differently organized than those constituting the neurofibrillary tangles (Wisniewski, 1983). In the normal aging brain and in Alzheimer's disease, plaques are most likely to be seen in the second and third layers of frontal and temporal association cortices and in the hippocampus, but may be particularly obvious in cerebellar cortex in other dementias like kuru and Creutzfeld-Jakob disease. Some, but not all, investigators stress the preferential perivascular position of plaques.

As with almost every other histological or histopathological component of the aging and/or dementing brain, there is no clearcut idea as to the pathogenesis of these structures. Some investigators believe that degenerating neurons and their processes release neurofilament proteins, which combine in the extracellular space with locally present glycoproteins and glycosaminoglycans to form amyloid. Others favor the possibility that microglia and pericytes of the brain's reticuloendothelial system either process the compo-

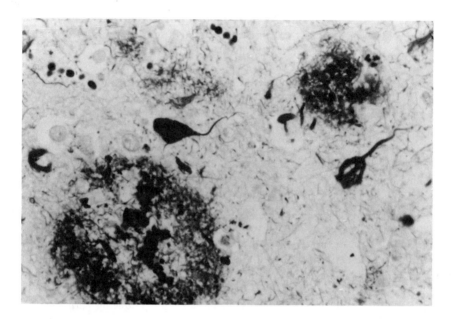

Figure 4   Entorhinal cortex of a patient with senile dementia of Alzheimer showing senile plaques and several neurons with neuro-fibrillary tangles. The larger plaque has an easily visible central core of amyloid. The black-staining neuron in the center of the field appears solidly filled with abnormal neurofibrillar material. Reduced silver stain. Original magnification ×440.

nents mentioned above or produce the amyloid, *de novo,* following stimulation by external antigens (Wisniewski, Vorhodt, Moretz, Lossinsky & Grundke-Igbal 1982; Wisniewski, 1983). In either case, microglia and pericytes would seem intimately involved in the ultimate processing of the protein(s) into the familiar β-pleated sheets characteristic of plaque amyloid (Glenner, 1980). A somewhat different hypothesis has been advanced by Miyakawa and Kuramoto (1989) who believe that amyloid fibrils are produced in the basement membrane of capillary endothelial cells in degenerating capillaries and are subsequently projected into the surrounding parenchyma where they become the nidus around which senile plaques develop. Such a pattern of pathogenesis could account for the apparent perivascular position of many plaques already mentioned.

For our purposes, the important thing to remember is that both plaques and tangles are present in limited numbers in the nondemented aged individual. Quantitative studies by Tomlinson, Blessed, and Roth (1968, 1970) stress their range of densities in brain tissue from older patients and have demonstrated an approximately linear relationship between increasing numbers of plaques and tangles per high-powered microscopic field and developing dementia.

C. Dendrite Systems

The dendrite arbors of neurons constitute 80 to 95% of the total synaptic receptive surface area of each neuron (Aitken & Bridger, 1967; Schade & Baxter, 1960). Anatomical and functional integrity of these structures is accordingly vital to every aspect of cognitive function and behavior. The number of synaptic terminals present in each neuronal soma–dendrite element varies enormously with the site and with the age of the organism, and probably with the intensity with which that particular neural subsystem is used. Computations by a number of investigators suggest that there may be as few as several thousand terminals on a small spinal cord neuron, and as many as 300,000 to 500,000 terminals on a cerebellar Purkinje cell. Dendritic growth begins shortly after the primitive neurons have assumed their final position in the central nervous system (e.g., the cortical plate of archicortex or neocortex, and the mantle layer of spinal cord) and continues during infancy, childhood, and puberty. The pace of development slows during maturity, and regression becomes manifest in the aged, particularly in the very old (i.e., beyond age 75). On the other hand, experimental data suggest that some degree of dendritic plasticity in response to environmental challenge may continue into very old age (Diamond, 1988). Accordingly, we must assume that although the growth–regression balance swings in favor of regression in the later stages of life, some capacity for growth and repair undoubtedly continues to exist if environmental conditions are optimal.

Both qualitative (Scheibel, Lindsay, Tomiyasu, & Scheibel, 1975, 1976; Scheibel, Tomiyasu, & Scheibel, 1977) and quantitative (Nakamura, Akiguchi, Kaneyama, & Mizuno, 1985; Coleman & Flood, 1987) studies of aging human cortices reveal dendritic regression in the very old. However, residual dendritic plasticity is dramatically demonstrated by the net dendritic growth in layer II pyramidal neurons of the parahippocampal gyrus (Buell & Coleman, 1979). Some of this increment may be responsive to limited loss of neurons, which Coleman and Flood (1986) postulate can reactively stimulate increased dendrite sprouting in adjacent cells. This would appear to provide dramatic demonstration of the maintenance of integrity of neuropil during a period of gradual neuronal loss. However, the differential sensitivity of such reparative phenomena to age and site is emphasized in studies comparing old (18–20 years) and very old (27–28 years) macaque neocortex and subiculum by Cupp and Uemura (1980) and Uemura (1985).

Maintenance of the enormous number of interneuronal connections that characterizes the central nervous system is critically dependent on the integrity of the neuronal dendrite ensembles. Those cognitive changes in processing speed and *style* that develop, benignly during the process of normal aging, and more catastrophically in dementias such as Alzheimer's disease, can be related in large measure to the loss of dendrite surface, with resultant disappearance of synaptic connections and progressive restriction in the computational power of the brain. There are as yet no clear data on the minimal amount of neuronal and dendritic loss that can be recognized in the cognitive and psychosocial behavior of the individual. However, dendritic alterations, while suggestive of developing functional changes in the neuron, almost certainly do not in themselves indicate a dead or dying cell. There appears to be a spectrum of structural alterations that presage failure, but with which the cell may probably continue to live in an at least partially functioning state for some time. This sequence of changes can be identified by the appearance of many neurons studied in a number of brain specimens from patients of different ages and different degrees of cognitive intactness.

The sequence of dendritic alterations that will be followed here is best visualized, in human brain material at least, by some modification of the impregnation methods of Golgi. These rely for their effect on deposition of heavy metal salts (i.e., silver, mercury, etc.) along and within the suitably prepared protein structure of neurons and their dendritic and axonal processes. Progressive autolytic changes in nerve cell structure following death rapidly alter the original *in vivo* appearance of the neurons, making rapid initial fixation of brain tissue a requirement. In addition, the natural tendency of Golgi impregnations to stain only a small fraction of the neurons (both a strength and a drawback of the technique) provide constraints on the interpretation of the data. More precise morphological information can be obtained by modern visualization methods such as vital intracellular injection of horse-radish peroxidase, but such techniques are obviously possible only in experimental animals. Nonetheless, with proper controls and a sufficiently broad sampling, the Golgi methods have contributed significantly to our conceptions of the early stages of neuronal failure.

The range of age-related histological changes that can be followed in this way include loss of dendritic spines, irregular swelling of the neuron soma and initial segments of apical dendrite, progressive loss of basilar dendrite systems beginning with the most peripheral branches and proceeding inward along the dendrite tree, and in the final stages of neuronal dissolution, shrivelling, and fragmentation of the apical shaft (Figure 5). The sequence and tempo of these changes show marked interindividual variation. The dendritic structure of neurons in a healthy octogenarian may appear more intact than that of an

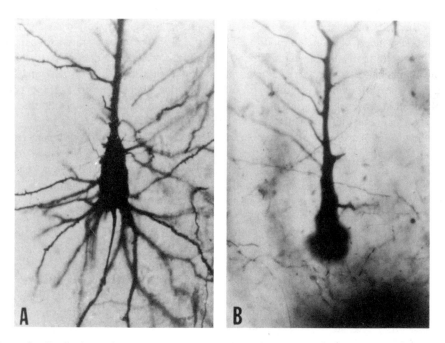

Figure 5   Comparison of a normal large cortical pyramidal neuron in a mature adult with a similar cell from an 80-year-old patient. Note the virtually complete loss of basilar dendrites, residual presence of apical dendrites and oblique branches, and globular misshapen cell body. Golgi method. Original magnification ×440.

apparently equally intact individual in the early sixties. The appearance of Alzheimer-type dementia, whether senile or presenile, accentuates the degree and compresses the timetable of the regressive process. With these provisos, the following description will serve as a model of late neuronal change, no matter what the age of onset, pace of progression, nor degree of involvement.

Early alterations include patchy loss of dendrite spines along various portions of the dendritic tree. These may be widespread or initially limited to a single dendrite branch. Portions of the dendrites become irregular and lumpy in outline, especially as they become denuded of spines. The lumpiness often appears initially at dendrite bifurcations and at the juncture of the apical shaft with the cell body. Dendrite changes are most obvious and appear to progress most quickly along the elements of the basilar dendrite ensemble. Structural changes in the apical dendrite system seem to progress more slowly, despite the progressive loss of oblique branches. The apical shaft is usually the last element of the neuron to undergo degenerative change before the disappearance of the neuron soma itself. This pattern of progression reverses that of dendritic growth and maturation in which the apical shaft appears earliest and the basilar system develops later. As the neuron undergoes degenerative changes, increased numbers of neuroglial cells surround the cell body and initial portions of the dendrites. These are mainly protoplasmic and fibrous astroglia, and the larger the neuron, the more obvious the glial involucrum (Scheibel *et al.*, 1977). The nerve cell body is progressively distorted in shape, an alteration that seems due to the development of intracellular inclusions like neurofibrillar tangles, granulovacuolar degeneration, and lipofuscins. In the Alzheimer patient, the neurons may finally disappear, leaving only the tangles and a few pigmented or radiopaque granules.

It is difficult to estimate the degree of dendritic change present in the various scenarios the aging brain may present. Quantitative studies by Buell and Coleman (1979) stress an actual net dendritic growth of layer II pyramids in the parahippocampal gyrus in the old (but not *very old*) individual, an increment which they assume may be compensatory to the loss of neighboring neurons. They also report "continuous decrease in dendritic extent of layer II pyramidal neurons in middle frontal gyrus (p. 855)" in similarly aged individuals, thereby emphasizing regional differences in the expression of age-related alterations. In our own experience, some of the most dramatic and widespread dendritic changes appear in the dendrite systems of the giant pyramidal cells of Betz in primary motor cortex of normally aging individuals. In these elements, dendritic alterations may appear as early as the fifth decade of life, and as many as 75% of the Betz cells may have been damaged or destroyed by the eighth decade (Scheibel *et al.*, 1977; Figure 6). This degree of involvement, however, seems unique to this neuronal population and is, to our present knowledge, matched by no other neuronal set in the normal aging brain.

When this picture is compared with that demonstrated by a patient suffering from Alzheimer's dementia, the most obvious change is the more widespread pattern of cellular damage in the latter. In many cases, 30 to 50% of all of the neurons in a field stained by the Golgi method and viewed at magnifications of 250x to 400x show moderate or widespread evidence of dendritic atrophy, and cell body swelling and distortion. Such fields are also richer in fibrous astroglia and in senile plaques, which can often be visualized simultaneously by this method.

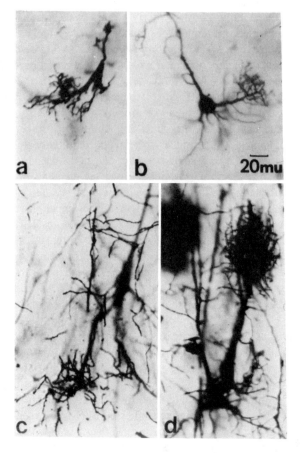

Figure 6   Degenerating neurons in the neocortex (a and b) and archicortex (c and d) of a patient with familial presenile Alzheimer's disease showing areas of newly developing dendritic tissue. Golgi stains. Original magnification ×440.

Two variations from this picture now appear to distinguish the neuropathological picture of presenile Alzheimer's disease from the more frequently occurring senile version:

1. In the former, which develops almost by definition in the late fifth or early sixth decade, the pace of the disease is often more rapid, and the neuropathology more florid. Dendritic damage is more widespread with often more than one half of the neurons in a Golgi-stained microscopic field involved in the process.
2. A more dramatic and idiosyncratic characteristic of the presenile form of the disease rests in the development along degenerating dendrite trees of dense clusters of new dendritic growth, the young shafts of which appear to be richly clothed in spines (Figure 6). This phenomenon of exuberant dendrite sprouting on an obviously dying neuron has been noted only in tissue from cases of familial

presenile dementia and in these cases, up to 25% of the neurons show the phenomenon (Scheibel and Tomiyasu, 1978). It has been seen in a number of areas of the cerebral neocortex, in the hippocampus and subiculum, and in the cerebellar cortex. Although the functional significance of this unexpected finding is at best speculative, it would appear to document the enormous potential for plasticity resident in even the most severely injured nerve cell.

The age- and senescence-related dendritic changes seen in the cerebral neocortices are reflected to varying degrees in cerebral archicortex, basal ganglia, and cerebellum. The dendrite systems of hippocampal granule cells demonstrate marked regression in the very old subject (Flood, Buell, DeFiore, Horwitz, & Coleman, 1985). In Alzheimer's disease, both hippocampus and dentate gyrus are severely affected, the latter losing 50–60% of its neurons. In the adjacent entorhinal cortex, the apical dendrite shafts of 20 to 30% of the deep pyramids show unusual persistence of dendrite spines and the development of spindle-like enlargements approximately one third to two thirds of the way along the shafts toward the pial surface (Scheibel *et al.*, 1976). Massive loss of dendrite arbors in the cerebellar Purkinje cells of dorsal vermis and posterior lobe have been described by Mehraein, Yamada, and Tarnowska-Dziduszko (1975). Somewhat similar changes have been noted in the basal forebrain, basal ganglia, and certain of the catecholaminergic nuclei of the brain stem, but these studies remain fragmentary and less completely documented.

V. Changes in the Vascular System

Age-related changes in the blood vessels of the central nervous system show as wide a range of inter-individual variation as do other components of the brain. One need only turn over the fixed brains from two 70-year-old patients and examine the vertebral–basilar arteries clinging to the inferior aspect of the brain stems. The one may be firm and irregularly distended, sclerotic, even *pipestem,* to palpation and studded with yellow or whitish plaques. In contrast, the other may be pliant and flexible, smooth-surfaced, and soft and mobile to palpation. To some extent, these contrasting appearances of a major vessel system provide some index to the state of the cerebral vasculature as a whole. On the other hand, despite the more obvious risks of cerebral infarction in the first patient, it is now clear that dementias of the Alzheimer type bear little or no relationship to this type of obvious cerebral arteriosclerosis. A close relationship may exist, however, with dementias of frankly vascular origin, e.g., multi-infarct and Binswanger types of lesions.

On the other hand, it should also be noted that gross vascular pathology in cerebral vessels is less marked and appears later than that of systemic vessels. "At age 60, the middle cerebral artery looks like the radial artery at age 40 and the coronary arteries at age 20 to 30" (Schneck, 1982; p. 42). With these provisos, certain generalizations can be made about age-related cerebrovascular alterations.

Blood vessels tend to become thicker and less pliable with increasing age. "The elastic lamina of the cerebral arteries ceases to grow by middle life but . . . the muscle continues to develop until the age of 60, after which the collagenous tissue alone continues to grow"

(Greenfield, 1976; p. 523). Fibrotic changes occur in the media of the vessel walls, and calcareous material is frequently deposited in the walls of arterioles and precapillaries. Congo red–positive material may appear within the walls of cerebral vessels of the very old patient, reminiscent of, though not in the same quantities as, that seen in patients with Alzheimer's disease.

A more dramatic group of changes is now known to exist in the cerebral capillary bed of most patients with Alzheimer's disease and in a few very old (> 85 years) but apparently not frankly demented individuals. Although general interest in this area has only developed recently, a number of antecedent observations can be noted. As early as 1873, Tuke called attention to changes in the structure of small blood vessels in brain tissue of certain types of *insane* patients (Tuke, 1873). Almost a century later, Hassler (1965) speculated on the possible role of vascular changes in impeding blood flow and thereby compromising cerebral nutrition. Shortly thereafter, Ravens (1978) and Bell and Ball (1981) suggested a possible relationship between alterations in the blood vessel walls with disturbances of the blood–brain barrier and altered transport mechanism. Putative functional correlates of such changes have been sought using *in vivo* visualization techniques such as PET and ^{133}Xenon radiography (Ingvar & Gustafson, 1970; Lassen & Ingvar, 1980; Reivich et al., 1979).

Scanning electron micrography has been especially useful in revealing both the normal structure of the capillary wall, and a group of alterations that appear most clearly in brain tissue from patients with clinically and pathologically documented Alzheimer's disease. In the mature and the healthy aged population, the cerebral capillary wall is thin and smooth, made up of a single row of endothelial lining cells bound to each other by tight junctions and surrounded by a single sheet of basement membrane, which forms the abluminal surface. Occasional oval pericytes with their branching cytoplasmic extensions are found along this surface, along with scattered astrocytic end feet which, in concert, make up the major part of the pericapillary milieu. Closely applied to the capillary abluminal surface is a plexus of very fine nodulated fibers that constitutes the capillary innervation. A number of immunocytochemical and pharmacophysiological studies (Rennels & Nelson, 1975; Hartman, 1973; Raichle, Hartman, Eichling, & Sharpe, 1975; Brayden & Bevan, 1985) have established the neurotransmitter-rich nature of this plexus and its almost certain origin in a group of subcortical nuclei including locus ceruleus, nucleus basalis of Meynert, etc.

The capillary bed in Alzheimer patients appears very different in structure. The vessel walls are studded with outpouchings and excrescences, which give each vessel an irregular, lumpy appearance (Scheibel, Duong, & Tomiyasu, 1987). The nodular profile seems to be due to the presence within reduplicated sheets of basement membrane of cells, possibly monocytes and/or pericytes, and rounded masses of amorphous material, composed of, although perhaps not limited to, amyloid and preamyloid (Figure 7). The outer surface of each vessel wall appears to have lost the fine pericapillary neural plexus that characterized the normal vessel. In addition, in approximately one half of the cases of Alzheimer's disease studied to date, lengths of capillary wall are pitted or cratered by openings ranging from 0.5 to 5 or 6 μm in diameter. These lacunae do not appear to penetrate the endothlial lining of the vessel and may represent sites from which the intramural inclusions and cell bodies already noted have disappeared. It is not clear at this

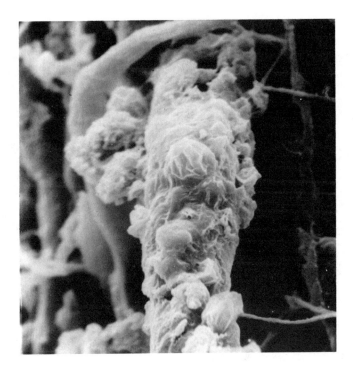

Figure 7 Small blood vessel (capillary arteriole) in parietal cortex of a patient with Alzheimer's disease showing lumpy wall (intramural inclusions) and wrinkling of the basement membrane. Scanning electron micrograph. Original magnification ×4000.

time whether these represent late stage *in vivo* alterations, or changes induced by postmortem tissue preparation. The latter is, of course the more conservative interpretation. However, since such changes have never been seen in the capillary walls of age-matched nondemented control patients, it argues for a structurally disturbed and enormously fragile vessel wall structure (Scheibel *et al.* 1987).

The relationship of these robust microvascular changes to the pathogenesis of Alzheimer's disease remains problematic. Several hypotheses have been advanced, each of which envisions the role of the vessel in a somewhat different light. Glenner (1980) called attention to the possible role of the blood vessel wall in facilitating the progression of some type of preamyloid component into the β-pleated amyloid sheets that appear characteristic of mature plaque amyloid. Peers, Lenders, Defossey, Delacourte and Mazzuca (1988) stress the importance of vessel size in relation to the parenchymal pathology that surrounds it. The walls of large vessels (> 100 μm) present a congophilic angiopathy without apparent reaction in the surrounding neuropil (Figure 8). Vessels of less than 100 μm in diameter are surrounded by a discontinuous sleeve of *dystrophic neurites,* rich in aggregated tau protein, and in close contact with the perimural amyloid. Very small vessels (10–15 μm) are frequently surrounded by structures similar to senile plaques. "Thus the exudation of these amyloid fibrils seems to induce the formation of dystrophic

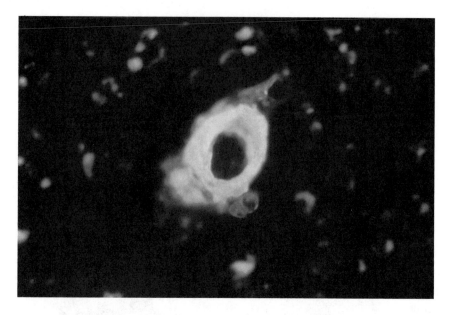

Figure 8   Cross-section through small cerebral vessel of patient with Alzheimer's disease showing presence of intramural amyloid. Thioflavine S. with ultraviolet stimulated fluorescence. Original magnification ×440.

neurons (neuritic reaction)" (Peers et al., 1988; p. 17). This pathogenic model appears to receive support from the ultra-microscopic studies of Miyakawa and Kuramoto (1989) and would appear to minimize the possible role of parenchymal elements themselves (neurons and neuroglia) in the production of amyloid. Such models remain noncommittal as to the original site and mechanisms of the pathological process.

A somewhat different scenario has been advanced by Scheibel *et al.* (1987), who emphasize the possible role of the pericapillary neural plexus in the pathogenesis of the disease process. They stress the delicate balance between brain metabolic needs and metabolic precursors, especially oxygen and glucose, and the likely connection between progressive structural changes in the vessel walls and developing incompetence of the blood–brain barrier. The presumed breakdown of the blood–brain barrier allows entry into the brain parenchyma of globulins (Nandy, Fritz, & Threatt, 1975) including IgG and albumen (Wisniewski & Koslowski, 1982) and the development of brain-reactive anti-bodies (BRA) (Makinodan, 1976; Nandy, 1972). Since BRAs have been shown to be cytotoxic to neurons (Nandy, 1983) another putative sequence of pathologic processes starting with vessel–wall alterations is provided. A possible model for the progressive and destructive changes in the capillary walls may exist in the experiments of Gunn (1971). He showed that surgical denervation of cardiac muscle tissue was regularly followed by hypertrophy and hyperplasia of cellular components in the cardiac vessel walls, including increased phospholipid synthesis and deposition of intramural lipids. "These data strongly suggest that the artery wall needs the trophic influence of neural stimulation to maintain morphological and functional integrity" (Gunn, 1971; p. 56). Although the vascular intramural pathology is obviously different, it is tempting to postulate that the cerebral microvasculature may also bear some type of trophic dependence on its own innervation. The absence of this perivascular neural plexus in brain specimens from Alzheimer patients has already been alluded to. If this innervational loss is primary, and cerebral micro-angiopathy follows, bringing with it all of the consequences of developing blood–brain barrier incompetence including penetration of the parenchyma by globulin, amyloids, etc., then the ultimate trigger for the entire pathogenic sequence may lie elsewhere. A likely site for the inception of the process should perhaps be sought in the nuclei of origin of the perivascular neural plexus, i.e., the locus ceruleus, nuclei basalis of Meynert, etc. Such a scenario implies that Alzheimer's disease may ultimately prove to be the long-term result of an initial subcortical insult!

VI. Structural Change and Behavioral Change: An Overview _____

The spectrum of structural changes reviewed in the preceding sections provide, at best, isolated clues to the dynamic interactive processes that accompany the impact of aging on brain tissue. The nature of the aging process itself remains enigmatic, although several recent reports provide some substance to those theories that favor the presence of *built in* biological instructions leading to involutional change, in contrast to those that argue for wear and tear, destructive environmental conditions, etc.

Seshadri and Campisi (1990) recently reported that senescent fibroblasts in tissue culture were unable to proliferate "because of, at least in part, repression of c-fos; moreover . . . multiple changes in gene expression support the view that cellular senescence is a process of terminal differentiation (p. 205)." Sugawara, Oshimura, Koi, Annab, and Barret (1990) examined the effects on cellular senescence of specific human chromosomes. Using hybrid fibroblasts, they found the introduction of human chromosome 1, but not chromosome 11 "caused typical signs of cellular senescence (p. 707)." Although studies such as these are subject to all of the problems and caveats of tissue and cell culture work, their implications are of considerable interest.

Granted that the structural changes we have reviewed provide only single *freeze-frame* views of cellular processes idiosyncratic to each individual, we may still suggest tentative correlations relating what we have seen to the cognitive and behavioral picture that aging individuals present. One specific example worth addressing involves the apparently selective, early disappearance of the giant pyramidal cells of Betz (Scheibel *et al.*, 1977).

These very large (50–100 μm), fifth-layer pyramids are peculiar to the primary cortical motor strip (area 4) and more specifically to those strip areas that control the major antigravity muscles (i.e., proximal portion of the arms, axial musculature of the trunk, back, and pelvis, and the lower extremities). They are characterized by their very small numbers, i.e., 30,000–40,000 per hemisphere (Lassek, 1954), the great length and development of their basilar dendrite systems (Scheibel & Scheibel, 1978) and their apparently remarkable sensitivity to the aging process (Scheibel *et al.*, 1977). Betz cells begin to show alterations as early as the fourth or fifth decade of life, as evidenced by patchy loss of dendrite spines, and irregular thickening of parts of the basilar and apical dendrite systems. By the seventh decade of life, virtually all of the cells show varying degrees of change and one third to two thirds of them may have disappeared. Although the cause for this precocious regression and loss is not known, the limited size of the Betz cell population suggests that functional consequences of so large a relative loss should be recognizable.

Unlike almost all of the deep pyramids that surround them, the functional role of the Betz cell appears to be in very large part an inhibitory one, i.e., the selective inhibition of their target extensor motor neurons with associated facilitation of the flexor antagonists (Lundberg and Voorhoeve, 1962). Their characteristic discharge pattern is a single phasic burst of action potentials, which arrives at the spinal motor neuron pool before the beginning of a discrete motor action (Evarts, 1965). This Betz cell–derived, large corticospinal fiber discharge has already ceased by the time the masses of somewhat smaller corticospinal neurons around them become active. It seems increasingly probable that the role of this discrete cell group of highly specialized elements is to prepare individual agonist–antagonist muscle pairs for action by diminishing their antigravity (extensor) tone immediately before the programmed action (Scheibel et al., 1977).

It seems not unlikely that the precocious loss of this type of control may produce subtle but profound effects on the smoothness and ease of motor activity. In the absence of the initial relaxation of extensor tone induced by Betz cell discharge, the imposed motor act is patterned onto a muscle system already tonically active in its antigravity role. The perceived result may well be one of some degree of muscle stiffness, and movement against mild resistance. The willed action is completed, but somewhat more slowly and with a residual sense of *soreness* across weight-bearing joints. This is a familiar complaint in those individuals in their sixties and beyond. The change in timing of the motor response accompanying such changes may be partly responsible for other problems that these individuals frequently notice in performing familiar acts like stepping off curbs or climbing a few stairs. The slowing and brief *hanging fire* on the follow-through across hip and knee may be sufficient to cause momentary balance problems and occasional falls. Clearly, other factors such as connective tissue and articular changes may also be involved, but this progressive age-related alteration in motor programming due to loss of Betz cell function deserves consideration.

Expressed in the broadest terms, structural alterations become significant to the individual only when they affect cognitive, motor, or psychosocial functioning. The remarkable plasticity that neural tissue appears to maintain, even into advanced age, and the redundancy of neuronal circuits provide, in most cases, a good deal of functional margin, even in the presence of age-related structural change. In the long run, it is the loss of interconnectivity among neurons, individually and collectively, that eventually compromises computational power and produces symptoms. Although there is compelling evidence to indicate that cognitive *styles* change with increasing age, there now seems little reason to doubt that accumulated experience can make up for age-related loss in the speed of cerebral processing or of memory recall. As a matter of fact, recognition and appreciation of this cognitive change of style is seen in most cultures. The wisdom of the elder, the senator envisioned as the embodiment of judicial restraint and balance, may have an important and as yet unexplored structurofunctional message for us to ponder. Neuronal populations in the language-involved superior temporal lobe decrease by 30% between the ages of 2 months and 18 years (Brody, 1955), precisely the period during which language develops and achieves its fullest repertoire. Furthermore, programmed cell death and axonal retraction now appear to be essential parts of early development of significant forebrain structures such as the corpus callosum (Innocenti, Koppel, & Clarke, 1981). Mesulam (1987) wonders "why neuronal attrition which is described as 'developmental' early in life should be called 'involutional' later on (p. 580)."

Is it possible that progressive diminution in size or loss of neuronal elements in later life represents an essential part of that *continuous developmental sequence* mentioned in the first sentence of this chapter? And could a significant outcome of this process lie in the continuing maturation of cognitive function where breadth and speed are sacrificed for depth and weight? Thus the process, perhaps describable as "enhancement of fidelity at expense of channel width" (Mesulam, 1987; p. 583) provides certain advantages, at a price. But the price paid in loss of agility, both cognitive and behavioral, comes at a time when those age-old biological functions of territorial defense, mating, and child-rearing are no longer individual imperatives. Perhaps what is lost matters less than what is gained!

The disabling age-related disease processes such as Alzheimer's dementia represent tremendous medical, social, and economic challenges. We must assume that further research will eventually lead the way toward treatment or prevention. However, everything we now know indicates that the aging process itself is part of the biological, and therefore, of the human condition. Here our main thrust must lie in the direction of maximizing the quality of life during a period of subtle but continuous change in brain structure and function. Today, increasing numbers of healthy individuals in their eighth and ninth decades and beyond, continue to work effectively in the business world, in the arts, and in the sciences. In every case, their lives are marked by activity, involvement, and purpose. Can we doubt that zest for life is the best single therapeutic agent for the later years?

References

Aitken, J. T., & Bridger, J. E. (1967). Neuron size and neuron population density in the lumbrosacral region of the cat's spinal cord. *Journal of Anatomy, 95*, 38–53.

Alzheimer, A. (1907). Über eine eigenartige Erkrankung der Hirnrinde. *Allgemeine Zeitschrift für Psychiatrie und Psychisch-Gerentliche Medizin, 64*, 146–148.

Anderson, J. M., Hubbard, B. M., Coghill, C. R., & Sliders, W. (1983). The effect of advanced old age on the neurone content of the central cortex. Observations with an automatic image analyzer point counting method. *Journal of Neurological Science, 58*, 233–244.

Baillie, M. (1977). *The morbid anatomy of some of the most important parts of the human body.* (American ed.) New York, Dabor.

Ball, M. J. (1983). Granulovacuolar degeneration. In B. Reisberg (Ed.), *Alzheimer's disease; the standard reference* (pp. 62–68). New York: The Free Press.

Beal, M. F., & Martin, J. B. (1986). Neuropeptides in neurological disease. *Annals of Neurology, 20*, 547–565.

Bell, M. A., & Bell, J. (1981). Morphometric comparison of hippocampal microvasculature in aging and demented people: Diameters and densities. *Acta Neuropathologica (Berlin), 53*, 299–318.

Bigler, E. D., Hubler, D. W., Cullum, M., & Turkheimer, E. (1985). Intellectual and memory impairment in dementia. *The Journal of Nervous and Mental Disease, 173*, 347–352.

Bondareff, W. (1987). Changes in the brain in aging and Alzheimer's disease assessed by neuronal counts. *Neurobiology of Aging, 8*, 562–563.

Borst, M. (Ed.) (1922). *Pathologische Histologie.* Leipzig: Vogel.

Brayden, J. E., & Bevan, J. A. (1985). Neurogenic muscarinic vasodilatation in the cat. *Circulation Research, 56*, 205–211.

Brinkman, S. D., Sarwar, M., Leven, H. S., & Morris, H. D. (1981). Quantitative indexes of computed tomography in dementia and normal aging. *Radiology, 138*, 89–92.

Brody, H. (1955). Organization of the cerebral cortex. III. A study of aging in the human cerebral cortex. *Journal of Comparative Neurology, 103*, 511–556.

Brody, H. (1970). Structural changes in the aging nervous system. In H. Blumenthal (Ed.), *The regulatory role of the nervous system in aging. (Vol. 7). Interdisciplinary topics in gerontology* (pp. 9–21). basal: Karger Press.

Brun, A. (1983). An overview of light and electron microscopic changes. In B. Reisberg (Ed.), *Alzheimer's disease, the standard reference* (pp. 37–47). New York: The Free Press.

Brun, A. (1988). White matter disease in the elderly demented. *Bulletin of Clinical Neurosciences, 53*, 125–127.

Buell, S. J., & Coleman, P. D. (1979). Dendritic growth in the aged human brain and failure of growth in senile dementia. *Science, 206*, 854–856.

Chui, H. C., Bondareff, W., Zarow, C., & Slazer, U. (1984). Stability of neuronal number in the human nucleus basalis of Meynert with age, *Neurobiology of Aging, 5*, 83–88.

Clouston, T. S. (1911). *Unsoundness of mind.* New York, NY: Dutton.

Coleman, P. D., & Flood, D. C. (1986). Dendritic proliferation in the aging brain as a compensatory repair mechanism. *Progress in Brain Research, 70*, 227–237.

Coleman, P. D., & Flood, D. C. (1987). Neuron numbers and dendritic extent in normal aging and Alzheimer's disease. *Neurobiology of Aging, 8*, 521–545.

Creasey, H., Schwartz, M., Frederickson, H., Hoxby, J. V., & Rapoport, S. F., (1986). Quantitative computed tomography in dementia of the Alzheimer type. *Neurology, 36*, 1563–1568.

Cupp, C. J., & Uemura, E. (1980). Age-related changes in prefrontal cortex of Macaca mulatta. Quantitative analysis of dendritic branching patterns. *Experimental Neurology, 69*, 143–146.

Cutler, R. G. (1982). The dysdifferentiative hypothesis of mammalian aging and longevity. In E. Giacobini, G. Filogamo, G. Giacobini & A. Vernadakis (Eds.), *The aging brain: Cellular and molecular mechanisms of aging in the nervous system* (pp. 1–19). New York: Raven Press.

Diamond, M. C. (1988). *Enriching heredity. The impact of the environment on the anatomy of the brain.* New York: The Free Press.

Diamond, M. C., Johnson, R. E., & Gold, M. W. (1977). Changes in neuron number and size and glia number in the young adult, and aging rat medial occipital cortex. *Behavioral Biology, 20*, 409–412.

Diamond, M. C., Johnson, R. E., & Ingham, C. A. (1975). Morphological changes in the young, adult, and aging cerebral cortex, hippocampus, and diencephalon. *Behavioral Biology, 148*, 163–179.

Englund, E., Brun, A., & Persson, B. (1987). Correlations between histopathologic white matter changes and proton MR relaxation times in dementia. *Alzheimer's Disease and Associated Disorders, 1*, 156–170.

Eslinger, P. J., Damasio, H., Graff-Radford, N., & Damasio, A. (1984). Examining the relationship between computed tomography and neuro-psycholotical measures in normal and demented elderly. *Journal of Neurology, Neurosurgery, and Psychiatry, 47*, 1319–1325.

Evarts, E. (1965). Relation of discharge frequency to conduction velocity in pyramidal tract neurons. *Journal of Neurophysiology, 28*, 216–228.

Flood, D. G., Buell, S. J., Defiore, C. H., Horwitz, G. J., & Coleman, P. D. (1985). Age-related dendritic growth in dentate gyrus of human brain is followed by regression in the "oldest old." *Brain Research, 345*, 366–368.

Gado, M., Hughes, C. P., Danziger, W., Chi, D., Jost, G., & Berg, L. (1982). Volumetric measurements of the cerebrospinal fluid spaces in demented subjects and controls. *Radiology, 144*, 535–538.

George, A. F., DeLeon, M. J., Rosenbloom, S., Ferris, H., Gentes, C., Emmerich, M., & Kricheff, I. I. (1983). Ventricular volume and cognitive deficit: a computed tomographic study. *Radiology, 149*, 493–498.

Glenner, G. G. (1980). Amyloid deposits and amyloidosis. *New England Journal of Medicine, 302*, 1283–1292.

Greenfield, J. P. (1967). *Neuropathology.* Baltimore: Williams & Wilkins.

Greenough, W. T., Juraska, J. M., & Volkmar, F. R. (1979). Maze training effects on dendritic branching in occipital cortex of adult rats. *Behavioral & Neural Biology, 26*, 287–297.

Gunn, C. G. (1971). Proliferative nature of arteriosclerosis and regulators of metabolism and movement. In S. Wolfe (Ed.), *The artery and the process of arteriosclerosis* (pp. 56 *et seq.*, 230 *et seq.*). New York: Plenum Press.

Gyldensted, C. (1977). Measurements of the normal ventricular system and hemispheric sulci of 100 adults with computed tomography. *Neuroradiology, 14,* 183–192.

Hall, T. C., Miller, A. K. C., & Corsellis, A. N. (1975). Variations in the human Purkinje cell population according to age and sex. *Neuropathology and Applied Neurobiology, 1,* 267–292.

Hartman, B. K. (1973). The innervation of cerebral blood vessels by central noradrenergic neurons. In E. Usden & S. Snyder (Eds.), *Frontiers in catecholamine research* (pp. 91–96). New York: Pergamon Press.

Hassler, O. (1965). Vascular changes in senile brains. *Acta Neuropathologica (Berlin), 5,* 40–53.

Haxby, J. V., & Rapoport, S. F. (1988). Alzheimer disease begins with altered metabolism in the parietal, frontal, and temporal association neocortices. *Bulletin of Clinical Neurosciences, 53* 43–50.

Henderson, V. W., Kortman, K. E., Chui, H. C., Mack, W., Bardolph, E. L., & Bradley, W. G. (1988). Alzheimer disease: High-intensity periventricular white matter alterations on magnetic resonance imaging. *Bulletin of Clinical Neurosciences, 53,* 137–147.

Hodge, C. F. (1894). Changes in ganglion cells from birth to senile death. Observations on man and honey-bee. *Journal of Physiology, London, 17,* 129–134.

Hubbard, B. M., & Anderson, J. M. (1981). A quantitative study of cerebral atrophy in old age and senile dementia. *Journal of Neurological Science, 50,* 135–145.

Hyden, H., & Lindstrom, B. (1950). *Discussions of the Faraday Society, 9,* 436.

Ihara, K., & Kondo, J. (1989). Polypeptide composition of paired helical filaments. *Annals of Medicine, 21,* 121–125.

Ingar, D. H., & Gustafson, L. (1970). Regional cerebral blood flow in organic dementia with early onset. *Acta Neurologica Scandinavica, (Suppl. 46), 43,* 42–73.

Innocenti, G. M., Koppel, H., & Clarke, S. (1981). Glial phagocytosis during the postnatal shaping of visual corpus callosum. *Neuroscience Letters (Suppl.), 7,* S160.

Iqbal, K., & Wisniewski, H. (1983). Neurofibrillary tangles. In B. Reisberg (Ed.), *Alzheimer's disease, the standard reference* (pp. 48–56). New York: The Free Press.

Kidd, M. (1963). Paired helical filaments in electron microscopy of Alzheimer's disease. *Nature, 197,* 192–193.

Kuhl, D. E. (1986). Determination of cerebral metabolic patterns in dementia using positron emission tomography. In A. Scheibel & A. Wechsler (Eds), *The biological substrates of Alzheimer's disease* (pp. 21–32). San Diego: Academic Press.

Lassek, A. M. (1954). *The pyramidal tract.* Springfield, IL: Thomas.

Lassen, N. A., & Inguar, D. H. (1980). Blood flow studies in the normal brain and in senile dementia. In L. Amaducci, A. N. Davison, & P. Artuono (Eds.), *Aging of the brain and dementia* (pp. 91–98). New York: Raven Press.

Lundberg, A., & Voorhoeve, P. (1962). Effects from the pyramidal tract on spinal reflex arcs. *Acta Physiologica Scandinavica, 56,* 201–219.

Makinodan, T. (1976). Immunobiology of aging. *Journal of the American Geriatrics Society, 2,* 249–252.

Mann, D. M. S., Yates, P. O., & Hawkes, J. (1983). The pathology of the human locus ceruleus. *Clinical Neuropathology, 2,* 1–7.

Mann, D. M. A., Yates, O., & Marcyniuk, B. (1984). Monoaminergic neurotransmitter systems in presenile Alzheimer type. *Clinical Neuropathology, 3,* 199–205.

McGeer, P. L. McGeer, E., & Suzuki, J. S. (1977). Aging and extra-pyramidal function. *Archives of Neurology, 34,* 33–35.

McGeer, P. L., McGeer, E. G., Suzuki, J., Dolman, C. E., & Nagai, T. (1984). Aging, Alzheimer's disease, and the cholinergic system of the basal forebrain. *Neurology, 34,* 741–745.

Mehraein, P., Yamado, M., & Tarnowska-Dzidnszko, E. (1975). Quantitative study on dendrites and dendritic spines in Alzheimer's disease and senile dementia. *Advances in Neurology, 12,* 453–458.

Mesulam, M.-Marcel (1987). Involutional and developmental implications of age-related neuronal changes: In search of an engram for wisdom. *Neurobiology of Aging, 8,* 581–583.

Miller, A. K. H., Alston, R. L., Mountjoy, C. Y., & Corsellis, J. A. N. (1984). Automated differential cell counting on a section of the normal human hippocampus. The influence of age. *Neuropathology and Applied Neurobiology, 10,* 123–141.

Miller, C., Haugh, M., Kahn, J., & Anderton, B. (1986). The cytoskeleton and neurofibrillary tangles in Alzheimer's disease. *Trends in Neuroscience, 9*, 76–81.

Minckler, J. (1968). *Pathology of the nervous system (Vol. 1).* New York: McGraw-Hill.

Miyakawa, T., & Kuramoto, R. (1989). Ultrastructural study of senile plaques and microvessels in the brain with Alzheimer's disease and Down's syndrome. *Annals of Medicine, 21*, 99–102.

Mouritzen Dam, A. (1979). The density of neurons in the human hippocampus. *Neuropathology and Applied Neurobiology, 5*, 249–264.

Nakamura, S., Akiguchi, I., Kameyama, M., & Mizuno, N. (1985). Age-related changes of pyramidal cell basal dendrites in layers III and IV of human motor cortex. A quantitative Golgi study. *Acta Neuropathologica (Berlin), 65*, 281–284.

Nandy, K. (1972). Brain-reactive antibodies in mouse serum as a function of age. *Journal of Gerontology, 30*, 412–416.

Nandy, K. (1983). Immunologic factors. In B. Reisberg (Ed.), *Alzheimer's disease, the standard reference* (pp. 135–138). New York: The Free Press.

Nandy, K., Fritz, R. B., & Threatt, J. (1975). Specificity of brain-reactive antibodies in serum in old mice. *Journal of Gerontology, 30*, 269–274.

Olszewski, J. (1962). Subcortical arteriosclerotic encephalopathy. Review of the literature on the so-called Binswanger's disease and presentation of two cases. *World Neurology, 3*, 359–375.

Peers, M. C., Lenders, M. B., Difossey, A., Delacourte, A. & Mazzuca, M. (1988). Cortical angiopathy in Alzheimer's disease. The formation of dystrophic perivascular neurites is related to the exudation of amyloid fibrils from the pathological vessels. *Virchows Archives A, Pathological Anatomy, 414*, 15–20.

Raichle, M. E. Hartman, B. K., Eichling, J. O., & Sharpe, L. G. (1975). Central noradrenergic regulation of cerebral blood flow and vascular permeability. *Proceedings of the National Academy of Science U.S.A, 72*, 3726–3730.

Ravens, J. R. (1978). Vascular changes in the human senile brain. In J. Cervos-Navarro, E. Betz, G. Eberhardt, R. Ferst, & R. Wiellenwebber (Eds.) *Advances in neurology* (Vol. 20, pp. 478–501). New York: Raven Press.

Reivich, M., Kuhl, D. E., Wolf, A. P., Greenberg, J., Phelps, M., Ido, T., Casella, V., Fowler, J., Hoffman, E., Alair, A., Som, P., & Sokoloff, L. (1979). The (18F) fluorodeoxyglucose method for the measurement of local cerebral glucose utilization in man. *Circulation Research, 44*, 127–137.

Sashadri, T., & Campisi, J. (1990). Repression of c-fos transcription and an altered genetic program in senescent human fibroblasts. *Science* 247: 205–209.

Rennels, M. L., & Nelson, E. (1975). Capillary innervation in the mammalian central nervous system, *American Journal of Anatomy, 144*, 233–241.

Schadé, J. P., & Baxter, C. F. (1960). Changes during growth in the volume and surface area of cortical neurons in the rabbit. *Experimental Neurology, 2*, 158–178.

Scheibel, A. B., Duong, T., & Tomiyasu, U. (1987). Denervation microangiopathy in senile dementia, Alzheimer type. *Alzheimer Disease & Associated Disorders, 1*, 19–37.

Scheibel, A. B., & Tomiyasu, U. (1978). Dendritic sprouting in Alzheimer's presenile dementia. *Experimental Neurology, 60*, 1–8.

Scheibel, M. E., Lindsay, R. D., Tomiyasu, U., & Scheibel, A. B. (1975). Progressive dendritic changes in aging human cortex. *Experiemental Neurology, 47*, 392–403.

Scheibel, M. E., Lindsay, R. D., Tomiyasu, U., & Scheibel, A. B. (1976). Progressive dendritic changes in the aging human limbic system. *Experimental Neurology, 53*, 420–430.

Scheibel, M. E., & Scheibel, A. B. (1978). The dendritic structure of the human Betz cell. In M. Brazier & H. Petsche (Eds.), *Architectonics of the cerebral cortex* (pp. 43–57). New York: Raven Press.

Scheibel, M.E., Tomiyasu, U., & Scheibel, A. B. (1977). The aging human Betz cell. *Experimental Neurology, 56*, 598–609.

Schneck, S. A. (1982). Aging of the nervous system and dementia. In R. W. Schrier, (Ed.), *Clinical internal medicine in the aged* (p. 42). Philadelphia, PA: W. B. Saunders.

Schwartz, M. Creasey, H., Grady, C. L., De Leo, J. M., Frederickson, H. A., Cutler, N. R. G., Rapaport S. J. (1985) Computed tomographic analysis of brain norphometrics in 30 healthy men aged 21 to 81 years. *Annals of Neurology, 17*, 146–157.

Shefer, V. F. (1973). Absolute number of neurons and thickness of the cerebral cortex during aging, senile, and vascular demential and Pick's and Alzheimer's disease. *Neuroscience and Behavioral biology, 6,* 319–324.

Simchowitz, T. (1910). *Histologische und Histopathologische Arbeiten R,* 267. Quoted from *Greenfield's Neuropathology* (1967). (pps. 526 & 575). Baltimore, MD: Williams & Wilkens.

Sugiwara, O., Oshimura, M., Koi, M., Annab, L. & Barrat, J. (1990). Induction of cellular senescence in immortalized cells by human chromosome I. *Science 247,* 707–710.

Terr, R. D., Gonatas, N. K., & Weiss, M. (1964). Ultrastructural studies in Alzheimer's presenile dementia. *American Journal of Pathology, 44,* 269–297.

Terry, R. D., De Teresa, R., & Hansen, L. N. (1987). Neocortical cell counts in normal human adult aging. *Annals of Neurology, 21,* 530–539.

Tomlinson, B. E., Blessed, G., & Roth, M. (1968) Observations on the brains of non-demented old people. *Journal of Neurological Science, 7,* 331–356.

Tomlinson, B. E., Blessed, G., & Roth, M. (1970). Observations on the brains of demented old people. Journal of Neurological Science, 11, 205–242.

Tomlinson, B. E., Irving, D., & Blessed, G. (1981). Cell loss in the locus coeruleus in senile dementia of Alzheimer type. *Journal of Neurobiological Science, 49,* 419–428.

Torvik, A., Torp, S., & Lindboe, C. F. (1968). Atrophy of the cerebellar vermis in aging. A morphometric and histologic study. *Journal of Neurological Science, 76,* 283–294.

Tuke, J. B. (1983). On the morbid anatomy of the brain and spinal cord as observed in the insane. *British Forensic Medical & Chirurgical Review, 51,* 450–460.

Uemura, E. (1985). Age-related changes in the subiculum of Macaca mulatta. Dendritic branching pattern. *Experimental Neurology, 87,* 412–427.

Vijayashankar, N., & Brody, H. (1977). A study of aging in the human abducens nucleus. *Journal of Comparative Neurology, 173,* 433–437.

Vijayashankar, N., & Brody, H. (1979). A quantitative study of the pigmented neurons in the nuclei locus coeruleus and subcoeruleus in man as related to aging. *Journal of Neuropathology and Experimental Neurology, 38,* 490–497.

Whitehouse, P. J., Parhad, J. M., Hedreen, J. C., Clark, A. W., White, C. L., Struble, R. G. & Price, D. L. (1983). Integrity of the nucleus basalis of Meynert in normal aging. *Neurology, 33, Suppl. 2,* 159.

Wilks, S. (1864). Clinical notes on atrophy of the brain. *Journal of Mental Science,* 10.

Wisniewski, H. M., & Koslowski, P. B. (1982). Evidence for blood–brain barrier changes in senile dementia of the Alzheimer type (SDAT). In F. M. Sinex & C. R. Merril (Eds.), *Alzheimer's disease, Down's syndrome, and aging.* (Vol. 396, pp. 119–129). New York: New York Academy of Science.

Wisniewski, H. (1983). Neuritic (senile) and amyloid plaques. In B. Reisberg (Ed.), *Alzheimer's disease, the standard reference* (pp. 57–61). New York: The Free Press.

Wisniewski, H. M., Vorhodt, A. W., Moretz, R. C., Lossinsky, A. S., & Gundke-Igbal, I. (1982). Pathogenesis of neuritic (senile) and amyloid plaque formation. *Exp. Brain Res.* Suppl. 5: 3–9.

Neurochemical Changes with Aging: Predisposition toward Age-Related Mental Disorders __

David G. Morgan

I. General Anatomical Changes in the Brain with Normal Aging
   A. The Absence of Neuron Loss with Age
   B. The Accumulation of Engrams
II. Aging Changes in Synaptic Neurochemistry
   A. The Dopamine System
   B. The Acetylcholine System
   C. The Noradrenaline System
   D. The Serotonin System
   E. Other Neurotransmitter Systems
III. Usual Aging in the Dopamine System, Schizophrenia, and Parkinson's Disease
IV. The Interaction of Aging with the Pathological Features of Alzheimer's Disease
   A. Age-Related Changes in the Anatomical Features of Alzheimer's Disease
   B. Age-Related Changes in the Neurochemical Features of Alzheimer's Disease
   C. Age of Onset versus Duration of Disease
   D. Age of Onset and Other Neurological Disorders
   E. Significance of Age of Onset to Alzheimer's Disease
V. Summary and Conclusions
   References

I. General Anatomical Changes in the Brain with Normal Aging __

Before considering neurochemical changes in the brain, it is of primary importance to understand the nature of anatomical changes with age. All neurochemicals must reside within some cellular structure (although secreted chemicals may be there only transiently), and changes in the numbers or phenotypes of cells will affect the neurochemical changes

Handbook of Mental Health and Aging, Second Edition

observed. While superficially this selective review may appear to overlap with other chapters of this volume, the perspective provided is different from most other summaries of this area.

A. The Absence of Neuron Loss with Age

One general concept about aging in the brain is that neuron loss proceeds at some inevitable and inexorable rate, resulting in a roughly 50% loss of neurons over the human life span. Much of this belief is based on research performed over 35 years ago by Brody (1955), in which a 50% decline in visual cortex neuron density was reported over the lifespan. A number frequently given for usual neuron loss in human brain is 100,000 per day. It is uncertain where this number originated, but if we multiply 100,000 neurons per day by the 36,500 days in a 100-year lifespan, we estimate a loss of 4 billion neurons, seemingly an overwhelming number, rendering all but the most resistant into a vegetative condition. However, our best present estimate of the total number of neurons in the human brain is one trillion (Kandel & Schwartz, 1985). Even if this estimate is high by an order of magnitude, 100,000 neurons per day would cause a 0.4 to 4% reduction in the total neuronal complement, hardly an insurmountable deficit.

Two recent studies have reported extensive analyses of human neuronal changes with age. The first of these (Haug, 1985) examined over 100 specimens obtained at autopsy ranging from 19 to 111 years. He reports a roughly 50-g loss in brain weight over the lifespan (3.5%), after correcting for secular changes in body size, and reports a 6% decline in overall brain volume. However, in four separate regions of the cerebral cortex, he reports no decline in neuron density; in fact, there is a slight increase in neuron density. Importantly, Haug does report a significant reduction in neuron size with age. This ranges from a 50% size reduction in those regions with the largest neurons, to no change for cortical regions with relatively small neurons. One important artifact in neurohistology was uncovered by Haug in these studies; brains of older individuals shrink less during fixation. Hence, because the neuron fields are less compressed during fixation, their density would appear to decline with age, unless the measurements were corrected for this fixation artifact. Haug's are the only data published thus far that account for this artifact.

A second study was recently published by Terry, DeTheresa, and Hansen (1987), examining over 50 brains from 24 to 100 years of age. These brains were carefully evaluated for infarcts, signs of preclinical Alzheimer's disease (AD), or other disease-related pathology, and only brains lacking pathology were included in the analysis. The results of Terry's study corroborate those of Haug and his collaborator's. Terry et al. (1987) found no change in total neuron number with age in the three cerebral cortical regions examined. However, they did observe a decrease in neuron size, expressed in these results as a loss of large neurons ($> 90 \ \mu m^2$), and an increase in small neurons (between 40 and 90 μm^2). Terry et al. (1987) also reported a decrease in brain weight and cortical thickness over the lifespan, and an increase (almost two fold) in the number of glial cells in the cerebral cortical regions.

This increase in glial cells with age now appears more consistently in the neuroanatomy literature on aging than does neuron loss. This author has reviewed this literature previously (Finch & Morgan, 1990). In summary, there appears with age in both rodent and human brain an increase in the total volume of grey matter occupied by glial cells, and more specifically the glial subtype called astrocytes. Some report an increase in the number of these cells, while others claim that the increase is primarily in the size of the astrocytes. Hansen, Armstrong, and Terry (1987) report that this increase in astrocyte number is as high as five fold in certain layers of the human cerebral cortex. Geinisman (1979) have detected an increase in the astrocytic compartment of the molecular layer of the rat dentate gyrus using areal measures of electron micrographs.

While we do not intend to review this area in detail, our understanding of changes in the brain with successful aging, particularly the cerebral cortex, is in transition. The notion of considerable neuron loss during the lifespan is being replaced by the concept of gradual neuron shrinkage, and concurrent increase in glial cells, particularly astrocytes. It should be emphasized that this interpretation of the present state of this field does not go unchallenged. Many contemporary reports of brain aging do report substantial neuron loss with age in areas of the cerebral cortex. However, these studies rarely include the rigorous pathological criteria of Terry and co-workers, nor the corrections for secular changes and fixation artifacts that Haug has performed. A more detailed account of this literature can be found in the reviews by Coleman and Flood (Coleman & Flood, 1987; Flood & Coleman, 1988). Hence, while there does appear to be neuron loss normally with aging in certain human brain regions such as locus ceruleus, subregions of the hippocampus, and the substantia nigra (discussed in Section III), the cerebral cortex, that region most intimately involved in those aspects of cognition peculiar to humans, does not appear to suffer inevitable loss of cells with age.

B. The Accumulation of Engrams

When interpreting neurochemical changes with aging, one must consider in addition to anatomical considerations, the undeniable requirement that mnemonic engrams, the permanent residual changes in brain encoding long-term memory, must accumulate over the lifespan. Thus, *those neurochemical changes we observe with aging in the brain need not necessarily indicate degenerative events,* a biological deficiency leading to cognitive decline, but may simply represent a lifetime of accumulated memories. The shrinkage of neurons normally with age may reflect a sculpting of the nervous system, an elimination of those input–output pathways that were never used, or detrimentally competed with an optimal input–output pathway. The possibility that synapse loss with age exceeds that of neuron loss (Geinisman, 1979; Matsumoto, Okada, Arai, 1982; Gibson, 1983a; Leuba, 1983; Adams, 1986; Bertoni-Freddari et al., 1986; Levine et al., 1988) is consistent with this notion. Knowing precisely those neurochemical and anatomical changes that appear in the brains of mammals progressively over the lifespan may provide the key to unlocking the mechanisms of learning and memory formation.

Assuming that engram accumulation occurs with age, it is conceivable that usual age-related memory problems (Poon, 1985) may be a necessary consequence of the biological constraints on memory accumulation with age, i.e., there is some limited capacity to long-term memory. The brain, as a repository of the engrams for memories, is a finite entity. If we accept the synaptic doctrine of brain function (that the synapse is the smallest functional unit of plasticity), at some time, a specific synapse must be recruited for involvement in more than one engram, as more and more permanent memories accumulate. (Transitory memories, such as those involved in sensory information stores and other short-term memories, may recycle synapses, but more enduring long-term memories would presumably be represented by more enduring changes.) This argument also assumes that memory engrams are distributed throughout the nervous system as multiple representations; a gain system linked to motivational and hedonic components of the experience would regulate the number of synapses involved in the engram for each memory. At some point, the strength of the memory (as measured by the total number of participating synapses) must be degraded by subsequent engrams, as synapses are switched from participating in memory A to memory B. In order to preserve some components of older engrams, the brain may be required to decrease the overall gain mechanism on engram size (in the synaptic space), leading to poorer acquisition. To some extent, this concept is a biological correlate of interference theory (Postman & Underwood 1973).

Thus, the memory-retrieval problems accompanying usual aging need not represent any dysfunction of the memory-forming or retrieval apparatus, but are a necessary pleiotropic consequence of a lifetime of accumulated memories (and their cognate engrams). Analogizing the brain to an attic, while the attic may not be completely full in advanced age, it is so crowded that finding exactly what you want becomes extremely difficult, and requires more time than when the attic was considerably less cluttered in youth. Yet at the same time, exercising one's memory, rooting through the synaptic attic, will increase the probability of knowing where a specific engram is when one goes to retrieve it (the mnemonic version of "use it or lose it"). It is within this context of neuronal shrinkage, but not loss, and the accumulation of engrams over the lifespan that we need to interpret age-related neurochemical changes in brain.

II. Aging Changes in Synaptic Neurochemistry

For roughly the last decade, the primary research focus of this author has been the delineation of normal age-related changes in biochemical markers of specific neurotransmitter pathways in the central nervous system (CNS) of rodents and humans. This interest has also led to a number of past summaries, detailing study by study the results of most published reports of aging brain synaptic neurochemistry, the most recent being in the latest edition of the *Handbook of the Biology of Aging* (Morgan & May, 1990). The goal of this chapter is not to reiterate a detailed and technical analysis of the field, but to summarize our present knowledge, and subsequently, indicate how this knowledge may interact with mental health disorders.

A. The Dopamine System

Of all neurotransmitter systems, the one that has been most extensively studied with aging is the dopamine system, particularly the nigrostriatal pathway. This is perhaps owing to the detection of age-related changes in this pathway early in the history of neurogerontology (Finch, 1973), and the large number of neurochemical tools for the examination of this system. In addition, it remains one of the few neurotransmitter pathways whose degeneration is tightly coupled to a specific neurological disorder, Parkinson's disease (see Section III below). A weighted average of the available studies suggests that the presynaptic markers of the dopamine system in mice, rats, and rabbits do appear to decline with age, but this decline begins late in the lifespan and is roughly a 10–30% reduction in mice and rats. Some studies fail to detect changes in dopamine with age, yet none report increases (reviewed in Morgan & Finch 1988; Morgan & May, 1990). Other indices of presynaptic dopamine function, dopamine metabolites, and the activity of the rate-limiting synthetic enzyme, tyrosine hydroxylase, are less likely to decline with aging.

Postsynaptically, the changes are most robust. The most consistent and universal age-related change in synaptic neurochemistry is a decline in the D2 dopamine receptor. This change appears progressive, and averages 50% over the lifespans of most species studied. This receptor also appears important in the etiology of schizophrenia (see Section III). The other dopamine receptor, the D1 subtype, also appears to decline with age in rats, but not in mice (although significantly fewer studies have examined this receptor). The activity of dopamine-sensitive adenylate cyclase, an index of D1 receptor function, also declines with age, but as an early event (up to 12 months in rats).

In humans, the presynaptic declines in dopamine levels are greater than those observed in rodents, averaging about 50% over the lifespan (however, some studies still fail to detect a difference, perhaps owing to the high variability in this measure from postmortem human samples). To some degree, these changes in presynaptic markers are paralleled by loss of the dopamine-containing neurons in the substantia nigra, although the cell loss is smaller than the dopamine loss (McGeer, McGeer, Suzuki, Dolman, & Nagai, 1977; Mann, Lincoln, Yates, Stamp, & Toper, 1980). Postsynaptically, the D2 receptor consistently declines in all studies, while the D1 receptor has been reported to increase (Morgan et al., 1987b), decrease (Seeman et al., 1987), or remain unchanged (Rinne 1987). The largest study to date is that of Seeman, Bzowej, and co-workers; hence, some minor decline in the D1 receptor is probable.

In summary, both humans and rodents exhibit pre- and postsynaptic declines in the dopamine system. Presynaptically these changes appear more severe in humans. Postsynaptically, there is almost universal agreement that the D2 receptor declines with age, and this change serves as a biomarker of brain aging. Dietary restriction, which retards the rate of aging in rodents, appears to similarly retard the age-related decline in the D2 receptor (Roth, Ingram & Joseph, 1984).

B. The Acetylcholine System

Rivaling the dopamine system in attention, age-related declines in the major presynaptic marker for acetylcholine, the synthetic enzyme choline acetyltransferase, are convincingly demonstrated in rat hippocampus and striatum (20–30%), with smaller declines in cerebral cortex (10%) (reviewed in Morgan & May, 1990). In mouse brain, there appears to be a surprising increase in choline acetyltransferase activity with age (Waller, Ingram, Reynolds, & London, 1983).

Postsynaptically, the muscarinic receptor declines by 20 to 40% in cerebral cortex and striatum, and by 10 to 30% in hippocampus. These changes appear smaller in the mouse than in the rat.

In human brain, there are very few studies of the cholinergic system with usual or successful aging (most studies have focused on AD). McGeer *et al.* (1984) report a 60% loss of cortical choline acetyltransferase activity over the human life span, associated with a 75–90% loss of cholinergic neurons in the nucleus basalis. Mann, Yates, & Marcyniak (1984) similarly report a loss of neurons (30%) in the nucleus basalis with age. Conversely, Chui, Bondareff, Zarow, & Slager (1984) and Bigl, Arendt, Fischer, Werner & Arendt (1987) report no change in nucleus basalis neuron density with usual aging. The cholinergic neurons of the nucleus basalis degenerate in a variety of neurological disorders that share a common symptom of cognitive dysfunction (AD, Parkinsonians with dementia, dementia pugilistica, Pick's disease, Korsakoff's disease: see Ezrin-Waters & Resch, 1986 for a review). This area is of critical importance for evaluation of some of the biological deficiency hypotheses of usual age-related memory dysfunction. One such hypothesis, termed the cholinergic hypothesis of geriatric memory dysfunction (Bartus, Dean, Beer & Lippa 1982) elegantly develops the concept that declines in cholinergic function using lesions and pharmacological manipulations produce changes in mnemonic function that mimic those observed with usual aging. However, the data reviewed by Bartus *et al.* concerning human aging and choline acetyltransferase activity suggest that this enzyme is stable over the human life span in the absence of neurological disease.

Postsynaptically, the data suggest a loss of muscarinic receptors with usual aging in human brain, yet not all studies report this change (see Morgan, May, & Finch 1988). A recent large study by Rinne (1987) reports losses of 50% in muscarinic receptors throughout the brain during the human lifespan.

In summary, rats appear to lose presynaptic markers of the acetylcholine system with aging, but the evidence is less compelling for mice and men. Postsynaptically, there is a loss of the muscarinic receptor in all species examined, but this loss is probably smaller than the D2 receptor loss.

C. The Noradrenaline System

In rodents, the data are fairly convincing that presynaptic markers of the noradrenaline system remain stable over the life span. While some studies do report declines, others actually report increases (see Morgan & May, 1990). One exception may be the hypothalamus, where age-related declines in noradrenergic markers are reported more frequently than in other brain regions. Postsynaptically, the data are presently insufficient to draw conclusions concerning either the α- or β-adrenergic receptors.

In human brain, a meager number of studies suggest no change in noradrenaline with age (see Rogers & Bloom, 1985). An equally small number report no change in beta-adrenergic receptors with age. This apparent stability of the neurochemical measures of the noradrenergic system are surprising in light of the sizeable loss of neurons in the locus ceruleus (the major noradrenergic nucleus in the brain; Vijayashankar & Brody, 1979; Tomlinson, Irving & Blessed, 1981). The paucity of studies in this system may explain the present discrepancy between neurochemical and anatomical results.

D. The Serotonin System

The data on the presynaptic markers of the serotonin system in rodents are very consistent and indicate no change in serotonin content with usual aging (reviewed by Morgan & May, 1990). The few studies on human samples confirm this conclusion.

Postsynaptically, there appear to be declines of 20 to 40% in both the S1 and S2 receptor classes (Morgan & May, 1990) As the S1 receptor class is now believed to consist of four discrete subtypes, further characterization is necessary to elucidate which of the subtypes is most affected. Similar results are found in human cerebral cortex and hippo-campus, with declines in both S1 and S2 sites, in some cases reaching 70% reductions (Morgan et al., 1988). A further loss of S2 receptors is a consistent finding in AD (see Section IV.B). Still, the number of studies is too few to make specific statements concerning the extent of the declines in specific brain regions.

E. Other Neurotransmitter Systems

Perhaps the most unfortunate circumstance concerning synaptic neurochemistry and brain aging is that the above-mentioned neurotransmitter systems, on which 90% of the research has been conducted, account for 5% of the total synapses in the brain. The two major neurotransmitters in the central nervous system are gamma aminobutyric acid (GABA) (inhibitory) and the excitatory amino acids (glutamate, aspartate, and related substances). The presynaptic marker for GABA is limited primarily to the activity of the synthetic enzyme glutamate decarboxylase, which in several studies does not change with age, but in others increases or decreases (see Morgan & May, 1990). No studies have yet been performed in human tissues. Postsynaptically, most studies have focused on the diazepam receptor, the binding site for the antianxiety drugs, which appears complexed with the $GABA_A$ receptor site around a chloride channel. The diazepam receptors decline by 20 to 40% with aging. In human brain, two small studies have reported a 100–300% increase in the $GABA_A$ receptor with aging. Further analyses are necessary to determine the validity of these findings which, if true, could have broad implications for aging and brain functions, since GABA is the major inhibitory transmitter in the brain. Virtually nothing is known concerning the excitatory amino acid transmitter systems with aging.

A smattering of reports is emerging concerning the neuropeptide systems with aging. In this context, the few available reports suggest that the receptors for the endogenous opiate transmitters decline with age. For other neuropeptides (substance P, somatostatin, neurotensin, vasopressin) there does not appear to be a significant age-related decline, although isolated changes in specific brain regions have been reported (Morgan & May, 1990).

In summary, the field of synaptic neurochemistry during aging is filled with inconsistencies and contradictory results. Rarely can these discrepancies be reconciled by differences in species or brain regions studied. Nonetheless, in some systems sufficient numbers of studies have been performed that tentative conclusions can be drawn based on weighted averages of all published studies. For these reasons, it is important that negative data also be reported. Those tentative conclusions are detailed above, and some of their implications will be discussed below. However, the most important neurotransmitter

Table I
Anatomical Comparisons of Pathological Differences
in Young and Old Alzheimer's Cases

A. Pathology in young AD > control; pathology in old AD = control (no change)

Study	Measure/region
Bowen *et al.* (1976)	Weight/temporal lobe[c]
Pro *et al.* (1980)	Plaque number/cerebellum
Bondareff *et al.* (1982)	Neuron loss/locus ceruleus[a]
Mountjoy *et al.* (1983)	Brain weight
	Brain volume
	Ventricular volume
	Neuron loss/frontal cortex
	Neuron loss/temporal cortex
Mann *et al.* (1984)	Plaque number/temporal cortex[c]
	Tangle number/temporal cortex[c]
Hubbard & Anderson (1985)	Neuron loss/frontal cortex
	Neuron loss/temporal cortex
Bondareff & Mountjoy (1986)	Neuron loss/locus ceruleus

B. Pathology in young AD > pathology in old AD

Study	Measure
Ball & Lo (1977)	Granulovacuolar degeneration/hippocampus
Gibson & Tomlinson (1977)	Hirano bodies/hippocampus
Bowen *et al.* (1979)	Atrophy/temporal lobe
	Neuron loss/temporal lobe
Gibson (1983b)	Plaque counts/cerebral cortex
Mountjoy *et al.* (1983)	Plaque counts/9 cortical regions
Mann *et al.* (1984)	Neuron loss/nucleus basalis
	Neuron loss/locus ceruleus
Mann *et al.* (1985)	Plaque number/temporal cortex
	Tangle number/temporal cortex
	Neuron loss/temporal cortex
	Nucleolar shrinkage/temporal cortex
	Neuron loss/hippocampus
	Nucleolar shrinkage/hippocampus
McDuff & Sumi (1985)	Diencephalic degeneration
Jellinger (1987)	Neuron loss/dorsal raphe
	Neuron loss/nucleus basalis
	Neuron loss/pedunculopontine nucleus
Alafuzoff *et al.* (1987)	Plaque number/frontal cortex, hippocampus
	Tangle number/frontal cortex, hippocampus

C. Pathology in young AD and old AD similar

Study	Measure
Hubbard & Anderson (1988)	Neuropil volume atrophy/frontal cortex, temporal cortex
	Neuron loss/subiculum

(*continued*)

Table I (*Continued*)

C. Pathology in young AD and old AD similar

Study	Measure
Mann *et al.* (1985)	Cortical thickness atrophy/temporal cortex
	Hippocampal atrophy
	Plaque number/hippocampus[b]
	Tangle number/hippocampus[b]
George *et al.* (1986)	Leukoencephalopathy/white matter

[a]Groups were divided on the basis of locus ceruleus neuron number from a bimodal distribution. Age was a significant predictor of the extent of neuron loss.

[b]Although not statistically different, the average pathology was still more severe in the younger cases.

[c]These conclusions are derived from the reviewers' interpretation of graphs of the data, and not a direct statistical comparison.

systems on a sheer numbers basis have been examined only superficially. In part this reflects the later development of research tools with which to study these systems. Yet from a global impact basis, these systems are probably the most important for the normal functioning of the brain; undoubtedly it is within the synapses containing these neurotransmitters that the engrams encoding memories reside. The goal of the next decade for the descriptive neurochemistry of aging should be to define the limits of lifespan changes in these systems with usual, successful, and ultimately diseased aging.

To some extent, it is conceivable that these losses in synaptic transmitters and receptors may represent biological deficiencies that develop over the lifespan and underlie some of the age-related cognitive changes described elsewhere in this volume. Unfortunately, even for the well-characterized markers, there is no simple hypothesis to explain the results. There are no general categories of markers that change in all systems (i.e., receptors or synthetic enzymes or transmitter levels), nor regions in which most systems demonstrate major declines, nor any systems reported to degenerate in all regions. All combinations of region by system by marker category declines can be found in the literature. Hence, these studies have failed to reveal a simplifying hypothesis of age-related neurotransmitter system changes.

However, the anatomical data summarized above suggest that some declines in all synaptic neurochemical markers would be expected owing to neuronal shrinkage and synapse loss. Importantly, the issue is complicated by the discovery of many purportedly synaptic markers (receptors, uptake systems, channels) on nonneuronal cells such as astrocytes (Murphy & Pearce, 1987), which increase in size with aging. Thus, because of neuronal shrinkage and expansion of the astrocytic compartment, the old brain contains a greater proportion of astrocytic protein (relative to neuronal protein) than does the young brain. Hence, even in the absence of changes in intraneuronal concentrations, the chemical markers found exclusively on neurons are expected to decrease with aging, those markers found on both neurons and astrocytes should remain stable, while those exclusively on astrocytes are expected to increase. For at least one astrocytic marker, glial fibrillary acidic protein, the results support the hypothesis (Goss, Finch, & Morgan,

1991), and additional markers are being evaluated with respect to this hypothesis. This argument is presented in greater detail in Finch and Morgan (1990).

III. Usual Aging in the Dopamine System, Schizophrenia, and Parkinson's Disease

As described in Section II, one of the few age-related changes about which some certainty exists is a decline in the markers for dopaminergic synapses. This author estimates there is a 50% decline in the overall dopaminergic tone (integrated presynaptic and postsynaptic function) during the typical human life span. Of interest for this handbook is the potential interaction of this usual age change with two neurological disorders involving the dopamine system, schizophrenia and parkinsonism.

Schizophrenia is the major form of psychosis in this country, and has an early age of onset such that first symptoms are rare after the age of 30 (Loranger, 1984). The dopaminergic hypothesis of schizophrenia has had a long history (Snyder, Banerjee, Yamamura, & Greenberg, 1974), and although not without competitors, is massively strengthened by the finding that the dose of neuroleptic drugs used to treat schizophrenics is correlated perfectly with the dose necessary to attain 70–80% blockade of the D2 dopamine receptor (Seeman, 1980). In fact, one disturbance in the brains of schizophrenics appears to be an increase in the number of D2 dopamine receptors (Reisine, Rossor, Spokes, Iverson, & Yamamuru 1980; Seeman *et al.,* 1984; Owen, Owen, Poulter, & Crow, 1984; Wong, Wagner, & Tune, 1985; Reynolds, Czudek, Bzowej, & Seeman, 1987) and even elevations in the levels of dopamine (Mackay *et al.,* 1982; Reynolds, 1983). Hence, one aspect of the problem in schizophrenia appears to be excess dopaminergic tone, and those symptoms successfully ameliorated by the neuroleptic drugs would be those mediated by overactivation of the D2 receptor.

Parkinsonism, on the other hand, is primarily a motor disorder, characterized by a resting tremor, and muscular rigidity. The major defect in parkinsonism is degeneration of dopaminergic neurons in the substantia nigra, although neuron loss and Lewy body formation can be found in other regions as well, including the noradrenergic locus ceruleus, serotonergic dorsal raphe nucleus, and the cholinergic nucleus basalis (Forno, 1988). Associated with the degeneration of the nigral neurons is a 75–90% loss of dopamine in the striatal regions (caudate nucleus, putamen); the primary therapy for parkinsonism involves replacement of the lost dopamine with its immediate precursor, L-dopa (Hornykiewicz, 1983). Thus, parkinsonism results from too little activity in the dopamine system, and in this regard may be thought of as the opposite of schizophrenia. However, it is important to consider that the motoric effects of dopamine deficiency, and the psychotic effects of dopamine excess need not be mediated in the same brain regions. Most likely, the motoric effects result from dopamine deficiencies in the extrapyramidal motor system of the striatum, while the psychosis-inducing effects of dopamine excess are mediated by dopaminergic innervation of the frontal and/or entorhinal cortices.

Further support for the linkage between schizophrenia and Parkinsonism is the side effects of the drugs used to treat these disorders. Nueroleptics are notorious for their iatrogenic induction of movement disorders, one of which is called pseudoparkinsonism.

L-Dopa, the primary therapy for advanced parkinsonism, also has a significant side effect; hallucinations (Pederzoli *et al.*, 1983).

How then does normal aging affect these disorders? It would seem likely that the typical early age of onset for schizophrenia, and the late age of onset for parkinsonism are directed by the usual age-related loss of dopamine (Figure 1). That is, early in the life span, when dopamine levels are high, a genetic or environmental condition that would elevate dopamine activity would be likely to push the dopamine tone in the brain above a theoretical threshold for the clinical expression of psychotic symptoms. However, the same event later in life would have a reduced probability of surpassing the threshold because of the age-related losses of dopamine. In this sense, usual aging is protective against the onset of psychosis. In addition, with usual aging there appears some

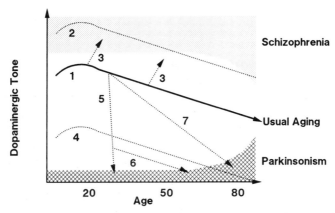

Figure 1 The interaction of usual aging in the dopamine system with the onset of schizophrenia and Parkinson's disease. Usual changes in the dopamine system proceed along the line indicated by (1) Usual Aging, with roughly 50% loss occurring over the life span. Dopaminergic Tone refers to the integrated pre-synaptic and post-synaptic activity in the dopamine system. The stippled region indicates excessive dopaminergic activity leading to some of the symptoms of schizophrenia. The cross-hatched region represents deficient dopaminergic activity leading to parkinsonism. Age is presented in years. Line (2) represents genetically excessive dopaminergic activity leading to schizophrenic symptoms, which tend to diminish with usual age-related reductions in dopaminergic tone. Lines labeled (3) represent environmental factors that elevate dopaminergic activity. At younger ages, these elevations are more likely to exceed the threshold for schizophrenic symptoms than at later ages. Line (4) represents a genetic model of parkinsonism (presently viewed as unlikely, see text) that also has been referred to as an *initial deficit* model. Here, a low level of dopaminergic activity to begin with leads to early symptoms of parkinsonism as usual aging changes proceed. Line (5) represents individuals exposed to dopaminotoxins in youth (such as MPTP) that rapidly cause degeneration in the dopamine system. Some individuals exposed to these toxins may have restricted degeneration that predisposes them to higher risk of parkinsonism as usual age-related reductions in dopaminergic tone continue (line 6). A final model by which parkinsonism might develop is *accelerated aging* of the dopamine system, in which the age-related reduction in dopaminergic tone proceeds at an accelerated rate. The changes in threshold values for the expression of parkinsonian and schizophrenic symptoms are derived from the age-related loss of compensatory capacity (see Section IV and Figure 2).

improvement in schizophrenic symptoms even in the absence of medication (Bleuler, 1974). This spontaneous improvement may reflect the underlying age-related reductions in dopaminergic tone.

However, at the same time that usual aging protects against schizophrenia, it increases the likelihood of parkinsonism. The precise causes of idiopathic parkinsonism are not clear, but most attention is now focused on environmental toxins. Part of the basis for this focus in the marvelous medical detective story of William Langston tracing down the compound methylphenyltetrahydropyridine (MPTP) as a contaminant in a batch of synthetic heroin (Langston, Ballard, Tetrud, & Irwin, 1983). Young heroin addicts were presenting in a northern California clinic with all the signs and symptoms of parkinsonism. Langston and colleagues traced the source of this disorder to a batch of synthetic heroin common to all these individuals. The condition produced by MPTP in these individuals is identical in virtually all aspects to idiopathic parkinsonism. Using positron emission tomography with [18F] fluorodopa, Calne et al. (1985) determined that there was massive loss of striatal dopamine terminals in the affected individuals. Moreover, other addicts, while presently asymptomatic, nonetheless had smaller losses of dopamine terminals as well. It is predicted that usual aging declines in the dopamine system will sum with these initial deficits to produce parkinsonian symptoms later in life.

It is now speculated that idiopathic parkinsonism derives from some environmental agent much like MPTP. Of interest is the fact that parkinsonism evidently did not exist before James Parkinson's description in 1817; no anecdotal reports of the symptoms are found before that time. There also does not appear to be a genetic link in parkinsonism, as identical twins have no greater concordance rates than the general population (Martilla, Kaprio, Koskenvuo, & Rinne, 1988), and the low incidence of parkinsonism in less-industrialized societies points to agents introduced into western societies with industrialization in the late 18th century (Tanner et al., 1989). Two scenarios have been proposed for how usual aging affects Parkinsonian symptomology. One model proposes an initial deficit in the dopamine system, by acute exposure to a dopaminotoxin (such as MPTP or some industrial pollutant). This initial deficit is insufficient for immediate clinical expression, but sums with the usual aging loss. A second mechanism assumes a more chronic exposure to the environmental toxin, which accelerates the rate at which dopaminergic function is usually lost with age (see Finch, 1981). A third possibility, which this author has yet to see suggested, is that in nonindustrialized societies, there may not be a usual age-related presynaptic loss in the dopamine system. Rats and mice have smaller changes presynaptically than humans (see Section II,A). Perhaps even the usual changes observed in the dopamine system of humans are pathological, in that they would not occur in the absence of exposure to an environmental toxin. Most rodent studies have also been conducted in western societies, where exposure to the same air- and water-borne toxins might variably influence age-related loss of dopamine tone. It remains to be determined whether even usual aging in the dopamine system might be effected by an environmental agent, with excessive exposure leading to the additional losses responsible for the primary symptoms of Parkinson's disease.

In summary, the data strongly support an overall loss of dopaminergic tone with age. This usual loss of dopamine function may interact with other genetic and extragenetic factors responsible for neurological disorders such as schizophrenia and Parkinson's disease. Specifically, the usual aging pattern may protect against the onset of schizophrenia (caused by excessive dopaminergic tone) by decreasing dopamine activity, thus restricting the onset of schizophrenia to younger ages. However, the protection against schizophrenia conferred by this decline may enhance the risk of developing parkinsonism, which is caused by 75 to 90% reductions in dopaminergic tone.

IV. The Interaction of Aging with the Pathological Features of Alzheimer's Disease

Alzheimer's disease is a devastating neurological disorder with dramatically increased incidence over the life span. Certain pathological aspects of this disorder will be covered in other chapters of this volume by Scheibel (6) and Grady and Rapoport (8). The focus of this section, however, is the dramatically different degrees of pathology in AD depending upon the age of onset of the dementing illness. In most studies comparing early- and late-onset AD, the extent of the neuropathology is greater in the early-onset cases. In fact, for the very oldest cases, the degree of pathology in demented and nondemented cases may not be distinguishable for many parameters. The basic tenet of this section is that *age results in a decreasing capacity to functionally compensate for the pathological changes caused by AD.* This decline in compensatory capacity effectively lowers the threshold amount of damage required for the clinical expression of dementia as individuals advance in years. This change in the capacity to compensate functionally may be a general feature of neurological disorders of aging, and not limited to AD.

A. Age-Related Changes in the Anatomical Features of Alzheimer's Disease

In Table I are listed a number of studies that have evaluated the neuritic plaque and neurofibrillary tangle densities in AD and control cases, as a function of patient age. While a few exceptions exist, most studies report that the degree of pathology is much less in older AD cases (Table IB), and in some studies there is no statistical difference between the AD and control cases in the older age groups (Table IA). Part of the reason for the lack of statistical significance in some studies is that older control cases to which the older AD cases are compared have some plaques and tangles, while younger control cases rarely present such changes. Still, the major difference is that the older AD cases have less severe pathology.

   The same is true for neuron loss. Bondareff and colleagues classified AD cases into two groups based on the number of neurons in the noradrenergic locus ceruleus (Bondareff, Mountjoy, & Roth, 1982). One distinguishing characteristic of these two populations is patient age; the AD cases with little noradrenergic neuron loss tend to be older. Even in the cerebral cortex, the focus of many of the changes in AD that appear most critical for the cognitive dysfunction in this disorder, the older cases fail to exhibit significant declines in neuron number in regions where statistically significant changes are present in younger cases (Mountjoy, Roth, Evans, & Evans, 1983). In the nucleus basalis of Meynert, the origin of the cholinergic neurons that project to the cerebral cortex, and which at one time was proposed to be *the* cause of dementia, the neuron loss in the older cases is less severe than in cases with earlier onset of the disorder (Mann *et al.*, 1984).

Table II

Biochemical Comparisons of Pathological Differences in Young and Old Alzheimer's Cases

A. Pathology in young AD > control; Pathology in old AD = control (no change)

Study	Measure/region[a]
Gottfries *et al.* (1969)	[Homovanillic acid]/CSF
Bowen *et al.* (1979)	Carbonic anhydrase/temporal lobe LSD binding (S1 + S2 serotonin receptors)/temporal lobe
Cross *et al.* (1984)	S1 receptors/temporal cortex, frontal cortex, amygdala
Rossor *et al.* (1982)	ChAT activity/7 cortical regions
Bird *et al.* (1983)	ChAT activity/frontal cortex, temporal cortex, cerebellum, nucleus basalis
Bowen *et al.* (1983)	S1 receptors/temporal cortex
Yates *et al.* (1983)	[Noradrenaline]/mammilary body ChAT activity/caudate nucleus AChE activity/temporal cortex, caudate nucleus
DeKosky *et al.* (1985)	ChAT activity/frontal cortex
Bowen & Davison (1986)	Phosphohexoisomerase/temporal cortex Aldolase/temporal cortex Phosphoglycerate mutase/temporal cortex Total protein/temporal cortex
Pierotti *et al.* (1986)	[Somatostatin]/temporal cortex

B. Pathology in young AD > pathology in old AD

Study	Measure
Gottfries *et al.* (1969)	[5-HIAA]/CSF
Bowen *et al.* (1979)	Phosphohexoisomerase/temporal lobe ChAT activity/temporal lobe
Bareggi *et al.* (1982)	[Homovanillic acid]/CSF
Bird *et al.* (1983)	ChAT activity/hippocampus
Francis *et al.* (1985)	[Serotonin]/temporal cortex [Noradrenaline]/temporal cortex
Volicer *et al.* (1985)	[DOPAC]/CSF
Bowen & Davison (1986)	ChAT activity/temporal cortex Ganglioside/temporal cortex ChAT activity/temporal cortex
Reinikainen *et al.* (1988)	ChAT activity/frontal cortex, temporal cortex, parietal cortex, hippocampus
Brane *et al.* (1989)	[Homovanillic acid]/CSF [5-HIAA]/CSF

C. Pathology in young AD and old AD similar

Study	Measure
Bowen *et al.* (1979)	[5-HIAA]/temporal lobe
Bowen *et al.* (1983)	ChAT activity/temporal lobe Imipramine binding/temporal lobe

(continued)

Table II (*Continued*)

C. Pathology in young AD and old AD similar

Study	Measure
Yates *et al.* (1983)	[Noradrenaline]/hypothalamus ChAT activity/temporal cortex
Reynolds *et al.* (1984)	S2 receptors/frontal cortex
Cross *et al.* (1984)	S2 receptors/frontal cortex, temporal cortex, amygdala
Palmer *et al.* (1984)	[Homovanillic acid]/CSF
Francis *et al.* (1985)	ChAT activity/temporal cortex

[a]CSF, cerebrospinal fluid; ChAT, choline acetyltransferase activity; 5-HIAA, 5-hydroxyindoleacetic acid; DOPAC, dihydroxyphenylacetic acid; [X], concentration of compound X.

B. Age-Related Changes in the Neurochemical Features of Alzheimer's Disease

A similar picture emerges from the neurochemical literature on AD; early-onset cases typically have the most severe neurochemical pathology. Studies comparing early- and late-onset AD cases are summarized in Table II. Even those neurochemical markers believed by some to be intimately involved with the cognitive dysfunction of AD, such as choline acetyltransferase, fail to differ significantly from control values in late onset cases (Table IIA). This is particularly true for frontal cortical choline acetyltransferase; activity in the temporal lobe is more consistently reduced in late onset cases (Table IIC), but often less than in the early onset cases (Table IIB). Of all the other neurochemical markers of AD, the only one that appears consistently reduced in both early- and late-onset AD is the S-2 serotonergic receptor (Cross *et al.*, 1984; Reynolds *et al.*, 1984).

C. Age of Onset versus Duration of Disease

One potential explanation for this young versus old difference in the severity of AD pathology is the duration of the disease. It would generally be thought that younger onset of the disease would be associated with greater duration before death, owing to the overall better health and lower death rates of younger humans. Surprisingly, the several studies that have compared duration of disease in early- and late-onset AD have failed to detect a significant difference in the duration of the disorder as a function of age of onset (Bird, Stranahan, Sumi, & Raskind, 1983; Mann *et al.*, 1984; Brane *et al.*, 1989). Two studies have directly compared the correlations between indices of AD pathology and age of onset versus duration of disease. *Age of onset correlates with the degree of pathology* for most variables; remarkably *duration of disease does not* correlate with the degree of pathology at death (Mann, Yates, & Marcyniuk, 1985; McDuff and Sumi, 1985).

D. Age of Onset and Other Neurological Disorders

The data for other neurodegenerative diseases with respect to age of onset is negligible. However, it is consistent with the overall trend of the data for AD. In Parkinson's disease, early onset cases (mean age, 65 years) have a roughly 90% reduction in dopamine in the neostriatum, while the later onset cases (mean age, 81 years) have only a 75% reduction in dopamine (both groups were compared to the same control group; Hornykiewicz, 1985). A similar picture emerges in Huntington's disease. Cases with onsets after 50 years tend to have less severe neuropathological involvement, and a slower rate of progression of the disorder (Myers *et al.*, 1985).

E. Significance of Age of Onset to Alzheimer's Disease

The data presented above would superficially suggest that late-onset neurological disorders are milder forms of the disease, because the underlying pathological changes are fewer in late-onset cases. However, it is important to consider another possibility, and that relates to the notion of thresholds for the expression of clinical symptoms of neurological disorders. The studies of parkinsonism have indicated that certain systems in the brain have considerable redundancy built into them. As mentioned in Section III, a 75–90% loss of dopamine is required before clinical symptoms become present. Other systems have similar or lesser degrees of functional redundancy (see examples in Finch & Morgan, 1987). The degree to which functional redundancy is a true excess or reserve capacity in the affected system, or a plasticity mechanism that recruits previously uninvolved systems to bear on the compromised function is unclear at present. However, another potential measure of functional redundancy is the ability to recover from acute damage to a system.

The neurodegenerative diseases are presumably chronic disorders with progressive deterioration occurring over years if not decades. However, other insults to the brain occur suddenly and massively; among these are stroke-induced ischemic damage and head injury. In both cases, some recovery of the initial deficit will occur, but the rate and extent of recovery is diminished as the age of the individual increases (Bannister, 1985; Jennett *et al.*, 1980). In experimental animal models of recovery after brain injury, it has been demonstrated that young animals initially lose synapses in target areas of the damaged brain regions, but the number of synapses returns to near normal in a phenomenon called reactive synaptogenesis. The mechanism involves the sprouting of new synapses from fibers in the vicinity of the degenerating synapses. Studies that examine synaptic sprouting in aged animals report a reduced amount of sprouting, or a delay in sprouting in both hippocampal (Scheff, Benardo, & Cotman, 1980; Hof, Scheff, Benardo, & Cotman, 1982; McWilliams & Lynch, 1984; Booze & Davis, 1987;) and neuromuscular junction lesion paradigms (Pestronk, Drachman, & Griffin, 1980; Fagg *et al.*, 1981). In young animals, brain lesions also induce the secretion of neuronotrophic factors (capable of stimulating neuron survival and neurite outgrowth *in vitro*) believed to play a role in the sprouting response. The secretion of these factors is greatly reduced in aged animals (Needels, Neito-Sampedro, & Cotman, 1986; Calderini *et al.*, 1987). These deficits in reactive synaptogenesis with aging suggest that recruitment of other systems to take over the function previously mediated by the lesioned area may be impaired with age.

Animal studies also suggest that age reduces the capability of the brain to withstand toxic insults. The dopaminergic neurotoxin MPTP produces permanent lesions only in old mice; young mice ultimately recover from its effects (Gupta et al., 1986; Ricaurte, Delanney, Irwin, & Langston, 1987). Old rats are also more sensitive to another dopamine neurotoxin, 6-hydroxydopamine (Marshall, Drew & Neve, 1983). Even the behavioral and neurochemical responses to thiamin deficiency are greater in old rats (Freeman, Nielsen, & Gibson, 1987). Importantly, young rats receiving 6-hydroxydopamine lesions initially recover from the behavioral deficits, but these behavioral abnormalities reappear 14 months after the lesion (Schallert, 1983). These studies imply that the aged brain is less resistant to toxic insults, and that with aging, there is a loss of the redundancy necessary for functional compensation from insults sustained early in life.

The greater susceptibility to damage and reduced plasticity of the aged brain suggest a novel hypothesis concerning the greater severity of pathology in early-onset AD. The key feature of this hypothesis is that the threshold amount of neurological damage required for the clinical expression of dementia is not constant over the lifespan, but declines with age. Because of the decrease in the ability of the brain to compensate for damage with age, the threshold amount of damage required for the expression of symptoms is not constant over the life span, but declines with age as shown in Figure 2. This decreasing compensatory capacity may result from a loss of reserve capacity in many brain systems with age, a loss of the ability to recruit other remaining systems into the function normally performed by the damaged tissue (presumably requiring plasticity), or both. Another important feature is that this loss of compensatory capacity would decline at different rates in different individuals, consistent with the increased variance of many physiological parameters with age. Hence, two individuals of advanced age may have similar amounts of neuropathology, yet one will be demented and the other, compensating successfully. While careful examination of the entire brain may allow pathologists to correctly identify dements from nondements, adherence to rigid criteria for plaque and tangle densities result in some misdiagnosis in cases where death occurs after 80 years (Crystal et al., 1988). To a large degree, this age-related decrease in brain compensation for damage is the neurobiological equivalent of impaired healing responses in other systems.

Assuming the threshold declines with age, the pathology in early-onset AD must be severe; individuals with small amounts of pathology would be asymptomatic owing to compensation (see Figure 2). Several researchers have remarked that even nondemented individuals show some plaque and tangle pathology at autopsy, particularly at advanced age (Ulrich, 1982; Miller, Hicks, D'Amato, & Landis, 1984; Ulrich, 1985; Mann, Tucker, & Yates, 1987). These are often interpreted as preclinical AD cases. While it is truly impossible to determine when the preclinical cases would become symptomatic (in part because they are already deceased), one can estimate the time that plaques and tangles take to develop from Down's syndrome, where Alzheimer-type behavioral changes appear in all cases by their late 40s and 50s. Almost all Down's cases have plaques and tangles after age 30 (Wisniewski, Wisniewski, & Wen, 1984) and preplaque deposits may precede even the formation of detectable plaques (Giaccone et al., 1989). Motte and Williams (1989) claim there are four stages of plaque development in Down's starting as early as 25 years, and completing their development no earlier than 48 years of age. It would seem likely that similar events occur in AD; that it requires 20 years or more for some of the pathological features to develop fully; this rate of development would vary

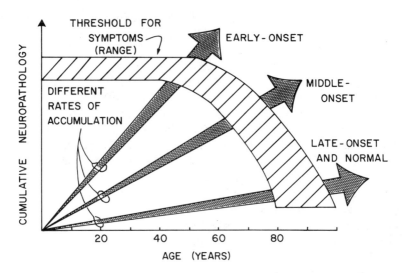

Figure 2 Adaptive capacity and neuropathology interact to produce the clinical symptoms of dementia. *Cumulative pathology* refers to the amount of neuronal damage, either from plaque and tangle pathology, infarcts, brain injury, congenital neuron degeneration, toxin exposure, or any other cause. In particular, damage to cortical structures (cerebral association cortices, hippocampus, amygdala) would be the most critical structures in this regard, but subcortical structures (nucleus basalis, locus ceruleus, raphe nuclei) may also be important. The hatched region represents the theoretical threshold amount of pathology required before clinical symptoms of dementia would become manifest. The decline in this threshold value with age reflects a decrease in the capacity to compensate functionally for accumulated pathology as chronological age proceeds. The width of this threshold represents individual variability in the capacity to tolerate certain levels of pathology. This variability in compensatory capacity across individuals is predicted to increase with the age of the population (like most physiological variables), hence the hatched zone widens as age progresses. The general decline in the severity of neuropathology in dements with age, and the fact that at advanced ages, dements and nondements do not differ significantly in the degree of neuropathology, are consistent with this model. The cross-hatched arrows represent three different rates at which neuropathology might accumulate to illustrate the relationship of age at onset with the change in threshold. The origin and linearity of these arrows is arbitrary, and not significant for the model proposed. The key feature is that early-onset dements are required to have severe pathology; otherwise, they would compensate successfully for the function lost, although a rare individual that had extreme losses of compensatory capacity at early ages might be demented with moderate to low amount of pathology. This model is proposed to apply to neurodegenerative disease in general, and is not restricted to Alzheimer's disease or other dementias.

among individuals. This is reflected in Figure 2 as three rates of acummulation of pathology starting at birth, although the time of initiation of the pathology cannot be known with confidence, and probably starts later. The lines are also drawn linear, although this need not be the case depending on whether environment or genetic causes of AD proceed in a continuous or discontinuous manner. The key feature is that the early-onset cases must have greater pathology to exceed the higher threshold for the expression of symptoms. Later onset cases probably accumulate the pathology at a slower rate, and fail to exceed the threshold until later in life, as the pathology becomes greater and the threshold declines. Finally, there are some who accumulate AD-type pathology at a slow rate. These individuals may never become demented, or they may ultimately lose their capacity to compensate for even this slight amount of pathology they possess, and clinically express the symptoms of dementia.

V. Summary and Conclusions

Aging and synaptic neurochemistry, like most of gerontology, is an infant discipline. Most research is still in a necessarily descriptive phase, although some more convincing hypotheses concerning those changes are beginning to emerge. Nonetheless, one dogma of brain aging that is being dispelled is that significant neuron loss is a necessary correlate of advanced age. This implies that the biological-deficiency hypotheses of age-related declines in cognitive function may need to be substantially revised, and the ensuing agism that is their natural correlate can be extinguished. Instead, those changes that do occur with usual and successful aging may not represent brain dysfunction, but the necessary consequences of a lifetime of information processing, with the gradual accumulation of mnemonic engrams. The cognitive dysfunctions of aging may represent the filling of the available synaptic space with multiple memories, rather than a loss of the biological mechanisms capable of such functions.

However, unsuccessful aging does occur. The specific ages of onset for certain neurological disorders may reflect independent changes in related systems as a typical part of brain aging. In this regard, the normal loss of dopamine in mesostriatal and mesocortical pathways may underlie the typically early age of onset for schizophrenia and the late age of onset of Parkinson's disease; schizophrenia resulting from dopamine excess and Parkinson's disease from severe dopamine deficiency.

Perhaps the most unsuccessful aging in brain function is that occurring in AD. Here neurodegeneration and brain atrophy are the norm (except at advanced ages, see Table I), unlike usual aging (see Section I). However, there are cases of dementia in which the degree of pathology is slight, and in many respects no different from age-matched nondements. These are typically cases in which death occurs after 80 years. Not only in AD, but also in other neurological disorders, the degree of pathology appears less in the later-onset forms of the disorder. This phenomenon reflects a second age-related process, independent of the disorder, referred to here as a loss of compensatory capacity. Such loss is most readily apparent in cases of acute brain injury, and may be the neurobiological equivalent of the loss of healing capacity elsewhere in the body.

Conceivably, the loss of compensatory capacity and learning and memory difficulties with aging may reflect the same process, an overall loss of synaptic plasticity with age. Evidence for this loss can be found in the neurochemical, anatomical, and behavioral literatures, but the precise mechanisms of synaptic plasticity have yet to be elucidated. However, one important question raised by this chapter is the degree to which these changes in plasticity should be thought of as biological deficiencies (avoidable pathologic changes) versus pleiotropic concomitants of a lifetime of accumulated memories.

Acknowledgments

I thank Marcia Gordon and Tuck Finch for helpful discussions during the preparation of this manuscript, and Russell Ruth, Tim Collier, and Richard Conway for constructive debates concerning engrams and aging. DGM was supported by the Anna Greenwall Award from the American Federation on Aging Research, NIA Grant AG-07892 and an Established Investigator Award from the American Heart Association.

References

Adams, I. (1986). Comparison of synaptic changes in the precentral and postcentral cerebral cortex of aging humans: A quantitative ultrastructural study. *Neurobiology of Aging, 8,* 203–212.

Alafuzoff, I., Iqbal, K., Friden, H., Adolfsson, R., & Winblad, B. (1987). Histopathological criteria for progressive dementia disorders: Clinical-pathological correlation and classification by multivariate data analysis. *Acta Neuropathologica, 74,* 209–225.

Ball, M. J., & Lo, P. (1977). Granulovacuolar degeneration in the ageing brain and in dementia. *Journal of Neuropathology and Experimental Neurology, 36,* 474–487.

Bannister, R. (1985). *Brain's Clinical Neurology.* London: Oxford University Press.

Bareggi, S. R., Franceschi, M., Bonini, L., Zecca, L., & Smirne, S. (1982). Decreased CSF concentrations of homovanillic acid and gamma-aminobutyric acid in Alzheimer's disease. *Archives of Neurology, 39,* 709–712.

Bartus, R. T., Dean, R. L., III, Beer, B., & Lippa, A. S. (1982). The cholinergic hypothesis of geriatric memory dysfunction. *Science, 217,* 408–417.

Bertoni-Freddari, C., Giuli, C., Pieri, C., Paci, D. Amadio, L. Ermini, M., & Dravid, A. (1987). The effect of chronic hydergine treatment on the plasticity of synaptic junctions in the dentate gyrus of rats. *Journal of Gerontology, 42,* 482–486.

Bigl, V., Arendt, T., Fischer, S., Werner, M., & Arendt, A. (1987). The cholinergic system in aging. *Gerontology, 33,* 172–180.

Bird, T. D., Stanahan, S., Sumi, S. M., & Raskind, M. (1983). Alzheimer's disease: Choline acetyltransferase activity in brain tissue from clinical and pathological subgroups. *Annals of Neurology, 14(3),* 284–293.

Bleuler, M. (1974). The long-term course of the schizophrenic psychoses. *Psychological Medicine, 4,* 244–254.

Bondareff, W., Mountjoy, C. Q., & Roth, M. (1982). Loss of neurons of origin of the adrenergic projection to cerebral cortex (nucleus locus ceruleus) in senile dementia. *Neurology, 32(2),* 164–168.

Bondareff, W., & Mountjoy, C. Q. (1986). Number of neurons in nucleus locus ceruleus in demented and non-demented patients: Rapid estimation and correlated parameters. *Neurobiology of Aging, 7,* 297–300.

Booze, R. M., & Davis, J. N. (1987). Persistence of sympathetic ingrowth fibers in aged rat hippocampus. *Neurobiology of Aging, 8,* 213–218.

Bowen, D. M., Allen, S. J. Benton, J. S., Goodhardt, M. J., Haan, E. A., Palmer, A. M., Sims, N. R., Smith, C. C. T., Spillane, J. A., Esiri, M. M., Neary, D., Snowdon, J. S., Wilcock, G. K., & Davison, A. N. (1983). Biochemical assessment of serotonergic and cholinergic dysfunction and cerebral atrophy in Alzheimer's disease. *Journal of Neurochemistry, 41(1),* 266–272.

Bowen, D. M., & Davison, A. N. (1986). Biochemical studies of nerve cells and energy metabolism in Alzheimer's disease. *British Medical Bulletin, 42(1),* 75–80.

Bowen, D. M., Smith, C. B., White P., & Davison, A. N. (1976). Neurotransmitter-related enzymes and indices of hypoxia in senile dementia and other abiotrophies. *Brain, 99,* 459–496.

Bowen, D. M. Spillane, J. A., Curzon, G., Meier-Ruge, W., White, P., Goodhardt, M. J., Iwangoff, P., & Davison, A. N. (1979). Accelerated aging or selective neuronal loss as an important cause of dementia? *Lancet, i(8106),* 11–14.

Brane, G. Gottfries, C. G., Blennow, K., Karlson, I., Lekman, A., Parnetti, L., Svennerholm, L., & Wallin, A. (1989). Monoamine metabolites in cerebrospinal fluid and behavioral ratings in patients with early and late onset of Alzheimer dementia. *Alzheimer Disease and Associated Disorders, 3,* 148–156.

Brody, H. (1955). Organization of the cerebral cortex. III. A study of aging in the human cerebral cortex. *Journal of Comparative Neurology, 102,* 511–556.

Calderini, G., Bellini, F., Consolazione, A., Dal Toso, R., Milan, F., & Toffano, G. (1987). Reparative processes in aged brain. *Gerontology, 33,* 227–233.

Calne, D., Langston, J. W., Martin, W., Stoessel, A., Ruth, T., Adam, J., Pate, B., & Schulzer, M. (1985). Observations relating to the cause of Parkinson's disease: PET scans after MPTP. *Nature, 317,* 246–248.

Chui, H. C., Bondareff, W., Zarow, C., & Slager, U. (1984). Stability of neuronal number in the human nucleus basalis of Meynert with age. *Neurobiology of Aging, 5,* 83–88.

Coleman, P. D., & Flood, D. G. (1987). Neuron numbers and dendritic extent in normal aging and Alzheimer's disease. *Neurobiology of Aging, 8,* 521–545.

Cross, A. J., Crow, T. J., Ferrier, I. N., Johnson, J. A., Bloom, S. R., & Corsellis, J. A. N. (1984). Serotonin receptor changes in dementia of Alzheimer type. *Journal of Neurochemistry, 43,* 1574–1581.

Crystal, H., Dickson, D., Fuld, P., Masur, D., Scott, R., Mehler, M., Masdeu, J., Kawas, C., Aronson, M., & Wolfson, L. (1988). Clinico-pathological studies in dementia: Nondemented subjects with pathologically confirmed Alzheimer's disease. *Neurology, 38,* 1682–1687.

DeKosky, S. T., Scheff, S. W., & Markesbery, W. R. (1985). Laminar organization of cholinergic circuits in human frontal cortex in Alzheimer's disease and aging. *Neurology, 35(10),* 1425–1431.

Ezrin-Waters, C., & Resch, L. (1986). The nucleus basalis of Meynert. *The Canadian Journal of Neurological Sciences, 13,* 8–14.

Fagg, G. E., Scheff, S. W., & Cotman, C. W. (1981). Axonal sprouting at the neuromuscular junction of adult and aged rats. *Experimental Neurology, 74,* 847–854.

Finch, C. E. (1973). Catecholamine metabolism in the brains of aging male mice. *Brain Research, 52,* 261–276.

Finch, C. E. (1981). Neural and endocrine mechanisms in aging. In R. T. Schimke (Ed.), *Biological mechanisms in aging* (pp. 537–557). (Publ. # 81-2194). Bethesda, MD: U.S. Department of Health & Human services.

Finch, C. E., & Morgan, D. G. (1987). Aging and schizophrenia: A hypothesis relating asynchrony in neural aging processes to the manifestations of schizophrenia and other neurologic diseases with age. In N. E. Miller & G. D. Cohen (Eds.), *Schizophrenia and aging* (pp. 97–108). New York: Guilford Publications.

Finch, C. E., & Morgan, D. G. (1987). Aging and schizophrenia: A hypothesis relating asynchrony in neural aging processes to the manifestations of schizophrenia and other neurologic diseases with age. In N. E. Miller & G. D. Cohen (Eds.), *Schizophrenia and aging* (pp. 97–108). New York: Guilford Publications.

Finch, C. E., & Morgan, D. G. (1990). RNA and protein metabolism in the aging brain. *Annual Review of Neuroscience, 13,* 75–87.

Flood, D. G., & Coleman, P. D. (1988). Neuron numbers and sizes in aging brain: Comparisons of human monkey and rodent data. *Neurobiology of Aging, 9,* 453–463.

Forno, L. S. (1988). The neuropathology of Parkinson's disease (The Lewy body as a clue to the nerve cell degeneration). In F. Hefti & W. J. Weiner (Eds.), *Progress in Parkinson research* (pp. 11–22). New York: Plenum.

Francis, P. T., Palmer, A. M., Sims, N. R., Bowen, D. M., Davison, A. N., Esiri, M. M., Neary, D., Snowden, J. S., & Wilcock, G. K. (1985). Neurochemical studies of early-onset Alzheimer's disease. *New England Journal of Medicine, 313,* 7–11.

Freeman, G. B., Nielsen, P. E., & Gibson, G. E. (1987). Effect of age on behavioral and enzymatic changes during thiamin deficiency. *Neurobiology of Aging, 8,* 429–434.

Geinisman, Y. (1979). Loss of axosomatic synapses in the dentate gyrus of aged rats. *Brain Research, 168,* 485–492.

George, A. E., de Leon, M. J., Gentes, C. I., Miller, J., London, E., Budzilovich, G. N., Ferris, S., & Chase, N. (1986). Leukoencephalopathy in normal and pathologic aging: 1. CT of brain lucencies. *American Journal of Neuroradiology, 7,* 561–566.

Giaccone, G., Tagliavini, F., Linoli, G., Bouras, C., Frigerio, L., Frangione, B., & Bugiani, O. (1989) Down patients: Extracellular preamyloid deposits precede neuritic degeneration and senile plaques. *Neuroscience Letters, 97,* 232–238.

Gibson, P. H. (1983a). EM study of the numbers of cortical synapses in the brains of aging people and people with Alzheimer-type dementia. *Acta Neuropathologica, 62,* 127–133.

Gibson, P. H. (1983b). Form and distribution of senile plaques seen in silver-impregnated sections in the brains of intellectually normal elderly people and people with Alzheimer-type dementia. *Neuropathology and Applied Neurobiology, 9,* 379–389.

Gibson, P. H., & Tomlinson, B. E. (1977). Numbers of Hirano bodies in the hippocampus of normal and demented people with Alzheimer's disease. *Journal of the Neurological Sciences, 33,* 199–206.

Goss, J. R., Finch, C. E., & Morgan, D. G. (1991). Age-related changes in glial fibrillary acidic protein RNA in the mouse brain. *Neurobiology of Aging, 12,* 165–170.

Gottfries, C. G., Gottfries, I., & Roos, B. E. (1969). Homovanillic acid and 5-hydroxyindoleacetic acid in the cerebrospinal fluid of patients with senile dementia, presenile dementia, and Parkinsonism. *Journal of Neurochemistry, 16,* 1341–1345.

Gupta, M., Gupta, B. K., Thomas, R., Bruemmer, V., Sladek, J. R., & Felten, D. L. (1986). Aged mice are more sensitive to 1-methyl-4-phenyl-1,2,3,6-tetrahydropyridine treatment than young adults. *Neuroscience Letters, 70,* 326–331.

Hansen, L. A. Armstrong, D. M., & Terry, R. D. (1987). An immunohistochemical quantification of fibrous astrocytes in the aging human cerebral cortex. *Neurobiology of Aging, 8,* 1–6.

Haug, H. (1985). Are neurons of the human cerebral cortex really lost during aging? A morphometric examination. In J. Traber & W. H. Gispen (Eds.)., *Senile dementia of the Alzheimer type* (pp. 150–163). Berlin: Springer-Verlag.

Hoff, S. F., Scheff, S. W., Benardo, L. S., & Cotman, C. W. (1982). Lesion-induced synaptogenesis in the dentate gyrus of aged rats: I. Loss and reacquisition of normal synaptic density. *Journal of Comparative Neurology, 205,* 246–252.

Hornykiewicz, O. (1983). Dopamine changes in the aging human brain: Functional considerations. In A. Agnoli (Ed.), *Aging (Vol. 23.): Aging brain and ergot alkaloids* (pp. 9–14). New York: Raven.

Hornykiewicz, O. (1985). Brain dopamine and ageing. *Interdisciplinary Topics in Gerontology, 19,* 143–155.

Hubbard, B. M., & Anderson, J. M. (1985). Age-related variations in the neuron content of the cerebral cortex in senile dementia of Alzheimer type. *Neuropathology and Applied Neurobiology, 11,* 369–382.

Jellinger, K. (1987). Quantitave changes in some subcortical nuclei in aging, Alzheimer's disease and Parkinson's disease. *Neurobiology of Aging, 8,* 556–561.

Jennett, B., Teasdale, G., Fry, J., Braakman, R., Minderhoud, J., Heiden, J., & Kurze, T., (1980). Treatment for severe head injury. *Journal of Neurology Neurosurgery and Psychiatry, 43,* 289–295.

Joseph, J. A., Bartus, R. T., Clody, D., Morgan, D., Finch, C., Beer, B., & Sesack, S. (1983). Psychomotor performance in the senescent rodent: Reduction of deficits via striatal dopamine receptor up-regulation. *Neurobiology of Aging, 4,* 313–319.

Kandel, E. R., & Schwartz, J. H. (1985). *Principles of neural science.* New York: Elsevier.

Langston, J. W., Ballard, P. A., Tetrud, J. W., & Irwin, I. (1983). Chronic Parkinsonism in humans due to a product of meperidine-analog synthesis. *Science, 219,* 979–980.

Leuba, G. (1983). Aging of dendrites in the cerebral cortex of the mouse. *Neuropathology and Applied Neurobiology, 9,* 467–475.

Levine, M. S., Adinolfi, A. M., Fisher, R. S., Hull, C. D., Guthrie, D., & Buchwald, N. A. (1988). Ultrastructural alterations in caudate nucleus in aged cat. *Brain Research, 440,* 267–279.

Loranger, A. W. (1984). Sex difference in age at onset of schizophrenia. *Archives of General Psychiatry, 41,* 157–161.

Mackay, A. V. P., Iverson, L. L., Rossor, M., Spokes, E., Bird, E., Arregui, A., Creese, I., & Snyder, S. H. (1982). Increased brain dopamine and dopamine receptors in schizophrenia. *Archives of General Psychiatry, 39,* 991–997.

Mann, D. M. A. (1985). The neuropathology of Alzheimer's disease: A review with pathogenetic, aetiological and therapeutic considerations. *Mechanisms of Ageing and Development, 31,* 213–255.

Mann, D. M., Lincoln, J., Yates, P. O., Stamp, J. E., & Toper, S. (1980). Changes in the monoamine-containing neurones of the human CNS in senile dementia. *British Journal of Psychiatry, 136,* 533–541.

Mann, D. M. A., Tucker, C. M., & Yates, P.O. (1987). The topographic distribution of senile plaques and neurofibrillary tangles in the brains of non-demented persons of different ages. *Neuropathology and Applied Neurobiology, 13,* 123–139.

Mann, D. M. A., Yates, P. O., & Marcyniuk, B. (1984). Alzheimer's presenile dementia, senile dementia of Alzheimer type, and Down's syndrome in middle age form an age-related continuum of pathological changes. *Neuropathology and Applied Neurobiology, 10,* 185–207.

Mann, D. M. A., Yates, P. O., & Marcyniuk, B. (1985). Some morphometric observations on the cerebral cortex and hippocampus in presenile Alzheimer's disease, senile dementia of Alzheimer type, and Down's syndrome in middle age. *Journal of Neurological Science, 69*, 139–159.

Marshall, J. F., Drew, M. C., & Neve, K. A. (1983). Recovery of function after mesotelencephalic dopaminergic injury in senescence. *Brain Research, 259*, 249–260.

Martilla, R. J., Kaprio, J., Koskenvuo, M., & Rinne, U. K. (1988). Parkinson's disease in a nationwide twin cohort. *Neurology, 38*, 1217–1219.

Matsumoto, A., Okada, R., & Arai, Y. (1982). Synaptic changes in the hypothalamic arcuate nucleus of old male rats. *Experimental Neurology, 78*, 583–590.

McDuff, T., & Sumi, S. M. (1985). Subcortical degeneration in Alzheimer's disease. *Neurology, 35(1)*, 123–126.

McGeer, P. L., McGeer, E. G., Suzuki, J., Dolman, C. E., & Nagai, T. (1984). Aging, Alzheimer's disease, and the cholinergic system of the basal forebrain. *Neurology, 34*, 741–745.

McGeer, P. L. McGeer, E. G., & Suzuki, J. S. (1977). Aging and extrapyramidal function. *Archives of Neurology, 34*, 33–35.

McWilliams, J. R., & Lynch, G. (1984). Synaptic density and axonal sprouting in rat hippocampus: Stability in adulthood and decline in late adulthood. *Brain Research, 294*, 152–156.

Miller, F. D., Hicks, S. P., D'Amato, C. J., & Landis, J. R. (1984). A descriptive study of neuritic plaques and neurofibrillary tangles in an autopsy population. *American Journal of Epidemiology, 120(3)*, 331–341.

Morgan, D. G., & Finch, C. E. (1988). Dopaminergic changes in the basal ganglia. *Annals of the New York Academy of Sciences, 515*, 145–160.

Morgan, D. G., & May, P. C. (1990). Age-related changes in synaptic neurochemistry. In E. L. Schneider & J. W. Rowe (Eds.), *Handbook of the biology of aging* (pp. 219–254). New York: Academic Press.

Morgan, D. G., May, P. C., & Finch, C. E. (1987a). Dopamine and serotonin systems in human and rodent brain: Effects of age and neurodegenerative disease. *Journal of the American Geriatrics Society, 35*, 334–345.

Morgan, D. G., Marcusson, J. O., Nyberg, P., Wester, P., Winblad, B., Gordon, M. N., & Finch, C. E. (1987b). Divergent changes in D-1 and D-2 dopamine binding sites in human brain during aging. *Neurobiology of Aging, 8*, 195–201.

Morgan, D. G., May, P. C., & Finch, C. E. (1988). Neurotransmitter receptors in human aging and Alzheimer's disease. In A. K. Sen & T. Lee (Eds.), *Receptors and ligands in neurological disorders* (pp. 120–147). Cambridge, England: Cambridge University Press.

Motte, J., & Williams, R. S. (1989). Age-related changes in the density and morphology of plaques and neurofibrillary tangles in Down syndrome brain. *Acta Neuropathologica, 77*, 536–546.

Mountjoy, C. Q., Roth, M., Evans, N. J. R., & Evans, H. M. (1983). Cortical neuronal counts in normal elderly controls and demented patients. *Neurobiology of Aging, 4*, 1–11.

Murphy, S., & Pearce, B. (1987). Functional receptors for neurotransmitters on astroglial cells. *Neuroscience, 22*, 381–394.

Myers, R. H., Sax, D. S., Schoenfeld, M., Bird, E. D., Wolf, P. A., Vonsattel, J. P., White, R., & Martin, J. B. (1985). Late onset of Huntington's disease. *Journal of Neurology, Neurosurgery, and Psychiatry, 48*, 530–534.

Needels, D. L., Neito-Sampedro, M., & Cotman, C. W. (1986). Induction of a neurite-promoting factor in rat brain following injury or deafferentation. *Neuroscience, 18(3)*, 517–526.

Owen, R., Owen, F., Poulter, M., & Crow, T. J. (1984). Dopamine D2 receptors in substantia nigra in schizophrenia. *Brain Research, 299*, 152–154.

Palmer, A. M., Sims, N. R., Bowen, D. M., Neary, D., Palo, J., Wikstrom, J., & Davison, A. N. (1984). Monoamine metabolite concentrations in lumbar cerebrospinal fluid of patients with histologically verified Alzheimer's dementia. *Journal of Neurology, Neurosurgery, and Psychiatry, 47*, 481–484.

Pederzoli, M., Girotti, F., Scigliano, G., Aiello, G., Carella, F., & Caraceni, T. (1983). L-dopa long-term treatment in Parkinson's disease: Age-related side effects. *Neurology, 33*, 1518–1522.

Pestronk, A., Drachman, D. B., & Griffin, J. W. (1980). Effects of aging on nerve sprouting and regeneration. *Experimental Neurology, 70*, 65–82.

Pierotti, A. R., Harmar, A. J., Simpson, J., & Yates, C. M. (1986). High-molecular-weight forms of somatostatin are reduced in Alzheimer's disease and Down's syndrome. *Neuroscience Letters, 63*, 141–146.

Poon, L. W. (1985). Differences in human memory with aging: Nature, causes and clinical implications. In J. E. Birren & K. W. Schaie (Eds.), *Handbook of the psychology of aging* (pp. 427–462). New York: Van Nostrand Reinhold.

Postman, L., & Underwood, B. J. (1973). Critical issues in interference theory. *Memory and Cognition, 1,* 19–40.

Pro, J. D., Smith, C. H., & Sumi, S. M. (1980). Presenile Alzheimer disease: Amyloid plaques in the cerebellum. *Neurology, 30,* 820–825.

Reinikainen, K.J., Riekkinen, P. J., Paljarvi, L., Soininen, H., Helkala, E-L., Jolkkonen, J., & Laakso, M. (1988). Cholinergic deficit in Alzheimer's disease: A study based on CSF and autopsy data. *Neurochemical Research, 13(2),* 135–146.

Reisine, T. D., Rossor, M., Spokes, E., Iversen, L. L., & Yamamura, H. I. (1980). Opiate and neuroleptic receptor alterations in human schizophrenic brain tissue. In G. Pepeu, M. J. Kuhar, & S. J. Enna (Eds.), *Receptors for neurotransmitters and peptide hormones* (pp. 443–450). New York: Raven.

Reynolds, G. P. (1983). Increased concentrations and lateral asymmetry of amygdala dopamine in schizophrenia. *Nature, 305,* 527–529.

Reynolds, G. P., Arnold, L., Rossor, M. N., Iversen, L. L., Mountjoy, C. Q., & Roth, M. (1984). Reduced binding of [3H]ketanserin to cortical 5-HT2 receptors in senile dementia of the Alzheimer type. *Neuroscience Letters, 44,* 47–51.

Reynolds, G. P., Czudek, C., Bzowej, N., & Seeman, P. (1987). Dopamine receptor asymmetry in schizophrenia. *Lancet, i,* 979–979.

Ricaurte, G. A., Delanney, L. E., Irwin, I., & Langston, J. W. (1987). Older dopaminergic neurons do not recover from the effects of MPTP. *Neuropharmacology, 26(1),* 97–99.

Rinne, J. O. (1987). Muscarinic and dopaminergic receptors in the aging human brain. *Brain Research, 404,* 162–168.

Rogers, J., & Bloom, F. E. (1985). Neurotransmitter metabolism and function in the aging central nervous system. In C. E. Finch & E. L. Schneider (Eds.), *Handbook of the biology of aging* (pp. 645–691). New York: Van Nostrand Reinhold.

Rossor, M. N., Garrett, N. J., Johnson, A. L., Mountjoy, C. Q., Roth, M., & Iversen, L. L. (1982). A postmortem study of the cholinergic and GABA systems in senile dementia. *Brain, 105,* 313–330.

Roth, G. S., Ingram, D. K., & Joseph, J. A. (1984). Delayed loss of striatal dopamine receptors during aging of dietarily restricted rats. *Brain Research, 300,* 27–32.

Schallert, T. (1983). Sensorimotor impairment and recovery of function in brain-damaged rats: Reappearance of symptoms during old age. *Behavioral Neuroscience, 97(1),* 159–164.

Scheff, S. W., Benardo, L. S., & Cotman, C. W. (1980). Decline in reactive fiber growth in the dentate gyrus of aged rats compared to young adult rats following entorhinal cortex removal. *Brain Research, 199,* 21–39.

Seeman, P. (1980). Brain dopamine receptors. *Pharmacology Reviews, 32,* 229–313.

Seeman, P., Bzowej, N. H., Guan, H.-C., Bergeron, C., Becker, L. E., Reynolds, G. P., Bird, E. D., Riederer, P., Jellinger, K., Watanabe, S., & Tourtellotte, W. (1987). Human brain dopamine receptors in children and aging adults. *Synapse, 1,* 399–404.

Seeman, P., Ulpian, C., Bergeron, C., Riederer, P., Jellinger, K., Gabriel, E., Reynolds, G. P., & Tourtellotte, W. W. (1984). Bimodal distribution of dopamine receptor densities in brains of schizophrenics. *Science, 225,* 728–731.

Snyder, S. H., Banerjee, S. P., Yamamura, H. I., & Greenberg, D. (1974). Drugs, neurotransmitters, and schizophrenia, *Science, 184,* 1243–1253.

Tanner, C. M., Chen, B., Wang, W., Peng, M., Liu, Z., Liang, X., Kao, L. C., Gilley, D. W., Goetz, C. G., & Schoenberg, B. S. (1989). Environmental factors in Parkinson's disease: A case-control study in China. *Neurology, 39,* 660–664.

Terry, R. D., DeTeresa, R., & Hansen, L. A. (1987). Neocortical cell counts in normal human adult aging. *Annals of Neurology, 21,* 530–539.

Tomlinson, B. E., Irving, D., & Blessed, G. (1981). Cell loss in the locus ceruleus in senile dementia of Alzheimer type. *Journal of Neurological Science, 49,* 419–428.

Ulrich, J. (1982). Senile plaques and neurofibrillary tangles of the Alzheimer type in nondemented individuals at presenile age. *Gerontology, 28,* 86–90.

Ulrich, J. (1985). Alzheimer changes in nondemented patients younger than sixty five: Possible early stages of Alzheimer's disease and senile dementia of Alzheimer type. *Annals of Neurology, 17(3)*, 273–277.

Vijayashankar, N., & Brody, H. (1979). A quantitative study of the pigmented neurons in the nuclei locus ceruleus and subceruleus in man as related to aging. *Journal of Neuropathology and Experimental Neurology, 37*, 490–497.

Volicer, L., Direnfeld, L. K., Langlais, P. J., Freedman, M., Bird, E. D., & Albert, M. . (1985). Catecholamine metabolites and cyclic nucleotides in cerebrospinal fluid in dementia of Alzheimer type. *Journal of Gerontology, 40(6)*, 708–713.

Waller, S. B., Ingram, D. K., Reynolds, M. A., & London, E. D. (1983). Age and strain comparisons of neurotransmitter synthetic enzyme activities in the mouse. *Journal of Neurochemistry, 41*, 1421–1428.

Wisniewski, K. E., Wisniewski, H. M., & Wen, G. Y. (1984). Occurrence of neuropathological changes and dementia of Alzheimer's disease in Down's syndrome. *Annals of Neurology, 17(3)*, 278–282.

Wong, D. F., Wagner, H. N., & Tune, L. E. (1986). Positron emission tomography reveals elevated D2 receptors in drug-naive schizophrenics. *Science, 234*, 1558–1563.

Yates, C. M., Simpson, J., Gordon, A., Maloney, A. F. J., Allison, Y., Ritchie, I. M., & Urquhart, A. (1983). Catecholamines and cholinergic enzymes in pre-senile and senile Alzheimer-type dementia and Down's syndrome. *Brain Research, 280*, 119–126.

8

Cerebral Metabolism in Aging and Dementia

Cheryl L. Grady and Stanley I. Rapoport

I. Introduction
   A. Early Methods of Measuring Cerebral Metabolism
   B. Positron Emission Tomography
II. Cerebral Metabolism and Aging
III. Dementia of the Alzheimer Type
   A. Cerebral Metabolism
   B. Cerebral Metabolism and Cognitive Function
IV. Other Dementias
   A. Cerebrovascular Dementia
   B. Depression
V. Future Directions
VI. Summary and Conclusions
   References

I. Introduction

According to current estimates as much as 10% of the population over the age of 65 has Alzheimer's disease (Evans, *et al.,* 1989), which is by far the most common form of dementia (Chui, 1989). As our population ages, dementia, as well as other age-related problems, will increase in importance as an issue of concern for workers in the fields of both medicine and mental health. One of the research areas in this field that has interested scientists for many years is the study of brain function in aging and dementia. In this chapter we will review the techniques that have been used to measure cerebral function and the contributions that have been made to our understanding of both age-related processes and dementia.

A. Early Methods of Measuring Cerebral Metabolism

The direct measurement of regional brain function has only recently been possible as techniques that allow the measurement of regional cerebral blood flow and metabolism have become available. These methods are designed to measure cerebral blood flow, the process by which nutrients are delivered to the brain, and oxidative metabolism, the process by which the energy necessary for neuronal activity is produced. The first procedure to be developed, known as the Kety-Schmidt technique after its creators (Kety & Schmidt, 1948), involved calculating whole-brain blood flow by measuring arterio–venous differences in the concentration of a freely diffusible gas, such as nitrous oxide, and using this clearance value to calculate flow. Similarly, cerebral glucose and oxygen consumption were calculated by measuring arterio–venous differences in the concentrations of these substances. Later techniques of intracarotid injection (Lassen, *et al.*, 1963) or inhalation (Obrist, Thompson, King, & Wang, 1967) of ^{133}Xenon allowed localization of blood flow to relatively large cortical areas in the two cerebral hemispheres. Although these methods were an improvement over the Kety-Schmidt technique in allowing regional measurements, the detectors could measure only radioactivity from relatively restricted areas of the lateral surface of the cortex and underlying white matter.

B. Positron Emission Tomography

With the advent of positron emission tomography (PET) it became possible to measure flow and metabolism in specific regions throughout the brain with a resolution approaching 5 mm. With PET, cross-sectional images of the brain are obtained that allow calculation of flow and metabolism in many areas of interest, both cortical and subcortical, using appropriate mathematical models. In addition to the ability to make more detailed measurements related to brain function and integrity, PET also allows the study of specific structure–function relationships between numerous brain regions and various physiological or cognitive processes thought to be mediated by those regions.

PET involves the injection into the blood of minute amounts (usually less than 10 mCi) of a radioactive isotope, a positron emitter, which is delivered by the blood to the brain. The most commonly used isotope for the PET measurement of cerebral metabolism is ^{18}fluorine labeled 2-fluoro-2-deoxy-D-glucose (^{18}FDG), which has a half-life of 110 min. Other isotopes and methods are available to measure cerebral oxygen metabolism (Frackowiack, Lenzi, Jones, & Heather, 1980), but are less widely used, particularly in the study of dementia, and so will not be presented here. The measurement of cerebral glucose metabolism is based on a model developed by Sokoloff and colleagues (1977) that makes use of the ^{18}FDG molecule as an analog of glucose. The ^{18}FDG is delivered by the blood to the brain where it crosses the blood–brain barrier via the glucose transport system, as if it were glucose. Once it enters the brain cells, the labeled molecule is phosphorylated to ^{18}FDG-6-P by hexokinase (Figure 1). The labeled molecule becomes *trapped* after this first step because the next enzyme in the pathway (phosphofructokinase) cannot act upon it, and because little phosphatase exists in brain to dephosphorylate ^{18}FDG-6-P and thus reform significant amounts of ^{18}FDG. The labeled substance remains

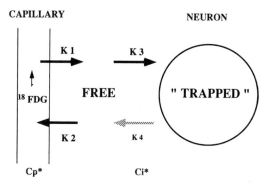

Figure 1   Schematic of the ^{18}FDG model. ^{18}FDG is delivered to the brain where it is taken up by the neurons (K1 is the rate constant for influx into the cells). From the free intracellular pool the ^{18}FDG is phosphorylated by hexokinase (K3 is the phosphorylation rate constant) and remains trapped in this state until dephosphorylated by phosphatase (K4), a slow process that has little effect during the time period of the scan. K2 is the rate constant for the efflux of ^{18}FDG out of the cells. Cp* is the concentration of ^{18}FDG in plasma and Ci* is the concentration in brain.

in the neurons in this phosphorylated state long enough for the emitted radioactivity to be measured by the PET imaging system and assigned to specific areas of the brain.

Once in the brain cells, the labeled ^{18}FDG emits its positrons (or positively charged electrons), each of which travel a short distance from the site of emission and collides with an electron. This collision results in annihilation of the two particles and the release of two annihilation photons (or gamma rays). These photons travel out of the head in opposite directions (180° apart) and impinge upon a ring of detectors in the PET imaging device, called a tomograph, that surrounds the subject's head. Since two photons are emitted for each positron annihilation, two detectors, on opposite sides of the subject's head, must register the presence of a photon simultaneously. This is known as coincidence detection (Figure 2). A computer linked to the tomograph collects these coincident events, and reconstructs horizontal images of brain radioactivity. The brain radioactivity, which is a measure of the amount of ^{18}FDG in various parts of the brain, then is converted into units of glucose utilization using the equation derived from the model (Sokoloff *et al.*, 1977), and making use of the fact that uptake of ^{18}FDG is proportional to the rate of glucose consumption for oxidative metabolism.

The different tomographs used for PET imaging and the experimental conditions under which the studies are done vary widely among the different PET groups. For example, the spatial resolution of tomographs routinely used for research can vary from 17 mm to 6 mm and is directly related to the size of the brain regions that can be imaged, with smaller regions being adequately imaged only with higher-resolution scanners. In addition, some studies of resting or baseline metabolism are conducted with the subjects in a state of reduced sensory input (eyes closed and ears occluded), whereas others make no attempt to reduce such stimulation, a fact that surely accounts for some of the variability in results reported among groups. These issues of methodology will not be discussed at great length

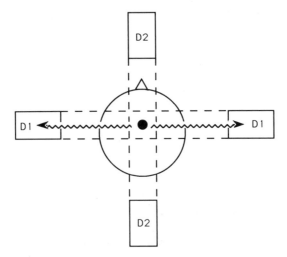

Figure 2 Schematic of a subject's head inside the tomograph, as viewed from the top of the head (facing up). The rectangles labeled D1 and D2 are detector pairs that are connected via a coincidence circuit. The dark circle within the subject's head represents an annihilation event, and the two wavy lines are the two photons from the event that impinge on the detector pair D1. The simultaneous interaction between the two detectors and the photons will cause a coincidence event to be registered in the location of the line joining the detectors. All such lines, or projections, are then assembled and reconstructed to produce the image for each tomographic plane.

in this chapter (see Horwitz, 1990), for a full review), but should be kept in mind when attempting to interpret different sets of PET data.

An additional methodological issue is the difficulty inherent in using PET to study demented patients. Some patients with dementing illnesses are agitated or are unable to cooperate with the procedure owing to other symptoms of the disease. Patients are generally studied while drug-free, which thus limits the study samples to those patients who are able to cooperate adequately. Foster and colleagues (1987) have shown that the metabolic patterns seen in a group of demented patients sedated with diazepam were similar to those seen when the patients were scanned unsedated. Although this finding suggests that difficult patients could be studied while under sedation, this is not routinely done.

II. Cerebral Metabolism and Aging ——————————————

All of the studies of cerebral metabolism and aging have been cross-sectional rather than longitudinal, and thus can address only age-related decreases and not declines in metabolism during the life span. Early studies of cerebral metabolism and aging using the Kety-Schmidt technique generally reported a decrease in whole-brain blood flow and oxygen consumption with age (Dastur *et al.*, 1963; Gottstein & Held, 1979; Kety, 1956; Lassen, Feinberg, & Lane, 1960), although no age-related changes in blood flow were found in one study (Shenkin, Novak, Goluboff, Soffe, & Bortin, 1953). Later studies using

[133]Xenon administration to measure regional cerebral blood flow reported a decrease in elderly subjects of 15% to 20% (Mamo, Meric, Luft, & Seylaz, 1983; Melamed, Lavy, Bentin, Cooper, & Rinot, 1980; Naritomi, Meyer, Sakai, Yamaguchi, & Shaw, 1979). Since 1980, numerous reports on the effects of age on brain metabolism as measured by PET have appeared, and are summarized in Table I. Frackowiack and colleagues (1980) originally reported that both cerebral blood flow and oxygen use fell with age, but, in a later study with more subjects, only a statistically significant fall in blood flow was found (Frackowiack & Gibbs, 1983). Others (Lebrun-Grandie, et al., 1983; Pantano, et al., 1984) also have reported a significant linear decrease with age in blood flow but not oxygen utilization, although when the older subjects as a group were compared to the younger subjects, a significant 17% decrease in oxygen consumption was noted (Pantano et al., 1984). A more recent study reported an age-related decrease in oxygen consumption as well as blood flow (Leenders et al., 1990). Studies of cerebral glucose metabolism also have reported conflicting results, with some finding an age-related decrease (Chawluk et al., 1987; Kuhl, Metter, Reige, & Phelps, 1982), and others finding no change with age (de Leon, et al., 1984; Duara et al., 1983; Duara et al., 1984), or a decrease in only a small percentage of brain regions (Hoffman et al., 1988). Thus, although the finding of a significant effect of age on cerebral metabolism has been elusive, the size of the metabolic decrease attributed to aging generally has been reported to be in the range of values reported for age-related decreases in blood flow, i.e., between 10 and 30%. Problems of subject selection and adequacy of health screening, in addition to differences between studies in the actual experimental conditions (e.g., eyes open versus eyes closed), and whether regional or global measures are examined, all may contribute to the variability of the published results.

To illustrate the relationship between cerebral glucose utilization and age, as well as some of the difficulties inherent in measuring this relationship, data from two samples of healthy subjects are shown in Figure 3. The relationship between global gray matter

Table I

Summary of Age-Related Changes in Cerebral Metabolism Using
Positron Emission Tomography

Authors	Year	CMRO$_2$	CMR$_{glc}$	Change (%)[a]
Kuhl et al.	1982		Decreased	−26
Duara et al.	1983		Unchanged	−17
Lebrun-Grandie et al.	1983	Unchanged		−32
Frackowiack et al.	1983	Unchanged		−23
Pantano et al.	1984	Decreased		−17
Duara et al.	1984		Unchanged	−2
DeLeon et al.	1984		Unchanged	+2
Chawluk et al.	1987		Decreased	−16
Grady et al.	1990		Decreased	−12
Leenders et al.	1990	Decreased		−19

[a]Percentage change over 20 to 80 years. (Some values estimated from published data.)
CMRO$_2$, cerebral metabolic rate for oxygen; CMR$_{glc}$, cerebral metabolic rate for glucose.

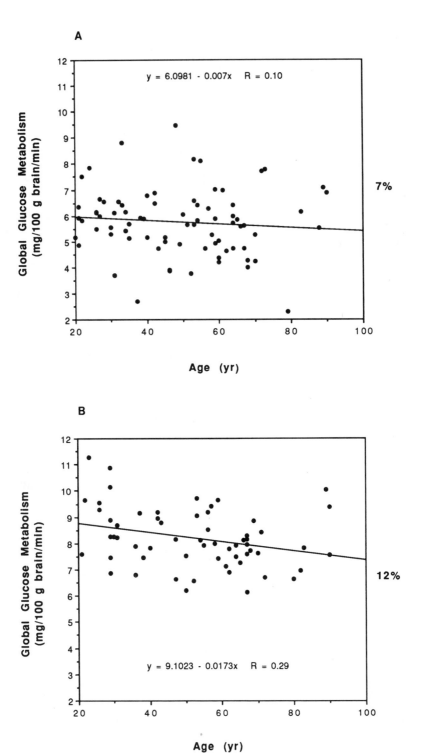

Figure 3 Global gray matter metabolic values from two samples of healthy subjects obtained from an ECAT II tomograph (17-mm resolution) (A) and a Scanditronix scanner (6-mm resolution) (B). The equation for the regression line is shown for each sample and the number to the right of each graph represents the percentage change in metabolism over the age range of 20 to 80 years.

glucose use and age seen in Figure 3A represents data from a series of studies that was performed using a low resolution PET tomograph (Duara *et al.*, 1984; Schlageter *et al.*, 1987). The decrease in glucose metabolism between 20 and 80 years seen in this cross-sectional sample is 7%, which is not statistically significant. In Figure 3B are shown data from a second group of subjects obtained with a high-resolution tomograph under the same set of experimental conditions (Grady, Horwitz, Schapiro, & Rapoport, 1990). The decrease in global metabolism over the same age range in this group of subjects is 12% and is statistically significant.

Several conclusions can be drawn from Figure 3. First, even if the subject-selection criteria and experimental paradigm are the same, the statistical significance of any relationship between metabolism and age will depend not only on the number of subjects but also on the variability of the data. The slopes presented in Figure 3 are not very different (0.01 mg of glucose per year versus 0.02 mg per year), but the data from the higher-resolution scanner show a considerably smaller coefficient of variation, and thus allow demonstration of a significant correlation with age. Second, regardless of how the data are collected, it would seem that the effect of age on cerebral glucose utilization is relatively small, and is most likely in the range of 10 to 20% over a 60-year range. The data in Figure 3 suggest a decrease of no more than 15%, and that age accounts for only a small percentage of the total variance found in cerebral metabolism (less than 10% in these subject groups). The effect of age on glucose metabolism may be even less, given the fact that cerebral atrophy, which increases with age, can lower estimates of metabolic rate obtained with PET through the partial volume artifact (Mazziotta, Phelps, Plummer, & Kuhl, 1981). Attempts to correct for this artifact have shown that the age effect is reduced when an atrophy correction is applied (Schlageter *et al.*, 1987; Yoshii *et al.*, 1988).

Additional information may be obtained from brain metabolic data using PET, aside from the metabolic rates themselves. For example, measurement of metabolic rates alone does not allow one to ascertain functional relations among regions, which might be altered under different experimental conditions, whereas absolute metabolic rates might not change from one condition to the other. In order to learn which brain regions function together during a particular experimental paradigm, a correlation method was developed (Clark, Kessler, Buchsbaum, Margolin, & Holcomb, 1984; Horwitz, Duara, & Rapoport, 1984; Metter, Riege, Kuhl, & Phelps, 1984), using glucose metabolism as the measure of functional activity. The theory behind this analysis is as follows: if two brain regions (A and B) are functionally coupled, so that activity in one depends on the activity in the other, a plot of glucose metabolism in region A against that of region B will show a statistically significant correlation. Conversely, if there is a large correlation between rates of metabolism in two regions, the hypothesis is that these two regions are functionally coupled in the particular experimental state being investigated.

This approach was used to compare the regional intercorrelations of glucose metabolic rates in a group of young subjects and a group of older subjects (Horwitz *et al.*, 1986). The pattern of correlations in the young group showed many correlations within and between the frontal and parietal lobes, a smaller number of correlations within and between the temporal and occipital lobes, and few correlations between the frontal–parietal and temporal–occipital domains. The older group had the same general pattern of intercorrelations, but there were significantly fewer correlations in the old group between metabolic rates in the frontal and parietal regions and between regions within the parietal areas bilaterally. The reduced number of correlations within the parietal lobes, and between the frontal and parietal areas, were interpreted as a decrease in the integrated function between these areas and may be associated with some of the neuropsychological deficits that are seen in the elderly, specifically those that may depend heavily on the integrated function of anterior and posterior brain regions, such as tasks of attention (Mesulam, 1981).

Correlations between resting cerebral metabolism and cognitive performance generally are not found in healthy subjects (Duara *et al.*, 1984; Haxby *et al.*, 1986), although significant relationships may be found if both cognitive performance and metabolism are compromised by systemic disease (Birren, Butler, Greenhouse, Sokoloff, & Yarrow, 1963). However, some aspects of memory performance may be related to resting metabolic measures in both young and old healthy subjects as reported by Berardi and col-

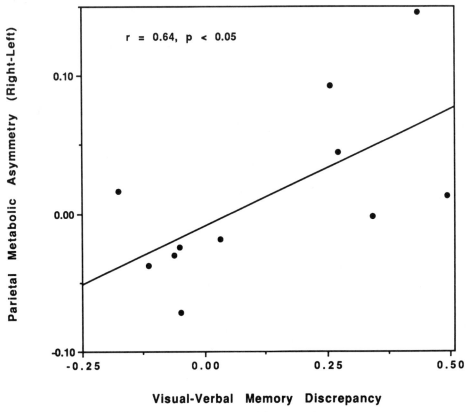

Figure 4   The relationship between parietal right–left metabolic asymmetry and visual–verbal differences in performance on memory tests for a sample of healthy elderly subjects. Points on the left of the graph represent subjects with better verbal memory and greater left than right parietal metabolic rates. Points on the right of the graph are subjects with better visual memory and greater right than left parietal metabolism.

leagues (Berardi, Haxby, Grady, & Rapoport, 1990 and 1991). In these studies, subjects performed continuous recognition tasks for both verbal and nonverbal visual stimuli, i.e., words and faces. Performance on these tasks was related to resting metabolic asymmetry in the parietal lobes in both age groups, such that those subjects with better verbal memory performance had greater left than right parietal metabolism and those with better memory for faces showed greater right than left parietal metabolism (Figure 4). Similarly, Miller *et al.* (1987) measured metabolism during performance of a verbal memory task and found an increase in left temporal metabolism compared to baseline measures in healthy elderly subjects. These results suggest that relationships between hemispheric lateralization of cognitive function and asymmetries of cerebral metabolism can be demonstrated in healthy subjects, and that these correlations are maintained during the aging process, although age-related differences may be elucidated with further research.

III. Dementia of the Alzheimer Type _____

A. Cerebral Metabolism

The most common cause of dementia is Alzheimer's disease (AD), which accounts for 50 to 80% of patients with dementia (Chui, 1989; Evans *et al.*, 1989). Cerebrovascular disease accounts for 4 to 10% of cases, and other diseases, such as Pick's disease, account for an even smaller percentage. Depression in the elderly can result in cognitive impairment (Cummings, Benson, & Lo Verma, 1980) which, although it is not a true dementia, can nevertheless be debilitating. Thus, it is not surprising that the majority of studies examining metabolic patterns in dementia have focused on dementia of the Alzheimer type (DAT). These will be reviewed in this section, and the findings in cerebrovascular dementia and depression will be reviewed in Section IV.

Postmortem studies of the neuropathology of AD have shown that all parts of the cortex are not affected equally. For example, association neocortex, hippocampus, and amygdala have been found to be more affected than primary neocortex (see Kemper, 1984 for a review), although within the affected neocortical areas there has been some disagreement as to which are most damaged, either parieto–temporal (Brun & Gustafson, 1976) or frontal (Jamada & Mehraein, 1968). One of the contributions of PET to the study of dementia has been to confirm this pattern of damage during life in patients with DAT, i.e., hypometabolism is seen disproportionately in association neocortex with relative sparing of metabolism in primary cortical and subcortical regions. One early study (Ferris *et al.*, 1980) that used PET to examine regional cerebral metabolic rates for glucose in patients with DAT reported equal degrees of metabolic reduction in both anterior and posterior association cortex compared to controls (about 35%). Other reports generally have found that the parietal and temporal lobes show the most diminution of glucose or oxygen utilization (Duara *et al.*, 1986; Foster *et al.*, 1984; Friedland *et al.*, 1983; Frackowiack *et al.*, 1981; McGeer *et al.*, 1986). These reductions were on the order of 30 to 40% for parieto–temporal areas and 10 to 20% for frontal and occipital regions. Primary cortical and subcortical regions were reported to be relatively spared (Benson *et al.*, 1983; Haxby *et al.*, 1988; Metter, Riege, Kameyama, & Phelps, 1984) In addition, a significant relationship between increasing dementia severity and decreasing metabolism was found by several groups (de Leon *et al.*, 1983; Ferris *et al.*, 1980; Foster *et al.*, 1984). Figure 5 shows the typical pattern of reduced glucose metabolism in association neocortex with relative sparing of primary cortical and subcortical regions in three DAT patients compared to a healthy control.

Measurement of absolute metabolic rates may not provide the best way of assessing metabolic disturbance in DAT. Dura *et al.* (1986) found that glucose metabolism in DAT patients was most markedly reduced in parietal and temporal regions, compared to control

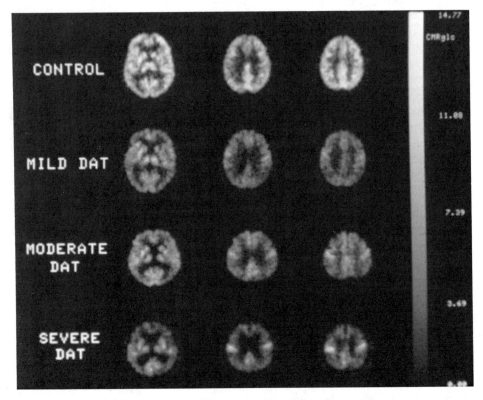

Figure 5 PET scan images from a healthy control (age 69), a mildly demented patient (age 53), a moderately demented patient (age 63), and a severely demented patient (age 72). All patients and the control are women. Scans were obtained using a Scanditronix PC1024-7B positron tomograph (6 mm in-plane resolution). Three brain levels above the inferior orbito–meatal line are shown: 45 mm on the left, 70 mm in the middle, and 90 mm on the right side of the figure. All of the patients show reduced metabolism in association neocortex (predominantly in the right hemisphere), with relative sparing in the primary cortical and subcortical regions. The glucose metabolic scale on the right is in mg/100g brain per min.

values, but that these reductions were statistically significant only in severely demented patients, and were on the order of 35 to 45%. Normalized metabolic measures (such as ratios) generally are more sensitive to small differences between groups of subjects (Haxby, 1986) because of the smaller variance of these measures compared to the variance of absolute metabolic rates (coefficient of variation less than 10% versus 20–30%). When normalized measures of metabolism (ratios of regional metabolism to whole brain metabolism) were examined (Duara et al., 1986), these were found to be reduced in parietal areas in even mildly affected patients, and also in frontal and temporal regions in both moderately and severely demented patients.

Much of the work on DAT has focused on describing the early manifestations of the disease in order to discern which brain regions are most vulnerable to the disease, and to establish criteria for early diagnosis. In addition, emphasis has been placed on the interrelations between metabolic rates in various brain regions. For example right–left asymmetries of metabolism in DAT patients have received considerable attention. Although Benson et al. (1983) reported no metabolic asymmetry between right and left hemispheres in DAT patients, Foster et al. (1983) examined patients chosen for either disproportionate aphasia or apraxia, and found that areas of reduced metabolism in these patients corresponded to the left and right hemispheres, respectively. In a more representative and unselected sample of patients, increased asymmetry in both directions (right lower than left and vice versa) would lead to increased variance of these measures in the patient group compared to control subjects. The variance of right–left asymmetry indices was found to be increased in frontal, parietal, and temporal association cortical regions in mildly to moderately demented patients compared to controls (Haxby, Duara, Grady, Rapoport, & Cutler, 1985; Friedland, Budinger, Koss, & Ober,1985; Kumar et al., 1991) (Figure 6). Asymmetry was not significantly increased in primary occipital or sensorimotor cortex. In general, no directional tendencies in these measures have been reported; i.e., there are equal numbers of patients with disproportionate left hemisphere abnormality as patients with disproportionate right hemisphere reductions. Only Duara and colleagues (1988) have found a predominance of left hemisphere abnormality in their patients.

In addition to interhemispheric heterogeneity, intrahemispheric (anterior–posterior) heterogeneity also is found in DAT patients (Chase, 1987; Haxby et al., 1988). When parietal–premotor and parietal–prefrontal metabolic ratios were calculated, an increased variance was demonstrated in DAT patients compared to controls, similar to the increased variance seen in right–left measures. This increased variance was seen in mildly, moderately, and severely demented patients, with some individuals showing greater reductions in parietal compared to frontal areas and others showing disproportionate frontal abnormality. One study used a type of cluster analysis to identify subgroups of patients with different metabolic patterns (Grady, et al., 1990) and found four distinct patterns of abnormality (Figure 7):

1. bilateral parieto-temporal hypometabolism with relative sparing of frontal cortex (45% of the patient sample);
2. metabolic deficit in paralimbic structures, including orbitofrontal and anterior cingulate (25%);

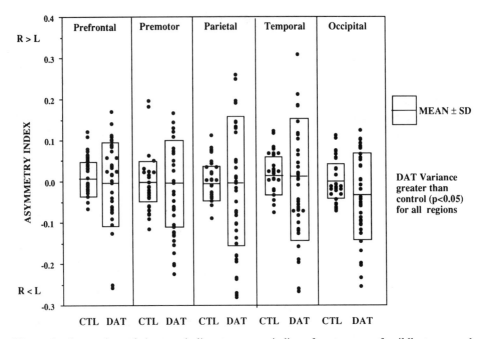

Figure 6 Scatterplots of the metabolic asymmetry indices for a group of mildly to severely demented DAT patients and an age-matched control group in five neocortical association regions. The asymmetry index is calculated as $(R-L/[(R+L)/2]$ where R is the metabolic value in a right hemisphere region and L is metabolism in the homologous region on the left. Positive values indicate that right hemisphere metabolism is greater than that in the left hemisphere, and negative values represent right metabolism lower than left. All regions showed an increased variance of asymmetry in the DAT patients compared to the control values.

3. left hemisphere hypometabolism in frontal, parietal, and temporal regions (15%); and

4. frontal and posterior metabolic defect of equal severity (15%).

Except for the fourth subgroup, which consisted of patients who were more severely demented, the patterns were not related to dementia severity, age at onset, or duration of illness. These findings demonstrate that metabolic deficits in DAT occur in a patchy distribution, and are heterogeneous both within and between hemispheres. In addition, frontal metabolism is not always spared in DAT, in contrast to earlier reports (Foster *et al.*, 1984; Kuhl, Metter, Riege, & Hawkins, 1985), but can be found as the primary metabolic deficit, as can paralimbic association cortical abnormalities.

There is some evidence that patients who have onset of dementia at a relatively early age have different clinical (Seltzer & Sherwin, 1983), neuropathological (Mountjoy, Roth, Evans, & Evans, 1983), and neurochemical characteristics (Rossor, Iverson, Reynolds, Mountjoy, & Roth, 1984) than do those patients with later onset of dementia. These differences have led to the suggestion that there are actually two disease processes in-

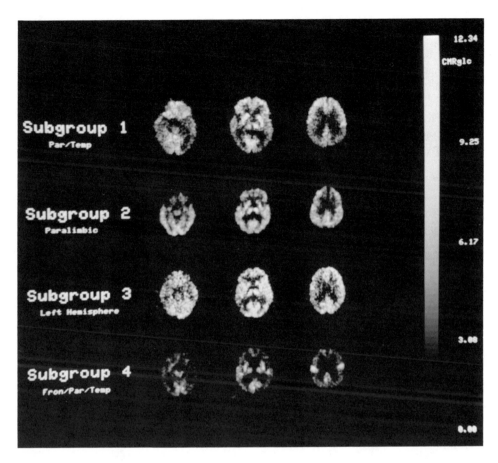

Figure 7 PET scan images from four DAT patients that characterize four metabolic subgroups identified with principal component analysis. Three planes are shown for each subject: left, at the level of the orbitofrontal cortex (30 mm above IOM line); middle, at the level of the basal ganglia (45 mm above IOM line), and right, at the level of the centrum semiovale (70 mm above IOM line). The subgroup numbers correspond to the subgroups described in the text. Metabolic rate is shown in mg/100 g brain per min (scale is on the right of the figure; CMRglc, cerebral metabolic rate for glucose). Data were obtained using a Scanditronix PC1024-7B tomograph.

volved (Seltzer, Burres, & Sherwin, 1984). One study examined right/left metabolic asymmetries in early-versus late-onset DAT patients and reported that the early-onset patients had a greater tendency toward disproportionate right hemisphere diminution of glucose use that was associated with poorer visuospatial performance (Koss, Friedland, Ober, & Jagust, 1985). In two later studies (Grady, Haxby, Horwitz, Berg, & Rapoport, 1987; Small *et al.*, 1989), no relation between metabolic asymmetry measures and age at onset was found. The early-onset patients did show significantly greater reductions in parietal regions, but these were not associated with greater reductions in performance on neuropsychological tests of parietal lobe function. These data suggest that younger DAT patients are better able to compensate cognitively for metabolic dysfunction than are older patients, but do not support the view that early- and late-onset DAT are two distinct disease entities.

Another clinical variable that has been used in attempts to differentiate among DAT patients is the presence of a family history of the disease. It is well known that in some families there is a genetic basis for AD that is manifested via autosomal dominant inheritance (Berg et al., 1986; Farrer, O'Sullivan, Cupples, Growdon, & Myers, 1989; Heston, Mastri, Anderson, & White, 1981; St. George-Hyslop et al., 1987). Although the effect of a positive family history on the metabolic defects seen with PET has not been examined in great detail, two preliminary studies have both shown that familial patients have metabolic patterns that are indistinguishable from those of patients with sporadic disease (Friedland et al., 1989; Hoffman et al., 1989). Thus, the pattern of metabolic brain dysfunction in an individual patient does not seem to depend on whether or not the disease in that patient has a genetic component. In addition, the validity of the metabolic patterns seen in sporadic patients is increased if similar patterns are seen in familial patients in whom the diagnosis is more certain.

Intercorrelations of regional metabolic rates also have been examined in patients with DAT. In one study that examined moderately to severely demented patients (Metter et al., 1984) inter-regional correlations were found to be elevated in the patients compared to controls, which may have been related to the diffuse nature of the hypometabolism seen in these patients who were in the severe stages of the disease. When mildly to moderately demented patients were compared to age-matched controls, the patient group showed fewer significant correlations between frontal and parietal regions, the number of which was already reduced in the older controls compared to younger subjects (Horwitz, Grady, Schlageter, Duara, & Rapoport, 1987). In addition, the number of significant correlations between glucose metabolism in right–left homologous regions was significantly reduced in DAT, which was of interest since these homologous correlations were among the largest correlations found in both the old and young healthy subjects (Horwitz et al., 1986). Thus, in DAT, there appears to be an alteration in the functional coupling of brain regions that is, in some ways, quantitatively different from the changes that are found in healthy aging (further reductions in the number of frontal–parietal correlations), and, in other ways, qualitatively different from age-related changes (reduced homologous correlations).

B. Cerebral Metabolism and Cognitive Function

The cerebral metabolic patterns that are found in DAT patients are correlated with the types of neuropsychological impairments that are shown by the patients. For example, metabolic right–left asymmetry measures in frontal and parietal cortices are significantly correlated with measures of right–left neuropsychological discrepancy, such that those patients with disproportionate left hemisphere hypometabolism have greater language impairment compared to visuospatial function, and those with disproportionate right hemisphere hypometabolism have more impairment of visuoconstructive abilities (Haxby et al., 1985; Foster et al., 1983; Friedland et al., 1985). One study examined metabolic and neuropsychologic patterns in mildly and moderately demented patients separately, and found that the mildly affected patients had abnormal memory performance, but scored in the normal range on neocortically mediated cognitive tests of attention, language, and visuospatial function (Haxby *et al.*, 1986). Moderately demented patients were significantly impaired on all neuropsychological tests. However, both mildly and moderately demented patients showed reductions in parietal–sensorimotor ratios of glucose metabolism, and had significantly increased metabolic asymmetry in frontal, parietal, and temporal association cortex. There was a significant correlation between right–left metabolic asymmetry and neuropsychological discrepancy measures only for those patients that had impaired performance on the cognitive tests, i.e., the moderately demented patients. Thus, in mildly affected DAT patients, metabolic changes in neocortex are seen before changes in neocortically mediated neuropsychological performance. A comparison of parietal–frontal metabolic measures and discrepancies between performance on neuropsychological tests mediated by parietal or frontal cortex revealed significant correlations between metabolic and cognitive discrepancies, but again only in the moderately demented patients, not in the mildly demented patients (Haxby *et al.*, 1988) Moderately demented patients with disproportionate parietal metabolic abnormality had more impairment on tests of calculations or visuoconstruction than on tests of sequencing or verbal fluency, whereas patients with disproportionate frontal metabolic defects showed the opposite pattern of neuropsychological impairments.

Followup of patients with DAT is vital in order to understand the evolution of cerebral metabolic and neuropsychological changes, as well as how the relationship between these measures changes as the disease progresses. The directions of the metabolic right/left asymmetries described in DAT patients are generally found to be stable over periods of several years (Figure 8), as are the correlations between these asymmetries and neuropsychological discrepancies (Grady, Haxby, Schlageter, Berg, & Rapoport, 1986; Haxby *et al.*, 1990; but see Jagust, Friedland, Budinger, Koss, & Ober, 1988). For example, patients with a disproportionate left hemisphere metabolic defect and poor language performance at the initial evaluation continue to show this pattern for long periods. In addition, these metabolic interhemispheric asymmetries are accentuated over time, but only in patients who are mildly affected at the initial evaluation (Grady, 1988). The intrahemispheric measures of parietal–frontal heterogeneity are not only directionally stable (Figure 9), but also become more pronounced over time in mildly, moderately, and severely demented patients (Haxby *et al.*, 1988). These results suggest that the metabolic patterns in individual patients are characteristic of the disease process in these patients and represent long-standing conditions that affect the behavioral manifestations of the disease. Also, the interhemispheric metabolic abnormalities appear to worsen in the early stages of the disease, whereas the intrahemispheric patterns continue to progress even in the later stages of DAT.

Mildly affected patients who initially show only progressive memory loss and yet have significantly abnormal metabolic patterns later demonstrate decline in other cognitive spheres (Haxby, Grady, Friedland, & Rapoport, 1987; Kuhl *et al.*, 1987), indicating that metabolic changes precede nonmemory cognitive changes. In addition, mildly demented patients show significant correlations between metabolic and neuropsychologic discrepancies after the development of nonmemory, neocortically mediated cognitive changes

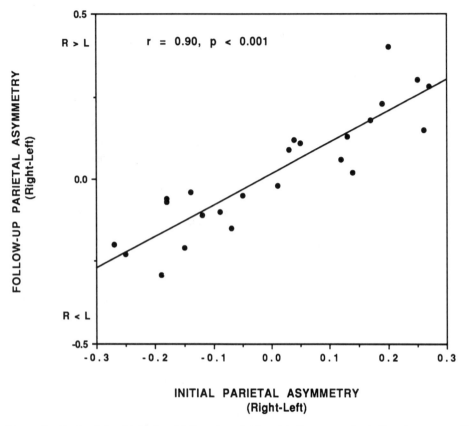

Figure 8   Scatterplots of initial and followup parietal metabolic asymmetry indices in a group of DAT patients (mean followup period was 15 months; range 9–25 months). A significant correlation is shown, indicating that the initial pattern of glucose use in individual patients is maintained over time.

(Haxby *et al.*, 1987). Thus the metabolic patterns not only precede the cognitive changes, but also predict the pattern of neuropsychological abnormalities seen at followup.

In a study that examined the development of these changes in a group of mildly demented DAT patients (Grady *et al.*, 1988), neocortical metabolic abnormalities preceded the appearance of neocortically mediated neuropsychological impairment by as few as 8 or as many as 36 months. This relationship between altered metabolic function and cognitive changes in DAT is illustrated in Figure 10, which shows the serial evaluations of a patient who was first seen in the early stages of the disease (Grady *et al.*, 1988). This patient (aged 45 years) presented initially with a progressive memory loss and a right parietal metabolic deficit, which became bilateral six months later. The first nonmemory neuropsychological impairments were seen in the areas of abstract reasoning and complex attention more than a year after the first evaluation. Finally, impairments in language and visuospatial function were noted almost two years after the appearance of bilateral parietal

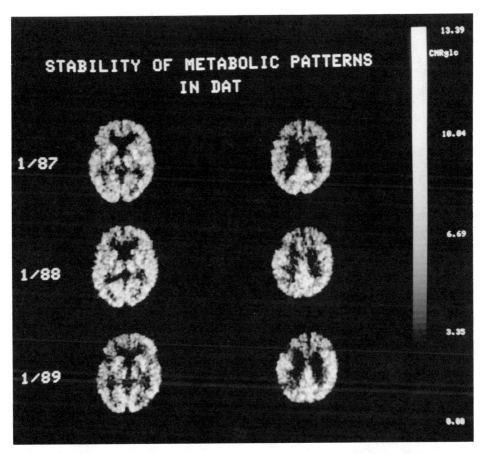

Figure 9   Three PET scans from a DAT patient seen over three consecutive years. At the first evaluation the patient was mildly demented, and was severely demented by the third evaluation. This patient showed a predominantly frontal distribution of metabolic defect at the initial evaluation, which persisted over the followup period, and eventually a left parietal abnormality also was seen. Data was obtained using a Scanditronix PC1024-7B tomograph.

metabolic changes. This patient demonstrates the typical finding in patients with DAT, i.e., significant and stable neocortical metabolic deficits before the appearance of any neocortically mediated cognitive dysfunction (Haxby *et al.*, 1986; Grady *et al.*, 1988). In addition, the first nonmemory impairments seen are in abstract reasoning and complex attention. These functions depend on the integrity of the frontal and parietal regions (Lezak, 1983), and probably involve the integrated function of these two brain areas (Mesulam, 1981). Changes in the functional connections between anterior and posterior brain regions early in the course of DAT, as indicated by the reductions in significant frontal–parietal correlations and the increased heterogeneity of parietal–frontal metabolic ratios (mentioned in the previous section), may impair the ability to attend to abstract and complex aspects of the environment. Thus, the longitudinal analysis of cerebral metabolic

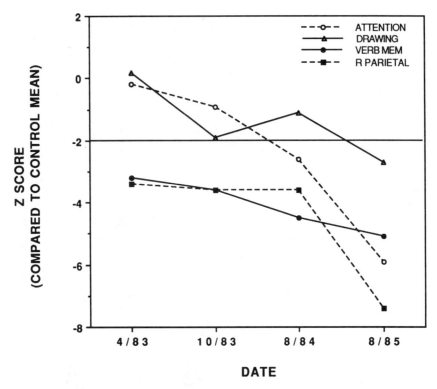

Figure 10   Data from one DAT patient seen over a period of 2 1/4 years. Scores on neuropsychological tests and the right parietal–sensorimotor metabolic ratio have been converted to Z scores based on the mean and standard deviation of an age-matched control group. The parietal metabolic measure and the memory score were significantly abnormal (Z score of −2 or less, $p < 0.05$) at the first evaluation and continued to deteriorate. Scores on tests of attention and drawing were not abnormal until over a year after the metabolic defect was first noted.

deficits in DAT has been useful not only in identifying those brain regions that are affected at different stages of the disease, but also in predicting the course of cognitive deterioration.

Studies of divided attention also have shown the importance of attentional deficits in the early stages of DAT. Performance on tests of dichotic listening, in which competing stimuli were delivered to the two ears simultaneously, was found to be deficient in DAT patients and related to hypometabolism in the left temporal region (Grimes, Grady, Foster, Sunderland, & Patronas, 1985). A subsequent study compared patients' performance on dichotic tests to performance on tests requiring discrimination of degraded monotic stimuli, and showed that dichotic performance was not only significantly more impaired than monotic performance, but that dichotic performance was again related to temporal lobe metabolism, whereas monotic performance was not (Grady *et al.,* 1989). This suggests that the dichotic impairment was directly related to the divided attention demands of the task, and was not due to an inability to make a difficult auditory discrimination among degraded speech stimuli. In addition, DAT patients are unable to selectively attend to either the right or the left ear during dichotic tasks, further indicating that the selective allocation of attention is impaired in this disease (Mohr, Cox, Williams, Chase, & Fedio, 1990). These studies combined with the results mentioned above, indicate that attentional mechanisms are disrupted in DAT and that these disruptions are related to abnormal metabolism in association neocortex.

IV. Other Dementias

A. Cerebrovascular Dementia

Cerebrovascular disease has long been known to cause dementia in older people (Hachinski et al., 1975), and, indeed, most if not all studies of DAT patients attempt to exclude a history of vascular disease in the patient sample. However, a history of vascular disease does not rule out the possibility of a mixed form of dementia involving AD and vascular disease. It is therefore important to examine the metabolic patterns in groups with different clinical diagnoses to try to differentiate among them and determine the specificity of the metabolic findings in DAT.

An early [133]Xenon study (Hachinski et al., 1975) found reduced global cerebral blood flow (CBF) in patients with cerebrovascular dementia (CVD). A later PET study (Frackowiack et al., 1981) compared CVD patients to DAT patients and controls and found that, although parieto–temporal metabolism was 23% lower in the CVD patients than in controls, this was not a significant reduction in oxygen metabolism. Benson et al., (1983) also compared CVD and DAT patients to controls and reported that whereas the DAT patients had reduced metabolism throughout the cortex, and particularly in parieto–temporal regions, the CVD patients had reduced metabolism in parieto–temporal regions, caudate, and thalamus. In CVD patients with evidence of infarcts on computed tomographic (CT) scans, areas of hypometabolism on PET images are reported to correspond well with the lesion sites on the CT images (Kuhl et al., 1985).

More recently, interest has focused on white matter lesions evident on CT or magnetic resonance imaging (MRI), which are associated with vascular disease and possibly with vascular dementia. DeCarli and colleagues (1990) examined a group of patients with dementia, a history of vascular disease, and white matter lesions on MRI, and compared metabolic patterns in these patients to those of a group of DAT patients. Whereas the DAT patients showed metabolic reductions primarily in parieto–temporal regions, the CVD patients showed more sparing of parietal metabolism and significantly reduced metabolism in the basal ganglia and thalamus compared to the DAT patients (Figure 11). Duara et al. (1989) found no difference in metabolic patterns between CVD and DAT patients, but a significant fraction of their DAT patients had evidence of white matter disease on MRI. Interestingly, another study showed that DAT patients with white matter lesions had less metabolic deficit in parieto–temporal areas than did those patients without such lesions (de Leon et al., 1988). This evidence suggests that vascular dementia is accompanied by

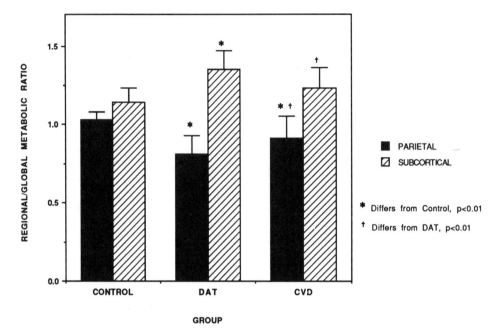

Figure 11 Metabolic ratios for DAT and CVD patients and age-matched controls. The parietal ratio is the mean value for superior and inferior parietal regions referenced to global metabolism, and the subcortical ratio is the mean value for caudate, thalamus, and putamen referenced to the global value. The DAT patients show reduced parietal ratios compared to controls and increased subcortical ratios, reflecting the relative sparing of metabolism in subcortical regions. The CVD patients also have reduced parietal ratios, but these are significantly less reduced than in the DAT patients. By contrast the CVD patients have lower subcortical ratios than the DAT patients, reflecting more involvement of these regions in CVD.

cortical metabolic abnormality similar to, but less severe than that seen in DAT, but, unlike DAT, is associated with metabolic dysfunction in basal ganglia and thalamus. This subcortical abnormality is probably the result of the white matter demyelination and may be found to contribute to some clinical features of CVD.

B. Depression

Studies of cerebral blood flow or metabolism in depression are few, and none has examined older patients with cognitive impairment secondary to the depression. PET studies of younger depressed patients have found that global metabolic measures are unchanged, but ratio measures of caudate and prefrontal to hemispheric metabolism are reduced compared to control values (Baxter *et al.*, 1985; Baxter *et al.*, 1989). The only two studies of older depressed patients were [133]Xenon studies, one that found no CBF differences compared to controls (Silfverskiold & Risberg, 1989), and one that reported both reduced global CBF and reduced CBF in prefrontal regions bilaterally (Sacheim *et al.*, 1990). In both studies reporting prefrontal metabolic abnormality, the metabolic values were significantly correlated with scores on rating scales for depression (Baxter *et al.*, 1989; Sackheim *et al.*, 1990) such that greater reduction of prefrontal values was associated with more severe depression. Involvement of the caudate and prefrontal cortex in depression is consistent with the hypothesis that dopamine plays a role in depression (McClure, 1973), because these brain regions are rich in dopaminergic innervation (Graybiel & Ragsdale, 1983). The caudate and prefrontal cortex also are part of several anatomical circuits, involving the thalamus and substantia nigra as well, which may be involved in memory processing (Alexander, DeLong, & Strick, 1986). How this caudate–frontal system is affected in elderly depressed subjects both with and without cognitive impairment and how this compares to the metabolic patterns found in DAT remain to be seen.

V. Future Directions

The majority of studies to date have examined cerebral metabolism and blood flow in aging and dementia in the resting or unstimulated state. Another approach is to examine metabolism under conditions of sensory or cognitive activation to determine the metabolic response to task performance (e.g., Fox, Miezin, Allman, Van Essen, & Raichle, 1987; Petersen, Fox, Posner, Mintun, & Raichle, 1989). This approach will become more important in the future as the short-lived radioisotopes that make it possible become more widely available. Measurement of regional CBF with $H_2{}^{15}O$ is particularly suited to this type of study, since the two-minute half-life of $H_2{}^{15}O$ allows multiple studies to be performed on the same individual. The ability to measure blood flow under activation conditions will allow the study of age-related differences in structure–function relationships, as well as the deterioration of these relationships in demented patients.

One activation paradigm that has been applied to the study of age-related changes in CBF is that of visual stimulation to examine the pathways involved in object discrimination and spatial location. These anatomically and functionally distinct pathways have been well defined in the extrastriate cortex of nonhuman primates (Ungerleider & Mishkin, 1982; Desimone & Ungerleider, 1989), and in humans, have been studied using $H_2{}^{15}O$ to measure brain blood flow during face matching (object) and dot-location matching (spatial) tasks (Haxby *et al.*, 1991). In young subjects, the face-matching task activates blood flow in occipito–temporal areas bilaterally, and the dot-location task selectively activates flow in superior parietal regions (Haxby *et al.*, 1991). Older subjects show a very similar pattern of activation in the two tasks, but have some parietal activation during the face-matching task that the young subjects do not show (Grady *et al.*, 1989). These results suggest that the functional dissociation of object and spatial vision in extrastriate cortex is preserved during aging, but that subtle changes occur, making the two systems less efficient or less functionally separate. Initial results suggest that DAT patients show activation of CBF during face matching that is similar in location and magnitude to that seen in the healthy elderly (Grady, *et al.*, 1990). Deustch and Halsey (1990) also have found a similar magnitude of activation in DAT patients and controls during a mental rotation task. Thus, the stimulation technique should prove very useful in shedding further light on the relation between metabolism and neuropsychological performance in both aging and dementia.

VI. Summary and Conclusions

The results with PET in aging have indicated that cross sectional, age-related changes in brain metabolism are relatively small in magnitude in healthy individuals. However, age-related reductions in the integrated activity among brain regions have been demonstrated and may be related to cognitive changes in the elderly. Nevertheless, preliminary comparisons of cognitive and metabolic relationships in young and old subjects suggest that these relationships are maintained in the elderly, with some fairly subtle alterations. This adds support to the notion that healthy aging is, in general, accompanied by smaller age-related changes than are found in a less optimally healthy population.

The use of PET to examine cerebral metabolism in patients with DAT has shown that the distribution of cortical metabolic abnormality seen during life is similar to that seen at postmortem, i.e., the finding of larger numbers of neurofibrillary tangles in association neocortex than in primary cortex (Lewis, Campbell, Terry, & Morrison, 1987) is mirrored by the marked metabolic decreases seen in association cortex and the relative sparing of glucose metabolism in primary cortical regions. This is important information for identifying which brain areas are most susceptible to the disease process, and can lead to hypotheses about disease mechanisms. One such hypothesis (Rapoport, 1988) is that the rapid evolution of the human brain by various genomic processes has made the newest areas, specifically the association neocortices and connected amygdaloid, hippocampal, and entorhinal areas, vulnerable to AD by increasing the value of a disease-specific genomic character function.

The use of PET also has shown that metabolic changes in the neocortex precede changes in the cognitive functions that depend on the integrity of the neocortex, sometimes by several years. This finding implies that there are cortical redundancies or compensatory mechanisms that allow cognitive processing to be maintained despite considerable metabolic dysfunction. One such mechanism might be axonal sprouting to compensate for cell loss and dysfunction during the period before neocortically mediated neuropsychological impairments are seen (Horwitz, 1988).

PET has proved to be a sensitive tool for measuring cerebral metabolic changes in even mildly demented patients. The ability to measure cerebral metabolism in DAT patients has increased further our understanding of the heterogeneous nature of this type of dementia by demonstrating both inter- and intra-hemispheric differences in metabolic deficit that are related to different patterns of neuropsychological impairment. Although it is probable that some variability is introduced from the inclusion of patients with diseases other than AD, owing to the small but inevitable uncertainty in the clinical diagnosis, much of the heterogeneity may be inherent in the variable way the disease begins in the neocortex. The findings to date suggest that medial structures involved in memory, such as the hippocampus and amygdala, are affected first in most patients, given that memory loss is usually the first symptom (Grady et al., 1988; Haxby et al., 1987; Rosen & Mohs, 1982). After that, however, the particular area of association neocortex that is affected (i.e., right versus left or frontal versus parietal) may be random, or attributable to regional differences in susceptibility, or to different etiologies. Whatever the cause of this heterogeneity in DAT, a full understanding of how it affects both cognitive impairments and patients' response to possible drug therapies will be important for the future. In addition, preliminary results suggest that other forms of dementia will be distinguishable from DAT in terms of metabolic patterns, but more work needs to be done to determine the specificity of the PET findings for DAT.

References

Alexander, G. E., DeLong, M. R., & Strick, P. L. (1986). Parallel organization of functionally segregated circuits linking basal ganglia and cortex. *Annual Review of Neuroscience, 9,* 357–381.

Baxter, L. R., Phelps, M. E., Mazziotta, J. C., Schwartz, J. M., Gerner, R. H., Selin, C. E., & Sumida, R. M. (1985). Cerebral metabolic rates for glucose in mood disorders. Studies with positron emission tomography and fluorodeoxyglucose F18. *Archives of General Psychiatry, 42,* 441–447.

Baxter, L. R., Schwartz, J. M., Phelps, M. E., Mazziotta, J. C., Guze, B. H., Selin, C. E., Gerner, R. H., & Sumida, R. M. (1989). Reduction of prefrontal cortex glucose metabolism common to three types of depression. *Archives of General Psychiatry, 46,* 243–250.

Benson, D. F., Kuhl, D. E., Hawkins, R. A., Phelps, M. E., Cummings, J. L., & Tsai, S. Y. (1983). The fluorodeoxyglucose 18F scan in Alzheimer's disease and multi-infarct dementia. *Archives of Neurology, 40,* 711–714.

Berardi, A., Haxby, J. V., Grady, C. L., & Rapoport, S. I. (1990). Memory performance in healthy young and old subjects correlates with resting state brain glucose utilization in the parietal lobe. *Journal of Nuclear Medicine, 31,* 879.

Berardi, A., Haxby, J. V., Grady, C. L., & Rapoport, S. I. (1991). Asymmetries of brain glucose metabolism and memory in the healthy elderly. *Developmental Neuropsychology, 7,* 87–97.

Berg, G., Grady, C. L., Sundaram, M., Haxby, J. V., Moore, A. M., White, J., Heston, L., Rapoport, S. I., & Avioli, L. V. (1986). Positron emission tomography in dementia of the Alzheimer type. A brief review with a case study. *Archives of Internal Medicine, 146,* 2045–2049.

Birren, J. E., Butler, R. M., Greenhouse, S. W., Sokoloff, L., & Yarrow, M. R. (1963). Interdisciplinary relationships: Interrelations of physiological, psychological, and psychiatric findings in healthy elderly men. In J.E. Birren, R. M. Butler, S. W. Greenhouse, L. Sokoloff, M. R. Yarrow (eds), *Human aging–A biological and behavioral study* (publication # 986, pp. 283–305). Bethesda, MD: US Department of Health, Education and Welfare.

Brun, A., & Gustafson, L. (1976). Distribution of cerebral degeneration in Alzheimer's disease. *Archiv fuer Psychiatrie und Nervenkrankheiten, 223,* 15–33.

Chase, T. N. (1987). Cortical glucose utilization patterns in primary degenerative dementia of the anterior and posterior types. *Archives of Gerontology and Geriatrics, 6,* 289–297.

Chawluk, J. B., Alavi, A., Jamieson, D. G., Hurtig, H. I., Gur, R. E., Resnick, S. M., Rosen, M., & Reivich, M. (1987). Changes in local cerebral glucose metabolism with normal aging: The effects of cardiovascular and systemic health factors. *Journal of Cerebral Blood Flow and Metabolism, 7 (Suppl. 1),* S411.

Chui, H. C., (1989). Dementia. A review emphasizing clinicopathologic correlation and brain-behavior relationships. *Archives of Neurology, 46,* 806–814.

Clark, C. M., Kessler, R., Buchsbaum, M. S., Margolin, R. A., & Holcomb, H. H. (1984). Correlational methods for determining regional coupling of cerebral glucose metabolism: A pilot study. *Biological Psychiatry, 19,* 663–678.

Cummings, J., Benson, D. F., & Lo Verma, S. (1980). Reversible dementia: Illustrative cases, definition and review. *Journal of the American Medical Association, 243,* 2434–2439.

Dastur, D. K., Lane, M. H., Hansen, D. B., Kety, S. S., Butler, R. N., Perlin, S., & Sokoloff, L. (1963). Effects of aging on cerebral circulation and metabolism in man. In J.E. Birren, R. N. Butler, S. W. Greenhouse, L. Sokoloff, & M. R. Yarrow (Eds.). *Human aging–A biological and behavioral study* (publication # 986, pp 59–76). Bethesda, MD: U.S. Department of Health, Education and Welfare.

DeCarli, C. S., Grady, C. L., Clark, C. M., Gouras, G., Schapiro, M. B., Haxby, J. V., Salerno, J. A., & Rapoport, S. I. (1990). Slowly progressive dementia with severe white matter changes (DWMC) on magnetic resonance imaging (MRI)—comparison to dementia of the Alzheimer type (DAT). *Neurology, 40 (Suppl. 1),* 176.

de Leon, M. J., Ferris, S. H., George, A. E., Reisberg, B., Christman, D. R., Kricheff, I. I., & Wolf, A. P. (1983). Computed tomography and positron emission transaxial tomography evaluations of normal aging and Alzheimer's disease. *Journal of Cerebral Blood Flow and Metabolism, 3,* 391–394.

de Leon, M. J., George, A. E., Ferris, S. H., Christman, D. R., Fowler, J. S., Gentes, C. I., Brodie, J., Reisberg, B., & Wolf, A. P. (1984) Positron emission tomography and computed tomography assessments of the aging human brain. *Journal of Computer Assisted Tomography, 8,* 88–94.

de Leon, M. J., George, A. E., Klinger, A., Miller, J., Franssen, E., Kluger, A., Ferris, S. H., Sachs, H., Christman, D., & Wolf, A. (1988). PET-11CDG studies of leukoencephalopathy in normal aging and Alzheimer's disease. *Neurology, 38 (Suppl. 1),* 372.

Desimone, R., & Ungerleider, L. G. (1989). Neural mechanisms of visual perception in monkeys. In F. Boller & J. Grafman (Eds.), *Handbook of Neuropsychology,* (Vol. 2, pp. 267–299). Amsterdam: Elsevier.

Deustch, G., & Halsey, H. (1990). Cortical blood flow effects of mental rotation in older subjects and Alzheimer patients. *Journal of Clinical and Experimental Neuropsychology, 12,* 31.

Duara, R., Barker, W., Loewenstein, D., Pascal, S., & Bowen, B. (1989). Sensitivity and specificity of positron emission tomography and magnetic resonance imaging studies in Alzheimer's disease and multi-infarct dementia. *European Neurology, 29 (Suppl. 3),* 9–15.

Duara, R., Grady, C. L., Haxby, J. V., Ingvar, D. H., Sokoloff, L., Margolin, R. A., Manning, R. G., Cutler, N. R., & Rapoport, S. (1984). Human brain glucose utilization and cognitive function in relation to age. *Annals of Neurology, 16,* 702–713.

Duara, R., Grady, C. L., Haxby, J. V., Sundaram, M., Cutler, N. R., Heston, L., Moore, A. M., Schlageter, N. L., Larson, S. & Rapoport, S. I. (1986). Positron emission tomography in Alzheimer's disease. *Neurology, 36,* 879–887.

Duara, R., Loewenstein, D. A., Barker, W. W., Chang, J. Y., & Kothari, P. (1988). Evidence for predominant left hemisphere dysfunction in FDG/PET scans of patients with Alzheimer's disease and multi-infarct dementia. *Journal of Nuclear Medicine, 29,* 912.

Duara, R., Margolin, R. A., Robertson-Tchabo, E. A., London, E. D., Schwartz, M., Renfrew, J. W., Koziarz, B. J., Sundaram, M., Grady, C. L., Moore, A. M., Ingvar, D. H., Sokoloff, L., Weingartner, H., Kessler, R. M., Manning, R. G., Channing, M. A., Cutler, N. R., & Rapoport, S. I. (1983). Cerebral glucose utilization, as measured with positron emission tomography in 21 healthy men between the ages of 21 and 83 years. *Brain, 106,* 761–775.

Evans, D. A., Funkenstein, H., Albert, M. S., Scherr, P. A., Cook, N. R., Chown, M. J., Hebert, L. E., Hennekens, C. H., & Taylor, J. O. (1989). Prevalence of Alzheimer's disease in a community population of older persons. Higher than previously reported. *Journal of the American Medical Association, 262,* 2551–2556.

Farrer, L. A., O'Sullivan, D. M., Cupples, L. A., Growdon, J. H., & Myers, R. H. (1989). Assessment of genetic risk for Alzheimer's disease among first-degree relatives. *Annals of Neurology, 25,* 485–493.

Ferris, S. H., de Leon, M. J., Wolf, A. P., Farkas, T., Christman, D. R., Reisberg, B., Fowler, J. S., MacGregor, R., Goldman, A., George, A. E., & Rampal, S. (1980). Positron emission tomography in the study of aging and senile dementia. *Neurobiology of Aging, 1,* 127–131.

Foster, N. L., Chase, T. N., Fedio, P., Patronas, N. J., Brooks, R. A., & DiChiro, G. (1983). Alzheimer's disease: Focal cortical changes shown by positron emission tomography. *Neurology, 33,* 961–965.

Foster, N. L., Chase, T. N., Mansi, L., Brooks, R., Fedio, P., Patronas, N. J., DiChiro, G. (1984). Cortical abnormalities in Alzheimer's disease. *Annals of Neurology, 16,* 649–654.

Foster, N. L., VanDerSpek, A. F. L., Aldrich, M. S., Berent, S., Hichwa, R. H., Sackellares, J. C., Gilman, S., & Agranoff, B. W. (1987). The effect of diazepam sedation on cerebral glucose metabolism in Alzheimer's disease as measured by positron emission tomography. *Journal of Cerebral Blood Flow and Metabolism, 7,* 415–420.

Fox, P. T., Miezin, F. M., Allman, J. M., Van Essen, D. C., & Raichle, M. E. (1987). Retinotopic organization of human visual cortex mapped with positron emission tomography. *Journal of Neuroscience, 7,* 913–922.

Frackowiak, R. S. J., & Gibbs, J. M. (1983). Cerebral metabolism and blood flow in normal and pathologic aging. In P. L. Magistretti (Ed.), *Functional radionuclide imaging of the brain.* (pp. 305–309). New York: Raven Press.

Frackowiak, R. S. J., Lenzi, G. L., Jones, T., & Heather, J. D. (1980). Quantitative measurement of regional cerebral blood flow and oxygen metabolism in man using [15]O and positron emission tomography: Theory, procedure, and normal values. *Journal of Computer Assisted Tomography, 4,* 727–736.

Frackowiak, R. S. J., Pozzilli, C., Legg, N. J., Du Boulay, G. H., Marshall, J., Lenzi, G. L., & Jones, T. (1981). Regional cerebral oxygen supply and utilization in dementia. A clinical and physiological study with oxygen-15 and positron tomography. *Brain, 104,* 753–778.

Friedland, R. P., Budinger, T. F., Koss, E., & Ober, B. A. (1985). Alzheimer's disease: Anterior-posterior and lateral hemispheric alterations in cortical glucose utilization. *Neuroscience Letters, 53,* 235–240.

Friedland, R. P., Budinger, T. F., Ganz, E., Yano, Y., Mathis, C. A., Koss, B., Ober, A. B., Heusman, R. H., & Derenzo, S. E. (1983). Regional cerebral metabolic alterations in dementia of the Alzheimer type: Positron emission tomography with (18F) fluoro-deoxyglucose. *Journal of Computer Assisted Tomography, 7,* 590–598.

Friedland, R. P., Grady, C. L., Schapiro, M. B., Moore, A. M., Kumar, A., & Kinsel, V. (1989). Family history of dementia and regional cerebral glucose utilization in dementia of the Alzheimer type. *Neurology, 39 (Suppl. 1),* 168.

Gottstein, U., & Held, K. (1979). Effects of aging on cerebral circulation and metabolism in man. *Acta Neurologica Scandinavica, 60 (Suppl. 72),* 54–55.

Grady, C. L. (1988). Longitudinal changes in brain metabolism. In R. P. Friedland (moderator): Alzheimer disease: Clinical and biological heterogeneity. *Annals of Internal Medicine, 109,* 302–304.

Grady, C. L., Grimes, A. M., Patronas, N., Sunderland, T., Foster, N. L., & Rapoport, S. I. (1989). Divided attention, as measured by dichotic speech performance, in dementia of the Alzheimer type. *Archives of Neurology, 46,* 317–320.

Grady, C. L., Haxby, J. V., Horwitz, B., Berg, G. W., & Rapoport, S. I. (1987). Neuropsychological and cerebral metabolic function in early versus late onset dementia of the Alzheimer type. *Neuropsychologia, 25,* 807–816.

Grady, C. L., Haxby, J.V., Horwitz, B., Schapiro, M. B., Carson, R. E., Herscovitch, P., & Rapoport, S. I. (1990). Activation of regional cerebral blood flow (rCBF) in extrastriate cortex during a face-matching task in patients with dementia of the Alzheimer type (DAT). *Society for Neuroscience Abstracts, 16,* 149.

Grady, C. L., Haxby, J. V., Horwitz, B., Schapiro, M. B., Carson, R. E., Herscovitch, P., Ungerleider, L. G., Mishkin, M., Friedland, R. P., & Rapoport, S. I. (1989). Mapping human visual systems for object recognition and spatial localization by measurement of regional cerebral blood flow. *Journal of Cerebral Blood Flow and Metabolism, 9 (Suppl. 1),* S574.

Grady, C. L., Haxby, J. V., Horwitz, B., Sundaram, M., Berg, G., Schapiro, M. B., Friedland, R. P., & Rapoport, S. I. (1988). Longitudinal study of the early neuropsychological and cerebral metabolic changes in dementia of the Alzheimer type. *Journal of Clinical and Experimental Neuropsychology, 10,* 576–596.

Grady, C. L., Haxby, J. V., Schapiro, M. B., Gonzalez-Aviles, A., Kumar, A., Ball, M. J., Heston, L., & Rapoport, S. I. (1990) Metabolic subgroups in dementia of the Alzheimer type identified using positron emission tomography. *Journal of Neuropsychiatry and Clinical Neurosciences, 2,* 373–384.

Grady, C. L., Haxby, J. V., Schlageter, N. L., Berg, G., & Rapoport, S. I. (1986). Stability of metabolic and neuropsychological asymmetries in dementia of the Alzheimer type. *Neurology, 36,* 1390–1392.

Grady, C. L., Horwitz, B., Schapiro, M. B., & Rapoport, S. I. (1990). Changes in the integrated activity of the brain with healthy aging and dementia of the Alzheimer type. In L. Battistin and F. Gerstenbrand (Eds.), *Aging brain and dementia. New trends in diagnosis and therapy* (pp. 355–370). New York: Wiley-Liss.

Graybiel, A., & Ragsdale, C. W. (1983). Biochemical anatomy of the striatum. In P. C. Emson (Ed.), *Chemical Neuroanatomy* (pp. 427–504). New York: Raven Press.

Grimes, A. M., Grady, C. L., Foster, N. L., Sunderland, T., & Patronas, N. (1985). Central auditory function in Alzheimer's disease. *Neurology, 35,* 352–358.

Hachinski, V. C., Iliff, L. D., Phil, M., Zilhka, E., Du Boulay, G. H., McAllister, V. L., Marshall, J., Russell, R. W. R., & Symon, L. (1975). Cerebral blood flow in dementia. *Archives of Neurology, 32,* 632–637.

Haxby, J. V. (1986). Letter to the editor. *Journal of Cerebral Blood Flow and Metabolism, 6,* 125–126.

Haxby, J. V., Duara, R., Grady, C. L., Rapoport, S. I., & Cutler, N. R. (1985). Relations between neuropsychological and cerebral metabolic asymmetries in early Alzheimer's disease. *Journal of Cerebral Blood Flow and Metabolism, 5,* 193–200.

Haxby, J. V., Grady, C. L., Duara, R., Robertson-Tchabo, E. A., Koziarz, B., Cutler, N. R., & Rapoport, S. I. (1986). Relations among age, visual memory, and resting cerebral metabolism in 40 healthy men. *Brain and Cognition, 5,* 412–427.

Haxby, J. V., Grady, C. L., Duara, R., Schlageter, N. L., Berg, G., & Rapoport, S. I. (1986). Neocortical metabolic abnormalities precede nonmemory cognitive defects in early Alzheimer's-type dementia. *Archives of Neurology, 43,* 882–885.

Haxby, J. V., Grady, C. L., Friedland, R. P., & Rapoport, S. I. (1987). Neocortical metabolic abnormalities precede nonmemory cognitive impairments in early dementia of the Alzheimer type: Longitudinal confirmation. *Journal of Neural Transmission, 24 (Suppl.),* 49–53.

Haxby, J. V., Grady, C. L., Horwitz, B., Ungerleider, L. G., Mishkin, M., Carson, R. E., Herscovitch, P., Schapiro, M. B., Rapoport, S. I., (1991). Dissociation of spatial and object visual processing pathways in human extrastriate cortex. *Proceedings of the National Academy of Science, 88,* 1621–1625.

Haxby, J. V., Grady, C. L., Koss, E., Horwitz, B., Heston, L. L., Schapiro, M. B., Friedland, R. P., & Rapoport, S. I. (1990). Longitudinal study of cerebral metabolic asymmetries and associated neuropsychological patterns in early dementia of the Alzheimer type. *Archives of Neurology, 47,* 753–760.

Haxby, J. V., Grady, C. L., Koss, E., Horwitz, B., Schapiro, M. B., Friedland, R. P., & Rapoport, S. I. (1988). Heterogeneous anterior–posterior metabolic patterns in Alzheimer's type dementia *Neurology, 38,* 1853–1863.

Heston, L. L., Mastri, A. R., Anderson, V. E., & White, J. (1981). Dementia of the Alzheimer type: Clinical genetics, natural history, and associated conditions. *Archives of General Psychiatry, 38,* 1085–1090.

Hoffman, J. M., Guze, B. H., Hawk, T. C., Pahl, J. P., Sumida, R., Baxter, L. R., Mazziotta, J. C., & Phelps, M. E. (1988). Cerebral glucose metabolism in normal individuals: Effects of aging, sex and handedness. *Neurology, 38 (Suppl. 1),* 371.

Hoffman, J. M., Guze, B. H., Baxter, L. R., Hawk, T. C.. Fujikawa, D. G., Dorsey, D., Maltese, A., Small, G., & Mazziotta, J. C. (1989). Metabolic homogeneity in familial and sporadic Alzheimer's disease: An FDG/PET study. *Neurology, 39 (Suppl. 1),* 167.

Horwitz, B., (1988). Neuroplasticity and the progression of Alzheimer's disease. *International Journal of Neuroscience, 41,* 1–14.

Horwitz, B. (1990). Quantification and analysis of positron emission tomography metabolic data. In R. Duara (Ed.), *Positron emission tomography in dementia* (pp. 19–76). New York: Willey-Liss.

Horwitz, B., Duara, R., & Rapoport, S. I. (1984). Intercorrelations of glucose metabolic rates between brain regions: Application to healthy males in a state of reduced sensory input. *Journal of Cerebral Blood Flow and Metabolism, 4,* 484–499.

Horwitz, B., Duara, R., & Rapoport, S. I. (1986). Age differences in intercorrelations between regional cerebral metabolic rates for glucose. *Annals of Neurology, 19,* 60–67.

Horwitz, B., Grady, C. L., Schlageter, N. L., Duara, R., & Rapoport, S. I. (1987). Intercorrelations of regional cerebral glucose metabolic rates in Alzheimer's disease. *Brain Research, 407,* 294–306.

Jagust, W. J., Friedland, R. P., Budinger, T. F., Koss, E., & Ober, B. (1988). Longitudinal studies of regional cerebral metabolism in Alzheimer's disease. *Neurology, 38,* 909–912.

Jamada, M., & Mehraein, P. (1968). Verteilungsmuster der senilen Veranderungen im Gehirn. *Arkiv fuer Psychiatrie und Nervenkrankheiten, 211,* 308–324.

Kemper, T. (1984). Neuroanatomical and neuropathological changes in normal aging and in dementia. In M. Albert (Ed.), *Clinical neurology of aging* (pp. 9–52) New York: Oxford University Press.

Kety, S. S. (1956). Human cerebral blood flow and oxygen consumption as related to aging. *Journal of Chronic Diseases, 3,* 478–486.

Kety, S. S., & Schmidt, C. F. (1948). The nitrous oxide method for the quantitative determination of cerebral blood flow in man: Theory, procedure and normal values. *Journal of Clinical Investigation, 27,* 476–483.

Koss, E., Friedland, R. P., Ober, B. A., & Jagust, W. J. (1985). Differences in lateral hemispheric asymmetries of glucose utilization between early- and late-onset Alzheimer-type dementia. *American Journal of Psychiatry, 142,* 638–640.

Kuhl, D. E., Metter, E. J., Riege, W. H., & Phelps, M.E. (1982). Effects of human aging on patterns of local cerebral glucose utilization determined by the [^{18}F]fluorodeoxyglucose method. *Journal of Cerebral Blood Flow and Metabolism, 2,* 163–171.

Kuhl, D. E., Metter, E. J., Riege, W. H., & Hawkins, R. A. (1985). Patterns of cerebral glucose utilization in dementia. In T. Greitz, D. H. Ingvar, and L. Widen (Eds.). *The metabolism of the human brain studied with positron emission tomography* (pp. 419–431). New York: Raven Press.

Kuhl, D. E., Small, G. W., Riege, W. H., Fujikawa, D. G., Metter, E. J., Benson, D. F., Ashford, J. W., Mazziotta, J. C., Maltese, A., & Dorsey, D. A. (1987). Cerebral metabolic patterns before the diagnosis of probable Alzheimer's disease. *Journal of Cerebral Blood Flow and Metabolism, 7 (Suppl. 1),* S406.

Kumar, A., Schapiro, M. B., Grady, C. L., Haxby, J. V., Wagner, E., Salerno, J. A., & Rapoport, S. I. (1991). High-resolution studies of cerebral glucose metabolism in Alzheimer's disease. *Neuropsychopharmocology, 4,* 35–46.

Lassen, N. A., Feinberg, I., & Lane, M. H. (1960). Bilateral studies of cerebral oxygen uptake in young and aged normal subjects and in patients with organic dementia. *Journal of Clinical Investigation, 39,* 491–500.

Lassen, N. A., Hoedt-Rasmussen, K., Sorensen, S. C., Skinhoj, E., Cronquist, S., Bodforss, B., Eng, E., & Ingvar, D. H. (1963). Regional cerebral blood flow in man determined by krypton 85. *Neurology, 13,* 719–727.

Lebrun-Grandie, P., Baron, J.-C., Soussaline, F., Loch'h, C., Sastre, J., & Bousser, M.-G. (1983). Coupling between regional blood flow and oxygen utilization in the normal human brain: A study with positron tomography and oxygen 15. *Archives of Neurology, 40,* 230–236.

Leenders, K. L., Perani, D., Lammertsma, A., Heather, J.D., Buckingham, P., Healy, M. J. R., Gibbs, J. M., Wise, R. J. S., Hatazawa, J., Herold, S., Beaney, R. P., Brooks, D. J., Spinks, T., Rhodes, C., Frackowiak, R. S. J., & Jones, T. (1990). Cerebral blood flow, blood volume, and oxygen utilization. Normal values and effect of age. *Brain, 113,* 27–47.

Lewis, D. A., Campbell, M. J., Terry, R. D., & Morrison, J. H. (1987). Laminar and regional distributions of neurofibrillary tangles and neuritic plaques in Alzheimer's disease: A quantitative study of visual and auditory cortices. *Journal of Neuroscience, 7,* 1799–1808.

Lezak, M. (1983). *Neuropsychological assessment* (2nd ed.). New York: Oxford University Press.

Mamo, H., Meric, P., Luft, A., & Seylaz, J. (1983). Hyperfrontal pattern of human cerebral circulation: Variations with age and atherosclerotic state. *Archives of Neurology, 40,* 626–632.

Mazziotta, J. C., Phelps, M. E., Plummer, M., & Kuhl, D. E. (1981). Quantitation in positron emission computed tomography: 5. Physical-anatomical effects. *Journal of Computer Assisted Tomography, 5,* 734–743.

McClure, D. J. (1973). The role of dopamine in depression. *Canadian Journal of Psychiatry, 18,* 309–312.

McGeer, P. L., Kamo, H., Harrop, R., Li, D. K. B., Tuokko, H., McGeer, E. G., Adam, M. J., Ammann, W., Beattie, B. L., Calne, D. B., Martin, W. R. W., Pate, B. D., Rogers, J. G., Ruth, T. J., Sayre, C. I., & Stoessl, A. J. (1986). Positron emission tomography in patients with clinically diagnosed Alzheimer's disease. *Canadian Medical Association Journal, 134,* 597–607.

Melamed, E., Lavy, S., Bentin, S., Cooper, G., & Rinot, Y. (1980). Reduction in regional cerebral blood flow during normal aging in man. *Stroke, 11,* 31–35.

Mesulam, M. M. (1981). A cortical network for directed attention and unilateral neglect. *Annals of Neurology, 10,* 309–325.

Metter, E. J., Riege, W. H., Kameyama, M., Kuhl, D. E., & Phelps, M. E. (1984). Cerebral metabolic relationships for selected brain regions in Alzheimer's, Huntington's and Parkinson's diseases. *Journal of Cerebral Blood Flow and Metabolism, 4,* 500–506.

Metter, E. J., Riege, W. H., Kuhl, D. E., & Phelps, M. E. (1984). Cerebral metabolic relationships for selected brain regions in healthy adults. *Journal of Cerebral Blood Flow and Metabolism, 4,* 1–7.

Miller, J. D., de Leon, M. J., Ferris, S. H., Kluger, A., George, A. E., Reisberg, B., Sachs, H. J., & Wolf, A. P. (1987). Abnormal temporal lobe response in Alzheimer's disease during cognitive processing as measured by ^{11}C-2-deoxy-D-glucose and PET. *Journal of Cerebral Blood Flow and Metabolism, 7,* 248–251.

Mohr, E., Cox, C., Williams, J., Chase, T. N., & Fedio, P. (1990). Impairment of central auditory function in Alzheimer's disease. *Journal of Clinical and Experimental Neuropsychology, 12,* 235–246.

Mountjoy, C. Q., Roth, M., Evans, N. J. R., & Evans, H. M. (1983). Cortical neuronal counts in normal elderly controls and demented patients. *Neurobiology of Aging, 4,* 1–11.

Naritomi, H., Meyer, J. S., Sakai, F., Yamaguchi, F., & Shaw, T. (1979). Effects of advancing age on regional cerebral blood flow: Studies in normal subjects and subjects with risk factors for atherothrombotic stroke. *Archives of Neurology, 36,* 410–416.

Obrist, W. D., Thompson, H. K., King, C. H., & Wang, H. S. (1967). Determination of regional cerebral blood flow by inhalation of 133-xenon. *Circulation Research, 20,* 124–135.

Pantano, P., Baron, J.-C., Lebrun-Grandie, P., Duquesnoy, N., Bousser, M.-G., & Comar, M. (1984) Regional cerebral blood flow and oxygen consumption in human aging. *Stroke, 15,* 635–641.

Petersen, S. E., Fox, P. T., Posner, M. I., Mintun, M., & Raichle, M. E. (1989). Positron emission tomographic studies of the processing of single words. *Journal of Cognitive Neuroscience, 1,* 153–170.

Rapoport, S. I. (1988). Brain evolution and Alzheimer's disease. *Revue Neurologique (Paris), 144,* 79–90.

Rosen, W. G., & Mohs, R. C. (1982). Evolution of cognitive decline in dementia. In S. Corkin, K. L. Davis, J. H. Growden, E. Usdin, & R. J. Wurtman (Eds.), *Aging, Vol. 19: Alzheimer's disease: A Report of progress* (pp. 183–188). New York: Raven Press.

Rossor, M. N., Iverson, L. L., Reynolds, G. P., Mountjoy, C. Q., & Roth, M. (1984). Neurochemical characteristics of early-and late-onset types of Alzheimer's disease. *British Medical Journal, 288,* 961–964.

Sackeim, H. A., Prohovnik, I., Moeller, J. R., Brown, R. P., Apter, S., Prudic, J., Devanand, D. P., & Mukherjee, S., (1990). Regional cerebral blood flow in mood disorders: I. Comparison of major depressives and normal controls at rest. *Archives of General Psychiatry, 47,* 60–70.

Schlageter, N. L., Horwitz, B., Creasey, H., Carson, R., Duara, R., Berg, G. W., & Rapoport, S. I., (1987). Relation of measured brain glucose utilisation and cerebral atrophy in man. *Journal of Neurology Neurosurgery and Psychiatry, 50,* 779–785.

Seltzer, B., Burres, M. J. K., & Sherwin, I. (1984). Left-handedness in early- and late-onset dementia. *Neurology, 34,* 367–369.

Seltzer, B., & Sherwin, I. (1983). A comparison of clinical features in early- and late-onset primary degenerative dementia. *Archives of Neurology, 40,* 143–146.

Shenkin, H. A., Novak, P., Goluboff, B., Soffe, A. M., & Bortin, L. (1953). The effects of aging, arteriosclerosis, and hypertension upon the cerebral circulation. *Journal of Clinical Investigation, 32,* 459–465.

Silfverskiold, P., & Risberg, J. (1989). Regional cerebral blood flow in depression and mania. *Archives of General Psychiatry, 46,* 253–259.

Sokoloff, L., Reivich, M., Kennedy, C., Desrosiers, M.H., Patlak, C. S., Pettigrew, K. D., Sakurada, O., & Shinohara, M. (1977). The [^{14}C]-deoxyglucose method for the measurement of local cerebral glucose utilization: Theory, procedure, and normal values in the conscious and anesthetized albino rat. *Journal of Neurochemistry, 28,* 897–916.

Small, G. W., Kuhl, D. E., Riege, W. H., Fujikawa, D. G., Ashford, J. W., Metter, E. J., & Mazziotta, J. C. (1989). Cerebral glucose metabolic patterns in Alzheimer's disease. Effect of gender and age at dementia onset. *Archives of General Psychiatry, 46,* 527–532.

St. George-Hyslop, P., Tanzi, R., Polinsky, R., Haines, J. L., Nee, L., Watkins, P. C., Myers, R. H., Feldman, R. G., Pollen, D., Drachman, D., Growdon, J., Bruni, A., Foncin, J.-F., Salmon, D., Frommelt, P., Amaducci, L., Sorbi, S., Piacentini, S., Stewart, G. D., Hobbs, W. J., Conneally, P. M., & Gusella, J. F. (1987). The genetic defect causing familial Alzheimer's disease maps on chromosome 21. *Science, 235,* 885–890.

Ungerleider, L. G., & Mishkin, M. (1982). Two cortical visual systems. In D. J. Ingle, M. A. Goodale, & R. J. W. Mansfield (Eds.), *Analysis of Visual Behavior* (pp. 549–584). Cambridge: MIT Press.

Yoshii, F., Barker, W. W., Chang, J. Y., Loewenstein, D., Apicella, A., Smith, D., Boothe, T., Ginsberg, M. D., Pascal, S., & Duara, R. (1988). Sensitivity of cerebral glucose metabolism to age, gender, brain, volume, brain atrophy, and cerebrovascular risk factors. *Journal of Cerebral Blood Flow and Metabolism, 8,* 654–661.

9

The Outcomes of Psychiatric Disorder in the Elderly: Relevance to Quality of Life

Barry Gurland and Sidney Katz

I. Centrality of the Quality of Life
   A. Definition
   B. Relevant Mental Health Problems
   C. Contrast with the Diagnosis of Disease
II. Domains
   A. Perspectives
   B. Subjective and Objective Perspectives
   C. Measurements of Domains
   D. Time
III. Interactions among Domains
   A. Depression and Disability
   B. Dementia and Disability
   C. Hierarchical Organization
   D. Biological and Psychological Links
   E. Context
   F. Incremental Impacts
   G. Integration
IV. Needed Developments
   A. Subjective versus Objective Dialectic
   B. Diagnosis and Quality of Life
   C. Difficulties with Global Assessments
   D. Adjustment of Scales
   E. Chronicity
   F. Evolution
   G. Interrelated Indicators
   H. Hierarchies
   I. Identification of Mechanisms
V. Prospect
  References

I. Centrality of the Quality of Life _____

Mental health professionals, in line with the mission of all disciplines serving the health of the elderly, are concerned with improving and protecting the quality of life of their clients. Such concerns carry the mental health professional into fields of expertise that may lie beyond the traditional scope of training and experience. Mental health in particular, and health in general are not the only determinants or indicators of quality of life. Other determinants arise from work, family, friends, leisure pursuits, finances, housing, and the like. Even the political climate and religious freedoms can influence the quality of a person's life. All these interact with the person's attitudes and values, instilled by upbringing and later experiences. The sources of quality of life can be summed up as emanating from the elder person (body, mind, and spirit), the world around (living and inanimate), and the person's experience in space and time (Katz & Gurland, 1990).

Yet no influence on quality of life is more powerful in old age than health. The prospect of repelling the threat to quality of life presented by ill-health, provides the central rationale for the role of the health professions. Mental health is no exception. There is a widely held belief that mental disorder has a more devastating impact on the quality of life of the victim than almost any other calamity could inflict. "Those whom God wishes to destroy, he first drives mad." (Bartlett, 1968, p. 86a).

Hopes and claims of success in the treatment of mental ill-health imply that treatment will prevent, ameliorate, or reverse mental ill-health's unfavorable impact on quality of life. Such expectations constitute the basis for well-meaning people to enter the mental health professions, for clients to come forward for treatment, and for society and legislation to support the mental health services.

In the past two decades, growing attention has been given to scientific study and documentation of the impact of physical ill-health on the quality of life of elders and their caregivers, and on the corresponding effectiveness of treatment. This direction of work has been given additional impetus by the challenges posed by the treatment of chronic, residual, and co-morbid illnesses, and the corresponding need to take account of the effects and side-effects of combined and extended treatments. This is of special interest to geriatrics. However, as yet little of this work has spilled over into mental ill-health. There is a vast literature on specific outcomes of mental illness and its treatment, but these are largely reductionist fragments of the picture of quality of life.

This chapter is one of the few to appear, in a text book of mental health, under an explicit *quality of life* title. It will cover concepts, definitions, and scope; domains and perspectives; and measurement techniques and empirical findings on quality of life in mental ill-health. The level of discourse will tread a fine line between the general and the particular. The main emphasis is on briefly outlining matters of general principle, but each principle will be illustrated by reference to particular problems of mental ill-health.

The issues raised here are more than of academic interest. Certain decisions in the field of mental health, of great consequence to the individual and society, are being made every day that are, or should be, based on estimates of quality of life in mental ill-health. These decisions are usually made without benefit of accurate or generally accepted information bearing upon a full and rounded view of quality of life.

A. Definition

To start with, there is no generally accepted meaning for the term quality of life in the context of mental ill-health, nor a salient consensual language. Therefore, in contrast to chapters on more conventional and established issues in mental health, this one cannot begin with a list of criteria for recognition of impairments in quality of life. Rather, a tentative definition and some clinical references must provide the framework for reviewing more precise fragments such as part measurement and isolated findings. As the chapter moves along, there will be a progressive integration of these fragments.

As an interim description, the term quality of life can be taken to refer to aspects of living which (1) can be evaluated: susceptible to description along such parameters as desirable, good, pleasurable and satisfying; or (2) are, in an immediate or an evolutionary sense, adaptive. The parameters are multiple, changing over time, and interactive. Their tone and substance may vary with context and perspective. Ideally (and perhaps only ideally), they can summate to form a single weighted and unitary value.

B. Relevant Mental Health Problems

A wide variety of mental conditions can critically impair the quality of life of the elderly. Depression and dementia are predominant, but also important are alcohol and drug abuse, anxiety (panic attacks, phobias, and chronic anxiety), obsessions, paranoid states, late effects of schizophrenia, personality disorder, and adjustment reactions.

There is an emphasis in this discussion on the accompaniments and consequences that are common to many mental and other types of diseases. The principles under consideration transcend disease categories. Nevertheless, it will be useful for purposes of illustration to refer to particular mental diseases: mainly depression, dementia, chronic schizophrenia, and panic attacks.

An extended range of mental health problems, not readily represented by diagnosable conditions, is also relevant to the quality of life of the elderly. Examples include maladaptive behaviors or distressing symptoms associated with health management (e.g., non-compliance with treatment, self-destructive health habits, side-effects of psychotropic medications, or mental symptoms due to non-psychotropic medications), and excessive stress (e.g., accumulated life events), or inadequacy of coping responses (e.g., learned helplessness and weakened social supports).

C. Contrast with the Diagnosis of Disease

One can draw from descriptive passages of the accompaniments of mental ill-health an empathic understanding of their potential impact on quality of life. That empathy would be much harder to derive from the diagnostic label alone, because of the fact, already mentioned, that there is no tight and invariant connection between a disease category and quality of life.

The same diagnostic (or disease) entity may have quite different implications for quality of life depending on the particulars of its presentation: severity, form, speed of onset, course, response to treatment, treatment side-effects, number of previous attacks, premorbid personality of the person affected, coexistence with other diseases, age of the person, family support, and so on. Within a given diagnostic category, these particulars may vary from one sufferer to another, or from one episode to another.

Conversely, the same profile of impaired qualities of life may proceed from quite different diagnostic entities. For example, loss of interests can be due to such diverse impairments as the apathy of depression or the intellectual erosion caused by dementia. Abandonment of usual activities can follow from the loss of interest that occurs in depression or dementia, or from many other sources. Among such sources are inhibition by the fears of phobic anxiety, panic attacks or paranoid states; the lack of initiative induced by the volitional deficit or thought disorganization found in the aging schizophrenic; or a sense of rejection imposed by others in response to the person's disturbing behaviors.

This tendency of different types and subtypes of diagnostic categories to impact the same cluster of impaired qualities of life, may offer a defining characteristic of what constitutes a psychiatric case. Thus, a broad spectrum of depressions, which are distinct subtypes according to a professional nomenclature (e.g. that of the American Psychiatric Association, DSM-III-R), all pervasively involve thoughts, attitudes and actions related to qualities of daily living (Gurland, Wilder, & Copeland, 1985). This pervasive impairment of quality of life could explain the behavior of the patient in seeking help from others and the motivation of others in giving help to the sufferer. From this vantage point, the definition of a case owes more to the non-specific impairment of quality of life than to specific criteria for recognition of a diagnostic category or subcategory.

II. Domains

The impact on quality of life of a variety of mental disorders can be parsimoniously explained by reference to a limited number of domains. These domains are final common pathways or outcomes leading from ill-health to impaired quality of life.

Some domains of particular relevance to mental ill-health are listed here. For clarity, illustrative examples are given below: these are taken, in this instance, from the area of depressive symptoms.

1. *Distress or psychic pain:* feelings of being depressed, unhappy, blue, sad, miserable, empty, tearful; or guilty, torn by doubts, tormented by scruples; or lonely; or self-depreciatory and low in self-esteem.
2. *Somatic discomforts:* lack of sleep, restlessness at night, early morning wakening, poor appetite, loss of weight, constipation, vague aches and pains, or a bad taste in the mouth.
3. *Incapacity or inefficiency in task performance:* basic functions (such as communication, continence, mobility, grooming and other aspects of self-care) or instrumental activities of daily living (such as maintenance of the household, shopping, cooking).

4. *Loss of self-control:* restraining one's own potentially disturbing or damaging behaviors.
5. *Perceived lack of incentives to live* on the part of the sufferer, to whom it seems as if there is no hope, the future is black, nothing is enjoyable, usual interests are pointless, sense of mastery is undermined, and energy cannot be summoned. Suicidal feelings and acts may indicate that the balance between valuation of life and desire to end pain has tipped unfavorably.
6. *Frustration of gratifications:* sexual, absence of appreciation and regard by others, failure of personal goals, interruption of leisure interests.
7. *Stress:* from a continuation of the stress that might have precipitated the mental condition or from added stress following the onset of illness.
8. *Indignities:* loss of privacy, independence and control.
9. *Side-effects:* problems superimposed by the nature of treatment.
10. *Pervasiveness of symptoms:* their presence is or seems endless, continuous, intruding on every thought and activity.
11. *Discontinuities in style of life:* loss of cherished traditions, insecurity and dreaded anticipation of the future, and regrets about lost opportunities.

Other domains might be added to this list in so far as they are consequences of mental ill-health rather than causes or coincidental situations. For examples, *reduced socio-economic circumstances:* loss of earning power, poverty, poor housing and other environmental deprivations, low social status, and diminished power; and *interpersonal deprivations:* isolation, unsatisfying social relationships, and interpersonal disharmony.

These domains are mostly characterized by their content, but some have a dynamic element (e.g., balance of positive and negative qualities; pervasiveness). They also span several perspectives: e.g., physical and mental, subjective and objective, and individual or societal. The domains and also the perspectives are interdependent and intersecting; they may interact with each other as causes or consequences. Thus, objective physical impairment can itself be a quality-of-life outcome, but is also an important cause of subjective distress.

There are a number of other ways of carving out and organizing the domains of quality of life; the classification presented above is mainly for the purpose of introducing appropriate language and fleshing out the scope. A classification geared to the impairments of dementia and expressed in terms of functioning has been detailed in a recent paper (Gurland and Katz, 1989).

The classification and selection of quality of life domains for studies of panic disorder has also been demonstrated (Markowitz *et al.*, 1989). These investigators chose as the indicators of quality of life, subjective feelings of poor physical and emotional health, increased likelihood of suicide attempts, impaired social and marital functioning, and financial dependency. They also included alcohol and drug abuse, increased use of psychoactive medications, and a raised frequency of attendance with complaints of emotional problems at health services and hospital emergency departments. Application of these indicators to their study enabled the investigators to point to a serious impairment of quality of life in persons with panic disorder, equal to or greater than that observed in major depression.

A. Perspectives

Katz (1987, p. 459) points out that quality of life "is a concept that is subject to multiple viewpoints." Others' views on the patient's quality of life are relevant because of the extent to which these will drive benign or harmful actions with respect to the patient. Differing values may be given to states of wellness or illness by the patient, family members, and various agents of society. Typically, a subjective sense of well-being has primacy for the individual. Often, the objective quality-of-life consequences of mental ill-health have primacy for society. Such relative values affect the success of a service program, since the individual must be motivated to cooperate, and society must usually be persuaded to foot part of the bill.

A psychiatric disorder has an effect on the functioning and quality of life not only of the one who has the disorder but also on others close to that person. Indeed, the family may suffer more than the patient in some cases. This is illustrated below by reference to dementia.

The great majority of patients with dementia are reported by families to have diminished initiative, disinterest in hobbies, and withdrawal, among other problems (Rabins, Mace, & Lucas, 1982). The withdrawal and isolation of the patient are particularly stressful to many caregivers (Deimling & Bass, 1984). Other problems of care emphasized by these families include the functional impairments of communication, eating, bathing, wandering (Rubin, Morris, Storandt, & Berg, in press; see Teri, Borson, Kayik, & Yamagishi, 1989) and incontinence.

The family may be forced to watch helplessly as the patient deteriorates and changes into someone whose personality they can barely recognize. At night, the patient's restless wandering may disturb the family's sleep. During the day the family caregivers may have to frequently clean up after the patient, answer the latter's endless and repetitive questions, tend to the patient's basic needs, and maintain constant vigilance and supervision to protect the patient. The family may receive in return little or no warmth and appreciation for these services. The patient's behavior may make it difficult to have visitors in the home. A family can become caught up in a dilemma: they need to answer to the call of their love and conscientious responsibility for the victim of mental ill-health, but at the same time must fulfill the competing demands of the ties and obligations that relate to other family, their job, and their accustomed style of life.

Corresponding scenarios could be constructed to portray the impacts of a mental ill-health on the functioning and quality of life of persons other than family: significant others, neighbors and friends, and health and social care workers. To stretch this point, even those distant and loosely linked to persons with mental ill-health may be affected: developers and urban planners, taxpayers and elected officials, regulators, and mentally ill people in general.

B. Subjective and Objective Perspectives

Some aspects of quality of life are subjective and knowable only from the complaints communicated by the one who suffers the psychiatric disorder; other domains can be observed with or without inferring the accompanying distress.

The extent of the damage to the fabric of life is only too clear in some cases. The older woman, who has previously successfully coped with several transitions in her life but is now depressed, may become unable to continue functioning as a wife, mother, grandmother, or homemaker. During the depths of her depression, she may refuse to see friends, give up her life-long intellectual, esthetic, and social interests, and restrict her activities to the minimum necessary for elementary survival. Outwardly and objectively, her life has become impoverished, while inwardly and subjectively it may be even worse.

A person with severe depression exemplifies a predominance of subjective distress. Unreasonable self-blame, shame, guilt, and remorse, unrelenting pessimism, restless insomnia, and continual torment may be viewed by the sufferer as more painful than death.

In contrast, some persons with a dementing illness may, from the objective viewpoint of children and other family, be stripped of everything previously valued in life, yet, as far as can be known, might not be inwardly distressed. There may be complete dependence on others for even the most private and basic actions. All personal interests may dissipate. Closeness to others may be attenuated by the person's inability to recognize even their own spouse or children, let alone friends. Awareness of self and identity might slip away. To outward appearances, a person might lose almost all the qualities of life once valued. Such impairments of functioning suggest an impoverishment of the quality of life of the mentally ill person whether or not the latter is sentient of the altered state.

Subjective and objective perspectives often converge. Afflicted persons may become distressed for reasons that are objectively evident, or the extent of inward distress may be so clearly expressed in speech and other behaviors that observers can accurately gauge the subjective state. However, the independence of the subjective and objective perspectives is apparent from the many occasions on which they can be discordant. The discordance may stem from the respective values given subjectivity and objectivity by the patient and others, or because there are different bodies of salient information. Subjective views are generally colored by a system of beliefs; objective approaches may acquire meaning from the accumulation of empirical experiences.

Third-party reports are not necessarily any more objective than the patient's own complaints. For this reason, researchers and clinicians may bypass the patient and informant, turning directly to laboratory (or consulting room) tests of functions within the quality-of-life scope. An example of a direct assessment of function is the Activities of Daily Living Situational Test (Skurla, Rogers, & Sunderland, 1988). This and similar performance tests correlate significantly but modestly with corresponding information from informants.

C. Measurements of Domains

There are a fair number of assessment instruments that bear upon psychopathology. To the extent that these instruments reflect quality of life, they attest to the feasibility of quantitative and reliable measurement in this area. However, instruments are often constructed to concentrate on diagnosis of mental disorder (i.e., a disease condition), and the quality of life of the person may be less well represented. Even severity ratings may not tap into the consequences of a condition in terms of quality of life.

Two illustrations (drawn from scales of depression and of cognitive impairment) can be offered to typify the ambiguities about quality of life, encountered in measures of psycho-pathology.

Measures of depression can be brief and reliable. Those couched in terms of altered mood (e.g., sadness, pessimism, self-depreciation) tend to be more directly expressive of impaired quality of life. Somatic symptoms (e.g., slowed movements, sluggish thinking, loss of weight) are often phrased to be useful as criteria for diagnostic subtypes. Complaints of sleep disturbance and loss of appetite may contribute to either quality or diagnostic assessments, depending on how the symptom characteristics are expanded and detailed.

The scales of depression demonstrate the range of styles that can be encompassed in quality-of-life measures. Some are self-rating forms (e.g., Zung, 1965; Yesavage, Brink, Terrence, & Adey, 1983) which can be filled out by any literate persons to reflect their own feelings; almost all can also be administered and completed by a rater with a modicum of training in the technique. Some are primarily rater administered; and a few require professional skills of a fairly high order (e.g., Hamilton, 1969). Inferences about the presence of depression may be attempted from observation of the patient by the rater or by nursing staff (Alexopoulos, 1988), and even from biomedical tests such as the dex-amethasone suppression test (Carrol, 1982).

Where an indicator of impaired quality of life is scaled, it can be analyzed as a continuous variable, or scores above a threshold value can be taken as forming a category of impaired quality of life. For instance, latent class analysis (Lazarsfeld & Henry, 1968; Golden, 1982) can be applied to produce a threshold score for a statistically abnormal category.

Correspondingly, the strength of the association between cognitive dysfunction and impaired quality of life will vary with the type of cognitive test employed. Different kinds of tests of cognitive dysfunction provide information that varies in its relevance to quality of life. Tests of cognitive dysfunction may emphasize:

1. a profile of mental deficits: e.g., in recognition, learning, and recall; attention, reasoning, calculating, coding and decoding language, and mental imaging;
2. indicators (symptoms and signs) of disorders affecting the brain; and
3. identification of impediments to adaptive tasks: e.g., orienting to time, place, and person; drawing upon recent and remote memory, using tools and objects, communicating, following instructions, problem solving, and comprehending. It is this third category that serves best the purposes of quality of life assessment.

Many of the measures of cognitive dysfunction are brief enough to be given in a primary care setting, embedded in a multidisciplinary assessment or used in epi-demiological research (e.g., Kahn et al., 1960; Katzman et al., 1983; Folstein, Folstein, & McHugh, 1975). Their reliability is generally high (Pfeffer et al., 1982); Vitaliano et al., 1984). However, salience to quality of life is most evident in those measures that assess the third category mentioned above; and especially in the measures that explore the consequences of cognitive dysfunction on functional tasks: the person's capacity to carry out their usual functions of work, chores, leisure activities, role responsibilities, and basic self-care; maintenance of interpersonal relationships and standards of decent behavior; avoidance of unnecessary danger, and control of behaviors that are unduly threatening or disturbing to others.

D. Time

The time dimension has a powerful effect in modifying the impact of mental health on quality of life. The expectation that an undesirable mental state will be time-limited makes all the difference to the impact on quality of life. Depressed patients may successfully act out suicidal impulses because they see no hope of recovery from black despair. The treatment team may see this as a tragic misunderstanding on the part of the patients and a failure on their part to convince the patients that such episodes respond to treatment.

A striking example of the intimate interlacing of time and quality of life is found in chronic conditions; schizophrenia or late onset paranoid disorders provide the illustration.

The onset of the frank symptoms of schizophrenia often occurs in the mid-twenties but the full story unfolds over a lifetime. Frequently an unusual personality can be traced back to high school days. The patient may never form a steady relationship and may keep dropping out of jobs. Still, it may come as a surprise when the patient eventually develops a florid episode. Hospitalization may follow and treatment with major tranquilizers to control hallucinations and delusions. After a few months, the patient may be released on medications. There may or may not again be an acute and dramatic episode of this nature, but many years may be spent in half-way homes, working in sheltered workshops and under constant medication. After a lengthy period of treatment the patient may develop a marked tremor of the hands, requiring discontinuation of medications. Perhaps by mid-life the patient may finally seem to settle down, find a routine, manageable job, and live in a boarding house. In old age there may be some remaining limitations and eccentricity.

When a mental disorder becomes chronic, it tends to profoundly alter the person's life–style. This stands in contrast to an acute condition, where the symptoms, dysfunction, and treatment are appropriately short term and for this reason need not involve substantial intrusion into the organization of the patient's life. The circumstances of a chronic condition inevitably change the nature of the patient's life. Life activities cannot be suspended and then resumed intact as in an acute condition, but must go forward with adjustments for the ongoing chronic processes: this involves compromises in jobs, career plans, interpersonal relations, and living arrangements, and sometimes acceptance of life dissatisfactions and symptom intensity for the foreseeable future. Ongoing treatment must become a fact of life, life must accommodate treatment as opposed to treatment's accommodating life.

The defining characteristic of chronicity in respect to mental disorder in old age is thus a blurring of the distinctions between quality of life, quality of care, and course of the disorder (Gurland & Toner, 1991). Chronicity arises where the course of the disorder or the treatment, over time, begins to displace, shape, or intrude upon the conduct or perceptions of the person's life:

1. The patient's quality of life is presently, retrospectively, and in prospect substantially determined by the course of the disorder; the history of the patient's quality of life may be characterized by the history of the mental condition;
2. Health care decisions are based on the expectation that active treatment will be needed for the foreseeable future and that some level of functional impairment will persist;
3. The patient has to spend considerable time each year and probably each day, in seeking or receiving health care;
4. The patient must make major changes in lifestyle, such as residential location, on the basis of the impaired functioning and/or the need to accommodate treatment; and
5. The family or other caregiver find their lives and plans altered by the course of the disorder.

Nevertheless, mapping fluctuations in the quality of life of persons with mental illness over time *to* old age does not necessarily provide information on the course of quality of life *in* old age. For that we need to track cases over the full lifespan: through old age to death. It is entirely possible that even illnesses with a long-standing course may subside in old age (as in the hypothetical case of schizophrenia described); if so, this may be a valuable salvation of a life previously blighted by chronic illness. Conversely, treatments that are successful at improving the quality of life during the adulthood of patients should not be finally judged until their impact and consequences have been evaluated during the later states of life; the latter should weigh in the balance as heavily as the results earlier in life.

The person's self-evaluation at a particular time may be shaped by considerations of their prior and anticipated life. Awareness of deficits incurred may be sharpened by memory of past enjoyable skills. Anxieties may revolve around the future progression of dysfunction including the implications for institutional admission, loss of supporting figures, impoverishment, premature death or long years of suffering.

III. Interactions among Domains

Dimensions of impaired function and quality of life interact with each other and summate. They are interconnected. As more of these connections are taken into account, a more complete and authentic picture of quality of life emerges. Because of their importance, the connections are touched upon in this section; however, only a limited number of connections are attempted.

A. Depression and Disability

Depression, as a disturbance of the function of mood (one domain of quality of life), is significantly increased in a wide range of impairments of physical function (another quality-of-life domain) (Blazer *et al*, 1982; Borson *et al.,* 1986). Disability is more likely to be associated with depression in old age than even such supposedly traumatic events as widowhood, isolation, retirement, financial hardship, unsatisfactory environment, and intellectual deterioration (Gurland, Wilder, & Berkman, 1988). The importance of physical functioning as a determinant of depression (as quality of life) in the elderly, may be universal. It has been found to prevail among elderly community subjects in several contrasting cultural and national groups (Wilder and Gurland, 1989).

The mechanisms that link the two domains of quality of life appear to include the neurotransmitter abnormalities that characterize major depression. The basis for this statement is that rates of major depression are probably substantially raised in elderly persons who have physical function impairment or chronic physical illnesses (Turner & Noh, 1988; Craig & Van Natta, 1983).

Impaired functional performance is also a direct psychological threat to quality of life. This provocation is evident from a microanalysis of a given task of daily living. For example, a subject who cannot dress herself without assistance may react to the undermining of pride in independence, to a sense of humiliation at failing to match expected standards of behavior, to the discomfort and strain of struggling to complete the task, to the attitudes of those assisting her, and to guilt about being a burden on others. There may also be anxiety and frustration from the loss of predictability and control over goal-directed behaviors that require dressing among the sequence of preparatory steps. Other potentially stressful costs and sacrifices are entailed in the obtaining of treatment, personal assistance, mechanical aids, and home restructuring, whether through outright purchase or receipt of favors. There are lost opportunities for economic gain through employment. All those qualities of life are at risk by virtue of the impairment of a single functional task. Yet in most instances, several functional impairments coexist, magnifying the effects on quality of life.

B. Dementia and Disability

With adequate care, persons with dementia will live for long periods, usually several years at least, while undergoing progressive encroachments into the quality of their lives.

Pathological processes can be closely tied to impairment of quality of life in dementia. Cognitive impairment may be highly correlated with structural changes in the brain. Associations (of the order of .53 to .83) have been noted with the characteristic neuropathology of Alzheimer's disease (Blessed *et al.,* 1968; Katzman, 1983), with the computerized tomography (CT) scan picture (ventricular dilatation and sulcal enlargement), and positron emission tomography (PET) scan changes (slow glucose utilization in the caudate, thalamic, and temporal regions) (De Leon *et al., 1980;* Ferris *et al.,* 1980). Nevertheless, the amount of unexplained variance leaves room for the possibility that personal, environmental, co-morbid, and psychosocial factors also influence the dementing patient's level of cognitive performance.

Similarly, levels of cognitive and functional impairment often do not coincide. Correlations are sometimes found to be high (around or above .70) (e.g., Knopman, Kitto, Deinard, & Heiring, 1988) but usually in the low to moderate range (e.g., Skurla, Rogers, & Sunderland, 1988; Weintraub, Baratz, & Marsel-Mesulam, 1982; Teri et al., 1989). Some reports of high intercorrelations between function and cognition are confounded by the inclusion of functional items in the cognitive tests (e.g., the Blessed Dementia Rating Scale) or items on cognition in the measure of function (e.g., the Clinical Dementia Rating). In clinical experience, certain patients may be capable of unexpectedly high functioning despite poor cognitive performance. Function helps to distinguish healthy from dementing persons among those with borderline scores of cognitive impairment (Pfeffer et al., 1982; Loewenstein et al., 1989).

Where functioning and quality of life in dementia are at issue, direct examination of these features is necessary; they cannot be completely inferred from diagnosis, neuropathology, or cognitive status.

C. Hierarchical Organization

The execution of adaptive tasks, essential to quality of life, can be viewed as the integration of component skills, each of which can be arranged in a hierarchy reflecting an increasing potential for adaptation. The successive level of adaptability requires that the lower-order skills be intact. The order of arrangement of the hierarchy of adaptation may replicate the sequence of development in childhood.

Certain aspects of functional disability fit a hierarchical organization quite well. This is exemplified in the studies by Katz and his colleagues on activities of daily living. The discovery of a hierarchy makes the staging and progress of impairment readily evident. Deterioration of functional skills may occur in reverse order to the hierarchy and to the developmental sequence (Constantinidis & Richard, 1978).

D. Biological and Psychological Links

In the discussion on interactions, several references were made to the mechanisms of the pathways between domains. The models suggested are eclectic. However, at the simplified level of connections reviewed, there is a dearth of solid evidence on the processes that affect quality of life.

E. Context

The context may alter the impact of psychiatric disorder on quality of life. Mental ill-health in the elderly usually occurs with co-morbidity. Beyond other mental and physical disorders, there may be concurrent states that modulate the consequences of mental ill-health. Accompanying anxiety and resentments may aggravate the impairments of quality of life (Viney and Westbrook, 1976); also, feelings of helplessness and hopelessness (Janis & Rodin, 1979), or an avalanche of life events and strains (Paykel, 1978; Pearlin, Lieberman, Menaghan, & Mullan, 1981). Conversely, quality may be sustained by a resilient personality (Billings & Moos, 1982), or the warmth and tenacity of the encouragement and assistance received from supporting family and the health care system, (Brown, Bhrolchain, & Harris, 1975). A rich variety of coping strategies may emerge to repulse assaults upon quality of life (Folkman & Lazarus, 1980).

These contextual influences also obtrude into the level of functioning (or, more generally, adaptation) that appears on assessment. Assessment may focus on actual performance or the potential for performance under challenge or assisted conditions (can do versus could do); the benchmark may be a demographically matched general population or the previous performance of that individual; severity may be parceled out to the assumed causes (e.g., due to dementia, physical causes, or customary life style); only completion of a task may be rated or the level of difficulty experienced in the process; use of assistive devices may be overlooked or regarded as evidence of partial failure; personal assistance may be counted only if used, or even if needed but not available; informal and professional assistance may be equally or differentially weighted; the surroundings might or might not be altered to make the accomplishment of tasks easier; and credit might or might not be given for partial achievement in a task.

F. Incremental Impacts

Even persons without health impairments have problems with the quality of their lives; what matters is the extent to which a given mental ill-health condition *incrementally* impairs quality of life. This is well shown in the oldest age strata where subjective complaints of memory impairment and physical impairments of function are common even in those who are mentally healthy. For example, only certain complaints of memory impairment are increased by dementia; where the complaints are pinned down to an effect of memory on the performance of daily tasks, then dementia *adds* considerably to an impaired quality of life (Gurland and Katz, 1989).

Cultural context also will alter the relationship between mental disorder and incremental impairments of quality of life. In a primary care setting, elderly Hispanics with dementia were found to report difficulties at a higher frequency than do whites for the tasks of finding words and finding the way in the neighborhood, but with a lower frequency for remembering the names of family and for managing business. However, when the nondementias were examined, more or less the same contrasts were noted between Hispanics and whites (Gurland and Katz, 1989).

G. Integration

The most challenging hypothesis in this field is that quality of life is a unitary concept. This would imply that the impact of mental ill-health could be expressed by a single quantitative statement. If so, the formula has not yet been discovered. Yet, intuition, clinical experience, and the momentum of research findings all point to an integrative concept of quality of life. A holistic concept of quality of life is syntonic with the major principles of mental health services for the elderly: multidisciplinary, interrelated, coordinated, extended, sensitive to social context, and client oriented.

Global ratings are one way of approximating an integrated measure of quality of life. In recognition of the limitations of diagnostic labels, the Diagnostic and Statistical Manual of the American Psychiatric Association incorporated (in 1980) a multiaxial system of classification. This enabled, among other advantages, the documentation of the patient's level of functioning (on axis V), as might be "useful for planning treatment and predicting outcome." It is an overall judgment covering psychological, social, and occupational functioning, on a nine-point scale; for current level (to indicate the present need for treatment) and for the highest sustained level during the previous year (to suggest the potential for recovery from the current episode). As an example of the content involved, highest functioning is indicated by evidence of interest and participation in a wide range of activities, occupational competence, meaningful family and other interpersonal relationships, social effectiveness, satisfaction with life, ability to communicate adequately, appropriate personal hygiene, no danger of injury to self and others, and no unusual problems, concerns, and symptoms.

The content of axis V is squarely within the territory of quality of life; the method of rating is global, as opposed to a profile of domains. The manual states that "Ratings of current functioning will generally reflect the current need for treatment or care (p. 20)." The nine-point scale, which is the basis for the rating, was originally developed for research purposes (the Global Assessment Scale) and tested under those conditions, then adopted for the nomenclature. (Endicott *et al.*, 1976).

IV. Needed Developments

The knowledge base on quality of life and mental ill-health is growing, but in an uneven manner. Some potentially productive directions for study and application are outlined here.

A. Subjective versus Objective Dialectic

There is need for a dialectic between subjective and objective vantage points on quality of life. One opportunity for this dialectic occurs in efforts to resolve differences of opinion about the usefulness of a service: between patients, service providers, and policy makers. The exhibition of objectively acquired data on quality-of-life outcomes in mental ill-health can reveal whether disagreements arise from lack of consensual information, or from discrepant values and priorities. Perhaps the objective indicators of outcomes meet with skeptical dismissal by some evaluators because they are regarded as too limited or tangential in scope; this can lead to the search for more sensitive and salient objective indicators. Alternatively, varying perspectives on outcomes, for instance by family members or policy makers, might be made concordant merely by sharing relevant information in which all have confidence. The extension of this iterative process can be seen to have the potential to improve both objective and subjective approaches.

B. Diagnosis and Quality of Life

The boundaries of diagnosis should be reconsidered in the light of quality of life accompaniments of mental disorders. The concepts of quality of life and of diagnosis can sometimes be usefully brought into closer apposition.

A case in point emerges from the conflicting reports on rates of dementia in the community-residing elderly population. A recent study (Evans et al., 1990) claimed that prevalence rates of dementia are twice as high as previously reported. To add to the confusion, widely differing screen positive rates for probable dementia were obtained in a study that applied five conventional scales to the same population of elderly (Gurland, Wilder, Cross, Teresi, & Barrett, in press). The most parsimonious explanation for differences in reported rates and diagnostic judgments about dementia is that different concepts are at play: a narrow (more stringent) and a broader (more inclusive) group.

Narrow and broad concepts of dementia were defined and examined in a large study of the general elderly community population (Gurland & Katz, 1989). The nonoverlapping group were called marginal dementias. With regard to such quality-of-life indicators as the ability to access one's memory store, subjective complaints of memory, depressive symptoms, and performance in the everyday tasks of living, the narrow-concept dementia group was substantially worse off than the marginals. There was no consistent distinction between the marginal dementias and the poorly performing normals.

Interpretation of the variously reported prevalence rates of dementia should make explicit the breadth of the concept of dementia chosen, and what implications it carries for quality of life. For most patients, and for their caregivers, the meaning of dementia, like any other disease, lies in its impact on quality of life. Similarly, projections of prevalence rates of dementia for the purposes of planning services and the prevention of human misery, have everything to do with quality of life. Moreover, the characterization of aging itself is closely tied to the expected rates of deterioration and the lifetime risk of developing dementia by a certain age. The devaluation of old age is a statement of the assumed decline in quality of life.

The choice between concepts of dementia obtrudes also into the act of making a diagnosis of dementia in the individual case. The meaning of the diagnosis for that patient and the family caregivers will reside in the relationship between the concept and quality of life.

C. Difficulties with Global Assessments

There are a number of unresolved dilemmas embedded in the current method of making global assessments of the impact of mental disorder on quality of life. There is no prescribed way of weighting, uniting, or comparing different but equally valid perspectives (e.g., of patient, provider, third-party insurers). Specific points or periods are generally taken into account (e.g., the present time or the past year) but not the longer and continuous evolution of past, present, and future time. Usually, there is little or no help offered in pinning down reported or observed impairments of quality of life (which are often overdetermined in the elderly) to mental health causes.

The norms against which to judge departures from quality-of-life standards are hardly ever stated; much less is the cultural relativity of these norms acknowledged. For example, a wide range of activities may be defined as desirable but the optimal breadth and depth is not specified. There is insufficient reference in mental measurement to the quality-of-life functions that are relevant to the elderly person (e.g., activities of daily living, independence, community tenure, continuity of life style). Above all, there is a glossing over of the need for a method of integrating (connecting, aggregating, forming a whole out of) all this information in order to rate a global score encompassing the whole person. For related reasons, severity categories in global scale may appear arbitrary.

D. Adjustment of Scales

Although numerous mental measures have been applied to the elderly, only a few have been developed especially with the elderly in mind. For example, where scales of depression have been developed on the elderly, empirical data on the elderly have shaped the content of the technique so that it reflects the way the elderly express symptoms of depression (Yesavage et al., 1983; Golden, Teresi, & Gurland, 1984; Gurland, 1989). Nevertheless, a concerted effort to bend these scales to the purposes of quality of life has not yet been attempted.

E. Chronicity

Measures of chronicity should be more sensitive to its bearing on quality of life. A drawback of widely used measures of chronicity is that they deal with chronicity as an administrative or demographic category rather than as a continuum (i.e., matter of degree). It is difficult to accept that those definitions that depend on a particular duration of illness or a specific number of hospitalizations or receipt of disability insurance are validly reflecting the intensity and extensiveness of chronicity. Nor can such categories as community tenure, employment, and marriage be adequate indicators of good quality of life: there is substantial variance of the quality of life within these categories. Institutional settings may vary widely in the degree to which they restrict or enhance the patient's life. Patients located in the community may or may not be considerably restricted or impaired by the treatment regimen they must follow.

F. Evolution

Reported outcomes of mental health problems often emphasize end points rather than interval status; where the patient ended up at a particular point in time, not the long period of time that it took to get there. Yet, it is the slow and continuous evolution of the patient's history that contains the best information on the quality of that life. Measurements of chronicity requires frequent follow-up evaluations and appropriate methods to portray the continuous consequences of the disorder.

G. Interrelated Indicators

The measurement of interrelated quality of life conditions (e.g., depression and disability) is complicated by their concurrence. The problem is that the indicators for the two qualities overlap. For example, fatigue occurs in both disability and depression. Indicators may be incorrectly assigned to a single condition when both coexist. Conversely, a depressed person who feels helpless may complain of a disability when insufficient objective physical reason for the impairment exists. The depression in this instance involves the subjective rather than objective aspect of disability.

H. Hierarchies

The existence, organization and applications of hierarchies in sectors of mental ill-health other than the dementias have not yet been established.

I. Identification of Mechanisms

The mechanisms by which function is affected should be elucidated in a way that facilitates management plans for caregiving, and improvements in quality of life of the patient and caregiver. For example, the cognitive deficits leading to impaired functioning may involve immediate memory, sequencing, judgment, volition, visuospatial ability, initiation and perseveration (Skurla et al., 1988; Teri et al., 1989). Identification of the mechanisms implicated in a patient's poor functioning could lead to an appropriate intervention.

Some investigators (viz., Reisberg, Ferris, & Fransson, 1985) have attempted to clinically exploit the observation that functional deterioration proceeds in a regular and orderly manner in dementia (of the Alzheimer's type). Any substantial variation from the typical progression is taken as a signal to look for some other disease process or complication. Others have focused on the patient's position in the hierarchy of functional performance in order to plan rehabilitation aimed at helping patients toward independence a step at a time, or to concentrate preventive efforts on the next step of deterioration predicted by the hierarchy (Asberg & Sonn, 1989).

V. Prospect ─────────────────────────────────

This chapter has spelled out some of the language that allows discussion and study of quality of life in relation to mental ill-health. The structure and processes of quality of life have been broached, as well as issues in measurement and applications. However, only a rough and tentative summary definition of quality of life has been attempted and the only mention of a global rating of mental ill-health was largely critical in tone.

For the present, quality of life in mental ill-health remains a dawning presence, dimly perceived. That does not diminish its growing importance. Quality-of-life issues should be a main reference point in consideration of planning of policy, service programs, clinical management and research aimed at care and relief of persons with mental ill-health, and support of their caregivers.

As impairments in quality of life imposed by mental-ill health become better understood, it will become possible to move on to considerations of positive mental health, enhanced well-being and enriched quality of life.

Acknowledgment

This work was supported by the Morris W. Stroud, III, Program on Scientific Approaches to Quality of Life in Health and Aging, of Columbia University Center for Geriatrics and Gerontology.

References

Alexopoulos, G. S., Abrams, R. C., Young, R. C., & Shamoian, C. A. (1988). Cornell scale for depression in dementia. *Biological Psychiatry, 23,* 271–284.

Asberg, K. H., & Sonn, U. (1988). The cumulative structure of personal and instrumental ADL. A study of elderly people in a health service district. *Scandinavian Journal of Rehabilitation Medicine.*

Bartlett, J. (1968). *Familiar Quotations,* fourteen Edition. (p. 86a). toronto: Little Brown and Co.

Billings, A. G., & Moos, R. H. (1982). Psychosocial theory and research on depression: An integrative framework and review. *Clinical Psychological Review, 2,* 213–237.

Blazer, D. (1982). Social support and mortality in an elderly community population. *American Journal of Epidemiology, 115,* 684–694.

Blessed, G., Tomlinson, B. E., & Roth, M. (1968). The association between qualitative measure of dementia and senile change with cerebral matter of elderly subjects. *British Journal of Psychiatry, 114,* 792–811.

Borson, S., Barnes, R. A., Kukull, W. A., Okimoto, J. T., Veith, R. C., Inui, T. S., Carter, W., & Raskind, M. A. (1986). Symptomatic depression in elderly medical outpatients I. Prevalence, demography and health service utilization. *Journal of the American Geriatric Society, 34,* 341–347.

Brown, G. W., Bhrolchain, M., & Harris, T. (1975). Social class and psychiatric disturbance among women in an urban population. *Sociology, 9,* 225–254.

Calman, K. (1987). Definition and dimensions of quality of life. In N. K. Aaronson & J. Beckman (Eds.), *The quality of life of cancer patients,* (p. 1–9). New York: Raven Press.

Carroll, B. J. (1982). The dexamethasone suppression test for melancholia. *British Journal of Psychiatry, 140,* 292–304.

Constantinidis, J., & Richard, J. (1978). Dementia with senile plaques and neurofibrillary changes. In A. D. Isaacs & F. Post (Eds.), *Studies in geriatric psychiatry.* New York: Wiley & Sons.

Craig, T. J., and Van Natta, P. A. (1983). Disability and depressive symptoms in two communities. *American Journal of Psychiatry, 140,* 598–601.

Deimling, G. T., and Bass, D. M. (1984). Mental status among the aged: Effect of spouse and adult-child caregivers. Presented at the Gerontological Society, San Antonio, Texas.

De Leon, M. J., Ferris, S. H., George, A. E., Reisberg, B., Kricheff, I. I., & Gershon, S. (1980). Computed tomography evaluations of brain–behavior relationships in senile dementia of the Alzheimer's type. *Neurobiology of Aging, 1,* 69–79.

Endicott, J., Spitzer, R. L., Fleiss, J., *et al.* (1976). The Global Assessment Scale: A procedure for measuring overall severity of psychiatric disturbance. *Archives of General Psychiatry, 33,* 766–771.

Evans, D. A., Funkenstein, H., Albert, M. S., Scherr, P. A., Cook, N. R., Chown, M. J., Hebert, L. E., Hennekens, C. H., & Taylor, J. O. (1989). Prevalence of Alzheimer's disease in a community population of older persons: higher than previously reported. *Journal of American Medical Association, 262(18)*, 2551–2556.

Ferris, S. H., de Leon, M. J., Wolf, A. P., *et al.*, (1980). Positron emission tomography in the study of aging and senile dementia. *Neurobiology of Aging, 1*, 127–131.

Folkman, S., & Lazarus, R. S.(1980). An analysis of coping in a middle-aged community sample. *Journal of Health and Social Behavior, 21*, 219–239.

Folstein, M. F., Folstein, S. E., & McHugh, P. R. (1975). "Mini-Mental State": a practical method for grading the cognitive state patients for the clinician. *Journal of Psychiatric Research, 12*, 189–198.

Golden, R. R. (1982). A taxometric model for the detection of a conjectured latent taxometric. *Multivariate Behavioral Research, 17*, 389–416.

Golden, R. R., Teresi, J. A., & Gurland, B. J. (1984). Development of indicator scales for the comprehensive assessment and referral evaluation (CARE) interview schedule. *Journal of Gerontology, 39*, 138–146.

Gurland, B. J. (1989). Mental health assessment: assessing mental health in the elderly. *Danish Medical Bulletin on Multidisciplinary Health Assessment of the Elderly.* Kellog Foundation, Special Supplement Series, *7*, 33–37.

Gurland, B. J., Wilder, D. E., Cross, P., Teresi, J., & Barrett, V. W. *Screening scales for dementia: reconciliation of conflicting cross-cultural findings.* Submitted to the International Journal of Geriatric Psychiatry.

Gurland, B., & Katz, S. (1990, October). Methods and uses of assessing function in Alzheimer's disease and related dementias. *Proceedings of the National Scientific Conference on the Care of Alzheimer's Disease Patients and Families,* Baltimore, Maryland.

Gurland, B., & Katz, S. *Quality of life in dementia: outline of a paper.* Presented at the New York State Office of Mental Health Research Conference, December 6th, 1989 in Albany, New York.

Gurland, B., & Toner, J. (1991). The chronically mentally ill elderly: Epidemiological perspectives on the nature of the population. In E. Light and B. Lebowitz (Eds.). *Chronically Mentally Ill Elderly: Directions for Research.* New York: Springer Publishing, 3–15.

Gurland, B. J., & Wilder, D. E. (1984). The CARE interview revisited: Development of an efficient, systematic, clinical assessment. *Journal of Gerontology, 39*, 129–137.

Gurland, B. J., Wilder, D. E., & Berkman, C. (1988). Depression and disability in the elderly: Reciprocal relations and changes with age. *International Journal of Geriatric Psychiatry, 3*, 163–179.

Gurland, B. J., Wilder, D. E., & Copeland, J. (1985). Concepts of depression in the elderly: Signposts to future mental health needs. In C. M. Gaitz & T. Samorajski (Eds.). *Aging 2000: Our Health Care Destiny, Vol I: Biomedical Issues.* (pp. 443–451). New York: Springer-Verlag.

Hamilton, M. (1969). Standardized assessment and recording of depressive symptoms. *Psychiatry, Neurology and Neurochir. 72(2)*, 201–205.

Janis, I. L., & Rodin, J. (1979). Attribution, control and decision making: social psychology and health. In G. C. Styone & N. E. Alder (Eds.). *A Handbook in Health Psychology.* San Francisco: Jossey-Bass.

Kahn, R. L., Goldfarb, A. I., Pollock, M., & Peck, A. (1960). Brief objective measures for the determination of mental status in the aged. *American Journal of Psychiatry, 117*, 326–328.

Katz, S. (1987). The science of the quality of life. *Journal Chronic Disorders, 40*, 459–463.

Katz, S., & Gurland, B. J. (in press). Science of quality of life of elders: challenges and opportunity. Chapter in *The Concept and Measurement of Quality of Life.* San Diego: Academic Press.

Katzman, R., Brown, T., Fuld, P., Peck, A., Schecter, R., Schimmel, H. (1983). Validation of a short orientation-memory-concentration test of cognitive impairment. *American Journal of Psychiatry, 140*, 734–739.

Knopman, D. S., Kitto, J., Deinard, S., & Heiring, J. (1988). Longitudinal study of death and institutionalization in patients with primary degenerative dementia. *Journal of the American Geriatric Society, 36*, 108–112.

Lazarsfeld, P., & Henry, N. (Eds.). (1968). *Latent structure analysis.* Boston: Houghton-Mifflin.

Loewenstein, D. A., Amigo, E., Duara, R., Guterman, A., Hurwitz, D., Berkowitz, N., Wilkie, F., Weinberg, G., Black, B., Gittleman, B., & Eisdorfer, C. (1989). A new scale for assessment of functional status in Alzheimer's Disease and Related Disorders. *Journal of Gerontology: Psychological Sciences, 44(4)*, 114–121.

Markowitz, J. S., Weissman, M. M., Ouellette, R., Lish, J. D., & Klerman, G. L. (1989). Quality of life in panic disorder. *Archives of General Psychiatry, 46*, 984–992.

Paykel, E. S. (1978). Contribution of life events to causation of psychiatric illness. *Psychological Medicine, 8,* 245–253.

Pearlin, L. I., Lieberman, M. A., Menaghan, E. G., & Mullan, J. T. (1981). The stress process. *Journal of Health and Social Behavior, 22,* 337–356.

Pfeffer, R. I., Kurosaki, T. T., Harrah, C. H., Chance, J. M., and Filos, S. (1982). Measurement of functional activities in older adults in the community. *Journal of Gerontology, 37(3),* 323–329.

Rabins, O. V., Mace, N. L., & Lucas, M. J. (1982). The impact of dementia on the family. *Journal of American Medical Association, 248,* 333–335.

Reisberg, B., Ferris, S. H., & Franssen, E. (1985). An ordinal functional assessment tool for Alzheimer's-type dementia. *Hospital and Community Psychiatry, 36(6),* 593–595.

Rubin, E. H., Morris, J. C., Storandt, M., & Berg, L. (in press). Behavioral changes in patients with mild senile dementia of the Alzheimer's type. *Psychiatric Research.*

Skurla, E., Rogers, J. C., & Sunderland, T. (1988). Direct assessment of activities of daily living in Alzheimer's Disease: A controlled study. *Journal of the American Geriatric Society, 36,* 97–103.

Teri, L., Borson, S., Kiyak, A., & Yamagishi, M. (1989). Behavioral disturbance, cognitive dysfunction, and functional skill. *Journal of the American Geriatric Society, 37,* 109–116.

Turner, R. J., & Noh, S. (1988). Physical disability and depression. *Journal of Health and Social Behavior, 29,* 23–37.

Viney, L. L., & Westbrook, M. T. (1976). Cognitive anxiety: A method of content analysis for verbal samples. *Journal of Personality Assessment, 40,* 140.

Vitaliano, P. P., Breen, A. R., Albert, M. S., Russo, J., & Prinz, P. N. (1984). Memory, attention and functional status in community residing Alzheimer's type dementia patients and optimally healthy aged individuals. *Journal of Gerontology, 39,* 58–54.

Weintraub, S., Baratz, R., & Marsel-Mesulam, M. (1982). Daily living activities in the assessment of dementia. In Corkin (Ed.). Alzheimer's Disease: A Report of Progress in Research. *Aging,* vol. 19, 189.

Wilder, D. E., & Gurland, B. J. (1989). Cross-cultural comparisons of disability and depression among older persons in four community-based probability samples. In L. Adler (Ed.). *Cross-cultural research in human development: focus on life span.* New York: Praeger-Greenwood, 223–233.

Yesavage, J. A., Brink, T. L., Terrence, L. R., and Adey, M. (1983). The Geriatric Depression Rating Scale: comparison with other self-report and psychiatric rating scales. In T. Crook, S. Ferris &R. Bartus (Eds.). *Assessment in geriatric psychopharmacology.* New Canaan, CT: Mark Powley Associates, 153–168.

Zung, W. W. K. (1965). A self-rating depression scale. *Archives of General Psychiatry, 12,* 63–70.

Behavioral Sciences
and Aging

Aging and the Senses

Frank Schieber

I. Vision
 A. Age-Related Structural Changes in the Visual System
 B. Psychophysical Studies of Visual Aging
 C. Spatial Resolution
 D. Temporal Resolution
 E. Color Sensitivity
 F. Common Age-Related Visual Pathologies
II. Hearing
 A. Structural Changes in the Auditory System
 B. Age-Related Changes in Auditory Functioning
III. Taste
 A. Age-Related Structural Changes in the Taste System
 B. Absolute Taste Sensitivity
 C. Suprathreshold Taste Perception
 D. Flavor Recognition
IV. Olfaction
 A. Age-Related Changes in the Olfactory System
 B. Absolute Olfactory Sensitivity
 C. Suprathreshold Odor Perception
 D. Compensating for Chemosensory Losses
V. Cutaneous Sensitivity
 A. Age-Related Changes in Cutaneous Sensory Structures
 B. Absolute Touch Sensitivity
 C. Vibrotactile Sensitivity
 D. Haptic Recognition
 E. Temperature Sensitivity
 F. Pain Sensitivity
VI. Future Considerations
 References

The purpose of this chapter is to describe the sensory and perceptual capacities of the aging adult and to relate these changes to one's ability to cope with the demands of the environment. Since little information is available that specifically links sensory capacity to mental health, the data presented in this chapter will focus upon normative aging. Thus, a foundation will be provided for comparing persons with mental health problems to normal aging individuals. As a consequence of this approach, topics such as sensory illusions and hallucinations will not be discussed. Similarly, the relationship between sensory–perceptual processes and specific mental disorders such as depression and Alzheimer's disease is beyond the scope of this report.

I. Vision

A. Age-Related Structural Changes in the Visual System

The clear anterior surface of the eye through which light first enters is known as the cornea. The cornea is the major refractive surface of the eye, accounting for most of its focusing power. The amount of light that actually enters the eye is controlled by the pupillary aperture of the pigmented iris muscle. Through the processes of constriction and dilation, the pupil can regulate the amount of light entering the eye over a 16:1 range (Geldard, 1972). After passing through the pupil, light rays from the visual stimulus next encounter the crystalline lens. In response to the contraction of the ciliary muscles, the lens can change its shape and, hence, alter its focusing power. This process is known as *accommodation* and enables the lens to dynamically increase the imaging power of the eye as required for tasks such as the viewing of near objects. Light next passes through the vitreous body, the transparent gel that enables the eye to maintain its constant spherical shape. Finally, the light composing the visual stimulus is imaged upon the retina. The millions of rods and cones of the retina transduce light energy into nervous system activity. The activity generated by these photoreceptors is collected and extensively processed by retinal ganglion cells, which subsequently converge to form the optic nerve. Visual information is carried from the retina via the optic nerve to the lateral geniculate nucleus of the thalamus, whose fibers ultimately project to the primary visual cortex.

Many of the optical and neural characteristics of the visual system change with increasing adult age. Changes in the cornea that accompany aging include an increased irregularity in its surface properties (Kuwabara, 1979), which may contribute to increased intraocular scatter or *stray* light. The cornea also has a tendency to flatten along the vertical meridian, contributing to the emergence of astigmatic refractive errors in older adults (Leighton & Tomlinson, 1972; Weale, 1963). Unlike increased intraocular scatter of light, most astigmatisms can be corrected with eyeglasses or contact lenses. Aging is also accompanied by a pronounced reduction in the diameter of the pupil (Birren, Casperson, & Botwinick, 1950; Weale, 1961). Known as *senile miosis,* this phenomenon results in a marked reduction in the amount of light reaching the senescent retina. This reduction in retinal illumination is most pronounced under low-luminance conditions, where the age differences in pupil size are most pronounced (Lowenfeld, 1979). Although senile miosis has typically been attributed to degenerative changes in the iris and its supporting structures (see Weale, 1963), recent evidence suggests that it may represent an adaptation to the development of ocular imperfections within the older eye (Sloane, Owsley, & Alvarez,

1988). Perhaps the major age-related changes in the eye occur at the level of the lens. The ability of the lens to accommodate and, hence, focus near objects decreases continuously from early childhood (Garner & Spector, 1978). By the fifth decade of life, the loss of accommodation becomes so great that most persons require optical correction to read text within arm's length (Hofstetter, 1965). This condition is known as *presbyopia*. As adult age increases, the lens also becomes less transparent (Sample, Esterson, Weinreb, & Boynton, 1988; Weale, 1988), differentially absorbs light in the blue-green end of the spectrum (Porkorny, Smith, & Lutze, 1987; Said & Weale, 1959), and begins to increasingly scatter light away from its principal axis (Allen & Vos, 1967). Owing to the combined effects of senile miosis and lenticular opacification, Weale (1961) has estimated, the retina of a typical 60-year-old receives less than one third the light of its 20-year-old counterpart.

Age-related changes in the neural elements of the visual system have also been documented. Gross examination of the retina reveals more narrow and sclerotic blood vessels, a progressive decrease in the pigmentation and apparent thickness of the retinal pigment epithelium (which provides metabolic support for the photoreceptors), and a diminished ophthalmoscopic light reflex from the central area of the retina (Marmor, 1982). Microscopic examination of the retina reveals more profound age-related changes such as the loss of rods and cones (Marshall, Grindle, Ansell, & Borwein, 1980; Youdelis & Hendrickson, 1986), atrophy of retinal ganglion cells (Vrabec, 1965; Kuwabara, 1979) and the degeneration of retinal capillaries (Kuwabara & Cogan, 1965). Changes beyond the retina are also apparent. The number of fibers composing the optic nerve has been shown to decline with age (Dolman, McCormick, & Drance, 1980). Finally, age-related changes in the visual cortex have also been noted. Devaney and Johnson (1980) reported that the number of cells in the primary visual cortex representing the central field of vision declined from approximately 40 million per gram of tissue at age 30 to about 30 million per gram at age 60—a 25% reduction. Qualitative changes such as shortened dendritic arborizations appear to characterize the cells of the visual cortex that survive the aging process (Schiebel & Schiebel, 1975). For a thorough review of age-related changes in the structures of the visual pathways refer to Ordy and Brizzee (1979), Corso (1981), and Weale (1984).

B. Psychophysical Studies of Visual Aging

Survey studies indicate that older adults demonstrate greater levels of dissatisfaction with their degree of visual functioning than do younger adults (e.g., Hakkinen, 1984; Kosnik, Winslow, Kline, Rasinski, & Sekuler, 1988). Among the principal visual complaints reported by older adults are problems with seeing under low light levels, difficulty processing rapidly changing displays, problems with near visual tasks, and searching for visual targets in the environment (Kosnik, *et al.*, 1988). Although some of these problems can be explained on the basis of age-related anatomical differences such as those outlined above, many of these complaints can be understood only after reviewing laboratory studies of higher-order visual processing based upon psychophysical experiments. An impressive database of psychophysical studies regarding human age differences in visual processing has accumulated over the past few decades. This literature is briefly reviewed below. Owing to space limitations, the discussion is selective rather than exhaustive. Readers interested in more extensive coverage of this rapidly expanding area are referred to Kline and Schieber (1985) and Sekuler, Kline, and Dismukes (1982). A discussion of the research literature published since these reviews can be found in Fozard (1990).

C. Spatial Resolution

1. Oculomotor Function

The ability to resolve fine visual detail is mediated by a very small, centrally located region of the retina known as the fovea. Hence, optimal spatial resolution depends upon the oculomotor system's capacity to track and image a visual stimulus upon the fovea. This task of maintaining fixation is accomplished by two distinct but interacting eye-movement systems. The saccadic eye-movement system generates short, high-velocity ballistic motions that move an image onto the fovea. The pursuit eye-movement system mediates large-amplitude, continuous motions that enhance visual function by extending the useful field of view and allowing the eye to accurately track rapidly moving or accelerating targets. There is consistent evidence that the time needed to initiate a saccadic eye movement following the onset of a visual stimulus increases with adult age. Whitaker, Shoptaugh, and Haywood (1986) found that 18 to 32-year-olds demonstrated saccadic latencies of 255 msec, while older adults (ages 57–72) exhibited a mean latency of 284 msec. Pitt and Rawles (1988) reported that saccadic latency increased by 0.76%/year, while saccadic velocity decreased by about .25%/year between the ages of 20 and 68 years. Other studies have reported findings that support these observations (e.g., Spooner, Skalka, & Baloh, 1980). Age-related declines in the pursuit eye-movement system have also been noted. Sharpe and Sylvester (1978) reported that young subjects could accurately track targets at velocities up to 30 degrees/sec, whereas the fixational accuracy of pursuit eye movements began to break down for older observers when target velocity exceeded 10 degrees/sec. Similar findings have been reported by Hutton, Nagel, and Lowenson (1983). Relatedly, Kaufman and Abel (1986) have demonstrated that age differences in pursuit accuracy are exacerbated in the presence of competing or distracting stimulus backgrounds. Although the age-related oculomotor changes described above may lead to functional limitations in dynamic viewing situations, there is evidence that older adults demonstrate no loss in the ability to maintain accurate fixation while viewing a small, stationary stimulus (Kosnik, Kline, Fikre, & Sekuler, 1987).

Investigating another aspect of oculomotor function, Chamberlain (1971) reported that old age is accompanied by a significant restriction in the range of upward gaze (i.e., the maximal vertical extent of vision without the aid of head movements). Although classic texts on ophthalmology place the limits of upward gaze between 40 and 45 degrees (Adler, 1933; Duke-Elder, 1949), Chamberlain's assessment of 367 persons ages 5–94 revealed that upward gaze declined linearly across the lifespan from a maximum of 40 degrees at ages 5–14 years to a minimum of 16 degrees at ages 75–84. Little or no age-related limitation in the extent of lateral or downward gaze was noted.

2. Acuity

Acuity refers to the ability of the visual system to resolve fine spatial detail. Visual-acuity assessments are most often quantified in terms of the *minimum angle of resolution;* that is, the visual angle of the smallest spatial target that can be identified. The ability to resolve well-illuminated, high-contrast spatial features, which subtend a visual angle of 1 minute of arc (minarc), represents *normal* visual acuity. Snellen decimal acuity is computed by taking the reciprocal of the minimal angle of resolution (e.g., a minimal angle of resolution of 2.0 minarc would yield a Snellen decimal acuity of 0.5). Since the crystalline lens of the eye must accommodate, or change shape, in order to focus near targets, separate visual acuities for near (40 cm) versus far (6 m) targets are often measured. Because small amounts of refractive error in the eye yield reliable decrements in acuity, the acuity test has been widely adopted as the basis for correcting optical abberations of the eye with spectacle lenses (Schieber, 1988).

Pitts (1982) reviewed several large-scale, cross-sectional studies that examined age differences in far acuity. Figure 1 represents a summary of his findings. The data show that

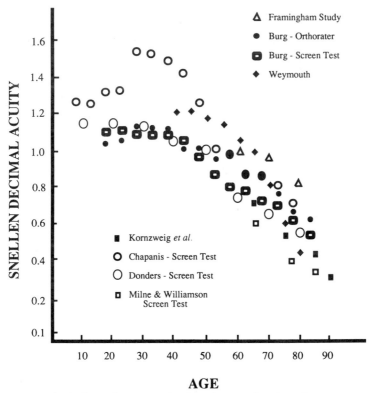

Figure 1   Composite indices of average visual acuity as a function of age as reported in eight major studies. (Adapted from D. G. Pitts, 1982. Reproduced by permission of Wiley-Liss, Inc.)

average corrected acuity is maintained to approximately age 50, declines only slightly from ages 50 to 60, and is then followed by a more accelerated loss through age 90. Data from the Framingham Eye Study (Kahn *et al.*, 1977), presented in Table I, show that the majority of adults maintain "good" corrected visual acuity (i.e., 20/25 (1.25 minarc) or better) through age 85. It is only after age 65 that a sizable proportion of the population begins to demonstrate significant acuity deficits. These age-related losses in acuity are observed even when factors such as refractive error and reduced retinal illumination due to senile miosis and increased optical density of the lens are factored out, and suggests that much of the acuity deficit in advanced age results from neural rather than optical degeneration (Weale, 1975; 1982). Recent findings that age differences in acuity are exacerbated under low-contrast testing conditions provide additional evidence suggestive of a neural mechanism of visual aging (Adams, Wong, Wong, & Gould, 1988).

Gittings and Fozard (1986) recently reported the results of a large-scale longitudinal study of age-related changes in visual acuity. Their data, collected from 577 male participants of the Baltimore Longitudinal Study of Aging, are summarized in Figure 2. These observations are based upon an average of seven repeated measurements of individuals spaced approximately two years apart. The numerous linear functions shown in the figure represent the best-fit regression lines for each age-stratified subgroup of the sample. The stereopsis findings (bottom panel) will be discussed below. These data indicate that uncorrected far (distance) acuity declines between ages 30 and 80. However, the falloff in corrected (presenting) far acuity is not readily noticeable until ages 55–60. This ability to maintain good far visual acuity [1.25 minarc (0.8 Snellen decimal) or better] until age 70 with the use of corrective eyeglasses supports the findings of cross-sectional studies (see Pitts, 1982). Gittings and Fozard's uncorrected near visual acuity data showed a marked decrement between the ages of 40 and 55 consistent with the well-known, age-related loss in the accommodative capacity of the lens (presbyopia), which occurs during the fifth decade of life. The age-related change in presenting (bifocal corrected) near acuity paral-

Table I
Age Distributions of Visual Acuity[a]

	Snellen acuity				
Age	20/25 or better	20/30 to 20/40	20/50 to 20/70	20/80 to 20/100	20/100 to 20/200
Age 52–64 (N = 1293)	98.4[b]	0.9	0.5	0.1	0.1
Age 65–74 (N = 786)	91.9	5.6	1.4	0.1	1.0
Age 75–85 (N = 392)	69.1	17.9	7.9	1.8	3.3

[a]Best-corrected acuity in the better eye as reported by the Framingham Eye Study (Kahn *et al.*, 1977).
[b]Percentage distribution.

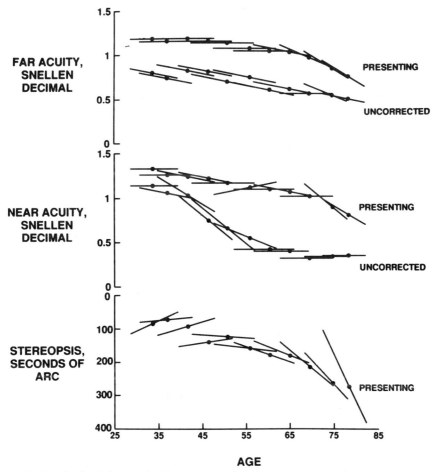

Figure 2 Longitudinal changes in binocular visual acuity and stereopsis from 577 male participants of the Baltimore Longitudinal Study of Aging. Each data point is located at the mean age for a particular subgroup, while the length of the lines represents the number of years the subgroup was followed. The slope of the lines represents the best-fit linear regression on age for each subgroup. (Adapted from J. L. Fozard, 1990. Reproduced with permission of the author and Academic Press.)

lels the pattern loss reported for far acuity. It is noteworthy that Gittings and Fozard (1986) reported that much of the longitudinal decline in acuity across increasing age was observed in persons who initially presented with good visual acuity. This pattern of results underscores the need for more frequent assessment of visual acuity where older populations are involved.

3. Contrast Sensitivity

Visual acuity measurements do not adequately describe the spatial sensitivity of an individual. Research has clearly demonstrated that the capacity to detect and identify spatial form varies widely as a function of target size, contrast, and spatial orientation (see Braddick, Campbell, & Atkinson, 1978; Olzak & Thomas, 1985). As a consequence, an assessment of visual acuity (i.e., the ability to resolve small, high-contrast targets) very often does not predict an individual's ability to detect objects of large size and/or diminished contrast (Ginsburg, Evans, Sekuler, & Harp, 1982; Watson, Barlow, & Robson, 1983). However, contrast-sensitivity testing complements and extends the assessment of visual function provided by acuity measures. At the cost of more complex and time-consuming procedures, contrast-sensitivity measurements yield information about an individual's ability to see low-contrast targets over an extended range of target size (and orientation).

Contrast-sensitivity tests use sine-wave gratings as targets instead of the letter optotypes typically used in acuity tests. Sine-wave gratings possess useful mathematical properties (Ginsburg, 1977), and researchers have discovered that early stages of visual processing are optimally sensitive to such targets (Maffei, 1978; Watson, et al., 1983). A conventional contrast-sensitivity assessment procedure consists of presenting the observer with a sine-wave grating of a given *spatial frequency* (i.e., number of sinusoidal luminance cycles per degree of visual angle). The contrast of the grating target is then varied while the observer's contrast-detection threshold is determined. Typically, contrast thresholds of this sort are collected using vertically oriented gratings that vary in spatial frequency from 0.5 cycles/degree (very wide) to 32 cycles/degree (very narrow). Because high levels of visual sensitivity are associated with low-contrast thresholds, a reciprocal measure (1/threshold) termed the contrast-sensitivity score is computed. These sensitivity scores are plotted across the range of spatial frequencies examined during the assessment procedure and constitute an individual's *contrast-sensitivity function* (CSF).

The Baltimore Longitudinal Study of Aging (BLSA) has recently initiated a long-term assessment of age-related changes in the contrast-sensitivity function (Schieber, Fozard, Dent, & Kline, 1989). Unlike previous studies of age and the CSF, the BLSA investigation employed rigorous forced-choice psychophysical procedures, large sample sizes, longitudinal followup, and the opportunity to cross-reference individual changes in the CSF with many other variables related to functional status (such as lens–retina health, self-reports of visual problems, driving behaviors, etc.). Preliminary data from 200+ participants in this study are presented in Figure 3. These data clearly reveal that contrast sensitivity for intermediate and high spatial-frequency targets declines significantly across age groups. These findings replicate and extend the results of previous studies (Kline, Schieber, Abusamra, & Coyne, 1983; Owsley, Sekuler, & Siemsen, 1983). Since older adults demonstrated losses at intermediate spatial frequencies, they would be expected to experience disproportionate losses in visual sensitivity for larger objects as well as smaller ones. In support of this conclusion, Owsley and Sloane (1987) found that older adults with poor contrast sensitivity for intermediate spatial frequencies demonstrated problems with detecting and identifying human faces presented at low contrast. This result was predicted by their contrast-sensitivity data but not by measurements of simple visual acuity. The superiority of contrast sensitivity over acuity in accounting for age differences in the ability to see large, real-world stimulus objects has also been demonstrated by Evans and Ginsburg (1985). It is interesting to note, however, that no age differences have been observed in tasks involving suprathreshold contrast matching across spatial frequencies (e.g., Tulunay-Keesey, Ver Hoeve, & Terkla-McGrane, 1988).

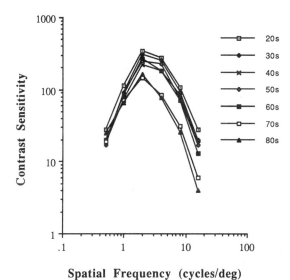

Spatial Frequency (cycles/deg)

Figure 3   Contrast sensitivity functions for several age groups.

Owsley *et al.*, (1983) found that age differences in contrast sensitivity were not eliminated when young subjects viewed the stimulus objects under conditions of simulated ocular aging (*viz.*, markedly reduced retinal illumination and refractive error induced via *plus* spherical defocusing lenses). These results indicate that the residual age difference in contrast sensitivity represented an age-related change in the neural, rather than optical, characteristics of the visual system. When laser interferometry is used to minimize the effects of age differences in the optics of the eye, substantial age differences in contrast sensitivity at intermediate and high spatial frequencies persist (Morrison & McGrath, 1985; Elliott, 1987). These findings also strongly indicate that much of the age-related change in contrast sensitivity results from neural differences in visual processing. For a timely discussion of ocular versus neural mediation of age differences in spatial vision see Elliott, Whitaker, and MacVeigh (1990).

4. Stereopsis

The images formed by our two eyes do not exactly overlap in terms of their relative retinal positions. As an object moves closer, the amount of this binocular retinal disparity increases. The ability of the visual cortex to detect and utilize changes in binocular retinal disparity to make inferences about depth is known as binocular depth perception, or *stereopsis*. Although stereopsis is only one of many visual cues used to make judgments of depth or distance, virtually all of the studies that have examined age differences in depth perception have been limited to the assessment of stereopsis via stereoacuity tests (Pitts, 1982). Gittings, Fozard, and Shock (1987) examined age changes in stereopsis over a period of 10 years in 577 male participants of the Baltimore Longitudinal Study. Age changes in the minimal amount of binocular disparity required to yield a perception of depth are summarized in the bottom panel of Figure 2. As can be seen in this figure, threshold stereopsis increases from a minimum of 100 sec of arc in the 30-year-olds to a maximum of approximately 300 sec in the 80-year-olds. This age-related loss in stereopsis ability did not correlate with age changes in acuity collected from these same individuals. Similar age-related increases in the threshold for stereopsis have been reported using cross-sectional techniques (Bell, Wolf, & Bernholz, 1972; Greene & Madden, 1987; Hofstetter & Bertsch, 1976). Although neural mechanisms are most often cited as the basis for age-related changes in stereopsis threshold, there is evidence from the general literature that optical factors may be involved. For example, reduced retinal contrast, a common effect of aging, is associated with diminished levels of stereopsis (Heckmann & Schor, 1989). Stereopsis has been found to be affected even more severely when interocular differences in retinal contrast exist, such as might be observed in the case of monocular cataract (Schor & Heckmann, 1989).

5. Visual Search

The ability to detect and orient to events that occur in the parafoveal and peripheral fields of vision is essential for many daily tasks. However, very little is known about nonfoveal visual functioning in the older adult. Wolf (1967) assessed the limits of far peripheral visual sensitivity for individuals ages 16 through 91 using a dim, 1mm² target. The maximal extent of peripheral vision remained relatively stable through age 55, followed by a small but progressive decrease in the width of the visual field through age 91. However, recent evidence suggests that perimetric measures such as those obtained by Wolf may severely underestimate age-related declines in the ability to utilize information presented to the noncentral areas of the retina. Sekuler and Ball (1986) measured age differences on a task that assessed how well a simple target could be localized when randomly positioned anywhere within the central 30 degrees of the visual field. This localization task was performed in the presence of distractor stimuli as well as under conditions of divided attention where the observer had to perform a concurrent central visual field task. In the absence of the distractor stimuli, observers of all ages did equally well at localizing the peripherally presented target. However, the presentation of the peripheral distractors resulted in a significant performance decrement for the old group (mean age, 68.8) but not the young group (mean age, 25.1). In a followup study, Ball, Beard, Roenker, Miller, and Griggs (1988) determined the range of parafoveal vision over which accurate localization performance could be maintained under conditions of divided attention with peripheral distractors. They determined that the *useful field of view*, the visual area over which information can be acquired within a single eye fixation under complex conditions, contracted significantly in size as age increased from 22 to 75 years. Findings consistent with an age-related reduction in the spatial extent of the working field of vision have been reported by other investigators (e.g., Cerella, 1985; Scialfa, Kline, & Lyman, 1987).

6. Visibility under Adverse Viewing Conditions

a. Low illumination.   When available light is decreased to low levels, visual functions such as acuity and contrast sensitivity become impaired (Lit, 1968; van Meeteren & Vos, 1972). There are many instances in which individuals must use their vision despite the fact that insufficient light is available (e.g., reading a label in a dimly lit store, or nighttime driving). In most of these cases the visual system is operating in the mesopic or low photopic range rather than in the fully dark-adapted state (Byrnes, 1962). Although limited, some data are available regarding age differences in visual function under mesopic and low photopic levels of light adaptation. These studies have revealed consistently that age-related declines in visual function become exacerbated under conditions of low illumination. Richards (1977) measured the acuity of individuals ranging in age from 16 to 90 using charts varying in luminance from 0.03 to 34 cd/m². Although the acuity of all individuals decreased as available light was diminished, the magnitude of this effect was much stronger for those individuals in their 70s and 80s. Relatedly, Rice and Jones (1984) examined corrected visual acuity under normal and reduced (i.e., nighttime) illumination conditions. Of 4038 drivers who passed the test (20/40 or better) under standard levels of illuminance, 267 (6.6%) were unable to pass the night vision version of the test. Older persons were disproportionately represented in this group as 36% of those ages 61–70, and 68% of those ages 81+ failed the nighttime version of the visual screening test. Vola, Cornu, Carruel, Gastaud, and Leid (1983) examined photopic (100 cd/m²) and mesopic (0.8 cd/m²) acuity in 221 persons ages 20 through 50. No age differences in photopic acuity were observed, but mesopic acuity was found to decline from 1.5 minarc at age 20 to approximately 2.0 minarc at age 50. A control study obtained the same pattern of results when the optics of the eye were *bypassed* using laser interferometry, suggesting that the disproportionate age difference at low luminance was mediated by changes in the nervous system. Sturr, G. E. Kline, and Taub (1990) also observed a disproportionate drop in acuity among observers over the age of 65 as target luminance fell from 245 to 0.2 cd/m². Relatedly, Sloane, Owsley, and Jackson (1988) reported that age differences in contrast sensitivity increased as target luminance was decreased from 107 to 0.107 cd/m². In fact, at the lowest luminance level, more than 50% of the older subjects failed to detect targets having a spatial frequency of 4 cycles/degree or higher at the maximal available contrast (70%). Field studies have also demonstrated that the performance of older adults suffers disproportionately under low luminance conditions. For example, Sivak and Olson (1982) found that older adults demonstrated nighttime legibility distances for highway signs that were only 65–77% of those obtained by their young counterparts. This age difference in legibility distance at night could be predicted on the basis of low-luminance acuity scores but not on the basis of acuity data collected under the high-luminance conditions traditionally employed by vision screening tests. Hence, standard tests of visual acuity may greatly underestimate the functional level of performance to be expected from older populations under impoverished viewing conditions.

b. Glare.   Age-related increases in susceptibility to the deleterious effects of glare have been demonstrated by numerous investigators. Bennett (1977) reported a threefold age-related decrease in the amount of glare that could be tolerated before significant levels of psychological discomfort were encountered. This decreased threshold for discomfort glare among the elderly was especially problematic at low levels of background illumination (i.e., those resembling nighttime driving conditions). Similarly, Pulling, Wolf, Sturgis, Vaillancourt, and Doliver (1980) observed a significant decline with age in headlight glare resistance when observers were tested in a driving simulator. Wolf (1960) examined the effects of a bright, central glare source on the luminance required to identify the orientation of an acuity target (Landolt-ring) in persons ages 5 through 85. The luminance increment required to overcome the glare-mediated reduction in acuity significantly increased with age, especially after age 45. Burg (1967) repeated Wolf's (1960) observations on a sample of 17,000+ drivers aged 16 to 92. In addition, he assessed the time needed to recover visual sensitivity lost following exposure to a glare source. The amount of luminance required to identify the acuity targets in the presence of the glare source increased systematically with age. Glare recovery was also greater in older adults: 3.9, 5.6, and 6.8 sec for drivers aged 20–24, 40–44 and 75–79, respectively. Other studies have also reported a similar age-related increase in the time required to recover lost visual sensitivity following exposure to a transient glare source (Elliott & Whitaker, 1990; Olson & Sivak, 1989). Although age differences in glare sensitivity have typically been ascribed to changes in light absorption and scatter by the crystalline lens (e.g., Ijspeert, de Waard, van den Berg, & de Jong, 1990), the magnitude of the age-related increase in glare-recovery times appears to implicate a neural mechanism. Recent studies of the disabling effects of glare suggest that contrast sensitivity may be more sensitive than acuity measures for assessing the magnitude and nature of age differences in the susceptibility to glare effects (e.g., Abrahamsson & Sjostrand, 1986; Elliott, 1987; Schieber, 1988).

D. Temporal Resolution

The visual system of older adults becomes diminished in its ability to detect temporal changes in the environment. Temporally contiguous visual events that would be seen as separate and distinct by young observers are often seen as fused or indistinguishable by older individuals (Kline & Schieber, 1982). This age-related *slowing* of the visual system affects not only higher-order events such as those revealed in sequential integration of form (e.g., Kline & Birren, 1975; Walsh, 1976), but also can be demonstrated in the form of age-related losses in flicker sensitivity, dynamic visual acuity, and motion perception.

1. Flicker Sensitivity

The classic index of the temporal resolving power of the visual system is the *critical flicker frequency* threshold (CFF). The CFF is the minimal frequency of a pulsating light source at which the light *appears* to be *fused* into a continuous, rather than flickering, stimulus. The CFF represents the point at which the visual system can no longer resolve rapid temporal changes in illumination. There is a well-documented decline with age in flicker sensitivity as revealed by the CFF (e.g., Brozek & Keys, 1945; Huntington & Simonson, 1965; Misiak, 1947). Wolf and Shaffra (1964) collected CFF measures from 302 observers aged 6 through 95. CFF thresholds increased (i.e., flicker sensitivity decreased) gradually to around age 60 and then rapidly thereafter. Although part of the age-related loss in flicker sensitivity appears to be due to a reduction in retinal illumination (i.e., an optical mechanism), experiments by McFarland, Warren, and Karis (1958) and Weekers and Roussel (1945) support the notion that much of the age difference in the CFF is due to changes in the senescent visual nervous system (Kline & Schieber, 1985).

A more recently developed tool for examining the temporal resolving power of the visual system is the *temporal contrast sensitivity function* (TCSF)—the so-called de Lange function. The TCSF is analogous to the spatial CSF described above. The contrast of a small illuminated target is sinusoidally modulated at a given temporal frequency. Then the minimal amplitude of contrast modulation required to detect the presence of flicker is determined for a range of temporal frequencies that usually extends from 1 to 50 Hz. Mayer, Kim, Svingos, and Glucs (1988) collected TCSFs in a group of 16 young (18–42) and 12 old (65–86) observers. Age differences in retinal illumination were minimized by using a long-wavelength test stimulus and by mathematically adjusting performance on the basis of each observer's pupil size. Significant age declines in flicker sensitivity were observed at temporal frequencies up to 40 Hz. Wright and Drasdo (1985) reported even larger age differences in the TCSF, but did not utilize the procedures for *equalizing* retinal illuminance described above.

2. Dynamic Visual Acuity

Dynamic visual acuity (DVA) refers to the ability to resolve fine detail in targets that are in motion relative to the observer. DVA is limited by a complex interaction between static visual acuity and oculomotor coordination. Individuals with identical static visual acuities can demonstrate markedly different DVA levels (Morrison, 1980). DVA performance declines as target velocity increases. This is apparently the result of errors in stimulus capture by the pursuit eye-movement system, which result in a *smearing* of the retinal image (Murphy, 1978). Since oculomotor accuracy appears to decline somewhat with advancing age, one would expect to observe a concomitant age-related change in DVA. Burg (1967) examined static and dynamic acuity in 17,000+ California drivers between the ages of 16 and 92. The ability to resolve fine detail in a moving target was found to decline more dramatically with age than did traditional static acuity measures. Similar patterns of results have been reported by other investigators (e.g., Farrimond, 1967; Reading, 1972; Scialfa, Garvey, Tyrell, & Leibowitz, 1989). Age-related declines in DVA performance may involve mechanisms other than oculomotor pursuit. For example, Long and Crambert (1990) recently reported large age differences in DVA even when stimulus-exposure times were too short to engage pursuit eye movements (i.e., 200 msec). Once more, Long and Crambert found that the DVA performance of their young (ages 17–23) and old (60–75) groups did not differ when the presumed age-related reduction in retinal illuminance was experimentally eliminated. However, the significance of these results is difficult to interpret, since the older subjects had poor static visual acuities (mean, 20/32) and the retinal-illuminance manipulation confounded stimulus luminance and contrast. Finally, Henderson and Burg (1974) found that, unlike static visual acuity, poor DVA performance among the elderly was predictive of poor traffic safety records. This increase in the number of traffic violations and accidents among older drivers with poor DVA scores may be related to the recent finding that oculomotor coordination is severely degraded by the onset of Alzheimer's disease (Hutton, Nagel, & Lowenson, 1984).

3. Motion Sensitivity

Several studies have demonstrated age-related declines in motion sensitivity. Buckingham, Whitaker, and Banford (1987) measured threshold sensitivity for the detection of horizontal oscillatory motion in a 2 cycle/degree sine-wave grating target as a function of age and temporal frequency (1–20 Hz). At all frequencies of oscillation, older (mean age, 69.7) observers were about a factor of 2 less sensitive to motion than middle-aged (mean age, 48.0) observers who, in turn, were only slightly less sensitive than the young (mean age, 20.7). When the grating oscillated at a frequency of 8 Hz, young, middle-aged, and older observers required oscillation amplitudes of approximately 39, 52, and 97 seconds of arc, respectively, to detect the occurrence of motion. Similar age-related losses in motion sensitivity have been demonstrated using a horizontally oscillating line segment (Whitaker & Elliott, 1989) and a small, vertically oscillating dot (Schieber, Hiris, White, & Williams, 1990). Controls implemented by these later studies clearly revealed that the age-related deficit was independent of refractive error and retinal illumination and was, hence, probably of neural origin. Shinar (1977) examined motion sensitivity in a sample of 890 drivers between the ages of 17 and 89. Threshold angular rates of change required to detect motion in depth (i.e., looming) and angular displacement across the central field of vision were collected from each observer. Motion sensitivity in both cases was found to decline only very slightly between the ages of 17 and 60, with an accelerated loss occurring thereafter. Using a somewhat different approach, Ball and Sekuler (1986) found that older adults were less able to discriminate among arrays of moving dots that drifted in slightly different directions. In another study demonstrating loss of motion sensitivity with age, Owsley, Sekuler, and Siemsen (1983) reported that older adults exhibited markedly attenuated contrast sensitivity for the detection of a 1.0 cycle/degree sine-wave grating, which drifted at a velocity of 4.3 degrees/sec, despite the fact that no age differences in sensitivity were observed for a stationary grating of the same spatial frequency. Finally, in a study that underscored the potential applied significance of an age-related change in motion perception, Scialfa et al. (1987) reported decrements in the accuracy with which older adults could estimate the speed of an approaching vehicle on a rudimentary driving-simulation task.

E. Color Sensitivity

The ability to discriminate between subtle differences in hue declines systematically with age. Dalderup and Fredericks (1969) observed age-related losses in color sensitivity that became particularly acute beyond the age of 70. Gilbert (1957) examined color sensitivity in 355 observers ranging in age from 10 to 93 using the Color Aptitude Test. Color discrimination ability peaked in the mid-20s and declined steadily thereafter. Although all observers demonstrated more errors of discrimination among the blues and greens (shorter wavelengths) as opposed to the reds and yellows (longer wavelengths), this tendency to confuse similar hues within the blue-green range became especially pronounced among the elderly. Similar findings have been reported using the more quantitatively rigorous Farnsworth-Munsell 100-Hue test (Knoblauch et al. 1987). Early studies attributed this pattern of age differences to the "yellowing" of the senescent lens (see Weale, 1986). However, recent investigations have provided evidence that adult aging is associated with a differential loss of sensitivity in the short-wavelength-sensitive (SWS) photoreceptors and/or their postreceptoral projections to the nervous system (e.g., Haegerstrom-Portnoy, 1988; Johnson, Adams, Twelker, & Quigg, 1988; Werner & Steele, 1988). A concise summary of these recent findings is presented by Owsley and Sloane (1990).

Table II

Prevalence of Major Visual Pathologies[a]

Age (years)	Cataract (%)	Age-related maculopathy (%)	Glaucoma (%)
52–64	5	2	1
65–74	18	11	5
75–85	46	28	7

[a]As reported by the Framingham Eye Study (Kahn *et al.*, 1977).

F. Common Age-Related Visual Pathologies

Profound visual impairment is more likely to be seen in the older population. The leading causes of severe visual impairment in the United States are cataract, age-related maculopathy, open-angle glaucoma, and diabetic retinopathy (Sekuler *et al.* 1982). All four of these visual pathologies become more prevalent after the age of 55 (Kahn & Milton, 1980); Sperduto & Siegel, 1980). Prevalence of these disorders as a function of age is presented in Table II. Loss of vision due to cataractous clouding of the lens may become severe but can be corrected in most cases via outpatient surgical procedures. Glaucoma gradually decreases sensitivity of the retina owing to increased intraocular pressure, which destroys the head of the optic nerve. Since the primary early symptoms of glaucoma are loss of peripheral vision, it often progresses to an advanced stage before it is noticed by the patient. Although vision lost to glaucoma cannot be recovered, once diagnosed, it often can be controlled via pharmacologic or surgical intervention. Age-related maculopathy and diabetic retinopathy are both progressive disorders that gradually destroy the central areas of the retina that subserve acuity and color vision. At present, neither of these disorders responds well to treatment.

II. Hearing

A. Structural Changes in the Auditory System

Sound pressure waves are captured by the outer ear and conducted by air through the auditory canal to the tympanic membrane, or eardrum. Sound pressure vibrations are then amplified and transferred from the eardrum to the fluid-filled cochlea of the inner ear by way of a mechanical linkage formed by three tiny bones in the middle ear (*viz.*, the ossicular chain consisting of the incus, malleus, and stapes). The waves of pressure introduced to the fluid within the cochlea cause a *shearing* motion to stimulate thousands of so-called hair cells situated between several membranes that medially bisect the cochlea along its full length. The mechanical stimulation of these hair cells results in the transduction of sound pressure waves into nervous system activity. Position-dependent changes in the mechanical properties of the cochlear membranes together with neural tuning mechanisms give rise to the differential frequency sensitivity of the auditory system. Neural activity generated by the hair cells is collected at the spiral ganglia and subsequently conducted along the auditory nerve to the central auditory pathway, beginning with a structure in the pons known as the trapezoid body. At this point, the nerve fibers ascend both ipsilateral and contralateral to the superior olivary body. The majority of these fibers ascend to the inferior colliculus of the midbrain. These fibers then synapse at the medial geniculate nucleus of the thalamus and ultimately project to the auditory cortex, which is located in the temporal lobe of the brain. Much neural information is exchanged and processed at the various sites along the ascending auditory pathway. Hence, the structural integrity of these sites is thought to be critical for the maintenance of optimal auditory function (for a detailed discussion of auditory pathways and processing see Gulick, Gescheider, & Frisina, 1989).

Anatomical studies of aging have tended to find degenerative changes at virtually every level of the auditory system. Atrophic changes in the outer ear noted to accompany aging include increased secretion of ear wax (cerumen) with excessive accumulation and blockage of the auditory canal (Corso, 1963) as well as a tendency for the auditory canal to collapse (Schow, Christensen, Hutchinson, & Nerbonne, 1978). In the middle ear, the joints of the ossicular bone chain have been noted to become calcified and less elastic with advancing age (Belal, 1975; Etholm & Belal, 1974). These changes in the auditory canal and the ossicular chain probably contribute to conductive hearing losses observed among the elderly (Olsho, Harkins, & Lehnhardt, 1985). At the level of the inner ear, many changes in the structure and metabolism of the cochlea have been reported, including reduced flexibility and responsiveness of the medial cochlear membranes (Hansen & Reske-Nelson, 1965; Wright & Schuknecht, 1972); profound losses among certain classes of hair cells (Bredberg, 1967; Johnsson & Hawkins, 1972); and diminished cochlear blood flow (Schuknecht, 1974). Many investigators have also demonstrated age-related degeneration in the structures of the central auditory pathway. Kirikae (1969) found atrophic changes at the cochlear nucleus (trapezoid body), superior olive, inferior colliculus, and medial geniculate nucleus of the thalamus. Similar findings were also reported by Hansen and Reske-Nielsen (1965). Dublin (1976) reported the development of vascular insufficiency in the tissues that attend to the metabolic needs of the ascending central auditory pathway. Brody (1955) found that the auditory cortex was among the areas of the brain most affected by age-related cell loss. These degenerative changes in the temporal lobe of the brain were corroborated by Samorajaski (1976). Many additional age-related changes in the physiology of the auditory system have been found and are expertly reviewed by Corso (1981), Olsho et al. (1985), and Ordy and Brizzee (1979).

Unfortunately, there are few data available that directly relate histological assessments of auditory structure to age-related changes in the ability to detect and utilize auditory information. There is a great need to perform post mortem histological examinations upon older individuals for whom auditory performance data are available. Large-scale research efforts such as the National Institute on Aging's Baltimore Longitudinal Study have just recently begun to implement an autopsy protocol for recently deceased participants. This work promises to contribute much to our knowledge regarding the relationship between structure and function in the elderly.

B. Age-Related Changes in Auditory Functioning

The anatomical changes that accompany aging suggest that older adults should experience a certain degree of hearing difficulty. Yet, in order to estimate the nature and magnitude of these problems, one must resort to the growing database of psychophysical studies. A highly selective review of the psychophysical literature regarding aging and human auditory function is presented below. More exhaustive accounts of this literature can be obtained by referring to Corso (1981), Hinchcliffe, (1983), and Olsho *et al.* (1985).

1. Prevalence of Hearing Problems

In 1981 the National Health Interview Survey (NHIS), conducted by the U.S. National Center for Health Statistics, estimated that 13.4 million noninstitutionalized adults older than 45 suffered from significant hearing impairment. NHIS prevalence estimates for hearing impairment as a function of age are presented in Table III. Reference to this table clearly indicates that the proportion of the population with hearing problems grows rapidly with advancing age. Beyond age 65, approximately one in four individuals is affected by hearing loss or significant levels of *tinnitis*—a persistent ringing in the ears. Population studies that have estimated the prevalence and magnitude of hearing loss using audiometric examinations yield results consistent with survey-based research (see Ries, 1985). Clearly, advancing adult age is associated with an ever-increasing risk of the development of significant hearing impairment, even among otherwise healthy, non-institutionalized persons.

2. Absolute Sensitivity for Pure Tones

Human observers demonstrate a characteristic absolute sensitivity for pure-tone stimuli, which varies as a function of stimulus frequency. The amount of sound pressure required to "just detect" the presence of a pure tone reaches a minimum at approximately 1000 Hz (Hz = Hertz = cycles per second). This absolute sensitivity then declines as stimulus frequency is either increased or decreased. Since the sound pressure required for the absolute detection threshold varies with frequency, it has become conventional to express an individual's hearing level in relative rather than absolute terms. Hence, the traditional

Table III

Prevalence of Hearing Impairment[a]

Age	Prevalence per 1000 population
Under 17	17.7
17–44	43.8
45–64	142.9
65 and older	283.8

[a]Including tinnitus. As reported by the 1981 U.S. National Health Interview Survey (Ries, 1985).

clinical audiogram consists of a plot of an individual's hearing threshold relative to a *standard observer* over a range of stimulus frequencies (e.g., ANSI Standard S3.6-1969—see American National Standards Institute, 1970).

Clinical audiograms typically sample hearing ability in the frequency range from 250 to 8000 Hz. Relative measures of auditory function (known as *hearing levels*) are usually expressed in terms of a logarithmic unit known as the *decibel* (dB). For example, a hearing level of 6 dB would mean that you required twice as much sound pressure as the standard observer to detect a tone, while a hearing level of 20 dB would indicate that you required 10 times more sound pressure than the standard observer [see Gulick *et al.* (1989) for a discussion of decibel scales].

The hearing loss for pure tones that usually accompanies aging is typically referred to as *presbycusis*. The early onset of presbycusis typically involves a loss of hearing sensitivity for only the very highest frequencies. Clinical audiometry tends to underestimate the magnitude of presbycotic hearing loss, as audiograms typically fail to sample frequencies above 8 KHz—a frequency well below the cutoff frequency of hearing in healthy, young adults (Møller, 1983). Spoor (1967) combined the results of eight classic studies to formulate the composite hearing curves for age, sex, and frequency, which are depicted in Figure 4. These curves represent the amount of hearing loss experienced by persons of increasing age relative to the average hearing level obtained from persons age 25. Several trends are apparent in these data. First, one can see the emergence of a high-frequency loss beginning at around age 40. Second, as age increases, the magnitude of this hearing loss becomes greater and begins to encroach upon the lower audio frequencies. Third, the nature of the hearing loss for high-frequency pure tones is greater among men than among women of comparable age.

Robinson and Sutton (1979) also reviewed the results of several large-scale, cross-sectional studies of hearing levels as a function of age. They developed a set of mathematical functions that related pure-tone hearing loss (relative to the average 18-year-old) to normal aging. Their mathematical model was especially useful because it provided an account of the wide range in variability seen among persons of the same age, both within and across studies. Some of the curves generated by their mathematical model that depict age-related hearing loss at 4 KHz appear in Figure 5. These curves extend the data presented by Spoor (1967) by demonstrating the relative aging functions for individuals falling at the 10th, 25th, 50th, 75th, and 90th percentiles of their respective age groups. Note that the amount of hearing loss accompanying aging is minimal for persons in the top 25% of the population. However, even among this most fortunate subset of the modeled population, a clear pattern of age-related loss is still apparent. These changes probably represent "pure" presbycusis; that is, age-related changes in hearing independent of pathology and/or exposure to environmental insults such as industrial noise.

Several longitudinal investigations of age-related changes in pure tone hearing sensitivity have been reported in the literature (e.g., Milne, 1977; Møller, 1981; Brandt & Fozard, 1990). These studies have tended to support the accounts derived from classic cross-sectional studies such as Corso (1963) and those outlined above. Brandt and Fozard (1990) collected data from 813 male participants of the Baltimore Longitudinal Study of Aging over a 20-year period from 1968 to 1987. The average testing interval was three years. They found that hearing thresholds in males declined across the entire adult life-

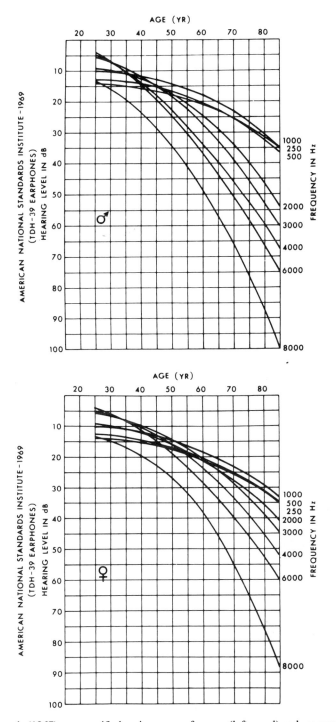

Figure 4 Spoor's (1967) age-specific hearing curves for men (left panel) and women (right panel). The original data was modified to conform to the ANSI-1969 standard, (TDH–39 earphones). (Adapted from C. P. Lebo and R. C. Reddell, 1971. Reproduced with the permission of the Triological Foundation, Inc.)

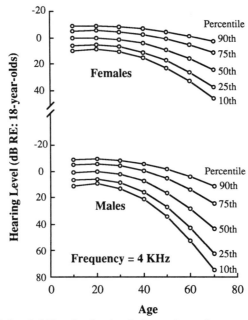

Figure 5   Predicted threshold hearing levels relative to the performance of the typical 18-year-old for females (top panel) and males (bottom panel). These curves are for a 4-KHz pure tone stimulus and represent the expected performance of persons at the 10th through 90th percentiles (numbers at right) across age.

span. For high-frequency stimuli (8 KHz), a continuous rate of decline of approximately 1 dB per year was observed between the ages of 20 and 80. However, for the range of frequencies that contribute most heavily to speech perception (500 to 2000 Hz), a different pattern was observed. These speech frequencies demonstrated a loss of about 0.3 dB per year through age 60 and then rapidly climbed to a rate of loss approaching 1.4 dB per year from ages 60 through 80. Møller (1981) collected audiograms from 261 randomly selected men and women at age 70 and again at age 75. Consistent with the results of the Baltimore Longitudinal Study, she reported that men showed a loss of approximately 1 dB per year at 8 KHz. However, the women in Møller's sample of Swedish adults showed a loss of approximately 2—3 dB per year. Møller (1981) suggested that women showed more high-frequency loss between the ages of 70 and 75 because their hearing at age 70 was better and, hence, they had more potential for subsequent loss than their male counterparts. That is, women of the 1901 to 1902 birth cohort in Sweden had probably been exposed to much less industrial noise than their male counterparts. As such, the potential impact of normal aging upon the males was lessened because they had already suffered considerable loss of their hearing potential due to prolonged exposure to environmental noise. This apparent gender difference in the rate of auditory aging needs to be examined more fully in future research endeavors [see Corso (1980) for an interesting discussion of gender by age interactions in hearing ability].

One of the fundamental issues of research into hearing and aging has centered upon the question: "To what extent does life-long exposure to environmental noise contribute to the development of presbycusis?" The results of several often-cited, cross-cultural studies have suggested that most of the age-related loss in hearing observed in Western societies results from accumulated damage due to prolonged exposure to high levels of environmental noise (e.g., noise from industrial machinery, highway traffic, etc.). The most well-known example of such a study is that of Rosen, Bergman, Plester, El-Mofty, & Satti (1962), who collected audiometry data from members of the Mabaan tribe in the Sudan. The Mabaans represented a nonindustrialized society that had not been exposed to the hazards of noise pollution. The audiograms collected from the older members of the tribe did not show the high-frequency hearing loss characteristic of presbycusis. This finding was interpreted as support for the notion that presbycusis results from exposure to noise. A study of inhabitants from remote regions of Cameroon also found a reduction (not absence) of presbycusis among older individuals who lived in low-noise environments (Siminetta, 1968; cited in Corso, 1981). Yet, other investigations of persons reared in environments free from industrial noise have failed to support the environmental noise model of presbycusis (e.g., Hinchcliffe, 1973; Kell, Pearson, & Taylor, 1970; Reynaud, Camara, & Basteris, 1969). However, these failures to replicate do not mean that noise does not play an important role in the mediation of age-related hearing loss. Corso's (1981) review of the cross-cultural literature regarding age-related hearing loss concluded that both noise and aging, *per se,* are significantly involved in the genesis of presbycusis. Once more, Corso (1980) has proposed a mathematical model that attempts to separate the covarying influences of age from noise exposure in late-life hearing loss. As discussed above, Møller (1981) has provided evidence that suggests that differential noise exposure histories may account for much of the typically observed sex difference in presbycusis. In a comparison of 197 females and 179 males aged 70, no sex differences were observed at low frequencies. However, males demonstrated greater levels of loss at higher frequencies. The magnitude of this sex difference was 15 and 10 dB at 4 and 8 KHz, respectively (Møller, 1981). This pattern of results suggests that the increased exposure risk of males to the damaging effects of noise has a direct impact upon the nature and magnitude of presbycusis, since the deleterious effects of prolonged exposure to industrial noise are known to elevate audiometric thresholds more at 4 KHz than at 8 KHz (National Institute for Occupational Safety, 1972). Relatedly, the distribution of hearing thresholds for the males at 4 KHz was bimodal rather than unimodal as is typically observed. This spread in the distribution of the data is consistent with an increased variability in male hearing thresholds due to differential exposure to noise within the male population. The sex differences in the spread of the hearing functions depicted in Figure 5 are consistent with this conclusion.

3. Auditory Frequency Analysis and Discrimination

The ability to discriminate between sounds of different frequencies is an important part of auditory processing and is thought to be critical for basic speech perception (Corso, 1981). Despite the potential significance of this ability, little research examining potential age differences is available. Konig (1957) investigated the ability to discriminate between pairs of 40 dB tones (i.e., well above threshold) on the basis of their frequency in males and females ranging in age from 20 through 90. Relative difference thresholds (frequency difference required at threshold divided by the frequency of the comparison stimulus) were found to vary systematically with age. Relative difference thresholds doubled between age 20 and 89 at intermediate stimulus frequencies (1 to 2 KHz). However, the magnitude of this age difference increased greatly at lower stimulus frequencies (125 to 500 Hz). In general, discrimination performance declined only slightly between the ages of 20 and 59, with an acceleration in the rate of the aging effect above age 60. The greater age-related loss in differential frequency sensitivity below 1000 Hz could not be predicted on the basis of normal presbycusis, which is characterized by high-frequency hearing loss. Hence, the nature and magnitude of the age decrement in differential frequency sensitivity is suggestive of neurological involvement. However, the nature of the mechanism mediating this phenomenon has yet to be established (Corso, 1981). Findings from studies of speech perception suggest that age differences in differential frequency sensitivity might be reduced or eliminated if test stimuli were presented at intensity levels of 80 dB or higher (Schieber, Fozard, Gordon-Salant, & Weiffenbach, in press).

4. Sound Localization

Localization of a sound source stems primarily from the auditory system's ability to process small differences in sound arrival time and intensity across the two ears (Geldard, 1972). Hence, the ability to localize sound is studied in the laboratory by determining the amount of interaural delay and intensity difference required to correctly lateralize the apparent spatial source of a stimulus. Using such techniques, several studies have found that sound-localization performance declines with advancing adult age (Tillman, Carhardt, & Nicholls, 1973; Herman, Warren, & Wagener, 1977; Warren, Wagener, & Herman, 1978). Herman et al. (1977) used a forced-choice procedure to reveal that men older than 60 required greater interaural time delays in order to successfully localize a sound stimulus. However, no age difference was observed in the amount of interaural intensity difference required for the localization of a sound. Since the localization of low-frequency stimuli is strongly mediated by the perception of interaural delays, while localization of high frequencies is dependent upon the processing of intensity differences between the ears, Olsho et al. (1985) have suggested that older adults will have problems localizing low-frequency sounds outside of the laboratory. This suggested deficit has important performance implications for tasks such as driving a car.

5. Speech Perception under Ideal Listening Conditions

A considerable amount of research has been conducted to demonstrate and explore the nature of age-related changes in the perception of speech. Taken together, these studies indicate that both peripheral and central mechanisms are involved in the declining levels of speech intelligibility that accompany old age. Many investigations have found support for the notion that speech perception in the elderly declines at a much faster rate than would be expected on the basis of age-related changes in pure-tone audiograms alone. Such *phonemic regression,* as it was termed by Gaeth (1948), has been demonstrated by Goetzinger, Proud, Dirks, & Embrey (1961), Jerger (1973), Plomp and Mimpen (1979),

Punch and McConnell (1969), and Stevenson (1975). The classic data regarding the loss of speech intelligibility with age are those of Jerger (1973), which are presented in Figure 6. Speech-recognition performance was assessed using monosyllabic words in over 2000 individuals sampled from a clinical population. Jerger found a disproportionate age deficit in older subjects, even when compared to younger subjects demonstrating pure-tone audiometric losses similar to those experienced by typical older adults. The existence of this disproportionate loss, which appears to be relatively independent of pure-tone hearing level, has typically been cited as support for a centrally mediated mechanism of aging.

However, not all researchers agree with this conclusion (Schieber *et al.*, in press). The classic studies on speech recognition and aging cited above employed low stimulus intensity levels, usually in the range of 20 to 40 dB (about 10 times less intense than normal conversation). When Gordon-Salant (1987) compared healthy young and old observers using more intense stimuli (about 10 times more intense than normal conversation), she failed to observe any systematic age-related decline in speech-recognition performance. Similarly, Møller (1981) found only very small reductions in speech-recognition performance among 376 randomly selected 70-year-olds. Females and males demonstrated mean recognition levels of 93 and 86%, respectively. Although worse than the performance of healthy young persons, these scores were far better than those that would be predicted by Jerger's (1973) data and are consistent with the degree of impairment observed among young patients with presbycotic-like high-frequency, pure-tone hearing loss (Møller, 1983). Hence, recent investigations using nonclinical samples and stimuli at or above conversational levels have failed to demonstrate support for phonemic regression under quiet testing conditions. These data are more consistent with a peripheral or patho-

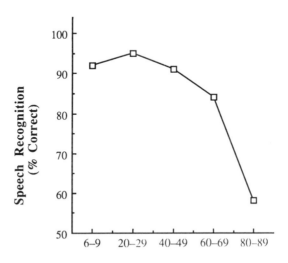

Age

Figure 6 Expected speech discrimination performance for phonetically balanced words as a function of age. (Adapted from J. Jerger, 1973. Reproduced with permission of S. Karger AG.)

genic explanation of age-related change in speech perception. Given recent advances in digital hearing aid technology, the potential role of peripheral loss in mediating changes in speech perception merits additional research attention (Schieber *et al.*, in press).

6. Speech Perception under Degraded Listening Conditions

Despite the controversy involving the magnitude and nature of age-related changes in speech perception observed under ideal laboratory or clinical conditions, much more robust, centrally mediated aging effects can be demonstrated under adverse listening conditions (Corso, 1981). Numerous studies have revealed that age-related performance deficits are exacerbated when speech stimuli are presented under challenging conditions. These conditions have included the addition of background noise and reverberation, alterations in the temporal rate of stimulus presentation, frequency filtering, and cyclic interruption of speech stimuli.

a. Noise.   Plomp and Mimpen (1979) found that the presence of background noise, rather than presbycusis, accounted for age differences in speech-recognition thresholds. Dubno, Dirks, and Morgan (1984) found age-related decrements in speech recognition when a 12-talker babble background was superimposed upon target-word stimuli (The babble simulated background conversations one might encounter in many real-world situations). When the test stimuli were presented without contextual information, older individuals required greater signal-to-noise ratios to recognize the target words. However, when the test stimuli were preceded by prompts that provided a rich linguistic context (or cues), the age differences were diminished. This finding suggests that in many situations, older adults may utilize cognitive processes to compensate for diminished sensory–perceptual functions such as extracting word stimuli from noisy backgrounds. This reliance upon cognitive compensatory processes could contribute to the age-related slowing in performance often observed upon behavioral tasks. Similar age-related decrements in performance have been observed when noise is characterized in terms of high levels of reverberation (e.g., Bergman, 1971; Nabelek & Robinson, 1982).

b. Time compression.   Increasing adult age is associated with a near universal slowing in the rate at which many higher-order cognitive processes are completed (Birren, Woods, & Williams, 1980; Salthouse, 1982). These centrally mediated constraints upon performance in the elderly clearly emerge when speech perception is studied under varying temporal presentation rates. Speech rates can be mechanically or electronically compressed so that the number of words per minute can be varied without affecting the frequency content of the words in a sentence. Such speeded speech is characterized acoustically by a reduction in the duration of both vowel and consonant phonetic segments as well as the duration of interword pauses (Picheny, Durlach, & Braida, 1986). As a result, the time available to process speeded speech is greatly diminished. Calearo and Lazzaroni (1957) found that speech-recognition performance among the young approached 100% at a rate of 350 words per minute while the performance of 6 persons aged 70 to 85 declined to 40%. Unlike the young subjects in this study, older adults failed to benefit in their perception of speeded speech when stimulus intensity level was increased. Stricht and Gray (1969) and Antonelli (1970) found similar age-related performance deficits for speeded speech using large groups of older persons with normal hearing. Møller (1981) tested 70-year-olds using 300-word-per-minute electronically speeded speech. Møller's older adults demonstrated speech recognition levels of 83% compared to near 100% performance for the young. Among the older subjects, but not younger ones, there was also a tendency for better performance when stimuli were delivered to the right ear (contralateral to the speech-dominant left cerebral hemisphere) as opposed to the left ear (Møller, 1983). Evidence for age-related changes in the lateralization of central auditory processing is also presented by Bergman (1983).

Young patients with high-frequency, pure-tone hearing losses show a deficit in the perception of speeded speech (Grimes, Mueller, & Williams, 1984). Since healthy older subjects show a similar hearing loss, it might be postulated that age differences in the perception of speeded speech are mediated by peripheral changes. However, the size and nature of this age-related deficit are more consistent with a centrally mediated loss. Older adults show much greater deficits than young adults with high-frequency impairment. In addition, unlike younger adults, performance deficits in the elderly stemming from increased presentation rate cannot be compensated for by increasing stimulus loudness levels (but see Otto & McCandless, 1982).

c. Interrupted speech. Studies employing interrupted speech stimuli have demonstrated remarkably large age effects. Interrupted speech consists of sentence-length passages that are cyclically turned on and off at a constant periodic rate. For example, 8 Hz interrupted speech would change between the signal "on" and "off" states every 62.5 msec. Individuals with lesions of the central auditory pathways and auditory cortex demonstrate disproportionate losses in speech-recognition performance under interrupted presentation conditions (Bocca & Colearo, 1963; Berlin & Lowe, 1972; Møller, 1983). Bergman (1971) measured speech-recognition performance in a large group of audiologically normal persons ranging in age from 20 to 89. Speech perception was tested using a variety of stimuli, including unaltered speech, reverberated speech (reverberation constant = 2.5 sec) and 8 Hz interrupted speech passages. The results of this study are presented in Figure 7. Exponential losses with age are seen for recognition performance in

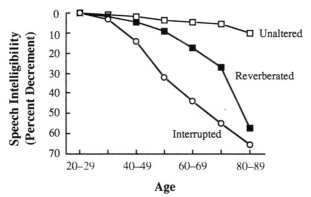

Figure 7 Relative speech intelligibility as a function of age for each of three listening conditions: unaltered speech, reverberated speech (tc, 2.5 sec), and speech interrupted at a rate of 8 Hz. (Adapted from M. Bergman, 1971. Reproduced with permission of S. Karger AG.)

both the unaltered and reverberated speech conditions. The nature of this exponential loss is much less severe for unaltered speech than for reverberated speech stimuli. However, the function depicting age-related performance under the interrupted speech condition is different in two important ways: first, the magnitude of the age-related loss is more pronounced; and, second, the aging function is linear rather than exponential in shape. The nature and magnitude of the age effect for interrupted speech suggests that this test may be tapping into a higher-order constraint or limiting process than the other measures of speech perception. Bergman (1980, 1983) reported additional evidence suggesting that age differences in the perception of interrupted speech are mediated by central mechanisms. Bergman varied the amount of time that the speech signal was on, in proportion to the silent time, while holding the rate of interruption constant. If performance of older persons were limited by the rate of higher-order information processing, then it was hypothesized that older subjects would improve less rapidly as the proportion of signal "on" time increased from low to high levels. The results of Bergman's study were consistent with the hypothesized age effect: the performance of young subjects improved rapidly with initial increments of stimulus "on" time while the performance of older adults improved little over the same temporal envelope. Bergman (1983) concluded that these findings were in agreement with Hicks and Birren's (1970) observation that degenerative changes of higher-order sites in the central nervous system limit processing speed and place constraints upon perceptual processing.

7. Social and Psychological Implications of Hearing Loss

The data reviewed above clearly suggest that older adults can expect to experience at least some hearing problems. In fact, between 30 and 40% of persons of retirement age will possess a degree of hearing loss that will lead to significant levels of functional disability (Gilhome-Herbst & Humphrey, 1980). A considerable volume of research has accumulated that has attempted to relate psychological health and social well-being to age-related hearing loss. These studies show that uncorrected mild to moderate hearing losses have little impact upon the social, emotional, and psychological health of elderly individuals (e.g., Norris & Cunningham, 1981; Thomas et al., 1983; Weinstein & Ventry, 1983). However, older individuals who have developed pure-tone hearing losses greater than 40 dB (in the speech frequency range) appear to be at increased risk of developing psychological and social problems (Gilhome-Herbst, 1983).

Gilhome-Herbst and Humphrey (1980) studied the effects of severe hearing impairment in a sample of 253 persons over the age of 70 who were fitted with hearing aids by the British National Health Service. Severe hearing impairment was defined as an average bilateral loss of at least 35 dB over the 1–4 KHz frequency range. Compared to age-matched subjects with normal hearing levels, the hearing-impaired elderly demonstrated statistically significant differences upon social and psychological rating scales, including decreased number and extent of trips out of the home; less satisfaction with trips from the home; fewer numbers of friends; perceived inability to contribute fully to a friendship; diminished enjoyment of life as a whole; and increased levels of depression. These differences remained even after factors such as age and general health status were statistically controlled. These findings mirror the results reported by other studies of older adults with severely impaired hearing (e.g., Alpiner, 1979; Jackson, 1979; von Leden, 1977). Many mental health researchers have repeatedly made an association between hearing loss and the development of depression (Denmark, 1976; Menninger, 1924; Ramsdell, 1978). Gilhome-Herbst and Humphrey (1980) found that fully 35% of their elderly hearing-impaired population were clinically depressed. This estimate exceeds the 25% prevalence rate of depression typically observed among the older population in general (Kay, Beamish, & Roth, 1964; Milne, Maule, & Williamson, 1971). An even stronger relationship was observed between hearing impairment and depression in a study of hearing aid patients of preretirement age. Thomas and Gilhome-Herbst (cited in Gilhome-Herbst, 1983) reported that employed persons with severe hearing impairment were four to five times more likely to be rated as depressed than were age-matched controls with normal hearing levels. It appears that the responsibilities associated with employment exacerbate adjustment problems associated with severe hearing loss. Conversely, retirement status may provide some degree of psychological protection following the onset of hearing impairment.

The characteristic response of the elderly to the development of adventitious hearing loss has long been described as one of *conscious denial* (e.g., Alpiner, 1979; Menninger, 1924; Glass, 1988; Ramsdell, 1978). Such denial is believed to greatly restrict the individual's range of behavioral responses and results in a state of *emotional numbing and ideational avoidance* (Horowitz, 1984). This notion of senescent denial, stemming from anecdotes and clinical observations, has recently received empirical support from a study reported by Gilhome-Herbst (1983). She attempted to administer a survey to 136 elderly persons with clinically confirmed severe hearing loss, but found that 27% refused to acknowledge that they suffered any problems with hearing. Hence, it would appear that active denial processes will have to be confronted when attempting to remediate hearing losses in many older individuals.

Finally, there has been a persistent belief that the presence of a hearing loss is associated with the onset of late-life paranoid psychosis and related paranoid disorders (e.g., Bromley, 1966; Post, 1966; Roth, 1976). In a review of the available literature, Cooper (1976) demonstrated that the risk of late-life paranoid psychosis may be associated with hearing loss, but only in cases in which the onset of the hearing loss occurred early in life. Hence, it would appear that late-life onset of hearing loss does not predispose an individual toward the development of paranoid mental illness. Moore (1981) also failed to find an association between age-related sensory loss and the development of paranoid psychopathologies.

8. Compensation for Severe Hearing Loss

Currently available techniques for compensating for severe hearing losses include the use of amplification through assistive listening devices and personal hearing aids, enhancement of environmental acoustic conditions, and participation in rehabilitation-oriented training programs. The most widely attempted remediation involves the use of personal hearing aids. These devices attempt to improve speech recognition and related tasks by amplifying sound. This approach often yields satisfactory results under ideal listening conditions. However, in situations where there is a significant level of background noise (such as in shops, restaurants, and many business locations) the effectiveness of hearing aids is often compromised. This is because conventional hearing aids amplify noise as well as the target sound. In fact, when the target source is distant, the background noise can be amplified to a greater extent than the source, thus reducing the signal-to-noise ratio. Because of such problems only about 50% of persons over the age of 65 who have been fitted with hearing aids use them on a continuous basis. In fact, upwards of 25% have discontinued the use of their hearing aids altogether (Upfold & Wilson, 1982). The most common reasons given for this failure of compliance include problems with the amplification of noise and the inability to tolerate the loudness levels required to restore speech intelligibility (Franks & Beckman, 1985). Research is needed to improve fitting and training procedures for the use of conventional hearing aids as well as the design of new hearing-aid technologies, which are better suited for operation in poor acoustic environments. The recent advent of the *digital* hearing aid represents a great potential for improving auditory function through techniques such as real-time phonetic power enhancement and dynamic noise suppression [see Levitt (1987) and Neuman (1987) for reviews]. These developments hold much promise for the realization of performance gains as well as improved acceptance by the elderly with severe hearing loss.

Much can be done to enhance environmental conditions in the service of improving speech recognition in the hearing-impaired elderly. Most of these techniques focus upon the reduction of background noise sources and reverberation (see Schieber, *et al.,* in press for a review). Speech-reception capacity can also be improved through participation in aural rehabilitation programs. These programs usually consist of a comprehensive combination of training in the use of assistive technology, applied acoustics, speechreading (if necessary) and counseling. Kaplan's (1985) review of the literature indicates that older adults can benefit much from such programs. In fact, the most significant factor limiting the effectiveness of aural rehabilitation programs for the elderly appears to be underutilization of such services. Fewer than 25% of elderly persons who could benefit from aural rehabilitative services actually receive them (McCarthy, 1985) probably owing to limited professional referral and lack of awareness that such services exist (Shadden & Raiford, 1984). It would appear that a public education program regarding the nature and availability of aural rehabilitative services is in order.

III. Taste

Cells lying within the mouth respond differentially to the presence and concentration of a wide variety of chemical compounds. Activity within these cells is transduced into neural information, which ultimately gives rise to our sense of taste. Gustatory perception has traditionally been described as having a quantitative dimension (i.e., intensity) and a qualitative aspect. This qualitative dimension consists of the four basic categories of taste, namely sweet, sour, salty, and bitter. However, human taste perception is complex, and the taste experience cannot be conceptualized as the simple additive mixture of these four basic categories in a manner analogous to the mixing of primary colors (Corso, 1981). Once more, as will be discussed below, human taste perception interacts highly with covarying stimulation received by the olfactory system. Together these senses play an important role in the regulation of eating behavior and, hence, the maintenance, health and pleasure of the individual.

A. Age-Related Structural Changes in the Taste System

Taste buds are the structures in the mouth that transduce concentrations of specific chemical compounds into a graded response within the nervous system. Although taste buds are found throughout the oral cavity, they are concentrated in clusters of tissue known as papillae on the upper surface of the tongue. Fungiform papillae hold one to five taste buds each and are distributed over the anterior two thirds of the tongue. Foliate papillae occupy the posterior edges of the tongue. Circumvallate papillae, which are few in number, hold 200–300 taste buds each and are located in the central posterior region of the tongue (Corso, 1981). Taste buds are highly specialized epithelial cells containing receptor sites that enable only specific classes of chemical compounds to serve as an effective stimulus. The intensity of the taste stimulus appears to depend upon the number of taste buds stimulated (Arvidson & Freiberg, 1980; Smith, 1971). The neural information generated by the taste buds' interaction with their chemical environment is conveyed along several functionally distinct pathways by cranial nerves VII and IX to the nucleus of the solitary tract in the medulla (Kinnamon, 1987). At this level in the brain, stimulation from the taste buds feeds into circuits involving various motor systems, which serve to mediate oral reflexes such as coughing, spitting, salivation, swallowing, and gastric motility (Finger, 1987). The gustatory pathway next ascends to the parabrachial nucleus in the pons, which then projects to the posteromedial nucleus of the thalamus and ultimately to the cortex. Some neural fibers diverge from this course and project to the lateral hypothalamus and the amygdala. A detailed account of the central taste pathways has been provided by Norgen (1976).

Classic studies have reported that both the number of papillae (fungiform) and the number of taste buds per papilla decline with adult age. Mochizuki (1937) reported a 40% reduction in the number of circumvallate taste buds by age 60, while Arey, Tremaine, and Monzingo (1935) reported a 60% loss beyond age 74. Mochizuki (1939) reported no loss in foliate taste buds between the ages of 20 and 60, but a 20% loss from age 60 to 90. Moses *et al.*, (1967) counted the number of fungiform papillae in 200 persons aged 5 to 55 and reported a systematic decline in their number as a function of age. However, Miller (1988) has criticized the validity of these findings on the basis of sampling and procedural problems. In fact, several recent studies have failed to find an age-related decline in taste bud numbers. For example, Arvidson (1979) performed a postmortem study in which subjects were carefully selected and autopsied within 12 hours after death. An examination of 22 individuals ranging in age from birth to 90 revealed no correlation between age and the number of taste buds in fungiform papillae. Miller (1988) autopsied 18 cadavers ranging in age from 22 to 90. A 2 log unit (100-fold) range in taste bud counts was observed across individuals. This variation did not appear to depend upon age or sex. That is, intersubject variability was so large as to preclude the detection of a slight to moderate age-related change. Other age-related changes in the oral cavity that may affect taste perception have been noted. The epithelial layer of the tongue's upper surface decreases in thickness with age, resulting in a flattening in its surface with a possible alteration in the aqueous access to the taste buds (Shklar, 1966). Probably of greater significance is the documented change in the saliva of older adults. Many foodstuffs must be dissolved in saliva before chemical access to the taste buds is made possible. Change in the quantity or qualitative properties of saliva could affect taste in many ways. Saliva production has been shown to decline with age (Balogh & Lelkes, 1961; Pickett, Appleby, & Osborn, 1972). This reduction in quantity appears to be accompanied by a chemical change in saliva content, together with an increase in its viscosity (Pickett, Appleby, & Osborn, 1972; Wainwright, 1943). Data regarding normative age-related changes in the ascending gustatory pathways are not currently available.

B. Absolute Taste Sensitivity

The absolute threshold for taste is defined by the minimal aqueous concentration of a chemical compound that can be detected reliably. Age-related increases in taste threshold for compounds in solution have been reported by numerous investigators (e.g., Cooper, Bilash, & Zubek, 1962; Harris & Kalmus, 1959; Hinchcliffe, 1962; Murphy, 1979; Richter & Campbell, 1940). In general, these studies found significant losses in threshold taste sensitivity, which grew exponentially larger across the adult lifespan. Murphy (1979) reported an average 1 log unit (10-fold) increase in taste thresholds between the ages of 30 and 80. Harris and Kalmus (1949) examined taste thresholds in 441 individuals ranging in age from 10 to 91. They reported that thresholds doubled with every 20-year increment in age. In a longitudinal followup of this study, Kalmus and Trotter (1962) retested many of the same individuals 10 to 15 years later and observed a 3% increment in threshold per year—a rate of loss that mirrored the cross-sectional findings. However, more recent studies (which used healthy noninstitutionalized samples and more rigorous psychophysical procedures) have demonstrated age-related losses that are less severe in magnitude and that vary as a function of the taste category being examined. For example, Weiffenbach, Baum, & Burghauser (1982) collected taste-threshold data from participants of the Baltimore Longitudinal Study on Aging who ranged in age from 23 to 88. Using a two-alternative, forced-choice procedure, thresholds representing all four taste categories were determined: viz., sweet (sucrose), salty (sodium chloride), sour (citric acid), and bitter (quinine sulfate). As in the classical studies, age was associated with a 1 log unit decline in threshold sensitivity for the salty solution. However, a much smaller age-related decline (half a log unit) was observed for the bitter solution, while no significant age-related change in threshold sensitivity was observed for the sweet or sour tastants. Perhaps the most interesting outcome of this study was the fact that very few persons demonstrated a general loss of sensitivity across taste categories. That is, while 38 of the 144 subjects had threshold sensitivities below the 10th percentile for one of the taste categories, only 6 of these individuals demonstrated reduced sensitivity for more than one taste category (see Schieber et al., in press). Similar findings of small or nonsignificant age-related declines in taste sensitivity among healthy, community-resident participants have been reported by others (e.g., Grzegorczyk, Jones, & Minstretta, 1979). All of these studies reported large between-subject variability among their older participants. That is, although sensitivity declined in many older adults, a large proportion of the elderly performed at or better than the average values obtained by their young counterparts. There is some evidence that significant reductions in taste sensitivity observed prior to age 60 may result from secondary, rather than primary, age-related mechanisms such as a prolonged history of cigarette smoking (e.g., Kaplan, Glanville, & Fischer, 1965; Smith & Davies, 1973) and the increased use of prescription drugs—especially medications associated with hypertension (see Schiffman, 1983; Spitzer, 1988).

C. Suprathreshold Taste Perception

Absolute threshold measures provide important information about the ultimate sensitivity and overall integrity of a sensory system. However, knowledge of one's absolute threshold level provides little information about the magnitude of one's sensory experience across the full range of stimulus intensities over which a given sense modality operates. For example, absolute threshold data would not be useful if you wanted to know how much sugar you needed to add to your coffee to make it taste twice as sweet. Using suprathreshold psychophysical scaling techniques, Stevens (1962) found that, in general, the magnitude of a sensation can be described as a power function of stimulus intensity

$$[\text{i.e., sensation} = k(\text{stimulus intensity})^n]$$

When such a power function is plotted with logarithmic stimulus and sensation coordinates, it forms a straight line whose slope is equivalent to the exponent n. If the exponent of such a scaled psychophysical function is less than 1.0, then the neurosensory system is compressing information. That is, to obtain a doubling in the magnitude of sensation one would have to *more than double* the intensity of the stimulus. The exact amount required would be given by the magnitude of the exponent. Psychophysical intensity functions for taste, like most sensory systems, yield exponents less than 1.0 (Geldard, 1972).

Magnitude estimation is the most commonly used procedure for scaling suprathreshold sensory intensity functions. Subjects are presented with a random series of stimuli that vary only along a single dimension. The first stimulus is assigned a number that reflects the intensity of the individual's concomitant perceptual experience. This procedure is repeated several times for each of many stimulus intensity levels over a broad continuum (usually several log units); the subjects are required to numerically rate the magnitude of the perceptual response accompanying each stimulus. For example, if the subject assigns a value of 10 to the first stimulus, and the magnitude of the second stimulus is perceived as being twice as strong, a value of 20 would be reported. If, instead, it appeared only half as strong, a value of 5 would be given. Numerous studies have revealed that observers are capable of giving reliable and meaningful numerical estimates to the magnitude of their perceptual experiences. These data are then normalized and fit to a standard mathematical function. An exponent representing the best fit of the data to this function is calculated for each individual [see Marks (1974) for a complete discussion of magnitude estimation]. When log sensory magnitude is plotted as a function of log stimulus intensity this exponent is proportional to the slope of the resulting psychophysical function. Several studies have demonstrated age differences in the slope of suprathreshold intensity functions based upon magnitude estimations of taste stimuli. Schiffman and Clark (1980) collected intensity functions from 106 young (18–22) female students and 42 older (65+) female residents of a retirement home. Magnitude estimations were made for 23 different amino acids (which tend to taste sweet) while participants wore a nose plug to minimize the confounding influence of odor. In general, the older participants yielded psychophysical intensity functions that were much flatter than those generated by the young subjects. Ratios of young-to-old slopes ranged from a high of 10.9 for L-aspartic acid to 1.1 for L-lysine. The average young-to-old ratio across all 23 tastants was 2.55. These results suggest that (at least for most amino acids) an older person would require a much greater increment in stimulus intensity in order to realize the equivalent increment of sensation magnitude experienced by a typical young person. Similar findings of an age-related flattening in the psychophysical intensity function for 10 artificial sweeteners was reported by Schiffman, Lindley, Clark, & Makins (1981).

Weiffenbach, Cowart, and Baum (1986, p. 461) argued that the findings of Schiffman and her associates could not be used to make generalizations about age differences in suprathreshold taste perception because (1) the number of subjects per tastant was small, (2) only tastants from the *sweet* category were tested, and (3) all of the subjects except one were female. In response, Weiffenbach *et al.* (1986) examined age differences in suprathreshold intensity functions across the four major taste categories using sucrose (sweet), sodium chloride (salty), citric acid (sour), and quinine sulfate (bitter). Ninety-one men and 79 women between the ages of 23 and 88 were sampled from the Baltimore Longitudinal Study on Aging. Rather than using numbers to estimate the magnitude of sensation, a cross-modality matching procedure was employed. Subjects matched the length of a retractable steel tape to the perceived intensity of each concentration of the taste stimuli. Responses were averaged across the multiple exposures of each taste category. Regression analyses of the slopes of the individual intensity functions resulted in a small but statistically significant age-related decrease in slope for citric acid and quinine. No age differences in slope were observed for sucrose and sodium chloride. Analyses of the group psychophysical intensity functions revealed a remarkable similarity in performance among the subjects older than 40, who as a group, demonstrated somewhat flatter functions than those younger than 40. On the basis of this finding, young : old (younger than 40 : older than 40) slope ratios analogous to those reported by Schiffman and her associates can be calculated. The resulting young : old ratios were 1.14, 1.13, 1.12 and 1.08 for the bitter, sweet, salty, and sour categories, respectively. These values yield a much different picture of age differences in suprathreshold taste perception from the great *flattening* of response revealed by Schiffman and Clark's (1980) finding of a mean young : old slope ratio of 2.55.

Bartoshuk, Rifkin, Marks, and Bars (1986) used magnitude estimation to collect concurrent suprathreshold intensity functions for loudness and taste in 18 young (mean age, 24.4) and 18 old (mean age, 82.8) subjects. The four basic taste categories were investigated using sodium chloride, sucrose, citric acid, and quinine hydrochloride. The intensity functions for loudness used low-frequency noise limited to a band where age differences in pure tone audiometry were minimal. The loudness functions of the two age groups were highly similar. Using a procedure known as magnitude matching (J. Stevens & Marks, 1980), the psychophysical intensity functions obtained for the various taste categories were normalized using each individual's loudness function. By standardizing the taste functions using the common psychophysical continuum of loudness, absolute age differences in the taste functions become more meaningful (see Murphy, 1987, p. 257). The normalized taste functions for all four categories tended to become somewhat flatter with age. The age difference in the intensity functions for the sour tastant (i.e., citric acid) is reproduced in Figure 8. Across most of the 2.25 log unit range of stimulus intensities, the functions for the two age groups overlapped. However, over the lower region of stimulus intensities (which extended about 0.5 log units above absolute threshold), the older subjects tended to report greater magnitudes of taste sensation than their younger counterparts. A similar age-related elevation of the lower portion of the intensity function was seen with the other three taste categories as well. Hence, it would appear that the primary reason for the age-related reduction in the slope of the psychophysical functions was the elevation of the lower portion of the curves. This suggests that age differences in taste intensity are minimal for stimulus levels 0.5–1.0 log units above threshold. The data of Weiffenbach *et al.* (1986) were not characterized by this upward shift at low intensities. However, it should be noted that the weakest stimulus levels used for each tastant in their study began at about 0.5 log units higher than the minima employed by Bartoshuk, Rifkin, Marks, and Bars (1986). It is interesting to note that the age group intensity functions of Bartoshuk *et al.* start to overlap at about the same stimulus levels where the data collection of Weiffenbach *et al.* began. Bartoshuk and her associates suggested that the intensity functions of their old subjects looked "as if a background taste had been added to the lower concentrations" (p. 56). Such a background taste attributed to water and dilute stimulus solutions may have reflected a mild form of *dysgeusia*—that is, a persistent taste in the mouth. Mild forms of dysguesia can affect taste thresholds and may result from

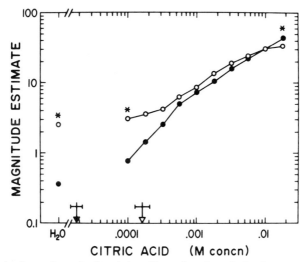

Figure 8   Perceived taste intensity for citric acid as a function of stimulus concentration for young (●, mean age of 24) and elderly (○, mean age of 83) participants. (Adapted from L. Bartoshuk *et al.* Reproduced with the permission of the Gerontological Society of America.)

chronic age-related conditions such as tooth decay, periodontal disease, and the use of dentures (e.g., Cimasoni, 1974; Henkin & Christiansen, 1967; Langan & Yearick, 1976).

Bartoshuk (1989) has recently presented data that may help explain further the conflicting findings obtained by studies investigating age differences in suprathreshold taste perception. She found when stimulus solutions were applied directly to *discrete* locations on the surface of the tongue that older persons demonstrated large reductions in perceived taste intensity at some sites but not at others. Apparently, aging is associated with the development of *localized taste losses* at various sites across the tongue. When the same subjects were tested by stimulating the whole mouth using the more traditional *sip-and-rinse* procedure, the age effect was greatly minimized. Despite localized losses in function, the aging taste system appears to compensate by integrating and normalizing information provided by the sensory regions of the tongue that remain intact.

D. Flavor Recognition

On the basis of the suprathreshold taste intensity data, one would expect to observe little or no age difference in the recognition of everyday foodstuffs and additives. Yet, the elderly often complain about the *odd* or *diminished* flavor of foods (e.g., Cohen & Gitman, 1959). Once more, there is ample experimental evidence that older adults possess major deficits in the recognition of common household flavorants and foods (e.g., Murphy, 1986; Schiffman, 1977). Schiffman (1977) examined food recognition ability in a sample of 27 young (18–22) and 29 old (67–93) persons. Twenty-four common foods (e.g., fruits, vegetables, meats, fish, nuts, dairy products, grains) were pureed to minimize texture cues and served at 160°F. Participants tasted the food samples while blindfolded to eliminate the effects of color cues. The young subjects demonstrated a remarkable superiority in their ability to recognize and correctly identify the food samples under these conditions. In fact, the young demonstrated significantly superior recognition for 21 of the 24 foods tested. How could such a large age difference in food-recognition performance be observed given the near age-equivalence of the suprathreshold taste intensity functions? The ability of Schiffman's subjects to recognize the flavor of foodstuffs was based upon the use of odor as well as taste information. Murphy (1979, 1986) reasoned that the large, unexpected deficit in food-recognition performance was not due to age differences in taste mechanisms but, instead, resulted from age-related losses in the sense of smell. Murphy (1986) repeated Schiffman's (1977) recognition experiment using 12 of the same food items and observed the same superiority among the young subjects. However, when the subjects' nostrils were obstructed so that olfactory information was minimized, the age difference in food recognition was eliminated, and the performance of the young subjects fell to the impoverished level of their older counterparts. These findings support the conclusion that age differences in suprathreshold taste perception are minimal and that age-related problems with the recognition and enjoyment of food items stem from a deficit in the olfactory system. Data supporting this view have been presented by numerous investigators (e.g., Schemper, Voss, & Cain, 1981; Stevens, Plantinga, & Cain, 1982).

IV. Olfaction

Olfaction, our ability to detect and identify airborne chemical substances as specific odors, plays an important role in determining the flavor and palatability of the food we eat. In addition, our sense of smell serves as an early warning system for the detection of fire and dangerous fumes stemming from polluted environments (Doty *et al.*, 1984). As seen above, evidence from research on flavor perception indicates that adult aging is accompanied by a precipitous loss of odor sensitivity. Additional evidence supporting this view is explored in the paragraphs that follow. For a detailed review of age-related changes in the chemical senses, the reader should refer to Murphy (1986).

A. Age-Related Structural Changes in the Olfactory System

The olfactory receptors that transduce airborne molecules of chemical stimuli into nervous system activity are located deep within the nasal cavity in an area known as the *olfactory epithelium*. These olfactory receptors are highly specialized neurons that possess a number of motile cilia, which are covered by a layer of mucous. These cilia agitate the mucous layer, which increases the likelihood of bringing a stimulus molecule in contact with the receptor cells (Bradley, 1979). The receptors contain specialized sites that interact with specific geometric properties of molecular stimuli. It is this *lock and key* interaction between receptor cells and stimuli that appears to give rise to the qualitative aspects of olfactory perception (Amoore, 1970). The human olfactory epithelium contains about 1 million receptor cells whose axons converge together to form the olfactory nerve, which projects directly to the *olfactory bulb* of the brain (Corso, 1981). Upon reaching the olfactory bulb, the axons of the receptor cells make their first synaptic connections within diffuse structures known as *glomeruli*. Olfactory information processed at the site of the glomeruli next is carried to the primary olfactory cortex, as well as being routed along secondary pathways to subcortical structures associated with memory and emotional functions (Schiffman, Orlandi, & Erickson, 1979).

Although little is known about the status of the ascending olfactory pathways in old age, several studies have documented age-related changes in the olfactory epithelium and olfactory bulb. Naessen (1971) used electron microscopy to examine age differences in the structure of the olfactory epithelium. By age 30, a clear degeneration in the olfactory receptors and their supporting cells was observed. Massive degeneration and receptor-cell loss was observed at age 60 (see Corso, 1981). Similar findings have been observed at the level of the olfactory bulb. Smith (1942) found that the number of atrophied glomeruli increased linearly with age. This atrophy advanced at a rate of approximately 1% per year until leveling off at age 75, when only about one quarter of the glomeruli remained intact. Liss and Gomez (1958) observed similar age-related changes in the olfactory bulb including a massive loss of neurons. They speculated that this loss resulted from environmental insult to the part of the olfactory neurons situated in the periphery, since viral and chronic nasal inflammatory diseases were known to adversely affect the olfactory epithelium. A comprehensive review of age-related changes in the olfactory anatomy can be found in Corso (1981).

B. Absolute Olfactory Sensitivity

The absolute threshold for the sense of smell is defined as the minimal number of stimulus molecules per volume of carrier gas that can be reliably detected. Early studies revealed that increasing adult age was associated with a general decline in absolute olfactory sensitivity (e.g., Chalke & Dewhurst, 1957; Joyner, 1963; Kimbrell & Furtchgott, 1963; Shiokawa, 1975). Recent studies, which have employed more rigorous psychophysical procedures and have sampled elderly participants from healthy, noninstitutionalized populations, have also demonstrated age-related losses in olfactory sensitivity. For example, Venstrom and Amoore (1968) used a forced-choice procedure to investigate age differences in detection thresholds for 18 commonly studied odorants. Overall relative sensitivity was reduced by a factor of 2 for each 20-year increment between the ages of 20 and 70. Although the magnitude of this age-related deficit varied across the stimuli, statistically significant age differences were observed for 15 of the 18 odor stimuli. Murphy (1983) found that old (mean age, 75) participants required a twofold increase in stimulus intensity to detect the presence of menthol. Stevens and Cain (1987) measured absolute olfactory thresholds for D-limonene (citrus), benzaldehyde (almond), and iso-amyl butyrate (fruity; e.g., apricot) in 20 young (18–24) and 20 old (70–90) adults. Significant age-related losses in sensitivity were observed for all three stimuli. However, the magnitude of the deficit varied across stimuli. Older adults demonstrated ninefold, threefold, and twofold sensitivity losses for D-limonene, benzaldehyde, and iso-amyl butyrate, respectively. This age by odorant interaction is consistent with the pattern of results reported by Kimbrell and Furtchgott (1963) and Venstrom and Amoore (1968). In general, there is strong evidence that olfactory thresholds increase with age. However, the magnitude of this loss has yet to be established and probably strongly interacts with the class of odor stimuli being examined (Murphy, 1986).

C. Suprathreshold Odor Perception

Numerous investigators have reported an age-related deficit in the ability to identify suprathreshold odor stimuli (e.g., Doty et al., 1984; Murphy, 1986; Schemper, Voss, & Cain, 1981; Stevens & Cain, 1987). Doty et al. (1984) administered a 40 odorant forced-choice smell identification test to 1955 individuals between the ages of 5 and 99. The relative performance of these individuals as a function of age and sex is depicted in Figure 9. The number of correct identifications reached a peak of 38 between the ages of 20 and 45 and then declined slightly to approximately 35 between the ages of 45 and 65. It is only after age 65 that a precipitous loss in the ability to identify odors was observed. More than half of those aged 65 to 80 evidenced major olfactory impairment. Beyond age 80, more than three quarters of the sample demonstrated major impairment. Females demonstrated a small but significant performance advantage at every age level. Of the 443 participants over the age of 60, 184 were residents of homes for the aged. Statistically significant losses were observed among these institutionalized subjects relative to age-matched community residents. This finding suggests that general health and/or cognitive factors exert a potentially significant role in odor perception among the elderly (Doty, 1989). Similar

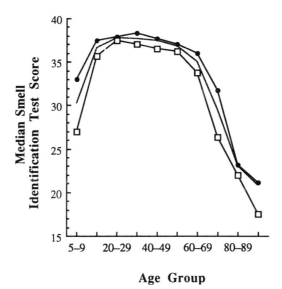

Figure 9   University of Pennsylvania Smell Identification Test (UPSIT) scores as a function of age and sex (—•— females, $n=1158$; —□— males, $n=797$; —— total group, $n=1955$) (Adapted from R. Doty *et al.* 1984. Reproduced with the permission of R. Doty and the American Association for the Advancement of Science.)

findings were obtained by the National Geographic Society Smell Survey, a "scratch and sniff" test that was completed by 1.42 million readers of *National Geographic* magazine (Wysocki & Gilbert, 1989). More severe age-related declines in odor-identification performance have been demonstrated using other types of stimuli. For example, Murphy (1986) administered a battery of 80 odorants to persons ranging in age from 19 to 68. She found that correct identification declined from approximately 70% at age 20 to 35% at age 65. Similar findings were reported by Stevens and Cain (1987) who observed a threefold decrease in odor identification performance with advancing adult age. The difference in the magnitude of the age effect across the Doty *et al.* (1984) and subsequent studies may be owing to the fact that the Doty *et al.* investigation required subjects to choose their responses from a list of alternatives (i.e., a multiple-choice test) rather than relying upon uncued recall (see Schonfield & Robertson, 1966). Nonetheless, the available evidence consistently reveals that significant age-related decrements in odor identification exist, at least for those aged 65 and older.

Several investigators have examined age differences in suprathreshold intensity functions for the sense of smell (e.g., Murphy, 1983; Stevens & Cain, 1987; Stevens *et al.*, 1982). Stevens and Cain (1987) determined suprathreshold intensity functions for three odorants using the magnitude-matching technique (discussed above). Perceived magnitude of odor sensation across a wide range of stimulus concentrations was normalized to each individual's magnitude estimation function for taste (sodium chloride). Expressing odor-intensity functions relative to a common scale of concurrent estimates for taste sensation enabled absolute comparisons of sensory experience across age groups for the olfactory modality (see Stevens & Marks, 1980). Absolute age-related declines in the magnitude of suprathreshold odor sensation were observed for all three odorants. No age differences in the slopes of the psychophysical intensity functions were obtained for D-limonene (citrus) or iso-amyl butyrate (apricot), suggesting that an age-related decrement in the perceived magnitude of these stimuli would be observed across all stimulus intensity levels. These results replicated the previous findings of Stevens et al. (1982). However, an age difference in the slope of the psychophysical intensity function for benzaldehyde (almond) was observed. That is, relative to the young, older subjects perceived benzaldehyde as less intense as stimulus concentrations increased above threshold. Murphy (1983) also observed some age-related flattening of the suprathreshold odor intensity function for menthol. Hence, studies of suprathreshold odor functions agree that there is a general decrease in the magnitude of odor sensation with age and that the magnitude of this effect across stimulus intensity and type varies as a function of the odorant being examined.

D. Compensating for Chemosensory Losses

The elderly often suffer from a chronic loss of appetite, which can lead to a state of malnutrition (Massler, 1980). Although geriatric anorexia is mediated by many cognitive and psychological variables (e.g., depression), there is evidence that eating behavior and the enjoyment of food can be enhanced by compensating for age-related losses in chemosensory sensitivity. Since age differences in pure taste sensitivity have been shown to be minimal, one would predict that age-related deficits in flavor perception would be mitigated through the amplification of the odor rather than taste components of food. Indeed, Schiffman (1979) found that older persons rated food as more palatable when flavor (olfactory) enhancing essences were added. Similar findings have been reported by Schiffman and Warwick (1988). Schiffman also noted that the reported improvements in the flavor of the odor-enhanced foods was also accompanied by a decrease in complaints regarding bitterness by the elderly. Schiffman speculated that the bitter components of many foods (such as certain vegetables and chocolate) may be masked when their concomitant odor components are sufficiently intense. It should be noted, however, that the food enhancements reported as improvements for the elderly were generally judged less pleasing by young subjects.

Some preventive measures can be adopted to enhance flavor perception in old age. For example, olfactory sensitivity can be optimized by avoiding smoking and by receiving timely treatment for inflammatory nasal diseases, which can affect the long-term status of the olfactory epithelium. A review of the factors which can be manipulated to optimize flavor perception in the elderly can be found in Schieber et al. (in press).

V. Cutaneous Sensitivity

The skin is a complex organ that covers the entire surface of the human body. It serves as a protective barrier against noxious environmental stimuli and disease, participates in thermal regulation via the sweat glands, and provides a rich source of sensory information. The sensory properties of the skin can be divided into three major functional subdivisions: mechanical sensitivity, temperature sensitivity, and pain. The major findings regarding age-related changes in these areas of cutaneous sensory function are reviewed in the sections that follow.

A. Age-Related Changes in Cutaneous Sensory Structures

A diffuse network of fine peripheral nerves extends throughout the various regions of the skin. Most of these nerves possess *free endings* that appear to be highly sensitive to thermal and noxious stimuli. However, many of the fibers enervating the skin have developed encapsulated endings, which appear to be highly specialized transducers for mechanical deformations of the skin. For example, the nonhairy (i.e., glabrous) skin of the hands, feet, and other bodily regions contain *Meissner's corpuscles*—cylindrical nerve endings that apparently mediate fine touch perception. *Pacinian corpuscles* represent another, more deeply located type of mechanical receptors, which mediate the perception of deep pressure and vibration (Geldard, 1972). The cutaneous receptors responsible for touch and vibration sensitivity converge to form the *lemniscal* system. These receptors are connected via long axons to their cell bodies, which congregate to form the *dorsal spinal roots* located near the spinal cord. These same cells ascend the spinal column to the medulla where they form their first synapse. At this point, the nerves cross over to the opposite side of the brain and project to the contralateral somatosensory cortex by way of the thalamus. The cutaneous receptors that play a dominant role in the mediation of temperature and pain perception converge to form the *extralemniscal* system. The ascent of this system is somewhat more diffuse. The long axons of the receptors project via their cell bodies in the dorsal spinal roots directly to the spinal cord. However, instead of traveling to the medulla, these axons immediately synapse with contralateral spinal neurons. Most of these cells then project to the thalamus and ultimately to the somatosensory cortex. However, many of these fibers bypass the cortical route and project directly to regions in the reticular formation and the cerebellum (Corso, 1981).

Numerous age-related changes in the properties of the skin and its receptors have been documented. Several investigators have noted that the skin becomes less elastic with age (e.g., Jackson, 1972; Pearce & Grimmer, 1972). Such a change could alter cutaneous sensitivity to mechanical stimuli. Systematic declines in the quantity and quality of Meissner's corpuscles also accompany adult aging (e.g., Bolton, Winkleman, & Dyck, 1966; Cauna, 1965; Quilliam & Ridley, 1971). Age-related atrophy of Pacinian corpuscles was reported by Cauna (1965). The ascending pathways carrying cutaneous information to the brain have also been found to suffer from age-related structural changes. Corbin and Gardner (1937) reported a significant age-related loss in the number of axons projecting from the dorsal spinal roots. Similar results were confirmed in a followup study by Gardner (1940). Changes in the myelinization of ascending cutaneous axons, which could potentially disrupt the temporal coding of sensory inputs, have been reported by Lascelles and Thomas (Kenshalo, 1977). Hence, anatomical findings suggest that age-related deficits in cutaneous sensitivity should be expected. The magnitude and nature of these deficits, as revealed by psychophysical investigations, are discussed below.

B. Absolute Touch Sensitivity

Classical studies have consistently reported that advancing age is associated with a loss in absolute touch sensitivity (e.g., Axelrod & Cohen, 1961; Howell, 1949; Ronge, 1943). Howell (949) found that 5% of 200 elderly participants failed to detect a criterion touch stimulus (e.g., the cotton-wool test). Using modified von Frey hairs, stimulus fibers designed to deliver calibrated levels of pressure to a point on the skin, Axelrod and Cohen (1961) examined age differences in touch sensitivity for the glabrous surfaces of the palm and thumb. They reported highly significant deficits in touch sensitivity for old (63–78) as compared to young (20–36) participants. More recent studies that have employed healthy older adults, as well as procedures to control response-bias effects, have tended to confirm the results of classical investigations. For example, Thornbury and Minstretta (1981) observed a continuous loss of sensitivity for punctate pressure stimulation upon the pad of the index finger between the ages of 19 and 88. Concomitant measures of skin temperature at the site of stimulation failed to account for any of this age difference. Hence, the investigators concluded that local decreases in blood flow were not responsible for age difference in cutaneous sensitivity. However, they did find that the data relating loss of Meissner's corpuscles to advancing age (Bolton et al., 1966) agreed well with the ob-served age-related decline in touch sensitivity. Kenshalo (1986) reported similar age differences for 0.5 sec ramp-and-hold deformations of the skin. Thresholds taken from the thenar eminence (glabrous base of the thumb) and the sole of the foot were sampled from 27 young (19–31) and 21 healthy older (55–84) adults. Age-related losses in sensitivity on the order of 0.5 and 1.0 log units were observed for the hand and foot locations, respectively. Again, the magnitude of the age difference in touch sensitivity was consis-tent with levels predicted by age-related losses in Meissner's corpuscles. However, age-related differences in touch sensitivity appear to involve more than the simple peripheral loss of a given class of cutaneous receptors. For example, both Boberg-Ans (1956) and Millodot (1977) have observed an accelerated loss in touch sensitivity at the cornea with advancing age. That is, a gradual loss of sensitivity between the ages of 10 and 50 followed by a rapid rate of decline between the ages of 60 and 90. The cornea, it should be noted, contains no Meissner's corpuscles and appears to be innervated only by a diffuse dermal nerve net.

C. Vibrotactile Sensitivity

The amplitude of oscillatory displacement of a stimulus on the skin that can just be detected yields the vibrotactile threshold. Vibrotactile sensitivity appears to involve mech-anisms other than those which limit absolute touch sensitivity (Verrillo & Verrillo, 1985). Classic experimental studies have demonstrated an age-related loss in vibration sensitivity that begins to emerge around age 50 and that appears to be more severe in the lower as opposed to the upper extremities (e.g., Cosh, 1953; Plumb & Meigs, 1961; Rosenberg, 1958; Steiness, 1957). More recent investigations have replicated and extended these findings (e.g., Era, Jokela, Suominen, & Heikkinen, 1986; Kenshalo, 1986; Petrosino, Fucci & Robey, 1982; Verrillo, 1980).

Vibrotactile sensitivity appears to be relatively independent of the rate of temporal modulation at frequencies below 50 Hz, but is highly influenced by changes in the rate of temporal modulation above this level. Hence, it appears that two distinct sensory systems mediate vibrotactile sensitivity: a high-frequency mechanism based upon the response of Pacinian corpuscles located deep within the dermal layer and a slower non-Pacinian system (Kenshalo, 1979). Verrillo (1980) examined vibrotactile sensitivity as a function of stimulus frequency in subjects ranging in age from 10 to 65. No adult age differences in sensitivity were reported for 25- and 40-Hz stimuli. However, an exponential age-related loss in vibrotactile sensitivity emerged and became more pronounced as stimulus frequency increased from 80 to 250 Hz. Similar findings were reported by Verrillo (1982). Verrillo and Verrillo (1985) have interpreted this *sparing* of sensitivity for low temporal frequency stimuli as evidence that age differences in mechanical sensitivity of the skin are due to systematic atrophy of Pacinian corpuscles. However, more recent findings reported by Kenshalo (1986) suggest that low-frequency, non-Pacinian mechanisms of vibrotactile perception may not be spared entirely during adult aging. Older adults (55–84) demonstrated a 0.5 log unit decline in 40 Hz (non-Pacinian) vibrotactile sensitivity of the hand relative to the young (19–31). It should be noted, however, that a larger age-related deficit (1.5 log) was observed when the stimulus oscillated at a rate of 250 Hz. Kenshalo (1986) also observed an additional log unit decline in sensitivity when the site of stimulation was moved from the hand to the foot, replicating the findings of earlier investigations.

Verrillo (1982) used a modification of the magnitude-estimation technique to investigate age differences in suprathreshold perception of vibrating stimuli. At 250 Hz, older adults demonstrated a constant loss in the perceived magnitude of vibratory stimuli across the full range of suprathreshold levels tested (i.e., no difference in the slope of the psychophysical function). The amount of this constant decrement in perceived magnitude of stimulation was approximately 1 log unit—a value similar to the size of the age difference in absolute vibrotactile threshold obtained at 250 Hz. Hence, older adults appear to experience high levels of vibration as less intense than younger adults to an extent that can be predicted by age differences in absolute vibration threshold.

D. Haptic Recognition

Haptic recognition refers to the ability to identify a stimulus on the basis of cutaneous information alone. Very little information regarding touch recognition in old age is currently available. Axelrod and Cohen (1961) had blindfolded young (20–36) and old (63–78) subjects use their hands to search for and identify geometric forms. Older adults identified many fewer targets and took significantly longer to do so. A similar pattern of results was obtained by Kleinman and Brodzinsky (1978) who had young (mean age, 18.8), middle-aged (mean age, 41.0) and old (mean age, 76.0) subjects perform 12 tactile match-to-comparison tasks. Compared to the young and middle-aged groups, the old demonstrate much less success in finding the match on the basis of tactile information alone. Additional analyses revealed that older adults demonstrated qualitative differences in their search behaviors and strategies, suggesting that an attentional and/or cognitive mechanism was responsible at least in part for the age-related performance deficit. Finally,

Kenshalo (1979, p. 210) has cited several studies that have demonstrated an age-related deterioration in the ability to identify geometric forms placed in the mouth.

E. Temperature Sensitivity

Temperature sensitivity refers to the ability to detect changes in the temperature of the skin. These changes may involve either increases (warming) or decreases (cooling) relative to the adapted temperature level of the skin. The temperature-sensation system appears to serve primarily as an *early warning* system. This alerting role of thermioception is evidenced by the finding that observers are more sensitive to temperature shifts away from the level of adaptation than toward it (Hensel, 1981). Little evidence regarding temperature sensitivity and aging is available. On the basis of the study of 3 older (70–74) adults, Kenshalo (1970) failed to find evidence for an age-related change in cutaneous temperature sensitivity. Clarke and Mehl (1971) investigated detection sensitivity for warming of the skin in young (mean age, 23.1; range: 18–30) and old (mean age, 46.6; range: 30–67) subjects. Only a very small difference in thermal sensitivity (d′) was observed. It should be noted that the so-called old sample primarily consisted of middle-aged adults. Kenshalo (1986) used a two-interval forced-choice procedure to assess potential age differences in cutaneous warming and cooling thresholds measured from both the hand and foot. No age differences were observed for the cooling thresholds collected at either the hand or foot. Negative age-related findings were also observed for the warming thresholds taken from the hand. A small but significant age-related decline for the warming threshold from the foot was observed. Taken together, the available evidence fails to demonstrate a general age-related change in the ability to detect the warming or cooling of the skin.

F. Pain Sensitivity

The evidence regarding age differences in cutaneous pain sensitivity remains inconclusive. Several studies that have employed radiant heat stimuli to elicit pain have reported an age-related decrease in pain sensitivity (e.g., Chapman & Jones, 1944; Procacci, Bozza, Buzzelli & Della Cort, 1970; Schluderman & Zubek, 1962; Sherman & Robillard, 1964). Procacci *et al.* (1970) found that the skin's ability to disperse thermal energy increased with age and attributed the age-related loss in thermal pain sensitivity to this peripheral change. Other investigators have attributed elevated cutaneous pain thresholds among the aged to more *stoic* response criteria (Clark & Mehl, 1971; Harkins, Kwentus, & Price, 1984). However, there are also studies of radiant-heat thresholds that have failed to demonstrate meaningful age differences in cutaneous pain sensitivity (e.g., Birren, Shapiro, & Miller, 1950; Hardy, Wolff, & Goodell, 1952; Kenshalo, 1986; Schumacher, Goodell, Hardy & Wolff, 1940). While radiant-heat studies have demonstrated both age-related declines as well as no age difference in pain sensitivity, investigations using electrical and pressure impulses to induce pain have reported age-related increases in pain sensitivity (e.g., Collins & Stone, 1965; Woodrow, Friedman, Siegelaub, & Collen, 1972). A thorough review and commentary regarding the factors contributing to the confusion regarding aging and pain perception can be found in Harkins *et al.* (1984).

VI. Future Considerations

A review of the literature on age-related changes in sensory-perceptual processes leads one to formulate recommendations regarding future research initiatives. Among the most critical considerations are a need to

1. account for the increased between-subject variability observed within older groups;
2. isolate peripheral versus central nervous system contributions to age-related sensory deficits;
3. explore more thoroughly suprathreshold sensory experience among the elderly;
4. explore how cognitive strategies are employed to compensate for reduced sensory abilities;
5. evaluate demonstrated opportunities for preventing age-related loss of sensory function due to environmental insult and disease; and
6. initiate remediation-based research aimed at optimizing the sensory-perceptual environment to the older individual.

Many researchers have noted the increased intersubject variability observed among samples of older adults. This trend has been found in virtually every one of the studies reviewed in this chapter. Yet, little systematic effort has been expended to identify and understand the factors underlying this increased variability. This characteristic of elderly populations represents more than a problem in meeting the basic assumptions required for our statistical analysis of the data. Instead, this increased variability holds much information that could help us evaluate the role of pathological versus "pure" aging mechanisms; identify factors amenable to preventive or remediation strategies; and/or provide important input toward choosing between *statistical* versus *deterministic* models of the aging process itself. Future attempts to understand the basis of this variability should yield rich results.

Across most of the sensory modalities, heated debate continues among researchers as to the *peripheral* versus *central* locus of age-related performance deficits. There is no doubt that peripheral degeneration of the sensory receptors and their supporting structures contribute to observed age differences. However, it is difficult to control the influence of these changes to an extent that the relative contribution of brain mechanisms can be evaluated unambiguously. Yet, when one examines age-related performance trends across the senses, it becomes apparent that central mechanisms must be playing an important role in the aging process. Figure 10 shows changes in visual, olfactory, and hearing performance across the lifespan. The basic shapes of these functions are the same despite the great differences in the nature and degree of peripheral atrophy observed across the three systems. The similarity of these curves suggests that a common, centrally mediated mechanism of sensory–perceptual aging is being manifest. The exponential nature of this

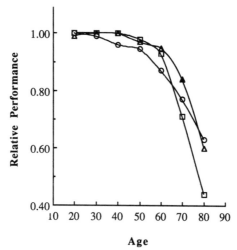

Figure 10   Life span losses in visual (□), olfactory (△), and hearing (○) ability. Based upon the visual-acuity data of Pitts (1972), the odor identification data of Doty *et al.* (1984), and the speech-recognition data of Jerger (1973).

aging effect is consistent with the pattern expected from a constant rate of random brain-cell loss with age. Such a mechanism is consistent with the histological findings.

Almost all of the research available regarding age differences in sensory–perceptual processes has been oriented toward the determination of detection, identification, and/or discrimination thresholds. Although threshold measures reveal much about the ultimate efficiency and integrity of a sensory system, they provide little information about sensory experience at the higher stimulus levels encountered in the real world. Research in the area of the chemical senses has revealed that age differences in suprathreshold sensory experience cannot be predicted on the basis of threshold data. In an attempt to better understand the potential impact of age-related sensory changes upon the ability to perform everyday tasks, future research efforts need to increase their focus upon suprathreshold stimulus levels. The need for evaluating suprathreshold performance functions is especially important in the area of vision research.

Applied research has revealed that age-related reductions in sensory capacity often are accompanied by the development of compensatory cognitive strategies that tend to minimize the functional impact of the sensory loss. For example, hearing-impaired elderly tend to rely upon contextual cues to "fill in the holes" of conversational speech. Similarly, older drivers with reduced visual function avoid driving at night or during rush hour traffic. Many such compensatory behaviors have been chronicled. Yet, the nature of these cognitive compensations for sensory losses and their impact upon psychological function have not been systematically explored. Many complex and important issues such as the impact of the additional cognitive load imposed by changing sensory capacities remain to be examined. It may be that cognitive capacity places the ultimate limit upon an individual's ability to adapt to age-related losses in sensory function. Investigations that focus upon such sensory-by-cognitive interactions promise to greatly increase our understanding of the dynamics of successful (as well as unsuccessful) aging.

Finally, there is a great need for researchers to consider factors that may be useful in terms of the prevention and remediation of common age-related sensory deficits. Important preventive measures have already been uncovered in many areas. For example, protection from the ultraviolet light of the sun across the lifespan promises to help maintain the integrity of the retina while reducing the risk of cataract. Recent laws requiring protection from work-related noise hold the potential of significantly preserving hearing ability well into old age. Yet, the recent proliferation of powerful, low-cost, personal stereo systems may do much to reverse this benefit. Similarly, timely treatment of common inflammatory infections of the nasal passages needs to be encouraged in the service of minimizing the lifespan declines observed for the appreciation of olfactory and flavor stimuli. As new ways to prevent and correct age-related deficits in sensory experience accrue, the real challenge will involve educating the public and their caregivers.

Acknowledgments

The author is indebted to previous reviews of the scientific literature on aging and the senses presented by Robert A. Weale, John F. Corso, James L. Fozard, and Claire Murphy. They illuminated the findings of the past and provided valuable insights regarding the future of aging research. Special acknowledgment must also be given to James E. Birren and again to John F. Corso for numerous comments and suggestions, which contributed immensely to improving this chapter.

References

Abrahamsson, M., & Sjostrand, J. (1986). Impairment of contrast sensitivity function as a measurement of disability glare. *Investigative Ophthalmology and Visual Science, 27,* 1131–1136.

Adams, A. J., Wong, L. S., Wong, L., & Gould, B. (1988). Visual acuity changes with age: Some new perspectives. *American Journal of Optometry and Physiological Optics, 65,* 403–406.

Adler, F. H. (1933). *Clinical physiology of the eye.* New York: Macmillan.

Allen, M. J., & Vos, J. J. (1967). Ocular scattered light and visual performance as a function of age. *American Journal of Optometry and Physiological Optics, 44,* 717–727.

Alpiner, J. G. (1979). Psychological and social aspects of aging as related to hearing rehabilitation of elderly clients. In M. A. Henoch (Ed.), *Aural rehabilitation for the elderly* (pp. 74–89). New York: Grune & Stratton.

American National Standards Institute (1970). *American National Standards specifications for audiometers (ANSI 53.6-1969).* New York: American National Standards Institute.

Amoore, J. E. (1970). *Molecular basis of odor.* Springfield, IL: Charles C Thomas.

Antonelli, A. R. (1970). Sensitized speech tests in aged people. In C. Rojskaer (Ed.), *Speech audiometry* (pp. 66–79). Copenhagen: Danavox, Borgergrade.

Arey, L., Tremaine, M. & Monzingo, F. (1935). The numerical and topographical relations of taste buds to human circumvallate papillae throughout the lifespan. *Anatomical Record, 64,* 9–25.

Arvidson, K. (1979). Location and variation in number of taste buds in human fungiform papillae. *Journal of Dental Research, 87,* 435–442.

Arvidson, K., & Freiberg, U. (1980). Human taste: Response and taste bud number in fungiform papillae. *Science, 209,* 807–808.

Axelrod, S., & Cohen, L. D. (1961). Senescence and embedded-figure performance in vision and touch. *Perceptual and Motor Skills, 12,* 283–288.

Ball, K., & Sekuler, R. (1986). Improving visual perception in older observers. *Journal of Gerontology, 41,* 176–182.

Ball, K., Beard, B. L., Roenker, D. L., Miller, R. L., & Griggs, D. S. (1988). Age and visual search: Expanding the useful field of view. *Journal of the Optical Society of America: A, 5,* 2210–2219.

Balough, K., & Lelkes, K. (1961). The tongue in old age. *Gerontologia Clinica (Suppl.), 3,* 38–54.

Bartoshuk, L. M. (1987). Taste: Robust across the age span? In C. Murphy, W. S. Cain, and D. M. Hegsted (Eds.), Nutrition and the chemical senses in aging: Recent advances and current research needs. *Annals of the New York Academy of Sciences, 561,* 65–75.

Bartoshuk, L. M., Rifkin, B., Marks, L. E., & Bars, P. (1986). Taste and aging. *Journal of Gerontology, 41,* 51–57.

Belal, A. (1975). Presbycusis: physiological or pathological. *Journal of Laryngology, 89,* 1011–1025.

Bell, B., Wolf, E., & Bernholz, C. D. (1972). Depth perception as a function of aging. *Aging and Human Development, 3,* 77–81.

Bennett, C. (1977). The demographic variables of discomfort glare. *Lighting Design and Application, 9,* 22–24.

Bergman, M. (1971). Hearing in aging. *Audiology, 10,* 164–171.

Bergman, M. (1980). *Aging and the perception of speech.* Baltimore, MD: University Park Press.

Bergman, M. (1983). Central disorders of hearing in the elderly. In R. Hinchcliffe (Ed.), *Hearing and balance in the elderly* (pp. 145–158). London: Churchill Livingstone.

Berlin, C. I., & Lowe, S. S. (1972). Temporal and dichotic factors in central auditory testing. In J. Katz (Ed.) *Handbook of clinical audiology* (pp. 280–312). Baltimore: Williams and Wilkins.

Birren, J. E., Casperson, R. C., & Botwinick, J. (1950). Age changes in pupil size. *Journal of Gerontology, 5,* 267–271.

Birren, J. E., Shapiro, H. B., & Miller, J. H. (1950). The effect of salicylate upon pain sensitivity. *Journal of Pharmacology and Experimental Therapy, 100,* 67–71.

Birren, J. E., Woods, A. M., & Williams, M. V. (1980). Behavioral slowing with age: Causes, organization, and consequences. In L. W. Poon (Ed.), *Aging in the 1980s: Psychological issues* (pp. 293–308). Washington, DC: American Psychological Association.

Boberg-Ans, J. (1956). On the corneal sensitivity. *Acta Ophthalmologica, 34,* 149–162.

Bocca, E., & Colearo, C. (1963). Central hearing processes. In J. Jerger (Ed.), *Modern developments in audiology* (pp. 337–370). New York: Academic Press.

Bolton, C. F., Winkelmann, R. K., & Dyck, P. J. (1966). A quantitative study of Meissner's corpuscles in man. *Neurology, 16,* 1–9.

Braddick, O., Campbell, F. W., & Atkinson, J. (1978). Channels in vision: Basic aspects. In R. Held, H. W. Leibowitz, & H. Teuber (Eds.), *Perception* (pp. 3–38). Berlin: Springer-Verlag.

Bradley, R. M. (1979). The effect of aging on the olfactory sense. In S. S. Han & D. H. Coons (Eds.), *Special senses in aging* (pp. 34–40). Ann Arbor, MI: Institute of Gerontology, University of Michigan.

Brandt, L. J., & Fozard, J. L. (1990). Age changes in pure-tone hearing thresholds in a longitudinal study of normal human aging. *Journal of the Acoustical Society of America, 88,* 813–820.

Bredberg, G. (1967). The human cochlea during development and aging. *Journal of Laryngology and Otology, 81:* 739–758.

Brody, H. (1955). Organization of the cerebral cortex. *Journal of Comparative Neurology, 102,* 511–556.

Bromley, D. B. (1966). *The Psychology of Human Ageing.* New York: Penguin Books.

Brozek, J. & Keys, A. (1945). Changes in flicker-fusion frequency with age. *Journal of Consulting Psychology, 9,* 87–90.

Buckingham, T., Whitaker, D., & Banford, D. (1987). Movement in decline? Oscillatory movement displacement thresholds increase with age. *Ophthalmic and Physiological Optics, 7,* 411–413.

Burg, A. (1967). *The relationship between vision test scores and driving record: General findings.* Los Angeles, CA: Institute of Transportation and Traffic Engineering, University of California.

Byrd, E., & Gertman, S. (1959). Taste sensitivity in aging persons. *Geriatrics, 14,* 381–384.

Byrnes, V. A. (1962). Visual factors in automobile driving. *Transactions of the American Ophthalmological Society, 60,* 60–84.

Calearo, C., & Lazzaroni, A. (1957). Speech intelligence in relation to the speed of the message. *Laryngoscope, 67,* 410–419.

Cauna, N. (1965). The effects of aging on the receptor organs of the human dermis. In W. Montagna (Ed.), *Advances in biology of skin. Vol. 6. Aging* (pp. 63–96). New York: Pergamon.

Cerella, J. (1985). Age-related decline in extra-foveal letter perception. *Journal of Gerontology, 40,* 727–736.

Chalke, H. D., & Dewhurst, J. R. (1957). Accidental coal-gas poisoning. *British Medical Journal, 2*, 915–917.

Chamberlain, W. (1971). Restriction of upward gaze with advancing age. *American Journal of Ophthalmology, 71,* 341–346.

Chapman, W. P., & Jones, C. M. (1944). Variations in cutaneous and visceral pain sensitivity in normal subjects. *Journal of Clinical Investigation, 23,* 81–91.

Cimasoni, G. (1974). *The crevicular fluid.* New York: S. Karger.

Clark, W. C., & Mehl, L. (1971). Thermal pain: A sensory decision theory analysis of the effects of age and sex on d', various response criteria, and 50-percent pain threshold. *Journal of Abnormal Psychology, 78,* 202–212.

Cohen, T., & Gitman, L. (1959). Oral complains and taste perception in the aged. *Journal of Gerontology, 14,* 294–298.

Collins, G., & Stone, L. A. (1965). Pain sensitivity, age, and activity level in chronic schizophrenia and normals. *British Journal of Psychiatry, 112,* 33–35.

Cooper, A. F. (1976). Deafness and psychiatric illness. *British Journal of Psychiatry. 129:* 215–226.

Corbin, K. B., & Gardner, E. D. (1937). Decrease in number of myelinated fibers in human spinal roots with age. *Anatomical Record, 68,* 63–74.

Corso, J. F. (1963). Age and sex differences in pure-tone thresholds. *Archives of Otolaryngology, 77,* 385–405.

Corso, J. F. (1980). Age correction factor in noise-induced hearing loss: A quantitative model. *Audiology, 19,* 221–232.

Corso, J. F. (1981). *Aging, sensory systems, and perception.* New York: Praeger.

Corso, J. F. (1987). Sensory–perceptual processes and aging. In K. W. Schiae (Ed.), *Annual review of gerontology and geriatrics.* (Vol. 7, pp. 29–55). New York: Springer.

Cosh, J. A. (1953). Studies on the nature of vibration sense. *Clinical Science, 12,* 131–151.

Dalderup, L. M., & Fredericks, M. L. C. (1969). Color sensitivity in old age. *Journal of the American Geriatrics Society, 17,* 388–390.

Denmark, J. C. (1976). The psycho-social implications of deafness. *Modern Perspectives in Psychiatry. 7,* 188–205.

Devaney, K. O., & Johnson, H. A. (1980). Neuron loss in the aging visual cortex of man. *Journal of Gerontology, 35,* 836–841.

Dolman, C. L., McCormick, A. Q., & Drance, S. M. (1980). Aging of the optic nerve. *Archives of Ophthalmology, 98,* 2053–2058.

Doty, R. L. (1989). The influence of age and age-related diseases on olfactory function. In C. Murphy, W. S. Cain, & D. M. Hegsted (Eds.), Nutrition and the chemical senses in aging: Recent advances and current research needs. *Annals of the New York Academy of Sciences, 561,* 76–86.

Doty, R. L., Shaman, P., Appelbaum, S. L., Giberson, R., Sikorski, L., & Rosenberg, L. (1984). Smell identification ability: Changes with age. *Science, 226,* 1441–1443.

Dublin, W. B. (1976). *Fundamentals of sensorineural auditory pathology.* Springfield, IL: Charles C Thomas.

Dubno, J. R., Dirks, D. D., & Morgan, D. E. (1984). Effects of age and mild hearing loss on speech recognition in noise. *Journal of the Acoustical Society of America, 76,* 87–96.

Duke-Elder, W. L. (1949). *Textbook of Ophthalmology.* St. Louis, MO: Mosby.

Elliott, D. B. (1987). Contrast sensitivity decline with aging: A neural or optical phenomenon? *Ophthalmic and Physiological Optics, 7,* 415–419.

Elliott, D. B., & Whitaker, D. (1990). Decline in retinal function with age. *Investigative Ophthalmology and Visual Science (Suppl.), 31*(4), 357.

Elliott, D., Whitaker, D., & MacVeigh, D. (1990). Neural contribution to spatiotemporal contrast sensitivity decline in healthy aging eyes. *Vision Research, 30,* 541–547.

Enns, M. P., Van Itallie, T. B., & Grinker, J. A. (1979). Contributions of age, sex, and degree of fatness on performance and magnitude estimations for sucrose in humans. *Physiology and Behavior, 22,* 999–1003.

Era, P., Jokela, J., Suominen, H., & Heikkinen, E. (1986). Correlates of vibrotactile thresholds in men of different ages. *Acta Neurologica Scandinavica, 74,* 210–217.

Etholm, B., & Belal, A., Jr. (1974). Senile changes in the middle ear joints. *Annals of Otology, Rhinology, and Laryngology, 83,* 49–64.

Evans, D. W., & Ginsburg, A. P. (1985). Contrast sensitivity predicts age differences in highway sign discriminability. *Human Factors, 27,* 637–642.

Farrimond, T. (1967). Visual and auditory performance variations with age: Some implications. *Australian Journal of Psychology, 19,* 193–201.

Finger, T. E. (1987). Gustatory nuclei and pathways in the central nervous system. In T. E. Finger & W. L. Silver (Eds.), *Neurobiology of taste and smell.* (pp. 331–335). New York: Wiley.

Fons, M. (1976). Electrically evoked taste threshold. *Annals of Otology, Rhinology, and Laryngology, 85,* 359–367.

Fozard, J. L. (1990). Vision and hearing in aging. In J. E. Birren & K. W. Schiae (Eds.), *Handbook of the psychology of aging. (Third ed.)* (pp. 150–170). New York: Academic Press.

Franks, J. R., & Beckman, N. (1985). Rejection of hearing aids: Attitudes of a geriatrics sample. *Ear and Hearing, 6,* 161–167.

Gaeth, J. (1948). A study of phonemic regression in relation to hearing loss. Unpublished doctoral dissertation, Northwestern University.

Gardiner, E. (1940). Decrease in human neurones with age. *Anatomical Record, 77,* 529–536.

Garner, W., & Spector, A. (1978). Racemization in human lens: Evidence of rapid insolubilization of specific polypeptides in cataract formation. *Proceedings of the National Academy of Sciences, 75,* 3618–3620.

Geldard, F. (1972). *The human senses.* (2nd ed.). New York: Wiley.

Gilbert, J. G. (1957). Age changes in color matching. *Journal of Gerontology, 12,* 210–215.

Gilhome-Herbst, K. (1983). Psychosocial consequences of disorders of hearing in the elderly. In R. Hinchcliffe (Ed.), *Hearing and balance in the elderly.* (pp. 174–200). London: Churchill Livingstone.

Gilhome-Herbst, K. R., & Humphrey, C. M. (1980). The prevalence of hearing impairment in the elderly living at home. *Journal of the Royal College of General Practitioners, 31,* 155–160.

Ginsburg, A. P. (1977). *Visual information processing based on spatial filters constrained by biological data. AMRL-TR-78-129.* Springfield, VA: National Technical Information Service.

Ginsburg, A. P., Evans, D., Sekuler, R., & Harp, S. (1982). Contrast sensitivity predicts pilots' performance in aircraft simulators. *American Journal of Optometry and Physiological Optics, 59,* 105–109.

Gittings, N. S., & Fozard, J. L. (1986). Age-related changes in visual acuity. *Experimental Gerontology, 21,* 423–433.

Gittings, N. S., Fozard, J. L., & Shock, N. W. (1987). Age changes in stereopsis, visual acuity, and color vision. *The Gerontologist (Special Issue), 27,* 167A.

Glass, L. E. (1988). Adventitious hearing loss: Some aspects of denial. In G. Lesnoff-Caravaglia (Ed.), *Aging in a technological society* (pp. 91–94). New York: Human Sciences Press.

Goetzinger, C. P., Proud, G. O., Dirks, D., and Embrey, J. (1961). A study of hearing in advanced age. *Archives of Otolaryngology. 73,* 662–674.

Gordon-Salant, S. (1987). Age-related differences in speech recognition performance as a function of test format and paradigm. *Ear and Hearing, 8,* 277–282.

Greene, H. A., & Madden, D. J. (1987). Adult age differences in visual acuity, stereopsis, and contrast sensitivity. *American Journal of Optometry and Physiological Optics, 64,* 749–753.

Grimes, A., Mueller, G., & Williams, D. L. (1984). Clinical considerations in the use of time-compressed speech. *Ear and Hearing, 5,* 114–117.

Grzegorczyk, P. B., Jones, S. W., & Minstretta, C. M. (1979). Age-related differences in salt taste acuity. *Journal of Gerontology, 34,* 834–840.

Gulick, W. L., Gescheider, G. A., & Frisina, R. D. (1989). *Hearing: physiological acoustics, neural coding and psychoacoustics.* New York: Oxford University Press.

Haegerstrom-Portnoy, G. (1988). Short-wavelength cone sensitivity loss with aging: A protective role for macular pigment. *Journal of the Optical Society of America: A, 5,* 2140–2144.

Hakkinen, L. (1984). Vision in the elderly and its use in the social environment. *Scandinavian Journal of Social Medicine, 35,* 5–60.

Hansen, C. C., & Reske-Nielson, E. (1965). Pathological studies in presbycusis. *Archives of Otolaryngology 82,* 115–132.

Hardy, J. D., Wolff, H. G., & Goodell, H. (1952). The pain threshold in man. *American Journal of Psychiatry, 99,* 744–751.

Harkins, S. W., Kwentus, J., & Price, D. D. (1984). Pain and the elderly. In C. Benedetti, C. R. Chapman, & G. Moricca (Eds.), *Recent advances in the management of pain* (pp. 103–121). New York: Raven Press.

Harris, H., & Kalmus, H. (1949). The measurement of taste sensitivity to phenylthiourea (PTC). *Annals of Human Genetics, 15,* 24–31.

Harris, R. W., & Reitz, M. I. (1985). Effects of room reverberation and noise on speech discrimination by the elderly. *Audiology, 24,* 319–324.

Heckmann, T., & Schor, C. M. (1989). Is edge information from stereoacuity spatially channeled? *Vision Research, 29,* 593–607.

Henderson, R. L., & Burg, A. (1974). *Vision and audition in driving. Report TM(L)-5297.* Washington, DC: U.S. Department of Transportation.

Henkins, R. I., & Christiansen, R. L. (1967). Taste thresholds in patients with dentures. *Journal of the American Dental Association, 75,* 118–120.

Hensel, H. (1981). *Thermoreception and temperature regulation.* New York: Academic Press.

Herman, G. E., Warren, L. R., & Wagener, J. W. (1977). Auditory lateralization: Age-differences in sensitivity to dichotic time and amplitude cues. *Journal of Gerontology, 32,* 187–191.

Hicks, L. H., & Birren, J. E. (1970). Aging, brain damage, and psychomotor slowing. *Psychological Bulletin, 74,* 377–396.

Hinchcliffe, R. (1962). Aging and sensory thresholds. *Journal of Gerontology, 17,* 45–50.

Hinchcliffe, R. (1973). Epidemiology of sensorineural hearing loss. *Audiology, 12,* 446–452.

Hinchcliffe, R. (Ed.) (1983). *Hearing and balance in the elderly.* New York: Churchill Livingstone.

Hofstetter, H. W. (1965). A longitudinal study of amplitude changes in presbyopia. *American Journal of Optometry, 42,* 3–8.

Hofstetter, H. W., & Bertsch, J. D. (1976). Does stereopsis change with age? *American Journal of Optometry and Physiological Optics, 53,* 664–667.

Horowitz, M. (1984). Stress and the mechanisms of defense. In H. H. Goldman (Ed.), *Review of general psychiatry* (p. 44). Lost Altos, CA: Lange Medical Publications.

Howell, T. H. (1949). Senile deterioration of the central nervous system: Clinical study. *British Medical Journal, 1,* 56–58.

Hughes, G. (1969). Changes in taste sensitivity with advancing age. *Gerontologia Clinica, 2,* 224–230.

Huntington, J. M. and Simonson, E. (1965). Critical flicker-fusion frequency as a function of exposure time in two different age groups. *Journal of Gerontology, 20,* 527–529.

Hutton, J. T., Nagel, J. A., & Lowenson, R. B. (1983). Variable affecting eye tracking performance. *Electroencephalography and Clinical Neurophysiology, 56,* 414–419.

Hutton, J. T., Nagel, J. A., & Lowenson, R. B. (1984). Eye-tracking dysfunction in Alzheimer-type dementia. *Neurology, 34,* 99–102.

Ijspeert, J. K., de Waard, van den Berg, T. J. T. P., & de Jong, P. T. V. M. (1990). The intraocular straylight function in 129 healthy volunteers; dependence on angle, age, and pigmentation. *Vision Research, 30,* 699–707.

Jackson, P. H. (1979). Special problems of the hard of hearing. *Journal of Rehabilitation of the Deaf, 12*(4), 13–26.

Jackson, R. (1972). Solar and senile skin: Changes caused by aging and habitual exposure to the sun. *Geriatrics, 27,* 106–112.

Jerger, J. (1973). Audiological findings in aging. *Advances in Otorhinolaryngology, 20,* 115–124.

Johnson, C. A., Adams, A. J., Twelker, J. C., & Quigg, J. M. (1988). Age-related changes of the central field for short-wavelength-sensitive (SWS) pathways. *Journal of the Optical Society of America, 5,* 2131–2139.

Johnsson, L. G., & Hawkins, J. E., Jr. (1972). Sensory and neural degeneration with aging, as seen in microdissections of the human inner ear. *Annals of Otology, Rhinology, and Laryngology, 81,* 179–193.

Joyner, R. E. (1963). Olfactory acuity in an industrial population. *Journal of Occupational Medicine, 5,* 37–42.

Kahn, H. A. Leibowitz, H. W., Ganley, S. P., Kini, M. M., Colton, J., Nickerson, R. S., & Dawber, T. R. (1977). Framingham eye study. I. Outlines and major prevalences and findings. *American Journal of Epidemiology, 106,* 17–32.

Kahn, H. A., & Milton, R. C. (1980). Revised Framingham Eye Study. Prevalence of glaucoma and diabetic retinopathy. *American Journal of Epidemiology, 11,* 769–776.

Kalmus, H., & Trotter, W. R. (1962). Direct assessment of the effect of age on PTC sensitivity. *Annals of Human Genetics, 26,* 145–149.

Kaplan, A. R., Glanville, E. V., & Fischer, R. (1965). Cumulative effect of age and smoking on taste sensitivity in males and females. *Journal of Gerontology, 20,* 334–337.

Kaplan, H. (1985). Benefits and limitations of amplification and speech reading for the elderly. In H. Orlans (Ed.), *Adjustment to adult hearing loss* (pp. 85–98). San Diego, CA: College-Hill Press.

Kaufman, S. R., & Abel, L. A. (1986). The effects of distraction on smooth pursuit in normal subjects. *Acta Otolaryngolica, 102*, 57–64.

Kay, D. W. K., Beamish, P., & Roth, M. (1964). Old age mental disorders in Newcastle upon Tyne. Pt. I: A study of prevalence. *British Journal of Psychiatry, 110*, 146–158.

Kell, R. L., Pearson, J. C. G., & Taylor, W. (1970). Hearing thresholds of an island population in north Scotland. *International Audiology, 9*, 334–349.

Kenshalo, D. R. (1970). Psychophysical studies of temperature sensitivity. In W. D. Neff (Ed.), *Contributions to sensory physiology* (pp. 19–74). New York: Academic Press.

Kenshalo, D. R. (1977). Age changes in touch, vibration, temperature, kinesthesis, and pain sensitivity. In J. E. Birren & K. W. Schaie (Eds.), *Handbook of the psychology of aging* (pp. 562–579). New York: Van Nostrand Reinhold.

Kenshalo, D. R. (1979). Aging effects on cutaneous and kinesthetic sensibilities. In S. S. Han & D. H. Coons (Eds.), *Special senses in aging* (pp. 189–217). Ann Arbor, MI: Institute of Gerontology, University of Michigan.

Kenshalo, D. R. (1986). Somesthetic sensitivity in young and elderly humans. *Journal of Gerontology, 41*, 732–742.

Kimbrell, C. M., & Furtchgott, E. (1963). The effect of aging on olfactory threshold. *Journal of Gerontology, 18*, 364–365.

Kinnamon, J. C. (1987). Organization and innervation of taste buds. In T. E. Finger & W. L. Silver (Eds.), *Neurobiology of taste and smell* (pp. 277–297). New York: Wiley.

Kirikae, I. (1969). Auditory function in advanced age with reference to histological changes in the central auditory system. *International Audiology, 8*, 221–230.

Kleinman, J. M., & Brodzinsky, D. M. (1978). Haptic exploration in young, middle-aged, and elderly adults. *Journal of Gerontology, 33*, 521–527.

Kline, D. W. (1987). Aging and the spatiotemporal discrimination performance of the visual system. *Eye, 1*, 323–329.

Kline, D. W., & Birren, J. E. (1975). Age differences in backward dichoptic masking. *Experimental Aging Research, 1*, 17–25.

Kline, D. W., & Orme-Rogers, C. (1978). Examination of stimulus persistence as the basis for superior visual identification performance among older adults. *Journal of Gerontology, 33*, 76–81.

Kline, D. W., & Schieber, F. (1980). What are the age differences in visual sensory memory? *Journal of Gerontology, 36*, 86–89.

Kline, D. W., & Schieber, F. (1982). Visual persistence and temporal resolution. In R. Sekuler, D. W. Kline, & K. Dismukes, (Eds.), *Aging and human visual function* (pp. 231–244). New York: Alan R. Liss.

Kline, D. W., & Schieber, F. (1985). Vision and aging. In J. E. Birren & K. W. Schaie (Eds.), *Handbook of the psychology of aging* (pp. 296–331). New York: Van Nostrand Reinhold.

Kline, D. W., Schieber, F., Abusaura, L. C., & Coyne, A. C. (1983). Age and the visual channels: Contrast sensitivity and response speed. *Journal of Gerontology, 38*, 211–216.

Knoblauch, K., Saunders, F., Kusuda, M., Hynes, R., Podgor, M., Higgins, K. E., & de Monasterio, F. M. (1987). Age and illuminance effects in Farnsworth-Munsell 100-hue test. *Applied Optics, 26*, 1441–1448.

Konig, E. (1957). Pitch discrimination and age. *Acta Otolaryngologica, 48*, 475–489.

Kosnik, W., Kline, D. W., Fikre, J., & Sekuler, R. (1987). Ocular fixation control as a function of age and exposure duration. *Psychology and Aging, 2*, 302–305.

Kosnik, W., Winslow, L., Kline, D. W., Rasinski, K., & Sekuler, R. (1988). Vision changes in daily life throughout adulthood. *Journal of Gerontology, 43*, 63–70.

Krarup, B. (1958). Electro-gustometry: A method for clinical taste examinations. *Acta Otolaryngologica, 49*, 294–305.

Kuwabara, T. (1979). Age-related changes in the eye. In S. S. Hain & D. H. Coons (Eds.), *Special senses in aging* (pp. 46–78). Ann Arbor, MI: Institute of Gerontology, University of Michigan.

Kuwabara, T., & Cogan, D. G. (1965). Retinal vascular patterns, VII. A cellular change. *Investigative Ophthalmology, 4*, 1049–1058.

Langan, M. J., & Yearick, E. S. (1976). The effects of improved oral hygiene on taste perception and nutrition of the elderly. *Journal of Gerontology, 31*, 413–418.

Leighton, D. A., & Tomlinson, A. (1972). Changes in axial length and other dimensions of the eyeball with increasing age. *Acta Ophthalmologica, 50*, 815–825.

Levitt, H. (1987). Digital hearing aids: A tutorial review. *Journal of Rehabilitation Research and Development, 24*, 7–20.

Liss, L., & Gomez, F. (1958). The nature of senile changes of the human olfactory bulb and tract. *Archives of Otolaryngology, 67*, 167–171.

Lit, A. (1968). Visual acuity. *Annual Review of Psychology, 19*, 22–54.

Long, G. M., & Crambert, R. F. (1990). The nature and basis of age-related changes in dynamic visual acuity. *Psychology and Aging, 5*, 138–143.

Lowenfeld, I. E. (1979). Pupillary changes related to age. In H. S. Thompson (Ed.), *Topics in neuro-ophthalmology* (pp. 124–150). Baltimore: Williams and Wilkins.

Maffei, L. (1978). Spatial frequency channels: Neural mechanisms. In R. Held, H. W. Leibowitz, & H. Teuber (Eds.), *Perception* (pp. 39–66). Berlin: Springer-Verlag.

Marks, L. E. (1974). *Sensory processes: The new psychophysics.* New York: Academic Press.

Marmor, M. F. (1982). Aging and the retina. In R. Sekuler, D. W. Kline, & K. Dismukes (Eds.), *Aging and human visual function* (pp. 59–78). New York: Alan R. Liss.

Marshall, J., Grindle, J., Ansell, P. L., & Borwein, B. (1980). Convolution in human rods: An aging process. *British Journal of Ophthalmology, 63*, 181–187.

Marston, E., & Goetzinger, C. P. (1972). A comparison of sensitized words and sentences for distinguishing nonperipheral auditory changes as a function of aging. *Cortex, 8*, 213–223.

Massler, M. (1980). Geriatric nutrition: The role of taste and smell in appetite. *Journal of Prosthetic Dentistry, 43*, 247–250.

Mayer, M. J., Kim, C. B. Y., Svingos, A., & Glucs, A. (1988). Foveal-flicker sensitivity in healthy aging eyes I. Compensating for pupil variation. *Journal of the Optical Society of America: A, 5*, 2201–2209.

McCarthy, P. (1985). Aural rehabilitation. In H. G. Mueller & V. C. Geoffrey (Eds.), *Communication disorders in aging* (pp. 437–463). Washington, DC: Gallaudet University Press.

McFarland, R. A., Warren, B., & Karis, C. (1958). Alterations in critical flicker frequency as a function of age and light: dark ratio. *Journal of Experimental Psychology, 56*, 529–538.

Menninger, K. A. (1924). The mental effects of deafness. *Psychoanalytic Review, 11*, 144–155.

Miller, I. J., Jr. (1988). Human taste-bud density across adult age groups. *Journal of Gerontology, 43*, B26–30.

Millodot, M. (1977). The influence of age on the sensitivity of the cornea. *Investigative Ophthalmology, 16*, 240–242.

Milne, J. S. (1977). A longitudinal study of hearing loss in older people. *British Journal of Audiology, 11*, 7–14.

Milne, J. S., Maule, M. M., & Williamson, J. (1971). Method of sampling in a study of older people with a comparison of respondents and nonrespondents. *British Journal of Preventive and Social Medicine, 25*, 37–41.

Misiak, H. (1947). Age and sex differences in critical flicker frequency. *Journal of Experimental Psychology, 37*, 318–332.

Mochizuki, Y. (1937). An observation on the numerical and topographical relations of the taste buds to circumvallate papillae of Japanese. *Okajimas Folia Anatomica Japonica, 15*, 595–608.

Mochizuki, Y. (1939). Studies on the papillae foliata. II. The number of taste buds. *Okajimas Folia Anatomica Japonica, 18*, 355–369.

Møller, M. B. (1981). Hearing in 70- to 75-year-old people: Results from a cross-sectional and longitudinal population study. *American Journal of Otolaryngology, 2*, 22–29.

Møller, M. B. (1983). Changes in hearing measures with increasing age. In R. Hinchcliffe, (Ed.), *Hearing and balance in the elderly* (pp. 97–122). London: Churchill Livingstone.

Moore, L. M., Nielsen, C. R., & Minstretta, C. M. (1982). Sucrose taste thresholds: Age-related differences. *Journal of Gerontology, 37*, 64–69.

Moore, N. C. (1981). Is paranoid illness associated with sensory deficits in the elderly? *Journal of Psychosomatic Research, 25*, 69–74.

Morrison, J. D., & McGrath, C. (1985). Assessment of optical contributions to the age-related deterioration in vision. *Quarterly Journal of Experimental Psychology, 70*, 249–269.

Morrison, T. R. (1980). *A review of dynamic visual acuity. NAMRL monograph 28.* Pensacola, FL: Naval Aerospace Medical Research Laboratory.

Moses, S., Rotem, Y., Jagoda, N., Talmor, N., Eichorn, F., & Levin, S. (1967). A clinical genetic and biochemical study of familial dysautonomia in Israel. *Israel Journal of Medical Science, 3*, 358–371.

Murphy, B. J. (1978). Pattern thresholds for moving and stationary gratings during smooth eye movements. *Vision Research, 18,* 521–530.

Murphy, C. (1979). The effect of age on taste sensitivity. In S. S. Han & D. H. Coons, (Eds.), *Special senses in aging* (pp. 21–33). Ann Arbor, MI: Institute of Gerontology, University of Michigan.

Murphy, C. (1983). Age-related effects on the threshold, psychophysical function, and pleasantness of menthol. *Journal of Gerontology, 38,* 217–222.

Murphy, C. (1986). Taste and smell in the elderly. In H. L. Meiselman & R. S. Rivlin (Eds.), *Clinical measures of taste and smell* (pp. 343–371). New York: Macmillan.

Murphy, C. (1987). Olfactory psychophysics. In T. E. Finger & W. L. Silver (Eds.), *Neurobiology of taste and smell* (pp. 251–273). New York: Wiley.

Nabelek, A. K., & Robinson, P. K. (1982). Monaural and binaural speech perception in reverberation for listeners of various ages. *Journal of the Acoustical Society of America, 71,* 1242–1248.

Naessen, R. (1971). An inquiry on the morphological characteristics of possible changes with age in the olfactory region of man. *Acta Otolaryngologica, 71,* 49–62.

National Institute for Occupational Safety and Health. (1972). *Occupational exposure to noise.* Washington, DC: U. S. Department of Health, Education and Welfare.

Neuman, A. C. (1987). Digital technology and clinical practice: The outlook for the future. *Journal of Rehabilitation Research and Development, 24,* 1–6.

Norgen, R. (1976). Central neural mechanisms of taste. In I. Darian-Smith, J. M. Brookhart, & V. B. Mountcastle (Eds.), *Handbook of Physiology: The Nervous System Sensory Processes.* (Vol. 2, Pt. 3, pp. 1087–1128). Bethesda, MD: American Physiological Society.

Norris, M. L., & Cunningham, D. R. (1981). Social impact of hearing loss in the aged. *Journal of Gerontology, 36,* 727–729.

Olsho, L. W., Harkins, S. W., & Lenhardt, M. L. (1985). Aging and the auditory system. In J. E. Birren & K. W. Schaie (Eds.), *Handbook of the psychology of aging. (2nd ed.)* (pp. 332–377). New York: Van Nostrand Reinhold.

Olson, P. L., & Sivak, M. (1989). Glare from automobile rear-vision mirrors. *Human Factors, 26,* 269–282.

Olzak, L. A., & Thomas, J. P. (1985). Seeing spatial patterns. In K. R. Boff, L. Kaufman, & J. P. Thomas (Eds.), *Handbook of perception and human performance* (pp. 7:1–7:56). New York: Wiley.

Ordy, J. M., & Brizzee, K. R. (1979). *Aging. Vol. 10. Sensory Systems and Communication in the Elderly.* New York: Raven Press.

Orlans, H. (Ed.) (1985). *Adjustment to adult hearing loss.* San Diego: College-Hill Press.

Otto, W. C., & McCandless, G. A. (1982). Aging and auditory site of lesion. *Ear and Hearing, 3,* 110–117.

Owsley, C., & Sloane, M. E. (1987). Contrast sensitivity, acuity, and the perception of real-world targets. *British Journal of Ophthalmology, 71,* 791–796.

Owsley, C., & Sloane, M. E. (1990). Vision and aging. In F. Boller & J. Grafman (Eds.), *Handbook of neuropsychology* (Vol. 4, pp. 229–249). Amsterdam: Elsevier.

Owsley, C., Sekuler, R., & Siemsen, D. (1983). Contrast sensitivity throughout adulthood. *Vision Research, 23,* 689–699.

Pearce, R. H., & Grimmer, B. J. (1972). Age and the chemical constitution of normal human dermis. *Journal of Investigative Dermatology, 58,* 347–361.

Petrosino, L., Fucci, D., & Robey, R. R. (1982). Changes in lingual sensitivity as a function of age and stimulus exposure time. *Perceptual and Motor Skills, 55,* 1083–1090.

Picheny, M. A., Durlach, N. I., & Braida, L. D. (1986). Speaking clearly for the hard of hearing II: Acoustic characteristics of clear and conversational speech. *Journal of Speech and Hearing Research, 29,* 434–446.

Pickett, H. G., Appleby, R. G., & Osborn, M. O. (1972). Changes in the denture-supporting tissues associated with the aging process. *Journal of Prosthetic Dentistry, 27,* 257–262.

Pitt, M. C., & Rawles, J. M. (1988). The effect of age on saccadic latency and velocity. *Neuro-ophthalmology, 8,* 123–129.

Pitts, D. G. (1982). The effects of aging upon selected visual functions: Dark adaptation, visual acuity, stereopsis, and brightness contrast. In R. Sekuler, D. W. Kline, & K. Dismukes (Eds.), *Aging and human visual function* (pp. 131–160). New York: Alan R. Liss.

Plomp, R., & Mimpen, A. M. (1979). Speech-reception threshold for sentences as a function of age and noise level. *Journal of the Acoustical Society of America, 66,* 1333–1342.

Plumb, C. S., & Meigs, J. W. (1961). Human vibration perception. Part I. Vibration perception at different ages. *Archives of General Psychiatry, 4,* 611–614.

Pokorny, J., Smith, V. C., & Lutze, M. (1987). Aging of the human lens. *Applied Optics, 26,* 1437–1440.

Post, F. (1966). *Persistent persecutory states of the elderly.* Oxford: Pergamon Press.

Procacci, P., Bozza, G., Buzzelli, G., & Della Court, M. (1970). The cutaneous pricking-pain threshold in old age. *Gerontologia Clinica, 12,* 213–218.

Pulling, N. H., Wolf, E., Sturgis, S. P., Vaillancourt, D. R., & Doliver, J. J. (1980). Headlight glare resistance and driver age. *Human Factors, 22,* 103–112.

Punch, J. L., & McConnell, F. (1969). The speech discrimination function of elderly adults. *Journal of Audiological Research, 9,* 159–166.

Quilliam, T. A., & Ridley, A. (1971). The receptor community in the finger tip. *Journal of Physiology (London), 216,* 15P–17P.

Ramsdell, D. A. (1978). Psychology of the hard-of-hearing and deafened adult. In H. Davis & S. R. Silverman (Eds.), *Hearing and deafness.* (4th ed.) (pp. 499–510). New York: Holt, Rinehart & Winston.

Reading, V. M. (1972). Visual resolution as measured by dynamic and static tests. *Pflugers Archives, 333,* 17–26.

Reynaud, J., Camara, M., & Basteris, L. (1969). An investigation into presbycusis in Africans from rural and nomadic environments. *International Audiology, 8,* 299–304.

Rice, D., & Jones, B. (1984). *Vision screening of driver's license renewal applicants.* Salem, OR: Department of Transportation, Motor Vehicle Division.

Richards, O. W. (1977). Effects of luminance and contrast on visual acuity, ages 16 to 90 years. *American Journal of Optometry and Physiological Optics, 54,* 178–184.

Richter, C. & Campbell, K. (1940). Sucrose taste thresholds in rats and humans. *American Journal of Physiology, 128,* 291–297.

Ries, P. W. (1985). The demography of hearing loss. In H. Orlans (Ed.) *Adjustment to adult hearing loss* (pp. 3–21). San Diego, CA: College-Hill Press.

Robinson, D. W., & Sutton, G. J. (1979). Age effect in hearing—a comparative analysis of published threshold data. *Audiology, 18,* 320–334.

Ronge, H. (1943). Altersveranderungen des Beruhrungssinnes I. Druckpunktschwellen und Brunchpunktfrequenz. *Acta Physiologica Scandinavica, 6,* 343–352.

Rosen, D. E., Bergman, M., Plester, D., El-Mofty, A., & Satti, M. H. (1962). Presbycusis study of a relatively noise-free population in the Sudan. *Annals of Otology, Rhinology, and Laryngology, 71,* 727–743.

Rosenberg, G. (1958). Effects of age on peripheral vibratory perception. *Journal of the American Geriatrics Society, 6,* 471–481.

Roth, M. (1976). The psychiatric disorders of later life. *Psychiatric Annals, 6,* 57–101.

Said, F. S., & Weale, R. A. (1959). The variation with age of the spectral transmissivity of the living human crystalline lens. *Gerontologia, 3,* 213–231.

Salthouse, T. A. (1982). *Adult cognition.* New York: Springer.

Samorajaski, T. (1976). How the brain responds to aging. *Journal of the American Geriatrics Society, 24,* 4–11.

Sample, P. A., Esterson, F. D., Weinreb, R. N., & Boynton, R. M. (1988). The aging lens: *In vivo* assessment of light absorption in 84 human eyes. *Investigative Ophthalmology and Visual Science, 29,* 1306–1311.

Schemper, T., Voss, S., & Cain, W. S. (1981). Odor identification in young and elderly persons: Sensory and cognitive limitations. *Journal of Gerontology, 36,* 446–452.

Schiebel, M. E., & Schiebel, A. B. (1975). Structural changes in the aging brain. In H. Brody, D. Harmon, & J. M. Ordy (Eds.), *Aging* (pp. 11–37). New York: Raven Press.

Schieber, F. (1988). Vision assessment technology and screening of older drivers: Past practices and emerging techniques. In National Research Council. *Transportation in an aging society: Improving mobility and safety of older persons. Special report No. 218, Vol. 2* (pp. 325–378). Washington, DC: Transportation Research Board.

Schieber, F., Fozard, J. L., Dent, D., & Kline, D. W. (1989). Age and contrast sensitivity. *The Gerontologist (Special Issue), 29,* 23A.

Schieber, F., Fozard, J. L., Gordon-Salant, S., & Weiffenbach, J. M. (in press). Optimizing sensation and perception in older adults. *International Journal of Industrial Ergonomics.*

Schieber, F., Hiris, E., White, J., & Williams, M. J. (1990). Assessing age differences in motion perception using simple oscillatory displacement versus random dot cinematography. *Investigative Ophthalmology and Visual Science, 31,* 355.

Schiffman, S. S. (1983). Taste and smell in disease. *New England Journal of Medicine, 308,* 1275–1279; 1337–1343.

Schiffman, S. (1979). Changes in taste and smell with age: Psychophysical aspects. In J. M. Ordy & K. R. Brizzee (Eds.), *Sensory systems and communication in the elderly* (pp. 227–246). New York: Raven Press.

Schiffman, S. S. (1977). Food recognition by the elderly. *Journal of Gerontology, 32,* 586–592.

Schiffman, S. S., & Clark, T. B. (1980). Magnitude estimates of amino acids for young and elderly subjects. *Neurobiology and Aging, 1,* 81–91.

Schiffman, S. S., Lindley, M. G., Clark, T. B., & Makins, C. (1981). Molecular mechanism of sweet taste: Relationship of hydrogen bonding to taste sensitivity for both young and elderly. *Neurobiology and Aging, 2,* 173–185.

Schiffman, S., Orlandi, M., & Erickson, R. P. (1979). Changes in taste and smell with age: Biological aspects. In J. M. Ordy & K. Brizzee (Eds.), *Sensory systems and communication in the elderly* (pp. 247–268). New York: Raven Press.

Schiffman, S. S., & Warwick, Z. S. (1988). Flavor enhancement of foods for the elderly can reverse anorexia. *Neurobiology of Aging, 9,* 24–26.

Schluderman, E., & Zubek, J. P. (1962). Effects of age on pain sensitivity. *Perceptual and Motor Skills, 14,* 295–301.

Schonfield, D., & Robertson, E. A. (1966). Memory storage and aging. *Canadian Journal of Psychology, 20,* 228–236.

Schor, D., & Heckmann, T. (1989). Interocular differences in contrast and spatial frequency: Effects on stereopsis and fusion. *Vision Research, 29,* 837–847.

Schow, R., Christensen, J., Hutchinson, J., & Nerbonne, M. (1978). *Communication disorders of the aged: A guide for health professions.* Baltimore, MD: University Park Press.

Schuknecht, H. (1974). *Pathology of the ear.* Cambridge, MA: Harvard University Press.

Schumacher, G. A., Goodell, H., Hardy, J. D., & Wolff, H. G. (1940). Uniformity of the pain threshold in man. *Science, 92,* 110–112.

Scialfa, C. T., Garvey, P. M., Tyrell, R. A., & Leibowitz, H. W. (1989). Age differences in dynamic contrast sensitivity. *Investigative Ophthalmology and Visual Science (Suppl.), 30,* 406.

Scialfa, C. T., Kline, D. W., & Lyman, B. J. (1987). Age differences in target identification as a function of retinal location and noise level: An examination of the useful field of view. *Psychology and Aging, 2,* 14–19.

Scialfa, C. T., Kline, D. W., Lyman, B. J., & Kosnik, W. (1987). Age differences in judgments of vehicle velocity and distance. *Proceedings of the Human Factors Society, 31st Annual Meeting* (pp. 558–561).

Sekuler, R., Kline, D. W., & Dismukes, K. (1982). *Aging and human visual function.* New York: Alan R. Liss.

Sekuler, R., & Ball, K. (1986). Visual localization: Age and practice. *Journal of the Optical Society of America: A, 3,* 864–867.

Shadden, B. B., & Raiford, C. A. (1984). Factors influencing service utilization by older individuals. *Journal of Communicative Disorders, 17,* 209–224.

Shafar, J. (1965). Dygeusia in the elderly. *Lancet, 1,* 83–84.

Sharp, J. A., & Sylvester, T. O. (1978). Effects of age on horizontal smooth pursuit. *Investigative Ophthalmology and Visual Science, 17,* 465–468.

Sherman, E. D., & Robilliard, E. (1964). Sensitivity to pain in relationship to age. *Journal of the American Geriatrics Society, 12,* 1037–1044.

Shinar, D. (1977). *Driver visual limitations: Diagnosis and treatment. Department of Transportation Contract DOT-HS-5-1275.* Bloomington, IN: Institute for Research in Public Safety, Indiana University.

Shiokawa, H. (1975). The clinical studies on the olfactory test using standard odorous substances: The change in olfactory acuity due to aging. *Journal of the Oto-Rhino-Laryngological Society of Japan, 78,* 1258–1270.

Shklar, G. (1966). The effects of aging upon oral mucosa. *Journal of Investigative Dermatology, 47,* 115–120.

Sivak, M., & Olson, P. L. (1982). Nighttime legibility of traffic signs: Conditions eliminating the effects of driver age and disability glare. *Accident Analysis and Prevention, 14,* 87–93.

Sloane, M. E., Owsley, C., & Alvarez, S. L. (1988). Aging, senile miosis, and spatial contrast sensitivity at low luminances. *Vision Research, 28,* 1235–1246.

Sloane, M. E., Owsley, C., & Jackson, C. (1988). Aging and luminance adaptation effects in spatial contrast sensitivity. *Journal of the Optical Society of America: A, 5,* 2181–2190.

Smith, C. G. (1942). Age incidence of atrophy of olfactory nerves in man. *Journal of Comparative Neurology, 77,* 589–595.

Smith, D. V. (1971). Taste intensity as a function of areas and concentration: Differentiation between compounds. *Journal of Experimental Psychology, 87,* 163–171.

Smith, S. E., & Davies, P. D. (1973). Quinine taste thresholds: A family study and a twin study. *Annals of Human Genetics, 37,* 227–232.

Sperduto, R. D., & Siegel, D. (1980). Senile lens and senile macular changes in a population-based sample. *American Journal of Ophthalmology, 90,* 86–91.

Spitzer, M. E. (1988). Taste acuity in institutionalized and noninstitutionalized elderly men. *Journal of Gerontology: Psychological Sciences, 43,* 71–74.

Spooner, J. W., Skalka, S. M., & Baloh, R. W. (1980). Effects of aging on eye tracking. *Archives of Neurology, 37,* 575–576.

Spoor, A. (1967). Presbycusis values in relation to noise-induced hearing loss. *International Audiology, 6,* 48–57.

Steiness, I. (1957). Vibratory perception in normal subjects. *Acta Medica Scandinavica, 158,* 315–325.

Stevens, S. S. (1962). The surprising simplicity of sensory metrics. *American Scientist, 48,* 226–252.

Stevens, J. C., & Cain, W. S. (1987). Old-age deficits in the sense of smell as gauged by thresholds, magnitude matching, and odor identification. *Psychology and Aging, 2,* 36–42.

Stevens, J. C., & Marks, L. E. (1980). Cross-modality matching functions generated by magnitude estimation. *Perception and Psychophysics, 27,* 379–389.

Stevens, J. C., Plantinga, A., & Cain, W. S. (1982). Reduction of odor and nasal pungency associated with aging. *Neurobiology of Aging, 3,* 125–132.

Stevenson, P. W. (1975). Responses to speech audiometry and phonemic discrimination patterns in the elderly. *Audiology, 14,* 185–231.

Stricht, R., & Gray, B. (1969). The intelligibility of time-compressed words as a function of age and hearing loss. *Journal of Speech and Hearing Research, 12,* 443–448.

Sturr, J. F., Kline, G. E., & Taub, H. A. (1990). Performance of young and older drivers on a static acuity test under photopic and mesopic luminance conditions. *Human Factors, 32,* 1–8.

Thomas, P. D., Hunt, W. C., Garry, P. S., Hood, R. B., Goodwin, J. M., & Goodwin, J. S. (1983). Hearing acuity in a healthy elderly population: Effects on emotional, cognitive and social status. *Journal of Gerontology, 38,* 321–325.

Thornbury, J. M., & Minstretta, C. M. (1981). Tactile sensitivity as a function of age. *Journal of Gerontology, 36,* 34–39.

Tillman, T. W., Carhardt, R., & Nicholls, S. (1973). Release from multiple maskers in elderly persons. *Journal of Speech and Hearing Research, 16,* 152–160.

Tulunay-Keesey, U., VerHoeve, J. N., & Terkla-McGrane, C. (1988). Threshold and suprathreshold spatiotemporal response throughout adulthood. *Journal of the Optical Society of America, 5,* 2191–2200.

Upfold, L., & Wilson, D. (1982). Factors associated with hearing aid use. *Australian Journal of Audiology, 5,* 20–26.

vanMeeteren, A., & Vos, J. J. (1972). Resolution and contrast sensitivity at low luminances. *Vision Research, 12,* 825–833.

Venstrom, D., & Amoore, J. E. (1968). Olfactory threshold in relation to age, sex, or smoking. *Journal of Food Science, 33,* 290–298.

Verrillo, R. T. (1980). Age-related changes in the sensitivity to vibration. *Journal of Gerontology, 35,* 185–193.

Verrillo, R. T. (1982). Effects of aging on the suprathreshold responses to vibration. *Perception and Psychophysics, 32,* 61–68.

Verrillo, R. T., & Verrillo, V. (1985). Sensory and perceptual performance. In N. Charness (Ed.), *Aging and human performance* (pp. 1–46). New York: Wiley.

Vola, J. L., Cornu, C., Carruel, P., Gastaud, P., & Leid, J. (1983). L'age et les acuites visuelles photopiques et mesopiques. *Journale Francaise Ophtalmolgie, 6,* 473–479.

Von Leden, H. (1977). Speech and hearing problems in the geriatric patient. *Journal of the American Geriatrics Society, 25*(9), 422–426.

Vrabec, F. (1965). Senile change in the ganglion cells of the human retina. *British Journal of Ophthalmology,* *49,* 561–572.

Wainwright, W. W. (1943). Inorganic phosphorus content of resting saliva of 650 healthy individuals. *Journal of Dental Research, 22,* 403–414.

Walsh, D. A. (1976). Age differences in central perceptual processing: A dichoptic backward masking investigation. *Journal of Gerontology, 31,* 178–185.

Warren, L. R., Wagener, J. W., & Herman, G. F. (1978). Binaural analysis in the aging auditory system. *Journal of Gerontology, 33,* 731–736.

Watson, A. B., Barlow, H. B., & Robson, J. G. (1983). What does the eye see best? *Nature, 302,* 419–422.

Weale, R. A. (1961). Retinal illumination and age. *Transactions of the Illuminating Engineering Society, 26,* 95–100.

Weale, R. A. (1963). *The aging eye.* London: H. K. Lewis.

Weale, R. A. (1975). Senile changes in visual acuity. *Transactions of the Ophthalmological Society (U.K.), 95,* 36–38.

Weale, R. A. (1982). Senile ocular changes, cell death, and vision. In R. Sekuler, D. W. Kline, & K. Dismukes (Eds.), *Aging and human visual function* (pp. 161–172). New York: Alan R. Liss.

Weale, R. A. (1984). The aging retina. In D. Platt (Ed.), *Geriatrics 3* (pp. 425–450). Berlin: Springer-Verlag.

Weale, R. A. (1986). Aging and vision. *Vision Research, 26,* 1507–1512.

Weale, R. A. (1988). Age and the transmittance of the human crystalline lens. *Journal of Physiology, 395,* 577–587.

Weekers, R., & Roussel, F. (1945). Introduction a l'etude de la frequence de fusion en clinique. *Opthalmalogica, 112,* 305–319.

Weiffenbach, J. M. (1984). Taste and smell perception in aging. *Gerontology, 3,* 137–146.

Weiffenbach, J. M., Baum, B. J., & Burghauser, R. (1982). Taste thresholds: Quality-specific variation with human aging. *Journal of Gerontology, 37,* 372–377.

Weiffenbach, J. M., Cowart, B. J., & Baum, B. J. (1986). Taste intensity perception in aging. *Journal of Gerontology, 41,* 460–468.

Weinstein, B., & Ventry, I. (1983). Audiometric correlates of the Hearing Handicap Inventory for the Elderly. *Journal of Speech and Hearing Disorders, 48,* 379–384.

Werner, J. S., & Steele, V. G. (1988). Sensitivity of human foveal color mechanisms throughout the lifespan. *Journal of the Optical Society of America: A, 5,* 2122–2130.

Whitaker, D., & Elliott, D. (1989). Toward establishing a clinical displacement threshold technique to evaluate visual function behind cataract. *Clinical Vision Science, 4,* 61–69.

Whitaker, L. S., Shoptaugh, C. F., & Haywood, K. M. (1986). Effect of age on horizontal eye movement latency. *American Journal of Optometry and Physiological Optics, 63,* 152–155.

Wolf, E. (1960). Glare and age. *Archives of Ophthalmology, 60,* 502–514.

Wolf, E. (1967). Studies in the shrinkage of the visual field with age. *American Journal of Ophthalmology, 167,* 1–7.

Wolf, E., & Shaffra, A. M. (1964). Relationship between critical flicker frequency and age in flicker perimetry. *Archives of Ophthalmology, 72,* 832–843.

Woodrow, K. M., Friedman, G. D., Siegelaub, A. B., & Collen, M. F. (1972). Pain tolerance: Differences according to age, sex, and race. *Psychosomatic Medicine, 34,* 548–556.

Wright, C. E., & Drasdo, N. (1985). The influence of age on the spatial and temporal contrast sensitivity function. *Documenta Ophthalmologica, 59,* 385–395.

Wright, J. L., & Schuknecht, H. F. (1972). Atrophy of the spiral ligament. *Archives of Otolaryngology, 96,* 16–21.

Wysocki, C. J., & Gilbert, A. N. (1989). National Geographic Smell Survey: Effects of age are heterogenous. In C. Murphy, W. S. Cain, & D. M. Hegsted (Eds.), Nutrition and the chemical senses in aging: Recent advances and current research needs. *Annals of the New York Academy of Sciences, 561,* 12–28.

Youdelis, C. & Hendrickson, A. (1986). A qualitative and quantitative analysis of the human fovea during development. *Vision Research, 26,* 847–855.

Memory, Learning, and Attention

Judith A. Sugar and Joan M. McDowd

I. Introduction
II. Memory and Learning
   A. Defining Memory, Learning, and Cognition
   B. Capacities, Opportunities, and Performance
   C. A Preliminary Model of Aging and Memory Performance
   D. Age-Related Differences in Memory and Learning
   E. Explanations for Age-Related Differences in Memory and Learning Performance
   F. Everyday Memory and Aging
   G. Interventions
III. Attention and Aging
   A. Defining Attention
   B. Selective Attention and Aging: Data
   C. Selective Attention and Aging: Theory
   D. Selective Attention: Facilitation and Inhibition
   E. Everyday Attentional Functioning and Aging
IV. Mental Health Issues
   A. Depression
   B. Dementia
V. Future Research Directions
   References

I. Introduction

Since the first edition of the *Handbook on Mental Health and Aging,* there have been many research developments in memory, learning, and attention in relation to aging. The change in the chapter title from "Learning, Memory, and Aging" (Schonfield, 1980) to

"Memory, Learning, and Attention" reflects two such developments—a shift in emphasis from learning to memory research, and an increased interest in attention and aging. Rather than attributing age-related memory problems to acquisition deficits, psychologists now increasingly emphasize the postacquisition phase, particularly retrieval deficits (Burke & Light, 1981). A corollary of this shift in emphasis is that there has been considerably less research activity in the area of learning, or acquisition of information. During the past decade, attention has re-emerged, and the title and discussion of this chapter reflect its increased importance in the research literature.

In the 1980s, researchers developed a new appreciation for the complexity of the relationship between aging, memory, learning, and attention. One outcome of this development is a new approach to cognitive functioning, viewing cognition from the standpoint of its adaptiveness (Anderson & Milson, 1989; Bjork & Bjork, 1988). The notion of the adaptiveness of memory is likely to provide important insights into cognitive aging research over the next decade.

As if in response to the decree that "future research in learning and remembering areas will benefit from the increased pressure for ecological validity" (Schonfield, 1980, p. 240), a new interest in everyday memory has surfaced. Although controversial (Banaji & Crowder, 1989; Neisser, 1978), the area of everyday memory, or ecological memory, has burgeoned over the past decade.

Finally, the surge of interest in Alzheimer's disease over the past decade has brought an enormous increase in research on dementia, including research on deficits in memory, learning, and attention and how tests of these processes may be of diagnostic value.

The first section of this chapter focuses on (1) distinguishing between *capacity* and *performance,* which has important consequences for interpreting and understanding research findings in memory, learning, and attention as they relate to mental health and aging; (2) discussing research findings within the context of a preliminary model of performance; and (3) presenting research on everyday memory, which, contrary to findings in the laboratory, often shows that older adults are as good as or better at remembering than are their younger counterparts. The second section of this chapter will be devoted to attention and aging, an area that, though related in important ways to memory and learning, has used different methodologies and has asked somewhat different questions. The third and fourth sections of this chapter will discuss mental health issues in the area of cognitive aging, and future research directions.

II. Memory and Learning

A. Defining Memory, Learning, and Cognition

The three topics of this chapter, memory, learning, and attention, are all aspects of cognition. Cognition is defined as the processes by which information is acquired, stored, and used. Memory, one of the most central aspects of cognition, has been defined as "the mental processes of retaining information for later use and retrieving such information" (Ashcraft, 1989, p. 703). Memory also involves the mental processes responsible for carrying out plans in the future. Learning, which is a relatively permanent change in behavior potential due to experience, clearly depends on memory, and similarly, both memory and learning depend on attention, which is the mechanism by which incoming information is ranked and passed on for further processing.

B. Capacities, Opportunities, and Performance

Many factors influence memory and learning performance, and capacity is certainly one of them. Capacity, however, can be demonstrated only when an opportunity exists to exercise the capacity. The distinction between capacity and performance is important, but it is often overlooked in the memory and learning literature. Being capable of performing well is not the same as performing well. Capacity refers to what individuals *can do,* whereas performance refers to what individuals *actually do,* given the opportunities their environments provide. Performance depends on capacity and the opportunity to express the capacity.

C. A Preliminary Model of Aging and Memory Performance

Although many data on aging and cognitive performance have been gathered over the past decade, models and theories to account for these data are still lacking (Hultsch & Dixon, 1990). In addition to guiding research, models and theories could help sort out the increasing number of contradictory results in the cognitive aging literature. The relationship between age, memory, learning, and attention is clearly very complex, and no one factor can account for all the existing data on memory performance, even within a particular domain of content (e.g., memory for text) or tasks (e.g., free recall).

Figure 1 presents a preliminary model of the relationships between aging and memory performance. The model could easily be extended to other domains of cognitive performance, including learning and attention. According to the model, changes in physiological capacity accompanying aging can directly affect memory performance. Aging can

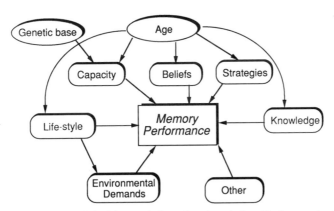

Figure 1   A preliminary model of factors influencing the relationship between aging and memory performance.

also, however, differentially affect other factors including environmental demands for memory, lifestyle, beliefs about memory and self-efficacy, strategy use, and the learner's knowledge base, which, in turn, can affect memory performance.

An important aspect of the preliminary model is that it emphasizes performance as opposed to capacity. A second important aspect of the model is that changes accompanying aging can have positive effects, as well as negative effects, on memory performance. For example, increases in knowledge can improve memory performance (Chi, 1978), and aging may bring with it an increase in knowledge. Hence, the model indicates that aging can have both direct and indirect effects as well as positive or negative effects on memory performance.

D. Age-Related Differences in Memory and Learning

What aspects of memory and learning seem to change with age? Reviews of the literature on this question are not in short supply. Between 1977 and 1982, there were 19 reviews of aging and memory research, which have been summarized by Poon (1985). Many of them discuss age effects in terms of sensory, primary, and secondary memory, or encoding, storage, and retrieval, or both.

Keeping in mind that inconsistent results are not uncommon in cognitive aging research, we nevertheless can discern patterns of age effects. Aging does not seem to appreciably affect sensory memory (very brief memory for visual and other sensory information) or primary memory (memory for events currently in consciousness). There is ample evidence, however, that secondary memory (memory for events that have already occurred) declines with age (Craik, 1977; Craik & McDowd, 1987; Poon, 1985).

Nevertheless, the conclusion that secondary memory declines with age must be tempered by several facts: (1) not all types of secondary memory tasks show a decline with age; for example, performance on simple recognition memory tasks appears to be similar across age (Hultsch, 1975); (2) age effects do not occur with some types of materials; for example, older adults recall more words than do younger adults when the words are more familiar to the older adults (Barrett & Wright, 1981); (3) older adults with high verbal ability perform as well as younger adults even on tasks, such as free recall, that otherwise show age effects (Cavanaugh, 1983); and (4) not all types of information show age effects favoring the young; for example, older adults may be better than younger adults at recalling the gist, as opposed to the details, of prose passages (Labouvie-Vief, Campbell, Weaver, & Tannenhaus, 1979). An excellent review and discussion of many of these findings can be found in Hultsch and Dixon (1990) and will not be repeated here.

As we enter the decade of the 1990s, several tentative conclusions about aging, memory, and learning can be drawn from the literature. First, aging does not produce a uniform decline in memory or learning processes. Second, there are some differences between younger and older adults in cognitive abilities, differences that generally favor younger adults. Third, age differences in cognitive performance are often small, and "the magnitudes of age differences reported in the research literature over the last three decades [seem to] have shrunk" (Poon, 1989, p. 129). Fourth, from a practical point of view, observed differences due to age may be insignificant, though theoretically interesting.

Fifth, some observed age differences disappear with practice or training or both. And last, but not least, on some memory and learning tasks, older adults sometimes simply perform better than some younger adults.

E. Explanations for Age-Related Differences in Memory and Learning Performance

Most explanations for age-related differences in memory and learning performance arise from one of two approaches. Some researchers attribute most of the observed age differences to endogenous factors. For example, Salthouse (1985) has theorized that an overall reduction in processing speed accounts for declining cognitive abilities in older adults. More recently, Hasher and Zacks (1988) have proposed that aging causes a decrease in the ability to inhibit irrelevant information. According to this notion, aging causes more environmental stimuli to impinge on us, and, consequently, we become slower at taking in new information and retrieving old information.

On the other hand, some researchers attribute most of the observed age differences to exogenous factors. For example, the argument has been made that younger and older adults may differ on educational, lifestyle, and personality variables that affect memory and learning performance (Schaie, 1983). Another argument has been that older adults are at an unfair disadvantage relative to young college students because the typical laboratory tasks and settings are less familiar and less relevant to them (Labouvie-Vief & Schell, 1982).

The new approach to cognitive functioning as adaptive has the potential to unite these previously disparate explanations for age-related differences in memory and learning performance. Craik (1986), for example, has proposed a functional approach to memory, which pays attention to the interaction between processing resources and the amount of environmental support available to the individual. We agree with Craik, Byrd, and Swanson (1987) that "theories of cognitive performance must model the interactions between mental processes and relevant aspects of the environment" (p. 85).

1. Environmental Demands

Most research studies compare the performance of older adults to that of young college students. In addition to age differences, then, such groups of old and young subjects may differ on other variables that could be the true source of any differences in their performance. One possible other variable is being *in school*. In order to investigate the importance of this variable, Zivian and Darjes (1983) tested recall and metamemory (awareness of one's memory) in four groups of subjects: young college students, middle-aged college students, middle-aged adults who were not students, and older adults who were not students. The young and middle-aged in-school groups performed equally well on an experimental task by recalling a similar number of words, which was significantly higher than the number of words recalled by the middle-aged and older *out-of-school* groups, who did not differ from each other. Furthermore, compared to the in-school adults, the out-of-school adults relied on fewer and less effective mnemonic strategies; out-of-school adults also did not appear to value strategies, such as organizing and grouping the material, that are considered optimal for learning and remembering categorized word lists. Zivian and Darjes concluded that "the combined results reveal that years of schooling, as well as actually being in school, may be better predictors than age of differences in metamemory and memory performance" (p. 513).

Studies in which older adults are compared to young adults who are not in college are rare. One such study was conducted by Ratner, Schell, Crimmins, Mittelman, and Baldinelli (1987). Ratner *et al.* tested prose recall and learning strategies in three groups of subjects: young college students, young adults who were not in college, and older adults who were not in college. Noncollege young adults and noncollege older adults recalled a similar amount of information and spent a similar length of time studying; young college students outperformed both noncollege groups, remembering more and studying for a longer period. One explanation for these results is that school may provide an environment in which students learn and practice effective memory strategies. Indeed, Rice and her colleagues (e.g., Rice, Meyer, & Miller, 1988) have suggested just such a *practice effect* to account for a relationship they have found between how well adults recall prose and the amount of time they spend on everyday activities that are similar to recalling prose. As Ratner *et al.* have concluded, "memory differences between old and young have been overattributed, perhaps, to the natural aging process" (p. 524).

Contrary to what might be expected on the basis of the results of the two studies just described, Hartley (1986) failed to find a difference between older adults who were students, and those who were not, in their memory for discourse. Clearly, the conditions under which student status may make a difference in performance for young and older adults have yet to be established. Differences between the samples or the measures may account for these apparently inconsistent findings.

2. Age Differences in Lifestyle

Adults of different ages have different lifestyles. Some of the age differences in lifestyles may contribute to observed age differences in memory and learning performance. For example, researchers have demonstrated a relationship between memory performance and the types of daily activities in which older adults engage (Arbuckle, Gold, & Andres, 1986; Craik, Byrd, & Swanson, 1987; Winocur, Moscovitch, & Freedman, 1987). In a sample of 285 adults ranging in age from 65 to 93 years, Arbuckle, Gold, and Andres found that the amount of involvement in intellectual activities was one of the best predictors of performance on memory tasks that included digit span, free recall, and recall and comprehension of prose. Older adults who participated in more intellectual activities did better on the memory tasks.

Clarkson-Smith and Hartley (1990) have hypothesized that "age-related deterioration of cognitive abilities, such as working memory, is delayed when individuals participate in activities requiring use of these abilities" (p. P236). Consistent with their hypothesis, they found that elderly bridge players performed significantly better on cognitive tasks related to bridge playing—working memory and reasoning tasks—than did elderly nonplayers. On the other hand, cognitive tasks unrelated to bridge playing—vocabulary and reaction time—yielded similar performance for bridge players and nonplayers, as expected. Everyday activities may involve more or fewer opportunities to use and, thus, practice, memory and learning skills. Individual differences in everyday activities, then, may account for differences in memory and learning performance.

Another aspect of lifestyles that may have consequences for cognitive functioning is regularity in the structure of daily life. To test the hypothesis that age differences in the structure of daily life may be associated with differences in memory functioning, Sugar (1989, 1990) asked young and older adults to keep daily diaries of instances of forgetting as they occurred, and to record their bedtimes. She found that higher incidences of forgetting were associated with greater variability in sleep patterns. Furthermore, older adults reported significantly fewer instances of forgetting and significantly less variability in their sleep patterns than did younger adults. Thus, a more regular structure to daily life appears to be associated with less forgetting. Compared to young college students, older adults lead more structured lives, and this seems to be related to the maintenance of their everyday cognitive functioning. The types of activities that people engage in and the structure of their daily life are aspects of lifestyle that differ with age and that influence memory performance. Other aspects of lifestyle that differ with age may also influence cognitive performance.

3. Age Differences in Beliefs

Of particular importance to mental health is people's beliefs about their memory and learning abilities and how these beliefs might affect their behavior. The past decade has seen an explosion of interest in measuring beliefs, perceptions, attitudes, and knowledge about personal memory abilities, as well as memory in general. Questionnaires typically ask respondents how frequently they forget names and events, how anxious they are about forgetting, what they know about how to improve memory, and what strategies they use in remembering. Instruments include the Subjective Memory Questionnaire (Bennett-Levy & Powell, 1980), the Cognitive Failures Questionnaire (Broadbent, Cooper, Fitzgerald, & Parkes, 1982), the Metamemory in Adulthood Questionnaire (Dixon & Hultsch, 1983), the Short Inventory of Memory Experiences (Herrmann & Neisser, 1978), the Memory Questionnaire (Perlmutter, 1978), the Error Proneness Questionnaire (Reason & My-cielska, 1982), and the Metamemory Questionnaire (Zelinski, Gilewski, & Thompson, 1980). Reviews of these questionnaires can be found in Herrmann (1982, 1984) and Dixon (1989).

A common belief, and one that is supported by some research (Cavanaugh, Grady, & Perlmutter, 1983; Gilewski & Zelinski, 1986; Perlmutter, 1978), is that older adults experience more difficulties with their memory than do younger adults. Compared to younger adults, older adults are also reportedly more upset by their memory failures (Zarit, Cole, & Guider, 1981). These beliefs and feelings of self-efficacy can influence how adults of different ages respond to memory tasks (Sehulster, 1981; West & Bramblett, 1990). In a sample of 60- to 80-year-old adults, for example, West and Bramblett found that memory self-evaluation predicted recall scores better than did age or depression scale scores.

Cultural beliefs about age-related declines in cognitive abilities may cause individual instances of cognitive failures to become more salient than they might otherwise be for older adults. In the case of forgetting, for example, increased salience of instances of forgetting could lead to beliefs that the frequency of forgetting is higher than it actually is. Older adults, then, may think they forget more than they actually do because they pay more attention when they forget something. However, there are some reasons to believe that memory failures may not always be more common among older adults than younger adults.

Even for middle-aged adults, "I must be getting Alzheimer's" has become a familiar refrain following an instance of forgetting. Furthermore, the popularity of self-help books for improving memory (Cermak, 1976; Herrmann, 1988; Higbee, 1977; West, 1985) indicates that the desire to maintain or enhance memory is not only a concern of the elderly. Although older adults' complaints about their inability to remember proper names has some empirical basis (Cohen & Faulkner, 1986), most people will readily admit that they are not, and never have been, good at remembering names. Indeed, almost half of one book on memory techniques for business people is devoted to improving memory for names and faces (Keith, 1989).

To assess the common belief that old age is always accompanied by declining memory abilities, Cutler and Grams (1988) examined responses to two questions about memory problems that were taken from the 1984 Supplement on Aging to the National Health Interview Study (National Center for Health Statistics, 1986). They found that

> memory problems are not universally experienced by community-residing elders. Only 15% of this national sample of [14,783] persons aged 55 and older said that they frequently had had problems forgetting things during the past year, whereas more than 25% said they had never had problems. Perhaps of even greater importance, less [sic] than 1 in 5 of the respondents said the trouble was happening with increasing frequency (p. S88).

Researchers have often commented that everyday memory failures may be less salient for younger adults than for older adults (Cavanaugh, 1986–1987; Perlmutter et al., 1987; Zelinski et al., 1980). An age difference in the salience of forgetting may explain why younger adults are not known for complaining about memory failures, but older adults are. In a diary study of everyday forgetting, Sugar (1989) found that older adults thought they forgot often, even when they reported half as many instances of forgetting as the younger adults.

Older adults may compare their current memory experiences with idealized notions of how good their memories used to be. Anecdotally, it seems that many people who complain about memory failures imagine that they never forgot anything when they were younger! Diary reports of forgetting collected from college students suggest that these perceptions are inaccurate. For example, Sugar (1988) found that the fewest number of instances of forgetting reported by 39 college students over the course of one week was 8, and one student reported 54 instances! Although this is likely to be an underestimate of the actual number of instances, it is certainly not an overestimate. Older adults may perceive a decrease in memory functioning with age that is, in part, due to an increased sensitivity to instances of cognitive failures.

4. Age Differences in Strategy Use

Learning and remembering require the use of strategies. The effectiveness of the strategies that are used in learning and remembering are likely to interact with the capacities of the individual in determining performance. Figure 2 shows theoretical relationships between capacity, strategy, and performance. Asterisks on each graph represent the performance of two hypothetical individuals, one who has a large memory capacity and another who is adept with memory strategies. In the top of the figure, capacity and strategy interact to enhance performance; the greater an individual's capacity, the greater will be effects due to the use of strategies to increase performance. In the middle of the figure, capacity and strategy are independent; each can affect performance, but they do so independent of one another. Finally, in the bottom of the figure, strategy is the major determinant of performance and improvements in capacity do not have much effect.

Theoretically, then, capacity is not the sole determinant of memory performance. Our two hypothetical individuals demonstrate that it is possible for someone who is adept with

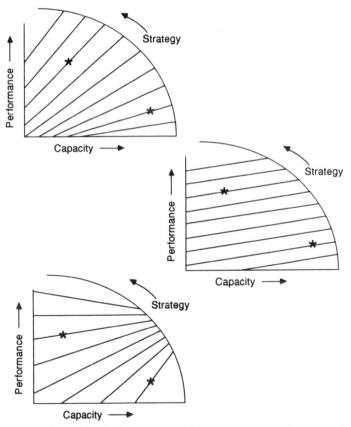

Figure 2   Theoretical relationships between capacity, strategy, and performance. Asterisks represent the performances of different individuals.

memory strategies to outperform someone with a large memory capacity. Regardless of the specific relationship, or relationships, they may exist between capacities and strategies, performance is likely to be enhanced when more numerous or more efficient strategies are used. The ways in which capacities and strategies interact for persons differing in age is likely to be an exciting area of research in the 1990s.

Strategies for learning and remembering can be categorized as primarily internal or external. Internal memory strategies are those that rely on the internal mental processes of the person. Repeating to yourself over and over again the items you want to buy at the grocery store is an example of an internal strategy. Harris (1978) describes these strategies as "automatic in the sense that they are not taught and that in many instances the user is probably not aware of using them" (p. 173). Harris differentiates internal strategies from internal aids, which are "techniques which often have to be consciously learned and used, such as the 'peg' and 'loci' methods" (p. 173). Both the peg method and the method of loci are mnemonic techniques in which items to be remembered are visually associated with something that is already familiar; in the peg method, the association is made to keywords (*pegs*) that have already been learned in a numbered sequence, and in the method of loci, the association is made to familiar locations. External memory strategies involve the use of aids that are external to the person. Writing out a list of the items you want to buy at the grocery store is an example of an external memory strategy.

There is evidence of age differences in the use of internal and external memory strategies. In laboratory environments, older adults often fail to spontaneously use the internal memory strategies that are likely to be most effective in learning and remembering the materials to which they are exposed in the laboratory (Craik, 1977), although they can use them successfully if they are so instructed (e.g., Hulicka & Grossman, 1967; Hultsch, 1969; Treat, Poon, & Fozard, 1978). Furthermore, studies have demonstrated that in their everyday lives, older adults seem to use external memory strategies more often and more effectively than do younger adults (Cavanaugh *et al.*, 1983; Loewen, Shaw, & Craik, 1990; Moscovitch, 1982; Poon & Shaffer, 1982; Sugar, 1989; but see West, 1988, for a different result). Age differences in the use of strategies for remembering appear to be an important factor in the age-related performance differences found in the laboratory and may also help to explain differences between performance in laboratory tasks and performance in everyday memory tasks.

F. Everyday Memory and Aging

Research on everyday memory has special significance for the field of mental health. After all, how people function in their everyday environments is the most important concern of mental health professionals. The memory abilities and skills required for everyday memory may differ from those required for laboratory tasks, and such differences could have practical, as well as theoretical, significance. Despite its importance, everyday memory has received little attention until recently.

Most research on aging and memory has investigated retrospective memory, remembering something that was learned in the past. Learning a list of 10 words and then recalling them five minutes later is an example of a retrospective memory task. Another kind of memory, however, forms a larger part of everyday experiences, namely, prospective memory, or remembering to carry out intended actions. Remembering that you have an appointment with your physician at 10 AM next Tuesday is an example of a prospective memory task. Whether prospective memory and retrospective memory are seen as two aspects of the same kind of memory system (Baddeley, 1989) or as two distinctly different kinds of memory (Einstein & McDaniel, 1990), people with good memories for events in the past do not necessarily have good memories for events that are to take place in the future (Kvavilashvili, 1987; Meacham & Lieman, 1982; Wilkins & Baddeley, 1978). Conclusions about everyday functioning, then, may be erroneous if they are based only on measures of retrospective memory. For example, an older adult who does less well than a younger adult on a retrospective memory task in the laboratory may, nevertheless, do much better on prospective memory tasks, which are much more abundant in our everyday lives.

Although few in number, studies of prospective memory in which old and young adults have been compared have generally found that older adults' memories are often at least equal to younger adults' memories (Sinnott, 1986), and sometimes better than younger adults' memories (Martin, 1986; Moscovitch, 1982; Poon & Schaffer, 1982). This finding will not be surprising to those who are familiar with the everyday behaviors of teenagers or young adults. Moscovitch (1982), for example, found that, compared to young college students, 65- to 75-year-olds were better at remembering to make phone calls at particular times.

Studies in which adults have been asked to keep diaries of their memory experiences also suggest that older adults' everyday memories may not be so poor as once thought. For example, Tenney (1984) found that young and older adults reported a similar number of incidents of losing objects over a two-week period, and Sugar (1989) found that older adults reported fewer instances of forgetting over a one-week period than did younger adults. Although there are methodological concerns about subjects keeping track of their own behavior (Morris, 1984), diary studies can provide valuable information not otherwise obtainable (Linton, 1978). Some confusions about how to interpret data collected from diaries can be avoided if it is remembered that diaries can never measure capacity. For example, some people may report very little forgetting because, in their lives, there are few occasions for forgetting to occur, whereas other people may forget very little because they work very hard at remembering. Phenomenological similarities in the amount of forgetting are not necessarily of interest from the point of view of memory capacity. They are of interest only from a performance point of view, and then they represent an index of the experience of everyday forgetting.

In everyday memory research, the most frequent criticism of diaries is that subjects are likely to fail to record all their forgetting. Failure to record instances of forgetting may occur as a consequence of a lack of recognition about what constitutes forgetting (a problem of definition), a lack of awareness that forgetting occurred (a problem of low sensitivity of salience to forgetting), or a lack of compliance with recording instructions (a problem in carrying out the investigator's instructions). Lack of recognition and lack of awareness, though, would not appear to be major sources of difficulty for older people, otherwise we have a paradox: If older adults are less likely to recognize instances of forgetting when they occur, or if they are less aware than younger adults of their forgetting, or both, then why do they complain about forgetting more than do younger adults? The importance of having completely accurate records of all instances of forgetting depends on what questions the investigator is trying to answer. The information obtained from diaries may be useful for many different questions, including what, if anything, to do about memory failures.

G. Interventions

1. Mnemonics Training

As mentioned previously, older adults can use internal strategies for remembering, though they may not often do so spontaneously. Cognitive aging researchers have successfully taught older adults how to use mnemonic devices to improve their performance. The mnemonic most often taught is the method of loci (Anschutz, Camp, Markley, & Kramer, 1985; Robertson-Tchabo, Hausman, & Arenberg, 1976; Rose & Yesavage, 1983). For example, Rose and Yesavage (1983) found that teaching older adults the method of loci significantly improved their recall for a list of words. But memory researchers themselves do not use these techniques. Memory researchers prefer to use external memory aids, aids they forbid their subject to use. Memory researchers' favorite technique for remembering is to *write things down* (Park, Smith, & Cavanaugh, 1990), a mnemonic that has been called "the greatest memory aid ever invented" (Gruneberg, 1978, p. 206).

An important lesson for mnemonics trainers is that programs need to be tailored to the individual; what works for one person may not work for another, and some techniques may be preferred, or disliked, by one or another individual or age group. For example, Poon and Walsh-Sweeney (1981) found that older adults did not like creating bizarre images to remember paired associates. Intervention programs should take into account the purposes to which the intervention will be put and the learner's abilities, existing knowledge, and preferences. Advice borrowed from the other end of the lifespan would seem to be equally appropriate for aging researchers:

> The types of cognitive activities . . . suitable for intensive intervention should have certain properties, (a) they should have trans-situational applicability, (b) they should readily be seen by the [learner] to be reasonable activities that work, (c) they should have some counterpart in real-life experiences, and (d) their component processes should be well understood so that effective training techniques can be devised (Brown & Campione, 1978, p. 36).

2. Exercise and Nutrition

A lack of physical activity may exacerbate older adults' declining physiological capacities. If this hypothesis is correct, then another intervention that might be successful in improving cognitive performance is exercise. The investigation of the effects of physical fitness on cognitive abilities is a relatively new area and is still plagued with methodological problems. Nevertheless, there are encouraging indications that physical exercise can improve cognitive performance (Dustman *et al.*, 1984; Elsayed, Ismail, & Young, 1980).

Aging has also been associated with decrements in nutritional status (O'Hanlon & Kohrs, 1978) which, in turn, may negatively affect cognitive functioning. For example, Cherkin (1984) found poor memory performance in older adults with thiamine deficiencies, and Goodwin, Goodwin, and Garry (1983) reported low scores on the Wechsler Memory Scale in older adults with low levels of vitamins C and B_{12} who otherwise seemed healthy. Because nutritional deficiencies may be readily ameliorated, more research in this area could lead to improvements in cognitive functioning for many older adults.

Maintaining or improving cognitive functioning in normal, healthy older adults is an important goal for mental health professionals. Another important goal is to be able to differentiate normal from pathological functioning. We will take up this issue after we review the data and theories about another cognitive process in aging, attention.

III. Attention and Aging

A. Defining Attention

One of the most comprehensive definitions of attention describes it as "the mechanism by which we prepare to process stimuli, focus on what to process, and determine how far it will be processed and whether it should call us to action" (Heilman, Watson, Valenstein, & Goldberg, 1987, p. 461). Attention is the mechanism by which incoming information is assigned priority and passed on for further processing. Broadly speaking, selective attention is the controller of information processing, in that in a given situation, priority is given to the signals required by the current goals and intentions of the individual. If performance in some situation deteriorates due to a failure of this control mechanism, a selective attention deficit is said to have occurred. The focus of the following sections will be on the selective nature of attention, and how selective processes may change with age.

B. Selective Attention and Aging: Data

The most frequently cited and perhaps first work in aging and selective attention was conducted by Rabbitt (1965). He had young and old adults sorting decks of cards according to the identity of target letters printed on them. In some cases, in addition to the target letters, extraneous letters were also printed on the cards. Rabbitt observed that the sorting times of all individuals increased as a function of the number of nontarget items present on the cards, and that this increase was greater for older than for young adults. This finding has been interpreted as indicating an age-related inability to ignore irrelevant information. Older adults are said to be distracted by the presence of irrelevant information; this distractibility slows older adults more than young; and this relative slowing increases as a function of the number of irrelevant items in a display.

A number of studies of aging and selective attention have appeared since Rabbitt's work, and have established important qualifications to early conclusions regarding age-related distractibility. For example, Wright and Elias (1979) questioned Rabbitt's notion that the nontarget information present on the to-be-sorted cards was strictly irrelevant. In fact, each of these items had to be scanned for the presence of the target item, and could be discarded as irrelevant only after its identity had been determined. Wright and Elias devised a task to look at distractibility in the face of irrelevant items that also eliminated the need for processing of those irrelevant items.

Their task was a two-choice, reaction-time task in which one of two target letters appeared in the center of a visual display. Subjects responded to the identity of the target, in this case, whether it was an *H* or an *S*. In one condition, the letter appeared by itself in the center of the screen, without distractors. In the distracting condition, the target letter again appeared in the center of the screen, but was flanked on both sides by extraneous, irrelevant letters. Wright and Elias observed reaction-time slowing to targets flanked by distractors relative to targets presented alone, but the magnitude of this slowing was equivalent for young and old adults. That is, when the requirement of search was eliminated, older adults were not differentially affected by the presence of irrelevant information.

Plude (1980) reported a study with similar results. He used a yes/no target-detection task in which target letters appeared either singly, or in an array of five letters arranged in a 3×3 grid. In the nonsearch condition, the target appeared only in the center position of the display. In the search condition, the target was equally probable in each display condition. In the nonsearch condition, young and old adults were comparably and only slightly affected by the presence of distracting letters. However, in the search condition, the presence of distracting letters slowed older adults significantly more than young adults. Plude and Hoyer (1986) have followed up on this finding in similar paradigms, taking care to control for any age differences in visual acuity, and have found the same result. In addition, Madden (1983) has reported a similar finding in his task condition, which reduced the search requirement from four to two possible locations. Again, reducing or eliminating the need for searching a display eliminated age differences in selective attention.

A study by Farkas and Hoyer (1980) examined the contribution of both uncertainty about target location and similarity between target and distractors to age differences in selective attention performance. Theirs was another card-sorting task, in which the subject was to sort cards on the basis of the orientation of the target letter *T*. Card-sorting was carried out in three conditions. In the first, no distractor items were present on the cards. In the second, the distractors were the letter *I*, oriented in a manner contrasting with that of the *T*s. Finally, the third condition contained distracting *I*s in the same orientation as the *T*s. In the search condition, targets were located with equal probability in any one of the four positions formed by a 2×2 grid. In the nonsearch condition, the subjects were informed where the target would appear in the array, and the location was kept constant across a given deck of cards.

The results show that in the nonsearch condition, only the older adults were slowed by the presence of irrelevant items, and only in the presence of similar targets. In the search condition, older adults, but not young adults, were slowed in the presence of dissimilar targets. With similar targets, both old and young were slowed, but the magnitude of the slowing was greater for old than for young adults. Together, these results indicate that age differences in distractibility or selective attention depend on the uncertainty about the location of relevant target information as well as the physical similarity of targets and distractors.

Nebes and Madden (1983) looked at the contribution of yet another physical feature, that of color, to age differences in selective attention. In their study, subjects made a yes/no decision about the presence of a target digit in a 2 × 3 array of digits. In this 6-item array, half of the digits were red and half were black. On half of the trials, a color cue specified the subset of items in which the target would appear. That is, a red cue indicated that the target, if present, would be among the red items. The items in the other color could be ignored as irrelevant. Nebes and Madden reported that both young and older adults were equally able to take advantage of the color cue to speed their responding. They concluded that "when stimulus relevance can be determined from a salient physical feature, such as color or location, the old can focus their attention as well as can the young" (p. 142).

C. Selective Attention and Aging: Theory

A number of studies have documented the conditions under which older adults do and do not seem to be affected by the presence of distracting or irrelevant information. How do we begin to understand these sets of data? Plude and Hoyer (1985) have postulated what they call the Spatial Localization Hypothesis. This hypothesis posits that age decrements in selective attention are due to a decline in the ability to locate task-relevant information in the visual field. Plude and Hoyer postulate that the operation of the selective attention mechanism in locating target information is more capacity-demanding for older adults than for young adults. The assumption is made that the capacity available for information processing is an inverse function of the amount of capacity required by the selective-attention mechanism, and that speed of information processing is a function of the amount of capacity available for carrying out those processes. Thus, older adults are slowed in processing relevant information in situations in which that information is not easily located.

Another attempt to synthesize existing data on age differences in selective attention was put forward by Rabbitt (1979). He distinguished between data-driven and memory-driven selective attention. The nature of selectivity might be thought of as the parameters of the filter through which information must pass. In the case of data-driven selective attention, the nature of the input processed at one moment determines the selection of input to be processed next. Memory-driven selectivity, on the other hand, is determined by information stored within the system (or individual).

Rabbitt contends that age differences are in memory-driven selectivity rather than data-driven selectivity. For example, he cites the results of a two-choice, reaction-time task in which a plus sign or a minus sign appeared on a to-be-ignored color patch. Subjects simply pressed one of two keys, depending on whether the stimulus was a plus or a minus. In cases in which immediately successive stimuli shared features, the response times of young and old were equally speeded. Rabbitt suggests that selectivity parameters remain set to match those of a previous stimulus; if repetition of stimulus features occurs, then processing is facilitated. If the stimulus changes, then the selectivity parameters are passively reset.

In contrast to data-driven selectivity, memory-driven selectivity depends on parameters set by processes internal to the organism. As an example, Rabbitt cites a study in which subjects are instructed to press a button if a visually presented digit is from the set 1,3,4, or 8, and to do nothing if some other digit is presented. The data indicate that old and young showed comparable facilitation when the identical digit was presented on suc-cessive trials. This is equivalent to the data-driven selectivity described in the previous experiment. However, young but not older adults exhibited facilitation when two mem-bers of the target *set* of items were presented on successive trials. Rabbitt suggests that the attentional selectivity of young adults could be set to a category held in memory, but not so for older adults. He goes on to suggest that "age decrements in selective attention may be related to failures in central control processes by means of which information stored in memory is used to optimize attentional selectivity from moment to moment during the course of continuous tasks" (p. 93).

Rabbitt's distinction between data-driven and memory-driven selectivity has received some support from related studies in the literature. For example, Nissen and Corkin (1985) reported that old and young adults were equally responsive to visual cues pertain-ing to the probable location of target items. A visual, simple reaction-time task was used in which a cue appeared at the beginning of each trial to indicate the probable location of the target stimulus. Subjects simply pressed a key as soon as they detected the target on the display screen. The cues could be either valid, neutral, or invalid with regard to the actual location of the target stimulus. Response times of both groups were shortest when the target stimulus appeared at the expected location and longest when it appeared in the unexpected location. In addition, the magnitude of these effects was comparable in the two age groups.

In contrast to the findings of Nissen and Corkin, an earlier series of studies by Sanford and Maule (e.g., 1973), in which subjects had to selectively attend to multiple inputs on the basis of learned probability information, indicated that older adults were less likely to use the probability information to guide their selective allocation of attention. Nissen and Corkin suggest that older adults may be more dependent on exogenous cues to control attention: the arrow is perhaps a more salient aid than memory-dependent probability information. This notion is also akin to one put forth by Craik (e.g., Craik & McDowd, 1987) in the literature on memory functioning and aging, that older adults do best when external cues are available to support retrieval, and do less well when memory depends on self-initiated processing.

Other studies of age differences in data-driven and memory-driven attention have provided only mixed support for Rabbitt's hypotheses. Nebes and Madden (1983) caution that "Rabbitt's distinction between data-driven and memory-driven forms of selective attention may well be valid, but other factors such as the reliability of subjects' expecta-tions, as well as the size and complexity of the memory requirements of the task, may interact to determine the degree to which an age decrement in selective attention is evident" (p. 142).

Although the vast majority of studies of age differences in selective attention have used visual search paradigms, other paradigms have occasionally been used. Kausler and Kleim (1978) investigated age-related distractibility in a multiple-item recognition memory task. In such a task, two or more items are presented, one of which is designated as relevant, or to-be-studied. This designation is made simply by underlining the relevant item. On subsequent trials following study, the subject's task is to identify which items had been previously designated relevant when re-presented in combination with other items but in the absence of any cues. Obviously, the most effective strategy at study is to focus on designated items and ignore the others. To the extent that attention is paid to irrelevant items, memory performance will deteriorate.

Kausler and Kleim predicted, based on a hypothesis of age-related distractibility, that the magnitude of age differences in performance would increase with the number of non-target items presented. That is, if older adults are more distracted by irrelevant information, they should pay more attention to the nontarget words at the expense of processing the target words for later retrieval. Kausler and Kleim's study paired target words with either one or three distractor words. At retrieval, older adults did less well than young even on items that had been paired with only one distractor, and this difference was magnified when three distractors had been present. Kausler and Kleim conclude from these results that older adults show a differential susceptibility to distraction.

In another study, Hoyer, Rebok, and Sved (1979) examined age-related distractibility in the problem-solving domain of concept formation. The concept-formation literature has demonstrated that the difficulty of concept acquisition increases with the number of irrelevant dimensions that may appear. Hoyer et al. hypothesized that if older adults are more distracted by irrelevant information, increasing the number of irrelevant dimensions in a concept-formation task should negatively affect older adults more than young. They tested young and old adults on a stimulus-matching task in which one dimension was relevant and three dimensions were irrelevant. In addition, the irrelevant dimensions were either variable or constant. Time to complete the match was the dependent variable.

The results of this study indicated that response time increased as the number of variable, irrelevant dimensions increased, and that this increase was greater for the old than for the young. In their analysis of the task, Hoyer et al. suggest that correct solution of the problem involves not only efficient processing of relevant information, but also the ability to mentally eliminate dimensions and stimuli that are irrelevant. They conclude that "age-associated problem-solving deficits in adulthood are due in part to an inability to efficiently discard irrelevant information" (p. 559).

D. Selective Attention: Facilitation and Inhibition

At the present time, there is no general model or theory of age differences in selective attention. One might postulate that older adults have leaky filters, in terms of structural models of attention (e.g., Broadbent, 1958), or that they have inefficient allocation policies, in terms of capacity models (e.g., Kahneman, 1973). However, filter and capacity models emphasize only the processes carried out on the selected information, and do not deal with the processes that might be carried out on the ignored information. Selective attention may be more complex than these models imply, requiring both an active facilitation of selected information and an active inhibition of nonselected, or ignored information. Posner and Snyder (1975) said that theories of attention must deal with both facilitatory and inhibitory effects, and that these are separate processes. Neill (1977) suggested that selectivity might be accomplished by the inhibition of undesired inputs, so that ignored information is *disattended* rather than *unattended*. These models indicate that attention is a complex process involving both facilitation and inhibition, and efficient behavior requires a delicate balance between the two.

It has been suggested that, for older adults, inhibitory processes are more compromised than are facilitatory processes, and this interrupts the balance required by efficient selective attention, producing in older adults a higher level of distractibility than is present in young adults. For example, Shaw (1990) recently presented some data examining age differences in the magnitude of a phenomenon known as the flanker effect. In such a task, subjects are presented with three words arranged vertically in a visual display. They are to make a two-choice categorization decision about the word appearing in the center of the display, and ignore the flanking items. Shaw designed the flankers such that they varied in their relationship to the target item. Flankers were either identical to the target word, semantically related to the target word, semantically unrelated to the target word, or from the other relevant category opposite to the target word. Response times indicated that older adults were more slowed by the presence of flankers, especially if the flankers produced response competition as in the case in which they were from the other relevant category. Shaw suggests that such a finding is due to a failure on the part of older adults to inhibit the processing of irrelevant items.

Shaw's result is reminiscent of Comalli's (1962) early finding with regard to age differences in Stroop task performance. The Stroop task requires the inhibition of an overlearned response, that of reading a color word, in favor of a color-naming response, naming the color of ink in which the word was printed. With advancing age, the time taken to output the desired color response increases to a significantly greater extent relative to the control condition of naming color patches. Again, such a finding has been interpreted as reflecting a reduction of inhibitory efficiency in older adults, which results in the lengthened response times.

In another recent study (Hasher, Connelly, & Zachs, 1990), young and older adults read short printed texts containing to-be-ignored material presented in italics. They then answered multiple-choice factual questions about the texts. Older adults were slower and less accurate on texts containing distracting information, and Hasher *et al.* attribute this to a difficulty in inhibiting the processing of irrelevant information.

The phenomenon of negative priming has been interpreted as a direct result of the inhibition of previously irrelevant information (Tipper, 1985). This finding with young adults allows the straightforward prediction that older adults should show reduced negative priming if indeed inhibitory processes undergo an age-related decline. McDowd and Oseas (1990) tested this prediction, and the data are consistent with the hypothesis of reduced inhibitory function in older adults. The same finding has also been reported by Hasher *et al.* (1990).

Yet another piece of the puzzle regarding facilitation and inhibition in selective attention is provided by the work of Rogers and Fisk (1988). Their interest has been in examining the development of automatic processing in a visual search paradigm. They propose a hybrid connectionist model in which the development of automaticity is composed of two separate processes: associative learning and priority learning. Associative learning changes the weights of the connections between input and output information such that after sufficient training, a given input will automatically evoke the proper output. Priority learning, on the other hand, modifies how strongly a given message will be transmitted through the system via a priority tag on the message. Consistent practice leads to the continual incrementing of the priority tag for target information and decrementing of the priority tag for distractor information. A combination of associative learning and priority learning allows stimuli to be filtered and messages transmitted in the most efficient manner. Rogers and Fisk conclude that the ability to differentially strengthen targets and weaken distractors is disrupted as a function of age, implicating deficient priority learning.

The data of Rogers and Fisk (1988) suggest that age deficits in selective attention have their source in a difficulty in discriminating relevant from irrelevant information. In the context of developing notions of an age-related decline in inhibitory function, if discrimination of relevant and irrelevant information is particularly difficult, then inhibitory mechanisms cannot work efficiently because there is uncertainty as to the information that should be inhibited. Such a view, isolating discrimination processes as the locus for the attentional deficit, is consistent with data reviewed earlier in the context of visual search and target detection paradigms. For example, when the demands to locate and identify task-relevant information are slight, fewer demands are made on inhibitory mechanisms as there is no uncertainty about where or what to inhibit. When fewer demands are put on inhibitory mechanisms as in the nonsearch conditions, older adults are able to perform more comparably to young adults. What is needed now are experiments designed explicitly to test such hypotheses. In addition, the domains for which an age-related decline in inhibitory processes can provide an acceptable account of age differences in performance need to be carefully delimited with continued research.

E. Everyday Attentional Functioning and Aging

Although the majority of laboratory studies of aging and attention show older adults to be at a disadvantage relative to young adults, there is some evidence to suggest that the magnitude of this deficit is mitigated in everyday life, as we have argued is the case for aging and memory. Taylor, McDowd, Birren, and Gutacker (1989) reported a study in which 364 individuals ranging in age from 17 to 84 were asked to complete the Error-Proneness Questionnaire (Reason & Mycielska, 1982). The questionnaire asks subjects to report the frequency with which they commit a series of lapses of attention and memory. The data revealed that young adults in their teens and twenties report more lapses than do adults in any other age group. The picture for adults across the middle and later decades of life was one of relatively stable levels of functioning with regard to everyday lapses of attention and memory. Perhaps the discrepancy between this finding and the findings of many laboratory studies reflects the positive ability of older adults to bring to bear life-long strategies in managing everyday lapses, whereas such compensatory strategies are not useful in most laboratory situations. An interesting question for future research will be how to reconcile these two findings.

IV. Mental Health Issues

Although much of the research reviewed in this chapter concerns the extent to which differences in performance between young and older adults might be attributed to factors other than biological aging, it is clear that performance is influenced by biological aging. Comparisons between young and older adults on standardized tests can be deceiving in this regard. Indeed, the norms for standardized tests adjust for decrements in performance with age so that, "having thus magically restored equality in achievement, we can now comfortably deny the existence of differences between young and old" (Jarvik, 1988, p. 741).

Mental health researchers and clinicians need to be able to distinguish between changes in performance one might expect from normal aging and those that could be symptomatic of pathological aging. Recently, a work group from the National Institute for Mental Health (NIMH) developed a preliminary set of criteria by which we can differentiate *age-associated memory impairment* (AAMI) from the kinds of memory losses that might be associated with depression or age-related disorders such as dementia (Crook *et al.*, 1986).

"AAMI is characterized by complaints of memory impairment in tasks of daily life, substantiated by evidence of such impairment on psychological performance tests with adequate normative data" (Crook *et al.*, 1986, p. 269). Proposed criteria for the diagnosis of AAMI include being older than 50 years, complaining of gradual worsening of every-day memory, performing at least one standard deviation below the mean on a measure of secondary memory for which adequate normative data are available, scoring adequately on a measure of intellectual functioning, and showing no evidence of neurologic disorders (such as dementia), consciousness disturbances (such as delirium), psychiatric disorders (such as depression), brain diseases or pathologies, head injury, or drug dependence. For the measure of secondary memory deficits, Buschke and Grober (1986) have suggested that a cued recall task be used to differentiate *genuine* memory impairment in healthy, elderly people from apparent memory impairment due to cognitive factors other than memory, such as inattention or language deficits.

As the proposed criteria for age-associated memory impairment suggest, many types of mental disorders may be accompanied by memory deficits. Depression and dementia are particularly important because they are two of the most prevalent disorders in older adults.

A. Depression

The most common form of depression, unipolar depression, can be defined as feelings of sadness that persist for several weeks or more and are often accompanied by physical symptoms including loss of appetite, insomnia, and fatigue (American Psychiatric Association, 1980). Although depression seems to be the most common emotional problem in older adults (Butler & Lewis, 1982), recent evidence suggests that, compared to other age groups, depression is much less common in the elderly than has previously been believed. For example, data from the NIMH Mental Health Statistics for 1980 show that "only 139 in 100,000 persons 65 years and older received a diagnosis of a Unipolar Depressive Disorder, compared to an average of 213 in 100,000 among 18- to 64-year-olds" (Nolen-Hoeksema, 1988, p. 214).

Consistent with the view that depression is primarily a mood disorder, most assessment instruments for depression focus on emotional and somatic symptoms. Nevertheless, difficulties in cognitive processes, such as memory, decision making, and concentrating or focusing attention are often cited as symptoms of depression, and some instruments do measure these symptoms. For example, the Geriatric Depression Scale (Yesavage *et al.*, 1983) asks respondents, "Do you feel you have more problems with memory than most?"

The literature on the relationship between depression and memory functioning, however, is equivocal. While researchers have sometimes found an association (e.g., Raskin, Friedman, & DiMascio, 1982), at other times they have not (e.g., Popkin, Gallagher, Thompson, & Moore, 1982). Some researchers have focused on the characteristics of patients that might account for the discrepant findings.

> In general, it appears that the impact of depression on cognitive function is more likely to be evident in patients who are hospitalized, who are outpatients with a severe episode of depression as opposed to a mild to moderate level of depression, who are in poor physical health, or who are in the lower socioeconomic brackets (Thompson, Gong, Haskins, & Gallagher, 1987, p. 307).

Others have focused on the efficacy of our methods for measuring memory when memory is confounded by other factors during depression. Weingartner and his associates (Cohen, Weingartner, Smallberg, Pickar, & Murphy, 1982; Weingartner, 1986), for example, have proposed that depression primarily affects arousal and activation, and consequently, differentially affects effort-demanding as opposed to automatic cognitive processes.

If difficulty in concentrating is a common symptom in depression, then attentional processes should be affected in depressives. Although little research has been conducted in this area, some investigators have implicated abnormal inhibitory functioning in depression among older adults. One hypothesis suggests that an inability to inhibit persistent negative thoughts may contribute to depressive symptomatology (e.g., Edwards & Dickerson, 1987), and that normal age-related declines in inhibitory processes may predispose older adults to depressive symptoms. While very provocative, this hypothesis regarding depression and aging awaits experimental verification. It must also be reconciled with the fact that, in reviewing the literature on depression and aging, Niederehe (1986) failed to find support for the belief that older adults are more likely than younger adults to suffer from cognitive impairments as a result of depression.

B. Dementia

Unlike depression, dementia is by definition a diagnosis that implicates deficits in cognitive processing, including memory, learning, attention, language abilities, and complex reasoning abilities such as decision making and problem solving. Assessment instruments for dementia—for example, the Mini-Mental Status Examination (Folstein, Folstein, & McHugh, 1975), the Alzheimer's Disease Assessment Scale (Rosen, Mohs, & Davis, 1984), and the Mattis Dementia Rating Scale (Mattis, 1976)—commonly include one or more measures of memory and attention.

Mental status tests provide a global index of a patient's cognitive functioning. However, these tests should be supplemented by other measures that can delineate the pattern of disrupted cognitive abilities. Additionally, these tests should be administered on several occasions to assess any progressive changes in cognitive abilities. Both the more detailed examination of cognitive deficits and repeated testings can help in identifying the underlying cause of the deficits. Indeed, Shimamura, Salmon, Squire, and Butters (1987) have argued that studying which aspects of memory are impaired in Alzheimer's "may help in determining the usual trajectory of the disease and in identifying which brain systems are first affected" (p. 350).

Accurately diagnosing dementia and distinguishing among types of dementia are critical for at least two other reasons. Of the more than 40 disorders that have been found to cause dementia (Katzman, Lasker, & Bernstein, 1986), several are currently treatable, and some, including infectious and toxic diseases, are preventable (Office of Technology Assessment, 1987). Secondly, evaluating the relative effectiveness of potential treatments for dementia depends on accurate diagnosis.

More than half of all dementia patients suffer from Alzheimer's disease (Smith & Kiloh, 1981). Perhaps because memory deficits are the most salient symptom of Alzheimer's, many different aspects of memory have been tested in Alzheimer's patients, and almost all of them have been shown to be impaired (Thompson, Gong, Haskins, & Gallagher, 1987). The Wechsler Memory Scale (Wechsler, 1945) and the Benton Test of Visual Retention (Benton, 1974) are two of the most common tests that have been used. Even relatively simple measures of memory, such as backward digit span, seem to be able to differentiate mildly demented Alzheimer's patients from healthy age-matched controls (Storandt, Botwinick, & Danziger, 1986).

Increasingly, researchers are using more sophisticated memory tests that have proven to be of significant value in the differential diagnosis of Alzheimer's. For example, Grober, Buschke, Crystal, Bang, and Dresner (1988) reported that a more complex cued recall task is better than simple free recall or recognition tasks at differentiating demented from nondemented elderly. Some newer standardized tests may also be helpful. For example, LaRue, D'Elia, Clark, Spar, and Jarvik (1986) were quite accurate at distinguishing between demented and healthy older adults with the Fuld Object–Memory Evaluation (Fuld, 1981).

In addition to memory deficits, researchers and clinicians can expect to find significant declines in attentional functioning in Alzheimer's disease. Freed, Corkin, Growdon, and Nissen (1988) have identified a group of patients with Alzheimer's disease who show an anomalous pattern of responding on an attentional cuing task similar to the pattern reported by Nissen and Corkin (1985) described earlier. Capitani, Sala, Lucchelli, Soave, and Spinnler (1988) have reported that performance on a selective attention task, the Hidden Figures Test, can discriminate with 90% accuracy between normal and demented older adults. Vitaliano and colleagues (1984a, 1984b) have reported a similar finding using attention items from the Mini-Mental Status Examination and the Dementia Rating Scale. They found attention items to be successful in discriminating severity of impairment of Alzheimer's disease patients. Thus, attentional functioning may prove to be a useful index of the central nervous system (cf, Gummow, Miller, & Dustman, 1983), and as such, may discriminate normal aging from pathological aging.

In addition to discriminating normal aging from pathological aging, tests of cognitive functioning can help us to differentiate among different pathologies. For example, previous studies have not been very successful in differentiating between dementia and depression in older adults (Feinberg & Goodman, 1984). Although *amount* of forgetting does not seem to be a good diagnostic tool, *rate* of forgetting may be better. Hart, Kwentus, Taylor, and Harkins (1987) found that even patients in the early stages of Alzheimer's could be distinguished from depressed patients by their more rapid rates of forgetting; within the first 10 minutes after viewing pictures of common objects, Alzheimer's patients recognized significantly fewer of the pictures than did depressed patients. Other candidates for good diagnostic tools include measures of qualitative differences in performance. There is some evidence, for example, that compared to depressed individuals, demented patients more often falsely "recognize" items that do not occur in the material on which they are tested (Thompson *et al.,* 1987). Given that depressed individuals are reportedly notorious for complaining of cognitive deficits when they do not exist, or for greatly exaggerating any cognitive declines that have occurred, a ratio comparing self-perceptions to actual performance might be very helpful in differentiating depression from other types of mental health disorders.

Tests of attentional function seem to be good candidates for distinguishing between dementia and delirium. According to Zisook and Braff (1986),

> the essential feature of delirium is reduced awareness and attentiveness to the environment. . . . The delirious person has decreased capacity to attend to environmental stimuli. As a result, the delirious patient is a victim of transient shifts of attention, is easily distracted by irrelevant stimuli, and senses an uneasy equilibrium with the environment" (p. 67).

Such severe attentional abnormalities probably indicate delirium rather than a dementing process, especially if they have an abrupt onset (Lipowski, 1982). Delirium is a reversible organic state, but if left untreated can result in permanent brain damage. One important area for future research is the development of reliable diagnostic measures of attentional function that can be easily used by physicians in nonlaboratory settings (Albert, 1988).

The ability to maintain and direct attention, to learn new information, and to remember events is vital to the mental health of aging adults and to their successful adaptation to the environmental demands they face in carrying out the activities of daily living (Gordon, 1985; Martin & Jones, 1983). For example, selective attention is required in driving an automobile, in pedestrian street crossing, as well as in walking and carrying out domestic activities in the household. Memory is required in keeping appointments, in keeping track of medication regimens, and in monitoring and planning everyday activities. The capacity to measure cognitive functioning is a prerequisite to the separation of reversible and irreversible performance deficits in memory, learning, and attention. Research in this area has great significance for the personal lives of older adults and for older adults' effectiveness in maintaining a high quality of life in the later years.

V. Future Research Directions

The difficulties in conducting research on cognitive aging cannot be overestimated. The research advances in cognitive aging over the last decade are promising, but at the same time they have been accompanied by some disappointments. A constructive approach to these disappointments is to suggest that over the next decade we turn these disappointments into an agenda for reaching new insights into the relationships between memory, learning, attention, and aging.

One disappointment has been the lack of theory about the relationships between aging and memory, learning, and attention. The development of theory to guide future research on cognitive aging would be a substantial contribution in the 1990s. With theory to guide us, we may also be able to understand the many research findings that currently seem to be contradictory.

Earlier research was criticized for relying on the *extreme group* design in which one group of subjects, called the young group, is compared to another group of subjects, called the old group. Data that we collected for this chapter from research reports on memory in the *Journal of Gerontology, Experimental Aging Research,* and *Psychology and Aging* for 1988 and 1989 reveal that the overwhelming majority of investigators (73%) still use the extreme group design. As Schonfield remarked in 1980, "if the term aging rather than the aged is to be taken seriously as the subject matter of gerontology, much more needs to be known about stability and change in learning and remembering during the middle adult years" (p. 216). Unfortunately, a decade later we still have very little data on those middle adult years (but see Camp & Pignatiello, 1988; Fisk, McGee, & Giambra, 1988; Foos, 1989; Hess, Donley, & Vandermaas, 1989; Hyland & Ackerman, 1988). The dearth of research on middle-aged people continues to be a major obstacle to our understanding of developmental processes in memory, learning, and attention. Including data from more age groups should be a goal of researchers over the next decade. We also need to know more about differences in cognitive functioning among older adults of different ability levels, and between young adults who are in college and those who are not.

Unfortunately, the earlier lessons of lifespan developmental psychologists (e.g., Baltes, 1968; Schaie, 1973, 1977) have not been heeded during the past decade. Rather than longitudinal or cross-sequential designs, researchers have used cross-sectional research designs in which birth cohort effects are confounded with age effects. Consequently, we still know very little about intraindividual changes with age in memory, learning, and attention processes. We need a variety of developmental research designs and innovative use of data-analysis techniques to tackle questions about intraindividual changes.

The hypothesis that forgetting is significantly more salient for older adults than for younger adults is intriguing and needs to be investigated further. We also need to know more about the effects of physical fitness and nutritional status on the cognitive functioning of aging adults. Other areas that may be important determinants of cognitive functioning but about which we know little or nothing include the effects of the aging adult's knowledge base on cognitive performance, and how the importance to the individual of remembering, learning, and attending might affect those cognitive processes.

Last, but not least, we need to increase the breadth of approaches for investigating cognitive functioning. Many of the most interesting and challenging issues regarding cognitive aging demand innovative methods. Structural equation models are a promising method but have yet to be appreciated by most researchers (Hertzog, 1987). Although "objective verifiability remains a paramount criterion of scientific truth, . . . it need not apply to the individual datum as long as it applies to the generalizations that are ultimately established by using a given method" (Bahrick & Karis, 1982, p. 461). Let us have an increased tolerance for diversity—of methods and theories—as we approach the 21st century (Hertzog, 1990)!

References

Albert, M. S. (1988). Cognitive function. In M. S. Albert & M. B. Moss (Eds.), *Geriatric neuropsychology* (pp. 33–56). New York: Guilford Press.

American Psychiatric Association. (1980). *Diagnostic and statistical manual of mental disorders* (3rd ed.). Washington, DC: Author.

Anderson, J. R., & Milson, R. (1989). Human memory: An adaptive perspective. *Psychological Review, 96*, 703–719.

Anschutz, L., Camp, C. J., Markley, R. P., & Kramer, J. J. (1985). Maintenance and generalization of mnemonics for grocery shopping by older adults. *Experimental Aging Research, 11*, 157–160.

Arbuckle, T. Y., Gold, D., & Andres, D. (1986). Cognitive functioning of older people in relation to social and personality variables. *Psychology and Aging, 1*, 55–62.

Ashcraft, M. H. (1989). *Human memory and cognition*. Glenview, IL: Scott, Foresman.

Baddeley, A. (1989). The psychology of remembering and forgetting. In T. Butler (Ed.), *Memory. History, culture and the mind* (pp. 33–60). New York: Basil Blackwell.

Bahrick, H. P., & Karis, D. (1982). Long-term ecological memory. In C. R. Puff (Ed.), *Handbook of research methods in human memory and cognition* (pp. 427–465). New York: Academic Press.

Baltes, P. B. (1968). Longitudinal and cross-sectional sequences in the study of age and generation effects. *Human Development, 11*, 145–171.

Banaji, M. R., & Crowder, R. G. (1989). The bankruptcy of everyday memory. *American Psychologist, 44*, 1185–1193.

Barrett, T. R., & Wright, M. (1981). Age-related facilitation in recall following semantic processing. *Journal of Gerontology, 36*, 194–199.

Bennett-Levy, J., & Powell, G. F. (1980). The Subjective Memory Questionnaire (SMQ): I: An investigation into the self-reporting of "real life" memory skills. *British Journal of Social and Clinical Psychology, 19*, 177–178.

Benton, A. L. (1974). *The Revised Visual Retention Test* (4th ed.). New York: Psychological Corporation.

Bjork, E. L., & Bjork, R. A. (1988). On the adaptive aspects of retrieval failure in autobiographical memory. In M. M. Gruneberg, P. E. Morris, & R. N. Sykes (Eds.), *Practical aspects of memory: Current research and issues:* (Vol. 1. *Memory in everyday life*) (pp. 283–288). New York: Wiley.

Broadbent, D. (1958). *Perception and communication*. New York: Holt.

Broadbent, D. E., Cooper, P. F., Fitzgerald, P., & Parkes, K. R. (1982). The Cognitive Failures Questionnaire (CFQ) and its correlates. *British Journal of Clinical Psychology, 21*, 1–16.

Brown, A. L., & Campione, J. C. (1978). Memory strategies in learning: Training children to study strategically. In H. Pick & H. Stevenson (Eds.), *Applications of basic research in psychology* (pp. 22–41). New York: Plenum Press.

Burke, D. M., & Light, L. L. (1981). Memory and aging: The role of retrieval processes. *Psychological Bulletin, 90*, 513–546.

Buschke, H., & Grober, E. (1986). Genuine memory impairment in age-associated memory impairment. *Developmental Neuropsychology, 2,* 287–307.

Butler, R. N., & Lewis, M. I. (1982). *Aging and mental health* (3rd ed.). St. Louis, MO: Mosby.

Camp, C. J., & Pignatiello, M. F. (1988). Beliefs about fact retrieval and inferential reasoning across the adult lifespan. *Experimental Aging Research, 14,* 89–97.

Capitani, E., Sala, S., Lucchelli, F., Soave, P., & Spinnler, H. (1988). Perceptual attention in aging and dementia measured by Gottschaldt's Hidden Figure Test. *Journal of Gerontology: Psychological Sciences, 43,* P157–163.

Cavanaugh, J. C. (1983). Comprehension and retention of television programs by 20- and 60-year-olds. *Journal of Gerontology, 38,* 190–196.

Cavanaugh, J. C. (1986–87). Age differences in adults' self-reports of memory ability: It depends on how and what you ask. *International Journal of Aging and Human Development, 24,* 271–277.

Cavanaugh, J. C., Grady, J. G., & Perlmutter, M. (1983). Forgetting and use of memory aids in 20- to 70-year-olds in everyday life. *International Journal of Aging and Human Development, 17,* 113–122.

Cermak, L. S. (1976). *Improving your memory.* New York: McGraw-Hill.

Cherkin, A. (1984). Effects of nutritional factors on memory function. In H. J. Armbrecht, J. M. Prendergast, & R. M. Coe (Eds.), *Nutritional intervention in the aging process* (pp. 229–249). New York: Springer-Verlag.

Chi, M. T. H. (1978). Knowledge structures and memory development. In R. S. Siegler (Ed.), *Children's thinking: What develops?* (pp. 73–96). Hillsdale, NJ: Erlbaum.

Clarkson-Smith, L., & Hartley, A. A. (1990). The game of bridge as an exercise in working memory and reasoning. *Journal of Gerontology: Psychological Sciences, 45,* P233–238.

Cohen, G., & Faulkner, D. (1986). Memory for proper names: Age differences in retrieval. *British Journal of Developmental Psychology, 4,* 187–197.

Cohen, R. M., Weingartner, H., Smallberg, S. A., Pickar, D., & Murphy, D. L. (1982). Effort and cognition in depression. *Archives of General Psychiatry, 39,* 593–597.

Comalli, P. (1962). Interference effects of Stroop color-word test in childhood, adulthood, and aging. *Journal of Genetic Psychology, 100,* 47–53.

Craik, F. I. M. (1977). Age differences in human memory. In J. E. Birren & K. W. Schaie (Eds.), *Handbook of the psychology of aging* (pp. 384–420). New York: Van Nostrand Reinhold.

Craik, F. I. M. (1986). A functional account of age differences in memory. In F. Klix & H. Hagendorf (Eds.), *Human memory and cognitive capabilities* (pp. 409–422). New York: Elsevier Science.

Craik, F. I. M., Byrd, M., & Swanson, J. M. (1987). Patterns of memory loss in three elderly samples. *Psychology and Aging, 2,* 79–86.

Craik, F. I. M., & McDowd, J. M. (1987). Age differences in recall and recognition. *Journal of Experimental Psychology: Learning, Memory, and Cognition, 13,* 474–479.

Crook, T., Bartus, R. T., & Ferris, S. H., Whitehouse, P., Cohen, G. D., & Gershon, S. (1986). Age-associated memory impairment: Proposed diagnostic criteria and measures of clinical change—Report of a National Institute of Mental Health work group. *Developmental Neuropsychology, 2,* 261–276.

Cutler, S. J., & Grams, A. E. (1988). Correlates of self-reported everyday memory problems. *Journal of Gerontology: Social Sciences, 43,* S82–90.

Dixon, R. A. (1989). Questionnaire research on metamemory and aging: Issues of structure and function. In L. W. Poon, D. C. Rubin, & B. A. Wilson (Eds.), *Everyday cognition in adulthood and late life* (pp. 394–415). New York: Cambridge University Press.

Dixon, R. A., & Hultsch, D. F. (1983). Structure and development of metamemory in adulthood. *Journal of Gerontology, 38,* 682–688.

Dixon, R. A., Hertzog, C., & Hultsch, D. F. (1986). The multiple relationships among Metamemory in Adulthood (MIA) scales and cognitive abilities in adulthood. *Human Learning, 5,* 165–177.

Dustman, R. E., Ruhling, E. M., Russell, D. E., Shearer, H. W., Bonekat, J. W., Shigeoka, J. S., Wood, J. S., & Bradford, D. C. (1984). Aerobic exercise training and improved neuropsychological function of older individuals. *Neurobiology of Aging, 5,* 35–42.

Edwards, S., & Dickerson, M. (1987). Intrusive unwanted thoughts: A two-stage model of control. *British Journal of Medical Psychology, 60,* 317–328.

Einstein, G. O., & McDaniel M. A. (1990). Normal aging and prospective memory. *Journal of Experimental Psychology: Learning, Memory, and Cognition, 16,* 717–726.

Elsayed, M., Ismail, A. H., & Young, R. J. (1980). Intellectual differences of adult men related to age and physical fitness before and after an exercise program. *Journal of Gerontology, 35,* 383–387.

Farkas, M., & Hoyer, W. (1980). Processing consequences of perceptual grouping in selective attention. *Journal of Gerontology, 35,* 207–216.

Feinberg, T., & Goodman, B. (1984). Affective illness, dementia, and pseudodementia. *Journal of Clinical Psychiatry, 45,* 100–103.

Fisk, A. D., McGee, N. D., & Giambra, L. M. (1988). The influence of age on consistent and varied semantic-category search performance. *Psychology and Aging, 3,* 323–333.

Folstein, M. R., Folstein, S., & McHugh, P. R. (1975). Mini-mental state: A practical method for grading the cognitive state of patients for the clinician. *Journal of Psychiatric Research, 12,* 189–198.

Foos, P. W. (1989). Adult age differences in working memory. *Psychology and Aging, 4,* 269–275.

Freed, D., Corkin, S., Growdon, J., & Nissen, M. J. (1988). Selective attention in Alzheimer's disease: Characterizing cognitive subgroups of patients. *Neuropsychologia, 27,* 325–339.

Fuld, P. A. (1981). *The Fuld Object-Memory Evaluation.* Chicago: Stoelting Instrument Company.

Gilewski, M. J., & Zelinski, E. M. (1986). Questionnaire assessment of memory complaints. In L. W. Poon (Ed.), *Handbook for clinical memory assessment of older adults* (pp. 93–107). Washington, DC: American Psychological Association.

Goodwin, J. S., Goodwin, J. M., & Garry, P. J. (1983). Association between nutritional status and cognitive functioning in a healthy elderly population. *Journal of the American Medical Association, 249,* 2917–2921.

Gordon, P. (1985). Allocation of attention in obsessional disorder. *British Journal of Clinical Psychology, 24,* 101–107.

Grober, E., Buschke, H., Crystal, H., Bang, S., & Dresner, R. (1988). Screening for dementia by memory testing. *Neurology, 38,* 900–903.

Gruneberg, M. M. (1978). The feeling of knowing, memory blocks and memory aids. In M. M. Gruneberg & P. Morris (Eds.), *Aspects of memory* (pp. 186–209). London: Methuen.

Gummow, L., Miller, P., & Dustman, R. E. (1983). Attention and brain injury. *Clinical Psychology Review, 3,* 255–274.

Harris, J. E. (1978). External memory aids. In M. M. Gruneberg, P. E. Morris, & R. N. Sykes (Eds.), *Practical aspects of memory* (pp. 172–179). NY: Academic Press.

Hart, R. P., Kwentus, J. A., Taylor, J. R., & Harkins, S. W. (1987). Rate of forgetting in dementia and depression. *Journal of Consulting and Clinical Psychology, 55,* 101–105.

Hartley, J. T. (1986). Reader and text variables as determinants of discourse memory in adulthood. *Psychology and Aging, 1,* 150–158.

Hasher, L., & Zacks, R. T. (1988). Working memory, comprehension, and aging: A review and a new view. In G. H. Bower (Ed.), *The psychology of learning and motivation* (Vol. 22, pp. 193–225). San Diego: Academic Press.

Hasher, L., Connelly, S., & Zacks, R. (1990, March). *Age and reading: The impact of distracting material.* Poster presented at the Cognitive Aging Conference, Atlanta, GA.

Heilman, K., Watson, R., Valenstein, E., & Goldberg, M. (1987). Attention: Behavior and neural mechanisms. In V. Mountcastle (Ed.), *Handbook of physiology: Sec. 1. The nervous system* (pp. 461–481). Bethesda, MD: American Physiological Society.

Herrrmann, D. J. (1982). Know thy memory: The use of questionnaires to assess and study memory. *Psychological Bulletin, 92,* 434–452.

Herrmann, D. J. (1984). Questionnaires about memory. In J. E. Harris & P. E. Morris (Eds.), *Everyday memory, actions, and absent-mindedness* (pp. 133–151). London: Academic Press.

Herrmann, D. J. (1988). *Memory improvement techniques.* New York: Ballantine.

Herrmann, D. J., & Neisser, U. (1978). An inventory of everyday memory experiences. In M. M. Gruneberg, P. E. Morris, & R. N. Sykes (Eds.), *Practical aspects of memory* (pp. 35–51). London: Academic Press.

Hertzog, C. (1987). Applications of structural equation models in gerontological research. *Annual Review of Gerontology and Geriatrics, 7,* 265–293.

Hertzog, C. (1990, March). *Methodological issues in cognitive aging research*. Invited address presented at the Cognitive Aging Conference, Atlanta, GA.

Hess, T. M., Donley, J., & Vandermaas, M. O. (1989). Aging-related changes in the processing and retention of script information. *Experimental Aging Research, 15,* 89–96.

Higbee, K. L. (1977). *Your memory: How it works and how to improve it*. Englewood Cliffs, NJ: Prentice-Hall.

Hoyer, W., Rebok, G., & Sved, S. (1979). Irrelevant information and problem-solving. *Journal of Gerontology, 34,* 553–560.

Hulicka, I. M., & Grossman, J. L. (1967). Age group comparisons for the use of mediators in paired-associate learning. *Journal of Gerontology, 22,* 46–51.

Hultsch, D. F. (1969). Adult age differences in the organization of free recall. *Developmental Psychology, 1,* 673–678.

Hultsch, D. F. (1975). Adult age differences in retrieval: Trace-dependent and cue-dependent forgetting. *Developmental Psychology, 11,* 197–201.

Hultsch, D. F., & Dixon, R. A. (1990). Learning and memory in aging. In J. E. Birren & K. W. Schaie (Eds.), *Handbook of the psychology of aging* (3rd ed., pp. 258–274). New York: Academic Press.

Hyland, D. T., & Ackerman, A. M. (1988). Reminiscence and autobiographical memory in the study of the personal past. *Journal of Gerontology: Psychological Sciences, 43,* P35–39.

Jarvik, L. F. (1988). Aging of the brain: How can we prevent it? *The Gerontologist, 28,* 739–747.

Kahneman, D. (1973). *Attention and effort*. Englewood Cliffs, NJ: Prentice-Hall.

Katzman, R., Lasker, B., & Bernstein, N. (1986). *Accuracy of diagnosis and consequences of misdiagnosis of disorders causing dementia*. Contract report for Office of Technology Assessment, U.S. Congress.

Kausler, D., & Kleim, D. (1978). Age differences in processing relevant versus irrelevant stimuli in multiple-item recognition learning. *Journal of Gerontology, 33,* 87–93.

Keith, J. (1989). *Executive memory techniques* (rev. ed). New York: Dell.

Kvavilashvili, L. (1987). Remembering intention as a distinct form of memory. *British Journal of Psychology, 78,* 507–518.

Labouvie-Vief, G., & Schell, D. A. (1982). Learning and memory in later life: A developmental view. In B. Wolman & G. Stricker (Eds.), *Handbook of developmental psychology* (pp. 828–846). Englewood Cliffs, NJ: Prentice-Hall.

Labouvie-Vief, G., Campbell, S., Weaver, S., & Tannenhaus, M. (1979, November). *Metaphoric processing in young and old adults*. Paper presented at the annual meeting of the Gerontological Society, Washington, DC.

LaRue, A. D., D'Elia, L. F., Clark, E. O., Spar, J. E., & Jarvik, L. F. (1986). Clinical tests of memory in dementia, depression, and healthy aging. *Psychology and Aging, 1,* 69–77.

Linton, M. (1978). Real-world memory after six years: An *in vivo* study of very long-term memory. In M. M. Gruneberg, P. E. Morris, & R. N. Sykes (Eds.), *Practical aspects of memory* (pp. 69–76). New York: Academic Press.

Lipowski, Z. J. (1982). Differentiating delirium from dementia in the elderly. *Clinical Gerontologist, 1,* 3–10.

Loewen, E. R., Shaw, R. J., & Craik, F. I. M. (1990). Age differences in components of metamemory. *Experimental Aging Research, 16,* 43–48.

Madden, D. J. (1983). Aging and distraction by highly familiar stimuli during visual search. *Developmental Psychology, 19,* 499–507.

Martin, M. (1986). Ageing and patterns of change in everyday memory and cognition. *Human Learning, 5,* 63–74.

Martin, M., & Jones, G. (1983). Distribution of attention in cognitive failure. *Human Learning, 2,* 221–226.

Mattis, S. (1976). Mental status examination for organic mental syndrome in the elderly patient. In L. Bellak & T. B. Karasu (Eds.), *Geriatric psychiatry*. New York: Grune & Stratton.

McDowd, J., & Oseas, D. (1990, March). *Aging, inhibitory processes, and negative priming*. Poster presented at the Cognitive Aging Conference, Atlanta, GA.

Meacham, J. A., & Lieman, B. (1982). Remembering to perform future actions. In U. Neisser (Ed.), *Memory observed. Remembering in natural contexts* (pp. 327–336). San Francisco: W. H. Freeman.

Morris, P. E. (1984). The validity of subjective reports of memory. In J. E. Harris & P. E. Morris (Eds.), *Everyday memory, actions and absentmindedness* (pp. 153–172). London: Academic Press.

Moscovitch, M. (1982). A neuropsychological approach to memory and perception in normal and pathological aging. In F. I. M. Craik & S. Trehub (Eds.), *Aging and cognitive processes* (pp. 55–78). New York: Plenum Press.

National Center for Health Statistics. (1986). Aging in the eighties: Preliminary data from the Supplement on Aging to the National Health Interview Study, United States, January–June 1984. *Advance Data From Vital and Health Statistics, 115,* 1–8.

Nebes, R., & Madden, D. (1983). The use of focused attention in visual search by young and old adults. *Experimental Aging Research, 9,* 139–143.

Neill, W. (1977). Inhibition and facilitation processes in selective attention. *Journal of Experimental Psychology: Human Perception and Performance, 3,* 444–450.

Neisser, U. (1978). Memory: What are the important questions? In M. M. Gruneberg, P. E. Morris, & R. N. Sykes (Eds.), *Practical aspects of memory* (pp. 3–24). London: Academic Press.

Niederehe, G. (1986). Depression and memory impairment in the aged. In L. W. Poon (Ed.), *Handbook for clinical memory assessment of older adults* (pp. 226–237). Washington, DC: American Psychological Association.

Nissen, M., & Corkin, S. (1985). Effectiveness of attentional cueing in older and younger adults. *Journal of Gerontology, 40,* 185–191.

Nolen-Hoeksema, S. (1988). Life-span views on depression. In P. B. Baltes, D. L. Featherman, & R. M. Lerner (Eds.), *Life-span development and behavior* (Vol. 9, pp. 203–241). NY: Academic Press.

Office of Technology Assessment. (1987). *Losing a million minds: Confronting the tragedy of Alzheimer's disease and other dementias.* Washington, DC: U.S. Government Printing Office.

O'Hanlon, P., & Kohrs, M. B. (1978). Dietary studies of older Americans. *The American Journal of Clinical Nutrition, 31,* 1257–1269.

Park, D. C., Smith, A. D., & Cavanaugh, J. C. (1990). Metamemories of memory researchers. *Memory & Cognition, 18,* 321–327.

Perlmutter, M. (1978). What is memory aging the aging of? *Developmental Psychology, 14,* 330–345.

Perlmutter, M., Adams, C., Berry, J., Kaplan, M., Person, D., & Verdonik, F. (1987). Aging and memory. *Annual Review of Gerontology and Geriatrics, 7,* 57–92.

Plude, D. J. (1980). *Adult age differences and equivalence in the selectivity of attention: search and focusing.* Unpublished doctoral dissertation, Syracuse University.

Plude, D., & Hoyer, W. (1985). Attention and performance: Identifying and localizing age deficits. In N. Charness (Ed.), *Aging and performance* (pp. 47–99). New York: Wiley.

Plude, D., & Hoyer, W. (1986). Age and the selectivity of visual information processing. *Psychology and Aging, 1,* 4–10.

Poon, L. W. (1985). Differences in human memory with aging: Nature, causes, and clinical implications. In J. E. Birren & K. W. Schaie (Eds.), *Handbook of the psychology of aging* (2nd ed., pp. 427–462). New York: Van Nostrand Reinhold.

Poon, L. W. (1989). What do we know about the aging of cognitive abilities in everyday life? In L. W. Poon, D. C. Rubin, & B. A. Wilson (Eds.), *Everyday cognition in adulthood and late life* (pp. 129–132). New York: Cambridge University Press.

Poon, L. W., & Schaffer, G. (1982, August). *Prospective memory in young and elderly adults.* Presented at the American Psychological Association, Washington, DC.

Poon, L. W., & Walsh-Sweeney, L. (1981). Effects of bizarre and interacting imagery on learning and retrieval of the aged. *Experimental Aging Research, 7,* 65–70.

Popkin, S. J., Gallagher, D., Thompson, L. W., & Moore, M. (1982). Memory complaint and performance in normal and depressed older adults. *Experimental Aging Research, 8,* 141–145.

Posner, M., & Snyder, C. (1975). Facilitation and inhibition in the processing of signals. In P. Rabbitt & S. Dornic (Eds.), *Attention and performance* (pp. 669–681). New York: Academic Press.

Rabbitt, P. (1965). An age-decrement in the ability to ignore irrelevant information. *Journal of Gerontology, 20,* 233–238.

Rabbitt, P. M. A. (1979). Some experiments and a model for changes in attentional selectivity with old age. In F. Hoffmeister & E. Muller (Eds.), *Bayer Symposium VII; Evaluation of Change.* Bonn: Springer-Verlag.

Raskin, A., Friedman, A. S., & DiMascio, A. (1982). Cognitive and performance deficits in depression. *Psychopharmacology Bulletin, 18*, 196–202.

Ratner, H. H., Schell, D. A., Crimmins, A., Mittelman, D., & Baldinelli, L. (1987). Changes in adults' prose recall: Aging or cognitive demands? *Developmental Psychology, 23*, 521–525.

Reason, J. (1984). Lapses of attention in everyday life. In R. Parasuraman & D. Davies (Eds.), *Varieties of attention* (pp. 515–549). London: Academic Press.

Reason, J., & Lucas, D. (1983). Using cognitive diaries to investigate naturally occurring memory blocks. In J. E. Harris & P. E. Morris (Eds.), *Everyday memory, actions, and absentmindedness* (pp. 53–70). London: Academic Press.

Reason, J., & Mycielska, K. (1982). *Absent-minded? The psychology of mental lapses and everyday errors.* Englewood Cliffs, NJ: Prentice-Hall.

Rice, G. E., Meyer, B. J. F., & Miller, D. C. (1988). Relation of everyday activities of adults to their prose-recall performance. *Educational Gerontology, 14*, 147–158.

Robertson-Tchabo, E. A., Hausman, C. P., & Arenberg, D. (1976). A classic mnemonic for older learners: A trip that works! *Educational Gerontology, 1*, 215–226.

Rogers, W. A., & Fisk, A. D. (1988). Age-related effects of stimulus-specific context on perceptual learning. *Proceedings of the Human Factors Society 32nd Annual Meeting.* Santa Monica, CA: Human Factors Society.

Rose, T. L., & Yesavage, J. A. (1983). Differential effects of a list-learning mnemonic in three age groups. *Gerontology, 29*, 293–298.

Rosen, W. G., Mohs, R. C., & Davis, K. L. (1984). A new rating scale for Alzheimer's disease. *American Journal of Psychiatry, 141*, 1356–1364.

Salthouse, T. A. (1985). *A theory of cognitive aging.* New York: Elsevier Science.

Sanford, A. J., & Maule, A. J. (1973). The allocation of attention in multisource monitoring behavior: Adult age differences. *Perception, 2*, 91–100.

Schaie, K. W. (1973). Methodological problems in descriptive developmental research on adulthood and aging. In J. Nesselroade & H. W. Reese (Eds.), *Life-span developmental psychology. Methodological issues* (pp. 253–280). New York: Academic Press.

Schaie, K. W. (1977). Quasi-experimental research designs in the psychology of aging. In J. E. Birren & K. W. Schaie (Eds.), *Handbook of the psychology of aging* (pp. 39–58). New York: Van Nostrand Reinhold.

Schaie, K. W. (1983). The Seattle longitudinal study: A 21-year exploration of psychometric intelligence in adulthood. In K. W. Schaie (Ed.), *Longitudinal studies of adult psychological development* (pp. 64–135). New York: Guilford.

Schonfield, A. E. D. (1980). Learning, memory, and aging. In J. E. Birren & R. B. Sloane (Eds.), *Handbook of mental health and aging* (pp. 214–244). Englewood Cliffs, NJ: Prentice-Hall.

Sehulster, J. R. (1981). Structure and pragmatics of a self-theory of memory. *Memory and Cognition, 9*, 263–278.

Shaw, R. (1990, March). *Age-related increases in the effects of semantic activation in a selective attention task.* Poster presented at the Cognitive Aging Conference, Atlanta, GA.

Shimamura, A. P., Salmon, D. P., Squire, L. R., & Butters, N. (1987). Memory dysfunction and word priming in dementia and amnesia. *Behavioral Neuroscience, 101*, 347–351.

Sinnott, J. D. (1986). Prospective/intentional and incidental memory: Effects of age and passage of time. *Psychology and Aging, 1*, 110–116.

Smith, J. S., & Kiloh, L. G. (1981). The investigation of dementia: Results of 200 consecutive admissions. *Lancet, 1*, 824–827.

Storandt, M., Botwinick, J., & Danziger, W. L. (1986). Longitudinal changes: Patients with mild SDAT and matched healthy controls. In L. W. Poon (Ed.), *Handbook for clinical memory assessment of older adults* (pp. 277–284). Washington, DC: American Psychological Association.

Sugar, J. A. (1988, November). *A comparison of questionnaire and diary methods for studying forgetting.* Presented at the meeting of the Psychonomic Society, Chicago.

Sugar, J. A. (1989, November). *Everyday experiences of forgetting in young and older adults.* Paper presented at the meeting of the Psychonomic Society, Atlanta, GA.

Sugar, J. A. (1990, March). *Forgetting in young and older adults: Memory strategies and structure of daily life.* Poster presented at the meeting of the Cognitive Aging Conference, Atlanta, GA.

Taylor, A. K., McDowd, J. M., Birren, J. E., & Gutacker, P. (1989, November). *Everyday lapses of attention and memory across the lifespan.* Paper presented at the annual meeting of the Gerontological Society of America, Minneapolis, MN.

Tenney, Y. J. (1984). Ageing and the misplacing of objects. *British Journal of Developmental Psychology, 2,* 43–50.

Thompson, L. W., Gong, V., Haskins, E., & Gallagher, D. (1987). Assessment of depression and dementia during the late years. *Annual Review of Gerontology and Geriatrics, 7,* 295–324.

Tipper, S. (1985). The negative priming effect: Inhibitory effects of ignored primes. *Quarterly Journal of Experimental Psychology, 37A,* 571–590.

Treat, N. J., Poon, L. W., & Fozard, J. L. (1978). From clinical and research findings on memory to intervention programs. *Experimental Aging Research, 4,* 235–253.

Vitaliano, P., Breen, A., Albert, M., Russo, J., & Prinz, P. (1984a). Memory, attention, and functional status in community-residing Alzheimer-type dementia patients and optimally healthy aged individuals. *Journal of Gerontology, 39,* 58–64.

Vitaliano, P., Breen, A., Russo, J., Albert, M., Vitiello, M., & Prinz, P. (1984b). The clinical utility of the dementia rating scale for assessing Alzheimer patients. *Journal of Chronic Diseases, 37,* 743–753.

Wechsler, D. (1945). A standardized memory scale for clinical use. *Journal of Psychology, 19,* 87–95.

Weingartner, H. (1986). Automatic and effort-demanding cognitive processes in depression. In L. W. Poon (Ed.), *Handbook for clinical memory assessment of older adults* (pp. 218–225). Washington, DC: American Psychological Association.

West, R. (1985). *Memory fitness over forty.* Gainsville, FL: Triad.

West, R. L. (1988). Prospective memory and aging. In M. M. Gruneberg, P. E. Morris, & R. N. Sykes (Eds.), *Practical aspects of memory: Current research and issues: Vol. 2. Clinical and educational implications* (pp. 119–125). New York: Wiley.

West, R. L., & Bramblett, P., Jr. (1990, March). *Path analysis of the relationships among aging, depression, memory performance, and memory self-evaluation.* Paper presented at the Cognitive Aging Conference, Atlanta, GA.

Wilkins, A. J., & Baddeley, A. D. (1978). Remembering to recall in everyday life: An approach to absent-mindedness. In M. M. Gruneberg, P. E. Morris, & R. N. Sykes (Eds.), *Practical aspects of memory* (pp. 27–34). New York: Academic Press.

Winocur, G., Moscovitch, M., & Freedman, J. (1987). An investigation of cognitive function in relation to psychosocial variables in institutionalized old people. *Canadian Journal of Psychology, 41,* 257–269.

Wright, L., & Elias, J. (1979). Age differences in the effects of perceptual noise. *Journal of Gerontology, 34,* 704–708.

Yesavage, J., Brink, T., Rose, T., Lum, O., Huand, O., Adey, V., & Leirer, V. (1983). Development and validation of a geriatric depression-screening scale: A preliminary report. *Journal of Psychiatric Research, 17,* 37–49.

Zarit, S. H., Cole, K. D., & Guider, R. L. (1981). Memory training strategies and subjective complaints of memory in the aged. *The Gerontologist, 21,* 158–164.

Zelinski, E. M., Gilewski, M. J., & Thompson, L. W. (1980). Do laboratory tests relate to self-assessments of memory ability in the young and old? In L. W. Poon, J. L. Fozard, L. S. Cermak, D. Arenberg, & L. W. Thompson (Eds.), *New directions in memory and aging* (pp. 519–544). Hillsdale, NJ: Erlbaum.

Zisook, S., & Braff, D. (1986). Delirium: Recognition and management in the older patient. *Geriatrics, 6,* 67–78.

Zivian, M. T., & Darjes, R. (1983). Free recall by in-school and out-of-school adults: Performance and metamemory. *Developmental Psychology, 19,* 513–520.

Intellectual Functioning in Relation to Mental Health ___

Walter R. Cunningham and Kirsten L. Haman

I. Studies of Structure
II. Change in Level
III. Extraneous Influences on Intellectual Performance in the Elderly
   A. Dementia
   B. Physical Health
   C. Depression
IV. Developing New Tests for the Elderly?
   References

Since the time of the ancient Greeks, a healthy mind in a healthy body has been a widely recognized ideal of human functioning. This is true for the old as well as the young. Competent intellectual functioning is essential for the positive mental health of the elderly. Humans generally, including the old, should be sensitive to their environments, aware of nuances in the reactions of others, should be able to remember the joys, the triumphs, and the accomplishments of a long life, as well as the sorrows and frustrations. They should be able to focus attention, and remember useful information to share with their children, now adults, as well as their peers. They should be able to carry out simple cognitive tasks with reasonable speed, and should be able to bring reasoning and insight to bear on intellectual as well as concrete problems. Information about intellectual functioning is often important to the clinician to allow selection of optimal therapy leading toward better mental health.

Valid conclusions regarding the intellectual functioning of elderly persons are not always easily achieved, however. First, there has been some controversy regarding the normal course of intellectual functioning with age. It is only in the last decade that a clear view regarding the nature of decline for different intellectual variables has emerged and been endorsed by leading researchers. Further, there are many hazards to gaining sound diagnostic information with individual elderly persons. In addition, the interpretation of such information is clouded by a surprisingly long list of extraneous variables. While such

Handbook of Mental Health and Aging, Second Edition

problems hover in the background of any clinical assessment, a number of such considerations are much more urgent in the old than in the young.

The purpose of this chapter is to briefly review what is known about normative decline at different age levels, the significance of decline, and also to consider various extraneous variables that may either affect intellectual functioning or complicate the interpretation of test data obtained from elderly persons. Comments will be made also on some practical issues of intellectual assessment and the possibility of further test development and construction with respect to the mature capacities of elderly people.

Research on aging and intellectual functioning may be divided into three broad categories: studies of structure, studies of change in level, and considerations of various antecedents or, for the purposes of this chapter, extraneous variables that may have an important impact on intellectual functioning in the elderly.

I. Studies of Structure

Two main issues in the study of structure in relation to age are (1) stability and change in structure in the elderly, and (2) whether mental speed should be viewed as a single, broad, general construct, or whether mental speed is best viewed as a collection of separate ability factors. Most of this work has been motivated by Birren's (1965) classic paper as well as further developments by Salthouse (e.g., 1985).

With regard to the first issue, most studies in the last two decades (with an adequate number of multiple indicators for hypothesized ability factors) have found the same number of factors, very similar factor-loading patterns (technically configural invariance) and in some cases even exact equivalence of factor loadings (technically metric invariance). However, factor covariances have usually been found to increase with age (e.g., Cunningham, 1980a; 1980b; 1981). See Cunningham (1987) for a review. The theoretically expected convergence of factors in later life has, however, never been convincingly demonstrated. Indeed, White and Cunningham (1987), in studying highly speeded tasks such as Choice, Sternberg, and Card Sorting reaction times actually showed an increased number of speed factors with age (see Cunningham & Tomer, 1990, for further discussion). Hertzog, Raskind, and Cannon (1986) also report a number of speed factors.

With regard to the second issue, recent findings suggest considerable complexity of structure and the possibility of increased complexity in late life. Cunningham (1988) had previously reported longitudinal data on eight separate highly speeded tasks, which showed considerable variety of age changes and cohort differences. Such variations in relationships to other variables serve to support further the construct validity of distinctions emanating from factor analytic studies. Hertzog (1989) found that answer-sheet speed and perceptual speed reliably predicted independent variances in subtests of the Primary Mental Abilities battery. Also, Tomer (1989) found that Figural Perceptual Speed and Choice Reaction Time independently mediated the relationship between age and fluid intelligence. Relationships to several other speed factors were less strong. The general thrust of this work is to emphasize the factorial complexity of speed of performance in the elderly.

Most studies of structure do, however, find the same number of factors and similar patterns of factor loadings relating variables to factors. This type of finding supports the idea that similar ability constructs are being measured in the same way in the elderly as in young adults. Thus, from the viewpoint of comparative construct validity, this work suggests that ability tests developed in the young tend to have similar validity in the old. However, the possibility of emergent abilities in the elderly, for which we lack adequate operationalizations always hovers in the background. This issue is considered at the end of this chapter.

II. Change in Level

Is decline normative? This question has been at the heart of several decades of research on intellectual functioning. It is complicated by the diversity of intellectual abilities and also by the fact that declines typically seem to begin during different decades for several different classes of variables.

Most individuals think in terms of intelligence as a *general intelligence*. A broad composite score (for example, a Wechsler Adult Intelligence Score (WAIS) Total Score) is useful (and from the point of view of efficiency, even optimal) in many applied psychology and practical decision-making situations. The "g" factor theory is popular in some theoretical circles as well.

However, such composites are of little use in studying aging because test scores showing roughly equivalent relationships to a g factor may vary widely in their age sensitivity (see Horn, 1970), for an extended discussion). A far more effective approach to studying aging or evaluating an individual client entails viewing intelligence as consisting of a variety of separate and distinct factors of intelligence. Indeed, in research on aging, it is absolutely essential to distinguish between various intellectual factors such as verbal comprehension, inductive reasoning, and numerical facility to name only a few. At least two dozen such factors have been well replicated in young adult samples, and most of these have been confirmed in elderly samples (Cunningham, 1980a, 1980b, 1981); (See also Cunningham and Brookbank, 1988; Cunningham, 1987, Cunningham and Tomer, 1990).

A point that should be emphasized is that different intellectual abilities show considerable variety of age sensitivity. Also, the timing of the onset of decline varies widely. Therefore, what constitutes normative decline must be considered from a multifactor viewpoint. This approach is essential to avoid false generalizations and to achieve an accurate and analytical understanding of the nature of aging and intellectual functioning.

Another complication in understanding intellectual functioning in older adults concerns individual differences. There is a natural tendency for researchers to focus on averages, but such indicators belie the diversity of both individual differences in level and also *intraindividual* differences in pattern of change over time (see Cunningham & Tomer, 1990, for a discussion). Examination of individual longitudinal data indicate that some 70-year-olds (for example) show relative stability over time, while some 50-year-olds may be showing important declines. Often these declines are known to be related to diagnosed health problems such as cardiovascular disease, and/or a series of strokes. However, it is emphasized that both researchers and clinicians should avoid underestimating the importance of individual differences. Usually, while patterns of stability or decline that are divergent from average functioning for a given age level are accounted for by health factors, at least some theorists in aging are inclined to think that there may be individual differences in genetic programming that may be expressed in variations in the onset and magnitude of declines, in sympathy with known inherited patterns of longevity. In any event, there are wide individual differences in level and change, and so a healthy skepticism regarding averages should be involved in any evaluation of an older person.

With these caveats in mind, typical age changes in different decades of adulthood will now be considered. In the 30s decade, the vast majority of variables show at least stability and gains in some variables are common for the average person. This is particularly true for verbal comprehension. The only exception to this generalization in terms of group averages concerns speed-of-response measures such as reaction time or perceptual speed factors, which may begin to decline even in the 20s (Tomer, 1989). However, losses in the 20s tend to be small and are usually detectable only by effecting statistical control by partialling out a number of key extraneous variables.

In the 40s and the 50s, stability is still the rule for most people on most abilities, but the exceptions in terms of abilities (usually high-speed demand tasks) increase, and the number of individual declines for variables usually showing stability also increases (e.g., Cunningham & Birren, 1976).

This pattern appears to spread in the late 50s and the early 60s, so that very small declines (sometimes trends and sometimes statistically significant effects with very large samples) are detected for many variables, including power tests in the vast majority of ability variables. For most abilities, these losses are quite small, however. They are often only a small fraction of a standard deviation over a 5- to 10-year span. But these declines are quite general, and only very age-insensitive tasks such as verbal comprehension (measured with no speed demands) escape this pattern of change (Cunningham, 1988).

By the 70s, some speeded variables (such as figural perceptual speed, e.g., Cunningham, 1989) appear to be showing accelerating declines, although this conclusion is based on a limited number of studies, and in many of these, the results are based on very modest sample sizes. And by this age level, almost all intellectual abilities are showing statistically significant declines.

While it is obvious at this point that declines are natural in the 70s and 80s, are they inevitable? The answer seems to be *probably not,* at least for specific abilities. It is quite clear that training studies can improve performance (e.g., Schaie & Willis, 1986) and that experience with a given task can do much to diminish age difference in both experts (Charness, 1985) and in ordinary work situations (Salthouse, 1984, 1985), even in high-speed demand tasks such as typing.

Most research is conducted on community-dwelling volunteers that typically constitute somewhat positively biased samples. It is important to bear in mind, however, that there are many, many extraneous variables other than normal aging that affect intellectual performance, and that such influences tend to be underrepresented (implicitly by self-selection) or explicitly by screening for various conditions. The focus now shifts to consideration of a long list of extraneous variables that may have an important impact on assessed abilities.

III. Extraneous Influences on Intellectual Performance in the Elderly

Certainly, some amount of the intellectual decline observed in the elderly may be the result of unavoidable age processes. Neural pathways may, for example, diminish in number or efficiency, or the wear and tear of time might decrease the functioning of brain structures. However, the elderly—more often than the young—exhibit health problems that typically also affect cognitive abilities. The effects of these health factors, both physical and emotional, on cognition must be considered when studying or assessing intellect in the elderly.

A. Dementia

The most devastating influence on cognitive performance in the elderly is clearly dementia. Organic brain dysfunction owing to dementia afflicts many aged. The 1980 Census stated that 11% of all Americans older than 65 have mild dementia, while 4.5% suffer severe dementia. According to the DSM-III-R, dementia is diagnosed only when the loss of intellectual function is severe enough to interfere with social or occupational functioning. This loss of capability is typically degenerative and irreversible. Dementia may mimic the symptoms of delirium, or acute brain dysfunction, but the latter is temporary and can be cured if detected early.

While behavioral, emotional, and motivational abnormalities may be associated with dementia, the primary characteristic is cognitive decline. Various types of dementia commonly affect older people; the most common dementia is Alzheimer's disease, or senile dementia of the Alzheimer's type (SDAT). Pfeffer, Afifi, and Chance (quoted in Davis, Morris, & Grant, 1990) estimate that perhaps 15% of those aged 65 and older suffer from SDAT. The etiology of the disease is unclear at this time, but the results are clear. In SDAT victims, the white matter of the brain shrinks and the brain's ventricles enlarge owing to massive neuronal loss. Senile plaques appear, as do neurofibrillary tangles that displace normal structures. The disorder has an insidious onset, and follows a gradual progression from debilitating cognitive losses to eventual disintegration of personality and finally death. Some characteristic signs of SDAT are impaired intellect, personality change, and visual hallucinations.

Another type of dementia is multi-infarct dementia. This disorder is less common than SDAT. Wells (1978) estimates that only 10% of the dementia cases diagnosed each year are of this type. This dementia is characterized by an acute onset and a stepwise progression, in which periods of apparent stabilization are followed by the exacerbation of symptoms.

Generally, those suffering from multi-infarct dementia demonstrate intact personalities and insight until late in the course of the disease. Typical characteristics are labile emotions, irritability, and cognitive deficits. Often the patient is hypertensive. The severity of multi-infarct dementia seems related to a series of small strokes, or infarcts, rather than to the extent of the cerebral arteriosclerosis.

Other types of dementia occur less frequently. For example, Korsakoff's syndrome or alcohol amnestic disorder, is seen primarily in alcoholics. A thiamine deficiency due to the excessive consumption of alcohol leads to neuronal deterioration and enlarged ventricles. This disorder often follows an acute episode of Wernicke's encephalopathy; the neurological symptoms (confusion and eye-movement abnormalities) usually associated with Wernicke's will subside, but memory impairment, the hallmark of Korsakoff's syndrome, remains.

Similarly, Pick's disease is an uncommon cause of dementia. Pick's involves the lobar atrophy of the brain, and its symptoms are so similar to those of Alzheimer's that positive diagnosis can be made only through an autopsy. The clinical picture of Pick's includes deficits in memory and judgment, which precede progressive dementia (McClearn & Foch, 1985).

Huntington's chorea is another relatively rare cause of dementia. McClearn and Foch (1985) assert that the first signs may be as minor as increased irritability, but the disorder later proceeds to more severe and overt personality changes and cognitive losses. If the dementia precedes the appearance of the typical motor dysfunction (according to Cunningham & Brookbank, 1988, sufferers demonstrate jerky, involuntary movements of the face, neck, and upper extremities), the behavioral symptoms are easily mistaken for schizophrenia. In dementia resulting from Huntington's chorea, specific brain lesions are found in the cerebrum. The disease is genetically transmitted, and symptoms generally appear in the 40s and 50s.

Still other rare causes of dementia in the elderly are Creutzfeldt-Jakob syndrome, which can be either familial or virally transmitted and involves rapidly progressive dementia, myoclonus, and slowed brain activity due to brain lesions; multiple sclerosis, involving a loss of cells in the spinal cord; Friederich's ataxia, in which nerve cells of the cerebellum are lost; dementia due to Parkinson's disease; kuru; and scrapie.

Dementia is a significant problem for the elderly because it produces severe intellectual dysfunction. Dementia impairs diverse aspects of cognition, producing deficits in memory, psychomotor speed, constructional ability, and communicatory abilities.

Memory loss, for example, is often the first sign of dementia, particularly Alzheimer's. The DSM-III-R considers memory dysfunction an essential feature for a dementia diagnosis. Memory should be viewed from a multivariate perspective: various different kinds of memory exist. A clearly useful distinction is between short-term and long-term memory. Jorm (1987) reviews studies on short-term digit span, revealing that while most normal elderly can manage six or seven digits in their working memories, mild to moderate Alzheimer's sufferers can only hold around five digits. Nonverbal short-term memory also seems to be impaired in demented elderly. When asked to reproduce a pattern of tapping movements, even mildly impaired Alzheimer's patients were worse at the task than normals, and severe cases were greatly impaired (Corkin, cited in Jorm, 1987).

Weingartner and colleagues (1981) found that SDAT sufferers inefficiently used categories to encode information for long-term memory storage. While normal controls were able to utilize categories to remember strings of words, Alzheimer's patients—even when given words prearranged into categories—could not encode properly and thus recall the words. While Kopelman (quoted in Jorm, 1987) found that already-stored memories were not affected by dementia, retrieval of memories is significantly altered by the disorder.

Other cognitive capabilities are impaired by organic brain dysfunction. The demented person may develop language disorders like agnosia or aphasia. Rissenberg and Glanzer (1987), for example, state that word-finding difficulty is a consistent feature of SDAT, and that the deficit is essentially in word retrieval. Kirshner, Webb, and Kelly (quoted in Jorm, 1987) studied agnosia, in which objects are seen but not recognized correctly. They gave demented and control subjects different types of visual cues, such as actual objects, photographs of the objects, line drawings of the objects, and masked drawings. SDAT patients were poorer overall in naming, and were significantly affected by the degree of perceptual information provided.

Psychomotor speed deficits are also observed in demented subjects. Reaction time seems especially affected (Ferris, Crook, Sathananthan, & Gershon, 1976). Dementia produces impairment of abstract thinking. Rissenberg and Glazer (1987) gave young subjects, old subjects, and Alzheimer's patients definitions for both abstract and concrete nouns. Subjects were to produce the word that went with the definition. The young and old normals showed relatively small differences between ability to find abstract and concrete nouns. However, the SDAT subjects were significantly impaired on word finding in general and were much worse on abstract nouns than on the concrete.

It is essential for a clinician to distinguish between the irreversible dementias and disorders exhibiting similar symptoms. Delirium and depression both may present as dementia. Criteria distinguishing dementias, particularly Alzheimer's, include a history of intellectual deterioration, a global cognitive disturbance, and no disturbance in the state of consciousness. There should also be no clearly depressive symptoms or history of affective episodes, and decline in intellect should be gradual as opposed to the rapid drop evinced by the elderly depressed (Folstein & McHugh, 1978).

B. Physical Health

The physical status of an older person also seems to have a significant impact on intellectual functioning. Schaie and Hertzog (1986) suggest that physical health is predictive of the maintenance of cognitive function. Horn and Donaldson (1976) state that *health* is the variable implicated in ability loss in Horn's fluid-crystallized intelligence theory. Exposure to more potentially physiologically harmful situations, the authors say, is an unavoidable characteristic of aging. Botwinick (1984) discusses a study in which extremely healthy older men were compared to a group of older men in *normal* health. The latter group performed less well than the super-healthy group on several tests, most particularly performance tests. As physical health has long been assumed to decline with age owing to inactivity, illness, and the aging process, health is probably an important extraneous influence on intellectual performance in the elderly.

Cardiovascular status appears to exert impressive influence on cognitive functioning. There seems to be a decrease in the maximal capacity of the system with age, either because of the aging process itself or because of the reduced activity associated, for various reasons, with advancing age (Seals, Hagborg, Hurley, Ehsani, & Holloszy, 1984). Botwinick and Storandt (1974) reveal that "even subclinical levels of cardiovascular changes might diminish blood oxygen supples to central neural mechanisms sufficient to result in slowed reaction time and in altered reaction-time set functions" (p. 543). Anderson (quoted in Spieth, 1965) found that middle-aged and older men with coronary heart disease were inferior to same-aged, nondiseased men in solving simple but "tricky" math problems. Spieth (1965) concluded that the studies he reviewed, "taken together, demonstrate quite conclusively that subjects suffering arteriosclerotic coronary heart disease or who show evidence of old myocardial infarctions, and those with essential hypertension, will perform more poorly than reasonably well-matched health subjects on a wide variety of self-paced tasks in which sheer physical effort is minimal" (pp. 374–375). Spieth's 1965 study found that cardiovascularly impaired groups were proportionately slower on more complex tests, and found that performance on the Halstead Tactual Performance Test was poorer for the impaired groups. He concluded that the problem was in the decision-making process. Spieth's study compared medicated hypertensives to nonmedicated hypertensives to normals, so the medication was probably not a factor in the results. Elias, Schultz, Robbins, and Elias (1989) used tests from the Halstead-Reitan battery with hypertensive and normotensive subjects, testing them three times over a decade. Hypertensives were significantly worse on tests involving categories, memory, and localization, and the Average Impairment Rating (AIR, obtained from transformed scores on the subtests) was significantly lower in the hypertensives. Additionally, Elias *et al.* concluded that medication was not a factor in their results. Hertzog, Schaie, and Gribben (1978) analyzed previously collected longitudinal data on the Primary Mental Abilities test in terms of cardiovascular status. They found that test scores were poorer among those with vascular problems. Those subjects with atherosclerosis and cerebrovascular disease were especially poor in the Psychomotor Speed test.

Exercise levels also affect cognitive function in the elderly. Exercise habits are related to cardiovascular status in that exercise will improve cardiovascular health by helping to maintain blood flow to the brain, which slows with age. Also, regular exercise allows older subjects to maintain a *motor recruitment capability,* resulting in shorter contractile times (Baylor & Spirduso, 1988). This may affect psychomotor skills, for example. Some evidence in support of physical activity's positive effects on cognitive capabilities comes from Botwinick and Thompson (1967). Their study measured three groups, two of young subjects and one of older. The younger subjects were subdivided into exercising and nonexercising conditions, and then all groups were tested on a reaction time (RT) measure. While the young who exercised were faster in RT than the elderly, the nonexercising young were not significantly faster than the older subjects. Exercise habits seemed to alter the age–reaction time relationship.

On the other hand, a later study by Botwinick and Storandt (1974) found that exercise and reaction time were significantly correlated only in a young group. Correlations were nonsignificant in all analyses involving the older subjects. However, this study had some drawbacks. Botwinick and Storandt excluded all subjects who exercised daily or near-daily from their analyses; their *regular* exercise group included those exercising at least 1 hr., 2 days a week, not the typical amount; and they neglected to define exercise. Exercise that improves cardiovascular functioning is probably the most helpful, but Cunningham and Brookbank (1988) state that fewer than 20% of those in their 60s exercise with enough intensity to so improve.

Spirduso (1975) found an age-by-activity level effect for simple reaction time and movement time. Old inactive subjects were significantly slower than old active, young inactive, and young active subjects. Baylor and Spirduso (1988) tested two different components of reaction time: premotor time, representing central nervous system effects, and muscle contractile time. In comparisons of aerobic exercisers to nonexercisers ranging from age 48 to 63, the exercisers were consistently faster in both total RT and the fractionated components of RT. In comparison, Blumenthal *et al.* (1989) found no significant improvements on various psychomotor, memory, and motor/strength tests after an aerobic-exercise training program. However, while the exercisers in Baylor and Spirduso's study had been exercising regularly for at least 5 years, Blumenthal *et al.* gave subjects 4 months of aerobic training. Perhaps the effects of exercise on cognitive abilities are cumulative over time. Similarly, Panton, Graves, Pollock, Hagberg, and Chen (1990) found that after a 6-month aerobic exercise training program, no significant differences appeared between aerobically trained, strength-trained, or control groups in either total reaction time or fractionated RT. More recently, Rogers, Meyers, and Mortel (1990) found that retirees who engaged in regular physical activities such as walking, aerobics, or housework sustained more constant cerebral blood flow rates over a 4-year period and scored better on a measure of general cognitive functioning after the fourth-year retest than did the inactive retirees.

The self-perception of health has also been related to cognitive performance in the elderly. Milligan, Powell, Harkey, and Furchtgott (1984) found that the subjective assessment of health, determined by the Older Americans Resources and Services inventory (OARS), was the major contributing variable for all measures of serial learning in their study. Subjective perception of health was more significant than either objective health or educational level. Cunningham, Smook, and Tomer (1986) utilized a longitudinal study to analyze antecedents of intellectual change in older subjects. They found that subjective health, as measured on a five-point scale, showed a significant relationship to two different aspects of psychomotor speed, figural and symbolic perceptual speed, at the second point of measurement.

Another health variable that might influence intellectual abilities in the aged is nutrition. Although few studies have found significant effects for malnutrition, Botwinick (1984) says that improper nutrition can result in delirium or make for cognitive deficits; when the proper diet is restored and any metabolic problems corrected, cognitive skills are also restored. Older people may be more prone to nutritional problems because of drugs that affect metabolism or appetite, physical inability to prepare meals, or apathy.

Additionally, neurological and non-brain-related disorders may contribute to cognitive problems in the elderly. For instance, Parkinson's disease—a motor disorder that typically appears in later middle ages—has been implicated in intellectual dysfunction. While older studies found that the effect seemed to be on psychomotor tasks rather than on initiating-response time (Talland, 1965), Wilson (quoted in Hart & Kwentus, 1987) found that nondemented Parkinson's sufferers had longer response latencies as a function of memory-set size on the Sternberg short-term memory scanning procedure.

Diabetes mellitus, often observed in elderly people, may accelerate age-related declines in blood flow to the brain, impairing cognitive abilities. Another physical disorder that might affect cognitive performance in the elderly is arthritis. However, Sands and Meredith (1989) found that the presence of, use of medication for, or practical effects of arthritis did not significantly affect results of psychomotor or perceptual speed tests like the WAIS Block Design and Digit Symbol subtests. Interestingly, Sands and Meredith did conclude that auditory functioning significantly predicted WAIS Information and Comprehension declines. Vision problems have also been linked to poor elderly performance on measures of intellectual ability.

It is important to note that poor performance by an elderly subject on a measure might not reflect true cognitive decline, but merely result from a physical disability like those mentioned above. A subject who cannot clearly read a question, or who cannot carry out the motor demands of a performance test, or who mis-hears instructions from an examiner and thus answers incorrectly is not necessarily evincing intellectual decline. Additionally, Anastasi (1982) points out that working under time constraints or in strange surroundings may increase motor problems in the orthopedically handicapped, and subjects so disabled can be more susceptible to fatigue. Subjects with severe motor problems, like Parkinson's or multiple sclerosis, are often unable to take common tests. The adjustments necessary to administer such tests can render results invalid. However, some measures of cognitive ability are suitable for disabled individuals—Anastasi mentions Raven'ŋ Progressive Matrices—and other tests have adapted versions available for persons with special handicaps.

C. Depression

With any discussion of depression, one must first define the term. Various aspects of the disorder have been identified, and one experimenter's definition may not be comparable to that of another. Dysphoria, for instance, is defined by the DSM-III-R as a chronic mood disturbance, present most of the day for more days than not. Somatic symptoms of dysphoria include sleep and appetite problems, as well as lowered energy. Psychological symptoms of dysphoria include low self-esteem, poor concentration and decision making, and hopelessness. Often dysphoria may be a consequence of a preexisting nonmood condition, like a substance-abuse disorder or arthritis. Dysphoria is relatively mild and apparently common, and is generally what community-living depressed subjects in studies will report.

Major depression, on the other hand, involves one or more major depressive episodes, characterized by persistent unhappy mood (a loss of interest in usual activities). This mood is associated with various dysphoric and physical symptoms and is incapacitating. While depressive episodes can be induced by outside factors, like heart medications, organic causes are excluded before making a diagnosis of major depression. Researchers using clinical populations typically obtain subjects with major depression.

Some researchers may also subdivide depression into *neurotic* and *endogenous* or *psychotic* depression. The important comparisons, however, are between the depressed subjects and the controls.

Cunningham and Brookbank (1988) called depression the most common psychological complaint of the elderly person. Klerman (1983) says the incidence of depression is especially significant in people aged 65 or older. Recent studies have reported that from 14 to 27% of the elderly populations reveal significant depressive symptoms (Blazer, Hughes, & George, 1987; Blazer & Williams, 1980; Eaton & Kessler, 1981; Murrell, Himmelfarb & Wright, 1983). Stenback (1980) concludes that because these and other studies indicate such high rates of depression in the elderly, the disorders should receive a special emphasis in research involving the aged.

Depressed elderly exhibit various impairments in intellectual abilities. Perhaps the aspect of cognition most affected is psychomotor speed. Numerous studies have examined the relationship of depression to speed components, such as reaction time, perceptual speed, and memory-scanning speed. For example, Knott and LaPierre (1987) found elevated scores for two elements of reaction time, decision time (DT) and movement time (MT), in depressed younger subjects. Similarly, Byrne (1976) used choice-reaction time, again fractionated into DT and MT. He measured reaction time in two depressed subgroups (neurotic and psychotic) and in normals. Both DT and MT were significantly longer in the depressed groups than in normals. The mean age of the neurotic depressives was 35, while the mean age of the psychotic depressives was 45. While Baribeau-Braun and Lasevre (quoted in Knott & LaPierre, 1987) state that choice-reaction time, not simple-reaction time, is what differentiates depressives and controls and is sensitive to improvement in symptom status, Botwinick and Storandt (1974) found a significant main effect for depression on simple reaction-time measures. Those subjects in the Botwinick and Storandt study scoring over 50 on the Zung self-report measure of depression had significantly slower reaction times than subjects scoring under 50. However, the authors pointed out that depressive affect accounted for relatively little of the variance in their results, and noted that the results might have been confounded with cardiovascular status.

Weckowicz, Nutter, Cruise, and Yonge (1972) suggested that depressive symptoms might have an important effect on speeded test performance, even more so than on power test results. They gave clinically depressed subjects and comparable age group, nondepressed controls tests of both power (WAIS Vocabulary, Information, and Word Fluency subtests) and speed (perceptual speed, using the WAIS Digit Symbol subtest and the Brengelmann Picture Series, and simple- and choice-reaction time). The depressed subjects, even when equated with controls on educational level, showed lowered speed of performance. While age also affected scores, the simple-reaction-time test consistently differentiated groups. In general, the authors concluded, depression affected speed measures more significantly than did age, and affected power-test performance less than speeded.

Cunningham, Tomer, Haman, and Fitzgerald (1989) found that the presence of dysphoric symptoms (low spirits, hopelessness) in older subjects corresponded to slower performance on measures of figural perceptual speed, as measured by speeded discrimination between similar pictures. In a path analysis, a composite score of dysphoria items actually better predicted performance on the ability of figural perceptual speed than did age. No significant relationships were found, however, for two other aspects of depression (cognitive complaints and worry).

Hart and Kwentus (1987) gave the WAIS Digit Symbol subtest to depressed and nondepressed elderly subjects. The depressed subjects demonstrated notable psychomotor slowing. Memory-scanning speed also seems to be affected by depression. The Hart and Kwentus study also employed the Sternberg memory-scanning procedure. Speed and accuracy of short-term memory were measured independently: motor demands stayed constant, while the amount of information to be processed varied. They found that the depressed subjects had longer response latencies than did controls. This suggests that inefficient decision-making contributes to the slowing seen in the depressed.

Depression also affects memory in older persons. A study discussion in Weingartner and Silberman's (1984) review gave moderately depressed subjects different lists of words to learn and remember. Compared to age-, sex-, and education-matched controls, the depressed recalled significantly fewer words and differed most from controls on random, unrelated words, recalling many fewer.

Causes of the intellectual deficits seen in the depressed elderly are unclear, but several viable hypotheses have been suggested. The hypotheses can be subdivided into two categories, based on either psychological or biological factors. Theories based on psychological factors attempt to explain the deficits commonly seen in all depressives regardless of age. For example, Miller (1974) proposes a learned-helplessness model based on Seligman, Klein, and Miller's (1975) work. According to this combined cognitive–motivational explanation, depressives have learned to see reinforcement as being unrelated to their responses. Such a perception then lessens the motivation for a future response, and impedes learning in new situations.

Miller (1975) also suggests a related theory based on reduced motivation. In this construct, depressives exhibit impaired performance because they either are not motivated to do well or are unable to sustain their motivation. Knott and LaPierre offer a different hypothesis based on an attention-deficit model. They proposed that the patient group in their 1987 study may not have exhibited the same degree of attention to the task stimuli as did controls, and thus may have shown slower responsivity. A final explanation of depression's effect on cognition, based on psychological factors, involves decision-making processes. Miller and Lewis (quoted in McAlister, 1981) believe their results support the hypothesis that poor depressive performance on memory tasks stems not from true memory impairment but instead reflects altered attitudes toward the decision-making processes.

Other theories incorporate organic factors often seen in the elderly. Jorm (1986) suggests that the depressed elderly could have a real impairment of cognitive function fundamental to the depression, as opposed to an inability to utilize preexisting mental capacities. Jorm mentions various studies as support for his hypothesis. Savard, Rey, and Post (1980), for instance, state that depression might involve biogenic amine deficiencies, which would affect cognitive function. They also reveal that the effects of depression could interfere with normal aging; neurotransmitter systems affected by depression might share partially overlapping neural pathways with those systems altered by aging, resulting in more debilitating deficits in the depressed elderly. McHugh and Folstein (1979) also mention that neuronal losses with age result in a magnified reaction to biogenic amine deficits for the elderly.

Finally, Hemsi, Whitehead, and Post (1968), Cawley, Post, and Whitehead (1973), and Davies, Hamilton, Hendrickson, Levy, and Post (1978) all implicate lowered cortical arousal as the common factor in aging, dementia, and depression deficiencies. They believe that the normal aging process involves a lowering of arousal, which produces cognitive deficits; the lowered arousal makes the elderly more prone to depression, in turn further lowering arousal.

Physical or emotional problems commonly associated with aging, like dementia, depression, cardiovascular problems, or sensory impairments, clearly influence aspects of cognitive performance in the elderly. Not all older individuals will demonstrate declines in all cognitive functions, and the losses of those who do may be mediated by extraneous factors. Researchers and clinicians need to take this into account when examining the intellectual abilities of older people or when generalizing about lowered intellectual functioning with age.

IV. Developing New Tests for the Elderly?

An enduring issue in the assessment of intellectual functioning concerns the comprehensiveness of measurement. Guilford (e.g., 1967) was one of the first psychologists to recognize the full complexity of human intellectual functioning and to draw the logical conclusions with regard to scientific inquiry and coordinated test development. The issue of comprehensiveness is probably even more urgent with regard to mature adults than with younger persons. One part of this issue concerns full representation of the major known factors of intellectual functioning in an assessment. For example, a serious and long-standing criticism of the traditional WAIS is that there are far too many (highly correlated) tests of verbal comprehension, and precious little in the way of tests sensitive to inductive reasoning. It is quite useful to supplement the WAIS with a test of inductive reasoning such as the Progressive Matrices test developed by the British psychologist Raven. Naturally, there are many other well-replicated factors that could be used to supplement the WAIS (see Ekstrom, French & Harmon, 1976).

This approach of using additional tests with prefabricated inventories takes one only so far and does not fully resolve a potentially more serious issue: do existing tests reflect the mature capacities of adults generally, and elderly persons in particular? Many psychometricians intuitively sense that existing tests may be too narrowly focused on academic topics and not reflective of intellectual demands in the real world. With the exception of sporadic attempts to develop various achievement tests in some practical content areas (e.g., Demming & Pressey, 1957), little has been done in the way of answering this issue. What seems to be needed is a sustained, comprehensive, and creative program that would seek to identify new factors of intellectual ability germane to old age. Recent efforts hold the possibility of advances in the future (e.g., Sternberg & Wagner, 1986). A potential hazard to this, however, is the possibility that such new tests would only be redundant measures of verbal comprehension expressing themselves in particular content areas. The logistical requirements of item development, item and reliability analysis, convergent and discriminant validation, as well as empirical predictive validation would imply a very long program of research with a potentially elusive goal. On the other hand, in the absence of such efforts, a sense of lack of fulfillment is apt to continue with regard to a comprehensive assessment of the mature capacities of older people.

References

Anastasi, A. (1982). *Psychological Testing* (5th ed.). New York: Macmillan.

Baylor, A. M., & Spirduso, W. W. (1988). Systematic aerobic exercise and components of reaction time in older women. *Journal of Gerontology, 43*(5), 121–126.

Birren, J. E. (1965). Age changes in speed of behavior: Its nature and psychological correlates. In A. T. Welford & J. E. Birren (Eds.), *Handbook of aging, behavior, and the nervous system* (pp. 191–216). Springfield, IL: Charles C Thomas.

Blazer, D., Hughes, D. C., & George, L. K. (1987). The epidemiology of depression in an elderly community population. *The Gerontologist, 27,*(3), 281–287.

Blazer, D., & Williams, C. D. (1980). Epidemiology of dysphoria and depression in an elderly population. *American Journal of Psychiatry, 137*(4), 439–444.

Blumenthal, J. A., Emery, C. F., Madden, D. J., George, L. K., Coleman, R. E., Riddle, M. W., McKee, D. C., Reasoner, J., & Williams, R. S. (1989). Cardiovascular and behavioral effects of aerobic exercise training in healthy older men and women. *Journal of Gerontology, 44*(5) 147–57.

Botwinick, J. (1984). *Aging and Behavior* (3rd ed.). New York: Springer.

Botwinick, J., & Storandt, M. (1974). Cardiovascular status, depressive affect, and other factors in reaction time. *Journal of Gerontology, 29*(5), 543–548.

Botwinick, J., & Thompson, L. W. (1967). Depressive affect, speed of response, and age. *Journal of Consulting Psychology, 31,* 106.

Byrne, D. G. (1976). Choice reaction times in depressive states. *British Journal of Clinical Psychology, 15,* 149–156.

Cawley, R. H., Post, F., & Whitehead, A. (1973). Barbiturate tolerance and psychological functioning in elderly depressed patients. *Psychological Medicine, 3,* 39–52.

Charness, N. (1985). Aging and problem-solving performance. In N. Charness (Ed.), *Aging and Human Performance* (pp. 225–259). London: Wiley.

Cunningham, W. R. (1980a). Age comparative factor analysis of ability variables in adulthood and old age. *Intelligence, 7,* 133–149.

Cunningham, W. R. (1980b). Speed, age, and qualitative differences in cognitive functioning. In L. W. Poon (Ed), *Aging in the 1980s: Selected contemporary issues in the psychology of aging.* Washington, DC: American Psychological Association.

Cunningham, W. R. (1981). Ability factor structure differences in adulthood and old age. *Multivariate Behavioral Research, 16,* 3–22.

Cunningham, W. R. (1987). Intellectual abilities and age. In K. W. Schaie (Ed.), *Annual Review of Gerontology and Geriatrics, 7.* New York: Springer.

Cunningham, W. R. (1988). *Perspectives on aging and abilities.* Division 20 Invited Address, Meetings of the American Psychological Association, Atlanta, Georgia, August.

Cunningham, W. R. (1989). Intellectual abilities and age. In V. L. Bengston & K. W. Schaie (Eds.), *The course of later life: Research and reflections* (pp. 93–106). New York: Springer.

Cunningham, W. R., & Birren, J. E. (1976). Age changes in human abilities: A 28-year longitudinal study. *Developmental Psychology, 12,* 81–82.

Cunningham, W. R., & Brookbank, J. (1988). *Gerontology.* New York: Harper & Row.

Cunningham, W. R., Smook, G., & Tomer, A. (1986). *Antecedents of intellectual change in old age.* Paper presented at the 39th Annual Scientific Meeting of the Gerontological Society of America in Chicago.

Cunningham, W. R., & Tomer, A. (1990). Intellectual abilities and age: Concepts, theories and analyses. In E. A. Lovelace (Ed.), *Aging and cognition: Mental processes, self-awareness and interventions.* Amsterdam: Elsevier Science Publishers B. V., North Holland.

Cunningham, W. R., Tomer, A., Haman, K. L., & Fitzgerald, D. (1989). *Depression: An antecedent of intellectual decline.* Paper presented at the 42nd Annual Scientific Meeting of the Gerontological Society of America in Minneapolis, November.

Davies, G., Hamilton, S., Hendrickson, D. E., Levy, R., & Post, F. (1978). Psychological test performance and sedation thresholds of elderly dements, depressives, and depressives with incipient brain damage. *Psychological Medicine, 8,* 103–109.

Davis, P. B., Morris, J. C., & Grant, E. (1990). Brief screening tests versus clinical staging in senile dementia of the Alzheimer type. *Journal of the American Geriatrics Society, 38*, 129–135.

Demming, J. A., & Pressey, S. L. (1957). Tests "indigenous" to the adult and older years. *Journal of Counseling Psychology, 2*, 144–148.

Donnelly, E. F., Waldman, I. N., Murphy, D. L., Wyatt, R. J., & Goodwin, F. K. (1980). Primary affective disorder: Thought disorder in depression. *Journal of Abnormal Psychology, 89*(3), 315–319.

Eaton, W. W., & Kessler, L. G. (1981). Rates of symptoms of depression in a national sample. *American Journal of Epidemiology, 114*, 528–538.

Ekstrom, R. B., French, J., & Harman, M. (1976). *Manual for kit of factor-referenced tests.* Princeton, NJ: Educational Testing Service.

Elias, M. F., Schultz, N. R., Robbins, M. A., & Elias, P. K. (1989). A longitudinal study of neuropsychological performance by hypertensives and normotensives: A third measurement point. *Journal of Gerontology, 44*(1), 24–28.

Ferris S., Crook, T., Sathananthan, G., & Gershon, S. (1976). Reaction time as a diagnostic measure in senility. *Journal of the American Geriatrics Society, 24*, 529–533.

Folstein, M. F., & McHugh, P. R. (1978). Dementia syndrome of depression. In R. Katzman, R. D. Terry, & K. L. Bick (Eds.), *Alzheimer's disease: Senile dementia and related disorders* (Aging, Vol. 7). New York: Raven Press.

Guilford, J. P. (1967). *The nature of human intelligence.* New York: McGraw-Hill.

Hart, R. P., & Kwentus, J. A. (1987). Psychomotor slowing and subcortical-type dysfunction in depression. *Journal of Neurology, Neurosurgery, and Psychiatry, 50*, 1263–1266.

Hemsi, L. K., Whitehead, A., & Post, F. (1968). Cognitive functioning and cerebral arousal in elderly depressives and dements. *Journal of Psychosomatic Research, 12*, 145–156.

Hertzog, C. (1989). The influence of cognitive slowing on age difference in intelligence. *Developmental Psychology, 25*, 636–651.

Hertzog, C., Raskind, C. C., & Cannon, C. J. (1986). Age-related slowing in semantic information processing speed: An individual differences analysis. *Journal of Gerontology, 41*, 500–502.

Hertzog, C., Schaie, K. W., & Gribben, K. (1978). Cardiovascular disease and changes in intellectual functioning from middle to old age. *Journal of Gerontology, 23*, 872–883.

Heston, L. L., Mastri, A. (1982). Age at onset of Pick's and Alzheimer's dementia: Implications for diagnosis and research. *Journal of Gerontology, 37*, 422–424.

Horn, J. L. (1970). Organization of data on life-span development of human abilities. In L. R. Goulet & P. B. Baltes (Eds.), *Life-span developmental psychology.* (pp. 423–466). New York: Academic Press.

Horn, J. L., & Donaldson, G. (1976). On the myth of intellectual decline in adulthood. *American Psychologist, 31*, 701–719.

Jorm, A. F. (1986). Cognitive deficit in the depressed elderly: A review of some basic unresolved issues. *Australian and New Zealand Journal of Psychiatry, 20*, 11–22.

Jorm, A. F. (1987). *A guide to the understanding of Alzheimer's disease and related disorders.* New York: New York University Press.

Klerman, G. (1983). Problems in the definition and diagnosis of depression in the elderly. In L. D. Breslau & M. R. Haug (Eds.), *Depression and aging: Causes, care and consequences.* New York: Springer.

Knott, V. J., & LaPierre, Y. D. (1987). Electrophysiological and behavioral correlates of psychomotor responsivity in depression. *Biological Psychiatry, 22*, 313–324.

McAllister, T. (1981). Cognitive functioning in the affective disorders. *Comprehensive Psychiatry, 22*(6), 572–86.

McClearn, G., & Foch, T. T. (1985). Behavioral genetics. In J. R. Birren & K. Schaie (Eds.), *Handbook of the Psychology of Aging* (2nd ed.). New York: Van Nostrand Reinhold.

McHugh, P. R., & Folstein, M. F. (1979). Psychopathology of dementia: Implications for neuropathology, in R. Katzman (Ed.), *Congenital and Acquired Cognitive Disorders.* New York: Raven.

Miller, W. R. (1974). Learned helplessness in depressed and nondepressed students. *Dissertation Abstracts International, 35*, 1921B.

Miller, W. R. (1975). Psychological deficit in depression. *Psychological Bulletin, 82*(2), 238–260.

Milligan, W. L., Powell, D. A., Harley, C., & Furchtgott, E. (1984). A comparison of physical health and psychosocial variables as predictors of reaction time and serial learning performance in elderly men. *Journal of Gerontology, 39*(6) 704–710.

Murrell, S. A., Himmelfarb, S., & Wright, K. (1983). Prevalence of depression and its correlates in older adults. *American Journal of Epidemiology, 117,* 173–185.

Panton, L. B., Graves, J. E., Pollock, M. L., Hagberg, J. M., & Chen, W. (1990). Effect of aerobic and resistance training on frationated reaction time and speed of movement. *Journal of Gerontology, 45*(1), 25–31.

Rissenberg, M., & Glanzer, M. (1987). Free recall and word-finding ability in normal aging and senile dementia of the Alzheimer's type: The effect of item concreteness. *Journal of Gerontology, 42*(3), 318–322.

Rogers, R. L., Meyer, J. S., & Mortel, K. F. (1990). After reaching retirement age physical activity sustains cerebral perfusion and cognition. *Journal of the American Geriatrics Society, 38,* 123–128.

Salthouse, T. A. (1984). The skill of typing. *Scientific American 250,* 128–136.

Salthouse, T. A. (1985). *A Theory of Cognitive Aging.* Amsterdam: Elsevier/North Holland.

Sands, L. P., & Meredith, W. (1989). Effects of sensory and motor functioning on adult intellectual performance. *Journal of Gerontology, 44*(2), 56–58.

Savard, R. J., Rey, A. C., and Post, R. M. (1980). Halstead-Reitan Category Test in bipolar and unipolar affective disorders: Relationship to age and phase of illness. *Journal of Nervous and Mental Disease, 168,* 297–304.

Schaie, K. W., & Hertzog, C. (1986). Toward a comprehensive model of adult intellectual development: Contributions of the Seattle Longitudinal Study. In R. J. Sternberg (Ed.), *Advances in human intelligence* (Vol. 3). Hillsdale, NJ: Erlbaum.

Schaie, K. W., & Willis, S. L. (1986). Can intellectual decline be reversed? *Developmental Psychology, 22,* 223–232.

Seals, D. R., Hagborg, J. M., Hurley, B. F., Ehsani, A. A., & Holloszy, J. O. (1984). Endurance training in older men and women I. Cardiovascular response to exercise. *Journal of Applied Physiology, 57*(4), 1024–1029.

Seligman, M. E. P., Klein, D. C., & Miller, W. R. (1975). Depression. In H. Leilenberg (Ed.), *Handbook of behavior therapy.* New York: Appleton-Century-Crofts.

Shapiro, M. B., Post, F., Lofving, B., & Inglis, J. (1956). Memory function in psychiatric patients over sixty: Some methodological and diagnostic implications. *Journal of Mental Science, 102,* 233–246.

Spieth, W. (1965). Slowness of task performance and cardiovascular diseases. In A. T. Welford & J. E. Birren (Eds.), *Behavior, aging, and the nervous system.* Springfield, ILL: Charles C. Thomas.

Spirduso, W. W. (1975). Reachon and movement time as a function of age and physical activity test. *Journal of Gerontology, 30,* 435–440.

Stenback, A. (1980). Depression and suicidal behavior in old age. In J. R. Birren & R. B. Sloane (Eds.), *Handbook of Mental Health and Aging.* Englewood Cliffs, NJ: Prentice-Hall.

Sternberg, R., & Wagner, R. (Eds.) (1986). *Practical Intelligence.* New York: Cambridge University Press.

Talland, G. A. (1965). Initiation of response, and reaction time in aging, and with brain damage. In A. T. Welford & J. R. Birren (Eds.), *Behavior, aging, and the nervous system.* Springfield, ILL: Charles C Thomas.

Teri, L. Hughes, J. P., & Larson, E. B. (1990). Cognitive deterioration in Alzheimer's disease: Behavioral and health factors. *Journal of Gerontology, 45*(2), 58–63.

Tomer, A. (1989). *Slowing with age as an explanation of age changes in fluid intelligence.* Unpublished doctoral dissertation, University of Florida.

Weckowicz, T. E., Nutter, R. W., Cruise, D. G., & Yonge, K. A. (1972). Speed in test performance in relation to depressive illness and age. *Canadian Psychiatric Association Journal, 17,* 241–250.

Weingartner, H., Kay, W., Smallberg, S. A., Ebert, M. H., Gillin, J. C., & Sitaram, N. (1981). Memory failures in progressive idiopathic dementia. *Journal of Abnormal Psychology, 90*(3), 187–196.

Weingartner, H., & Silberman, E. (1984). Cognitive changes in depression. In R. M. Post & J. C. Ballenger (Eds.), *Neurobiology of mood disorders.* Baltimore MD: William & Wilkins.

Wells, C. E. (1978). Chronic brain disease: An overview. *American Journal of Psychiatry, 135*(1), 1–12.

White, N. A., & Cunningham, W. R. (1987). The age comparative construct validity of speeded cognitive factors. *Multivariate Behavioral Research, 22,* 249–265.

13

Emotion and Personality ⸻

Hans Thomae

I. Stability and Change of Emotional and Behavioral Dispositions
   A. Activity
   B. Affect
   C. Anxiety
   D. Extroversion–Introversion
   E. Neuroticism
   F. Rigidity
   G. Subjective Well-Being
II. Cognition: Emotion Interactions and Research on Personality and Aging
   A. Future Time Perspective
   B. Control Beliefs
   C. Beliefs in Possibility of Changing Life in Old Age
   D. Personality and Adjustment to Aging
III. Conclusions
   References

From reviews on developments in the field of personality and emotion like that of Shanan and Jacobowitz (1982), Singer and Kolligian (1987), and Carson (1989), it seems likely that the relationships between aging, personality, and related fields no longer can be discussed in the context of trait theories. Carson (1989) refers to a much-needed caution against enthusiasm about the renovation of personality factors like introversion–extroversion or neuroticism. Singer and Koligian (1987) predicted development of research on personality in agreement with the increased interest in emotion, fantasy, and imagination, especially in the interaction between cognition and emotion.

As research on personality and aging is still focusing on trait concepts, the first section of this chapter will report briefly some recent findings on consistency and change of selected trait variables. It also includes information on relationships between aging and emotion. A second part follows Singer's and Kolligian's (1987) recommendation and will discuss the issue of cognition–emotion interaction on the basis of cognitive constructs like time perspective and control belief as well as on that of different approaches to a cognitive but anticognitivistic theory of adjustment to aging.

I. Stability and Change of Emotional and Behavioral Dispositions __

In several studies and reviews, previous beliefs could not be confirmed regarding close relationships between advancing age on the one hand and decline in activity, emotional responsiveness, and adjustment as well as an increase of depressive states and maladjustive behaviors on the other. This finding is independent of the instruments used in the study, such as the Cattell 16 Personality Factor Inventory (Costa, McCrae & Arenberg, 1983; Siegler, George, & Okun, 1985) or the Guilford–Zimmermann Temperament Scales (Costa, McCrae & Arenberg, 1984) or other tests. Due to lack of space we can give only data on some of the major dispositions in alphabetical order.

A. Activity

In the Baltimore Longitudinal Study on Aging (BLSA), retest coefficients Guilford–Zimmerman–Temperament–Scale (GZTS)–Subscale General *activity* over a period of 6 years were .86 and .83 for middle and late adulthood (Costa & McCrae, 1984). In the Bonn Longitudinal Study on Aging (BOLSA) scores for social activities, active coping in daily life, and for activities observed during the 5-day stay of the participants at the center were used for the classification of the sample into groups of high-, medium-, and low-active women and men (Schmitz-Scherzer & Thomae, 1983; Thomae, 1983). These groups differed during a period of 12 years, in an highly significant way, in their tendencies to maintain the range of their own interests, and to expand the range of their social contacts, with high-active persons always scoring high in these variables. This was also true for WAIS scores (Performance and Verbal) and for perceived and objective health. In coping with problems in daily life, achievement-related behavior and cultivation of social contacts were preferred more often by the high-active elderly.

B. Affect

Using Izard's differential theory of emotion focusing on seven basic emotions (anger, fear, etc.), Malatesta and Kalnok (1984) showed that older people, in comparison to a young and middle-aged subsample, were not affectively impoverished or egocentric. Older subjects also did not experience more negative or fewer positive emotions than did younger ones (see Table 1).

C. Anxiety

Although there are reasons for the expectation that anxiety increases with advancing age, a critical review of the literature does not support this view (Schultz, 1986). It should be

Table I

Percentage of Responses in Each Thematic Category[a]

		Age group			Sex	
Affect	Theme	Young	Middle	Old	Men	Women
Happy	Personal gains	0.75	0.75	0.57	0.71	0.68
	Location change	0.25	0.25	0.43	0.29	0.32
Excited	Personal gains	0.60	0.74	0.78	0.71	0.70
	Location change	0.40	0.26	0.22	0.29	0.30
Sad[b]	Personal losses	0.45	0.34	0.21	0.37	0.30
	Physical problems	0.55	0.66	0.79	0.63	0.70
Anxious	Personal losses	0.50	0.42	0.39	0.42	0.45
	Physical problems	0.29	0.38	0.44	0.34	0.39
	Location change	0.17	0.16	0.11	0.19	0.12
	Meeting/not meeting responsibilities	0.04	0.04	0.06	0.05	0.04
Angry[b]	Unpleasant interpersonal encounters	0.16	0.10	0.18	0.16	0.15
	Personal losses	0.21	0.32	0.47	0.40	0.27
	Meeting/not meeting responsibilities	0.63	0.58	0.35	0.44	0.58
Shame	Unpleasant interpersonal encounters	0.27	0.27	0.10	0.19	0.22
	Personal losses	0.11	0.11	0.20	0.15	0.15
	Location change	0.16	0.16	0.20	0.19	0.132
	Meeting/not meeting responsibilities	0.32	0.32	0.34	0.32	0.35
	Personal appearance	0.14	0.14	0.16	0.15	0.15
Disgust[c]	Unpleasant interpersonal encounters	0.12	0.10	0.17	0.08	0.17
	Personal losses	0.61	0.47	0.31	0.62	0.37
	Physical problems	0.09	0.08	0.09	0.05	0.11
	Meeting/not meeting responsibilities	0.18	0.35	0.43	0.25	0.35

[a]From Malatesta and Zalnok (1984).
[b]Significant age effect, $p < 0.05$.
[c]Significant sex effect, $p < 0.05$.

emphasized that this statement refers only to trait anxiety and to general states of anxiety. Fears of becoming a victim of crime (Cutler, 1979, 1980) or of elderly abuse (Podnieks, 1989) certainly are more prevalent in elderly persons.

Special forms of anxiety like death anxiety were related to anxiety about aging and to negative attitudes toward aged persons in a sample of nursing home employees (Vickio & Cavanaugh, 1985). The level of death anxiety was not related to death experience generally, but to repeated exposure to deaths of nursing home residents. Findings like these emphasize the study of specific forms of anxiety and their correlates.

D. Extroversion–Introversion

C. G. Jung's (1924) personality types have been used in different approaches to the study of age changes. The operationalization of the constructs differs, however, in different studies. Using the Minnesota Multiphasic Personality Inventory (MMPI) Social Introversion Scale, Leon, Gillum, Gillum and Gouze (1979) found a stability coefficient of .74

over a period of 30 years in a sample tested originally in middle adulthood. Using GZTS, Costa and McCrae (1984a,c) also found highly significant retest correlates in BOLSA subjects for the period 1959–1966 to 1980, ranging from 59 to 70.

E. Neuroticism

The same degree of stability over time was found for the dimension of neuroticism. Retest correlation coefficients for the periods 1959–1966 on the one hand and 1979–1980 on the other hand ranged from .27 to .66. From different longitudinal as well as cross-sectional data, Costa & McCrae (1984b) point to close relationships between subjective well-being and low scores for neuroticism. From these data they conclude that higher scores for neuroticism result in low scores for subjective well-being in old age.

F. Rigidity

Riegel and Riegel (1960) found higher scores for rigidity in older people. Schaie (1983, 1986) discriminates between psychomotor, motor–cognitive, and attitudinal rigidity. Only the last component usually is discussed in the context of personality and aging. From his Seattle studies, Schaie (1983) concluded that attitudinal rigidity is lowest in young adulthood, highest in middle-aged people, and declining after age 60. In BOLSA, the Riegel scales for measuring rigidity were used for 15 years. From an analysis of the data from the first 5 years of the study, Angleitner (1987) rejected hypotheses regarding rising scores for rigidity with increasing age. Stability coefficients between measurement point I (1965) and IV (1970) ranged from .19 to .86 for the different rigidity scales. The lowest degree of stability was found for a scale measuring intolerance, and the highest, for personal rigidity.

G. Subjective Well-Being

Unlike the constructs of extroversion and anxiety, that of subjective well-being does not come from traditional trait-centered approaches to the study of personality. Its roots within the mental health movement and in social gerontology have been delineated by George (1981). She suggested defining life satisfaction as the cognitive assessment of well-being, and happiness as the affective assessment. Costa et al. (1987) found high stability of scores on the General Well-Being Schedule in a national sample over a period of 9 years. The authors emphasize that subjective well-being is independent not only of age but also of health and variables like present life circumstances.

This conclusion is contradictory to a great body of research that was summarized for the first time 20 years ago (Adams, 1971) and that pointed to many physical, psychological, and social correlates of life satisfaction or happiness. Diener (1984) added new information on social and psychological influences on subjective well-being. As in many other studies, Willits and Crider (1988) found evidence for a close association between health as perceived by their elderly sample and responses to direct questions about global and specific aspects of well-being. This association was evident for men and women, for those with low or high income, and for other groups.

Many studies are related to the influence of social networks and subjective well-being. According to Chappell and Badger (1989), having no confidants and no companions were the decisive correlates of low degrees of subjective well-being in a random sample in Canada. But overall in this study, health had the greatest explanatory power for life satisfaction. The authors emphasize from their findings the need to distinguish between social isolation and psychological isolation (or perceived isolation).

Other psychological predictors or correlates of subjective well-being were identified by Reker, Peacock and Wong (1987) in terms of *meaning and purpose in life*. These existentialistic constructs are derived from Viktor Frankl's humanistic psychology. They were used in seven scales, including one related to *goal seeking,* another to *future meaning,* etc. Well-being was assessed by the authors' own scale. Aside from age differences for the different measures of perceived meaningfulness of life, there were significant correlations between six of the existentialistic scales and subjective well-being. Perceived control over life was especially associated with subjective well-being.

The complexity of early antecedents of subjective well-being in old age was demonstrated by Mussen (1985) by an analysis of data from the parents of the children sampled for the Berkeley Guidance study (Jones, 1958). Very detailed information on the home environment of these children gathered in the 1930s could be compared with data obtained from these parents 40 years later.

For the prediction of the Berkeley fathers' happiness at age 70, both person and environment in early adulthood were effective. Characteristics of their spouses and the marital situation around the age of 30 were especially related to happiness in old age. If these fathers had healthy, even-tempered, and self-confident wives and enjoyed marriage without tension and worry, they were likely to become happy grandfathers. But the fathers' own personalities and careers were important also. Good health, emotional stability, energy, self-confidence, and job satisfaction were predictive for subjective well-being in old age.

For the women, the marital situation and their home environment in young adulthood were related especially closely to happiness in old age. A sufficient family income, enough leisure time, sexual satisfaction, mutual understanding between the couple, agreement between husband and wife on expenditures, cultural standards, and educational matters were the main predictors of happiness in old age.

The data of this unique study clearly support an interactionistic approach in the person–situation debate such as applied by Magnusson (1988) in his longitudinal studies on Swedish children. Following this approach, Rudinger and Thomae (1991) used structural equation models for the prediction of subjective well-being in BOLSA subjects. This analysis points especially to the impact of the present and past life situation of the individual and is in support of cognitive theories of personality and aging that hold that behavior and subjective well-being are dependent on the cognitive representation or construction of the situation rather than on its objective quality (Thomae, 1990).

II. Cognition: Emotion Interactions and Research on Personality and Aging

Cognitive theories of personality have been in vogue since Kelly's book on personal constructs (1955). Many other concepts have been introduced to utilize cognitions of self and situation and to trace their influences on behavior. Generalized expectancies, belief systems, schemata, prototypes, scripts, and plans—these are just some of the many constructs developed for linking cognition and behavior.

In the same way that Kelly believed motivational variables can be replaced by cognitive ones like future time perspective, many of his followers apparently agreed with Birch, Atkinson and Bongort (1974), that *thought directs action* without any emotional or motivational intervening processes. These cognitivistic developments are detrimental to the future development of cognitive theories, which can contribute greatly to the understanding of the relationships between aging, emotion, and personality. This will be shown on the basis of theories and research related to the study of future time perspective, control beliefs, and to adjustment to stress or problems in daily life.

A. Future Time Perspective

Kuhlen (1956), one of the pioneers of psychogerontology stated that "the changing time experience as age increases (p. 25)" is one of the most important aspects in the aging process. As shown by Thomae (1983), extension and quality of future time perspective were closely related to active coping with health problems, compliant behavior to active coping with health problems, compliant behavior regarding lifestyle, openmindedness, emotional responsiveness, and good adjustment. Shifflett (1987) showed that a positive future outlook had favorable effects on the health behavior of elderly people. If, for example, a grandchild, were expected, the readiness to comply with doctor's advice regarding weight control increased significantly. A negative personal future often resulted in nonadherence or excessively strict adherence to a diet, dependent on past influences.

According to Kastenbaum (1982) time perspective in any age group is the outcome of the person's construction and reconstruction of time. Cognitive acts, according to this statement, are the producers of different time perspectives and their behavioral outcomes. From this point of view, an emphasis on cognitive processes or productions seems to be valid for Kastenbaum. On the other hand, he refers to many social and biological variables and their relationships with different qualities and extensions of time perspective such as social class, unemployment, isolating and frustrating life conditions, and illness. Therefore it would be more valid to state that time perspectives are the outcome of cognitive emotional interactions in the person, rather than his or her constructions.

A complex network of interactions between future time perspective on the one hand and social as well as psychological variables was shown by Fooken (1985). This study compared the future time perspectives of elderly women (see Figure 1).

Married women with a negative attitude to the future were socially isolated by their husbands and children, who did not care very much about them; therefore, general satisfaction with life and feeling of being needed scored very low in this group. An

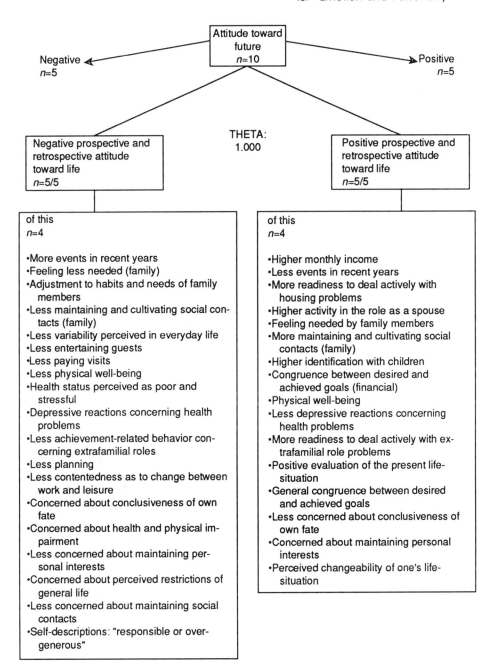

Figure 1 Multivariate analysis concerning married women's attitudes toward the future (Fooken, 1985).

objective unsatisfactory social and marital situation results in negative emotions about life generally and one's usefulness to others especially. These feelings, however, have their impact on their outlook for the future. These women's time perspectives developed in a situation of growing feelings of isolation and uselessness.

The same could be demonstrated by the longitudinal analysis of the development of a positive future outlook in a group of married elderly women who felt integrated into their families and the social world outside the family. Fooken's sample also included a group of long-widowed women, most of whom had lost their husbands in World War II. Those with positive attitudes toward the future had, during the long years of their widowhood, developed some skills in making use of their remaining social and personal resources to get something from their lives.

Within this context, a positive outcome could be developed, whereas long-widowed women with a negative future had to struggle with so many complications during their lives, that resources of this kind were not available. The main component of these resources was a feeling of satisfaction with the present situation, which was present in the first group and absent in those with a negative future outlook. Cognitive representations of situations grow mainly out of an emotional context. Without any reference to this context, cognitive theories are rationalistic and miss contact with the lives of average people.

A somewhat rationalistic interpretation of an attitude of negative future concern in a group of old-old persons is given by Kulys and Tobin (1980). This negative future concern is explained by a hypothesized strategy of not planning and caring before a crisis becomes evident. In a study of 35 survivors of BOLSA 20 years after its beginning, Schneider (1989) found an avoidant attitude in all of them when he approached them with the question about their future outlook. None of them agreed that they had a future. As the author had interviewed them before about their present and recent past, he knew about plans they had. Therefore it was possible to complete an in-depth interview in which realistic and unrealistic plans were closely interrelated with each other. Very clear, however, were the different representations of this future: one defined by a hopefully far-extended independent present situation, another one characterized by thoughts and worries about forthcoming dependency, and thoughts, not worries, about death as an immanent aspect of this future.

Schneider was able also to identify different longitudinal patterns of future time perspective over a period of 18 years. Men showed more positive feelings toward the future at the beginning, which became neutralized at the end. Women on the other hand, were more neutral at the beginning, as well at the end, with some positive trends in the intermediate time. These and other changes point to very complex processes characterized by complex cognitive emotional interactions.

B. Control Beliefs

As aging very often is evaluated as a process of gradual decline in competencies, psychologists not informed about the findings of population studies or of those of BOLSA, the Duke Studies (Busse & Maddox, 1986) hypothesized that the situation of aged persons can be defined as one of learned helplessness (Seligman, 1975). From these stereotypes, many authors believe that aging can be conceptualized as a process of increasing belief in external control of the life situation.

Another origin of the growing interest on control beliefs in old age (see Baltes & Baltes, 1986) goes back to social-learning theories of personality, linking behavior with cognitive systems like *generalized expectancies* (Rotter, 1966). Rodin, Timko, and Harris (1985) speak of *feelings of control* this way, stressing the close interaction of cognitive and emotional processes or systems in these beliefs. Life-span psychologists who expected a sequence from complete dependency on external control in infancy, through increasing internality in younger and middle adulthood, to more or less external control beliefs face many problems in the present state of research. Siegler and Gatz (1985), in a cross-sectional study, found that their oldest subjects were the most internally controlled, whereas a control group of college students scored highest in the external direction. In a longitudinal sample, the initially high degree of internality decreased during the 6 years of observation. Some writers emphasize the need for more domain-specific measures of perceived control. In aged subjects, beliefs concerning the maintenance of cognitive competencies were more external, and in younger subjects, more internal (Lachman, 1983). Regarding maintenance of health, elderly people also believed more often that it depended on the control of *powerful others*. This finding is not quoted as an argument for a critical assessment of the situation, although these powerful others, in relation to health risks, consist mainly of doctors with their readiness to come in case of extreme risk and helplessness.

Aside from a shift from generalized expectancies regarding internal versus external control, there is a tendency to focus on the elicitation of different beliefs in relation to different situational aspects. Krause (1987) measured perceived control and the amount of received social support in a sample of community aged. Those reporting more support scored more in the internal direction. This was true, however, only to one standard deviation above the mean level of emotional support (32.556). Further increases in emotional support are associated with decreased feelings of control ($b^x = -0.078$). At the highest observed value of emotional support, belief in a person's control decreased dramatically.

Another study of the same author (Krause, 1987b) hypothesized that persons with extreme values for external or internal control would be equally vulnerable to effects of high stress. This hypothesis was confirmed in a study of community aged. Extreme internality apparently causes self-blame in case of failure, whereas extreme externality can be linked with higher arousal as possibly negative events could not be managed. The whole emphasis in research on control beliefs apparently lacks information on the daily life of elderly people. Coping with partially predictable, but more frequently less predictable events requires flexibility in the belief system. Those with rigid beliefs in their own competence or those unable to master situations would be at risk in different ways. The translation of good cognitive theory into trait language and orientation blinds psychologists to the real challenges of daily life.

C. Beliefs in Possibility of Changing Life in Old Age

A belief system related to the possibility of depriving, unsatisfying conditions in old age became visible in the analyses of semistructured interviews administered in BOLSA. Contrary to beliefs in internal versus external control, this system is concerned with the chances of humankind or of society to improve certain conditions. No attributional processes are involved. An appraisal of the chance to improve conditions of life generally, and those of the reporting person especially, is at stake here.

Fisseni (1985) analyzed data from a 12-yr period and identified four patterns of consistency and change in this belief system. Consistency of this belief system was higher in persons with a more restricted and limited life space owing to low income, poor health, widowhood, etc.

Persons low in this belief were mainly men who had a better income, better subjective health status, stronger feelings of being needed by others, and better mood.

This is another example how cognitive systems develop in the context of well-defined social and physical conditions and their emotional and motivational concomitants. From some of the clusters analyzed by Fisseni, it became evident that this belief system functioned also as a matter of major concern, as a *theme* of thoughts and feelings. The close interaction between cognitions and emotions is the main challenge for cognitive theories of personality, especially in old age.

D. Personality and Adjustment to Aging

Problems in the life of the aged often are conceptualized as divergences from an optimal state of well-being, whether these divergences are caused by health problems, by loss of social roles, economic resources, or of significant others (Kuypers & Bengtson, 1974; Atchley, 1989). Therefore many sociogerontologic theories of aging try to answer the question about the best solution for adjustment to aging. Disengagement theory, activity theory, or continuity theory are examples of this. Another choice is a cognitive theory of adjustment to aging, which integrates findings on the impact of cognitions on emotions and behavior and those related to the influence of emotions and motivations on cognitions. We shall try to show the contribution of this theory in the context of three problem areas:

1. maintenance or reorganization of the self-concept;
2. adjustment to *daily hassles;* and
3. adjustment to dependency, bereavement, and other stresses.

1. Maintaining or Reorganizing the Self-Concept

Although research of the last decade does not support previous beliefs that *ageism* is the dominant attitude toward the aged in the United States as well in most other Western countries, (Crockett & Hummert, 1987; Lutsky, 1980; Neugarten, 1980), there still remains the problem of maintaining or restoring a continuity of the self-concept in a situation in which society assigns different roles and labels (Nuessel, 1982) to the aged. Atchley (1989) used many psychological arguments to defend his view of continuity in the aging person as the best strategy for successful aging. Erikson's (1950) concepts of identity and identity crisis were applied in this context in order to explain how old people can maintain or restore a concept (or a feeling?) of continuity in their own personality in the transition into the socially still rigidly defined status of an aged person. Many arguments of cognitive theories of personality were used by Atchley (1989), also, especially the principle that cognitive representations of a situation are more decisive than their objective qualities. As a matter of fact, who defines the objective quality of the self?

For trait theorists, the problems of maintaining or restoring continuity do not exist, as the structure of the self-concept remains invariant across age groups (McCrae, 1986). But apparently there are other findings, as Bengtson, Reedy, and Gordon (1985) summarized their review of research on the relationships between self-concept and aging, by stating that there is evidence for both stability and change in self-concept. The methodological problems involved in the assessment of self-concepts were stated very clearly by George and Okun (1985). Especially important is their emphasis on the supplementation of forced-choice techniques by open-ended instruments.

From data derived from semistructured interviews, Fisseni (1986) analyzed responses of aged persons mainly to perceived changes in themselves during the last year. Fisseni could identify two consistent patterns of self-concepts in terms of perceived change generally, and of perceived symptoms of the aging processes. One group reported less change and fewer age-related symptoms over several years; the second group, as the first one conceptualized by cluster-analyses, always reported more change and more symptoms of aging. The first group differed from the *high-change perceivers,* who also had mainly an old-age self-concept, with a higher degree of consistency of scores in cognitive tests, greater ego-control, more stability in mood, activity, and satisfaction in different social roles.

These different self-concepts and their correlates could be conceptualized from the longitudinal nature of the data as an outcome of a complex process of self-interpretation, in which were involved not only constructive actions and rational theory building (Epstein, 1973), but also feelings of satisfaction, dissatisfaction, frustration, or happiness.

2. Adjustment to Daily Hassles

Research on coping and stress attracted the attention of many scientists under the influence of the *critical-life-event* approach. Renner and Birren (1980) argued that events like death of a spouse or a friend, divorce, or loss of job are not frequent enough to instigate processes leading to disease. Lazarus and his co-workers introduced the construct of *daily hassles* as a more deleterious event type in the lives of elderly people. Lazarus' and Folkman's (1984) transactional theory of stress and coping assumes validity for both daily hassles and greater burdens and stresses.

His approach was consistent in emphasizing the role of cognitive appraisal of the situation in the whole transaction between the instigating situation and the person's reaction. After a period in which field research was more important (Lazarus, 1974), the group introduced trait-oriented methodology by developing the Ways-of-Coping Questionnaire.

On the basis of it, McCrae (1982, 1989) could show that immature and *emotional* responses decrease, and mature responses increase in the higher age groups.

By use of projective techniques and semistructured interviews, Shanan (1985) studied types of coping in the immigrants to Israel of the birth cohorts from 1902 to 1927. Shanan's theoretical orientation is determined by ego-psychology, trait theory, and

Lazarus' model. Using cluster analyses, he distinguished between different types of active and passive coping. A *modal* person from this point of view approaches problems in dangerous segments of the past as during the acculturation process and its hassles via high achievement orientation, high moral standards, high engagement in family life, and little complaint about losses and stresses. Following this group in the Jerusalem Study of Psychological Development (JESMA), Shanan (1985) found a slight drop in achievement motivation after 8 years, increased involvement in family life, and emphasis on consistency as a strategy of survival when Israel had to survive two wars.

Other types of coping with life in Israel were conceptualized as *active integrative coping, dependent passive coping, failing overcoping,* and *self-negating undercoping.* After 8 years, half of the active integrative copers stayed in the same group, almost one third of them, however, changed in the direction of dependent passive coping. Of the originally dependent passive copers, 60% preserved the same pattern, and 15% changed into the passive integrative way.

These findings reflect not only a unique historical period but also the different ways aged people adjust to different aspects of a new culture.

The findings from JESMA regarding a high prevalence of consistency and moderate degrees of change in dealing with problems in old age can be confirmed by those of BOLSA. This analysis is related to the period from 1965 to 1980, during which the political and economic situation in Western Germany had been stabilized considerably. From this point of view, even more consistency could be expected. The approach to the problem of providing information on dealing with problems in everyday life and with major burdens and stresses was similar to that of Shanan (1985) or Haan (1985), as far as the use of structured interviews is concerned. We structured the interview schedule in terms of typical problem areas of life in old age like problems in housing, income, health, family, and self. The analysis of the interview data was done by a classification system developed in studies on persons from adolescence to old age (Thomae, 1987a, 1987b, 1990). From the frequencies of well-defined response patterns in the *response hierarchies* (Thomae, 1987a) related to the problems of family, health, housing, and income, we conceptualized a General Psychological Adaptation System (Lehr & Thomae, 1991). This includes overt behaviors like achievement-related behavior, adjustment to institutional aspects of the situation, adjustment to characteristics and needs of others, and cultivating social contacts. The General Psychological Adaptation System includes covert also behaviors or cognitive appraisals and reappraisals, such as accepting the situation as it is or emphasizing positive aspects of the situation. Most of these response patterns rank higher in dealing with the problem areas. There are some divergences from this principle, however. For health problems, subjects from different cross-sectional and longitudinal samples very often adjusted to the institutional aspects of the situation by using the services proved by the German Health Care System, with obligatory health insurance, for most of the employees, free choice of a doctor, and biannual medical treatments in a spa.

The same response pattern was not applied regarding family problems, although the general structure of it, namely using the services of institutions, refers to family affairs, too. In all the aged people we interviewed in Germany, going to a child-guidance clinic to solve conflicts between a daughter and grandson, or attending a marriage counseling service, was no alternative because the social norm for these cohorts prescribed not involving any stranger in the affairs of the family.

It is not possible to outline the nature of all of these response classes. It should be mentioned that *accepting a situation as it is* does not refer to *passive behavior*. It is, in most cases, the outcome of efforts to make an unfavorable, but not controllable situation—like the divorce of a son—internally acceptable.

In dealing with the same problem area, aged persons showed a high degree of consistency up to age 85 and more, if their health enabled them to live independently. But even in cases of minor dependency, the main components of the General Psychological Adaptation System were preserved by emphasizing those coping devices that were functional in providing or maintaining social support, like adjustment to needs and habits of others or cultivating social contacts.

The comparison of response patterns of the same subjects in different problem areas is important because it can test, e.g., psychopathological opinions regarding a general decline of situation-specific response patterns in old age, like that formulated by Pfeiffer (1977). Social norms are effective in the avoidance of institutional adjustment for solving problems and conflict in the family, and the expected efficiency of some response classes can become a criterion. Prosocial behaviors like adjustment to the characteristics and needs of others or cultivating social contacts are helpful in dealing with problems within the family. Therefore they rank highest in this context from early adulthood into old-old age (Thomae, 1987b). Regarding health problems, they are evaluated as less valuable at least by community aged with health that enables them to enjoy a rather independent life. In poor health or dependency, these behaviors are ranked higher.

The situation-specific selection of response classes could be demonstrated especially by discussing the different status of more specific responses like hope, taking chances, revision of expectancies, or depressive reactions.

Depression ranked rather high in the BOLSA subjects during a period of 19 years in the problem areas of family and health, whereas depression was observed rather infrequently regarding housing or income problems. This difference certainly cannot be explained by reference to some coping strategy. The higher frequency of depressive states—in a non-psychiatric meaning of the term—in dealing with family and health problems is an expression of the central nature of these problems and the limitations of the aged person in coping with these problems. The whole process of dealing with problems of everyday life in any age group includes spontaneous emotional and affective reactions, rational thought, and efforts following trial and error.

All these reactions to challenging, frustrating, threatening, and sometimes boring situations are included in the term response, and all of them can be construed in a response hierarchy (Thomae, 1987a). Coping as a group of efforts to master the situation (Lazarus & Folkman, 1984) is part of this system. The choice between these different response classes is not always a matter of rational calculation as hypothesized by Lazarus (Laux & Weber, 1987). Responses similar to those expected can be elicited e.g., in neo-behavioristic models of behavior (Hull, 1952).

This unselected classification system is especially important for the understanding of processes involved in dealing with deprivation, disease, and dependency. This can be shown by an analysis of Kruse and Lehr (1989) of the longitudinal patterns in dealing with chronic disease. Seven years after the start of BOLSA, a clinical checkup of the survivors in the University Clinic for Internal Medicine showed that about one third of the originally rather healthy sample had at least one more or less serious diagnosis (cancer, heart attack, stroke, renal insufficiency, etc.). A comparison of these chronically ill women and men with control twins from the same study showed different *developmental trends* in responding to life stress. At the beginning, the group of later ill persons showed a preference for *accepting the situation as it is* and for avoidance of conflicts and tensions. In the following years—before the manifestation of the disease—they became more active in dealing with daily hassles of any kind.

After the manifestation of the illness, a high degree of planning for the future and a complete application of the General Psychological Adaptation System could be observed. They did not exhibit more depressive reactions than did the control group. Four to five years after the clinical checkup, the two groups differed in an opposite direction. Now the group of chronically ill persons was more active, engaged, busy in several extrafamilial roles, and more involved in family affairs than before. The formerly healthy group now responded more often by depressive and evasive reactions, as quite a few of them now had become chronically ill. The longitudinal analysis traces a developmental process that cannot be explained by reference to rational strategies.

3. Struggling with Major Crises and Threats

We shall review a small selection of studies related to coping with severe illness, with dependency as patient as well as caregiver, and to response patterns related to bereavement and death. The selection is from a theoretical point of view with an emphasis on a cognitive, but anticognitivistic theory of personality.

Coping behaviors are studied mainly in the context of health psychology (Rodin & Salovey, 1989). Problems and response patterns related to long-term care usually are the topic of research in applied social gerontology (Barusch, 1988). Any study of persons involved in these difficult and harmful situations can be justified only if it tries to improve the psychosocial situation in these stresses and crises.

On the other hand, research into the ways people deal with these major crises, burdens, or threats can contribute to theory building and testing as well as to applied sociogerontological research.

The association between major health problems and daily hassles was shown by Cohen (1990) in a longitudinal study of mentally ill elderly persons. *Little problems* can make life even more difficult for these women and men, and if they are *mounting* they can endanger the rehabilitation effect. Nerenz and Leventhal (1983) presented a theory of how individuals adapt to acute illness episodes emphasizing, among other topics, the phenomenon of *appraisal delay* in the initial illness episodes. They also trace other delay episodes in the illness process. Systematic research on response structures such as the General Psychological Adaptation System can point to the status of such behaviors and to similar behaviors in nonpatient populations. In a study on patterns of women coping with their partners' alcohol addiction, it was shown how many arguments and rationalizations can be produced by both partners of the couple before the right diagnosis has a chance to become accepted at least by the wife (Klasses, 1986).

Molleman, Pruyn, and Van Knippenberg (1986) report comparison processes in cancer patients that—according to the authors—bolster the patients in their feelings about their progress. The same kind of comparative reactions is mentioned in studies on other patient groups. A 55-year-old widow who was paralyzed by an accident and adjusted extremely well after years of struggle compared herself with blind or poor people. They could not see the pyramids, whereas, she could afford a trip and was physically able to see the structures.

From experiences like these, we would avoid the term bolstering, which according to Janis and Mann (1977) is a symptom of *hot cognitive processes* associated with wrong decision making and maladjustment. In the context of systematic and theoretically based research on response patterns, these comparative processes are (psychologically) good arguments in preparation for the acceptance of the situation, which belongs to the General Psychological Adaptation System.

In a study on the problems and response patterns of stroke patients who had been in home care at least 5 years, Kruse (1987) could trace a developmental process during this long time of dependency. In this process there grew—in the interaction with the care person or other persons—a personal view of the patient's situation, a *cognitive representation* of it, and in close connection with this view, a *personal response style*. By cluster analysis, the variety of these styles could be assigned to four clusters, ranging from tendencies to improve the external situation, to efforts to change the internal situation by cognitive restructuring, to clusters in which depressive or aggressive states prevailed.

The close relationship between specific clusters of the cognitive representation of the situation on the one hand, and specific response clusters on the other, could be used as argument by cognitivistic psychologists. The content of the cognitive representations directs the choice of the responses. But at the basis of these cognitive representations, there are different themes or *main concerns* like concern about survival as the basis for perceiving the situation as changeable. This perception elicits efforts to cooperate actively with the caregiver, which will result in this person's rewarding these efforts. The same association between a basic motivational unit (theme or concern), a cognitive system (the cognitive representation of the situation), and the selection of a specific response pattern was shown by Kruse (1986, 1987). This is one of the ways a cognitive, anticognitivistic theory of personality can be tested. Its application consists of the advice to change the perception of the situation by taking regard of some basic concerns. Rewarding or punishing isolated behaviors will not be effective in the long run.

The situation of caregivers has received attention (Brody, 1981). Using in-depth interviews, Barusch (1988) was able to identify problems of those caring for their spouses, which are similar to those described in other studies. Of the six coping strategies she identified, almost all were effective, but always for different types of problems. Most effective, according to this study, are caregivers who provide the whole repertoire of techniques.

In the study of Kruse (1987), the patient as well as the caregiver was interviewed. Achievement-related behaviors were dominant, but also a specific response class labeled

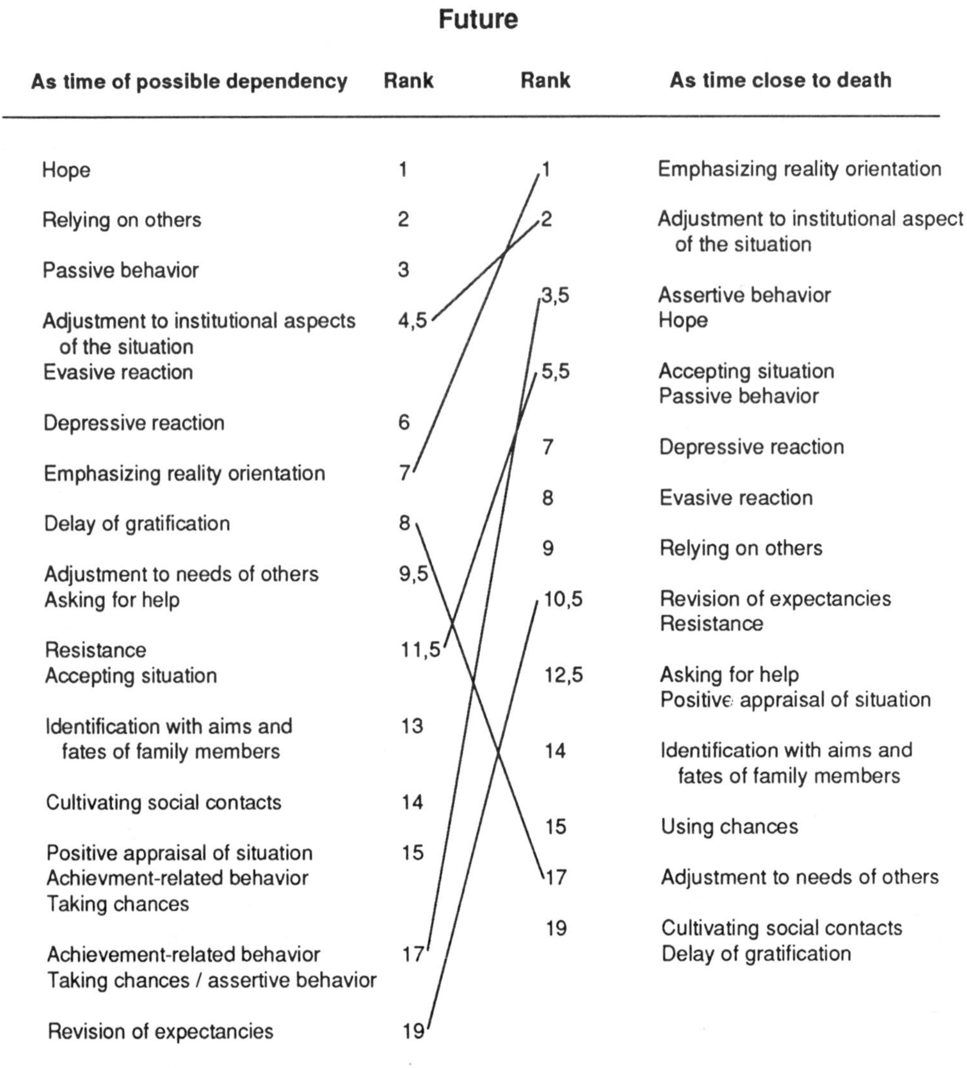

Future

As time of possible dependency	Rank	Rank	As time close to death
Hope	1	1	Emphasizing reality orientation
Relying on others	2	2	Adjustment to institutional aspect of the situation
Passive behavior	3		
Adjustment to institutional aspects of the situation	4,5	3,5	Assertive behavior Hope
Evasive reaction		5,5	Accepting situation Passive behavior
Depressive reaction	6		
Emphasizing reality orientation	7	7	Depressive reaction
Delay of gratification	8	8	Evasive reaction
Adjustment to needs of others	9,5	9	Relying on others
Asking for help		10,5	Revision of expectancies Resistance
Resistance	11,5		
Accepting situation		12,5	Asking for help Positive appraisal of situation
Identification with aims and fates of family members	13	14	Identification with aims and fates of family members
Cultivating social contacts	14		
Positive appraisal of situation	15	15	Using chances
Achievment-related behavior Taking chances		17	Adjustment to needs of others
Achievement-related behavior Taking chances / assertive behavior	17	19	Cultivating social contacts Delay of gratification
Revision of expectancies	19		

Figure 2 Response hierarchies of old-old BOLSA participants, related to two aspects of the future (from data of Schneider, 1989).

by us as *identification with the aims and fates of others*. This response pattern helps to motivate the caregiver and may change the perception of the situation for some time. Over a long duration, depressive reactions and revisions of expectancies were reported with increasing frequency. In some cases, this could lead to burn-out and, although not observed in this study, to elderly abuse. This sequence, however, is dependent on the history of the relationships between patient and caregiver. In a study on elderly daughters who care for their parents, conflicts from a remote past became acute again in complicated situations during the care process (Wand & Lehr, 1986).

As a final argument for the suggested interactionistic view of emotion–cognition relationships, some findings of studies on responses to anticipation of death will be mentioned briefly. Kalish (1985) found new evidence for previously stated hypotheses according to which death for the elderly is less frightening but more salient than for younger groups. In the study of Schneider (1989) on the future time perspective of old-old women and men, anticipation of dependency elicited more evasive and rationalizing responses than did anticipation of their own death (see Figure 2).

Two response classes were especially used for the construction of a mental wall against death anxiety. One of these consisted of an emphasis on reality orientation ("Of course, I know that everybody has to die. That's quite natural.") The other of these defensive responses (assertive behavior) was defined by an accumulation of arguments against any possible frightening effect of thoughts about death. Examples for this were responses like "As a soldier I faced death many times when I was young," or "I always obeyed the commands of God, so why should I care?" There were many variations of this technique of confirming oneself about competence in dealing with an unknown future. These techniques are mainly different ways to cognitively restructure the situation. The efficiency of these cognitive processes in maintaining or restoring at least some temporary emotional balance points to the decisive role of cognitions in the regulation of human behavior. On the other hand, there is evidence that the prevalence as well as the efficiency of these cognitive components of this behavior is dependent on the degree of emotional—affective arousal and the lifelong learning history of these and other responses. This history, however, includes experiences of reward and frustrations, of success and failure, of surprise and disappointment. Therefore this learning history is a continuous sequence of cognition–emotion interactions. The study of the aging and aged personality offers one of the most promising opportunities for the testing of hypotheses or models on cognition–emotion interactions as the basis of human adaptation.

III. Conclusions

Research on the problem of consistency and change of personality with increasing age made some decisive progress during the last decade. This is especially true regarding findings of high consistency in basic personality traits as found in longitudinal studies on healthy elderly people. At least of the same value are approaches to the study of the dynamics by which consistency in behavior and emotional states is preserved under changing social conditions as associated with aging.

The kinds of relationships between affect and emotion on the one hand and aging on the other need further clarification. Relationships between the content of cognitive systems like control beliefs or self-concept and affective–emotional changes should especially be studied in the context of the daily lives of elderly people.

References

Adams, D. L. (1971). Correlates of life satisfaction among the elderly. *The Gerontologist, 1.4* (Part II), 64–68.

Angleitner, A. (1987). Zur Konstanz und Veränderlichkeit von Rigidität im höheren Alter am Beispiel des

Riegelfragebogens. In U. Lehr & H. Thomae (Eds.), *Formen seelischen Alterns.* (pp. 115–212). Stuttgart, FRG: Enke.

Atchley, R. C. (1989). A continuity theory of normal aging. *The Gerontologist, 29,* 183–190.

Baltes, M. M., & Baltes, P. B. (Eds.) (1986). *The psychology of control and aging.* Hillsdale, NJ: Lawrence Erlbaum.

Barusch, A. S. (1988). Problems and coping strategies of elderly spouse caregivers. *The Gerontologist, 28,* 677–681.

Bengtson, V. L., Reedy, M. N., & Gordon, C. (1985). Aging and self-conceptions. In J. E. Birren & K. W. Schaie (Eds.), *Handbook of the psychology of aging* (2nd ed., pp. 544–593). New York: Van Nostrand Reinhold.

Birch, D., Atkinson, J. W., & Bongort, K. (1974). Cognitive control of action. In B. Weiner (Ed.), *Cognitive views on motivation* (pp. 85–90). New York: Academic Press.

Brody, E. (1981). The "woman in the middle" and family help to older people. *The Gerontologist, 21,* 471–480.

Busse, E. W., & Maddox, G. (Ed.) (1986). *The Duke Longitudinal studies on normal aging. 1955–1980.* New York: Springer.

Carson, R. C. (1989). Personality. *Annual Review of Psychology, 40,* 227–248.

Chappell, N. L., & Badger, M. (1989). Social isolation and well-being. *Journal of Gerontology, 44,* S169–176.

Cohen, G. (1990). Lessons from longitudinal studies of mentally ill and mentally healthy elderly: A 17-year prospective. In M. Bergener & S. Finkel (Eds.), *Clinical and scientific psychogeriatrics* (Vol. 1, pp. 135–148). New York: Springer.

Costa, P. T., Jr., & McCrae, R. R. (1984a). Concurrent validation after 20 years: The implications of personality stability for its assessment. In N. Shock, Greulich, R. C., P. T. Costa, Jr., R. Andres, E. G. Lakatta, D. Arenberg, & J. D. Tobin (Eds.), *Normal human aging. The Baltimore longitudinal study of aging* (pp. 105–128). NIH Publ. No 84-2450 Washington, DC: National Institutes of Health.

Costa, P. T., Jr., & McCrae, R. R. (1984b). Personality as a life-long determinant of well-being. In C. Z. Malatesta & C. E. Izard (Eds.), *Emotion in adult development* (pp. 141–157). Beverly Hills, CA: Sage.

Costa, P. T., Jr., McCrae, R. R., & Arenberg, D. (1984c). Enduring dispositions in adult males. In N. Shock, R. C. Greulich, P. T. Costa, Jr., R. Andres, E. G. Lakatta, D. Arenberg, & J. D. Tobin (Eds.), *Normal human aging. The Baltimore longitudinal study of aging.* (pp. 163–170) Publ. No. 84-12450. Washington, D.C.: National Institutes of Health.

Costa, P. T., Jr., McCrae, R. R., & Arenberg, D. (1983). Recent longitudinal research on personality and aging. In K. W. Schaie (Ed.) *Longitudinal studies of adult psychological development* (pp. 222–265). New York-London: The Guilford Press.

Costa, P. T., Jr., Zonderman, A. B., McCrae, R. R., Cornoni-Huntley, J., Locke, B. Z., & Barbano, H. E. (1987). Longitudinal analysis of psychological well-being in a national sample: Stability of mean levels. *Journal of Gerontology, 42,* 50–55.

Crockett, W. H., & Hummert, M. L. (1987). Perceptions of aging and the elderly. *Annual Review of Gerontology and Geriatrics, 7,* 217–242.

Cutler, S. J. (1979/80). Safety on the streets: Cohort changes in fear. *International Journal of Aging and Human Development, 10,* 373–384.

Diener, E. (1984). Psychological well-being. *Psychological Bulletin, 95,* 542–575.

Epstein, S. (1973). The self-concept revisited: Or a theory of a theory. *American Psychologist, 28,* 404–416.

Erikson, H. E. (1950). Growth and crises of the healthy personality. In M. Senn (Ed.), *Symposium on the healthy personality* (pp. 91–146). New York: J. Macey Foundation.

Fisseni, H. J. (1985). Perceived unchangeability of life and some biographical correlates. In M. J. A. Munnichs, P. Mussen, E. Olbrich, & P. Coleman (Eds.), *Life span and change in a gerontological perspective* (pp. 105–131). Orlando: Academic Press.

Fisseni, H. J. (1986). *Selbstinterpretation und Verhaltens-regulation.* Göttingen, FRG: Verlag für Psychologie Dr. Hogrefe.

Fooken, I. (1985). Old and female: psychosocial concomitants of the aging process in a group of older women. In J. M. A. Munnichs, P. Mussen, E. Olbrich, & P. Coleman (Eds.), *Life span and change in a gerontological perspective* (pp. 77–102). Orlando: Academic Press.

George, L. (1981). Subjective well-being. *Annual Review of Gerontology and Geriatrics, 2,* 346–382.

George, L., & Okun, M. A. (1985). Self-concept content. In E. Palmore, E. W. Busse, G. L. Maddox, J. B. Nowlin, & I. C. Siegler (Eds.), *Normal aging III* (pp. 267–287). Durham, NC: Duke University Press.

Haan, N. (1985). Common personality dimensions or common organisations across the life-span? In J. M. A. Munnichs, P. Mussen, E. Olbrich, & P. Coleman (Eds.), *Lifespan and change in a gerontological perspective* (pp. 17–44). Orlando: Academic Press.

Hull, C. L. (1952). *A behavior system*. New Haven, CT: Yale University Press.

Janis, I. L., & Mann, L. (1977). *Decision making*. New York: The Free Press.

Jones, H. E. (1958). Problems of method in longitudinal research. *Vita Humana, 1,* 93–99.

Jung, C. G. (1924). *Psychological types, or the psychology of individuation* (Trans. by H. G. Baynes). New York: Harcourt Brace Jovanovich.

Kalish, R. A. (1985). *Death, grief, and caring relationships* (2nd ed.). Monterey, CA: Brooks/Cole.

Kastenbaum, R. (1982). Time course and time perspective in later years. *Annual Review of Gerontology and Geriatrics, 3,* 80–101.

Kelly, G. A. (1955). *The psychology of personal constructs* Vol. 2 New York: Norton.

Klasses, I. (1986). *Coping of women with alcohol addiction of their partners.* Unpublished diploma thesis. Department of Psychology, University of Bonn.

Krause, N. (1987a). Understanding the stress process: Linking social support with locus of control beliefs. *Journal of Gerontology, 42,* 589–593.

Krause, N. (1987b). Life stress, social support, and self-esteem in an elderly population. *Psychology and Aging, 2,* 349–356.

Kruse, A. (1986). Strukturen des Erlebens und Verhaltens bei chronischer Erkrankung im Altrer. Bonn: Doctoral Dissertation, Univ. of Bonn. pp. 605

Kruse, A. (1987). Coping with chronic disease, dying, and death. A contribution to competence in old age. *Comprehensive Gerontology, 1,* 1–11.

Kruse, A., & Lehr, U. (1989). Longitudinal analysis of psychological development of chronically ill and healthy elderly. *International Psychogeriatrics, 1,* 73–87.

Kuhlen, G. A. (1956). Changing personal adjustment during the adult years. In J. E. Anderson (Ed.), *Psychological aspects of aging* (pp. 21–29). Washington, DC: American Psychological Association.

Kulys, R., & Tobin, S. S. (1980). Interpreting the lack of future concerns among the elderly. *International Journal of Aging and Human Development, 11,* 111–126.

Kuypers, J. A., & Bengtson, V. L. (1974). Social breakdown and competence: a model of normal aging. *Human Development, 16,* 181–201.

Lachman, M. E. (1983). Perceptions of intellectual aging: Antecedent or consequence of intellectual functioning? *Developmental Psychology, 19,* 482–498.

Laux, L., & Weber, H. (1987). Person-centered coping research. *European Journal of Personality Psychology, 1,* 193–214.

Lazarus, R. S. (1974). Cognitive and coping processes in emotion. In B. Weiner (Ed.), *Cognitive views on motivation* (pp. 21–32). New York: Academic Press.

Lazarus, R. S., & Folkman, S. (1984). *Stress, appraisal, and coping.* New York: Springer.

Lehr, U., & Thomae, H. (1991). *Alltagspsychologie.* Darmstadt, FRG: Wissenschaftliche Buchgesellschaft.

Leon, R., Gillum, B., Gillum, R., & Gonze, M. (1979). Personality stability over a thirty-year period—middle age to old age. *Journal of Consulting and Clinical Psychology, 23,* 245–259.

Lutsky, N. S. (1980). Attitudes toward old age and elderly persons. *Annual Review of Gerontology and Geriatrics, 1,* 287–336.

Magnusson, D. (1988). *Individual development from an interactional perspective.* Hillsdale, NJ: Lawrence Erlbaum.

Malatesta, C. Z., & Kalnok, M. (1984). Emotional experience in younger and older adults. *Journal of Gerontology, 39,* 301–308.

McCrae, R. R. (1982). Age differences in the use of coping mechanisms. *Journal of Gerontology, 37,* 454–460.

McCrae, R. R. (1986). Self-concept. In G. L. Maddox (Ed.), *Encyclopedia of aging* (pp. 590–91). New York: Springer.

McCrae, R. R. (1989). Age differences and changes in the use of coping mechanisms. *Journal of Gerontology, 44,* 161–169.

Molleman, E., Pruyn, J., van Knippenberg, A. (1986). Social comparison processes among cancer patients. *British Journal of Social Psychology, 1,* 1–13.

Mussen, P. (1985). Early adult antecedents of life satisfaction at age 70. In J. M. A. Munnichs, P. Mussen, E. Olbrich, & P. Coleman (Eds.), *Life span and change in gerontological perspective* (pp. 45–61). Orlando, FL: Academic Press.

Nerenz, D. R., & Leventhal, H. (1983). Self-regulation theory in chronic illness. In T. Burish & L. Bradley (Eds.), *Coping with chronic disease: Research and applications.* New York: Academic Press.

Neugarten, B. L. (1980). Acting one's age: New rules for old age. *Psychology Today, 4,* 66–80.

Nuessel, F. H. (1982). The language of age-ism. *The Gerontologist, 22,* 273–276.

Pfeiffer, E. (1977). Psychopathology and social pathology. In J. E. Birren & K. W. Schaie (Eds.), *Handbook of the psychology of aging* (pp. 650–671). New York: Van Nostrand Reinhold.

Podnieks, E. (1989). Elder abuse: A Canadian perspective. In R. S. Wolf & S. Bergman (Eds.), *Stress, conflict, and elder abuse* (pp. 111–140). Jerusalem: JDC-Brookdale Institute of Gerontology and Adult Development.

Reker, G. T., Peacock, E. J., & Wong, P. T. P. (1987). Meaning and purpose in life and well-being: A lifespan perspective. *Journal of Gerontology, 42,* 44–49.

Renner, V. J., & Birren, J. E. (1980). Stress: Physiological and psychological mechanisms. In J. E. Birren & B. Sloane (Eds.), *Handbook of mental health and aging* (pp. 310–336). Englewood Cliffs, NJ: Prentice-Hall.

Riegel, K. F., & Riegel, R. M. (1960). A study on changes of attitudes and interests during later years of life. *Viata Humana, 3,* 177–206.

Rodin, J., & Salovey, P. (1989). Health psychology. *Annual Review of Psychology, 40,* 533–580.

Rodin, J., Timko, C., & Harris, S. (1985). The construct of control: Biological and psychosocial correlates. *Annual Review of Gerontology and Geriatrics, 5,* 3–55.

Rotter, J. B. (1966). Generalized expectancies for internal vs. external control of reinforcement. *Psychological Monographs, 80* (Whole No. 609).

Rudinger, G., & Thomae, H. (1991). The Bonn longitudinal study: coping, life adjustment, and life satisfaction: In P. B. Baltes & M. M. Baltes (Eds.) *Successful aging: perspectives from the Behavioral Sciences* (pp. 265–295). New York: Cambridge University Press.

Schaie, K. W. (Ed.). (1983). *Longitudinal studies of adult psychological development.* New York: Guilford Press.

Schaie, K. W. (1986). Rigidity. In G. L. Maddox (Ed.), *Encyclopedia of aging* (p. 586). New York: Springer.

Schmitz-Scherzer, R., & Thomae, H. (1983). Constancy and change of behavior in old age: Findings from the Bonn Longitudinal Study on Aging. In K. W. Schaie (Ed.), *Longitudinal studies of adult psychological development* (pp. 191–221). New York: Guilford Press.

Schneider, W. (1989). *Zukunftsbezogene Zeitperspektive bei Hochbetagten* (Future time perspective in the old old) Regensburg, FRG: S. Roderer.

Schreiner, M. (1969). *Zur zukunftsbezogenen Zeitperspektive älterer Menschen.* Doctoral dissertation, University of Bonn, FRG.

Seligman, H. P. (1975). *Learned helplessness.* San Francisco: Freeman, Cooper.

Shanan, J. (1985). *Personality types and culture in later adulthood.* Basel–New York: Karger.

Shanan, J., & Jacobowitz, J. (1982). Personality and aging. *Annual Review of Gerontology and Geriatrics, 3,* 148–180.

Shifflett, P. A. (1987). Future time perspective, past experience, and negotiation of food patterns among the aged. *The Gerontologist, 27,* 611–615.

Siegler, I. C., George, L., & Okun, M. A. (1985). Cross-sequential analysis of adult personality. In E. Palmore, E. W. Busse, G. L. Maddox, J. B. Nowlin, & I. C. Siegler (Eds.), *Normal Aging III* (pp. 246–249). Durham NC: Duke University Press.

Siegler, I. C., & Gatz, M. (1985). Age patterns in locus of control. In E. Palmore, E. W. Busse, G. L. Maddox, J. B. Nowlin, & I. C. Siegler (Eds.), *Normal aging III* (pp. 259–266). Durham NC: Duke University Press.

Singer, J., & Kolligian, J., Jr. (1987). Personality: Developments in the study of private experience. *Annual Review of Psychology, 38,* 533–574.

Stappen, B. (1988). *Formen der Auseinandersetzung mit Verwitwung imhöhleren Alter.* Regensburg, FRG: Roderer.

Thomae, H. (1983). *Alternsstile und Altersschicksale*. Bern, Switzerland: Huber.

Thomae, H. (1987a). Conceptualizations of responses to stress. *European Journal of Personality Psychology, 1*, 171–192.

Thomae, H. (1987b). Responses to health and social problems in old age. In S. di Gregorio (Ed.), *Social gerontology: New directions* (pp. 161–176). London: Croom-Helm.

Thomae, H. (1990). Stress, satisfaction, competence: Findings from the Bonn Longitudinal Study of Aging. In M. Bergener & S. Finkel (Eds.), *Clinical and Scientific Psychogeriatrics* (Vol. 1, pp. 117–134). New York: Springer.

Vickio, C. J., & Cavanough, I. C. (1985). Relationships between death anxiety, attitudes toward aging, and experience with death in nursing home employees. *Journal of Gerontology, 40*, 347–349.

Wand, E., & Lehr, U. (1986). *Ältere Töchter alter Eltern*. Stuttgart, FRG: Kohlhammer.

Willits, F. K., & Crider, D. M. (1988). Health rating and life satisfaction in later years. *Journal of Gerontology, 43*, S172–176.

Psychopathology of Later Life

14

Mood Disorders and Suicide ___

Harold G. Koenig and Dan G. Blazer

I. Introduction
II. Classification and Clinical Presentation
    A. Continuous Classification
    B. Categorical Classification
    C. Late-Onset Depression
    D. Mania
III. Epidemiology
    A. Community
    B. Institutional
IV. Prognosis and Course
    A. Natural History
    B. All-Cause Mortality
V. Differential Diagnosis
    A. Dementia
    B. Physical Illness and Medications
    C. Other Psychiatric Disorders
VI. Laboratory Evaluation
    A. General Lab Tests
    B. Dexamethasone-Suppression Test
    C. Neuroradiological Studies
VII. Management
    A. General Measures
    B. Psychotherapy
    C. Pharmacotherapy
    D. Electroconvulsive Therapy
    E. Social and Family Therapies
VIII. Suicide
    A. Epidemiology
    B. Assessment of Risk Factors
    C. Management
    References

I. Introduction

Depression is a common syndrome that, along with the organic brain syndromes, is among the most prevalent of psychiatric disorders in late life and is undoubtedly the most treatable. Galen, in the second century, proclaimed an association between melancholia and aging, noting it to be most prevalent in old age (Jackson, 1969). Despite both ancient and popular opinion, however, depressive disorders with marked symptomatology are not more common among the elderly than among the young in today's society. This is surprising, given that elders appear to have many reasons to be depressed: declining physical health and functional status, death of friends and family, dwindling financial resources for some, and a decreased range of coping options. Nevertheless, recent epidemiological studies have demonstrated that major depressive disorder (MDD) is nearly four times more common in persons aged 18 to 44 than in those age 65 or older; bipolar disorder is 16 times more common among younger than older individuals (Weissman *et al.* 1988). While MDD and dysthymia are less common in later life, depressive symptoms and adjustment disorders are quite prevalent and understandably linked with social and health changes (Blazer, Hughes, & George, 1987). Even depressive syndromes with only minor symptoms may have significant clinical ramifications.

II. Classification and Clinical Presentation

A. Continuous Classification

Classification is particularly relevant to late-life depression because, while there is little difference in frequency of depressive symptoms across the life cycle, the prevalence of depressions with marked symptomatology is much lower in the elderly. The differences in the way investigators view mood disorders, then, is of substantial importance. Well-being, life-satisfaction, coping, and adjustment are terms frequently used to describe mental states by social scientists, and these are typically measured by subject report (self-completed or interview-administered surveys). If mood is construed in terms of a continuum or spectrum measured by the number of depressive symptoms, then the construct overlaps constructs of morale and life-satisfaction measured by frequency of responses indicating positive attitudes and enjoyment of life. This overlap is demonstrated by the high correlation between depression scales such as the Geriatric Depression Scale or Zung Depression Scale and the Philadelphia Geriatric Center Morale Scale, which are typically in the range of .75 to 0.80 (Koenig, 1989; Morris, Wolf, & Klerman, 1975). Alterations of mood and emotion in later life, regardless of terminology employed, are of great interest to mental health specialists and social scientists alike. The major difference in focus is a matter of severity of symptoms, with psychiatrists and psychologists more concerned with mood problems at the disabling end of the spectrum.

B. Categorical Classification

The current diagnostic classification in American psychiatry, DSM-III-R (Diagnostic and Statistical Manual, 3rd ed., rev.), provides different categories of depressive and manic states based on type and duration of symptom. A *major depressive episode* is diagnosed when a depressed mood or anhedonia has been present for at least 2 weeks and is associated with four of the following eight symptoms: significant weight loss or gain (> 5% of body weight), insomnia or hypersomnia, psychomotor agitation or retardation, fatigue or loss of energy, loss of interest, feelings of worthlessness or excessive guilt, decreased concentration, and recurrent suicidal ideation.

The *melancholic subtype* of major depression is present when at least five of the following nine symptoms are present: anhedonia (loss of interest or ability to experience pleasure), lack of reactivity to usually pleasurable stimuli, depression worse in morning, early morning awakening, psychomotor agitation or retardation, anorexia or weight loss, no significant personality disturbance, recovery from a previous major depressive episode, and good response to somatic antidepressant therapy. The validity of the melancholic subtype in the elderly has been demonstrated (Blazer, Bachar, & Hughes, 1987). When delusions or hallucinations complicate the clinical picture, then the diagnosis is *major depression with psychotic features* (mood congruent or incongruent). Meyers and colleagues found delusions to occur more commonly in late-life depressions (Meyers & Greenberg, 1986; Meyers, Kalayam, & Mei-Tal, 1984). It is estimated that 60% of women and 50% of men with their first major depressive episode after age 60 experience delusions (Charney & Nelson, 1981; Glassman & Roose, 1981; Meyers, Greenberg, & Mei-Tal, 1985). Delusions of nonexistence of the self or parts of the self, as well as those focused on the abdomen or gastrointestinal tract, may be particularly common in late life.

Chronic depressions lasting 2 years or longer, but not meeting criteria for major depression, are termed *dysthymic disorders* in DSM-III-R; these are further divided by age of onset, with the late variety beginning after age 21. The diagnosis of *adjustment disorder* with depressed mood is made when an identifiable psychosocial stressor has occurred within 3 months of onset of the depression, and either (1) there is impairment of functioning or (2) the symptoms are in excess of a normal or expectable reaction to the stressor. *Bereavement* is a normal expectable reaction to the death of a loved one. An *organic affective disorder* is the diagnosis made when evidence from the history, physical exam, or lab tests indicates a specific organic factor is responsible for the mood disturbance. When a depression is atypical or does not fit into any of the aforementioned categories, *depression not otherwise specified* is the diagnosis.

C. Late-Onset Depression

Late-onset MDD, a category not included in DSM-III-R, is defined as a major depressive episode that occurs for the first time in patients age 60 or older. There has been considerable debate over whether there are symptoms and signs that distinguish late-onset depression as a distinct mood syndrome separate from early-onset depression (Brown, Sweeney, Loutsch, Kocsis, & Frances, 1984; Mendlewicz & Baron, 1981; Meyers et al., 1984). The argument to do so centers around the clinical manifestations and the special role that biologic dysfunctions may have in the etiology of depression in late life (Alexopoulos, Young, Meyers, Abrams, & Shamoian, 1988; Meyers & Alexopoulos, 1988). Supporting this view are the correlations between late-onset depression and increased brain ventricular size, cortical atrophy, subcortical hyperintensity (Coffey, 1990; Jacoby & Levy,

1980), and a higher level of brain monoamine oxidase (MAO) activity (Alexopoulos *et al.*, 1988).

Unlike that with early-onset depression, a family history of affective disorder is less common in the late-onset variety (Baron, Mendlewicz, & Klotz, 1981; Brown *et al.*, 1984). This suggests that genetics plays a less vital role than do situational or illness-related biological factors. *Reactive* or *situational* depressions are reported to be frequent in later life, and depressive neuroses (chronic depressions with underlying personality disorder), less common (Verwoerdt, 1976). The psychological mechanism for depression may differ in late-onset and early-onset depression (Busse, Barnes, & Silverman, 1954). Rather than originating from the inward turning of hostile feelings toward the self (introjection), late-life depressions more often arise from a loss of self-esteem resulting from an inability to supply needs and fulfill drives owing to declining health, social, and financial resources with aging.

Brown and colleagues report a higher prevalence of hypochondriacal complaints, difficulty falling asleep at night, and agitation in depressed patients aged 50 or older (Brown *et al.*, 1984). De Alarcon (1964) also reported a higher prevalence of hypochondriacal symptoms in the elderly. Others have noted higher rates of lethargy (Gatz & Scott, 1972), agitation (Avery & Silverman, 1984), and lower rates of guilt (Winokur, Behan, & Schlesser, 1980). Decreased concentration and memory is a problem in elderly depressives, particularly those with more severe illness.

On the other hand, some investigators have not found a difference in symptoms in late-onset versus early-onset depressions. A recent study by Blazer *et al.*, (1987) in hospitalized depressives found that symptoms of depression, including those for melancholia, did not differ between older and younger patients. Others have noted that the clinical presentation of elderly depressives without central nervous system (CNS) dysfunction or medical illness is no different from that of younger depressives (Himmelhoch, Auchenbach, & Fuchs, 1982). The changes between early- and late-onset depression may be related to age of illness, rather than to the presence of two separate illnesses (Pichot & Pull, 1981; Rinieris, 1982). Hence, while there are data accumulating to support a distinct subtype of late-onset depression, this category is not yet firmly established.

D. Mania

At the other end of the mood-disorder spectrum is mania. A manic episode is defined as a distinct period of abnormally elevated or expansive mood (including irritability) associated with at least three of the following symptoms: grandiosity, decreased sleep, pressured speech, flight of ideas, distractibility, increased activity, and excessive involvement in pleasurable activities (DSM-III-R). When there has been a manic episode either alone or alternating with depressive episodes, the diagnosis of *bipolar disorder* is made. Less-severe mood swings that have lasted for 2 years or more are termed *cyclothymia*, and other states not meeting any of the criteria for a specific bipolar disorder are *bipolar disorder not otherwise specified.*

Bipolar disorder is less common in persons age 65 or older than in younger age groups. When bipolar disorder occurs in later life, the presentation may be atypical with a mixture of manic and dysphoric symptoms (Post, 1978; Spar, Ford, & Liston, 1979), with euphoria less common. Mania may be associated with significant changes in cognitive functioning, and the term manic delirium has been used to describe a state of altered consciousness that may be difficult to distinguish from organic conditions and schizophrenia (Shulman, 1986). Long-term followup of early-onset mania has shown that after a period of increasing episodes, there is a tendency for the disorder to burn out (Winokur, 1975). Likewise, Shulman and Post's (1980) study of elderly bipolars found only 8% of such cases had their first manic episode before age 40. Unfortunately, no long-term prospective studies of early-onset cases have been followed into old age.

There is some controversy over the differences in presentation and response to treatment of bipolar disorder in early and late life. While Glasser and Rabins (1984) reported few differences between early- and late-onset manics, a study by Young and Falk (1989) has found notable differences in presentation and treatment response. Increasing age was associated with less-intense levels of overactivity, sexual drive, and less-disturbed thought processes, differences similar to those found by Post (1982). Longer hospitalization, greater residual psychopathology, and a diminished response to pharmacotherapy were also associated with older age. Ameblas (1987) has reported a relationship between life events and the onset of a first manic episode; this association with life events is not so strong in later life, when *increased cerebral vulnerability* from stroke, head trauma, or other neurological disorders may be a more important factor (Shulman, 1989).

III. Epidemiology

A. Community

Kraeplin (1921) described melancholia as closely associated with the aging process. He noted that severe depressions in the elderly were similar to manic-depressive insanity and that such illness "demonstrates an almost continuous increase from the 20th to the 70th year." Recent surveys demonstrate that the prevalence of significant depressive *symptoms* in community-dwelling elderly populations has ranged from 11 to 44%, with an average of about 20% (Blazer, 1982). In contrast to Kraeplin's view, most studies today report that the elderly are generally more satisfied with their daily life than are younger persons, and cope with losses relatively well. Depressive symptoms, however, are still quite prevalent in later life, as demonstrated by the above rates.

The high rate of depressive symptoms contrasts with a relatively low rate for depressive disorders in later life. An explanation set forth for this seemingly contradictory finding is that the atypical presentation of depression in later life does not allow easy categorization into a specific disorder such as MDD. Using the Diagnostic Interview Schedule (DIS), the NIMH Epidemiologic Catchment Area (ECA) Survey has examined rates of depressive disorders in community-dwelling adults in five sites in the United States. The prevalence rate for all depressive disorders in persons aged 65 or older at the Piedmont, North Carolina site (N = 1304) was 27%; for MDD it was .8%; mixed depression and anxiety syndrome, 1.2%, dysthymia, 2%; symptomatic depression, 4%; and mild dysphoria, 19% (Blazer, Hughes, & George, 1987). MDD at the four other ECA sites in elderly participants ranged from .1 to .8% in men and .6 to 1.8% in women (Weissman *et al.,* 1988). In comparison, prevalence rates of MDD in persons aged 18–44 ranged from .7 to 2.7% in men and 3.1 to 6.1% in women. Sociodemographic and health correlates of depression among elders in the Piedmont survey were sex (female), educational status (low), marital status (unmarried), and socioeconomic status (low). Bipolar disorder was relatively rare among elders at all ECA sites, ranging from 0 to .4%, and contrast with rates of .8 to 2.1% in adults aged 18–44 (Weissman *et al.,* 1988).

B. Institutional

Rates of depression among institutionalized elderly in nursing homes and those hospitalized with medical illness far surpass rates in the community. A study of 958 older persons living in nursing homes and congregate housing reported a rate of 11.3% for major depression and 21.3% for minor depression using RDC criteria (Parmalee, Katz, & Lawton, 1987). Using onsite diagnoses by psychiatrists, a group from Johns Hopkins (Kafonek *et al.,* 1989) reported a lower prevalence of 21% for MDD, dysthymia, or adjustment disorder in a smaller population (N = 70) of nursing home patients.

Depressive disorders among the medically ill adults are particularly common. Schulberg and colleagues diagnosed MDD in 6.2% of adult medical outpatients (all ages) using the DIS (Schulberg, McClelland, & Gooding, 1987). Rates are even higher in medical inpatients with more severe illness and greater functional disability. In hospitalized men aged 65 or older, the prevalence of MDD ranges from 6 to 44% (Koenig, Meador, Cohen, & Blazer, 1988; Koenig *et al.,* 1991a; Rapp, Parisi, & Walsh, 1988; Kitchell, Barnes, Veith, Okimoto, & Raskind, 1982), averaging about 12% using the DIS. Simple dysphoria and adjustment disorders are present in an additional 18 to 26% of patients aged 65 or older (Koenig *et al.,* 1988; Koenig *et al.,* 1991a). Sociodemographic and health correlates of depression in this setting are young age (under 40), history of psychiatric problems, chronic respiratory illness, and severe medical illness or low functional status; a high level of social support and use of religion as a coping style are inversely related to depression (Koenig *et al.,* 1991a; Koenig *et al.,* 1991b). Much of the data on depressive disorders in medical inpatients comes from studies of hospitalized male veterans. Future studies are needed from community and private settings that also include women.

IV. Prognosis and Course

A. Natural History

The natural history of MDD is characterized by relapse and remission. Older persons are less likely than younger to have an episodic course, but more likely to have lengthy episodes and a high rate of chronicity (Angst *et al.,* 1973; Lundquist, 1945; MacDonald, 1918). The issue of whether the elderly are less likely than younger persons to recover completely from a depressive episode, however, is currently in dispute. In favor of this view are two British studies. Post (1972), following 92 depressed elders for 3 years, found that only 26% had a complete recovery from their index episode, 37% had further attacks with good recoveries, and 37% remained either continuously ill or experienced recurrent attacks on a baseline of chronic depression. Similarly, Murphy (1983) followed 124 depressed elders for 1 year and reported 35% with complete recovery, 19% with recovery but relapse, 29% continuously ill, 3% demented, and 14% dead. Prognosis was especially poor for those presenting with depressive delusions; only one in 10 such patients recovered. Based upon these studies, Millard (1983) was led to conclude that "no matter what is done, a third get better, a third stay the same, and a third get worse (p. 376)."

In contrast to the above studies, a more favorable prognosis for depressed elders in Great Britain was reported by Baldwin and Jolley (1986). Following up 100 psychiatric inpatients (mean age 74) with severe unipolar depression for 3 to 8 years, they found that after initial recovery, 60% remained well throughout or had further episodes followed by complete recovery, while only 7% suffered from continuous depression. Baldwin and Jolley concluded that "treatment with well established methods achieves worthwhile and sustained improvement for most patients" (p. 574), and that there was little basis for pessimism and nihilism in the treatment of depression in old age. Blazer and colleagues, in a North Carolina study, compared the outcome of MDD in middle-aged and elderly groups after 1 to 2 years of followup (Blazer, Fowler, & Hughes, 1987). Recovery from MDD determined by psychiatric evaluation was found in 27% of the elderly group compared with only 9% of the middle-aged group; however, residual symptoms (as indicated by a CES-D score of greater than 15) were more common in the elderly compared with middle-aged adults (59 versus 43%).

While much less is known about the natural history of depression in older adults hospitalized with medical illness, the prognosis in this group may be particularly poor. A short-term followup of 53 medically ill elders with major depressive disorder found that 31% had died after a mean followup time of 2 months; of those alive at psychiatric followup, 64% had persistent depression, 18% improved somewhat, and only 18% had completely recovered (Koenig et al., 1991c). Physical illness and impaired cognition have been noted by several other investigators as poor prognostic factors in late-life depression (Baldwin & Jolley, 1986; Ciompi, 1969; Cole, 1983; Murphy, Smith, Lindesay, & Slatter, 1988; Post, 1972).

Treatment with antidepressants has been shown to improve the long-term prognosis in the depressed elderly (Cole, 1985; Cook, Helms, Smith, & Tsai, 1986). Other factors associated with better outcome have been a family history of depression, absence of severe symptomatology, female sex, a history of recovery from prior attacks, extroverted personality, employment, not being in an institution, no substance or alcohol abuse, no prior history of other major psychiatric disorder, minimal life changes, and high levels of social support (Baldwin & Jolley, 1986; George, Blazer, & Hughes, 1989; Post, 1972). A followup study of 104 inpatients (half older than 60) found that those who perceived their social support to be adequate were over twice as likely to recover as those reporting inadequate support (George et al., 1989). This association persisted after controlling for baseline depressive symptoms, age, and sex.

B. All-Cause Mortality

The impact of depression on survival in later life is controversial. The mortality risk in older adults with depression would theoretically be high for a number of reasons—decreased immune response associated with both depression and advanced age, accidents, suicide, medication misuse, poor nutrition, and failure to seek prompt medical attention. In a 4-year followup of 120 depressed elders discharged from an inpatient psychiatric setting, Murphy and colleagues reported a significantly higher all-cause mortality in this group compared with a group of 197 age- and sex-matched controls (Murphy, Smith, Lindesay, & Slatter, 1988). Mortality rates were twice that expected for women and three times that expected for men. When stratifying the analysis by health status, however, the only group in which the difference in mortality remained significant was older men with health problems. In a 5-month followup study of 41 older medically ill hospitalized patients with MDD, inhospital mortality was significantly higher among depressed compared with nondepressed patients matched for age, sex, severity, and type of medical illness; however, there was no difference in mortality after hospital discharge (Koenig, Shelp, Goli, Cohen, & Blazer, 1989).

Five prospective studies have examined the relationship between depression and all-cause mortality in the community-dwelling elderly; four of these found a higher risk of mortality in depressed elders (Kay & Bergmann, 1966; Markush, Schwab, Farris, Present, & Holzer, 1977; Nielsen, Homma, & Biorn-Henriksen, 1977; Persson, 1981). Preliminary followup data on 1606 elderly patients involved in the NIMH ECA–Piedmont Health Survey revealed no increase in mortality for depressed patients after 2 years of followup regardless of sex, chronic disease, widowhood status, or age group (Fredman et al., 1989). Long-term survival data on this elderly cohort will be of considerable interest in the future.

V. Differential Diagnosis

A. Dementia

Intermittent depressive symptoms have been reported in up to 50% of demented patients (Ernst, Badash, Beran, Kosovsky, & Kleinhauz, 1977) and MDD in 20 to 30% of geriatric patients with Alzheimer's disease (Reifler, Larson, Teri, & Poulsen, 1986). Conversely, depression with cognitive impairment is common and particularly prevalent among the elderly (Wells, 1979). The relationship between depression and dementia makes distinction between these primary disorders difficult, and has given rise to the term pseudodementia to refer to patients with depression who have reversible cognitive impairment (Wells, 1979). Studies have shown that for both nondemented and demented depressed elderly, the treatment of the depression results in an improvement of cognitive impairment (Cohen, Weingartner, Smallberg, Pickar, & Murphy, 1982; Greenwald et al., 1989). Pseudodementia, however, is rare in later life; more common is dementia with concomitant depression (Blazer, 1989). Alexopoulos, Abrams, and Young (1987) followed up a group of elderly depressives with initially reversible cognitive impairment; many developed irreversible dementia in 2 to 4 years. There is currently a debate concerning whether cognitive dysfunction is a result of affective symptoms (i.e., impaired motivation–effort), whether it exists independent of affective symptoms as an intrinsic part of the depressive disorder itself, or whether a subclinical dementing disorder may predispose such patients to cognitive dysfunction during depression (Alexopoulos, 1989).

Despite the difficulties noted above, certain clinical features of pseudodementia may help in its recognition and separation from irreversible dementia. In depression, the onset of cognitive impairment is usually rapid and of short duration. Depressed mood is typically prominent, and patients will emphasize and complain about cognitive dysfunction rather than conceal or disguise it. Cognitive performance may fluctuate over time as depressive symptoms wax and wane, while a more constant disability is expected in dementia. While demented depressed patients treated with antidepressants may have some improvement in mentation, cognitive function typically remains in the demented range (Greenwald et al., 1989) and the reversal of affective symptoms is more prominent (Reifler et al., 1989).

The association between depression and cognitive impairment is not so notable in elderly medical inpatients as in elderly psychiatric inpatients; the former often have a significant level of cognitive dysfunction with the prevalence of delirium at about 20% (Cavanaugh & Wettstein, 1983; Koenig et al., 1991a; Rapp et al., 1988). The reason for the weaker association is not clear. It does, however, underscore the fact that one should not assume that cognitive dysfunction in depressed medical inpatients is due to their depression, but rather pursue medical evaluation to rule out reversible organic factors.

B. Physical Illness and Medication

It is important to make the distinction between (1) depression of a psychosocial nature secondary to medical illness (reactive or situational depression), (2) depression that presents with physical symptoms (masked depression), and (3) depression resulting from physiological or biological derangements induced by physical illness or drugs (organic mood syndrome). First, and most common, depression may be a psychological reaction to the disability and discomfort associated with severe medical illness. In this instance, the clinical diagnosis of depression depends heavily on the *psychological* symptoms of depression, such as feelings of worthlessness, decreased social interest, withdrawal or decreased talkativeness, crying, guilt, brooding or self-pity, pessimism, and suicidal ideation, or loss of the will to live (Endicott, 1984). Understandably, less emphasis is placed on appetite, sleep, cognitive function, energy level, and psychomotor changes.

In masked depression, the elderly person with depression will complain of multiple somatic complaints such as difficulty sleeping, loss of energy, loss of appetite, while completely denying a depressed mood. In an elderly population with a high prevalence of chronic often undetected physical illness, this is the most difficult depression to diagnose. It can be entertained only after a comprehensive medical evaluation and longitudinal followup reveals no organic cause for the symptoms.

Finally, organic mood disorder is an affective syndrome resulting from physiological or metabolic changes in the body, induced by disease or drugs. Here, an undiagnosed or untreated physical illness causes loss of energy, decreased appetite or weight loss, cognitive changes, psychomotor retardation, and may also cause psychological symptoms such as depressed mood, loss of interest, and even suicidal ideation in an agitated, delirious patient. This mood disorder is notable in that correction of the underlying illness or removal of the offending drug results in a complete reversal of depressive symptomatology. Sometimes, however, the underlying illness cannot be corrected, as in stroke, other neurological disorders, invasive cancer, or end-stage heart, lung, or renal disease. Biological treatments for depression may be helpful in such cases, although data supporting efficacy is quite limited (see Management).

A close association between depression and severity of physical illness or disability in medical inpatients has been reported by many investigators (Koenig et al., 1988; Moffic & Paykel, 1975; Rapp et al., 1988; Schwab, Bialow, Brown, & Holzer, 1967; Stewart, Drake, & Winokur, 1965; Yang, Zuo, Su, & Eaton, 1987). There is some data to suggest that this relationship may be particularly strong in older rather than younger inpatients (Koenig et al., 1991a). An association between depression and a number of specific medical disorders has been reported. These include Parkinson's disease (Mayeux et al., 1986), Huntington's disease (Folstein, Abbott, Chase, Jensen, & Folstein, 1983), pancreatic cancer (Holland et al., 1986; Pomara & Gershon, 1984), stroke (Robinson, Lipsey, & Price, 1985), multiple sclerosis (Joffe, Lippert, Gray, Sawa, & Horvath, 1987), acquired immunodeficiency syndrome (AIDS) (Holland & Tross, 1985), Cushing's disease (Haskett, 1985), postmyocardial infarction (Schleifer et al., 1989), and epilepsy (Mendez, Cummings, & Benson, 1986).

While much has been written about depression and specific medical disorders, many of these studies either did not control for level of functional disability or did not have control groups of patients with other medical illnesses. Those studies that have included a spectrum of chronic disorders and/or controlled for severity of illness have generally not found patients with any specific disorder to be particularly vulnerable to depression (Kitchell et al., 1982; Cassileth et al., 1984; Koenig et al., 1990; Moffic & Paykel, 1975; Schwab et al., 1967; Stewart et al., 1965; Yang et al., 1987). Rather than specific diagnosis, it is the level of functional disability and impairment of life activities that seem to be the crucial factors. This probably holds true for poststroke depression as well, where investigators have not yet clearly and consistently shown that organic brain changes, rather than the psychosocial reaction to functional disability, underlie the depression that is seen (Koenig & Studenski, 1988).

C. Other Psychiatric Disorders

Late-life schizophrenic disorder, when it presents for the first time with paranoid ideation and delusions may be confused with MDD with psychotic features, particularly since depression with delusions is especially common in later life. Nearly 10% of admissions to psychiatric hospitals for patients older than 60 are for late-life psychoses. Late-onset schizophrenia, however, usually presents with less depressive affect, evolves more insidiously, involves bizarre paranoid behaviors and complaints such as covering over or barring windows, placing elaborate locks on doors, or making other unusual preparations to ward off imagined pursuers.

Anxiety is frequently associated with depression, and the differentiation of depression from primary anxiety syndromes such as generalized anxiety disorder or adjustment disorder with anxious mood can be challenging. Blazer, Hughes, and Fowler (1989) found the presence of early-morning anxiety as a symptom in nearly a third of elderly and middle-aged patients 1 to 2 years after hospitalization for depression; nearly two thirds of these patients also had anxiety at other times during the day. Anxiety disorders are common among older persons with medical illness, particularly cancer (Derogatis *et al.*, 1983). Primary anxiety syndromes can generally be distinguished from depression in having less depressed mood and more symptoms of motor tension (such as shakiness, restlessness), autonomic hyperactivity (palpitations, dizziness), feelings of fear, apprehension or worry, and irritability or hypervigilance.

Chronic pain and depression often coexist, and they may be difficult to distinguish (Krishnan *et al.*, 1985). Furthermore, there is an overlap in biological markers for both chronic pain and depression. There is some evidence that the dexamethasone-suppression test (DST) may be helpful in separating these two entities (France, Krishnan, Houpt, & Maltbie, 1984), although further study is clearly needed. Because many elderly persons who have severe arthritis, chronic gastrointestinal problems, or advanced malignancies are often disabled with chronic pain, a diagnosis of depressive disorder in this group can be challenging. Fortunately, antidepressants may be quite effective in symptom relief for both disorders.

Hypochondriasis and other somatization disorders are not uncommon in later life, and may confound the diagnosis of depression (De Alarcon, 1964). Hypochondriasis is defined as excessive concern about disease, an unreasonable preoccupation with one's health, or unrealistic interpretation of physical sensations as indicative of a serious disease, when in fact there is no underlying medical illness present. De Alarcon, in a study of 152 patients with depression, noted that over 60% of both men and women reported hypochondriacal complaints, mostly centered around the gastrointestinal system. Hypochondriasis as a distinct disorder can be distinguished from depression by the duration of symptoms (usually present for many years) and the general lack of exacerbations and remissions that characterize depressive illness. Response to antidepressants may be another distinguishing factor; elderly with hypochondriasis tolerate the side-effects of these drugs poorly, whereas those with depression tolerate them better because of the relief from suffering that they afford (Blazer, 1984).

Sleep disorders may often be accompanied by depressive symptoms. Sleep-phase syndromes result from a shift in the hours of usual sleep either forward or backward. Elders may feel tired in the early evening and thus retire to bed at 8 PM, to find themselves waking up at 2 AM and unable to go back to sleep. On the other hand, they may have difficulty falling asleep at night, lying awake well after midnight, only to have great difficulty getting up at their usual waking time. Sleep apnea is another problem that may disturb sleep for the elderly with chronic lung disease, decreased oropharyngeal muscle tone, or extreme obesity. Periodic obstruction to airflow can result in deoxygenation of the blood and multiple "mini" awakenings throughout the night, which impair normal sleep and result in fatigue and disinterest during the day.

Alcoholism, while less prevalent in later than in earlier life, is nonetheless a frequent problem in the aged (3–10%) (Myers *et al.,* 1984; Adams *et al.,* 1990). Alcohol abuse can mimic depression by causing chronic fatigue, weight loss, disturbed sleep pattern, cognitive changes, and is a risk factor for suicide. Heavy alcohol use may disrupt families, social-support networks, occupation, and lead to financial ruin—factors that may contribute to the onset of depression in later life. Furthermore, depressed elders may self-medicate themselves with alcohol in attempts to alleviate their suffering. The diagnosis of depression in patients with alcohol abuse should be withheld until a 2-week period of sobriety has elapsed, since withdrawal symptoms often include dysphoria and other depressive symptomatology.

VI. Laboratory Evaluation

A. General Lab Tests

The laboratory workup of elderly adults with mood disorders should include a chemistry panel, serum test for syphilis, serum B_{12}, sedimentation rate, thyroid profile, complete blood count, urine analysis, human immunodeficiency virus (HIV) antibody (in persons receiving blood from 1977 to 1983), arterial blood gases (when hypoxia is likely), electrocardiogram, and chest x-ray. Metabolic disturbances from electrolyte abnormalities, or renal or liver dysfunction may cause or contribute to depression. A TSH along with a T_4 and T_3 uptake is helpful in ruling out hypothyroidism; TSH values above 10 are particularly significant. The presentation of thyroid disorder in later life may differ from that at younger ages; hence, hyperthyroidism may present with symptoms of decreased energy and disinterest (apathetic hyperthyroidism). Vitamin deficiencies (B_{12}) present with depression as well as dementia. Psychological testing may help distinguish depression from dementia, but usually adds little to the diagnostic workup in the presence of clear-cut depression.

B. Dexamethasone-Suppression Test

Carroll introduced the Dexamethasone-Suppression Test (DST) in 1981 to assist in the diagnosis of depression. This test is based on the hyperactivity of the hypothalamic–pituitary–adrenal (HPA) axis known to occur in severe depression. It is particularly useful for detecting biologically driven depression such as MDD with melancholia; however, the present view is that the DST is *not* specific to MDD, but is more likely to be increased in MDD than in other psychiatric illnesses. The test is performed by administering a 1 mg dose of dexamethasone at 11 PM and taking samples of serum cortisol at 11 AM and 4 PM the following day. A positive test occurs when either of the serum cortisols exceed 5 μm/ml. A false positive test may occur with various physical illnesses (particularly infectious diseases), certain medications, weight loss, and psychiatric disorders other than depression.

Unfortunately, nondepressed elderly persons may be particularly susceptible to HPA axis abnormalities. Rosenbaum (1984) found a higher prevalence of positive DSTs in adults aged 65 or older compared with those under age 65 (18 versus 9%), suggesting that the DST may be less specific in the elderly, especially after age 75. On the other hand, Magni and coworkers reported a sensitivity of 78% for the DST in depressed elderly medical inpatients (Magni *et al.*, 1986), and others have found it useful in distinguishing depressed from nondepressed elders in the early stages of Alzheimer's disease (Jenike & Albert, 1984). While useful from a research perspective, the DST is not currently being advocated for clinical screening of older adults for depression.

C. Neuroradiological Studies

Imaging studies such as computed tomography (CT) and magnetic resonance imaging (MRI) are being investigated for their usefulness in detecting structural brain changes in late-life depression. Using CT, investigators have found greater enlargement of the lateral ventricles in geriatric patients with late-onset depression compared to those in elders with the early-onset variety or nondepressed controls (Dolan, Calloway, & Mann, 1985; Jacoby, Dolan, Levy, & Baldy, 1983; Jacoby & Levy, 1980; Yates, Jacoby, & Andreasen, 1987). In retrospective studies using both CT and MRI, a high prevalence of structural brain abnormalities were found in elderly depressed patients referred for ECT (Coffey *et al.*, 1987; Coffey *et al.*, 1988a; Coffey *et al.*, 1988b).

In a prospective study using high-field-strength MRI, Coffey (1991) and colleagues have now confirmed a significantly higher prevalence of cortical atrophy, lateral ventricular enlargement, and subcortical hyperintensity in depressed elders compared with nondepressed controls. These findings persisted even after excluding patients with known neurological disease from the sample. In ongoing studies by this group, quantitative volume determinations of different brain structures in depressed and nondepressed elderly is now being performed. Preliminary data suggest that total frontal lobe volume is significantly smaller in elders with late-onset depression (excluding those with a history of neurological disease); no difference, however, has been found in other parts of the brain such as the temporal lobes (Coffey, 1991). These findings suggest that atrophy may be relatively specific for the frontal lobes in depressed elders, and the hypothesis has been generated that diffuse cortical and subcortical lesions are etiologically related to late-onset depression by disrupting neurotransmitter pathways that course through these areas (neurochemical disconnection syndrome).

VII. Management

A. General Measures

Because of the greater likelihood that mood disorders in later life will be accompanied by physical illness, the diagnostic evaluation should be thorough and comprehensive. Of foremost importance are a complete physical examination with particular emphasis on neurological systems, a review of the patient's current medication, and a comprehensive laboratory workup (as above). Once a diagnosis has been made, treatment typically includes one or more of the following: psychotherapy, pharmacotherapy, electrocon-vulsive therapy, and family–social therapies, apart from treatment of any associated physical illness.

B. Psychotherapy

Because of underlying chronic illness and concomitant medical treatments, older adults are often less tolerant than younger persons to the side-effects of biological therapies (Strauss & Solomon, 1983). In some cases psychotherapy may be called on to supplement or replace biological interventions, especially in the frail elderly. A wide variety of psychotherapies is available to the clinician for use in elderly depressed patients; only a few, however, have proven efficacy in late-life depression. Insight-oriented and psycho-analytic psychotherapy have not been studied systematically with depressed elders. Thus, the focus of this section will be on cognitive, behavioral, and time-limited dynamic therapies whose efficacy has been evaluated in elderly samples.

1. Cognitive, Behavioral, Brief Psychodynamic Therapies

Cognitive therapy (CT) is a psychological treatment designed to train patients to identify and correct the negative thinking in depression that has been hypothesized to contribute to its maintenance (Beck, Rush, & Shaw, 1979). *Behavioral therapy* (BT) involves positive reinforcement for those behaviors that are depression alleviating (increased social or occupational activity) and/or negative reinforcement for behaviors that are depression inducing (withdrawal, etc.) (Gallagher & Thompson, 1981; Lewinsohn, 1974). BT may include a weekly activity schedule, mastery and pleasure logs, and assignments that are graded by the therapist. *Brief dynamic therapy* (BDT) stresses the importance of the patient–therapist relationship, emphasizing realistic collaborative aspects of the therapeu-tic or working alliance, while de-emphasizing manipulation of the transference (Horowitz & Kaltreider, 1979).

Thompson, Gallagher, and Breckenridge (1987) treated 91 elders with major depres-sion using 16 to 20 sessions of CT, BT, or BDT, while assigning an additional 20 patients to a control group. Overall, 52% of treated patients were in full remission and 18% showed significant improvement at the end of 6 weeks. All therapies were equally effec-tive and superior to the control group, thus supporting the efficacy of short-term psycho-therapy in the treatment of MDD in elderly patients. These results were consistent with earlier work by the same investigators (Gallagher & Thompson, 1982) and others as well (Steuer *et al.*, 1984).

For depressed elders, the cognitive–behavioral approach is optimal because it is time-limited and directive. Typically only 15 to 20 sessions are required for good results. Depressed patients often overgeneralize, catastrophize, and think in terms of extremes. After a while, this negative thinking convinces patients that they are inadequate and ineffective, and dissipates all hope that their situation will ever improve. Cognitive restructuring and assigned tasks with reinforcement help to break this vicious cycle of depressive thinking and behavior.

2. Supportive Therapy

Elderly patients with minor depressions, such as adjustment disorder or dysphoria appropriate to the situation, require less-intensive psychotherapy. Supportive care alone is often sufficient to assist elders to adapt to minor losses or stressors. Often a concerned primary care physician, nurse, or social worker may provide such care. Because of the important role that religion plays in the lives of many older adults (Koenig, Smiley, & Gonzales, 1988), one readily available source of counseling and encouragement may be the clergy.

C. Pharmacotherapy

Antidepressants available for treatment of MDE may be subdivided into several classes. These include the older tricyclics (divided into tertiary and secondary amines), second-generation antidepressants, MAO inhibitors, mood-stabilizing drugs such as lithium or tegretol, and psychostimulants. Among older tricyclics are the tertiary amines amitriptyline, imipramine, trimipramine, and doxepin, and the secondary amines desipramine, nortriptyline, and protriptyline. The newer second-generation antidepressants include maprotiline, amoxapine, trazodone, fluoxetine and bupropion. Traditional MAO inhibitors such as phenelzine, isocarboxazid, tranylcypromine and pargyline, are inhibitors of both MAO-A and MAO-B isoenzymes. Newer agents include those that specifically inhibit MAO-A (clorgyline) or MAO-B (deprenyl).

1. Cyclic Antidepressants

A recent review noted that there were only 16 controlled studies of cyclic antidepressants in the past 15 years that dealt specifically with their use in the elderly (Rockwell, Lam, & Zisook, 1988). Most of the studies compared second-generation antidepressants with tricyclic antidepressants or placebo. In the majority of these studies, response rate was similar to those obtained with younger samples (i.e., 50 to 80%). Trazadone was found to be as effective as amytriptyline (Ather, Ankier, & Middleton, 1985) and imipramine (Gerner, Estabrook, Steuer, & Jarvik, 1980). Maprotiline was as effective as imipramine (Middleton, 1975) and superior to doxepin (Gwirtsman, Ahles, Halaris, DeMet, & Hill, 1983). Five studies examined nomifensine (recently taken off the market owing to hemolytic anemia), finding it as efficacious as amitriptyline and imipramine. Fluoxetine, a specific serotonin reuptake inhibitor, was compared with doxepin and placebo in a sample of 157 elderly outpatients, although only half of patients on either drug or placebo completed the trial; fluoxetine had fewer side-effects while being equally effective (Feighner & Cohn, 1985). Eight other studies examined drugs not yet available in United States, such as mianserin, fluvoxamine, and viloxazine, and again found them as effective as the older tricyclic antidepressants. Side-effects of antidepressants in these studies were not a limiting factor in treatment; however, elderly patients chosen for such clinical trials are typically free of major medical illnesses.

Secondary amines such as nortriptyline and desipramine are currently the agents of first choice for melancholic depression. Because of their anticholinergic, sedative, and hypotensive side-effects, tertiary amines should be avoided. Most concerning in elderly patients are orthostasis and anticholinergic side-effects, with the latter causing or worsening constipation or bladder-outlet obstruction. Drug-induced delirium is a particular problem in elderly patients (Davies, Tucker, Harrow, & Detre, 1971) and in those with CNS disease (Fullerton, 1984). The dose for nortriptyline should start at 10 to 25 mg/day and then increase gradually to 75 to 100 mg/day over several weeks. Some elders respond to as little as 25 to 50 mg/day. Drug levels are a helpful guide to therapy when compliance is questionable or side-effects appear. A therapeutic window exists for nortriptyline between 50 and 150 ng/ml and a response to desipramine is usually not seen until a level of at least 125 ng/ml is reached; however, the relevance of these levels in the elderly has not been established.

Trazadone is an alternative drug if side-effects to the secondary amines are intolerable; daytime sedation and occasional priapism, however, may cause problems. Fluoxetine and bupropion are virtually void of anticholinergic or sedative side-effects; however, gastrointestinal effects such as nausea and stomach fullness, sleep disturbances, and agitation have been quite distressing for some elderly patients on these drugs. In treating older patients with fluoxetine, the dose should begin at 5 to 20 mg (given in the morning) and should probably not exceed 40 mg/day. An advantage of the newer second-generation antidepressants is that the risk of toxicity from overdose is lower than in older tricyclics (Beaumont, 1989).

Elderly patients with Alzheimer's disease and MDD should probably be treated with antidepressants, although data on efficacy from double-blind, controlled studies is controversial (Greenwald et al., 1989; Reifler et al., 1989). While antidepressant efficacy has been established in the physical healthy elderly, it is not yet proven in frail medically ill hospitalized patients (Koenig et al., 1989; Koenig & Breitner, 1990). Interactions with physical illnesses and the drugs used to treat them increase the risk of side-effects in this population. When depression is detected in hospitalized seriously ill elders, the primary care physician's first impulse may be to start antidepressants; however, this decision should be made cautiously with the help of psychiatric consultation and sometimes only after nonpharmacologic therapies have been tried unsuccessfully.

2. MAO Inhibitors

MAO inhibitors are another alternative to cyclic antidepressants, particularly in atypical depression. One study in depressed elders has shown a clear superiority of an MAO inhibitor over a tricyclic for maintenance therapy (Georgotas, McCue, & Cooper, 1989); they report 13% recurrences with phenelzine, 54% with nortriptyline, and 65% with placebo over 1 year of followup. Elders, however, do not usually tolerate MAO inhibitors any better than tricyclic antidepressants. In cases of severe depression where electroconvulsive therapy (ECT) is a consideration, a 10- to 14-day period must elapse between discontinuation of an MAO inhibitor and the institution of ECT, making emergent therapy difficult. Furthermore, dietary restrictions and potential interactions with other medications make MAO inhibitor use less preferable in the elderly. The newer specific MAO-A and MAO-B inhibitors (clorgyline and deprenyl) have not been shown to have a therapeutic advantage over traditional mixed MAO inhibitors in depression.

3. Mood Stabilizers

Mood stabilizers such as lithium and tegretol help to dampen or prevent relapses in bipolar disorder and occasionally in unipolar depression. Age differences in pharmacokinetics with regard to brain sensitivity and elimination half-life must be considered when using these drugs in the elderly (Hardy, Shulman, MacKenzie, Kutcher, & Silverberg, 1987). Elderly patients may not respond as vigorously or as quickly to lithium as do younger patients (Young & Falk, 1989). Because these drugs have little immediate impact on symptoms, elderly bipolar patients in an acute depressive or manic episode may require supplemental therapy with either a cyclic antidepressant or an antipsychotic. In refractory cases of unipolar depression, in which cyclic antidepressants and ECT are ineffective, augmentation with lithium may be attempted. A small retrospective study by Finch and Katona (1989), found that lithium augmentation was successful in six of nine refractory depressions; followup over 3 to 20 months demonstrated that this regimen was relatively well tolerated in older patients.

4. Psychostimulants and Benzodiazepines

Psychostimulants, prescribed in low doses (methylphenidate 5 mg each morning), may be helpful and generally safe in some elders with retarded depression or coexisting major medical illness (Askinazi, Weintraub, & Karamouz, 1986; Kaplitz, 1975; Katon & Raskind, 1980; Woods, Tesar, Murray, & Cassem, 1986). Data on efficacy in the elderly from prospective, double-blind, controlled studies, however, are lacking.

Most clinicians prefer to avoid benzodiazepines when treating depression in the elderly. Reasons given for this reluctance are the need for increasing doses to maintain therapeutic effect, problems with drug withdrawal (alprazolam), effects on respiration, and excessive sedation (Miller & Whitcup, 1986). Because of their relative lack of other side-effects, however, benzodiazepines would appear to be a consideration in some highly anxious, depressed elders who have medical contraindications to antidepressants or ECT. One prospective, randomized, double-blind, 8-week comparison study of diazepam and a tricyclic in atypical depression found them to be equally efficacious; diazepam, however, had a more rapid onset of effect (Tiller, Schweitzer, Maguire, & Davies, 1989). Further studies comparing benzodiazepines and antidepressants are needed in the elderly, especially those in whom physical illness complicates the use of traditional antidepressants.

D. Electroconvulsive Therapy

There are few epidemiological data on the prevalence of ECT use in the elderly; however, one study from California found that 37% of all patients receiving ECT were aged 65 or older (Kramer, 1985). Early studies of ECT suggested that the elderly respond better than younger patients (Kalinowsky & Hoch, 1946), and later work has supported this observation (Carney & Sheffield, 1974; Coryell & Zimmerman, 1984; Mendels, 1965). Greenblatt and colleagues compared ECT to phenelzine and imipramine in patients with depression and an assortment of other psychiatric disorders; the largest difference in efficacy (ECT > drugs) was found in the bipolar depressed and involutional psychotic group (Greenblatt, Grosser, & Wechsler, 1964). A recent study by Wesner and Winokur (1989), which examined the influence of age on the natural history of unipolar depressive disorder, found that ECT reduced the rate of chronicity in older patients (aged 40 or older), but was associated with an increase in the frequency of episodes of depression in patients younger than 40.

Price and McAllister (1989) have examined the safety of ECT in elderly depressed patients with dementia. They reported an overall 86% response rate, with 21% experiencing significant cognitive or memory side-effects (mostly transient); 49% showed improvement in memory function after treatment. Clinical reports of ECT in patients with Parkinson's disease–dementia–depression complex, however, have suggested a poor therapeutic outcome in this group (Brown, Wilson, & Green, 1973; Young, Alexopoulous, & Shamoian, 1985). All studies thus far, however, have been retrospective in design, and there is not yet a single prospective, controlled study of ECT in the elderly.

Despite its proven effectiveness, however, ECT is generally not the first treatment of choice in elderly patients with MDD, and should probably not be utilized until one or more other treatments have proven ineffective. Because of its rapid therapeutic effect and generally less cardiovascular toxicity, ECT may be preferred over antidepressants in some elderly patients, particularly those with melancholia, with delusions, or at high risk for suicide. Patients with depression usually require ECT three times per week for a total of 7 to 9 treatments. Patients with either depression or mania are candidates, and major considerations for treatment lie in whether the patient can tolerate the effects of general anesthesia, muscle relaxation, and a major motor seizure. Elderly patients with pulmonary or cardiac disorders should receive evaluation by medical specialists before treatment.

Adverse effects of ECT may include hypoxia due to inadequate ventilation, cardiac arrythmias from vagal hyperactivity, cardiovascular effects from transient hypertension during the seizure, and both retrograde and anterograde memory disturbances (usually reversible by 6 weeks) (Burke, Rutherford, Zorumski, & Reich, 1985). The risk of side-effects may be considerably reduced in the elderly by adequate pre-ECT evaluation, ventilation with 100% oxygen before treatment, appropriate muscle relaxation, unilateral nondominant electrode placement and low-stimulus wave forms. The reported death rate from ECT using the latter precautions is only 1/60,000 patients. For further discussion of the role of ECT in the treatment of depression in later life, see Benlow's recent comprehensive review (1989).

E. Social and Family Support

While social withdrawal is a common part of depressive syndromes in later life, loneliness or isolation may themselves contribute to the onset of a depressive disorder. A number of investigators have shown that the quality of social support is inversely related to depression in older community-dwelling, psychiatric and medical inpatient populations (Blazer, 1983; George *et al.*, 1989; Goldberg, Van Natta, & Comstock, 1985; Koenig *et al.*, 1991a; Murphy, 1982; Surtees, 1980; Winefield, 1989). The tendency of depressed persons to lose interest in others and withdraw into themselves may be partly counteracted by encouragement and support from friends and family members. While depressed older persons may superficially shun contact with others, they typically feel intensely lonely and isolated from the world, and may not feel worthy of attention by others.

Because of the heavy burden of support that lies on the depressed person's family, there is often a need for respite from the caregiving role. One of the most common sources of support for most elderly outside their family comes from religious organizations (Tobin, Ellor, & Anderson-Ray, 1986). The elderly person is more likely to be involved in church groups than in all other voluntary social groups combined (Cutler, 1987; Mayo, 1951), and a study of patients attending a geriatric medicine clinic found that four of the five closest friends of patients were often from church congregations (Koenig, Moberg, & Kvale, 1988). The church, then, is a readily available, acceptable, and inexpensive source of support for many elderly. Senior centers are another outlet for social involvement and provide a source of age-matched peers with whom relationships may be obtained.

For example, an innovative and rapidly spreading concept that incorporates religious activities is the Shepherds' Center (Koenig, 1986). This program is not dependent on government funding, but instead is supported by donations from business and churches in the local community. Typical services include respite care, education and health information, meals on wheels, transportation for medical visits, exercise, and health maintenance. Shepherds' Centers are operated and managed entirely by older volunteers, and have as their goal the utilization of the talents and abilities of healthy elderly to provide services to needy, sick, or poor elderly. These programs give older adults a feeling of purpose and self-esteem as they provide a valuable and needed service to their community. The original Shepherds' Center (started 1972) located in Kansas City, Missouri, is supported by 26 churches and synagogues, and currently serves more than 6000 older adults through 400 elderly volunteers; centers now exist in 75 communities in 24 states.

In the end, the responsibility of providing emotional and material support often falls on family members, who may be reluctant or poorly prepared to take on this role. An important task of the clinician is encouragement and education of persons in the elder patient's family. Inquiry about other stresses impinging on the lives of family members or close friends may allow them to ventilate feelings of frustration, anger, or resentment that impede their ability to give the depressed elder the emotional support needed.

VIII. Suicide

A. Epidemiology

An association between age and suicide was noted by Seneca almost 2000 years ago, when he remarked that he would rather die than live in pain in his later years. Others have pictured later life as a time fraught with inevitable difficulties and carrying few prospects for happiness. If accepted by elders themselves, such a philosophy would foster suicide.

In fact, cross-sectional epidemiological studies have shown that suicide rates in later life are higher than at younger ages. The elderly commit 17% of all suicides, while making up only 11 or 12% of the population, and suicide ranks among the top ten causes of death in persons aged 65 or older.

When longitudinal data are examined, however, a different picture emerges. Since World War II, the rate of suicide in this country has remained relatively stable, despite an aging population. When examined by age group, the rate of suicide over the past 20 years in younger persons has been increasing, while that in the elderly has been decreasing. In the NIMH Epidemiological Catchment Area survey conducted in the Piedmont area of North Carolina, the prevalence of suicidal ideation in the past 2 weeks for 1622 randomly selected community-dwelling adults aged 60 or older, was .3%; 3.5% had contemplated suicide at some time in their lives, and .3% had actually attempted to take their lives (Blazer, Bachar, & Manton, 1986). These figures were lower than for younger adults in that study.

To understand the impact of age on suicide rates, both period and cohort effects must be considered. *Period effects* denote the impact of a unique stressor on the suicide rates for a particular age group at a particular point in time. For instance, if a law banning handgun control in the United States should come about, it would affect suicide rates especially in the elderly, because elders are more likely to use violent methods to commit suicide than are younger individuals. On the other hand, *cohort effects* on suicide rate result from stressors that affect a particular age group because of the generation into which they were born. For instance, Haas and Hendin (1983) examined suicide rates for persons aged 15 to 24 in 1908 and those aged 15 to 24 in 1923; they found rates of 13.5 per 100,000 and 6.3 per 100,000 respectively. Similarly, for 70-year-olds born in 1892, the suicide rate was 43.5 per 100,000, compared with 30.7 for 70-year-olds born in 1922. If one examines suicide rates for such cohorts throughout the life cycle, the rates for each cohort remain relatively stable (Blazer, Bachar, & Manton, 1986).

Several hypotheses have emerged to explain the differences in suicide rates between cohorts. The relative size of the birth cohort has been one explanation (Murphy & Wetzel, 1980). For example, the current "baby boom" cohort has an especially high rate of suicide, which may be attributable to a number of reasons including increased competition for jobs (Hendin, 1982). The current cohort of elderly has experienced fewer financial pressures and better health since World War II and, as noted earlier, a lower rate of depressive disorders than any other age cohort. However, this relatively bright outlook may be coming to an end, according to Nancy Osgood, who has recently calculated suicide rates from data collected by the National Center for Health Statistics. While suicide rates for elders declined from 1933 through 1980 (45.3 to 17.7 per 100,000), between 1981 and 1986 these rates have increased almost 25%. The reversal in the trend of declining suicide rates in the elderly is not easily explained and underscores the fact that suicide is still a serious problem of major concern in this age group.

B. Assessment of Risk Factors

Risk factors for suicide in later life include sex, race, marital status, economic status, mental illness, previous suicide attempts, and health. Age interacts with sex in its relationship with suicide rate. While men of all ages have a higher suicide rate than women, older men have a higher rate than any other age by sex group (Blazer, Bachar, & Manton, 1986). The difference between male and female suicides has remained constant throughout this past century. While the rate of suicide in white males aged 85 or older continues to be nearly three times that of black males in this age group, the rate for elderly black males has tripled since the 1960s for unknown reasons. Married persons, regardless of age, have the lowest risk of suicide, and widowed or divorced have the highest. This marital advantage, however, narrows among the elderly. The loss of a spouse in later life may be more expected than at other times in the life cycle; elderly widowed females in particular seem to be at a low risk for suicide. High-income status buffers against the risk of suicide in aged white males, even after controlling for other social variables.

Elderly patients with mental illness, particularly depression, alcohol dependence, and schizophrenia, are at high risk for suicide. When depression coexists with other mental disorders, especially in men, the risk increases. Well known as a risk factor for suicide is a history of a previous suicidal attempt. Dorpat, Anderson, and Ripley (1968) found that rates of successful suicide increased 100-fold in persons with a prior attempt. While the increased in suicide risk in previous attempters does not vary with age, the ratio of attempts to completed suicides changes from 20 to 1 in younger persons to 4 to 1 in persons aged 60 or over (Parkin & Stengal, 1965).

Poor health status is another major risk factor for suicide in later life. Cavan (1928) noted that physical illness led to suicide when a person's capacity to endure severe pain was exceeded. In a review of 391 cases of suicide, she found that 23% had physical illness; in two thirds of this group, the suicide was directly related to the illness. The close relationship between physical illness and suicide has been repeatedly demonstrated by other investigators (Abram, Moore, & Westervelt, 1971; Dorpat et al., 1968; Fawcett, 1972; Reich & Kelly, 1976; Sainsbury, 1956), particularly in men and patients with coexisting depression or organic brain syndrome. In an excellent review of the topic, MacKenzie and Popkin (1987) reported that there was strong epidemiological evidence to support an increased rate of suicide in patients with cancer, head injury, and peptic ulcer. There was also some evidence for increased risk in patients with neurological disorders, any painful or terminal illness, dyspnea, or other symptoms unresponsive to treatment. The high prevalence of chronic physical illness and disability in later life, and coexisting depression in elderly medically ill patients, underscores the suicide risk in this particular group.

Of great concern is that suicide rates in the medically ill elderly may considerably underestimate the true prevalence. Medication noncompliance, refusal of life-saving surgical therapies, or neglect in seeking timely medical care, may account for a substantial number of intentional deaths in the elderly that are now recorded as resulting from natural causes (Rodin et al., 1981).

C. Management

While knowledge of epidemiological data cannot replace a comprehensive psychiatric evaluation that acquires information on suicidal ideation, impulsivity, and severity of symptoms, it may help the clinician better assess a older patient for suicide risk. For instance, consider a 75-year-old divorced white man who has a major depressive disorder, periodically abuses alcohol, has financial and health problems, and lacks a friend or family member he can confide in. Even if the patient strongly denies suicidal ideation, he remains at high risk and must be monitored carefully, giving hospitalization serious consideration.

Involvement of family in helping to monitor the patient at home is vital when sending a potentially suicidal elderly patient back out in the community. Inquiry about a *plan* often reveals the means by which suicide might be attempted; the family should be instructed to remove from the house weapons such as guns, large knives, and all but necessary medications. If the family cannot assure the physician that at least one family member can be with the patient at all times until the risk of suicide has passed, then hospitalization is the safest course. The clinician must take care, however, not to place too much responsibility upon the family for the patient's safety.

While in hospital, the patient should be placed in an environment with windows of shatter-proof glass or safety screens, and should be protected from open stairwells or laundry chutes. All potentially harmful devices such as razors, scissors, knives, forks, ropes, and breakable glass bottles or glasses, should be closely monitored or removed from accessibility. When the suicidal risk is high, one-on-one supervision may be necessary; even q 15 min checks by nursing staff may be inadequate in such cases. For the confused or severely psychotic patient, adequate doses of psychotropic medication should be utilized. ECT may be the quickest and safest form of treatment in the severely depressed elder intending to harm himself. For suicidal elderly inpatients in the rehabilitation setting, Missel (1978) has provided an excellent review of management techniques. Providing terminally ill patients with some control over their circumstances may be helpful in averting suicide in such cases (Dubovsky, 1978).

References

Abram, H. S., Moore, G. L., & Westervelt, F. B. (1971). Suicidal behavior in chronic dialysis patients. *American Journal of Psychiatry, 127,* 119–224.

Alexopoulos, G. S. (1989). Late-life depression and neurological brain disease. *International Journal of Geriatric Psychiatry, 4,* 187–190.

Alexopoulos, G. S., Abrams, R. C., & Young, R. C. (1987). Late-life depression and dementing disorders. Abstract. Puerto Rico, American College of Neuropsychopharmacology.

Alexopoulos, G. S., Young, R. C., Meyers, B. S., Abrams, R. C. & Shamoian, C. A. (1988). Late-onset depression. *Psychiatric Clinics of North America, 11,* 101–115.

Ameblas, A. (1987). Life events and mania. *British Journal of Psychiatry, 150,* 235–240.

Angst, J., Baastrup, P., Grof, P., Hippius, H., Poldinger, W., & Weis, P. (1973). The course of monopolar depression and bipolar psychosis. *Psychiatrie, Neurologie, und Neurochirurgerie, 76,* 489–500.

Askinazi, C., Weintraub, R. J., & Karamouz, N. (1986). Elderly depressed females as a possible subgroup of patients responsive to methylphenidate. *Journal of Clinical Psychiatry, 47,* 467–469.

Ather, S. A., Ankier, S. I., & Middleton, R. S. W. (1985). A double-blind evaluation of trazodone in the treatment of depression in the elderly. *British Journal of Clinical Practice, 39,* 192–199.

Adams, W. L., Garry, P. J., Rhyne, R., Hunt, W. C., Goodwin, J. S. (1990). Alcohol intake in the healthy elderly. *Journal of the American Geriatrics Society 38,* 211–216.

Avery, D., & Silverman, J. (1984). Psychomotor retardation and agitation in depression. Relationship to age, sex and response to treatment. *Journal of Affective Disorders, 7,* 67–76.

Baldwin, R. C., & Jolley, D. J. (1986). The prognosis of depression in old age. *British Journal of Psychiatry, 149,* 574–583.

Baron, M., Mendlewicz, J., & Klotz, J. (1981). Age-of-onset and genetic transmission in affective disorders. *Acta Psychiatrica Scandinavica, 64,* 373–380.

Beaumont, G. (1989). The toxicity of antidepressants. *British Journal of Psychiatry, 154,* 454–458.

Beck, A. T., Rush, J., Shaw, B., & Emery, G. (1979). *Cognitive therapy of depression.* New York: Guilford.

Benbow, S. M. (1989). The role of ECT in the treatment of depressive illness in old age. *British Journal of Psychiatry, 155,* 147–152.

Blazer, D. G. (1982). *Depression in late life.* St. Louis, MO: Mosby.

Blazer, D. G. (1983). Impact of late-life depression on the social network. *American Journal of Psychiatry, 140,* 162–166.

Blazer, D. G. (1984). Hypochondriasis. In D. G. Blazer, & I. C. Siegler *A family approach to health care in the elderly.* Menlo Park, CA: Addison-Wesley.

Blazer, D. G. (1989). Depression in the elderly. *New England Journal of Medicine, 320,* 164–166.

Blazer, D. G., Bachar, J. R., & Hughes, D. C. (1987). Major depression with melancholia: A comparison of middle-aged and elderly adults. *Journal of the American Geriatrics Society, 35,* 927–932.

Blazer, D. G., Bachar, J. R., & Manton, K. G. (1986). Suicide in late life: review and commentary. *Journal of the American Geriatrics Society, 34,* 519–525.

Blazer, D. G., Fowler, N., & Hughes, D. C. (1987). [Followup of hospitalized depressed patients: An age comparison]. Unpublished data.

Blazer, D. G., Hughes, D. C., & Fowler, N. (1989). Anxiety as an outcome symptom of depression in elderly and middle-aged adults. *International Journal of Geriatric Psychiatry, 4,* 273–278.

Blazer, D., Hughes, D. C., & George, L. K. (1987). The epidemiology of depression in an elderly community population *Gerontologist, 27,* 281–287.

Brown, R., Sweeney, J., Loutsch, E., Kocsis, J., & Frances, A. (1984). Involutional melancholia revisited. *American Journal of Psychiatry, 141,* 24–28.

Brown, G. L., Wilson, W. P., & Green, R. L. (1973). Mental aspects of parkinsonism and their management. In S. J. Bern (Ed.), *Parkinson's disease—rigidity, akinesia and behavior* (Vol. 2, Selected communications on topic, pp. 265–278). New York; Verlag Hans Huber.

Burke, W. J., Rutherford, J. L., Zorumski, C. F., & Reich, T. (1985). Electroconvulsive therapy and the elderly. *Comprehensive Psychiatry, 26,* 480–486.

Busse, E. W., Barnes, R. H., & Silverman, A. J. (1954). Studies of the processes of aging: Factors that influence the psyche of elderly persons. *American Journal of Psychiatry, 110,* 897–903.

Carney, M., & Sheffield, B. (1974). The effects of pulse ECT in neurotic and endogenous depression. *British Journal of Psychiatry, 125,* 91–94.

Carroll, B. J., Feinberg, M., Greden, J. F., Tarika, J. Albala, A. A., Haskett, R. F., James, N. M., Kronfol, Z., Lohr, N., Steiner, M., De Vigne, J. P., Young, E. (1981). A specific laboratory test for the diagnosis of melancholia: Standardization, validity, and clinical utility. *Archives of General Psychiatry, 38,* 15–22.

Cassileth, B. R., Lusk, E. J., Strouse, T. B., Miller, D. S., Brown, L. L., Cross, P. A., & Tenaglia, A. N. (1984). Psychosocial status in chronic illness: A comparative analysis of six diagnostic groups. *New England Journal of Medicine, 311,* 506–511.

Cavanaugh, S. V., & Wettstein, R. M. (1983). The relationship between severity of depression, cognitive dysfunction, and age in medical inpatients. *American Journal of Psychiatry, 140,* 495–496.

Cavan, R. S. (1928). *Suicide.* Chicago: University of Chicago Press.

Charney, D. S., & Nelson, J. C. (1981). Delusional and nondelusional unipolar depression: Further evidence for distinct subtypes. *American Journal of Psychiatry, 138,* 328–333.

Ciompi, L. (1969). Followup studies on the evolution of former neurotic and depressive states in old age. *Journal of Geriatric Psychiatry, 3,* 90–100.

Coffey, C. E. (1991). Structural brain abnormalities in the depressed elderly. In P. Hauser (Ed.), *Brain imaging in affective disorders.* (in press).

Coffey, C. E., Figiel, G. S., Djang, W. T., Cress, M., Saunders, W. B., & Weiner, R. D. (1988a). Leukoencephalopathy in elderly depressed patients referred for ECT. *Biological Psychiatry, 24,* 143–161.

Coffey, C. E., Figiel, G. S., Djang, W. T., Sullivan, D. C., Herfkens, R. F., & Weiner, R. D. (1988b). Effects of ECT upon brain structure: A pilot prospective magnetic resonance imaging study. *American Journal of Psychiatry, 145,* 701–706.

Coffey, C. E., Hinkle, P. E., Weiner, R. D., Nemeroff, C. B., Krishnan, K. R. R., Varia, I., & Sullivan, D. C. (1987). Electroconvulsive therapy of depression in patients with white matter hyperintensity. *Biological Psychiatry, 22,* 626–629.

Cohen, R. M., Weingartner, H. W., Smallberg, A., Pickar, D., & Murphy, D. L. (1982). Effort and cognition in depression. *Archives of General Psychiatry, 39,* 593–597.

Cole, M. G. (1983). Age, age of onset, and course of primary depressive illness in the elderly. *Canadian Journal of Psychiatry, 28,* 102–104.

Cole, M. G. (1985). The course of elderly depressed outpatients. *Canadian Journal of Psychiatry, 30,* 217–220.

Cook, B. L., Helms, P. M., Smith, R. E., & Tsai, M. (1986). Unipolar depression in the elderly: Reoccurrence on discontinuation of tricyclic antidepressants. *Journal of Affective Disorders, 10,* 91–94.

Coryell, W., & Zimmerman, M. (1984). Outcome following ECT for primary unipolar depression: A test of newly proposed response predictors. *American Journal of Psychiatry, 141,* 862–867.

Cutler, S. J. (1976). Membership in different types of voluntary associations and psychological well-being. *Gerontologist, 16,* 335–339.

Davies, R. K., Tucker, G. J., Harrow, M., Detre, T. P. (1971). Confusional episodes and antidepressant medication. *American Journal of Psychiatry, 128,* 127–131.

De Alarcon, R. (1964). Hypochondriasis and depression in the aged. *Gerontologia Clinica, 6,* 266–277.

Derogatis, L. R., Morrow, G. R., Fetting, J., Penman, D., Piasetsky, S., Schmale, A. M., Henrichs, M., & Carnicke, C. L. M. (1983). The prevalence of psychiatric disorders among cancer patients. *Journal of the American Medical Association, 249,* 751–757.

Dolan, R. J., Calloway, S. P., & Mann, A. H. (1985). Cerebral ventricular size in depressed subjects. *Psychological Medicine, 15,* 873–878.

Dorpat, T. L., Anderson, W. F., & Ripley, H. S. (1968). The relationship of physical illness to suicide. In H. L. P. Resnik (Ed.), *Suicidal behaviors* (pp. 209–219). Boston: Little, Brown.

Dubovsky, S. L. (1978). Averting suicide in terminally ill patients. *Psychosomatics, 19,* 113–115.

Endicott, J. (1984). Measurement of depression in patients with cancer. *Cancer 53,* 2243–2249.

Enzell, K. (1984). Mortality among persons with depressive symptoms and among responders in a health check-up. *Acta Psychiatrica Scandinavica, 69,* 89–102.

Ernst, P., Badash, D., Beran, B., Kosovsky, R., & Kleinhauz, M. (1977). Incidence of mental illness in the aged: Unmasking the effects of chronic brain syndrome. *Journal of the American Geriatrics Society, 8,* 371–375.

Fawcett, J. (1972). Suicidal depression and physical illness. *Journal of the American Medical Association, 219,* 1303–1306.

Feighner, J. P., & Cohn, J. B. (1985). Double-blind comparative trials of fluoxetine and doxepin in geriatric patients with major depressive disorder. *Journal of Clinical Psychiatry, 46,* 20–25.

Figel, G. S., Coffey, C. E., & Weiner, R. D. (1989). Brain magnetic resonance imaging in elderly depressed patients receiving electroconvulsive therapy. *Convulsive Therapy, 5,* 26–34.

Finch, E. J. L., & Katona, C. L. E. (1989). Lithium augmentation in the treatment of refractory depression in old age. *International Journal of Geriatric Psychiatry, 4,* 41–46.

Folstein, S. E., Abbott, M. H., Chase, G. A., Jensen, B. A., & Folstein, M. F. (1983). The association of affective disorder with Huntington's disease in a case series and in families. *Psychological Medicine, 13,* 537–542.

France, R. D., Krishnan, K. R. R., Houpt, J. L., & Maltbie, A. A. (1984). Differentiation of depression from chronic pain with the dexamethasone suppression test and DSM-III. *American Journal of Psychiatry, 141,* 1577–1578.

Fredman, L., Schoenback, V. J., Kaplan, B. H., Blazer, D. G., James, S. A., Kleinbaum, D. G., & Yankaskas, B. (1989). The association between depressed symptoms and mortality among older participants in the Epidemiologic Catchment Area—Piedmont Health Survey. *Journal of Gerontology, 44,* S149–156.

Fullerton, A. G. (1984). Side-effects of nortriptyline treatment for post-stroke depression. *Lancet, i,* 519.

Gatz, C., & Scott, J. (1972). Age and measurement of mental health. *Journal of Health and Social Behavior, 13,* 55–67.

Gallagher, D., & Thompson, L. W. (1981). *Depression in the elderly: A behavioral treatment manual.* Los Angeles: University of Southern California Press.

Gallagher, D., & Thompson, L. W. (1982). Differential effectiveness of psychotherapies for the treatment of major depressive disorder in older adult patients. *Psychotherapy: Theory, Research, and Practice, 19,* 482–490.

George, L. K., Blazer, D. G., Hughes, D. C., & Fowler, N. (1989). Social support and the outcome of major depression. *British Journal of Psychiatry, 154,* 478–485.

Georgotas, A., McCue, R. E., & Cooper, T. B. (1989). A placebo-controlled comparison of nortriptyline and phenelzine in maintenance therapy of elderly depressed patients. *Archives of General Psychiatry, 46,* 783–786.

Gerner, R., Estabrook, W., Steuer, J., & Jarvik, L. (1980). Treatment of geriatric depression with trazodone, imipramine, and placebo: A double-blind study. *Journal of Clinical Psychiatry, 41,* 216–220.

Glaser, M., & Rabins, P. (1984). Mania in the elderly. *Age and Ageing, 13,* 210–213.

Glassman, A. H., & Roose, S. P. (1981). Delusional depression. A distinct clinical entity? *Archives of General Psychiatry, 38,* 424–427.

Goldberg, E. L., Van Natta, P., & Comstock, G. W. (1985). Depressive symptoms, social networks, and social support of elderly women. *American Journal of Epidemiology, 121,* 448–456.

Greenblatt, M., Grosser, G. H., & Wechsler, H. (1964). Differential response to hospitalized depressed patients to somatic therapy. *American Journal of Psychiatry, 120,* 935–943.

Greenwald, B. S., Kramer-Ginsberg, E., Marin, D. B., Laitman, L. B., Hermann, C. K., Mohs, R. C., & Davis, K. L. (1989). Dementia with coexistent major depression. *American Journal of Psychiatry, 146,* 1472–1477.

Gwirtsman, H. E., Ahles, S., Halaris, A., De Met, E., & Hill, M. A. (1983). Therapeutic superiority of maprotiline versus doxepin in geriatric depression. *Journal of Clinical Psychiatry, 44,* 449–453.

Hardy, B., Shulman, K., MacKenzie, S., Kutcher, S. P., & Silverberg, J. D. (1987). Pharmacokinetics of lithium in the elderly. *Journal of Clinical Psychopharmacology, 7,* 153–158.

Haskett, R. F. (1985). Diagnostic categorization of psychiatric disturbance in Cushing's syndrome. *American Journal of Psychiatry, 142,* 911–916.

Haas, A. P., & Hendin, H. (1983). Suicide among older people: Projections for the future. *Suicide and Life-Threatening Behavior, 13,* 147–154.

Hendin, H. (1982). *Suicide in America.* New York: Norton.

Himmelhoch, J. M., Auchenbach, R., & Fuchs, C. Z. (1982). The dilemma of depression in the elderly. *Journal of Clinical Psychiatry, 43*(9)(Sec. 2):26–34.

Holland, J. C., & Tross, S. (1985). The psychosocial and neuropsychiatric sequelae of the acquired immunodeficiency syndrome and related disorders. *Annals of Internal Medicine, 103,* 760–764.

Holland, J. C., Korzun, A. H., Tross, S., Siberfarb, P., Perry, M., Comis, R., & Oster, M. (1986). Comparative psychological disturbance in patients with pancreatic and gastric cancer. *American Journal of Psychiatry, 143,* 982–986.

Horowitz, M., & Kaltreider, N. (1979). Brief therapy of the stress response syndrome. *Psychiatric Clinics of North America, 2,* 365–377.

Jackson, S. W. (1969). Galen on mental disorders. *Journal of the History of the Behavioral Sciences, 5,* 365.

Jacoby, R. J., & Levy, R. (1980). Computed tomography in the elderly. 3. Affective disorders. *British Journal of Psychiatry, 136,* 270–275.

Jacoby, R. J., Dolan, R. J., Levy, R., & Baldy, R. (1983). Quantitative computed tomography in elderly depressed patients. *British Journal of Psychiatry, 143,* 124–127.

Jenike, M. A., & Albert, M. S. (1984). The dexamethasone suppression test in patients with presenile and senile dementia of the Alzheimer's type. *Journal of the American Geriatrics Society, 32,* 441–444.

Joffe, R. T., Lippert, G. P., Gray, T. A., Sawa, G., & Horvath, Z. (1987). Mood disorder and multiple sclerosis. *Archives of Neurology, 44,* 376–378.

Kafonek, S., Ettinger, W. H., Roca, R., Kittner, S., Taylor, N., & German, P. S. (1989). Instruments for screening for depression and dementia in a long-term care facility. *Journal of the American Geriatrics Society, 37,* 29–34.

Kalinowsky, L., & Hoch, P. (1946). *Shock treatments and other somatic procedures in psychiatry.* New York: Grune & Stratton.

Kaplitz, S. E. (1975). Withdrawn, apathetic geriatric patients responsive to methylphenidate. *Journal of the American Geriatrics Society, 23,* 271–276.

Katon, W., Raskind, M. (1980). Treatment of depression in the medically ill elderly with methylphenidate. *American Journal of Psychiatry, 137,* 963–965.

Kay, D. W. K., and Bergman, K. (1966). Physical disability and mental health in old age: a followup of a random sample of elderly people seen at home. *Journal of Psychosomatic Research 10,* 3–12.

Kitchell, M. A., Barnes, R. F., Veith, R. C., Okimoto, J. T., & Raskind, M. A. (1982). Screening for depression in hospitalized geriatric patients. *Journal of the American Geriatrics Society, 30,* 174–177.

Koenig, H. G. (1986). Shepherds' Centers: elderly people helping themselves. *Journal of the American Geriatrics Society, 34,* 73.

Koenig, H. G., & Breitner, J. C. S. (1990). Use of antidepressants in medically ill older patients. A review and commentary. *Psychosomatics, 31,* 22–32.

Koenig, H. G., & Studenski, S. (1988). Post-stroke depression in the elderly. *Journal of General Internal Medicine, 3,* 508–517.

Koenig, H. G., Moberg, D. D., & Kvale, J. N. (1988). Religious activities and attitudes of older adults in a geriatric assessment clinic. *Journal of the American Geriatrics Society, 36,* 362–374.

Koenig, H. G., Smiley, M., & Gonzales, J. (1988). *Religion, health and aging: A review and theoretical integration.* Westport, CT: Greenwood Press.

Koenig, H. G., Meador, K. G., Cohen, H. J., & Blazer, D. G. (1988). Depression in elderly hospitalized patients with medical illness. *Archives of Internal Medicine, 148,* 1929–1936.

Koenig, H. G., Shelp, F., Goli, V., Cohen, H. J., & Blazer, D. G. (1989). Survival and healthcare utilization in elderly medical inpatients with major depression. *Journal of the American Geriatrics Society, 37,* 599–606.

Koenig, H. G., Meador, K. G., Shelp, F., Goli, V., Cohen, H. J., & Blazer, D. G. (1991a). Depressive disorders in hospitalized medically ill patients. A comparison of young and elderly veterans. *Journal American Geriatric Society* (in press).

Koenig, H. G., Meador, K. G., Shelp, F., Golgi, V., Cohen, H. J., Blazer, D. G., & Dipasquale, R. (1991b). Religious coping and depression in hospitalization medically ill men. Manuscript submitted for publication.

Koenig, H. G., Goli, V., Shelp, F., Kudler, H. S., Cohen, H. J., & Blazer, D. G. (1991c). Major depression in hospitalized medically ill older patients: documentation, management, and prognosis. *International Journal of Geriatric Psychiatry* (in press).

Koenig, H. G., Goli, V., Shelp, F., Kudler, H. S., Cohen, H. J., Meador, K. G., & Blazer, D. G. (1989). Antidepressant use in elderly medical inpatients: Lessons from an attempted clinical trial. *Journal of General Internal Medicine, 4,* 498–505.

Kraepelin, E. (1921). Manic depressive insanity and paranoia (Trans. by R. M. Barclay from the 8th German ed., *Textbook of psychiatry*). Edinburgh: E.A. Livingstone.

Kramer, B. A. (1985). Use of ECT in California. *American Journal of Psychiatry, 142,* 1190–1192.

Krishnan, K. R. R., France, R. D., Pelton, S., McCann, U. D., Davidson, J., & Urban, B. J. (1985). Chronic pain and depression I: Classification of depression in chronic low back pain patients. *Pain, 22,* 279–287.

Lewinsohn, P. (1974). A behavioral approach to depression. In R. Friedman & M. Katz (Eds.), *The psychology of depression: Contemporary theory and research* (pp. 157–176). New York: Wiley.

Lundquist, G. (1945). Prognosis and course in manic depressive psychoses: A followup study of 319 first admissions. *Acta Psychiatrica Neurologica* (Suppl. 1), *35,* 1–96.

MacDonald, J. (1918). Prognosis in manic-depressive insanity. *Journal of Nervous and Mental Disorders, 47,* 20–30.

MacKenzie, T. B., & Popkin, M. K. (1987). Suicide in the medical patient. *International Journal of Psychiatry in Medicine, 17,* 3–22.

Magni, G., Schifano, F., De Leo, D., De Dominicis, G., Garbin, A., & Zangaglia, O. (1986). The dexamethasone suppression test in depressed and nondepressed geriatric medical inpatients. *Acta Psychiatrica Scandinavica, 73,* 511–514.

Markush, R. E., Schwab, J. J., Farris, P., Present, P. A., & Holzer, C. E. (1977). Mortality and community mental health, the Alachua County, Florida, Mortality Study. *Archives of General Psychiatry, 34,* 1393–1401.

Mayeux, R., Stern, Y., Williams, J. B. W., Cote, L., Frantz, A., & Dyrenfurth, I. (1986). Clinical and biochemical features of depression in Parkinson's disease. *American Journal of Psychiatry, 143,* 756–759.

Mayo, S. C. (1951). Social participation among the older population in rural areas of Wake County, NC. *Social Forces, 30,* 53–59.

Mendels, J. (1965). Electroconvulsive therapy and depression. I. The prognostic significance of clinical factors. *British Journal of Psychiatry, 111,* 675–681.

Mendez, M. F., Cummings, J. L., & Benson, D. F., (1986). Depression in epilepsy. *Archives of Neurology, 43,* 766–770.

Mendlewicz, J., & Baron, M. (1981). Morbidity risks in subtypes of unipolar depressive illness: Differences between early and late onset forms. *British Journal of Psychiatry, 139,* 463–466.

Meyers, B. S., & Alexopoulos, G. (1988). Age of onset and studies of late-life depression. *International Journal of Geriatric Psychiatry, 3,* 219–228.

Meyers, B. S., & Greenberg, R. (1986). Late-life delusional depression. *Journal of Affective Disorders, 11,* 133–137.

Meyers, B. S., Greenberg, R., & Mei-Tal, V. (1985). Delusional depression in the elderly. In C. A. Shamoian (Ed.), Progress in Psychiatry Series (pp. 19–28). Washington, DC: American Psychiatric Press.

Meyers, B. S., Kalayam, B., & Mei-Tal, V. (1984). Late-onset delusional depression: A distinct clinical entity? *Journal of Clinical Psychiatry, 45,* 347–349.

Middleton, R. S. W. (1975). A comparison between maprotiline (Ludiomil) and imipramine in treatment of depressive illness in the elderly. *Journal of Internal Medical Research, 3* (suppl.), 79–83.

Millard, P. H. (1983). Depression in old age. *British Medical Journal, 287,* 375–376.

Miller, F., & Whitcup, S. (1986). Benzodiazepine use in psychiatrically hospitalized elderly patients. *Journal of Clinical Psychopharmacology, 6,* 384–385.

Missel, J. (1978). Suicide risk in the medical rehabilitation setting. *Archives of Physical Medicine and Rehabilitation, 59,* 371–376.

Moffic, H. S., & Paykel, E. S. (1975). Depression in medical inpatients. *British Journal of Psychiatry, 126,* 346–353.

Morris, J. N., Wolf, R. S., & Klerman, L. V. (1975). Common themes among morale and depression scales. *Journal of Gerontology, 30,* 209–215.

Murphy, E. (1982). Social origins of depression in old age. *British Journal of Psychiatry, 141,* 135–142.

Murphy, E. (1983). The prognosis of depression in old age. *British Journal of Psychiatry, 142,* 111–119.

Murphy, E., Smith, R., Lindesay, J., & Slatter, J. (1988). Increased mortality rates in late-life depression. *British Journal of Psychiatry, 152,* 347–353.

Murphy, J., & Wetzel, R. (1980). Suicide risks birth cohort in the United States, 1949–1974. *Archives of General Psychiatry, 37,* 519–523.

Myers, J. K., Weissman, M. M., Tischler, G. L., Holzer, C. E., Leaf, P. J., Orvaschel, H., Anthony, J. C., Boyd, J. H., Burke, J. D., Kramer, M., & Stoltzman, R. (1984). Six-month prevalence of psychiatric disorders in three communities. *Archives of General Psychiatry 41,* 959–967.

Nielsen, J., Homma, A., & Biorn-Henriksen, T. (1977). Followup of 15 years after a gerontopsychiatric prevalence study. *Journal of Gerontology, 32,* 554–561.

Parmalee, P. A., Katz, I. R., & Lawton, M. P. (1989). Depression among institutionalized aged: Assessment and prevalence estimation. *Journal of Gerontology, 44,* M22–29.

Parkin, D., & Stengal, E. (1965). Incidence of suicide attempts in an urban community. *British Medical Journal, 2,* 133–134.

Persson, G. (1981). Five-year mortality in a 70-year-old urban population in relation to psychiatric diagnosis, personality, sexuality and early parental death. *Acta Psychiatrica Scandinavica, 64,* 244–253.

Pichot, P., & Pull, C. (1981). Is there an involutional melancholia? *Comprehensive Psychiatry, 22,* 2–10.

Pomara, N., & Gerson, S. (1984). Treatment-resistant depression in an elderly patients with pancreatic carcinoma: Case report. *Journal of Clinical Psychiatry, 45,* 439–440.

Post, F. (1972). The management and nature of depressive illness in late life: A follow-through study. *British Journal of Psychiatry, 121,* 393–404.

Post, F. (1978). The functional psychoses. In A. D. Isaacs & F. Post (Eds.), *Studies in geriatric psychiatry (p. 77)*. New York: John Wiley.

Post, F. (1982). Functional disorders II. Treatment and its relationship to causation. In R. Levy & F. Post (Eds.), The psychiatry of late life. London: Blackwell Scientific Publications.

Price, T. R. P., & McAllister, T. W. (1989). Safety and efficacy of ECT in depressed patients with dementia: A review of clinical experience. *Convulsive Therapy, 5,* 61–74.

Rapp, S. R., Parisi, S. A., & Walsh, D. A. (1988). Psychological dysfunction and physical health among elderly medical inpatients. *Journal of Consulting and Clinical Psychology, 56,* 851–855.

Reich, P., & Kelly, M. J. (1976). Suicide attempts by hospitalized medical and surgical patients. *New England Journal of Medicine, 294,* 298–301.

Reifler, B. V. (1982). Arguments for abandoning the term pseudo-dementia. *Journal of the American Geriatrics Society, 30,* 665–668.

Reifler, B. V., Larson, E., Teri, L., & Poulsen, M. (1986). Dementia of the Alzheimer's type and depression. *Journal of the American Geriatrics Society, 34,* 855–859.

Reifler, B. V., Teri, L., Raskind, M., Veith, R., Barnes, R., White, E., & McLean, P. (1989). Double-blind trial of imipramine in Alzheimer's disease patients with and without depression. *American Journal of Psychiatry, 146,* 45–49.

Rinieris, P. (1982). The "myth" of involutional melancholia. *Neuropsychobiology, 8,* 140–143.

Robinson, R. G., Lipsey, J. R., & Price, T. R. (1985). Diagnosis and clinical management of post-stroke depression. *Psychosomatics, 26,* 769–778.

Rockwell, E., Lam, R. W., & Zisook, S. (1988). Antidepressant drug studies in the elderly. *Psychiatric Clinics of North America, 11,* 215–233.

Rodin, G. M., Chmara, J., Ennis, J., Fenton, S., Locking, H., & Steinhouse, K. (1981). Stopping life-sustaining medical treatment: Psychiatric considerations in the termination of renal dialysis. *Canadian Journal of Psychiatry, 26,* 540–44.

Rosenbaum, A. H., Schatzberg, A. F., MacLaughlin, R. A., Snyder, K., Jiang, N., Ilstrup, D., Rothschild, A. J., & Kliman, B. (1984). The DST in normal control subjects: A comparison of two assays and the effects of age. *American Journal of Psychiatry, 141,* 1550–1555.

Sainsbury, P. (1956). *Suicide in London.* NY: Basic Books.

Schleifer, S. J., Macari-Hinson, M. M., Coyle, D. A., Slater, W. R., Kahn, M., Gorlin, R., & Zucker, H. D. (1989). The nature and course of depression following myocardial infarction. *Archives of Internal Medicine, 149,* 1785–1789.

Schulberg, H. C., McClelland, M., & Gooding, W. (1987). Six-month outcomes for medical patients with major depressive disorders. *Journal of Gen Intern Med, 2,* 312–317.

Schwab, J. J., Bialow, M., Brown, J. M., & Holzer, C. E. (1967). Diagnosing depression in medical inpatients. *Annals of Internal Medicine, 67,* 695–706.

Shulman, K. I., and Post, F. (1980). Bipolar affective disorder in old age. *British Journal of Psychiatry 136,* 26–32.

Shulman, K. I. (1986). Mania in old age. In E. Murphy (Ed.), *Affective disorders in the elderly* Edinburgh: Churchill Livingstone.

Shulman, K. I. (1989). The influence of age and ageing on manic disorder. *International Journal of Geriatric Psychiatry, 4,* 63–65.

Spar, J. E., Ford, C. V., & Liston, E. H. (1979). Bipolar affective disorders in aged patients. *Journal of Clinical Psychiatry, 40,* 504–507.

Steuer, J., Mintz, J., Hammen, C., Hill, M. A., Jarvik, L. F., McCarley, T., Motoike, P., & Rosen, R. (1984). Cognitive–behavioral and psychodynamic group psychotherapy in treatment of geriatric depression. *Journal of Consulting Clinical Psychology, 52,* 180–189.

Stewart, M. A., Drake, F., & Winokur, G. (1965). Depression among medically ill patients. *Diseases of the Nervous System, 26,* 479–85.

Strauss, D., & Solomon, K. (1983). Psychopharmacologic interventions for depression in the elderly. *Clinical Gerontologist, 2,* 3–29.

Surtees, P. G. (1980). Social support, residual adversity, and depressive outcome. *Social Psychiatry, 15,* 71–80.

Thompson, L. W., Gallagher, D., & Breckenridge, J. S. (1987). Comparative effectiveness of psychotherapies for depressed elders. *Journal of Consulting Clinical Psychology, 55,* 385–390.

Tiller, J., Schweitzer, I., Maguire, K., & Davies, B. (1989). Is diazepam an antidepressant? *British Journal of Psychiatry, 155,* 483–489.

Tobin, S. S., Ellor, J., Anderson-Ray, S. M. (1986). *Enabling the elderly: Religious institutions within the community service system.* Albany: State University of New York Press.

Verwoerdt, A. (1976). *Geropsychiatry.* Baltimore, MD: Williams & Wilkins.

Weissman, M. M., Leaf, P. J., Tischler, G. L., Blazer, D. G., Karno, M., Bruce, M. L., & Florio, L. P. (1988). Affective disorders in five United States communities. *Psychological Medicine, 18,* 141–153.

Wells, C. E. (1979). Pseudodementia. *American Journal of Psychiatry, 136,* 896–900.

Wesner, R. B., & Winokur, G. (1989). The influence of age on the natural history of unipolar depression when treated with ECT. *European Archives of Psychiatry and Neurological Science, 238,* 149–154.

Winefield, H. R. (1979). Social support and social environment of depressed and normal women. *Australian and New Zealand Journal of Psychiatry, 13,* 35–39.

Winokur, G. (1975). The Iowa 500: Heterogeneity and course in manic-depressive illness (bipolar). *Comprehensive Psychiatry, 16,* 125–131.

Winokur, G. (1985). The validity of neurotic–reactive depression. *Archives of General Psychiatry, 42,* 1116–1122.

Winokur, G., Behan, D., & Schlesser, M. (1980). Clinical and biological aspects of depression in the elderly. In J. O. Cole, J. E. Barrett (Eds.), *Psychopathology in the aged.* (p. 145). New York: Raven Press.

Woods, S. W., Tesar, G. E., Murray, G. B., & Cassem, N. H. (1986). Psychostimulant treatment of depressive disorders secondary to medical illness. *Journal of Clinical Psychiatry, 47,* 12–15.

Yang, L., Zuo, C., Su, L., & Eaton, M. T. (1987). Depression in Chinese medical inpatients. *American Journal of Psychiatry, 144,* 226–8.

Yates, W. R., Jacoby, C. G., & Andreasen, N. C. (1987). Cerebellar atrophy in schizophrenia and affective disorder. *American Journal of Psychiatry, 144,* 465–467.

Young, R. C., Alexopoulous, G. S., & Schamoian, C. A. (1985). Dissociation of motor response from mood and cognition in a parkinsonian patient treated with ECT. *Biological Psychiatry, 20,* 566–569.

Young, R. C., & Falk, J. R. (1989). Age, manic psychopathology, and treatment response. *International Journal of Geriatric Psychiatry, 4,* 73–78.

15

Anxiety and Its Disorders in Old Age

Javaid I. Sheikh

I. Introduction
II. Epidemiological Studies
    A. Surveys of Symptoms of Anxiety
    B. Surveys of Anxiety Syndromes
III. Classification and Phenomenology of Anxiety Disorders
    A. Panic Disorder
    B. Agoraphobia without History of Panic Disorder
    C. Social Phobia
    D. Simple Phobia
    E. Posttraumatic Stress Disorder
    F. Obsessive-Compulsive Disorder
    G. Generalized Anxiety Disorder
IV. Models of Anxiety and Phobias
    A. Psychological Models
    B. Biological Models
V. Evaluation of Anxiety
VI. Mixed Anxiety–Depression Syndromes
VII. Anxiety and Medical Illness
    A. Cardiovascular Illness
    B. Dietary Causes
    C. Drug-Related Causes
    D. Endocrine Conditions
    E. Pulmonary Causes
VIII. Psychological Treatments
IX. Pharmacological Treatments
X. Knowledge Gaps and Future Directions
    A. Need for Studies Using DSM-III-R Criteria
    B. Validation of Assessment Instruments in the Elderly
    C. Relationship of Anxiety States with Medical Conditions

Handbook of Mental Health and Aging, Second Edition

D. Studies of Panic Disorders and Phobias
E. Need to Establish Safe Guidelines for Drugs
F. Developing Nonpharmacological Treatments
XI. Conclusion
References

I. Introduction

The 1980s could be considered the decade of anxiety, with a plethora of articles addressing various aspects of anxiety disorders. A prominent exception to this trend, however, has been the lack of such studies in old age. It becomes obvious on examining various journals reporting geriatric studies that dementia and depression have received most of the attention during the last decade, and studies of anxiety have been virtually missing. This lack of attention to geriatric anxiety is hard to explain, considering that many prominent geriatricians such as Busse and Pfeiffer (1969), Butler and Lewis (1973), Bromley (1975), Blumenthal (1977), and Jarvik (1986) contend that anxiety is an important problem in old age. There is also evidence that such inattention can not be attributed to the infrequent occurrence of anxiety in the elderly. For example, a review of the literature (Sheikh, 1986) finds that various epidemiologic surveys estimate between 10 and 20% of elderly experience clinically significant symptoms of anxiety. In addition, more specific data about various anxiety disorders based on the Epidemiological Catchment Area (ECA) studies (Myers *et al.,* 1984) suggest that phobias alone may be the commonest psychiatric syndrome in elderly women and the second most common in elderly men. Such findings indicate that anxiety remains probably the most underaddressed psychiatric problem of old age.

A few words to clarify terminology may be in order here. The word *anxiety* is used in everyday language to describe a normal human emotion associated with a subjective sense of apprehension or nervousness about some future event. This emotion, however, can become unjustifiedly excessive, at which point it can be considered morbid or clinically significant. Examples of such clinically significant anxiety can range from excessive worry about everyday problems regarding job, relationships, or finances, or intense episodes of fear (panic attacks), usually accompanied by a multitude of cognitive, behavioral, and physiological symptoms. In this chapter, *anxiety* will be used to signify this pathological or clinically significant anxiety unless specifically mentioned otherwise. The terms anxiety disorder (s) and anxiety syndrome (s) will be used interchangeably to refer to a constellation of symptoms characterized as diagnostic entities in the revised version of the Diagnostic and Statistical Manual-III (DSM-III-R) [American Psychiatric Association (APA), 1987]. The term elderly is usually used in the literature to describe people aged 65 and older, though some surveys have used people 60 and older as well as 55 and older to describe that category. In this text this term will mean people 65 plus unless specified otherwise. Studies describing people 55 or 60 and older will be identified as such.

This chapter will begin with a review of epidemiological surveys; describe classification and phenomenology of various anxiety syndromes based on the DSM-III-R (1987), while pointing out any differential presentations in the elderly; present recent conceptualizations about anxiety; discuss assessment of anxiety in the elderly and its overlap with depression; and provide an overview of treatment methods with a particular focus on treatments suited for the elderly. Finally, knowledge gaps will be delineated and implications for future research, discussed.

II. Epidemiological Studies

Anxiety is variously described in clinical literature as a symptom of psychopathology, and a clinical syndrome or disorder (e.g., generalized anxiety disorder, panic disorder). This distinction between symptoms and disorders will be maintained in this chapter to minimize confusion.

A. Surveys of Symptoms of Anxiety

In the United States, the first large-scale survey of anxiety symptoms in an elderly population was reported by Gurin, Verhoff, and Feld (1963) as part of a nationwide sample of 2460 community-dwelling adults who were classified as young (21–44), middle-aged (45–64), and elderly (65 and older). A 22-item, self-report, mental health screening scale used in this survey also included questions pertaining to both cognitive (nervousness and insomnia) and somatic (shortness of breath and rapid heartbeat) components of anxiety. The results indicated a strong trend toward symptoms of both cognitive and somatic anxiety increasing across age groups. Specifically, the investigators found cognitive anxiety to be 2.9 times more frequent and somatic anxiety 6.5 times more frequent in the elderly (65 and older age group) compared to the young (21–44 age group). In this survey, the combined prevalence for cognitive and somatic anxiety in elderly subjects was 21.7%. In another survey, Gaitz and Scott (1972) used the above-mentioned self-rating instrument in a sample of 1441 Houston residents. The sample population was divided into young (20–39), middle-aged (40–64), and old (65 and older). The investigators found a linear increase in somatic anxiety with increasing age, almost four times greater in the oldest compared to the youngest age group. Unlike the above-mentioned survey by Gurin et al. (1963), these researchers did not find a significant increase in cognitive anxiety with increasing age. The combined prevalence for cognitive and somatic anxiety in the elderly was 19%. In retrospect, questions regarding the validity of the instrument used for rating symptoms of anxiety make it hard to rely on data from these two studies.

   In another large-scale survey of 1010 residents of a Canadian county, Leighton, Harding, Macklin, Macmillan, and Leighton (1963) used structured interviews to document psychiatric symptoms. Their results indicated that approximately 10% of the population from all age groups suffered from clinical anxiety, with no significant differences between age groups. Thus, their results do not seem to support the studies of Gurin et al. (1963) and Gaitz and Scott (1972). However, these investigators did not make a distinction between cognitive and somatic anxiety. In view of differences in methodology, it is difficult to compare the results of this study with those of Gurin *et al.* (1963), and Gaitz and Scott (1972).

During the last decade, Himmelfarb and Murrell (1984) conducted a survey of anxiety symptoms in a Kentucky community sample of 713 males and 1338 females aged 55 and older. This sample closely resembled the U.S. population in this age range on a number of demographic variables. The self-rating anxiety instrument used was the trait half of the State-Trait Anxiety Inventory (STAI) (Spielberger, Gorsuch, & Lushene, 1970). A score of 44 (of a maximum score of 80) on the trait version of the STAI was considered by the investigators as a cut-off point indicating sufficient anxiety and psychological distress to require intervention. They found that 17.1% of the males and 21.5% of the females fell into this category. In addition, a significant ($p < .05$) association of high anxiety with the presence of high blood pressure, kidney or bladder disease, heart trouble, stomach ulcers, hardening of arteries, stroke, and diabetes was found.

Keeping in mind that it is hard to compare the above-mentioned surveys owing to differences in demographics, instruments, and methodologies used, the prevalence of anxiety symptoms seems to range from 10% to 20% in the elderly.

B. Surveys of Anxiety Syndromes

Some of the studies of anxiety syndromes in the elderly were conceptualized in the era before the Diagnostic and Statistical Manual-III (DSM-III) (APA, 1980) was put into effect, and have tended to categorize anxiety and depression into a mixed, anxious–depressive neurosis following the tradition in that time. Early studies in this area were carried out in the United Kingdom. For example, Bergman (1971) reported a systematic investigation for the presence of mixed anxiety–depression neurosis in 300 randomly selected community-dwelling elderly (aged 61 and older). Of the 133 people he found to be suffering from neurosis, 61 had the onset of their illness before the age of 61 and 72, after that age. Furthermore, a majority of the early-onset neuroses consisted of anxiety states, whereas a majority of late-onset neuroses were found to be depressive. In another British study of 92 elderly patients admitted for complaints of depression, Post (1972) found that 75% of the *neurotic depressives* belonged to an intermediate affective group, presenting with clear symptoms of anxiety, restlessness, and hypochondriacal symptoms.

It is obviously quite difficult to discern from these studies the prevalence of different anxiety disorders as we classify them presently based on descriptive criteria of the revised version of DSM-III (DSM-III-R) (1987). Data from the ECA studies (Myers *et al.*, 1984) can be considered a first step in this direction. This survey found that the combined prevalence of panic disorder, obsessive-compulsive disorder, and phobias ranged between 5.7 and 33% for the three investigation sites. Phobias were found to be the most common psychiatric disorder in elderly women and the second most common in elderly men. More recently, in an age comparison of the ECA data between age groups of 45 to 64 (middle-aged) and 65 plus (older-aged), Blazer, George, and Hughes (1991) have reported the 6-month and lifetime prevalence in the Duke Community Sample for all anxiety disorders excluding posttraumatic stress disorder. They document that both 6-month and lifetime prevalence of all anxiety disorders declines somewhat from the middle-aged to the older group, though it still stands at a formidable combined prevalence of 19.7% for the 6-

Table I

Prevalence of Anxiety Disorders by Age[a]

Diagnosis	Six-month		Lifetime	
	45–64	65+	45–64	65+
Simple phobia	13.29	9.63	18.11	16.10
Social phobia	2.04	1.37	3.18	2.64
Agoraphobia	7.30	5.22	9.40	8.44
Panic disorder	1.10	0.04	2.04	0.29
OCD[b]	2.01	1.54	3.33	1.98
GAD[c]	3.10	1.90	6.70	4.60

[a]Duke ECA Community Sample. From Blazer, George, and Hughes (1991). Reproduced by permission.
[b]Obsessive-compulsive disorder.
[c]Generalized anxiety disorder.

month period and 34.05% for the lifetime for all anxiety disorders (See Table I). The investigators further document that people in the older age group are more likely to use outpatient mental health services and/or benzodiazepines when they do report symptoms of generalized anxiety. The authors also suggest that there is a possibility of under-reporting in the older age group owing to a higher threshold for reporting generalized anxiety symptoms. They hypothesize that if and when that threshold is reached, the elderly are prone to seek assistance.

It appears thus that anxiety symptoms and disorders are among the most common psychiatric afflictions experienced by the elderly.

III. Classification and Phenomenology of Anxiety Disorders

Presently accepted classification of anxiety disorders as described in the DSM-III-R is based on operationally defined, phenomenologically oriented, diagnostic criteria for various anxiety disorders. Though an atheoretical philosophy is usually subscribed to in the area of anxiety disorders, there are a few exceptions. For example, panic disorders has been given a central place, and agoraphobia is relegated to a secondary role, with the implication that over a period of time, avoidance behavior constituting agoraphobia usually follows recurrent panic attacks. In the following sections brief phenomenologic descriptions of various anxiety disorders are presented based on the DSM-III-R criteria, along with any features specific to the elderly population.

A. Panic Disorder

The central feature of this syndrome is recurrent episodes of severe anxiety or fear (panic attacks) manifested by a multitude of somatic and cognitive symptoms. Examples of these symptoms include palpitations, shortness of breath, chest pain or discomfort, sweating, hot and cold flashes, tingling in hands or feet, fear of dying, fear of losing control, and fear of going crazy. The panic attacks can occur either unexpectedly (spontaneous panic attacks) or in specific feared situations, though one or more panic attacks should be spontaneous in order to fulfill the DSM-III-R criteria of the syndrome. It is generally accepted that many patients with recurrent panic attacks go on to develop fear of being in places from where escape might be difficult in case of incapacitating panic attacks. Such a fear of panic may lead over time to multiple avoidance responses (agoraphobia). The severity of the agoraphobic syndrome can itself be classified into mild, moderate, or severe, depending upon the degree of avoidance. Some of the patients do not seem to develop agoraphobic symptoms. Panic disorder is thus differentiated into two subtypes, with or without agoraphobia. It is being diagnosed more frequently since modifications in the DSM-III-R have expanded this category to include most cases previously diagnosed as agoraphobia, and possibly many cases previously diagnosed as generalized anxiety disorder.

Panic disorder is typically chronic in its course, with frequent recurrences and remissions. With the exception of some recent reports (Luchins & Rose, 1989, Sheikh, 1991a, Sheikh, Taylor, King, Roth, & Agras, 1988), panic disorder still remains as especially neglected syndrome in older adults. It is of interest to note that there appears to be some phenomenological differences in early- versus late-onset panic disorder patients. Specifically, it appears that late-onset panic disorder (LOPD) patients report fewer panic symptoms, less avoidance, and score lower on somatization measures than the early-onset panic disorder (EOPD) patients (Sheikh & Bail, 1990). Implications of such findings for future research will be discussed in a later section.

B. Agoraphobia without History of Panic Disorder

The central feature of this relatively rare disorder is a fear of being in public places or situations from which escape might be difficult, in the absence of a history of panic attacks. It is not clear whether some of these patients are presenting with a variant of panic disorder.

C. Social Phobia

The diagnostic feature of this disorder is a persistent fear of one or more social situations. Common examples include fear of public speaking, inability to eat food in the presence of others, inability to write in public, and being unable to urinate in a public lavatory. Attempts to enter the phobic situation are typically accompanied by marked anticipatory anxiety. Clinical experience and epidemiologic evidence (Blazer et al., 1991) suggests that this disorder is chronic and persists in old age.

D. Simple Phobia

The characteristic feature here is a persistent fear of a circumscribed stimulus (object or situation) other than a fear of experiencing a panic attack or a fear of social situations, as is the case in panic disorder and social phobia, respectively. To fulfill the diagnostic criteria, the fear should be severe enough to produce distress or dysfunction. Example of simple phobias include fear of animals (dogs, snakes, insects, etc.), closed spaces (claustrophobia), flying, or heights. In urban settings, fear of crime seems to be particularly prevalent in the elderly population. For example, in a survey of elderly people in an English urban setting, Clarke and Lewis (1982) reported that 66% of the sample stated that they did not go out after dark for fear of victimization, and 15% reported this fear to be a primary concern. There is also indication that a nocturnal neurosis may develop in the elderly as a result of fear of crime (Cohen, 1976). It appears from the foregoing that the elderly may be the age group most anxious about crime, though they are apparently the least likely to be victimized (Clarke & Lewis, 1982).

E. Posttraumatic Stress Disorder

The diagnostic feature of this syndrome is the development of characteristic symptoms after a markedly distressing psychological trauma that is outside the range of usual human experience. The symptoms experienced are usually a combination of three categories:

1. re-experiencing of the traumatic event;
2. avoidance of stimuli associated with the trauma or numbing of general responsiveness (depression-like symptoms) ; and
3. symptoms of increased arousal (anxiety-like symptoms).

Examples of traumata might include a serious threat to one's life or physical integrity, serious threat or harm to one's children, spouse, or other close relatives and friends, or sudden destruction of one's home or community. The symptoms usually begin soon after the trauma but can be delayed for a number of months or years. Clinical experience with the elderly suggests presentations similar to those of younger people, though systematic studies of this syndrome in the elderly are lacking.

F. Obsessive-Compulsive Disorder

This disorder is characterized by recurrent obsessions or compulsions sufficiently severe to cause marked distress or dysfunction in occupational or personal matters. Obsessions are ideas, thoughts, impulses, or images that are experienced as senseless or intrusive and persist despite attempts to suppress them. Examples of common obsessions are repetitive thoughts of violence toward a loved one, contamination by germs or dirt, and doubts about injuring or offending someone. Compulsions are repetitive, purposeful, deliberate, and goal-directed behavior, performed in response to an obsession, according to certain rules, or a stereotyped fashion. Usually the compulsive behavior is designed to avoid discomfort or some dreaded situation and is often recognized by the individual as being either excessive or unrealistic. Attempting to resist a compulsion produces tension, which can be relieved by yielding to the compulsion. Examples of common compulsions include hand-washing, counting, checking, and touching. Depression, anxiety, and avoidance of situations that involve the content of obsessions, such as dirt or contamination, are common in this disorder. Differential manifestations of this disorder in the elderly are unknown.

G. Generalized Anxiety Disorder

The central feature of this syndrome is excessive or unrealistic anxiety on most days for 6 months or longer. The symptoms cluster into the following three categories:

1. Motor tension—trembling, muscle tension, restlessness, fatigability;
2. Autonomic hyperactivity—shortness of breath, rapid heart rate, sweating or cold clammy hands, dry mouth, dizziness, digestive disturbances, hot flashes or chills, frequent urination, and trouble swallowing or "lump in throat"; and
3. Vigilance and scanning—feeling on edge, exaggerated startle response, difficulty concentrating, insomnia, and irritability.

Since symptoms of generalized anxiety disorder do not qualitatively differ from everyday anxieties, it is the number of symptoms (at least 6 of 18) and duration (at least 6 months) that are essential to fulfill the diagnostic criteria. Many elderly patients with this syndrome may also present with features of depression, thus making the diagnosis and therapeutic decisions difficult at times.

IV. Models of Anxiety and Phobias

Generally accepted models of anxiety and phobias can be divided into psychological and biological models for the sake of simplicity. This is admittedly reductionistic, and readers are forewarned that it would be presumptuous to expect such a conceptualization to fully explain a phenomenon as complex as anxiety. Only a summary of these models is presented here, as a detailed discussion of this area is beyond the scope of this chapter.

A. Psychological Models

Three major schools of thought have dominated psychological theories of anxiety and phobias; psychoanalytic, classical conditioning models, and cognitive–behavioral models. The first two were quite popular in the past, and the third is presently in vogue.

The psychoanalytic model is based on Freud's theories. According to him, anxiety signals danger, and neurotic anxiety differs from everyday anxiety in signaling pressure from forbidden, repressed, and conflictual unconscious impulses that strive to become conscious (Freud, 1926). Thus, anxiety is considered a defense against such unacceptable impulses or ideas. Freud's phenomenological descriptions of anxiety included emotional, cognitive, physiological, and behavioral components, which are very similar to modern multidimensional approaches to anxiety. Further, his description of anxiety neurosis, which he separated from generalized diffuse anxiety and phobic anxiety, resembles re-markably the modern descriptions of panic attacks contained in the DSM-III-R. His etiological implications of sexual conflicts underlying phobias are, however, not accepted by most present-day scholars, and the treatment methods based on his theory have not been very effective (Roth, 1988).

The other major school of thought quite popular in the past has been a derivative of classical conditioning theories of Pavlov (1941). Such thinking espouses that phobias develop by classical conditioning and are reinforced by relief of anxiety that the patients experience by avoiding phobic situations. Again, this line of thinking is not generally accepted today since the settings of first panic attacks or phobic experiences are usually very different from subsequent feared situations (Roth, 1988).

The third model, which has aroused considerable interest lately, combines cognitive theories with somewhat modified conditioning paradigms to explain anxiety, panic at-tacks, and agoraphobia. Barlow (1988), Beck (1988), and Clark (1986) are the leading theorists in this area of cognitive–behavioral model of anxiety. In its simplest form, such a model assumes that individuals prone to anxiety states and particularly panic attacks misinterpret normal body sensations (Beck, Emery, & Greenberg, 1985) or sensations involved in normal anxiety responses (Clark, 1986) and create *catastrophic* cognitions about such sensations, which may spiral into full-blown panic attacks. There is further theorizing, based on the classical learning models, that fear can be conditioned to internal physiological stimuli resulting in a *learned alarm,* thus setting the stage of recurrent panic attacks (Barlow, 1988). There is increasing evidence that treatments based on such con-ceptualization are quite effective in the treatment of panic attacks and phobias (Barlow, 1988; Beck, 1988; Clark, Salkovskis, & Chalkley, 1985).

B. Biological Models

Darwin (1872) might have pointed to neurobiological origins of anxiety by suggesting the adaptive importance of anxiety for evolutionary development. Further theorizing by James (1890) and empirical work by Cannon (1929) might have paved the way for further inquiry into peripheral and central nervous system involvement in anxiety states, respec-tively. More recent biological work was stimulated in part by Klein's (1964) theorizing about anxiety attacks as being distinct from generalized anxiety, and reports that panic attacks could be precipitated by lactic acid infusions (Klein, 1981). Since then, many lines of inquiry have looked into physiological bases of panic attacks. Redmond's work sug-gested that the *locus ceruleus* may be implicated (Redmond & Haung, 1979), and Reiman *et al.,* (1984) documented increased parahippocampal activity during panic attacks provoked by lactic acid. Finally, there is a recent suggestion that panic disorder might be linked to a specific Mendelian gene (Crowe, 1988).

As can be seen, it is difficult to favor either the biological or the psychological model in explaining the phenomena of anxiety. Not surprisingly, there are attempts underway to integrate these various models (Ballenger, 1989). None of the psychological or biological theories has addressed the issue of anxiety in old age so far. Their relevance to our target population thus remains unproven at present.

V. Evaluation of Anxiety _____

Anxiety can be evaluated via clinical assessment as well as by rating scales. In addition to a history of present and past symptomatology, clinical assessment should include inquiry regarding various medical conditions and drugs that can be associated with symptoms of anxiety (see Table II). A detailed mental status examination will typically reveal many of the cognitive and behavioral manifestations of various anxiety disorders. A physical examination can be useful in observing physiological signs and symptoms of anxiety, including increased pulse rate, blood pressure, rapid breathing, and sweating.

Rating scales can be useful for screening, assessing severity of symptoms, and documenting effectiveness of various psychological and pharmacological interventions for anxiety. Various anxiety scales, their specific usage, and limitations are described in detail elsewhere (Sheikh, 1991b) and will be only briefly touched upon here. These scales are primarily of two kinds: observer-rated and self-rated. The most popular observer-rated scale is the Hamilton Anxiety Rating Scale (HARS), which was designed to measure the severity of anxiety in patients already diagnosed as having an anxiety disorder (Hamilton, 1959). It has 14 items consisting of 89 symptoms measuring psychic and somatic components of anxiety with each item rated on five levels of severity from *none* (0) to *very severe* (4). Though HARS is presently the standard in the field as a measure of change in clinical situations and in pharmacological research, published studies in geriatrics are infrequent and seem to indicate limited sensitivity to change with active drug treatment (Kochansky,

Table II

Physical Disorders Often Presenting with Anxiety[a]

Cardiovascular	*Endocrinologic (continued)*
Myocardial infarction	Cardinoid syndrome
Paroxysmal atrial tachycardia	Hypothermia
Mitral valve prolapse	Cushing's disease
Dietary	Hyperkalemia
Caffeine	*Hematologic*
Vitamin deficiencies	Anemia
Drug-related	*Immunologic*
Akathisia	Systemic lupus erythematosus
Anticholinergic toxicity	*Neurologic*
Antihypertensive side-effects	CNS infections
Digitalis toxicity	CNS masses
Withdrawal syndromes: alcohol,	Toxins
sedative–hypnotics	Temporal lobe epilepsy
Endocrinologic	Postconcussion syndrome
Insulinoma	*Pulmonary*
Hypoglycemia	Chronic obstructive lung disease
Hypo- or hyperthyroidism	Pneumonia
Hypo- or hypercalcemia	Hypoxia
Pheochromocytoma	

[a]Reproduced with permission from Jenike (1985, p. 98).

1979; Salzman, 1977). Experience with the elderly suggests that it is cumbersome to go through the list of 89 symptoms, and they tend to overendorse the somatic items. The usefulness of HARS in elders thus remains questionable. The most frequently used self-rated scale is the STAI (Spielberger, *et al.*, 1970). It seems particularly suited as a general measure of anxiety and in studies of psychological interventions, though its use in pharmacological studies is limited. A modified form for geriatric populations has been described by Patterson, Sullivan, and Spielberger (1980). Other commonly used scales include Hopkins Symptom Checklist (Derogatis, 1975) and Beck Anxiety Inventory (Beck, Epstein, Brown, & Steer, 1988).

Anxiety scales have some drawbacks that should be mentioned here. A major problem is that typically these measures were developed for and validated in younger populations, and empirical data documenting their applicability in the elderly are often lacking. It is possible that certain manifestations of anxiety states in the elderly might be different from these in younger people. This is clearly the case for depression in the elderly, which might present as *pseudodementia* (Wells, 1979). Additionally, somatic symptoms including sleep disturbances, decreased sexual desire, aches and pains, and decreased energy might not indicate depression in the elderly as they do in younger people (Yesavage *et al.*, 1983). As for anxiety states, though empirical data are lacking in general to draw any conclusions, there are preliminary indications that there may be differences in phenomenology between patients with LOPD and patients with EOPD (Sheikh, 1991a). Specifically, patients with LOPD seem to have fewer symptoms during panic attacks and are less avoidant. Another limitation of anxiety scales is that they show strongly positive correlations with scales for depression in older adults (Sheikh, Kilcourse, Gallagher, Thompson, & Tanke, 1989), thus making it difficult to differentiate anxiety from depression. Another potential problem is that increased medical comorbidity in the elderly may lead to overendorsement of items on anxiety scales related to cardiac and respiratory problems. Clinicians and researchers alike should be cognizant of these problems when interpreting scores of the elderly on anxiety scales.

VI. Mixed Anxiety–Depression Syndromes

The unresolved and somewhat controversial issue of mixed anxiety–depression is a recurring theme in the psychiatric literature. Debate is still on as to whether depression and anxiety lie on the same continuum or whether they are distinct psychiatric syndromes. A more detailed discussion of this issue has been provided elsewhere (Sheikh, 1991a) and will only be summarized here. After a review of several empirical studies, McNair and Fisher (1978) concluded that the distinction between anxiety and depressive neuroses was at best difficult. Prusoff and Klerman (1974) reported that approximately 40% of their neurotic outpatients showed mixed anxiety–depression and could not be classified into either diagnostic category through discriminant function analysis. There is also some evidence for the presence of a common neurobiological substrate for some forms of anxiety and depression (Paul, 1988). Klerman (1985) also points out that 80% of depressed patients may manifest symptoms of anxiety, whereas 35% of anxious individuals may experience secondary depression.

Many researchers come down on the side of *distinct syndromes* point of view. Gurney, Roth, Garside, Kerr and Schapira (1972) documented significant differences in symptomatology and mood, as well as histories of previous adjustment between patients diagnosed as having anxiety states and those termed depressive neuroses. They also documented a significant prognostic difference in favor of the depressed group on a follow-up study. Other investigators have also suggested that these syndromes are distinct. For example, Sir Martin Roth (Roth, Gurney, Garside, & Kerr, 1972) presented data suggesting that a 95% discrimination rate on 13 variables of anxiety and depression (e.g., panic attacks, agoraphobia, early-morning awakening, and retardation) was possible. This study was criticized by McNair and Fisher (1978) on the grounds that it was based on selected cases in which patients presented with clear symptoms of either panic attacks or endogenous depression. DSM-III clearly takes the stance that anxiety and depression are distinct syndromes.

Clinicians working with the elderly know that we see this mixed-symptom picture quite frequently in this population. There is some suggestion that the distinction between anxiety and depression may be harder to make in older populations (Kay, 1988). Controversy aside, it is particularly important in the elderly to make as fine a distinction between anxiety and depression as possible, not only for theoretical and diagnostic reasons, but also for practical therapeutic issues. This is because medications used for these categories may have different side-effect profiles. For example, tricyclic antidepressants have many undesirable side-effects like cardiotoxicity, anticholinergic side-effects, and orthostasis, compared to the relatively safer profile of anxiolytics, such as benzodiazepines and buspirone.

VII. Anxiety and Medical Illness

One of the unresolved issues facing the clinicians and researchers in the area of anxiety is that of its short- and long-term effects on physical health. This issue may be of particular relevance to the elderly populations owing to their relatively increased susceptibility to developing physical illness. A strong association of anxiety states with certain medical conditions has been mentioned in the literature. For example, researchers have documented that asthma (Alexander, 1972), hypertension (Whitehead, Blackwell, DeSilva, & Robinson, 1977), and duodenal ulcer (Sandberg & Bliding, 1976) are associated with high anxiety. There is also the suggestion that anxiety can give rise to potentially lethal arrhythmias (Jenkins, 1971) and a recommendation to use diazepam in such cases. Such contentions are considered controversial, however. This is partly owing to a lack of knowledge about the specific mechanism by which anxiety and autonomic arousal can cause tissue damage. Of course, the relationship between anxiety and heart disease is complicated, and anxiety seems to contribute to heart disease, while the disease in itself increases anxiety (Jenike, 1989), thus producing a vicious cycle. Of special relevance to the elderly, Nowlin, Williams, and Wilkie (1973) reported in a prospective study that high anxiety predicted the future occurrence of myocardial infarction in older men. As mentioned previously, in a survey of older adults, Himmelfarb and Murrell (1984) found a significant ($p < .05$) association of high anxiety with the presence of certain medical conditions including high blood pressure, kidney or bladder disease, heart trouble, stomach ulcers, hardening of the arteries, stroke, and diabetes. Cause-or-effect issues aside, such association warrants further studies. Finally, one should not forget that many medical conditions can produce anxietylike symptoms, which may confound the clinical picture at times. A list of such conditions is presented in Table II followed by a brief discussion of anxiety as it presents with the most common of these clinical syndromes.

A. Cardiovascular Illness

Certain cardiovascular syndromes like angina pectoris and myocardial infarction can present with a picture very similar to that of a panic attack with dyspnea, chest tightness, sweating, and a fear of dying. Needless to say, such episodes in older patients should always prompt thorough investigation of the cardiac status of the patient, unless a diagnosis of panic disorder is already established after proper investigations. The relationship of mitral valve prolapse with panic disorder remains controversial at best, with some of the studies suggesting a higher-than-normal incidence (Gorman, *et al.*, 1981; Kantor, Zitrin & Zeldis, 1980) and others refuting such evidence (Margraf, Ehlers & Roth, 1988; Mazza *et al.*, 1986).

B. Dietary Causes

Caffeine intake in the form of coffee, tea, and sodas can be a common cause of anxietylike symptoms in doses as little as 200 mg (one cup of coffee, 150 mg) (Victor, Lubersky, & Greden, 1981). There are also reports of caffeine inducing full-blown panic attacks (Charney, Heninger & Jatlow, 1985; Lee, 1985; Uhde *et al.*, 1984). It is thus a good idea to obtain a careful history of caffeine use in patients with symptoms of anxiety to rule out any temporal relationship. Cutting down on daily caffeine consumption can be a simple and effective intervention in some cases.

C. Drug-Related Causes

Akathisia, a very common side-effect of neuroleptics (Baldessraini, 1985), is a subjective sense of restlessness often indistinguishable from anxiety. Management techniques for this condition include cutting down the neuroleptic dose, adding anticholinergics or beta blockers, or short-term benzodiazepine use (Baldessraini, 1985; Ratey & Salzman, 1984). Another common cause of anxietylike symptoms are the adrenergic agonists like ephedrine and pseudoephedrine, which are quite commonly present in over-the-counter preparations for common colds and allergic conditions. Since older people seem to use over-the-counter medications quite frequently, it is a good idea to inquire about a history of intake of such preparations. Alcohol withdrawal is a well-recognized cause of anxiety and agitation among hospitalized patients (Lerner & Fallen, 1985). Sedative–hypnotic withdrawal, however, might be somewhat underestimated as a cause of anxiety syndromes in older populations in which hypnotic use is quite frequent (Schweizer, Case, & Rickels, 1989). It might behoove clinicians to inquire about any such use at the beginning of the hospitalizations and to cover with appropriate medications for withdrawal. Other drugs that can produce anxiety include amphetamines, bronchodilators like isoproterenol, theophylline, and some calcium channel blockers (e.g., verapamil, nifedipine).

D. Endocrine Conditions

Hyperthyroidism is probably the most common endocrine disorder that can masquerade as a generalized anxiety disorder in young patients. Kathol, Turner, and Delahunt (1986) thus report that two thirds or more of these patients will meet DSM-III criteria for an anxiety disorder. In patients older than 60, however, hyperthyroidism is usually due to a toxic nodular goiter (Hurley, 1983) and is more insidious in presentation, sometimes labeled as apathetic as opposed to anxious or agitated hyperthyroidism of younger people. Other endocrine causes like hypoparathyroidism, hypoglycemia, and Cushing's syndrome are relatively uncommon.

E. Pulmonary Causes

For elderly patients at bed rest, pulmonary embolism might be the most common pulmonary cause of sudden anxiety. A ventilation–perfusion scan and a phlebogram can be diagnostic. There is also some evidence of unusually high numbers of panic disorder cases among patients with chronic obstructive pulmonary disease (Karajgi et al., 1990; Yellowees et al., 1987).

VII. Psychological Treatments

Little empirical research has been done on the use of nonpharmacologic methods for management of anxiety in the elderly. This is somewhat surprising considering that cognitive–behavior therapy literature is full of reports describing anxiety-management procedures of demonstrated efficacy in a younger population. A number of cognitive and behavioral interventions are efficacious for the treatment of anxiety and depression in the general population (Barlow, 1988; Marks, 1981). Such procedures generally fall into three main categories—relaxation training, cognitive restructuring, and activity structuring. Relaxation procedures consist primarily of progressive relaxation of Bernstein and Borkovec (1973), whereas cognitive restructuring techniques to overcome anxiety are adaptations from Meichenbaum (1974), Mahoney (1974), and Beck et al., (1985). The principles of activity structuring for management of anxiety have been derived from chronic pain and depression literatures (Fordyce, 1976; Lewinsohn, 1975). Finally, there is increasing evidence (Barlow, 1988; Clark, 1985) that cognitive–behavior therapy is quite effective in panic disorder also.

It must be mentioned that a study by Sallis, Lichstein, Clarkson, Stalgaitis, and Campbell (1983) failed to confirm the efficacy of nonpharmacologic anxiety-management techniques in the anxious elderly. The number of subjects in this study was quite small, however, and one has to be quite cautious in interpreting their findings. There is some evidence from the memory-training literature that relaxation techniques can improve performance in the anxious elderly, possibly by reducing their anxiety (Yesavage, Sheikh, Tanke, & Hill, 1988). Given the sensitivity of elderly to any medications, non-pharmacologic anxiety-management techniques should always be considered as alternatives.

IX. Pharmacological Treatments

Before describing different types of medications, it will be helpful to briefly review the physiological changes occurring as part of normal aging. Age-related changes in absorption, distribution, protein binding, metabolism, and excretion of drugs can significantly alter plasma levels of drugs and make the elderly particularly prone to experience toxic effects, even at average dose ranges for the general population. Briefly, drug absorption may be altered due to decreases in splanchnic blood flow, increases in gastric pH, and changes in active and passive transport (Omslander, 1981). An increase in proportion of body fat with aging may prolong the half-life of lipophilic drugs like diazepam (Jenike, 1989). A reduction in serum albumin may mean more free drug in the plasma and greater chances of toxicity (Greenblatt, 1979). A decrease in hepatic metabolism may further increase the levels of unmetabolized drug. Finally, a gradual decrease in glomerular filtration rate and renal blood flow to 50% by the age of 70, as compared to that of a 40-year-old, means higher chances of toxicity (Paper, 1978). With this background in mind, we can now proceed to descriptions of different classes of compounds found effective in anxiety disorders.

Benzodiazepines have been the mainstay of anxiolytics for more than two decades now and have shown their superiority as anxiolytics over placebo, barbiturates, meprobamate, and antihistamines in most clinical trials (Jenike, 1989). They are the most frequently used antianxiety drugs in the elderly; as many as one third of elderly patients hospitalized for a medical illness receive a benzodiazepine (Shaw & Opit, 1976). Though effectiveness of these agents is presumably comparable, one must keep in mind the potentially serious problems of long-acting benzodiazepines like diazepam or chlordiazepoxide in this age group. These medications possess long-acting active metabolites, and may linger in the body of an elderly patient for long periods. Rosenbaum (1979) documents that the half-life of diazepam's metabolites increases from 20 hr in a 20-year-old to 90 hr in an 80-year-old. Studies have also documented several undesirable side-effects of diazepam in the elderly, including fatigue and drowsiness (Boston Collaborative Drug Surveillance Program, 1973) and memory impairment (Salzman, Shader, Harmatz, & Robertson, 1975). It has also been documented that female patients with symptoms of dementia are especially prone to confusion, impaired concentration, and memory problems with this drug (Hall & Joffee, 1972). Alprazolam, which has proved to be quite effective in panic disorder (Ballenger, Burrows, & Dupont, 1988), is an intermediate-acting drug whose metabolites seem to clear rapidly (Abernathy *et al.*, 1983). Greenblatt *et al.*, (1983) document that the mean half-life for alprazolam increases from 11 hours for young people to 19 hours in elderly men, but not in women. There is an insufficient body of knowledge as yet to suggest advantages or disadvantages of alprazolam in the elderly. Short-acting benzodiazepines like oxazepam and lorazepam seem preferable in the elderly, especially since they do not have active metabolites. These medications are probably safer in the presence of liver disease, and it appears that lorazepam is the drug of choice in lung disease (Jenike, 1989). It is important to remember, however, that long-term use of benzodiazepines in the elderly may be fraught with several complications, including psychomotor and cognitive impairment and a potential for abuse–dependence (Pomara *et al.*, 1991; Sheikh, in press). Time-limited use for specific indications thus cannot be overemphasized.

Buspirone is an anxiolytic with partial serotonin-agonist properties, which appears to have efficacy comparable to that of diazepam (Rickles *et al.*, 1982). Clinical experience in geriatric populations indicates that it is well tolerated and effective for remediation of chronic anxiety symptoms. Buspirone does not have any cross-tolerance with benzodiazepines, does not appear to be fraught with abuse or dependency potential, and may not be well accepted by patients who have become dependent on benzodiazepines. It takes 3–4 weeks for a therapeutic effect, has a good margin of safety, and even long-term use does not appear to cause psychomotor impairment commonly seen with benzodiazepines (Smiley & Moskowitz, 1986). Buspirone may be particularly indicated in chronic anxiety conditions in which use of benzodiazepines may be fraught with abuse and dependence potential. Preliminary, nonplacebo-controlled studies in geriatric populations indicate that it is well tolerated, does not cause adverse effects when coprescribed with a variety of other medications including antihypertensives, cardiac glycosides, and bronchodilators, and is effective for remediation of chronic anxiety symptoms in this population (Napoliello, 1986). It also appears that in both acute and chronic dosing, the pharmacokinetics of buspirone in the elderly is very similar to that in younger people (Gammans, Westrick, & Shea, 1989). Such a profile seems to suggest that buspirone may be a particularly desirable anxiolytic for the elderly, though further confirmatory data are needed to make the determinations.

Antidepressants are considered the treatment of choice in mixed anxiety–depression syndromes (Crook, 1982). Imipramine and phenelzine (a monoamine oxidase inhibitor) have been shown to be particularly effective in panic disorder (Klien, 1981; Kahn *et al.*, 1981; Sheehan, 1984). Well-controlled studies in the elderly are lacking, but preliminary data from our program suggest that imipramine is quite effective and well tolerated in elderly panic disorder patients if started in low doses (10mg/day) with a gradual increase in 3 to 4 weeks to between 100 and 150 mg/day on average. Antidepressants like desipramine or nortriptyline, which may be preferable in the elderly owing to their lower anticholinergic properties, have not been systematically studied in anxiety conditions of the elderly, and thus their efficacy in these disorders remain unknown.

Miscellaneous drugs: there is some evidence that beta blockers like propranolol and oxprenolol may be quite suitable for geriatric patients with anxiety and agitation (Petrie, 1983). Petrie and Ban (1981) have also shown that propranolol may be effective in the agitation and behavioral problems of demented individuals who are refractory to antipsychotic or benzodiazepine therapy. Antihistamines like hydroxyzine and diphenhydramine are also used sometimes to manage mild anxiety. Finally, our clinical experience suggests that low-dose, high-potency neuroleptics like p-18 haloperidol and fluphenazine hydrochloride are quite effective in anxiety and agitation associated with organic brain syndromes.

X. Knowledge Gaps and Future Directions

The following section will delineate the information gaps in the field of anxiety disorders of the aged and suggest directions for future studies.

A. Need for Studies Using DSM-III-R Criteria

As is evident from the literature review, most studies have not used the clearly defined, phenomenologically oriented, descriptive criteria laid down by the DSM-III-R. In the absence of an uniformly accepted neurophysiological, biochemical, psychosocial, or etiological theory, clinical practice and research studies must be based upon empirically validated clinical criteria. It is thus imperative that we conduct studies of anxiety disorders in the elderly using DSM-III-R criteria to obtain reliable information regarding prevalence and phenomenology. Such studies will eventually indicate whether the criteria of anxiety states need to be modified in the elderly and whether syndromes like obsessive-compulsive disorder really are rare in this population.

B. Validation of Assessment Instruments in the Elderly

There is a clear need to carry out validation studies of the existing measures of anxiety in the elderly, which may in turn lead to the development of better instruments specifically geared to measure anxiety in the elderly. Progress needs to be made in various directions at this time. To begin with, a large-scale validation study of the more popular existing anxiety scales can be carried out in anxious older people using various structured diagnostic interviews as external criteria. Second, we need to develop measures that can differentiate anxiety from depression on the one hand, and generalized anxiety from panic anxiety on the other. Finally, we need to develop measures that can accurately assess the severity of phobias in the elderly.

C. Relationship of Anxiety States with Medical Conditions

As mentioned earlier, there is enough evidence in the literature of various medical conditions' being frequently associated with anxiety disorders. Whether anxiety is a cause or effect of these illnesses is not clear at this time. The association with anxiety is, however, strong enough to suggest a need for further studies to clarify these issues.

D. Studies of Panic Disorders and Phobias

With the changes in the DSM-III-R from its predecessor DSM-III, and growing awareness of health care providers about these disorders, panic disorders and phobias are becoming more frequently diagnosed and thus increasingly important. The questions of differential phenomenology and clinical response to antipanic treatments in elderly patients thus warrant studies.

E. Need to Establish Safe Guidelines for Drugs

We need to carry out more studies of different anxiety syndromes of the elderly with the short-acting benzodiazepines such as oxazepam, lorazepam, and with non-benzodiazepines, such as buspirone, in order to establish empirically derived guidelines for safety, efficacy, and specificity of these drugs for this population. Such studies are a priority for the field.

F. Developing Nonpharmacological Treatments

As mentioned earlier, behavior-therapy literature is full of reports describing anxiety-management procedures of demonstrated efficacy in a younger population. Owing to the special vulnerability of the elderly to the multiple, undesirable side-effects of medications, there is clearly a need to study the efficacy of nonpharmacological methods for the management of anxiety in this population.

XI. Conclusion

Despite increasing research interest in the area of anxiety, few systematic studies of phenomenology and treatment of anxiety disorders in the elderly have been reported. The pervasive myth is that anxiety is usually an epiphenomenon of depression in old age. Among the contributing factors to such a folklore may be the model of *learned helplessness* (Seligman, 1975), which seems to indicate that anxiety is an initial reaction to threat, succeeded by depression if the threat persists for a long time. The implications of such a theory may be that old age, stereotyped by the usually irreversible nature of its multiple losses, ultimately leads to depression, with symptoms of anxiety being a temporary phenomenon on the way to that outcome. Empirical studies of anxiety symptoms and syndromes in the elderly population, however, tend to negate such a belief and suggest that point prevalence of symptoms of anxiety is around 10 to 20% and 6-month prevalence of all anxiety disorders is 19.7% (Blazer *et al.*, 1991). Geriatric anxiety thus remains woefully underaddressed.

It appears that short-acting benzodiazepines, such as oxazepam and lorazepam, and nonbenzodiazepines, such as buspirone, are the treatments of choice for symptoms of anxiety uncomplicated by depression. Antidepressants seem preferable in cases of mixed anxiety–depression or panic disorder. Finally, proven nonpharmacological methods for managing anxiety need to be modified to fit the needs of this population.

References

Abernethy, D. R., Greenblatt, D. J., Divoll, M., & Shader, R. I. (1983). Pharmacokinetics of alprazolam. *Journal of Clinical Psychiatry, 44,* 45–47.

Alexander, A. B. (1972). Systematic relaxation and flow rates in asthmatic children: Relationship to emotional precipitants and anxiety. *Journal of Psychosomatic Research, 16,* 405–410.

American Psychiatric Association, Committee on Nomenclature and Statistics. (1980). *Diagnostic and statistical manual of mental disorders. DSM-III (3rd ed).* Washington, DC: American Psychiatric Association.

American Psychiatric Association, Committee on Nomenclature and Statistics. (1987). *Diagnostic and statistical manual of mental disorders. DSM-III-R (3rd ed., rev.)* Washington DC: American Psychiatric Association.

Baldessraini, R. J. (1985). *Chemotherapy in psychiatry: Principles and practice (rev. ed.).* Cambridge, MA: Harvard University Press.

Ballenger, J. C. (1989). Toward an integrated model of panic disorder. *American Journal of Orthopsychiatry, 59,* 284–293.

Ballenger, J. C., Burrows, G. D., & Dupont, R. L. (1988). Alprazolam in panic disorder and agoraphobia: Results from a multicenter trial. *Archives of General Psychiatry, 45,* 413–422.

Barlow, D. H. (1988). *Anxiety and its disorders: The nature and treatment of anxiety and panic.* New York: Guilford Press.

Beber, C. (1965). Management of behavior in the institutionalized aged. *Diseases of the Nervous System, 26,* 591–595.

Beck, A. T., Emery, G., & Greenberg, R. L. (1985). *Anxiety disorders and phobias: A cognitive perspective.* New York: Basic Books.

Beck, A. T. (1988). Cognitive approaches to panic disorder: Theory and therapy. In S. Rachman & J. D. Maser (Eds.), *Panic: Psychological perspectives.* (pp. 91–109). Hillsdale, NJ: Erlbaum.

Beck, A. T., Epstein, N., Brown, G., & Steer, R. (1988). An inventory for measuring clinical anxiety: Psychometric properties. *Journal of Consulting and Clinical Psychology, 56,* 893–897.

Bergmann, K. (1971). The neuroses of old age. In D. W. K. Kay & A. Walk (Eds.), *Recent developments in psychogeriatrics: British Journal of Psychiatry, Special Publication No. 6.* (pp. 35–90). Ashford, England: Headley.

Bernstein, D. A., & Borkovec, T. D. (1973). *Progressive relaxation: A Manual for the helping professions.* Champaign, IL: Research Press.

Blazer, D., George, L., & Hughes, D. (1991). The epidemiology of anxiety disorders: An age comparison. In C. Salzman & B. Liebowitz (Eds.), *Anxiety Disorders in the Elderly.* New York: Springer Publishing Company, Inc., pp. 17–30.

Blumenthal, M. D. (1977). Anxiety in the elderly: problem and promises. *Proceedings of a conference on anxiety in the elderly.* (pp. 9–28). Tucson, AZ: Co-Sponsored by Roche Laboratories & University of Arizona College of Medicine.

Borkovec, T. D. (1976). Physiological and cognitive processes in the regulation of anxiety. In G. E. Schwartz & D. Shapiro (Eds.), *Consciousness and self-regulation: Advances in research* (Vol. 1, pp.). New York: Plenum.

Boston Collaborative Drug Surveillance Program (1973). Clinical depression of the central nervous system due to diazepam and chlordiazepoxide in relation to cigarette smoking and age. *New England Journal of Medicine, 288,* 277–280.

Brodsky, L., Zuniga, J. S., & Casenas, E. R. (1983). Refractory anxiety: A masked epileptiform disorder. *Psychiatric Medicine of the University of Ottawa, 8,* 42–45.

Bromley, D. B. (1975). *The psychology of human aging* (2nd ed.). Baltimore MD: Penguin.

Busse, E. W., & Pfeiffer, E. (1969). Functional and psychiatric disorders in old age. In E. W. Busse & E. Pfeiffer (Eds.), *Behavior and Adaptation in Late Life* Boston MA: Little, Brown.

Butler, R. N., & Lewis, I. L. (1973). *Aging and mental health: Positive psychological approaches.* St. Louis MD: Mosby.

Cannon, W. B. (1929). *Bodily changes in pain, hunger, fear and rage: An account of recent researches into the function of emotional excitement.* New York: Appleton-Century-Crofts.

Charney, D. S., Heninger, G. R., & Jatlow, P. L. (1985). Increased anxiogenic effects of caffeine in panic disorder. *Archives of General Psychiatry, 42,* 233–243.

Clark, D. M. (1986). A cognitive approach to panic. *Behavior Research and Therapy, 24,* 461–470.

Clark, D. M., Salkovskis, P. M., & Chalkley, A. J. (1985). Respiratory control as a treatment for panic attacks. *Journal of Behavior Therapy and Experimental Psychiatry, 16,* 23–30.

Clarke, A. H., & Lewis, M. J. (1982). Fear of crime among the elderly. *British Journal of Criminology, 232,* 49.

Cohen, C. I. (1976). Nocturnal neurosis of the elderly: Failure of agencies to cope with the problem. *Journal of American Geriatrics Society, 24,* 86.

Crook, T. (1982). Diagnosis and treatment of mixed anxiety–depression in the elderly. *Journal of Clinical Psychiatry, 43,* 35–43.

Crowe, R. R. (1988). Family and twin studies of panic disorder and agoraphobia. In M. Roth, R. Noyes, Jr., & G. D. Burrows (Eds.), *Handbook of Anxiety, Vol. 1: Biological, Clinical, and Cultural Perspectives* (pp. 101–114). Amsterdam: Elsevier/North Holland Science Publishers.

Darwin, C. (1872). *The expression of the emotions in man and animals.* London: John Murray.

Derogatis, L. R. (1975). *The SCL-90-R.* Baltimore: Clinical Psychometric Research.

Derogatis, L. R., Lipman, R. S., Covi, L., & Rickels, K. (1972). Factorial invariance of symptom dimensions in anxious and depressive neuroses. *Archives of General Psychiatry, 27,* 659–665.

Edlund, M. J., Swan, A. C., & Clothier, J. (1987). Patients with panic attacks and abnormal EEG results. *American Journal of Psychiatry, 144,* 508–509.

Eisdorder, C., & Raskind, M. A. (1970). *Improvement in learning in the aged by modification of autonomic nervous system activity. Science '70,* 1327–1329.

Feigenbrum, E. M. (1971). *Assessment of behavioral changes and emotional disturbance in a custodial geriatric facility.* Paper read at the 124th Annual Meeting of the American Psychiatric Association, Washington, DC.

Fordyce, W. E. (1976). *Behavioral methods for chronic pain and illness.* St. Louis, MO: Mosby.

Freud, S. (1926). Inhibitions, symptoms, and anxiety.In J. Strachey, (Ed.), *The Complete Psychological works of Sigmund Freud,* (Vol. XX.) London: Hogarth Press.

Gaitz, C. M., & Scott, J. (1972). Age and the measurement of mental health. *Journal of Health and Social Behavior, 13,* 55–67.

Gammans, R. E., Westrick, M. L., Shea, J. P., Mayol, R. F., & LaBudde, J. A. (1989). Phamacokinetics of buspirone in elderly subjects. *Journal of Clinical Pharmacology, 29,* 72–78.

Garmany, G. (1956). Anxiety states. *British Medical Journal, 1,* 943–946.

Garmany, G. (1958). Depressive states: Their etiology and treatment. *British Medical Journal, 8,* 341–344.

Gorman, J. M., Fyer, A. J., Gliklich, J. M. (1981). Mitral valve prolapse and panic disorders: Effect of imipramine. In D. F. Klein & J. G. Rabkin (Eds.). *Anxiety: New research and changing concepts* New York: Raven Press.

Greenblatt, D. J. (1979). Reduced serum albumin concentration in the elderly: A report from the Boston Collaborative Drug Surveillance Program. *Journal of the American Geriatrics Society, 27,* 20–22.

Greenblatt, D. J., & Shader, R. I. (1974) *Benzodiazepines in clinical practice.* New York: Raven.

Greenblatt, D. J., Divoll, M., Abernethy, D. R., Moschitto, L. J., Smith, R. B., & Shader, R. I. (1983). Alprazolam kinetics in the elderly: Relation to antipyrine disposition. *Archives of General Psychiatry, 40,* 287–290.

Gurin, G., Veroff, J., & Feld, S. (1963). *Americans view their mental health.* New York: Basic Books.

Gurney, C., Roth, M., Garside R. F., Kerr, T. A., & Schapira K. (1972). Studies in the classification of affective disorders: The relationship between anxiety states and depressive illness - II. *British Journal of Psychiatry, 121,* 162–166.

Hamilton, M. (1959). The assessment of anxiety states by rating. *British Journal of Medical Psychology, 32,* 50–55.

Hall, R. W. C., & Joffee, F. R. (1972). Aberrant response to diazepam: A new syndrome. *American Journal of Psychiatry, 126,* 738–742.

Himmelfarb, S., & Murrel, S. A. (1984). The prevalence and correlates of anxiety symptoms in older adults. *Journal of Psychology, 116,* 159–167.

Holliday, A. R., & Mihlayi, E. (1966). A controlled evaluation of two dose levels of oxazepam compared to placebo. *Journal of New Drugs, 6,* 124.

Hurley, J. R. (1983). Thyroid diseases in the elderly. *Medical Clinics of North America, 1983, 67,* 497–516.

James, W. (1890). *Principles of psychology.* New York: Holt, Rinehart & Winston.

Jarvik, L. (1986). *Anxiety in the elderly: A conceptual framework.* Paper presented in a symposium at the 39th Annual Meeting of the Gerontological Society of America. New Orleans, Louisiana, November, 1986.

Jenike, M. A. (1989). Anxiety disorders of old age. In M. A. Jenike (Ed.), *Geriatric psychiatry and psychopharmacology* (pp. 248–271). Chicago: Year Book Medical Publishers.

Jenkins, C. D. (1971). Psychological and social precursors of coronary disease. *New England Journal of Medicine, 284,* 244–255.

Kahn, R., McNair, D., Covi, L., Downing, R. W., Fisher, S., Lipman, R. S., Rickels, K., & Smith, V. K. (1981). Effects of psychotropic agents on high-anxiety subjects. *Psychopharmacology Bulletin, 17,* 97–100.

Kalish, R. A. (1977). *The later years.* Belmont, CA: Wadsworth.

Kantor, J. S., Zitrin, C. M., & Zeldis, S. M. (1980). Mitral valve prolapse syndrome in agoraphobic patients. *American Journal of Psychiatry, 137,* 467–469.

Karajgi, B., Rifkin, A., Doddi, S., & Kolli, R. (1990). The prevalence of anxiety disorders in patients with chronic obstructive pulmonary disease. *American Journal of Psychiatry, 147(2),* 200–201.

Kathol, R. G., Turner, R., & Delahunt, J. (1986). Depression and anxiety associated with hyperthyroidism: Response to antithyroid therapy. *Psychosomatics, 27,* 501–505.

Kay, D. W. K. (1988). Anxiety in the elderly. In M. Roth, R. Noyes, Jr., and G. D. Burrows (Eds.). *Handbook of Anxiety, Volume 1: Biological, Clinical and Cultural Perspectives.* (pp. 289–310).Amsterdam: Elsevier/North Holland Science Publishers.

Klein, D. F. (1964). Delineation of two drug-responsive anxiety syndromes. *Psychopharmacologia, 5,* 397–408.

Klein, D. F. (1981). Anxiety reconceptualized. In D. Klein & J. Rabkin (Eds.), *Anxiety: New research and changing concepts* (pp. 235–263). New York: Raven Press.

Klerman, G. L. (1985). *Internal Medicine for the Specialist (Special Issue),* 2–12.

Kochansky, G. E. (1979). Psychiatric rating scales for assessing psychopathology in the elderly: A critical review. In A. Raskin & L. Jarvik (Eds.), *Psychiatric symptoms and cognitive loss in the elderly.* Washington, DC: Hemisphere.

Lader, M. (1982). Differential diagnosis of anxiety in the elderly. *Journal of Clinical Psychiatry, 43,* 4–7.

Lader, M. (1974). The peripheral and central role of the catecholamines in the mechanism of anxiety. *International Pharmacopsychiatry, 9,* 125–137.

Lee, M. A. (1985). Anxiety and caffeine consumption in people with anxiety disorders. *Psychiatry Research, 15,* 211–217.

Leigh, D. (1979). Psychiatric aspects of head injury. *Psychiatry Digest, 40,* 21–32.

Leighton, D. C., Harding, J. S., Macklin, D. B., MacMillan, A. M., & Leighton, A. H. (1963). *The character of danger: Psychiatric symptoms in selected communities, III.* New York: Basic Books.

Lerner, W. D., & Fallen, H. J. (1985). The alcohol withdrawal syndrome. *New England Journal of Medicine, 313,* 511–515.

Lewinsohn, P. M. (1975). The behavioral study and treatment of depression. In M. Hersen, R. Eisler, & P. Miller (Eds.), *Progress in Behavior Modification* (Vol. 1). New York: Academic Press.

Luchins, D. J., & Rose, R. P. (1989). Late-life onset of panic disorder with agoraphobia in three patients. *American Journal of Psychiatry, 146,* 920–921.

Mahoney, M. J. (1974). *Cognition and behavior modification.* Cambridge, MA: Ballinger.

Margraf J., Ehlers A., & Roth, W. T. (1988). Mitral valve prolapse and panic disorder: A review of their relationship. *Psychosomatic Medicine, 50,* 93–113.

Marks, I. M. (1981). *Cure and care of neuroses: Theory and practice of behavioral psychotherapy.* New York: Wiley.

Mazza, D. L., Martin, D., Spacavento, L., Jacobsen, J. & Gibbs, H. (1986). Prevalence of anxiety disorders in patients with mitral valve prolapse. *American Journal of Psychiatry, 143,* 349–352.

McDonald, R. J., & Speilberger, C. D. (1978). *Measuring anxiety in hospitalized geriatric patients.* Berlin: Schering.

McNair, D. M., & Fisher, S. E. (1978). Separating anxiety from depression. In M. A., Lipton, A. DiMoscio, & K. Killam (Eds.), *Psychopharmacology: A Generation of Progress* New York: Raven Press.

Meichenbaum, D. (1974). Self-instructional strategy training: A cognitive prosthesis for the aged. *Human Development, 17,* 273–280.

Mellinger, G. D., & Balter, M. B. (1982). Prevalence and patterns of use of psychotherapeutic drugs: Results from a 1979 national survey of American adults. In G. Tognoni, C. Bellantuono, & M. Lader, (Eds.), *Epidemiological Impact of Psychotropic Drugs: Proceedings of International Seminar on Epidemiological Impact of Psychotropic Drugs* Amsterdam: Elsevier/North Holland.

Myers, J. K., Weissman, M. M., Tischler, G. L., Holzer, C. E., Leaf, P. J., Orvaschel, H., Anthony, J. C., Boyd, J. H., Burke, J. D., Kramer, M., & Stoltzman, R. (1984). Six-month prevalence of psychiatric disorders in three communities, 1980 to 1982. *Archives of General Psychiatry, 41,* 959–967.

Napoliello, M. J. (1986). An interim multicenter report on 677 anxious geriatric outpatients treated with buspirone. *British Journal of Clinical Practice, 40,* 71–73.

Nowlin, J. B., Williams, R., & Wilkie, F. (1973). Prospective study of physical and psychological factors in elderly men who subsequently suffer acute myocardial infarction (AMI). *Clinical Research, 21,* 465.

Omslander, J. G. (1981). Drug therapy in the elderly. *Annals of Internal Medicine, 94,* 711–722.

Papper, S. (1978). *Clinical nephrology.* Boston: Little, Brown.

Parry, H. J., Balter, M. B., Mellinger, G. D., Cisin, I. H., & Manheimer, D. I. (1973). National patterns of psychotherapeutic drug use. *Archives of General Psychiatry, 28,* 769–783.

Patterson, R. L., Sullivan, M. J., & Spielberger, C. D. (1980). Measurement of state and trait anxiety in elderly mental health clients. *Journal of Behavioral Assessment, 2,* 89–96.

Paul, S. M. (1988). Anxiety and depression: A common neurobiological substrate? *Journal of Clinical Psychiatry, 49,* (10 Suppl.), 13–16.

Pavlov, I. P. (1941). *Conditioned reflexes and psychiatry.* Translated by W. H. Ganto. London: Lawrence and Wishart.

Petrie, W. M. (1983). Drug treatment of anxiety and agitation in the aged. *Psychopharmacology Bulletin, 19,* 238–246.

Petrie, W. M., & Ban, T. A. (1981). Propranolol in organic citation. *Lancet, 1* (8215), 324.

Pomara, N., Deptula, D., Singh, R. (1991). Cognitive toxicity of benzodiazepines in the elderly. C. L. Salzman & B. Liebowitz (Eds.), *Anxiety disorders in the elderly.* New York: Springer Publishing Company, Inc., pp. 175–196.

Post, F. (1972). The management and nature of depressive illnesses in late life: A follow through study. *British Journal of Psychiatry, 121,* 394–404.

Prusoff, B., & Klerman, G. (1974). Differentiating depressed from anxious neurotic outpatients. *Archives of General Psychiatry, 30,* 302–309.

Ratey, J. J., & Salzman, C. (1984). Recognizing and managing akathisia. *Hospital & Community Psychiatry, 35,* 975–977.

Redmond, D. E., & Huang, H. Y. (1979). New evidence for a locus coeruleus norepinephrine connection with anxiety. *Life Sciences, 25,* 2149–2162.

Reiman, E. M., Raichle, M. E., Butler, F. K., Herscowitch, P., & Robins, E. (1984). A focal brain abnormality in panic disorder: A severe form of anxiety. *Nature, 310,* 683–685.

Rickles, K., Weisman, K.,Norstad, N., (1982). Buspirone and diazepam in anxiety: A controlled study. *Journal of Clinical Psychiatry, 43,* 81–86.

Rosenbaum, J. (1979). Anxiety. In A. Lazare (Ed.), *Outpatient Psychiatry* (pp. 252–256). Baltimore, MD: Williams & Wilkins.

Roth, M. (1988). Anxiety and anxiety disorders—general overview. In M. Roth, R. Noyes Jr., & G. D. Burrows (Eds.), *Handbook of anxiety, Vol. 1: Biological, clinical, and cultural perspectives* (pp. 1–44). Amsterdam: Elsevier/North Holland, Science Publishers.

Roth, M., Gurney, C., Garside, R. F., & Kerr, T. A. (1972). Studies in the classification of affective disorders: The relationship between anxiety states and depressive illness. *British Journal of Psychiatry, 121,* 147–161.

Roth, M., & Mountjoy, C. (1980). States of anxiety in late life: Prevalence of anxiety and related emotional disorders in the elderly. In G. Burrows & B. Davies (Eds.), *Handbook of studies on anxiety* (pp. 193–215). Amsterdam: Elsevier/North-Holland Biomedical Press.

Sallis, J. F., & Lichstein, K. L. (1982). Analysis and management of geriatric anxiety. *International Journal of Aging & Human Development 15*, 197–211.

Sallis, J. F., Lichstein, K. L., Clarkson, A. D., Stalgaitis, S., & Campbell, M. (1983). Anxiety and depression management for the elderly. *International Journal of Behavioral Geriatrics, 1(4)*, 3–12.

Salzman, C., Shader, R. I., Harmatz, J., & Robertson, L. (1975). Psychopharmacologic investigations in elderly volunteers. Diazepam in males. *Journal of American Geriatrics Society, 23*, 451–457.

Salzman, C. (1977). Psychometric rating of anxiety in the elderly. *Proceedings of a conference on anxiety in the elderly*. Tucson, AZ: Co-sponsored by Roche Laboratories & University of Arizona College of Medicine.

Sandberg, B., & Bliding, A. (1976). Duodenal ulcer in army trainees during basic military training. *Journal of Psychosomatic Research, 20*, 61–74.

Seligman, M. E. P. (1975). *Helplessness. On depression, development, and death*. San Francisco: W. H. Freeman.

Schweizer, E., Case, W. G., & Rickels, K. (1989). Benzodiazepine dependence and withdrawal in elderly patients. *American Journal of Psychiatry, 145(4)*, 529–531.

Shader, R. I., & Greenblatt, D. J. (1982). Management of anxiety in the elderly: The balance between therapeutic and adverse effects. *Journal of Clinical Psychiatry, 43*, 8–18.

Shaw, S. M., & Opit, L. J. (1976). Need for supervision in the elderly receiving long-term prescribed medication. *British Medical Journal, 1*, 505–507.

Sheehan, D. V. (1984). The treatment of panic and phobic disorders. In. J. G. Bernstein (Ed.), *Clinical Psychopharmacology* (2nd ed.), Boston: John Wright.

Sheikh, J. I. (1986). Anxiety disorder in the elderly: A literature review and future directions. Paper presented in a symposium at the 39th Annual Meeting of the Gerontological Society of America, New Orleans, LA, November 1986.

Sheikh, J. I. (1991a). Anxiety Disorders in the Elderly. In D. G. Blazer & W. R. Hazzard (Eds.): *Current Problems in Geriatrics*. Littleton, Massachusetts: Mosby-Year Book, Inc., Vol. 1 (1).

Sheikh, J. I. (1991b). Anxiety rating scales for the elderly. In Salzman C. & Leibowitz, B. (Eds.), *Anxiety in the Elderly*, New York: Springer Publishing Company, Inc., pp. 251–265.

Sheikh, J. I. (In press). Complications of long-term anxiolytic use in the elderly. In C. Shamoian (Ed.). *Treatment Complications in the Elderly*. Washington D.C.: American Psychiatric Press, Inc.

Sheikh, J. I., Taylor, C. B., King, R. J., Roth, W. T., Agras, W. S. (1988). Panic attacks and avoidance behavior in the elderly. *Proceedings of the 141st Annual Meeting of the American Psychiatric Assocation, Montreal, Quebec*, May, 1988.

Sheikh, J. I., & Bail, G. (1990). Somatization in older panic disorder patients. *Proceedings of the 143rd Annual Meeting of the American Psychiatric Association*, New York, May 1990.

Sheikh, J. I., Kilcourse, J., Gallagher, D., Thompson, L., & Tanke, E. (1989). Can we improve the specificity of anxiety and depression scales? *Proceedings of the 2nd Annual Meeting of American Association for Geriatric Psychiatry*, Orlando, FL., February 1989.

Smiley, A., & Moskowitz, H. (1986). Effects of long-term administration of buspirone and diazepam on driver steering control. *American Journal of Medicine, 80* (3b), 22–29.

Speilberger, C., Gorsuch, R., & Lushene, R. (1970). *STAI manual for the state-trait anxiety inventory*. Palo Alto, CA: Consulting Psychologists Press.

Turnbull, J. M.,& Turnbull, S. K. (1985). Management of specific anxiety disorders in the elderly. *Geriatrics, 40*, 75–82.

Uhde, T. W., Roy-Byrne, P., Gillin, J. C. (1984). The sleep of patients with panic disorders: A preliminary report. *Psychiatry Research, 12*, 251.

Victor, B. S., Lubersky, M., & Greden, F. (1981). Somatic manifestations of caffeinism. *Journal of Clinical Psychiatry, 42*, 185–188.

Wells, C. E. (1979). Pseudodementia. *American Journal of Psychiatry, 136*, 895–900.

Whitehead, W. E., Blackwell, B., DeSilva, H., & Robinson, A. (1977). Anxiety and anger in hypertension. *Journal of Psychosomatic Research, 21*, 383–389.

Yellowees, P. M., Alpers, J. H., Bowden, J. J., Bryant, G. O., & Raffin, R. E. (1987). Psychiatric morbidity in subjects with chronic airflow obstruction. *Medical Journal of Australia, 146,* 305–307.

Yesavage, J. A., Brink, T. L., Rose, T. L., Lum, O., Huang, V., Adey, M., & Leirer, V. O. (1983). Development and validation of a geriatric depression screening scale: A preliminary report. *Journal of Psychiatric research, 17,* 33–49.

Yesavage, J. A., Sheikh, J. I., Tanke, E. D., & Hill, R. (1988). Individual differences in response to memory training: Verbal intelligence and state anxiety predict improvement. *American Journal of Psychiatry, 145,* 636–639.

Personality Disorders in Old Age

Joel Sadavoy and Barry Fogel

I. Background
II. Classification of Personality Disorders
III. Stability of Personality
IV. Epidemiology of Personality Disorder in Old Age
V. Evolution of Personality Disorder Symptoms with Age
VI. Symptom Expression in the Elderly
VII. Residual and Emergent Personality Disorders
VIII. Special Considerations
    A. Organic Factors
    B. Institutionalization
    C. Forced Intimacy
    D. Personality Disorder and Depression
    E. Treatment Issues
IX. Research Directions
    A. Structural Assessment of Personality Disorders in the Elderly
    B. Future Research
    References

I. Background

The study of personality disorder (PD) is fraught with imprecision and plagued by an absence of data. This is true across all age categories but is especially evident in the old-age cohort—arbitrarily defined for the purpose of this chapter and in keeping with convention, as those older than 65. Parenthetically one should take note of the unsatisfactory nature of this definition of old age, since the stressors inherent in the young-old population are often very different from the normative stressors of the old-old cohort. For example, because white, North American women outlive men, on average, by 8 years, a woman in

Handbook of Mental Health and Aging, Second Edition

the old-old cohort (older than 75 years), will often have to contend with widowhood and bereavement, a normative, age-specific development that is likely to affect the expression of characteristics that relate to personality disorder, among other things (Fries 1987).

Definitions of personality and by extension, disorders of personality, do not provide satisfactory and specific criteria, although it seems clear that a stable identifiable core or self, expressed in a stable pattern of behavior, remains evident for much of one's adult life. The Diagnostic and Statistical Manual III-Revised (DSM-III-R) [American Psychiatric Association (APA), 1987] distinguishes personality traits from disorders. Traits are defined as "enduring patterns of perceiving, relating to, and thinking about the environment and oneself, and are exhibited in a wide range of important social and personal contexts. It is only when personality traits are inflexible and maladaptive and cause either significant functional impairment or subjective distress that they constitute personality disorders (p. 335)." Disorders are said to begin early in life and endure through most of adult life, often becoming less evident in middle-age or old age. The diagnosis depends on identification of specific behaviors or traits evident within the past year as well as throughout adult life. One important element in the definition is the need to identify either behavior or trait. While behaviors are subject to direct observation, traits are not, since aspects of a trait are internal processes of thought and reaction. Hence, as Livesley (1986), has pointed out, and as is acknowledged in DSM-III-R, a high degree of inference is necessary in transcribing observed behavior into a global trait category, for example, marked and persistent identity disturbance (a borderline-personality-disorder diagnostic criterion). In applying such labels, the observer must infer the presence of urges, needs, perceptions, etc., which are inherent elements of the individual's make-up or personality. This leap from behavioral observation to inference of internal state obviously leads to diagnostic pitfalls, since behavior may not be consistent, influenced by various life factors such as environmental factors or physical or mental capacity.

Botwinick quotes Costa and McCrae (1984, p. 80) in this regard. "Admittedly many things do change with age" . . . (i.e., social roles, bereavement) "And it can be admitted that there are unmistakable age changes in the specific behaviors that express enduring traits". . . . (e.g., activity level) "But all these changes do not amount to change in personality" (p. 80). This implies that personality is dependent primarily on the stability of the individual's inner psychobiological make-up rather than on observable behavior.

As the changes that accompany old age begin to impinge, the individual's behavioral responses become less-reliable measures of personality (i.e., internal) processes or disorder. For example, long-bereaved, socially isolated individuals at the age of 85 may well fulfill criteria for schizoid personality based on behavioral observation: does not appear to desire or enjoy close relationships, chooses solitary activities, is indifferent to praise or criticism of others, absence of close friends or confidants, and displays constricted affect. Longitudinal evaluation using ancillary sources of data may prove difficult, perhaps leaving the diagnostician with an erroneous conclusion about the patient's personality. Hence, personality diagnosis is problematic for any age, but is further confounded in old age.

Beyond questions of reliability and validity of diagnosis of personality disorder in old age, is the question of utility. Is there any reason to make such a diagnosis? Michels (1987) has suggested that no critical therapeutic decisions depend upon the current diagnostic criteria for personality disorder, stating that because no differential therapeutics or prognoses are inherent in these categories, they are of little value to the clinician. One could argue in contrast, however, that clinical utility would be enhanced if diagnosis were also tied to a theoretical etiological construct. For example, if the behavior of the borderline personality stems from primitive abandonment anxiety, then therapeutic intervention could be targeted to deal with this specific factor.

There is some consensus in the clinical literature, supported by studies of personality stability, that the intrapsychic structure of the individual remains consistent throughout life. The clinician (in contrast, perhaps, to the researcher) must take into account both behavioral clues to internal function and reaction, as well as other evidence of intrapsychic function (e.g., transference behaviors) if a full and utilitarian diagnosis is to be arrived at. While somewhat less reproducible between observers, this approach nevertheless helps to reduce the bias that derives from adhering solely to the behavior observational framework. The DSM-III-R recognizes this fact in asserting the importance of etiological theories to guide treatment or stimulate research. It is important, however, that when a theoretical perspective is in use, it be clearly labeled as such and identified.

II. Classification of Personality Disorders

While various approaches may be taken to labeling and grouping PD, the classification used in this chapter will be that of the DSM-III-R. Because specificity of diagnosis is often difficult with PD, the DSM-III-R has taken the appropriate measure of grouping PDs into three clusters, A, B, and C.

1. Cluster A, the odd or eccentric group, includes paranoid, schizoid, and schizotypal PDs;
2. Cluster B, the dramatic, emotional, and erratic group includes antisocial, borderline, histrionic, and narcissistic PDs; and
3. Cluster C, the anxious, fearful group includes avoidant, dependent, obsessive-compulsive, and passive-aggressive PDs.

III. Stability of Personality

The definition of personality and its disorders depends on the demonstration of enduring characteristics throughout adult life. The data on the stability of personality traits strongly favor a concept that underlying reactions to the environment, motivations, and self-perceptions remain relatively unvarying throughout most or all of adult life.

Studies of age-related factors in personality have been of three main types:

1. cross-sectional, examining specific age categories, comparing the traits found to the same factors in another age group;

2. longitudinal, examining personality traits at one time and retesting the same individuals some years later; and
3. cross-sequential, a combination of the longitudinal and cross-sectional designs. This is the more recent technique. A major criticism of the cross-sectional design is that it may be heavily biased by a cohort effect.

Schaie and Parham (1976) suggest that personality is a "function of specific early socialization experiences, commonly shared, generation-specific environmental impact and particular sociocultural transitions, that may affect individuals of all ages" (p. 157). Based on this view, personality changes that arise across the lifespan do so because of sociocultural influences. The concept that personality evolves with age because of biological or maturational forces is not a widely held view according to Botwinick (1984).

The so-called stage theories of development propose that life development occurs on a continuum, with a series of steps or stages that must be negotiated in turn. At each level there is a new task or accomplishment, and a biological force propels each individual along this pathway. The most widely known stage theory is that of Erikson (1963). He proposed eight stages. The first five cover the time between birth and adolescence. Adult stages include intimacy, stage 6 (including tasks of marriage, children, work, and play) generativity, stage 7, (including the task of teaching or guiding the next generation), and ego integrity, stage 8, (which includes the task of acceptance of the natural order of life's successes and failures, followed by inevitable death).

Schaie (1977), has suggested 4 stages of development: independence, goal-oriented behavior, responsibility (age 30 to 60), and the reintegrative stage. This latter stage is reached when life becomes so complicated that it needs to be simplified through retirement, disengagement and selective attention. Schaie postulates that the cognitive skills necessary for the first three stages are different from those needed for the last. However, the measures for the assessment of competence in the final stage are lacking.

In contrast to stage theory, Costa and McCrae (1980), state a widely held view that basic personality, as measured by a variety of standard instruments, remains essentially stable throughout adult life. Schaie and Parham (1976) reported stability of personality in longitudinal age comparisons but found differences in cross-sectional age comparisons. Hence, with regard to maturational theories of personality change, these authors suggest that such change is not the result of intrinsic maturational forces, but rather, arises from differences in the environment of the old and the young, which, therefore, shape personality differently.

Stoner and Panek (1985), using the Comrey Personality Scales in a cross-sectional study of a rural sample, showed that older subjects had significantly higher scores on scales of orderliness, social conformity, and emotional stability, and significantly lower scores on a scale measuring activity and energy. Johnson et al., (1985) studied Hawaiian parents and children of varying ages and ethnicities using the 16 PF (personality factors) (Cattell 1965) and Comrey scales, and found their older subjects to be more orderly, stable, and conscientious, and less active than their younger subjects. Eysenck, Pearson, Easting, & Allsopp (1985) conducted a normative study of 1320 subjects, 271 of whom were 60 or older, using an impulsiveness questionnaire. Mean ratings for impulsiveness and venturesomeness tended to decline with age. Reifman, Klein, and Murphy (1989) found that self-monitoring—the tendency to emphasize social cues over personal feelings—decreased with age in two nonclinical adult samples. Costa *et al.* (1986) observed small but significant decreases with age in extroversion, neuroticism, and openness to experience in a cross-sectional analysis of an epidemiologic sample of 10,063 adults. Analysis of 13-year longitudinal data from the Veterans Administration Longitudinal Study using a short form of the Eysenck Personality Inventory showed that aggregate mean levels of extroversion declined with aging (Spiro, 1990).

Some elements of personality may change over time, but results are conflicting. Overall, it is most striking how little change seems to occur. Conflicting results are difficult to interpret, since many appear to arise because of differences in the study techniques and possibly measuring instruments. The one personality construct that shows replicated change with age, introversion, tends to increase in the older age group (Gutman, 1966; Heron & Chown, 1967; Sealey & Cattell, 1965).

Vaillant and Vaillant (1990) reported on a further followup of a population of healthy college students recruited in 1940 to 1942. There were 204 subjects in the original sample. They were interviewed at the ages of 25, 30, 47, and 57. Interestingly, in this group, when examined prior to the age of 50, the best predictors of psychological health were childhood cohesiveness of the home, relationships with parents that were conducive to trust, autonomy, and initiative. Factors that predicted good psychosocial adjustment in young adulthood, i.e., childhood socioeconomic class, orphanhood, scholastic aptitude, were not correlated with late life outcome. The factors that predicted good psychosocial outcome in late life were good psychosocial adjustment in young adulthood. In Vaillant and Vaillant's opinion, the maturity of ego defenses that evolved in earlier life made the greatest contribution to psychosocial adjustment in late midlife. The most significant predictor of physical and mental health was the use of mood-altering drugs before the age of 50. This finding is particularly relevant to a discussion of PD, because it is the PD group, particularly the cluster B group, that has a high propensity for the aberrant use of drugs. The acting out and self-destructive drug abuse evident in cluster B disorders may be an important predictor of increased vulnerability of this group to a poor psychosocial adaptation with advancing age. Interestingly, psychopathic (antisocial) behavior during college years was not associated with any important outcome variable in psychosocial adjustment at age 65. This finding fits with other data but still does not shed much light on how these traits change, and what new behaviors may evolve, for example, alcoholism, affective disorder, or death. However, based on the data, the authors suggest that the study offers hope that PD, like adolescence, may be a self-limiting disorder.

IV. Epidemiology of Personality Disorder in Old Age _____

While studies of normal personality are important, they cannot be taken as definitive indications when it comes to the study of personality *disorder*. Disorder implies pathology, which may derive from a variety of sources and follow a pathway different from that of normal personality development and expression.

Unfortunately, data in this area are sparse indeed. Even when longitudinal studies have been undertaken, generally they have not taken into account the group older than 65. The studies of personality in aging all trace normal development. However, those results beg the question of what happens to individuals who are already vulnerable and who then experience chronic developmentally expectable stressors, which are normative in human old age. Such stressors include increasing dependency, physical disability, and various other forms of loss and bereavement.

The NIMH longitudinal study as described by Butler (1987) found the same psychiatric disorders in the aged as in the young, with apparently similar genesis and structure. Self-starters, who could establish new contacts and carry out new activities and involvement, had the least disease and longest survival rates. The healthy group was characterized by flexibility, resourcefulness, and optimism, whereas manifestations of mental illness were attributed to medical illness, personality factors, and sociocultural effects rather than the aging process *per se*.

McCrae (1987) has suggested that those elderly subjects who display neurotic characteristics (defined as maladaptive behaviors and proneness to negative emotions including anxiety, anger, depression, and shame) were probably neurotic throughout their adult lives. He further points out that longitudinal and cross-sectional studies show that non-institutionalized elderly score no higher than young adults on measures of neuroticism. Similarly, Schultz (1987) points out that the incidence of clinically significant anxiety is relatively low among older adults. Schaie and Geiwitz (1982) reported a linear decline in anxiety from age 20 to age 70, contrary to theoretical expectations. However, the vulnerable subpopulations such as PD individuals, were not discriminated. Hence, we still do not know the effect of aging on anxiety in this more specific subpopulation. Data from clinical populations perhaps would be more enlightening, but this work, while sorely needed, is still sparse.

Interpreting epidemiologial data on PD is complicated by evolving patterns of diagnosis and by variabilities in populations studied. For example, studies conducted before the publication of DSM-III were limited by the fact that diagnosis was restricted to the index psychiatric disorder. Multiaxial diagnoses, permitting both Axis I and Axis II diagnosis concurrently, led to substantial increases in estimates of PD.

Casey (1988), in reviewing community studies of the epidemiology of PD, makes almost no reference to old age. In studies of community-dwelling adults, a life-time prevalence of PD of 2.1 to 18% has been found (Casey, 1988). Robins *et al.* (1984) reporting on the Epidemiological Catchment Area (ECA) study, found a prevalence rate of .8% for PD in those older than 65 years. However, the instrument used (Diagnostic Interview Schedule), while sensitive to antisocial personalities, was not sensitive to other personality disorders. Hence this estimate is not representative of the true overall incidence of PD in the aged. Blazer *et al.* (1985) found that the prevalence of antisocial personality declined with age.

Personality diagnosis may be missed unless diligently sought. Casey, Dillon, & Tyrer (1984) found that on clinical interview alone, a diagnosis of PD was made by general practitioners in 8.9% of their patients. Psychiatrists examining the same group found a rate of 6.4%. When a formal, structured interview was used however, the rate jumped to 33.9%. This discrepancy was explained by the fact that the clinical diagnosis referred only to the primary diagnosis, while the structured interview made a PD diagnosis independent of any other diagnosis.

Overall, according to Casey (1988), PD is a primary diagnosis in the primary care setting in 5 to 8% of patients, more common in men than in women. Estimates of prevalence of PD in psychiatric hospital populations using multiaxial diagnoses are 30–40% for outpatients and 40–50% for inpatients (Bowman & Sturgeon, 1977; Casey, 1988; Cutting, Cowan, Mann, & Jenkins, 1986; Tyrer, Casey, & Gall, 1983).

Kastrup (1985) studied a Danish cohort of 12,737 first-time admitted psychiatric patients. Of the first-time admitted elderly (17.6% of the first-time admitted cohort was older than 65), she found that presenting complaints, while predominantly in the *senile and organic disorders* group, showed a substantial representation from *reactive disorders* (manic depressive, psychogenic psychosis, neurosis, and personality disorders). Of the males .7%, and of the females, 2.8% had diagnosed personality disorder; 1.9% of males, and 6.9% of females had diagnosed neurotic disorder. Unfortunately, the diagnostic criteria for this large-scale epidemiological study were not identified. Hence it is difficult to make comparisons.

V. Evolution of Personality Disorder Symptoms with Age

The evolution of symptoms into old age is accompanied by change in presentation. Tyrer and Seivewright (1988) go so far as to suggest that "personality disorders seen in early adult life do not present in anything like the same degree, if they present at all, in the elderly" (p. 119). This view, if somewhat overstated, conveys the error inherent in the requirement of the definition of PD that symptoms be enduring or persistent.

The literature makes sparse reference to old age when considering the evolution of symptoms. Solomon departs from the DSM-III-R definition of PD, suggesting that preexisting disorders may become manifest for the first time in old age. Abrams (in press) also suggests that a late-onset variant of PD may present in old age, despite the absence of evidence at this time.

McGlashan (1986), reported on followup data on 94 carefully diagnosed borderline personality disorders 2 to 32 years after treatment. He found that many middle-aged patients developed stable instrumental functioning but did not develop close social and personal relationships. He suggested that "the latter deficit appears not to change with time and may 'haunt' the patients in a symptom-exacerbating fashion as they age and lose their work capacities and opportunities." Patients examined 10–19 years after admission showed improvement, some demonstrating few or no symptoms of personality difficulties. However, after 20 years, there was a suggestion that improvement was less marked.

Snyder, Goodpaster, Pitts, Porkorny, and Gustin (1985) studied 4800 consecutive psychiatric admissions to a Veterans Administration hospital (4691 males, 109 females). They were rated on a 42-item Brief Psychiatric Rating scale from which a seven-item borderline subscale was developed. Results showed a moderate number of borderline traits in 20.7% and severe borderline characteristics in 5.1%. Traits clustered significantly in the under-29 age group with lessening of symptom expression with advancing age (although this study focused on a predominantly middle-aged male population, a weakness in the study acknowledged by the authors). The authors referred to another paper (Synder, Pitts, & Sajadi, 1982) in which it was suggested that the symptoms of borderline PD may reflect cortical immaturity, improving with advancing age. This same group in yet another paper (Gustin, Snyder, & Pitts, 1982) compared Minnesota Multiphasic Personality Inventory (MMPI) profiles of 27 nonborderlines, aged approximately 20–40 years, with a similar group of 21 patients older than 41 years. While both groups showed *borderline* profiles, the younger group had much higher mania-scale scores. They inferred that lower energy levels may be characteristic of older borderlines and that, with advancing age, older borderlines may begin to fulfill few DSM-III criteria because of relative *anergia*.

Just as borderline symptoms evolve with age, so do antisocial traits.. However, despite conventional wisdom that such traits "burn out" by the fifth decade, the evidence is inconsistent. Some authors indeed support this position (Curran & Partridge, 1963; Davis, 1972; Sargeant & Slater, 1962). Maddocks (1970) reviewed the literature on the course of psychopathic personality (now subsumed under the label antisocial) and found a range of opinion largely supportive of improvement of symptoms in the third and fourth decades of life. He studied 57 psychopaths over a period of 5 to 6 years on average. Of this group, 39 (66%) had not settled down, 15 of these developed alcohol abuse, and 15 showed marked hypochondriacal traits.

More recent evidence reported by Arboleda-Florez (1990) throws doubt on the belief that antisocial behavior inevitably declines with age. In examining a cohort of 38 patients aged 41 to 67, conviction data suggested that, while criminality diminished after the age of 27, a significant proportion of the cohort remained criminally active throughout most of their adult lives. He suggested that there may be a subtype of antisocial personality that does not burn out.

Solomon (1981), supports this view in asserting that impulsive traits diminish with age, an opinion confirmed by other clinicians (Verwoerdt 1980). Tyrer and Seivewright (1988) point out that histrionic personality is the female gender equivalent of antisocial personality in men and suggest that the outcome of histrionic PD parallels that of antisocial PD. Data for the elderly do not yet exist.

Schizotypal PD, unassociated with borderline features on long-term followup, frequently leads to schizophrenia (McGlashan 1983), although mixed borderline and schizotypal features tended to follow the borderline pattern of outcome mentioned above. Hence, it is the schizotypal PD that appears to be the less stable of the two disorders over time. Once again, however, data for the elderly age-group are unavailable.

In a group of 928 psychiatric patients (aged approximately 25–50 years), investigated by Casey and Tyrer (1986), Tyrer and Seivewright (1988) describe the relationship of age to personality-trait expression. "The key trait scores for each of the personality categories on the Personality Assessment Schedule (PAS) were calculated. . . . All the categories showed a negative slope, so that the older the patient, the lower the key trait scores" (p. 122). The antisocial and histrionic group showed the clearest decline with age, while the obsessive-compulsive, hypochondriacal, dysthymic, and anxious disorders were more or less independent of age. Fogel and Westlake (1990), reporting on the occurrence of Axis II diagnoses in psychiatric inpatients with major depression, similarly noted that antisocial and histrionic personality diagnoses decreased dramatically with age. Reich, Nduaguba, and Yates (1988), randomly sampled 500 households by questionnaire including the PDQ (Personality Diagnostic Questionnaire). Of the sample, 235 completed the PDQ. Schizoid, schizotypal, and paranoid trait prevalence showed no association with age.

Tyrer and Seivewright suggest that PDs be divided into two groups—the mature (obsessive-compulsive, schizotypal, schizoid, and paranoid) and the immature (borderline, antisocial, narcissistic, histrionic, and passive-aggressive). They justify this division, in part, on the differential outcome, over time, of these disorders. The mature group shows little variation with increasing age, while the immature group are characterized by earlier age of onset (often in childhood or adolescence) and improvement with time. According to these authors, the latter PDs are unusual in the elderly, while the former persist to old age. Solomon (1981) broadly supports this view, asserting that what he calls stable disorders (paranoid, compulsive, and schizotypal) remain stable or get worse with age. Compulsive individuals may become more rigid and demanding; paranoid, more suspicious; and schizoid and schizotypal, more withdrawn and anxious. These statements require the confirmation of careful studies, which are not available to date.

VI. Symptom Expression in the Elderly

Because the term old age is imprecise, it does not specifically define its components. In particular, while stressors are associated with aging, they are not unique to any age group. Rather, various events tend to cluster more frequently in old age. Many of these are associated with loss—decline in physical health, bereavement, role transitions, economic decline, environmental changes, and cognitive disruption. The impact of these events is compounded by the likelihood that more than one event will occur at a time. Hence, the coping capacities of aging individuals who encounter these often severe life stressors are strained. Many elderly individuals cope well or adequately; however, the PD subpopulation is burdened by additional vulnerabilities leading to failure in defensive and coping abilities in the very areas where strength is most required.

Environmental and interpersonal factors will play an important role in determining the expression of PD-related symptoms. Hence, in addition to evaluating the various strengths and weaknesses of the individual as well as the stressors being encountered, a full understanding of the evolution of behavior in PD of old age requires that these elements be placed within the context of the individual's milieu.

Simon (1980) asserted that stress will determine the form and extent of PD symptom expression in old age. The ICD-10 (preliminary draft of September 1988) makes a useful distinction between personality disorder and personality change. In the former, the definition is similar to that in DSM-III-R. Personality change, in contrast to PD, is seen as an acquired disturbance, usually developing in adult life, following severe or prolonged stresses, extreme environmental deprivation, serious psychiatric disorder, or brain disease or injury. Enduring personality change (not attributable to gross brain damage or disease) occurs in individuals with no previous PD following severe prolonged stress, catastrophe, or severe psychiatric illness. To make the diagnosis, the personality change should be significant and associated with inflexible and maladaptive behavior, which had not been present before the pathologic experience. However, the manual acknowledges that the differentiation between an acquired personality change and the unmasking or exacerbation of an existing PD may be very difficult. Importantly, the manual recognizes that enduring personality change may derive from, among other things, bereavement.

The importance of these concepts in the ICD-10 is the recognition that environmental impact may have a profound and long-standing mutagenic effect on personality, lending support to the view that the symptoms of PD, especially in old age, should not be separated from the wider environmental considerations. These may operate either positively or negatively. It is widely accepted by clinicians that the loss of a spouse, impoverishment, chronic physical illness, or institutionalization may aggravate maladaptive personality traits, although the work of Costa and his colleagues shows that these effects may be hard to detect on an epidemiologic basis using standardized tests (Costa, McCrae, & Zonderman, 1987; McCrae & Costa, 1988).

On the positive side, life experience accumulated by old age may have corrective effects on narcissistic personality traits. Ronningstam and Gunderson (1990) observed improvements over 3 years on clinically diagnosed narcissistic personality disorders, and attributed them to achievements, disillusionments, and relationships that had corrective effects on the subjects' narcissistic attitudes. The likelihood of having a corrective experience increases with age. Evidence that current environment could influence the expression of avoidant and dependent traits in elderly individuals is offered in a recent study by Berkowitz, Waxman, and Yaffe (1988). In a controlled study of residents of senior housing, those receiving a special self-help program showed greater self-esteem, social involvement, and sense of control.

Simon (1980) suggests that sensitive, restrictive, phobic, and obsessive-compulsive symptomatology all become more overt because of age-associated tendencies to withdraw from outward concerns. This coincides with the findings of increased introversion with aging, mentioned above. Overall, Simon felt that depressive, paranoid, obsessive-compulsive, dependent, and schizoid personalities are more likely to be seen in old age. Interestingly, in contrast to Tyrer and Seivewright (1988), he also includes histrionic personality in this group of more common PD in old age. The traits of obsessive-compulsive PD may become more overt and, under the stress of aging, "may reach the proportions of a neurosis" (Simon 1980, p. 661). Similarly, dependency characteristics may become more exaggerated when dependence is likely to have more basis in reality. Schizoid PD will be enhanced according to Simon because of the surrounding feelings of loneliness, isolation, and suspiciousness.

Verwoerdt (1981) divides PD into *high-energy* and *low-energy* categories. High-energy personality types include obsessive-compulsive, narcissistic, *paranoid,* and passive-aggressive. Low-energy personality types include passive-dependent and schizoid. He asserts that the high-energy types result in problems with aging, while the opposite is true for low-energy types. He concludes that histrionic and narcissistic personalities will manifest symptoms of depression as their defenses can no longer operate effectively in old age.

Straker (1982) is in broad agreement with others in asserting that paranoid, compulsive, narcissistic, or dependent personalities are more likely to seek assistance because of their "increased vulnerability to changes that are typically associated with aging" (p. 124). He includes dependent personalities in this vulnerable group, unlike Verwoerdt, who views this low-energy disorder as less likely to be assaulted by old age. Paranoid disorders, he suggests, may become more frankly psychotic, while compulsive disorders decompensate into withdrawal and depression. Clinical experience, however, often conflicts with this view. Obsessive-compulsive behavior may become more overt in the face of stress, and the rigidity of rituals, more extreme. Only with the more overwhelming assaults do these defenses crumble into the picture suggested by Straker.

Vaillant and Perry (1985) are less definitive in their conclusions about PD expression in old age. Paranoid PD may take several pathways including no change, schizophrenia, or improvement. They concur with the consensus that histrionic, antisocial, and borderline PD seem to improve with age.

Sadavoy (1987) has proposed that the underlying psychodynamic features of the Cluster B disorders remain relatively unmodified by aging processes. However, the manifestation of symptoms changes. Rather than burning out with age, these individuals remain vulnerable. He proposed that there are five core psychodynamically determined features of personality disorder.

1. the fear or experience of abandonment or internal, empty aloneness;
2. real or fantasized narcissistic injury and loss of self–self–object relationship (Lazarus, 1980);
3. impaired affect tolerance (Krystal, 1987);
4. constitutional failures in development of modulators of rage leading to overreliance on the defence of splitting (Kernberg, 1975); and
5. the fear and experience of loss of self-cohesion (sometimes leading to loss of reality, e.g., minipsychotic states) (Frosch, 1964).

These five vulnerabilities often come under assault from age-relevant stressors, which include interpersonal loss; physical incapacity; physical changes in prized features of the self; role loss and/or transition; loss of defensive outlets (especially those requiring high energy such as sexuality, aggression, and dramatic self-harm); forced intimacy secondary to increased dependency needs; and confrontation with the reality of time, mortality, and death.

As noted above, several authors have commented on the predominance of more passive modes of coping in aging PD. Sadavoy (1987) suggests that these manifest along four pathways in the aging Cluster B group: (1) depressive withdrawal; (2) overreliance on narcissistic defences; (3) somatic (hypochondriacal) preoccupations; and (4) intense interpersonal chaos, especially in high-dependent family or institutional situations. Some research has supported the increase in hypochondriacal symptoms in old age. Calden and Hokanson (1959), and Sevensen (1961), using the MMPI, both reported increased hypochondriacal traits in the elderly.

While dramatic behavioral manifestations diminish with age (although they clearly do not disappear), (Sadavoy, in press), the continued vulnerability of these patients to altered manifestations of underlying vulnerability to stress is probable. Sadavoy (1987), in agreement with others (Solomon, 1981; Verwoerdt, 1981), suggests that it is possible, and perhaps likely, that the alteration of dramatic symptoms to more internally focused symptoms gives the appearance that these patients improve with age. Clinical experience suggests that this is an erroneous idea and may lead the clinician to fail to make an appropriate diagnosis when confronted with the altered, but still aberrant, presentation of symptoms in this group of patients.

A primary symptom presentation is ongoing major problems in interpersonal relationships. The essential nature of these will be described below when considering factors of institutionalization.

A second major pathway of symptom expression is somatic preoccupation. The younger patient with an Axis II diagnosis will often somatize complaints. However, generally there is little objective confirmation of physical disability. In contrast, the older patient must face realistic frailty, which creates a fertile environment for somatization. Such bodily concerns cannot be dismissed as fantasy, making it difficult for the clinician to sort out the fact of physical illness from the patient's inherent anxiety and distortions. As Verwoerdt (1987), has pointed out with regard to the paranoid patient, illness behavior may become a mechanism for maintaining interpersonal contact and, for the Cluster B personality disorder, a method of extracting needed emotional supplies of caring, time, and attention from caregivers. Clinicians should beware, however, of responding to these behaviors as mere manipulation. An important perspective is to recognize that the patient is responding to largely unconscious fears of loss of control, fragmentation, and abandonment. As Gittelson (1948), has pointed out when referring to the elderly in general, "one must consider that the patient's own body may be the only vehicle remaining to him to express the intensity of his inner emotional pain and anxiety" (p. 11).

The third major pathway of expression of PD in old age is depressive withdrawal. This derives from three possible major dynamics. The first is the loss, to the patient, of avenues of acting out, which may lead to the inward expression of affective drive. Often, in the place of acting out, patients express evidence of the inner, empty hopelessness, which they may experience as the events of old age supervene. This withdrawal may follow a period of active protest when the patient's symptoms may have been more vigorous and dramatic. Once the environment fails to respond, however, depressive withdrawal may occur. Such withdrawal may resemble syndrome depression and may be the precipitant for psychiatric referral. Clinicians must take care to establish whether a depressive disorder is indeed present, or whether the symptoms have their roots in rejection sensitivity and abandonment anxiety. It is worth noting, parenthetically, that even if depression seems to be associated with underlying personality vulnerability, primary treatment with antidepressant medication or other forms of therapy may well be in order. Unfortunately, many of these patients remain refractory to intervention (Akiskal 1983).

Another feature of old age that often drives the expression of feelings inward into a depressive picture, is the forced dependency relationships referred to below, as well as societal attitudes. Caregivers may begin to view the regressed or anxious behavior of the vulnerable patient as a normal outcome of aging, thereby failing to understand and respond to the patient's protestations or acting out as expressions of personality pathology that need specific treatment and understanding. Finally, institutionalization, as noted below, may lead to a variety of factors that promote a depressive response in these patients.

In summary, clinical descriptions and sparse research data all support the view that the expression of cluster B disorders changes with aging, the dramatic, high-energy symptoms diminishing or disappearing, while the depressive, anxious–dependent, and hypochrondiacal symptoms become more evident. As Abrams (1991) asserts, the cluster B diagnoses are assigned to geriatric patients especially infrequently, possibly because they are truly immature syndromes that prove unstable over long periods. Opinion on the disorders of clusters A and C is less uniform, preventing a clear consensus statement at this time. If the clinical writings are taken as a group, it is evident that all of these personality disorders are vulnerable to the stresses of old age, often leading to impaired function in the aged patient. However, several authors have emphasized the need to distinguish regressive behavior, even if long-standing, precipitated by illness, institutionalization, or loss and abandonment from true personality disorder (Fogel & Martin, 1987).

VII. Residual and Emergent Personality Disorders

Emergent and residual catagories in PD diagnosis were first suggested by the authors at a meeting of the DSM-IV Geriatric Workshop. The terms are not yet in common usage but may serve as a useful shorthand to describe possible or probable evolutions in the expression of PD in old age, as will be described below.

As noted above, personality, in the sense of general behavioral dispositions measurable by standard personality tests, shows considerable stability over the life course (Costa *et al.*, 1987; Costa *et al.*, 1986). This observation must be reconciled with the decline in clinical personality disorder diagnoses with age (Casey & Schrodt, 1989; Fogel & Westlake, 1990; Kastrup, 1985; Mezzich, Fabrega, Coffman, & Glavin, 1987; Snyder, Goodpaster, Pitts, Pokorny, & Gustin, 1985), as well as with clinical impressions of age-related aggravation of unpleasant or maladaptive personality traits in some older persons. The apparent discrepancy probably has multiple explanations, beginning with the point that personality stability in general adult populations is certainly compatible with clinical instability in individuals and subpopulations. Other relevant phenomena of normal aging may include *changes toward decreased impulsivity, activity, extroversion, and self-monitoring, and toward greater orderliness and conscientiousness* (Stoner & Panek, 1985; Eysenck *et al.*, 1985; Reifman *et al.*, 1989; Costa *et al.*, 1986).

Declines in activity, impulsiveness, and extroversion with age may be related to age-related decrease in diagnosed personality disorders of the dramatic cluster. Increases in orderliness and conscientiousness may help explain the high rate of diagnoses of compulsive personality disorder reported among elderly depressed inpatients by Fogel and Westlake (1990). Self-monitoring changes could be relevant to a greater expression of maladaptive or deviant traits in some individuals, provided that they did not require a high level of energy or activity for their expression.

Age-related changes in circumstances, especially significant losses, are widely believed by clinicians to influence the behavioral expression of personality traits (Myers, 1990). *Depression, a widely prevalent and often chronic axis I disorder in old age, may influence both the expression and the rating of maladaptive personality traits* (Hirschfeld *et al.,* 1983; Thompson, Gallagher, & Czirr 1988; Zimmerman, Pfohl, Coryell, Corenthal, & Stangl, 1990). *Early dementia is often associated with personality change, with altered personality at times more prominent than initial cognitive changes.*

Recent studies by Petry and colleagues (Petry, Cummings, Hill, & Shapira, 1988; Petry, Cummings, Hill, & Shapira, 1989) showed increases in passive and self-centered behavior, which were strongly correlated with the course of Alzheimer-type dementia. Rubin and Kinscherf (1989) reported that patients with questionable dementia [Clinical Dementia Rating (CDR) of .5] showed significantly more passive, self-centered, and agitated behavior than controls; personality changes were similar to those seen in mild but definite dementia (CDR of 1.0). The early personality changes of the type described could aggravate pre-existing, dependent, or narcissistic traits, and initially present as a personality disorder, before cognitive deficits became predominant. This issue is discussed more fully below.

Changes in neurotransmitter function associated with aging may alter basic behavioral dispositions, leading to alterations in personality. Diseases and medications prevalent among older persons that affect neurotransmitter function may have similar effects.

Cloninger (1987) presented a speculative relationship between three crucial dimensions of personality, and the activity of three major neurotransmitter systems. Behavioral activation (novelty seeking) was linked to dopamine, behavioral inhibition (harm avoidance) was linked to serotonin, and behavioral maintenance (reward dependence) was linked to norepinephrine. Traditional personality categories were mapped by Cloninger onto stimulus–response characteristics. For example, an antisocial personality would be seen as high on novelty seeking and low on harm avoidance and reward dependence. A common feature of antisocial, histrionic, and explosive personalities in the Cloninger scheme is a high level of novelty seeking. It is tempting to speculate that the decline in dopaminergic function with normal aging (Finch & Morgan, 1987) could be linked to a reduced prevalence of these disorders in late life.

More broadly, changes in the noradrenergic and serotonergic systems are also known to occur in late life (Veith & Raskind, 1988), and may be aggravated by common diseases, such as Alzheimer's disease or Parkinson's disease. The applicability of Cloninger's theory to late-life PD could be empirically tested in studies of personality change in the setting of disease with measurable neurochemical correlates.

As already stated above, PD, according to DSM-III-R, are pervasive patterns of behavior that begin by early adulthood (APA, 1987, pp. 335–336). However, in DSM-III-R, it is implied that while attainment of a criterion number of behaviors is needed for diagnosis, not all criteria were *necessarily* present continuously since early adulthood. Thus, the door is open for DSM-III-R personality disorders to *remit* in later life, as well as for them to *emerge* from long-standing traits if behavioral manifestations become more florid in later years. Although borderline (Gunderson, 1989) and narcissistic (Plakun, 1990) PD may remit over time, they are often left with persistence of many maladaptive traits. Such individuals with *remitted* PD may respond differently to the vicissitudes of old age than those who never had PD. For this reason, the category of *residual personality disorder* deserves consideration to describe patients who once met full Axis II criteria but currently have only subsyndromal traits. Diagnoses of residual PD could have clinical value in identifying patients who might require different therapeutic or environmental management to reduce the possibility of acting out or malignant regression. In research, systematic identification of residual PD would permit a better understanding of the relationship between prior PD and the occurrence of emotional and behavioral problems relatively specific to old age, such as maladaptive relationships with caretaking children, or malignant regression in long-term care facilities.

Similarly, a category of *emergent personality disorder* deserves consideration, to describe those individuals who, in old age, meet full Axis II criteria, but whose traits were subsyndromal before late life. The application of this category in epidemiologic research would aid in the identification of both individual and social factors that lead to late-life aggravation of personality traits. Further, it would allow more precise diagnoses in cases in which mild organic disease appeared to produce disproportionate behavioral abnormalities, by identifying the subset of patients in whom aggravation of long-standing personality difficulties was the primary issue.

VIII. Special Considerations

Special emphasis is due certain of the age-relevant factors that alter the intensity or nature of the presentation of PD-related symptoms. These include the effect of institutionalization and associated dependency, the relationship between affective disorder and PD, and the impact of dementia and cognitive disorders on the syndrome.

A. Organic Factors

A large number of neurologic diseases and focal brain lesions may produce characteristic disturbances of personality. Two well-known examples are the interictal personality disorder of complex partial epilepsy, and the disinhibited, facetious behavior of patients with severe frontal lobe damage. A classic perspective on organic PD is offered in Lishman's (1987) work on organic psychiatry and will not be further discussed here. This section will address how commonly occurring brain diseases of later life might modify the expression of the traditional *non organic* personality disorders.

Dysfunction of the orbital frontal region may impair inhibition and reduce empathy (Stuss & Benson, 1986). This may aggravate antisocial, narcissistic, histrionic, or borderline traits. Highly prevalent causes of orbital–frontal dysfunction in later life include dementia (including Alzheimer's disease and Pick's disease), and drugs, particularly benzodiazepines and barbiturates (Fogel & Eslinger, in press).

Dorso–lateral frontal lobe dysfunction leads to impaired planning and motivation, and reduces appreciation of social circumstances (Stuss & Benson, 1986). Lack of planning and motivation may aggravate dependent and passive-aggressive traits. Decreased appreciation of social circumstances could also increase the oddness or eccentricity of a schizotypal patient's behavior, or the coolness or aloofness of a schizoid or narcissistic personality. Common causes of dorso–lateral frontal dysfunction are similar to those of orbital–frontal dysfunction, with the added point that the dorso–lateral frontal regions are heavily dependent on dopaminergic input, and thus subject to functional disruption by Parkinson's disease or neuroleptic drug therapy (Fogel & Eslinger, in press).

Parietal and temporal lobe dysfunction may cause misperception of sensory stimuli (Mesulam, 1985). In paranoid personalities, these might aggravate suspiciousness. In avoidant individuals, perplexing sensory misperceptions could promote further withdrawal. Right-hemisphere damage leading to misperceptions of the emotional content of speech and gestures may aggravate the empathic deficits of narcissistic, antisocial, and paranoid patients. Common causes of temporal- and parietal-lobe dysfunction in later life include cerebrovascular disease and Alzheimer's disease.

Subcortical diseases, including Parkinson's disease, can reduce overall activity, energy, and motivation (Freedman & Albert, 1985). These changes lead to diminished expression of all energy-dependent traits, from the dramatic expressions of histrionic personalities to the perfectionism and hard work of the compulsive personality. These behavioral traits are thus attenuated. However, affective reactions, such as depression or anxiety, could be provoked by the loss of habitual, energy-dependent defenses. Dependent and avoidant traits could be aggravated, the former by increased passivity and the latter by patients' avoidance of the increased subjective effort required for social interaction.

In all of these situations, the behavioral correlates of the organic disorders are well established, but the frequency and magnitude of effects on personality traits have not been systematically studied using standardized measures of personality. It is not known to what extent organic factors account for personality traits' crossing the line from the syndromal to the subsyndromal in either direction. It is to be hoped that the deficit of systematic knowledge in this area would be remedied by the more systemic use of standardized dimensional personality measures in geriatric studies. Also, the concepts of residual and emergent PD may prove valuable in research employing categorical personality diagnosis.

B. Institutionalization

Some authors have addressed the interaction of the PD patient within the institutional setting, in particular the impact of the institution on narcissistic pathology (Breslau, 1980; Sadavoy, 1987; Sadavoy & Dorian, 1983). However, no larger-scale studies, even of an uncontrolled nature, have yet been undertaken in this age group. Conversely, we know little about the effect that PD individuals have on the institution, although clinical case examples have been published (Sadavoy & Dorian, 1983; Sadavoy 1987; Sadavoy, in press).

Bennett (1983) reported finding that residents who experienced isolation before entering a home had difficulty becoming socialized. This finding is relevant to PD, in that an examination of the unsocialized group revealed that 45% of 100 consecutive admissions to the home for the aged that was studied were lifelong isolates, a figure that (the author points out) parallels the national institutional surveys, which show that about 50% of the elderly in institutions fall into this category of lifelong isolation. A cautious conclusion may be considered that the isolated group is made up, in part, of Cluster A PDs who, by virtue of their isolated lifestyles, may be more vulnerable to premature institutionalization. Once admitted to the institution, they may fail to integrate adequately, and the forced interactions inherent in institutional life may exacerbate symptoms of anxiety, agitation, or paranoia. Absence of data makes it necessary to explore these interactive factors in a more organized fashion.

C. Forced Intimacy

It is clear, regardless of the specific category of PD, that interpersonal dysfunction is a central and core characteristic of the syndromes. Perhaps the most difficult group in this regard are the Cluster B personality disorders, characterized by a sensitivity to rejection, intense affective responsiveness when disappointed, highly ambivalent, *love–hate* relationships, and related defensive processes characterized by splitting. The cause of these behaviors is not known. However, certain factors, based on psychodynamic theory, seem relevant particularly for the institutionalized PD elderly. Silver (1985), has suggested that the underlying dynamic structure of the Cluster B personality disorder is based in part on a primitive development that requires maximal mobility in relationships in order for defensive maneuvers to be most effective. The patient's control over the intensity of or distance in the relationship permits the patient to modulate feelings, protecting the patient from being overwhelmed, either by fears of merging or engulfment, or by anxiety engendered by poorly controlled internal feelings of rage, which are often mobilized in relationships in this patient group. This relationship ambivalence is often at the root of the interpersonal chaos seen in the young-adult years when symptomatology is most intense. Using this model, it is evident that the more restricted the patient is in modulating the intensity of her or his relationships with others, the greater the danger of exacerbation of personality pathology.

These factors become highly relevant when this type of patient enters the more-dependent phases of old age. In this group, as dependency needs, both real and fantasized, become more intense, and the potential for controlling the relationship becomes increasingly less likely because of the patient's actual reliance on others, the relationships of the PD individual become *emotional traps* (Sadavoy, 1987). While in younger patients, if the intensity of the therapeutic relationship becomes overwhelming, distance may be permitted or promoted (Silver, 1985), in the elderly this strategy may be either impractical or impossible. Whatever the vulnerability of the patient or the skill of the therapist, no matter whether one ideally should titrate the intensity of the relationship in order to attend to the fragility of the patient's intrapsychic structure, each of these factors may be overridden by the unavoidable fact of the patient's need to have someone do for him what, in reality, he cannot do for himself.

As the patient's tension rises without the possibility of distance or separation, which would permit some reintegration, all members of the system including other patients, as well as staff, are enmeshed in an interactive system that may lead to a chaotic breakdown of institutional structure (Sadavoy & Dorian, 1983). Staff anger may begin to develop, often leading to scapegoating of one member of the team. Staff may become demoralized and depressed by the unyielding intensity of a patient's emotional barrage, leading to increased absences, sick leave, and so on. When conflicts arise with families, members of the team are prone to feel accused and may become defensive in the way that they approach and deal with the patient. This is particularly evident when the patient and/or family becomes litigious. In these circumstances the patient's and families' complaints often are passed on to the administrative level of the institution. Subsequent enquiries that may carry a tone of blaming or nonsupport of the staff will increase the tensions.

Staff, under these circumstances, are often unaware of the source of the conflict and increased ward tensions. These feelings can permeate all aspects of the work and lead to marked alterations in the atmosphere of caring and help-provision on a unit.

The reaction of staff, particularly untrained or unsophisticated staff, will often aggravate rather than ameliorate the pathological situation. These reactions can lead staff to become overly solicitous, attempting to fulfill the unending needs of the patient, leading then only to increased levels of anger and frustration or guilt. Additionally, in the escalating efforts to control the patient's behavior, the therapeutic element inherent in appropriate limit setting may evolve into a punitive angry and unfeeling stance toward the patient. The manipulativeness and overt hostility of such patients, which is often evident, may lead staff to view them as bad rather than troubled. Many of these responses are not specific to the aged population and have been described by many authors (Main, 1957; Ploye, 1977).

However, the caregivers of the institutionalized elderly are in a somewhat unique position, in contrast to the caregivers of the younger, PD patient. The main difference is that the caregivers of the institutionalized elderly are *trapped* in a long-term indefinite contract. The staff do not have ready access to alternative methods of management, such as that suggested by Friedman (1969), who proposed that transferring the difficult patient off the unit may be the most appropriate method of intervention. Undoubtedly, the aged PD patient who creates major difficulties for staff in a long-term care institution, is at risk for transfer to a psychiatric institution. The realities of modern psychiatric practice, perhaps in contrast to years past, makes it highly likely that psychiatric facilities will be unable and unwilling to accept the long-term care of these troubled patients. Hence, even if transfer is considered, it will likely be a short-term intervention leading the patient to be returned to the unit, generally without much basic alteration in behavior. In the main, staff of long-term care facilities have to tolerate the often chaotic ward situations these patients may produce. Under such circumstances, when the staff are helplessly enmeshed with the patient, feelings of rage may emerge, leading the caregivers to fantasize the patient's death, as a mechanism of releasing them from the unbearable situation. These feelings may produce conscious or unconscious feelings of guilt in the staff, who may respond in a variety of fashions, sometimes with angry rejection of the patient, and at other times with oversolicitious and inappropriate attempts to rescue them. As Sadavoy and Dorian (1983) pointed out, the unacknowledged rage that may evolve can promote an abandonment of therapeutic optimism and balanced intervention so necessary in the care of these patients, sometimes increasing the danger of suicidal acting-out by the patient (Maltsberger & Buie, 1974).

Another central feature of care of the PD elderly in the institution is the necessity for the caregiver to provide intimate, personal, hands-on treatment and support. In light of the highly ambivalent feelings that arise both in patient and caregiver under such circumstances, this enforced intimacy can further exacerbate feelings of agitation, anxiety, and sometimes chaos in all members of the system. Just as the caregivers are in a situation different from that of treatment of the younger patient, so the patient is in a different situation. The environment of the long-term care institution tends to homogenize the identity of the older individual, often leading to a failure of the caregivers to know the patient as a separate, well-defined individual. Hamilton, Book, Sadavoy, & Silver, (1979) have shown that the attractiveness of the patient to the therapist is a factor in promoting a positive outcome in long-term psychotherapy of characterologically disturbed younger patients. This attractiveness may be inherent in the patient's physical appearance, intelligence, occupational ability, record of accomplishment, productivity, or wealth. The elderly institutionalized patient, in contrast, often has little or no evidence of these attributes. Under such circumstances, the attractiveness of the patient is redefined, and comprises behavior characterized as compliant, pleasant, and even cute. Individuality, intelligence, and a sense of uniqueness are not highly valued in institutional life, in which it is often necessary to deal with groups of patients as a unit. Hence, patients who are agitatedly attempting to maintain a fragile sense of self, a situation common to the PD individual, are often viewed as disruptive. Conversely, patients who withdraw and attempt to conform to the perceived norm of the environment, may become viewed by the staff as somewhat childlike objects, treated in a kind but condescending way. Either response may lead the patient to experience a sense of further loss of narcissistic supplies as well as further fragmentation in the internal perception of self.

D. Personality Disorder and Depression

As noted above, several authors have commented on the vulnerability of patients with PD, particularly Clusters B and C, to manifestations of depression under the stress of old age. Conversely, depressive disorder is often associated with features of PD, which makes it difficult, and at times impossible, to separate the two diagnoses until the affective disorder has been effectively treated (Hirschfeld et al., 1983; Koenigsberg, Kaplan, Gilmore, & Cooper, 1985; Liebowitz et al., 1979). A number of studies have established that patients in the midst of major depression show more maladaptive personality traits than when in remission, whether they are rated by questionnaire or by interview (Hirschfeld et al., 1983; Thompson et al., 1988; Zimmerman et al., 1990). Avoidant and dependent traits are particularly accentuated by depression. Chronic depression in particular might be expected to persistently aggravate maladaptive traits, at times beyond the threshold for diagnosis of an Axis II disorder. As Abrams (1991) has pointed out, dependency, helplessness, somatic preoccupation, and negative self-evaluation, which are frequent symptoms in elderly depressives, may represent either depressive phenomena or PD. Parenthetically, the difficulty in making this diagnosis also highlights the importance of avoiding a definitive Axis II diagnosis when acute depressive episodes or chronic dysthymia are evident or suspected. Similar caution may be expressed with regard to acute anxiety states, which also seem to distort personality assessment (Reich, 1985; Reich et al., 1987).

It is still uncertain how much of the chronic depressive syndromes should be or may be attributable to PD. In the elderly, there is a high degree of depressive dysphoria (15% in Blazer & Williams study, 1980). While the clinician may suspect that a proportion of these patients, perhaps the majority, become dysphoric because of pre-existing personality vulnerabilities that lead them to be more vulnerable to the stresses of aging, there are no strong data one way or the other. Attempts to differentiate this group have led to other terminology, such as that of double depression or depressive invalidism. The incomplete remissions often inherent in treatment of these patients may be attributable to concurrent PD that confounds the treatment process. Abrams (1991) suggests that masked depression (in which cognitive or somatic symptoms are more prominent than sadness, tearfulness, or other affective manifestations) may be a presentation of PD in the elderly.

The unreliability of the self-report of symptoms in depressed patients with regard to the assessment of personality has been reported by Hirschfeld, Klerman, Clayton, Keller, McDonald-Scott, and Larkin (1983). In their sample of 114 patients, 40 recovered depressions, 48 unrecovered depressions, and 26 partially recovered depressions, rated on scales of emotional strength and interpersonal dependency, there was a significant shift toward the healthier direction once patients recovered from depression, compared to their scores when assessed during the depressive episode. They showed consistently lower scores on scales of neuroticism, orality, emotional reliance on another person, and lack of social self-confidence. Scores were higher on scales of emotional stability and objectivity in the recovered phase. Overall, the study reveals that depression alters self-perception and may skew the assessment process in the direction of a greater appearance of pathology based on the patient's self-report. This finding has been supported by the work of Reich *et al.*, (1987). Zimmerman, Pfohl, Stangl, & Corenthal (1986), have shown that collateral information is crucial in making PD diagnosis. In another study, Zimmerman, Pfohl, Coryell, Stangl, & Corenthal (1988), interviewed a group of 66 depressed patients and conducted parallel informant interviews. Informants described much more personality-related psychopathology in the patients than did the patients themselves on self-report.

E. Treatment Issues

Very little specific information is available on treatment of PD patients in old age. In part, clinicians are inevitably to be confused by the diagnostic dilemmas that plague Axis II disorders. One is often left puzzling whether there is an underlying physical or Axis I disorder that is leading to an apparent Axis II picture. Moreover, collateral histories are often difficult to obtain even though, as Zimmerman has shown, they are likely to be essential if one is to make an accurate retrospective evaluation of the patient's personality functioning (Zimmerman *et al.*, 1986). Fogel and Martin (1987) have highlighted the importance of avoiding a diagnosis of personality disorder in the institutionalized medically ill elderly. Patients in this situation, as well as in other institutional settings, are often prone to regressive behaviors, which are difficult or impossible to sort out from PD. It is only by careful retrospective evaluation, looking for consistent lifelong patterns in the patient's behavior, that appropriate diagnoses may be made. As is shown elsewhere in this chapter,use of standard PD rating scales may be unreliable in this age group. Despite these difficulties, however, PD should be diligently sought out. As Casey's (1984) work suggests, failure to actively consider PD diagnosis will probably lead to underdiagnosis.

The treatment of disorders such as depression or anxiety may be slowed or frustrated by the presence of coexistent personality. Hence, the clinician must be diligent in efforts to diagnose this component of the patient's disorder and institute appropriate measures to deal with it. Various strategies have been employed and include individual psychotherapy, family system intervention, staff education and environmental change, and involvement of representatives of institutional administration in the overall treatment plan, if necessary (Sadavoy, in press; Sadavoy, 1987; Sadavoy & Dorian, 1983).

This section deals primarily with cluster B disorders as they present in the institution. To date little may said about age-relevant issues in treatment of the A and C clusters or about outpatient treatment that is not purely speculative, unsupported by either clinical or empirical data. Treatment that has been applied to younger adults patients may be equally effective (for many normative aging PD individuals) in the 65–75 age range. However, the ego-depletions of the older aged, including cognitive change, make it likely that new approaches will have to be developed for that group.

Sadavoy (1987), speaking of the Cluster B patients, identifies 4 goals of treatment:

1. containing and limiting pathological behavior;
2. establishing a working alliance between patient, staff, and family;
3. developing a cohesive team approach to the patient; and
4. reducing the patient's reliance on primitive pathological behaviour by reducing inner tension levels, altering interpersonal stresses and, infrequently, changing or modifying defense mechanisms.

Containment of pathological behavior utilizes a basic psychodynamic understanding of the patient's psychological state and behavior, to inform the introduction of cognitive behavioral interventions. Once a careful formulation has been developed and understood by all staff members, a conceptual model is formed, which becomes the basis of the treatment plan. In the treatment of younger patients, a formal written contract may be useful, and this form of intervention has been described for the elderly (Sadavoy, 1987; Sadavoy & Dorian, 1983). The treatment plan is often most effective if the staff can construct a mechanism for permitting the patient to maintain a sense of control over certain elements in the environment, while the staff takes control of those aspects of the patient's behavior that are causing major disruption, and that need to be settled in order for the patient to live in the milieu and maintain relationships. These treatment plans should be highly specific and detail the items of behavior to be focused upon, the milieu programs that must be attended by the patient, visiting hours, medications, and so forth. Such plans are most effective if written out to reduce confusion for both patient and staff. Such an approach helps to limit staff splitting, as do ongoing staff conferences to discuss the treatment program, a most important strategy, especially in the early phases of treatment.

Formation of a working alliance helps to identify the need for patient and therapist to define and work toward a mutual goal on behalf of the patient. Such an alliance is often difficult to establish with PD patients, and indeed, may be impossible. When families are present, it is crucial to involve them in the treatment planning. Failure to do so will leave the patient a frequently used avenue to split staff and family, creating situations in which the family members ally themselves with the patient's pathological responses to the environment, leading to heightened family-staff conflict.

IX. Research Directions

The study of PD and related disorders in old age offers an important opportunity to investigate their lifelong outcome. However, clearly the methodology will suffer from the restrictions of retrospective data, cohort effects, and the confounders posed by the multiple illnesses and stressors that are the norm in late life. Research into this aspect of psychiatric disorder, therefore, will require imaginative research strategies and the use of longitudinal prospective studies, which extend from younger years into old age. Cross-sectional studies, while most practical, must be examined critically, because the available data have shown that the patient's report of past behaviors associated with PD may be suspect, that current symptoms may be distorted by other Axis I disorders, most notably affective states, and that collateral informants may have inherent biases.

Perhaps the first task for researchers in this area is to develop reliable, valid measures of PD in old age. This is a formidable task, but essential since the currently employed measures are unlikely to tap the more age-specific behaviors and/or dynamics associated with old age.

The initial stage of scale construction, i.e., determining the items to be inquired about, is itself difficult. Little consensus exists among therapists about the expression of PD in old age. Hence, a preliminary stage to be encouraged is publication of carefully diagnosed cases of PDs in old age to help develop an empirical database for the development of valid items.

A. Structured Assessment of Personality Disorders in the Elderly

The 1980s were a time of intensive development of questionnaires and structured interviews for the categorical assessment of PDs based on DSM-III or ICD-9 classification schemes. Questionnaires included the Millon Clinical Multiaxial Inventory (MCMI) (Millon, 1982) and the Personality Disorder Questionnaire (PDQ) (Hyler, Reider, Spitzer, & Williams, 1982). Structured interview schedules included the Structured Interview for the DSM-III Personality Disorders (SID-P) (Stangl, Pfohl, Zimmerman, Bowers, & Corenthal, 1985), the Structured Clinical Interview for DSM-III-R Personality Disorder (SCID-II) (Spitzer, Williams, & Gibbon, 1987), the Personality Disorder Examination (PDE) (Loranger, Susman, Oldham, & Russakoff, 1985), the Personality Assessment Schedule (PAS) (Tyrer, Alexander, & Ferguson, 1988), and the Standardized Assessment of Personality (SAP) (Mann, Jenkins, Cutting, & Cowen, 1981).

These instruments were compared by Ferguson and Tyrer (1988), and more extensively by Reich (1985). They noted that all questionnaires, including the PDQ and the MCMI, are particularly vulnerable to contamination by the patient's present mood state. Zimmerman et al., (1990) observed that depressed inpatients showed generally higher rates of PD than did controls when assessed with the PDQ, but not with the SID-P. More generally, questionnaire and interview scales for DSM-III PDs show limited agreement. For example, in one study that compared the SID-P with both the MCMI and the PDQ, kappa correlations for several disorders were low, with agreement between interview and questionnaire poorest for compulsive personality (Reich, Noyes, & Troughton, 1987). Similarly, Hyler *et al.*, (1989) showed relatively poor agreement for PD diagnoses made using the PDQ and those made by clinicians, on a sample of 552 patients aged 14 to 77 (maximum kappa of .46).

In the reliability and validity studies of these instruments, aged subjects were included, but to our knowledge, no specific analysis of reliability and validity of any structured personality instrument has been carried out on an elderly sample.

Of the interview-based instruments, the SID-P, the SCID-II, and the PDE take more than an hour each to administer. This potentially limits their applicability to aged subjects with diminished stamina, and their suitability for inclusion in broad, diagnostic test batteries that might be used in general geriatric settings. (Commonly used mental measures in general geriatric batteries, such as the Geriatric Depression Scale (Yesavage *et al.*, 1983), can be administered in 10 minutes or less.) Aside from practical constraints on administration, the foundation of structured instruments on DSM-III-R may be particularly problematic for the elderly, in that DSM-III-R criteria may be based on somewhat age-specific *manifestations* of disordered personality, rather than enduring behavioral dispositions. Both manifestations and dispositions deserve scientific study, and it is too early to say which are most relevant to the understanding of life course and illness outcome in old age.

B. Future Research

It is not known the extent to which PDs of the dramatic cluster actually remit in old age, as opposed to changing their form. The issue would be addressed best by longitudinal studies combining categorical and dimensional assessments of personality at multiple time points. Evidence that such an approach might reveal substantial differences between categorical and dimensional evaluations is provided by Levenson, who studied change in alcohol consumption and problem drinking over a 9-year interval in a sample of 1498 men in the Veterans Administration Longitudinal Study (Levenson, 1990). He found that while the correlation in mean annual alcohol consumption between baseline and followup was .62, there was nearly complete turnover in the problem-drinking category, with 91% of problem drinkers at baseline and not such at follow-up. Thus, overt *problem behaviors* of the kind used to make DSM-III-R dramatic cluster diagnoses, may be more unstable than underlying behavioral dispositions.

In the meantime, investigators interested in PD as a covariate in geriatric studies might consider including at least one well-established dimensional measure of personality in their assessment batteries. This strategy would both improve the interpretability of their results and add to the currently sparse validation literature on structured assessments for PD in old age.

As is evident throughout this chapter, little systematic study, either clinical or empirical, exists with reference to outpatients with PD. This is a fertile area of inquiry.

An area of inquiry of essential importance is the relationship between Axis II disorders in old age, and affective disorders. As noted above, in this chapter, the presence of affective disorder often mobilizes behaviors that may resemble PD. Conversely, the presence of such disorders is a probable interacting variable that will promote refractoriness to the pharmacological treatment of depression. While firm data is lacking, the authors' clinical experience in chronic care institutions suggests that patients who are referred for behavioral and interpersonal difficulties and who have accompanying depressive features, often have evidence of depressive disorder earlier in life. However, it has yet to be determined whether such a history is actually revealing of a recurrent depressive disorder, or whether the *depressive episodes* were actually environmentally and interpersonally provoked reactions reflective of personality pathology, rather than affective spectrum disorder. An answer to this question is important in light of the frequency of depressive illness among institutionalized, particularly chronically ill, elderly (Sadavoy *et al.*, 1990), since the approach to treatment may be quite different depending on whether a predominantly Axis I or Axis II diagnosis is made.

In general, suicide is an important problem in geriatric psychiatry. Many studies have shown that there is a high correlation between the presence of PD and suicide attempts. (Lukianowcz, 1973; Philip & McCulloch, 1968; Vinoda, 1969). Evidence is strong that suicide attempters are in the younger age group. In Philip's (1970) study, 74% of all attempters were in the 21- to 50-year-old age group. This was confirmed by Whitlock and Schapira (1967), who found that two thirds of their sample of 274 patients were younger than 40 years. These authors suggested that the 30- to 39-year-old age group is the most suicide prone. They were speaking here about suicide *attempters,* who show a high rate among male adolescents and a peak in the rate among 30- to 39-year-old females. There is a significant decline in suicide attempts after the age of 50. Of great importance, however, is that there is a low *completer* incidence in adolescence, which rises in the third and fourth decades, but peaks between the ages of 50 and 70 before declining again. (McCarthy & Walsh, 1966). It is evident from these studies that the young-old age group is more likely to complete suicide, while the younger age group is more likely to attempt but not complete suicide. While it is well known that personality disorder is associated with attempters, we still do not know very much about suicide attempters and completers in old age. While aberrant personality traits or PD may predispose to a greater degree of vulnerability to intense depressive ideation and perhaps suicidal impulsivity in later life, there are no hard investigational data at this time. In light of the public health implications of this issue, it is of obvious importance to geriatric psychiatry research.

The clinical descriptions of PD patients in the institution makes it clear that in some and perhaps many circumstances, these patients create major difficulties that have a profound impact on staff, other patients, and overall institutional life. Because of the difficulties that such patients pose, as well as the possibility that PD in itself may be a predisposing factor to institutionalization, it is important that the role of PD in the preinstitutional and institutional phase of the geriatric patients' life be investigated. In particular, it would be of great interest to know more about the relationship between the family difficulties often inherent in the relationships of PD patients and the impetus which these difficulties may provide toward premature institutionalization of the patient.

Similar research efforts will be important in the relationship of PD to alcoholism and prescription drug use in the elderly, each of which has profound effects on both economic aspects of health care for the elderly and on human misery.

Finally, we know very little about the relationship between PD and medical illness in old age. Does the presence of personality or significant trait disorder earlier in life alter the likelihood of later life illness and/or morbidity? As noted above, these issues may be especially relevant to the nature of the symptomatology associated with organic brain disease, particularly the dementias.

References

Abrams, R. (1991). Anxiety and personality disorders. In J. Sadavoy, L. Lazarus, & L. Jarvik (Eds.), *Comprehensive Review of Geriatric Psychiatry* (pp. 369–386). Washington DC: American Psychiatric Press Inc.

American Psychiatric Association (1987). *Diagnostic and statistical manual of mental disorders* (3rd ed., rev.). (DSM-III-R). Washington, DC: American Psychiatric Association.

Akiskal, H. S. (1983). Dysthymic disorder: psychopathology of proposed chronic depressive subtypes. *American Journal of Psychiatry, 140,* 11–20.

Arboleda-Florez, J. (1990). *Antisocial burnout: An exploratory study.* Presented at the Annual Meeting of the American Psychiatric Association, New York.

Bennett, R. (1983). The socially isolated elderly. In M. K. Arenson, R. Bennett, & B. Gurland (Eds.), *The acting-out elderly* (p. 45–54). New York: Haworth Press.

Berkowitz, M. W., Waxman, R., & Yaffe, L. (1988). The effects of a resident self-help model on control, social involvement, and self-esteem among the elderly. *The Gerontologist, 28,* 620–624.

Blazer, D., & Williams, C. D. (1980). The epidemiology of dysphoria and depression in an elderly population. *American Journal of Psychiatry, 137* (4), 439.

Blazer, D., George, L. K., Landeman, R., Pennybacker, M., Melville, M. L., Woodbury, M., Manton, K. G., Jordan, K., & Lake, B. (1985). Psychiatric disorders. A rural urban Comparison. *Archives of General Psychiatry, 42,* 651–656.

Botwinick, J. (1984). *Aging and behaviour. A comprehensive integration of research findings* (3rd ed., pp. 143–165). New York: Springer.

Bowman, M. J., & Sturgeon, D. A. (1977). A clinic within a general hospital for the assessment of urgent psychiatric problems. *Lancet, II,* 1067–1068.

Breslau, L. (1987). Exaggerated helplessness syndrome. In J. Sadavoy & M. Leszcz (Eds.), *Treating the elderly with psychotherapy* (pp. 157–173). Madison, CT: International Universities Press.

Breslau, L. (1980). The faltering therapeutic perspective toward the narcissistically wounded institutionalized aged. *Journal of Geriatric Psychiatry, 13,* 193–206.

Butler, R. N. (1987). NIMH Human Aging Study. In G. L. Maddox (Ed.), *Encyclopedia of Aging* (pp. 484–485). New York: Springer.

Calden, G., & Hokanson, J. E. (1959). The influence of age on MMPI responses. *Journal of Clinical Psychology, 15,* 194–195.

Casey, P. (1988). The epidemiology of personality disorder. P. Tyrer (Ed.), *Personality disorders: Diagnosis, management, and care* (pp. 74–81). London: Wright.

Casey, D. A., & Schrodt, C. J. (1989). Axis II diagnoses in geriatric inpatients. *Journal of Geriatric Psychiatry and Neurology, 2,* 87–88.

Casey, P. R., Dillon, S., & Tyrer, P. J. (1984). The diagnostic status of patients with conspicious psychiatric morbidity in primary care. *Psychological Medicine, 14,* 673–681.

Casey, P., & Tyrer P. (1986). Personality, functioning and symptomatology. *Journal of Psychiatric Research, 20,* 363–374.

Cattell, R. B. (1965). *The scientific analysis of personality.* Harmondsworth, Mddx: Penguin Books.

Cloninger, C. R. (1987). A systematic method for clinical description and classification of personality variants. *Archives of General Psychiatry, 44,* 573–588.

Costa, P. T., & McCrae, R. R. (1980). Still stable after all these years: Personality as a key to some issues in adulthood and old age. In P. B. Baltes & O. G. Brim (Eds.), *Lifespan development and behaviour* (pp. 65–102). New York: Academic Press.

Costa, P. T., Jr., McCrae, R. R., & Zonderman, A. B. (1987). Environmental and dispositional influences on well-being: Longitudinal follow-up of an American national sample. *British Journal of Psychology, 78,* 299–306.

Costa, P. T., McCrae, R. R., Zonderman, A. B., Barbano, H. E., Lebowitz, B., & Larson, D. M. (1986).

Cross-sectional studies of personality in a national sample: 2. Stability in neuroticism, extroversion, and openness. *Psychology and Aging, 1,* 144–149.

Costa, P. T., Zonderman, A. B., McCrae, R. R., Cornoni-Huntley, J., Locke, B. Z., & Barbano, H. E. (1987). Longitudinal analyses of psychological well-being in a national sample: Stability of mean levels. *Journal of Gerontology, 42,* 50–55.

Curran, D., & Partridge, M. (1963). *Psychological medicine: an introduction to psychiatry.* (5th ed.). Edinburgh: E & S Livingstone.

Cutting, J., Cowen, P. J., Mann, A., Jenkins, R. (1986). Personality and psychosis. Use of the standardized assessment of personality. *Acta Psychiatrica Scandinavica, 73,* 87–92.

Davis, D. R. (1972). *Introduction to psychopathology* (3rd ed.). Oxford: Oxford University Press.

Erikson, E. H. (1963). *Childhood and society* (2nd ed.). New York: Norton.

Eysenck, S. B. G., Pearson, P. R., Easting, G., & Allsopp, J. F. (1985). Age norms for impulsiveness, venturesomeness, and empathy in adults. *Personality and Individual Differences, 6,* 613–619.

Ferguson, B., & Tyrer, P. (1988). Classifying personality disorder. In P. Tyrer (Eds.), *Personality disorders: Diagnosis, management and course* (pp. 12–32). London: Wright.

Finch, C. E., & Morgan, D. (1987). Aging and schizophrenia: A hypothesis relating asynchrony in neural aging processes to the manifestations of schizophrenia and other neurologic diseases with age. In N. E. Miller & G. D. Cohen (Eds.), *Schizophrenia and aging* (pp. 97–108). New York: Guilford Press.

Fogel, B. S., & Eslinger, P. (in press). Diagnosis and management of patients with frontal lobe syndromes. In A. Stoudemire & B. S. Fogel (Eds.), *Advanced medical psychiatric practice* Washington, DC: American Psychiatric Press.

Fogel, B., & Martin, K. (1987). Personality disorders. In A. Stoudemire & B. S. Fogel (Eds.) *The medical setting in Principles of Medical Psychiatry* (pp. 253–270). New York: Grune & Stratton.

Fogel, B. S., & Westlake, R. (1990). Age and personality diagnosis in inpatients with major depression. Manuscript submitted for publication.

Freedman, M., & Albert, M. L. (1985). Subcortical dementia. In J. A. M. Frederiks (Ed.), *Handbook of clinical neurology: Neurobehavioural disorders* (Vol. 2, pp. 311–321). Amsterdam: Elsevier.

Friedman, J. H. (1969). Some problems of inpatient management with borderline patients. *American Journal of Psychiatry, 126,* 299–304.

Fries, L. (1987). Life expectancy. In G. L. Maddoz (Ed.), *Encyclopedia of Aging* (pp. 393–395). New York: Springer.

Frosch, J. (1964). The psychotic character. *Psychiatric Quarterly 38,* 81–96.

Gitelson, M. (1948). The emotional problems of elderly persons. In S. Steury & M. L. Blank (Eds.), *Readings in psychotherapy with older people* (1981). (pp. 8–17). Washington, DC: U.S. Department of Health and Human Sciences.

Gunderson, J. (Ed.). (1989). *American psychiatric press annual review* (Vol. VIII, *The course in borderline personality disorder*). Washington, DC: American Psychiatric Press.

Gustin, Q., Snyder, S., & Pitts, W. M. (1982). *The DSM-III borderline personality disorder: Issues in diagnosis and treatment.* Presented at the Annual Meeting Southeastern Psychological Association, New Orleans.

Gutman, G. M. (1966). A note on the MMPI: Age and sex differences in extroversion and neurotisism in a Canadian sample. *British Journal of Social & Clinical Psychology, 5,* 128–129.

Hamilton, J., Book, H., Sadavoy, J., & Silver, S. (1979). *Prognostic factors in treatment of the borderline patient.* Presented in June at Research Day, University of Toronto Department of Psychiatry, Queen St. Mental Health Centre, Toronto, Canada.

Heron, A., & Chown, S. M. (1967). *Age and function.* London: Churchill Livingstone.

Heumann, K. A., & Morey, L. C. (1990). Reliability of categorical and dimensional judgments of personality disorder. *American Journal of Psychiatry, 147,* 498–500.

Hirschfeld, R. M. A., Klerman, G. L., Clayton, P. J., Keller, M. B., McDonald-Scott, P., & Larkin, B. H. (1983). Assessing personality: Effects of the depressive state on trait measurement. *American Journal of Psychiatry, 140,* 695–699.

Hyler, S. E., & Lyons, M. (1988). Factor analysis of the DSM-III personality disorder clusters: A replication. *Comprehensive Psychiatry, 29,* 304–308.

Hyler, S., Reider, R., Spitzer, R., & Williams, J. B. W. (1982). *Personality Diagnostic Questionnaire (PDQ).* New York: New York State Psychiatric Institute.

Hyler, S. E., Rieder, R. O., Williams, J. B. W., Spitzer, R. L., Lyons, M., & Hendler, J. (1989). A comparison of clinical and self-report diagnoses of DSM-III personality disorders in 552 patients. *Comprehensive Psychiatry, 30,* 170–178.

ICD-10 (1988). *Draft of Chapter V Categories F00-F99, Mental, Behavioural and Developmental Disorders, Clinical Descriptions and Diagnostic Guidelines.* Geneva: World Health Organization Division of Mental Health.

Johnson, R. C., Ahern, F. M., Nagoshi, C. T., McClearn, G. E., Vandenberg, S. G., & Wilson, J. R. (1985). Age- and group-specific cohort effects on personality test scores: A study of three Hawaiian populations. *Journal of Cross-Cultural Psychology, 16,* 467–481.

Kastrup, M. (1985). Characteristics of a nationwide cohort of psychiatric patients—with special reference to the elderly and the chronically admitted. *Acta Psychiatrica Scandinavica,* (Suppl. 319), *71,* 107–115.

Kernberg, O. (1975). *Borderline conditions and pathological narcissism.* New York: Aronson.

Koenigsberg, H. W., Kaplan, R. D., Gilmore, M. M., & Cooper, A. M. (1985). The relationship between syndrome and personality disorder in DSM-III: Experience with 2462 patients. *American Journal of Psychiatry, 142,* 207–212.

Krystal, H. (1987). The impact of massive psychic trauma and the capacity to grieve effectively: Later life sequelae. In J. Sadavoy & M. Leszcz (Eds.), *Treating the elderly with psychotherapy* (pp. 95–155). Madison, CT: International Universities Press.

Lazarus, L. W. (1980). Self-psychology and psychotherapy with the elderly: Theory and practice. *Journal of Geriatric Psychiatry, 13,* 69–88.

Leirer, V. O. (1983). Development and validation of a geriatric depression rating scale: A preliminary report. *Journal of Psychiatric Research, 17,* 37.

Levensen, M. R. (1990). *Change in Stability in alcohol consumption and problem drinking.* Abstract submitted to Gerontological Society of America Annual Meeting, Boston, MA November 16, 1990.

Lishman, W. A. (1987). *Organic psychiatry.* Oxford: Blackwell Scientific.

Livesley, W. J. (1986). Trait and behavioural prototypes of personality disorder. *American Journal of Psychiatry, 143,* 728–732.

Loranger, A. W., Susman, V. L., Oldham, J. M., & Russakoff, L. M. (1985). *Personality Disorder Examination (PDE). A structured interview for DSM-III-R and ICD-9 personality disorders. WHO/ADAMHA pilot version.* White Plains, New York: The New York Hospital, Cornell Medical Center, Westchester Division.

Lukianowicz, N. (1973). Suicidal behaviour: An attempt to modify the environment. *Psychiatric Clinics, 6,* 171–190.

Maddocks, P. D. (1970). A five-year followup of untreated psychopaths. *British Journal of Psychiatry, 116,* 511–575.

Liebowitz, M. R., Stallone, F., Dunner, D. L., *et al.* (1979). Personality features of patients with primary affective disorder. *Acta Psychiatrica Scand. 60,* 214–224.

Main, T. F. (1987). The ailment. *British Journal of Medical Psychology, 30,* 129–145.

Maltsberger, J. T., & Buie, D. H. (1974). Countertransference hate in the treatment of suicidal patients. Archives of General Psychiatry, 30, 625–633.

Mann, A. H., Jenkins, R., Cutting, J. C., & Cowen, P. J. (1981). The development and use of a standardized assessment of abnormal personality. *Psychological Medicine, 11,* 839–847.

McCarthy, P. D., & Walsh, D. (1966). Suicide in Dublin. *British Medical Journal 1,* 1395–1396.

McCrae, R. R. (1987). Neuroticism. In G. L. Maddox (Ed.), *Encyclopedia of aging* (pp. 482–483).

McCrae, R. R., & Costa, P. T., Jr. (1988). Psychological resilience among widowed men and women: A 10-year followup of a national sample. *Journal of Social Issues, 44,* 129–142.

McGlashan, T. H. (1983). The borderline syndrome: ii. Is borderline a variant of schizophrenia or affective disorder? *Archives of General Psychiatry, 40,* 1319–1323.

McGlashan, T. H. (1986). The Chestnut Lodge followup study: 3: Long-term outcome of borderline personalities. *Archives of General Psychiatry, 43,* 20–30.

Mesulam, M. M. (1985). *Principles of behavioral neurology.* Philadelphia, PA: F. A. Davis.

Mezzich, T. E., Fabrega, H., Coffman, G. A., & Glavin, Y. (1987). Comprehensively diagnosing geriatric patients. *Comprehensive Psychiatry, 28,* 68–76.

Michels, R. (1987). How should the criteria for personality disorders be formulated? *Journal of Personality Disorders, 1,* 95–99.

Millon, T. (1982). *Millon Clinical Multiaxial Inventory* (2nd ed.). Minneapolis, MN: Interpretive Scoring Systems.

Myers, W. A. (1990). Psychotherapy and the elderly patient. In A. Tasman, S. Goldinger, & C. A. Kaufmann (Eds.), *Review of psychiatry* (Vol. 9, pp. 263–278). Washington DC: American Psychiatric Press.

Petry, S., Cummings, J. L., Hill, M. A., & Shapira, J. (1988). Personality alterations in dementia of the Alzheimer type. *Archives of Neurology, 45,* 1187–1190.

Petry, S., Cummings, J. L., Hill, M. A., & Shapira, J. (1989). Personality alterations in dementia of the Alzheimer type: A three-year followup study. *Journal of Geriatric Psychiatry and Neurology, 2,* 203–207.

Pfohl, B., Coryell, W., Zimmerman, M., & Stangl, D. (1986). DSM-III personality disorders: Diagnostic overlap and internal consistency of individual DSM-III criteria. *Comprehensive Psychiatry, 27(1),* 21–34.

Philip, A. E., & McCulloch, J. W. (1968). Some psychological features of persons who have attempted suicide. *British Journal of Psychiatry, 114,* 1299–1300.

Plakun, E. M. (1990). Longitudinal course and outcome of narcissistic personality disorders. Symposium presented at the American Psychiatric Association 143 Annual Meeting, New York, New York.

Ploye, P. M. (1977). On some difficulties of inpatient individual psychoanalytically oriented therapy. *Psychiatry, 40,* 133–145.

Reich, J. (1985). Measurement of DSM-III, Axis II. *Comprehensive Psychiatry, 26,* 352–363.

Reich J., Noyes R., Hirschfeld R., Coryell W., & O'Gorman T. (1987). State and personality in depressed and panic patients. *American Journal of Psychiatry, 144,* 181–187.

Reich, J., Noyes, R., Jr., & Troughton, E. (1987). Lack of agreement between instruments assessing DSM-III personality disorders. *Proceedings of the first Millon Clinical Multiaxial Inventory Conference.*

Reich J., Nduaguba M., Yates W. (1988). Age and sex distribution of DSM-III personality cluster traits in a community population. *Comprehensive Psychiatry, 29,* 298–303.

Reifman, L., Klein, J. G., & Murphy, S. T. (1989). Self-monitoring and age. *Psychology and Aging, 4,* 245–246.

Robins L. N., Helzer J. C., Weissman M. M., Owaschel H., Bruenberg E., Burke, J. O., & Regier, D. A. (1984). Lifetime prevalence of specific psychiatric disorders in three sites. *Archives of General Psychiatry, 41,* 949–958.

Ronningstam, E. F., & Gunderson, J. G. (1990). *Changes in level of pathological narcissism.* (Abstract #92C.) Paper presented at American Psychiatric Association 143rd Annual Meeting, May, New York, New York.

Rubin, E. H., & Kinscherf, D. A. (1989). Psychopathology of very mild dementia of the Alzheimer type. *American Journal of Psychiatry, 146,* 1017–1020.

Sadavoy, J. (in press). The aging borderline. In D. Silver & M. Rosenbluth (Eds.), *The handbook of borderline disorders.* Madison, CT: International Universities Press.

Sadavoy, J., Smith, I., Conn, D. K., & Richards, B. (1990). Depression in geriatric patients with chronic medical illness. International Journal of Geriatric Psychiatry. *5,* 187–192.

Sadavoy, J. (1987a). Character disorders in the elderly: An overview. In J. Sadavoy & M. Leszcz, (Eds.), Treating the elderly with psychotherapy: the scope for change in later life. (pp. 175–229). Madison, CT: International Universities Press.

Sadavoy, J. (1987b). Character pathology in the elderly. *Journal of Geriatric Psychiatry, 20,* 167.

Sadavoy, J., & Dorian, B. (1983). Treatment of the elderly characterologically disturbed patient in the chronic care institution. Journal of Geriatric Psychiatry, *16,* 233–240.

Sargeant, W., & Slater, E. (1962). An introduction to physical methods of treatment in psychiatry (5th ed.). Edinburgh: Churchill Livingstone.

Schaie, K. W. (1977). Toward a stage theory of adult cognitive development. *Journal of Aging and Human Development, 8,* 129–138.

Schaie, K. W., & Geiwitz, J. (1982). *Adult Development and Aging.* Boston, MA: Little, Brown.

Schaie, K. W., & Parham, I. A. (1976). Stability of adult personality traits: Fact or fable? *Journal of Personality and Social Psychology, 34,* 146–158.

Schultz, N. R. (1987). Anxiety. In G. L. Maddox (Ed.), *Encyclopedia of aging* (pp. 34–45). New York: Springer.

Sealey, A. P., & Cattell, R. B. (1965, April). *Standard trends in personality development in men and women of*

16 to 70 years, determined by 16 PF measurements. Read at the British Psychological Society conference, April 1965.

Sevensen, W. H. (1961). Structured personality testing in the aged: An MMPI study of the gerontic population. *Journal of Clincial Psychology, 17,* 302–304.

Siegler, J. C. (1987). Personality. In G. L. Maddox (Ed.). *Encyclopedia of aging.* (p. 520). New York: Springer.

Simon A. (1980). The neuroses, personality disorders, alcoholism, drug abuse and misuse, and crime in the aged. In J. Birren & R. Sloan (Eds.), *Handbook of Mental Health and Aging* (pp. 653–670). Englewood Cliffs, NJ: Prentice-Hall.

Snyder S., Pitts W. M., & Sajadi C. (1982). *Electroencephalography of DSM-III borderline personality.* Presented at the Annual Meeting, American Psychiatric Association, May, Toronto.

Snyder S., Goodpaster, W. A., Pitts, W. M., Pokorny, A. D., & Gustin, Q. L. (1985). Demography of psychiatric patients with borderline traits. *Psychopathology, 18,* 38–49.

Solomon K. Personality disorders in the elderly. In J. R. Lion (Ed.), *Personality disorders: Diagnosis and management* (2nd ed., pp. 310–338). Baltimore, MD: Williams & Wilkins.

Spiro, A. (1990). Change and stability in personality. Abstract submitted to the Gerontological Society of America Annual Meeting, November 16, Boston, MA.

Spitzer, R., Williams, J. B. W., & Gibbon, M. (1987). *Structured interview for DSM-III-R personality disorders.* New York: Biometrics Research Department, New York State Psychiatric Institute.

Stangl, D., Pfohl, B., Zimmerman, M., Bowers, W., & Corenthal, C. (1985). Structured interview for DSM-III personality disorders. *Archives of General Psychiatry, 42,* 591–596.

Stoner, S. B., & Panek, P. E. (1985). Age and sex differences with the Comrey Personality Scales. *Journal of Psychology, 119,* 137–142.

Straker, M. (1982). Adjustment disorder and personality disorders in the aged. *Psychiatric Clinics of North America, 5,* 121–129.

Stuss, D. T., & Benson, D. F. (1986). *The frontal lobes.* New York: Raven.

Thompson, L. W., Gallagher, D., & Czirr, R. (1988). Personality disorder and outcome in the treatment of late-life depression. *Journal of Geriatric Psychiatry, 21,* 133–153.

Tyrer, P., & Seivewright, H. (1988). Studies of outcome. In P. Tyrer (Ed.), *Personality Disorders: Diagnosis, Management and Course* (pp. 119–136). London: Wright.

Tyrer, P., Alexander, J., & Ferguson, B. (1988). Personality assessment schedule. In P. Tyrer (Ed.), *Personality disorders: Diagnosis, management and course* (pp. 140–167). London: Wright.

Tyrer, P., Casey, P., & Gall, J. (1983). The relationship between neurosis and personality disorders. *British Journal of Psychiatry, 142,* 404–408.

Vaillant, G. E., & Perry, J. P. (1985). Personality disorders. In H. Kaplan, A. Freedman, & B. Sadock (Eds.), *Comprehensive textbook of psychiatry* (4th ed.). Baltimore, MD: Williams & Wilkins.

Vaillant, G. E., & Vaillant, C. O. (1990). Natural history of male psychosocial health, XII: A 45-year study of predictors of successful aging at age 65. *American Journal of Psychiatry, 147,* 31–37.

Veith, R. C., & Raskind, M. A. (1988). The neurobiology of aging: Does it predispose to depression? *Neurobiology of Aging, 9,* 101–117.

Verwoerdt, A. (1980). Anxiety, dissociative and personality disorders in the elderly. In E. W. Busse & D. E. Blazer (Eds.), *Handbook of geriatric psychiatry* (pp. 368–380). New York: Van Nostrand Reinhold.

Verwoerdt, A. (1981). *Clinical geropsychiatry.* Baltimore, MD: Williams & Wilkins.

Verwoerdt A. (1987). Psychodynamics of paranoid phenomenon in the aged. In J. Sadavoy & M. Leszcz (Eds.) *Treating Elderly with Psychotherapy* (pp. 67–93). Madison, Connecticut: Universities Press.

Vinoda, M. N. (1969). Personality and the nature of suicidal attempts. *British Journal of Psychiatry, 115,* 791–795.

Volkan, V. (1976). Primitive internalized object relations. New York: International Universities Press.

Whitlock, F. A., & Shapira, K. (1967). Attempted suicide in Newcastle Upon Tyne. *British Journal of Psychiatry, 113,* 423–434.

Yesavage, J. A., Brink, T. L., Rose, T. L., Lum, O., Huang, V., Adey, M. B., & Leirer, V. O. (1983). Development and validation of a geriatric depression rating scale: A preliminary report. *Journal of Psychiatric Research, 17,* 37.

Zimmerman, M., Pfohl, B. M., Coryell, W., Corenthal, C., & Stangl, D. (1990). *Major depression and personality disorder*. (Abstract #NR667). Paper presented at American Psychiatric Association 143rd Annual Meeting, May, New York, NY.

Zimmerman, M., Pfohl, B., Coryell, W., Stangl, D., & Corenthal, C. (1988). Diagnosing personality disorder in depressed patients. *Archives of General Psychiatry, 45,* 733–737.

Zimmerman, M., Pfohl, B., Stangl, D., & Corenthal, C. (1986). Assessment of DSM-III personality disorders: The importance of interviewing an informant. *Journal of Clinical Psychiatry, 47,* 261–263.

Schizophrenia and Psychotic States

Peter V. Rabins

I. Schizophrenia
II. Late-Life-Onset Schizophrenia
   A. Similarities and Differences between Early- and Late-Onset
      Schizophrenia
   B. Risk Factors for Developing Late-Onset Schizophrenia
   C. Treatment
III. Chronic Schizophrenia with Early-Life Onset
IV. Other Conditions
   A. Delusional Disorder
   B. Isolated Paranoia or Suspiciousness
   C. Suspiciousness as Part of Nonschizophrenic Syndromes
   D. Suspiciousness in Dementia and Delirium
   E. Organic Hallucinoses and Organic Delusional Disorders
   F. Hallucinations in Grief
   G. The Diogenes or Senile Recluse Syndrome
   References

This chapter will discuss conditions that have hallucinations, delusions, suspiciousness, or unusual behavior as core symptoms. It will be organized around a discussion of various *syndromes* (defined as groups of symptoms that frequently cluster together) in which so-called psychotic symptoms occur. This syndromic approach asserts that a single symptom can be a manifestation of several or many disorders. The clustering together of certain symptoms in patients and families, the response of a specific cluster of symptoms to specific treatments, and the identification of a specific prognosis for the cluster, all support the idea that a syndrome discussed can be treated as a disease entity, even though it may have several causes or etiologies.

Handbook of Mental Health and Aging, Second Edition
Copyright © 1992 by Academic Press, Inc. All rights of reproduction in any form reserved.

I. Schizophrenia ————————————————————————————————

Schizophrenia is a difficult condition to define succinctly, primarily because the symptoms are experiences that are alien to most people. In the broadest terms, schizophrenia is a syndrome of disordered mental processes in which there are abnormalities of (1) the form of a person's thinking (thought disorder); (2) fixed, false, idiosyncratic beliefs (delusions); and (3) perceptual experiences without stimuli (hallucinations); but (4) no evidence of cognitive (organic) or affective disorder.

The criteria for diagnosing schizophrenia from the Diagnostic and Statistical Manual (DSM-III-R) of the American Psychiatric Association (1987) are listed in Table I. These criteria are derived from the work of three individuals, Emil Kraepelin (1971), Eugen Bleuler (1950), and Kurt Schneider (Mellor, 1982). A brief review of their ideas may help the reader understand the complexities of diagnosing schizophrenia, the limitations of the current criteria, and the controversies that still exist.

Kraepelin is generally credited with recognizing that one set of mental symptoms frequently clustered together had as a unifying feature a *deterioration* of psychological and social function. He named the condition *dementia precox* to emphasize this deterioration (dementia) and its frequent early-life onset (precocious or precox). Bleuler, on the other hand, emphasized the *split from reality* experienced by patients. He suggested that the symptoms of the disorder were the core features, and deterioration was not a necessary outcome. The signs and symptoms he thought were keys to the diagnosis are referred to as the four As: flat *a*ffect (emotional expression incongruous with or inappropriate to the situation), *a*mbivalence (having opposite feelings or holding opposing beliefs about an issue), loose *a*ssociations (an abnormality of the form of speech in which the links between two adjacent thoughts are unclear to an observer) and *a*utism (meaning both to think idiosyncratically and to behave in an isolated manner). Schneider also emphasized the diagnostic importance of specific symptoms. The symptoms he believed most characteristic of schizophrenia have come to be called *first-rank symptoms*. They include *passivity experiences* (believing and feeling that thoughts are being put into or taken out of one's head; believing and feeling that one's body is being moved by an outside force; feeling shocks or other unpleasant sensations coming from outside the body); *auditory hallucinations,* which come from outside the head, consist of a group of voices that talk to one another, and that discuss the patient in the third person); *thought broadcasting* and *reception* (being able to send or receive thoughts through the air; and *delusional perceptions* (the sudden development of a delusional system from an actual perception: for example, seeing a car that exists and immediately developing a delusional system or interpretation).

As is shown in the table, the DSM-III-R criteria merge these disparate approaches. Criterion A lists some the specific symptoms emphasized by Bleuler and Schneider, while Criteria C and E emphasize that no identifiable somatic lesion or other psychiatric condition such as depression be present. Criterion D reflects the Kraepelinian view that schizophrenia is a chronic condition. It is important to note that the DSM-III-R approach requires that both inclusion and exclusion criteria be fulfilled.

A number of studies published in the last 20 years suggest that Kraepelin was wrong in limiting the diagnosis of schizophrenia to those who suffer a progressive downhill course.

Table I
DSM-III-R Criteria[a]

Schizophrenia	Delusional disorder

A. Presence of characteristic psychotic symptoms in the active phase: either 1, 2, or 3, for at least one week unless successfully treated:
  1. Two of the following:
    a. Delusions
    b. Prominent hallucinations (throughout the day for several days or several times a week for several weeks, each hallucinatory experience not being limited to a few brief moments)
    c. Incoherence or marked loosening of associations
    d. Catatonic behavior
    e. Flat or grossly inappropriate affect
  2. Bizarre delusions (i.e., involving a phenomenon that the person's culture would regard as totally implausible, e.g., thought broadcasting, being controlled by a dead person)
  3. Prominent hallucinations (as defined in 1b. above) of a voice with content having no apparent relation to depression or elation, or a voice keeping up a running commentary on the person's behavior or thoughts, or two or more voices conversing with one another.
	A. Nonbizarre delusion(s) (i.e., involving situations that occur in real life, such as being followed, poisoned, infected, loved at a distance, having a disease, being deceived by one's spouse or lover) of at least one month's duration

B. During the course of the disturbance, functioning in such areas as work, social relations, and self-care is markedly below the highest level achieved before onset of the disturbance (or, when the onset is in childhood or adolescence, failure to achieve expected level of social development)	B. Auditory or visual hallucinations, if present, are not prominent (as defined in schizophrenia, A, 1, b)
C. Schizoaffective disorder and mood disorder with psychotic features have been ruled out, i.e., if a major depressive or manic syndrome has ever been present during an active phase of the disturbance, the total duration of all episodes of a mood syndrome has been brief relative to the total duration of the active and residual phases of the disturbance	C. Apart from the delusion(s) or its ramifications, behavior is not obviously odd or bizarre
D. Continuous signs of the disturbance for at least six months	D. If a major depressive or manic syndrome has been present during the delusional disturbance, the total duration of all episodes of the mood syndrome has been brief, relative to the total duration of the delusional disturbance
E. It cannot be established that an organic factor initiated and maintained the disturbance	E. Has never met criterion A for schizophrenia, and it cannot be established that an organic factor initiated and maintained the disturbance
F. If there is a history of autistic disorder, the additional diagnosis of schizophrenia is made only if prominent delusions or hallucinations are also present	

[a]From American Psychiatric Association (1987).

For example, three European longitudinal studies reviewed by Ciompi (1987) reported that between 49 and 57% of individuals with a diagnosis of schizophrenia had a remission of symptoms or were left with "mild" residual symptoms. In the United States, Harding, Brooks, Ashikaga, Strauss, and Brier (1987) have done careful followup studies of a cohort of individuals hospitalized in the state hospitals of Vermont. Patients' charts were reviewed and were rediagnosed by current DSM-III-R standards. Even after excluding individuals who were likely to have been misdiagnosed, 30% of those alive at follow-up were reported to have a moderately good or good prognosis. Thus schizophrenia is not necessarily a dilapidating illness, but many patients have persistent hallucinations as well as residual apathy, social dilapidation, or subtle declines in interpersonal skills.

Another controversy in the diagnosis of schizophrenia, which has recently been resolved, is whether schizophrenia can begin in late life. This controversy can also be traced back to Kraepelin, who initially thought that the intact personality of later-onset cases meant that it was a different disorder. However, convinced by follow-up studies and his own clinical experience that many later-onset cases did have an illness that followed the dilapidating course of schizophrenia, Kraepelin states in the last edition of his textbook that late-onset cases resembled early-onset cases in all important ways. The DSM-III-R states that late onset be specified if the condition begins after age 45.

One other minor controversy related to the label used to identify the late-onset condition, Kraepelin originally used the word paraphrenia to refer to cases in which primary symptoms (hallucinations and delusions) occurred without social dilapidation. He used the term to describe cases with intact personality at any age. The term was later incorporated by the British psychogeriatrician Roth (1952) into the phrase late-onset paraphrenia. While this phrase is now used interchangeably with the phrase late-onset schizophrenia, we will use the latter, since the two phrases are similar in meaning, and schizophrenia is the term used in DSM-III-R.

II. Late-Life-Onset Schizophrenia

While the peak age of onset of a schizophrenic disorder is the late teens in males and late 20s in females, some individuals do develop the disorder later in life. In a consecutive clinical series of patients admitted to the Phipps Clinic of the Johns Hopkins Hospital with a diagnosis of schizophrenia (Pearlson and Rabins, 1988), 4% of males and 26% of females had the onset of their symptoms after age 45. Because these data come from a single inpatient service, they cannot be considered more than an indication of the low percentage of cases that do begin in late life.

Whether the schizophreniclike conditions that begin in late life are the same as those that begin in early life bears review. It is important to appreciate that because we currently rely only on identifying the clinical syndrome of schizophrenia it is quite possible that schizophrenia has several or many etiologies at any age. Even in the young, schizophrenia is quite likely a syndrome with multiple causes. E. Bleuler (1950) himself made this point when he subtitled his classic book, *The Group of Schizophrenias*.

A. Similarities and Differences between Early- and Late-Onset Schizophrenia

Schizophrenia beginning in late life presents with many of the same symptoms as in the young. The prevalence of delusions and hallucinations is the same, as is the prevalence of Schneiderian first-rank symptoms (Pearlson et al., 1989). Nonetheless, several notable differences between early- and late-onset cases have been consistently found. The delusions and hallucinations experienced by patients are often more florid in the elderly (Marneros and Deister, 1984; Pearlson and Rabins, 1988; Roth, 1952). For example, late-onset patients often vividly describe hearing groups of people or animals walk on their roof, see people walk through walls, feel electric pulses shoot through room walls into their sex organs or their brain, or feel shocks that inflict pain and make their body move. These symptoms cause both emotional and physical distress. Individuals experiencing such symptoms frequently call the police or other authorities with stories that they are being harassed by children, neighbors, or professionals. When assessing such complaints, it is always important to determine that harassment is not taking place.

Late-onset cases have less thought disorder (Marneros and Deister, 1984; Pearlson et al., 1989) and less affective flattening than earlier-onset individuals (Pearlson et al., 1989). Since these are core symptoms of schizophrenia, according to E. Bleuler (1950), their lower prevalence leads some to conclude that individuals without them have a different disorder. Also, in late-onset cases, hallucinations are more likely to be visual, olfactory, tactile, or gustatory. Smelling gas coming through the walls or under a door, and tactile hallucinations such as feeling electric shocks are common (Herbert & Jacobsen, 1967; Rabins, Pauker, & Thomas, 1984). Because nonauditory hallucinations are common in organic disorders, it is important to rule out identifiable focal central nervous system (CNS) lesions or systemic disorders such as brain tumor, peripheral neuropathy, metabolic or toxic encephalopathy, or hereditofamilial disorders as the cause of these experiences (as criterion E of the DSM-III-R emphasizes).

Follow-up studies have been an important means of validating diagnostic concepts in psychiatry since the turn of the 20th century (e.g., Roth, 1952). In general, they caution us not to overemphasize cross-sectional differences between early- and late-onset cases. For example, followup studies led Kraepelin to change his opinion and include paraphrenia as a schizophrenic disorder. The followup studies of Harding et al. (1987) and those reviewed by Ciompi (1987) support Kraepelin's view that dilapidation occurs in a majority of persons whose schizophrenia begins before midlife, but do not clarify the etiology of these changes. Likewise, short-term followup studies of elderly later-onset subjects by Levy and co-workers (Hymas, Naguib, & Levy, 1989; Naguib & Levy, 1987) show that late-onset cases frequently become or remain cognitively abnormal, although they do not deteriorate in a manner suggesting Alzheimer's disease or multi-infarct dementia. Whether this is the same volitional and social deterioration characteristic of the form of schizophrenia that begins earlier in life or is indicative of some other CNS degenerative condition must be determined by longer-term follow-up and autopsy studies. Subtle medication side-effects should be ruled out whenever a patient declines cognitively.

Patients with early-onset schizophrenia (Pearlson, 1988) and late-life onset schizophrenia (Breitner, Husain, Figiel, Krishnan, and Boyko, 1990); Naguib & Levy, 1987; Rabins, Pearlson, Jayaram, Steele & Tune, 1987) are similar in having larger lateral ventricles on computerized tomography (CT) head scan than age-similar normal controls. This ventricular enlargement is less than the ventriculomegaly seen in Alzheimer's disease patients of the same age (Rabins *et al.*, 1987).

B. Risk Factors for Developing Late-Onset Schizophrenia

A number of risk factors for developing schizophrenia later in life have been identified. Late-life-onset schizophrenia occurs more commonly in women than in men (Kay & Roth, 1961; Rabins *et al.*, 1984). This difference is not fully explained by the longer life expectancy of women. It is of interest that, even in the young, schizophrenia begins in women a mean of 10 years later than in men (Eaton, 1985). This may mean that some factor (for example, estrogen binding of dopamine receptors) might partially protect against or delay the development of schizophrenia (Seeman, 1981; Seeman, 1986). Hearing loss has generally been shown to be more common in late-onset schizophrenics than in patients with affective disorder (Cooper, Curry, Kay, Garside & Roth, 1974), although there is some controversy over this finding (Moore, 1981). This intriguing association is the best evidence that environmental or psychological factors (here *sensory deprivation*) could be risk factors of or precipitants to schizophrenia.

Patients with late-life-onset schizophrenia are frequently described as having had unusual or abnormal premorbid personalities (Kay, 1972; Marneros & Deister, 1984; Pearlson *et al.*, 1989). The most frequent pattern is a history of eccentricity and isolation. Nonetheless, they often have been successful at work. Late-onset patients are less likely to have ever married or to have had children (Kay & Roth, 1961; Kay, 1972; Rabins *et al.*, 1984) than similarly aged persons. This could reflect early-life social isolation, reflect different sex hormone activity, or indicate that marriage and childbearing are protections against developing schizophrenia. It seems most plausible that the unusual personality characteristics and the low fertility are subtle early-life manifestations of a disorder that presents with florid symptoms only late in life.

Several studies suggest a genetic or familial diathesis in late-onset schizophrenia (Kay & Roth, 1961; Rabins *et al.*, 1984). The association is weaker than that reported in early-onset cases.

C. Treatment

Neuroleptic medications are the treatment of choice for the primary symptoms of schizophrenia. These drugs treat the *active* or *positive* symptoms such as hallucinations and delusions, but do little to alleviate the *negative* symptoms of apathy and social isolation. The choice of which neuroleptic to prescribe is usually made on the basis of which side-effects can be best tolerated by an individual patient. Low-potency, high-dose drugs such as thioridazine and chlorpromazine are sedating and cause orthostatic hypotension. Beginning doses are from 10 m q.d. or b.i.d. to 25 mg b.i.d. High-potency, low-dose drugs such as haloperidol, thiothixene and fluphenazine are more likely to cause extrapyramidal symptoms. Beginning doses usually range from 1 to 3 mg daily.

The neuroleptic drugs also have long-term, persistent side-effects. Among the most serious is tardive dyskinesia (TD), an involuntary movement disorder that occurs months or years after neuroleptics have begun (thus the term tardy or tardive) and consists of abnormal repetitive (*dyskinetic*) movements of the lips, tongue, mouth, limbs, or trunk. Tardive dyskinesia can be permanent but resolves over a period of months in at least 50% of cases. It is particularly important to be vigilant about TD in the elderly, since old age is one of the risk factors for developing the disorder (Kane and Smith, 1982). Being female, having cognitive dysfunction (Waddington, Youssef, Dolphin, & Kinsella, 1987), and exposure to larger amounts of dopamine-blocking agents are also risk factors. Because of the risk of TD, neuroleptic medication should be discontinued in schizophrenic patients who are not benefiting. Patients taking neuroleptic drugs should be assessed for the presence of tardive dyskinesia on a regular basis. If signs of tardive dyskinesia develop, the clinician must then discuss with the patient whether he or she wishes to continue with the medication in spite of this. Current practice suggests that informed consent, at least of a verbal nature, be obtained from all patients put on neuroleptic drugs.

The neuroleptic clozapine appears to be particularly useful for younger patients who have not responded to other neuroleptic drugs (Kane, Honigfeld, Singer, Meltzer, & the Clorazil Collaborative Study Group, 1988) and might uniquely be effective for persons with negative symptoms. Most studies have excluded elderly patients, but there is no reason to suspect that they would not respond as well. Clozapine may not cause tardive dyskinesia or at least has a much-diminished likelihood of doing so. Its one serious side-effect is that it causes bone marrow suppression in 4 per 1000 individuals. Precautions against this must be taken, and informed consent about this risk obtained from the patient.

No well-designed, double-blind trials of neuroleptic therapy for late-life-onset schizophrenia exist. Unblinded clinical series (Post, 1965; Post, 1980; Rabins *et al.*, 1984) suggest that response rates are approximately the same as those in young individuals. Most clinicians recommend considering discontinuance of neuroleptic drugs if a patient remains symptom free for a year after a single episode. Informed consent should be obtained at regular intervals when neuroleptics are continued.

In addition to tardive dyskinesia, the elderly are particularly prone to develop the parkinsonian or extrapyramidal side-effects of neuroleptic drugs. One form of this, truncal dystonia (in which the patient leans to one side due to unilateral contraction of erector spinae muscles—hence the name "Pisa syndrome"), is seen almost exclusively in the elderly. The elderly are prone to develop orthostatic hypotension as well.

III. Chronic Schizophrenia with Early-Life Onset

In many ways elderly individuals with chronic schizophrenia should be viewed as survivors. They have not succumbed to suicide or other causes of mortality that lead to a shorter life expectancy for individuals with schizophrenia (Tsuang and Woolan, 1977). As Harding *et al.* (1987) have demonstrated, many patients with chronic schizophrenia have residual positive symptoms of hallucinations and delusions and persisting negative symptoms of apathy and isolation. A majority are living in the community and are partly self-sufficient, nonetheless.

Neuroleptic drugs, (except, perhaps, for clozapine), are used only for active treatment of positive symptoms or to prevent relapse. Patients who are no longer symptomatic should generally not be on neuroleptic drugs, unless they are being used in a prophylactic fashion.

IV. Other Conditions

A. Delusional Disorder

The classification of disorders characterized by single, circumscribed delusions or prominent delusions and minimal associated psychopathology has vexed practitioners and diagnosticians alike. Many specific syndromes have been described including a belief of parasite infestation (delusional parasitosis or Ekbom's syndrome) (Anonymous, 1977), dysmorphophobia (the delusions that a body part is distorted), erotomania (delusions of love at a distance) (Segal, 1989) and monosymptomatic hypochondriasis (Bishop, 1980). The DSM-III-R groups these disorders under the category delusional (paranoid) disorders (Table I). This diagnosis has as its primary but not only manifestation the presence of a *non bizarre* (defined as not "involving a phenomenon that in the person's culture would be regarded as totally implausible" (American Psychiatric Association, 1987, p. 188) delusion without identifiable organic etiology. Five specific subtypes, erotomania, grandiose, jealous, persecutory, and somatic are listed. Delusional disorders are rare. The DSM-III-R lists a point prevalence of .03% and a lifetime prevalence of less than .1%. Mean age of onset is between 40 and 55 (American Psychiatric Association, 1987). Patients with delusional disorder have a better prognosis than those with schizophrenia (Winokur, 1977; Jorgensen & Monk-Jorgensen 1985), although residual symptoms are present in two thirds of individuals at 22- to 39-year followup (Opjordsmoen, 1988). Some cases described in the literature as being examples of late-onset schizophrenia better fit the criteria for delusional disorder.

B. Isolated Paranoia or Suspiciousness

Suspiciousness is the tendency to view individuals or agencies as having harmful intents. It is a universal trait. While the term paranoid has popularly evolved into a synonym for paranoia, it is used clinically as an adjective indicating suspicion (Lewis, 1970) or as a synonym for the phrase delusional disorder. Lowenthal (1964) reported a prevalence of 2.5% among the elderly living in San Francisco, while Christenson and Blazer (1984) found a 4% prevalence in Durham County, North Carolina.

When suspiciousness presents as a clinical issue it is important first to determine whether the complaint is valid. Elder abuse can be subtle or overt and range from financial exploitation to physical abuse. The clinician should review the issue with the patient and, if indicated, seek corroborating or refuting support through other historians.

There is little written about the treatment of isolated suspiciousness. If the concerns are unfounded or exaggerated and are interfering with the patient's life, the therapist can offer to review with the patient whether psychogenic sources exist. Many patients do not see the suspiciousness as a problem and are not interested in formal psychotherapy. At times, the clinician can play the role of a neutral sounding board. At other times, the clinician can directly identify misperceptions or misinterpretations for the patient. The latter can usually take place only after a trusting, therapeutic relationship has developed. The goal of treatment is to prevent the belief from interfering with their lives. Rarely the therapist can help the patient see the falsity of an isolated paranoid belief. Psychotherapy thus focuses on limiting the distress and disability that is caused by the symptom.

While neuroleptic drugs are used to treat isolated paranoid delusions, clinical experience suggests that they are often ineffective. It is usually difficult to convince patients with isolated paranoid delusions to take medication even when the indications of danger and distress are present.

C. Suspiciousness as Part of Nonschizophrenic Syndromes

Because suspiciousness can be part of many *organic* and *functional* syndromes, disorders of these categories must be ruled out before concluding that it is an isolated symptom. All patients in whom suspiciousness presents as causing a clinical problem should be assessed for the presence of cognitive disorder (dementia or delirium), depression, and schizophrenia.

D. Suspiciousness in Dementia and Delirium

Hallucinations and delusions can be symptoms of focal or generalized brain disease (Berrios & Brook, 1985; Cummings, 1985; Rabins, Mace & Lucas, 1982). These disorders are discussed in detail in Chapter 14. Suspiciousness, paranoia, hallucinations, or other nonparanoid delusions can be the earliest or most prominent manifestation of some other disorder such as Alzheimer's disease (Shuttleworth, 1984). Treatment by pharmacologic, behavioral, or environmental means is appropriate even when an identifiable etiology is present, when these symptoms cause problems for either the patient or caregiver.

Hallucinations and delusions are common in delirium (Cutting, 1980; Lipowski, 1989). Underlying dementia is a significant risk factor for developing an acute delirium (Erkinjuntti, Wikstrom, Palo, & Autio, 1986) from a superimposed acute illness or as a medication side-effect. Indeed, the development of a delirium with hallucinations and delusions may first bring attention to the fact that an individual has been suffering from a long-standing dementia. One of the few studies showing that an underlying dementia can predispose to the development of hallucinations and delusions characteristic of a delirium is evidence from the earliest studies of L-dopa (Celesia and Barr, 1970), demonstrating that patients with preexisting cognitive impairment are more likely to develop *psychotic* symptoms from L-dopa.

E. Organic Hallucinoses and Organic Delusional Disorders

The DSM-III-R categorizes hallucinations and delusions that occur as a manifestation of an identifiable brain disease in the absence of dementia as organic hallucinoses and delusional syndromes. Parkinson's disease is one condition in which isolated delusions or hallucinations are frequent. For example, visual hallucinations occur in 9% of nondemented patients treated with antiparkinsonian drugs (Rabins, 1991). Rare cases of hallucinations in Parkinson's disease were reported before any treatment was available (Mjones, 1949), but they have become common only since dopamine-precursor loading and agonist therapies have become available (Moskowitz, Moses, & Klawans, 1978).

The visual hallucinations of Parkinson's disease are phenomenologically similar to the hallucinations seen in patients with lesions of the intracerebral peduncles (peduncular hallucinosis of Lhermitte), and it is possible that involvement of the ventral tegmental or pedunculopontine nucleus (Zweig, Jankel, Hedreen, Mayeux, & Price 1989) dopamine cells may cause these symptoms.

Frequently the parkinsonian patient is not distressed by the visual hallucinations, and no treatment is indicated. When the hallucinations are a source of distress to the patient (and this distress is unrelieved by reassurance), or if the patient acts upon them and endangers himself, then several options are present. First the anti-Parkinson's medication(s) can be decreased in dosage. This may lead to a diminution of hallucinations without marked decline in physical state. Sometimes, however, a choice must be made between a lower dose that results in poorer physical performance and fewer mental symptoms and a higher dose that results in more mental symptoms but better physical performance. The cautious use of neuroleptic drugs in very low doses can diminish or abolish the hallucinations. Unfortunately, it is quite likely that the neuroleptics will worsen the underlying parkinsonian syndrome.

Isolated visual hallucinations in otherwise healthy older individuals were reported more than 200 years ago by Charles Bonnet (Berrios & Brook, 1982), whose grandfather had the condition. He lived with the hallucinations for 25 years and showed no development of dementia or other serious mental illness. Bonnet speculated that his grandfather's cataracts had etiologic significance, and many individuals with isolated visual hallucinations have coexisting eye disease (Damas-Mora, Skelton-Robinson, & Jenner, 1982). Over time, many individuals develop difficulties in distinguishing between these hallucinatory states and normal life and sometimes became fearful of them or upset by their presence.

No studies of the treatment of individuals with lesion-induced hallucinations or delusions exist. Psychotherapeutic support, bright lights, and explanation to patient and family should be the primary focus of treatment unless the patient is becoming markedly or upset or incorporating symptoms into daily life. If the latter occurs, a trial of neuroleptic drugs can be initiated, but many patients do not respond, and the side-effects may outweigh any potential benefit.

F. Hallucinations in Grief

Isolated hallucinations or illusions (false perceptions that result from misinterpretations of actual stimuli) are common in the recently widowed. One study reported that 61% of widows experience visual or auditory manifestation of the dead person (Olson, Suddeth, Peterson, & Egelhoff, 1985). Most commonly the widow or widower reports seeing the deceased person's shape, having the feeling that the deceased was in the room, or actually feeling the person's presence, but are aware that they did not actually see the person. Some individuals experience the actual visualization of the dead person. In contrast to organic hallucinoses, the visualizations of the grief-stricken are often brief and not stereotyped (that is, not the same each time). These should be recognized as a normal phenomenon occuring in grief. The person who is distressed by them can be reassured that they are not pathological.

G. The Diogenes or Senile Recluse Syndrome

Elderly individuals have been described who show little interest in cleanliness or social activity, who collect, hoard, or pile up garbage, newspapers, or useless objects, and yet have no other evidence of cognitive or functional psychiatric disorder. MacMillan and Shaw (1966) described 22 individuals suffering the *senile breakdown in standard*. Their mean age was approximately 78; most were women and widowed. These individuals live in squalor, but many were cognitively psychiatrically normal. In a descriptive study from Sydney, Australia, Snowdon (1987) found 12 of 83 individuals living in squalor had no identifiable psychiatric or medical disorder.

An adequate premorbid history is sometimes difficult to obtain, but some of these individuals appear to have been eccentric and isolated in their youths. There has been some speculation that this might be a frontal lobe syndrome in some individuals (Orrell, Sahakian, & Bergman, 1989), but some patients with these behaviors have no identifiable abnormality on neuropsychological tests of frontal lobe function. Individuals with this symptom complex often resist all mental health interventions, but may respond if housing or public health authorities start legal action.

References

American Psychiatric Association. (1987). *Diagnostic and Statistical Manual of Mental Disorders* (3rd ed., rev.). Washington, DC: American Psychiatric Press.

Anon, (1977). Delusions of Parasitosis. *British Medical Journal*. 6064: 790–791. (Editorial).

Berrios, G. E., & Brook, P. (1982). The Charles Bonnet syndrome and the problem of visual perceptual disorders in the elderly. *Age and Aging, 11*, 17–23.

Berrios, G. E., & Brook, P. (1985). Delusions and the psychopathology of the elderly with dementia. *Acta Psychiatrica Scandinavica, 72*, 296–301.

Bishop, E. R. (1980). Monosymptomatic hypochondriasis. *Psychosomatics, 21*, 731–747.

Bleuler, E. (1950). (J. Zinking, Trans.) *Dementia praecox or the group of schizophrenias.* New York: International Universities Press.

Breitner, J., Husain, M. M., Figiel, G. S., Krishnan, K. R. R., & Boyko, R. B. (1990). Cerebral white matter disease in late-onset paranoid psychosis. *Biological Psychiatry, 28*, 266–274.

Celesia, G. G., & Barr, A. N. (1970). Psychosis and other psychiatric manifestations of levodopa therapy. *Archives of Neurology, 23*, 193–200.

Ciompi, L. (1987). Review of follow-up studies on long-term evolution and aging in schizophrenia. In N. E. Miller & G. D. Cohen (eds.), *Schizophrenia and aging.* New York: Guilford Press.

Christenson, R., & Blazer, D. (1984). Epidemiology of persecutory ideation in an elderly population in the community. *American Journal of Psychiatry, 141*, 1088–1091.

Cooper, A. F., Curry, A. F., Kay, D. W. K., Garside, R. F., & Roth, M. (1974). Hearing loss in paranoid and affective psychoses of the elderly. *Lancet, 2*, 851–854.

Cummings, J. L. (1985). Organic delusions: Phenomenology, anatomical correlations, and review. *British Journal of Psychiatry, 146*, 184–197.

Cutting, J. (1980). Physical illness and psychosis. *British Journal of Psychiatry, 136*, 109–119.

Damas-Mora, J., Skelton-Robinson, M., & Jenner, F. A. (1982). The Charles Bonnet syndrome in perspective. *Psychological Medicine, 12*, 251–261.

Eaton, W. W. (1985). Epidemiology of schizophrenia. *Epidemiologic Reviews, 7*, 105–126.

Editorial (1977). Delusions of parasitosis. *British Medical Journal, March 26*, 790–791.

Erkinjuntti, T., Wikstrom, J., Palo, J., & Autio, L. (1986). Dementia among medical inpatients. *Archives of Internal Medicine, 146*, 1923–1926.

Harding, C. M., Brooks, G. W., Ashikaga, T., Strauss, J. S., & Breier, A. (1987). The Vermont longitudinal study of persons with severe mental illness, I. Methodology, study sample, and overall status 32 years later. *American Journal of Psychiatry, 144*, 18–26.

Herbert, M. E., & Jacobson, S. (1967). Late paraphrenia. *British Journal of Psychiatry, 113*, 461–469.

Hymas, N., Naguib, M., & Levy, R. (1989). Late paraphrenia—A follow-up study. *International Journal of Geriatric Psychiatry, 4*, 23–29.

Jorgensen, P., Munk-Jorgensen, P. (1985). Paranoid psychosis in the elderly. *Acta Psychiatrica Scandinavica, 72*, 358–363.

Kane, J., Honigfeld, G., Singer, J., Meltzer, & the Clorazil Collaborative Study Group. (1988). Clozapine for the treatment-resistant schizophrenic. *Archives of General Psychiatry, 45*, 789–796.

Kane, J. M., & Smith, J. M. (1982). Tardive dyskinesia: Prevalence and risk factors, 1959 to 1979. *Archives of General Psychiatry, 39*, 473–481.

Kay, D. W. K. (1972). Schizophrenia and schizophrenia-like states in the elderly. *British Journal of Hospital Medicine, 8*, 369–376.

Kay, D. W. K., & Roth, M. (1961). Environmental and hereditary factors in the schizophrenias of old age ("late paraphrenia") and their bearing on the general problem of causation in schizophrenia. *Journal of Mental Science, 107*, 649–686.

Kraepelin, E. (1971). (R. M. Barclay, Trans. Originally published 1919). *Dementia Praecox and Paraphrenia.* Huntington, NY, Krieger.

Lewis, A. (1970). Paranoia and paranoid: A historical perspective. *Psychological Medicine, 1*, 2–12.

Lipowski, Z. J. (1989). Delirium in the elderly. *New England Journal of Medicine, 320*, 578–582.

Lowenthal, M. F. (1964). *Lives in Distress.* New York, Basic Books.

Macmillan, D., & Shaw, P. (1966). Senile breakdown in standards of personal and environmental cleanliness. *British Medical Journal, 2*, 1032–1037.

Marneros, A., & Deister, A. (1984). The psychopathology of "late schizophrenia." *Psychopathology, 17*, 264–274.

Mellor, C. S. (1982). The present status of first rank symptoms. *British Journal of Psychiatry, 140*, 423–4.

Mjones, H. (1949) (E. Oldelberg, Trans.). Paralysis agitans: A clinical and genetic study. *Acta Psychiatrica Et Neurologica, Supplementum 54.*

Moore, N. C. (1981), Is paranoid illness associated with sensory defects in the elderly? *Journal of Psychosomatic Research, 25*, 69–74.

Moskovitz, C., Moses, H., & Klawans, H. L. (1978). Levodopa-induced psychosis: A kindling phenomenon. *American Journal of Psychiatry, 135,* 669–675.

Naguib, M., & Levy, R. (1987). Late paraphrenia: Neuropsychological impairment and structural brain abnormalities on computed tomography. *International Journal of Geriatric Psychiatry, 2,* 83–90.

Olson, P. R., Suddeth, J. A., Peterson, P. J., & Egelhoff, C. (1985). Hallucinations of widowhood. *Journal of the American Geriatrics Society, 33,* 543–547.

Opjordsmoen, S. (1988). Long-term course and outcome in delusional disorder. *Acta Psychiatrica Scandinavica, 78,* 576–586.

Orrell, M. W., Sahakian, B. J., & Bergmann, K. (1989). Self-neglect and frontal lobe dysfunction. *British Journal of Psychiatry, 155,* 101–105.

Pearlson, G. D., & Rabins, P. (1988). The late-onset psychoses: Possible risk factors. In D. V. Jeste & S. Zisook (Eds.), *The psychiatric clinics of North America* (pp. 15–32). Philadelphia: W. B. Saunders.

Pearlson, G. D., Kreger, L., Rabins, P. V., Chase, G. A., Cohen, B., Wirth, J. B., Schlaepfer, T. B., and Tune, L. E. (1989). A chart review study of late-onset and early-onset schizophrenia. *American Journal of Psychiatry, 146,* 1568–1574.

Post, F. (1965). *Paranoid syndromes: The clinical psychiatry of late life.* Oxford: Pergamon Press.

Post, F. (1980). Paranoid, schizophrenia-like, and schizophrenia states in the aged. In J. E. Birren & R. B. Sloane (Eds.), *Handbook of mental health and aging* (pp. 591–615). Englewood Cliffs, NJ: Prentice-Hall.

Rabins, P. V., Mace, N. L., & Lucas, M. J. (1982). The impact of dementia on the family. *Journal of the American Medical Association, 248,* 333–335.

Rabins, P. V., Pauker, S., & Thomas J. (1984). Can schizophrenia begin after age 44? *Comprehensive Psychiatry, 25,* 290–295.

Rabins, P. V., Pearlson, G. D., Jayaram, G., Steele, C., & Tune, L. (1987). Elevated ventricle to brain ratio in late-onset schizophrenia. *American Journal of Psychiatry, 144,* 1216–1218.

Roth, M. (1952). The natural history of mental disorder in old age. *Journal of Mental Science, 101,* 281–292.

Seeman, M. V. (1981). Gender and the onset of schizophrenia: Neurohumoral influences. *The Psychiatric Journal of the University of Ottawa, 6,* 136–138.

Seeman, M. V. (1986). Current outcome in schizophrenia: Women vs. men. *Acta Psychiatrica Scandinavica, 73,* 609–617.

Segal, J. H. (1989). Erotomania revisited: From Kraepelin to DSM-III-R. *American Journal of Psychiatry, 146,* 1261–1266.

Shuttleworth, E. C. (1984). Atypical presentation of dementia of the Alzheimer type. *Journal of the American Geriatrics Society, 32,* 485–490.

Snowdon, J. (1987). Uncleanliness among persons seen by community health workers. *Hospital and Community Psychiatry, 38,* 491–494.

Tsuang, M. T., & Woolson, R. F. (1977). Mortality in patients with schizophrenia, mania, depression, and surgical conditions: A comparison with general population mortality. *British Journal of Psychiatry, 130,* 162–166.

Waddington, J. L., Youssef, H. A., Dolphin, C., & Kinsella, A. (1987). Cognitive dysfunction, negative symptoms, and tardive dyskinesia in schizophrenia. *Archives of General Psychiatry, 44,* 907–912.

Winokur, G. (1977). Delusional disorder (paranoia). *Comprehensive Psychiatry, 18,* 511–521.

Zweig, R. M., Jankel, W. R., Hedreen, J. C., Mayeux, R., & Price, D. L. (1989). The pedunculopontine nucleus in Parkinson's disease. *Annals of Neurology, 26,* 41–46.

18

Alzheimer's Disease and Other Dementing Disorders

Murray A. Raskind and Elaine R. Peskind

    I. Dementia
   II. Alzheimer's Disease
      A. Clinical Presentation of AD
      B. Epidemiology
      C. Pathogenesis of AD
      D. Genetics
      E. Amyloid and Other Abnormal Proteins
      F. Environmental Toxins
      G. Pathophysiology of AD
   III. Dementia in Parkinson's Disease and the Spectrum of Lewy Body Diseases
   IV. Multi-Infarct Dementia
    V. Pick's Disease
   VI. Normal-Pressure Hydrocephalus
  VII. Metabolic Dementing Disorders
 VIII. Infectious Dementing Disorders
      A. AIDS
      B. Creutzfeldt-Jakob Disease
      C. Neurosyphilis
   IX. Alcoholic Dementia
    X. Treatment of Secondary Behavioral Problems in Dementia
   XI. Dementia and Depression
  XII. The Relationship of Depression in Parkinson's Disease to Dementia in Parkinson's Disease
 XIII. Delirium
 XIV. Conclusion
      References

Handbook of Mental Health and Aging, Second Edition
Copyright © 1992 by Academic Press, Inc. All rights reserved.

This chapter discusses the organic mental disorders that produce the dementia syndrome in older adults. Because Alzheimer's disease (AD) is the most common and devastating of these disorders, AD is emphasized. For each disorder, clinical phenomenology, epidemiology, pathophysiology, and pathogenesis are reviewed. Delirium and depression, both of which can mimic or complicate the dementing disorders, are discussed as they relate to differential diagnosis and treatment, and general treatment approaches to the dementia patient and his or her caregiver are also reviewed. Particular emphasis is given to recent research findings.

I. Dementia

Dementia is a syndrome; that is, a group of signs and symptoms that cluster together without a specific identified causative disorder. Many specific disorders produce the dementia syndrome. The DSM-III-R provides criteria for diagnosing dementia. The central feature is demonstrable evidence of impairment in short- and long-term memory. In addition, at least one of the following four problems must be present: impairment in abstract thinking, impaired judgment, personality change, or other disturbances of higher cortical functions such as aphasia, apraxia, agnosia, and constructional difficulty. These disturbances must significantly interfere with work, usual social activities, and relationships with others, and not occur exclusively during the course of a delirium (see below). Furthermore, there must be evidence of a specific organic etiology, or an etiologic organic factor can be presumed if the disturbance cannot be accounted for by a nonorganic mental disorder such as major depression.

The course of the dementia syndrome depends on the nature of the underlying dementing disorder. An insidious onset with a gradually deteriorating course is typical of many of the common dementing disorders of later life, such as AD and the dementia of Parkinson's disease. However, dementia can have an acute onset as in dementia secondary to acute hypoxia, and the course of the dementia syndrome in this case can be stable or even improve. In unusual but fortunate patients, the dementia syndrome may be reversible and cognitive function, restored to levels approximating previous function. Such an optimal course is possible following successful surgical treatment of normal-pressure hydrocephalus or a benign intracranial mass lesion such as a meningioma.

II. Alzheimer's Disease

Most patients with dementia of insidious onset and a progressive deteriorating course in late life are suffering from AD. In this chapter, the term AD is used rather than the DSM-III-R term *primary degenerative dementia of the Alzheimer type* for simplicity and concordance with the usage in the general medical and neurological literature. DSM-III-R (APA, 1987) criteria for this disorder are straightforward. They include the presence of the dementia syndrome, an insidious onset with a generally progressive deteriorating course, and reasonable exclusion of all other specific causes of the dementia syndrome by history, physical examination, and laboratory tests.

Another set of widely used criteria for the diagnosis of probable AD in the living patient is that proposed by a work group on the diagnosis of Alzheimer's disease established by the National Institute of Neurological and Communicative Disorders and Stroke (NINCDS) and the Alzheimer's Disease and Related Disorders Association (ADRDA) (McKhann *et al.*, 1984). The six criteria are as follows:

1. the dementia syndrome as established by clinical examination and confirmed by neuropsychological tests;
2. deficits in two or more areas of cognition;
3. progressive worsening of memory and other cognitive functions;
4. no disturbance of consciousness;
5. onset between the ages of 40 and 90 and most often after age 65; and
6. absence of systemic disorders or other brain diseases that could account for the progressive deficits in memory and cognition.

The diagnosis becomes definite AD when postmortem neuropathologic examination reveals numerous neuritic plaques and neurofibrillary tangles in neocortex and hippocampus. In practice, a diagnosis of primary degenerative dementia of the Alzheimer's type by DSM-III-R criteria usually agrees nicely with a diagnosis of probable AD by NINCDS/ADRDA criteria.

A. Clinical Presentation of AD

AD begins insidiously. Subtle difficulties in memory are almost always the first symptom. Early in the course of the disease, memory loss tends to be more marked for recent events. The patient may be obviously repetitious in conversation, become disoriented in unfamiliar settings, and fail to remember appointments and obligations. As the disease progresses, remote and highly learned memory traces become lost or inaccessible, and the patient may eventually be unable to recognize even immediate family members. Other cognitive impairments affect judgment, abstract reasoning, calculation, and visual–spatial skills. In the middle stages of AD, a fluent type of aphasia usually appears, and the patient develops difficulty in properly naming objects or choosing the appropriate word to express an idea. In many patients, this aphasia is gradually progressive, and some patients totally lose useful speech. Apraxia (the inability to perform well-learned activities despite understanding the nature of the task and having intact motor function) often occurs coincidentally with the aphasia. Both aphasia and apraxia present major problems for care providers. The most common personality change in AD is apathy. A previously caring and responsive spouse, parent, or friend becomes increasingly self-centered and loses interest in and empathy for the needs of others. Other personality changes include increased dependency with anxious clinging behavior and exaggeration of premorbid personality traits. Angry outbursts are common when the patient does not comprehend why his or her activities are being limited. In the late stages of the illness, the sleep–wake cycle becomes disrupted; patients frequently pace and wander and lose the ability to attend to their own dressing, feeding, and personal hygiene. In the very advanced stages of the disorder, motor deficits include rigidity and bradykinesia. Both of these signs occur in Parkinson's disease, but the tremor characteristic of Parkinson's disease is uncommon in AD. Myoclonic jerks develop in a substantial number of patients and seizures of several types may occur in the late stages of the illness (Risse *et al.*, 1990). The terminal stages of the illness are manifested by mutism, inability to ambulate, loss of sphincter control, and cachexia. Death is usually from pneumonia. The course of AD can range from 3 to more than 20 years from the onset of early signs and symptoms. The *terminal* phase of illness can be prolonged for years with good nursing care and tube feeding. The proper approach to such terminally demented patients raises important ethical and medicolegal questions, which will have to be addressed as the number of such patients grows.

B. Epidemiology

Prevalence studies of dementia in later life have suggested that about 4% of persons older than 65 and 20% of persons older than 80 suffer from a dementing illness severe enough to impair their ability to live independently (Mortimer, 1983). Among these at least two thirds are demented secondary to AD. However, a recent carefully done study (Evens *et al.*, 1989) suggests the prevalence of AD may be much higher. All noninstitutionalized persons 65 or older in a geographically defined community of 32,000 in East Boston, MA were asked to respond to a structured questionnaire containing a range of items concerning medical and social problems of older persons as well as several brief cognitive screening tests. Of the 4485 age-eligible residents, 81% responded and underwent the above screening. A sample of individuals was selected from the intermediate- and poor-performance groups for further intensive neuropsychological and clinical evaluations, and another informant was interviewed for each participant. NINCDS and DSM-III criteria were used to make the clinical diagnosis of probable AD.

Of the 467 persons who underwent the intensive clinical evaluation, 134 had probable AD and 166, possible AD; the remainder had no evidence of AD. Of those with probable AD, 77% had moderate to severe cogntive impairment. Taking the sampling procedure into account, the prevalence rate for probable AD was 10.3% among those older than 65 years and 47% for those 85 years or older. Approximately 8% of persons older than 65 and 36% over 85 had moderate to severe cognitive impairment, limiting their ability to live independently. These data suggest that AD may even be more common than previously reported.

C. Pathogenesis of AD

The search for the cause or pathogenesis of AD has focused on three areas: genetics, the beta-amyloid protein, and potential environmental toxins. Research in these and other areas, such as the nature of the intracellular neurofibrillary tangle, or the possibility of an infectious cause, has increased exponentially during the past 10 years. It should be kept in mind that AD may have more than one cause. For example, one of several genetic defects could interact with one or more environmental toxins to produce the disease.

D. Genetics

The genetics of AD is complex, but several lines of evidence suggest opportunities for defining the pathogenesis of the disorder. First, it has become clear that the neuropathologic lesions of AD occur in almost all persons with Down's syndrome older than 40 (Lai & Williams, 1989). Because Down's syndrome (trisomy 21) is caused by an extra copy of genes on chromosome 21, it has been hypothesized that AD similarly may be caused by extra copies of genes on chromosome 21. Second, a large number of family pedigrees have been described in which multiple persons are affected by AD in several consecutive generations. In many of these families approximately 50% of the at-risk members are affected, and most of genetic inheritance is consistent with an autosomal dominant gene. The availability of these unusual familial AD (FAD) families has prompted several groups to use genetic linkage–analysis techniques to identify the chromosomal region containing the FAD gene, with the ultimate goal of identifying the gene itself. An initial report using this approach created great optimism that the gene for FAD had been mapped to chromosome 21, but subsequent findings from other groups suggest that the genetics of FAD is more complex. Specifically, in 1987, St. George-Hyslop et al. reported positive linkage results in four large FAD kindreds, all of whom had early-onset AD, to two markers (D21S1/11 and D21S16) close to the centromere on the long arm of chromosome 21. Adding to the interest in this finding was the discovery that the region containing the putative FAD gene was close to the region on chromosome 21 that encoded the gene for the amyloid found in the neuritic plaque lesions of AD. All of these findings appeared to support the hypothesis that an abnormal gene, in this case the one encoding amyloid, on chromosome 21, was present in excess quantity (as in Down's syndrome) and was etiologically involved in FAD. However, complicating data soon emerged. Tanzi et al. (1987) reported that the putative gene for FAD as reported by St. George-Hyslop et al. (1987) was not tightly linked to the amyloid gene, although both were mapped to the same chromosome. Furthermore, it has become clear that duplication of the amyloid gene is not observed in AD, and no other duplication on chromosome 21 has been identified in AD. Further doubt has resulted from attempts to replicate the St. George-Hyslop et al. findings. Although Goate et al. (1989) did find evidence for linkage of D21S1/11 and D21S16, the bulk of evidence for linkage came from a single family of the six families with early-onset FAD who were studied. Two other groups have failed to replicate the St. George-Hyslop et al. findings. Pericak-Vance et al. (1988) also have reported negative results for linkage to these chromosome 21 markers in both late-onset and early-onset FAD kindreds. Schellenberg et al. (1988) using a different set of FAD families, excluded linkage of the FAD gene from the region of interest on chromosome 21. Much of the data for exclusion in this latter study came from a group of families referred to as the Volga German kindreds. These families are part of an ethnic isolate, a group of ethnic Germans who migrated to southwestern Russia in the 18th century and subsequently immigrated to the United States during the past 100 years. These affected Volga German families are probably descended from a common founder or single person, who developed a mutation for the genetic abnormality and passed it on to his progeny. These families are thus genetically homogenous for the AD abnormality and can be pooled for genetic linkage analysis. Recently, Roses et al. (1990) presented data demonstrating linkage to markers on chromosome 19 in the late-onset AD kindreds. It is clear that finding the gene or genes for FAD will be difficult. However, the exciting results obtained from linkage analysis in Huntington's disease, cystic fibrosis, and Duchenne's muscular dystrophy make genetic linkage studies high priority for ultimately discovering the cause of AD. An antemortem marker for AD would enhance the chance for successful linkage analysis. Recent description of a platelet-membrane abnormality in AD (Zubenko, 1988) is a promising ante-mortem-marker candidate.

Detecting a genetic pattern of transmission in late-onset AD is complicated by the very real possibility that most relatives at risk will die of some other disorder before AD will ever be expressed. This phenomenon might make truly late-onset FAD kindreds appear to be *sporadic*. Two epidemiologic studies have used Kaplan-Meyer table methods to esti-mate a specific cumulative incidence of AD in relatives of AD probands. Breitner and Folstein (1984) found the 90-year lifetime risk of AD among pooled first-degree relatives of AD probands to exceed 50%, which they interpreted as suggesting autosomal dominant transmission. Mohs, Breitner, Silverman, and Davis (1987) demonstrated that first-degree relatives of patients of AD probands showed a 46% cumulative incidence of probable AD by 86 years of age. However, it must be kept in mind that the recent East Boston epidemiologic study (see above) demonstrated a prevalence of AD approaching 50% by age 85 in a community-based population (Evans *et al.*, 1989).

E. Amyloid and Other Abnormal Proteins

If one accepts that neuritic plaques are basic to the pathobiology of AD, then it is reasonable to explore the biochemical composition of neuritic plaques to gain insight into the pathogenesis of the disorder. Because amyloid is the major component of neuritic plaques and is also present in cerebral blood vessels (amyloid angiopathy) in many patients with AD, intense interest has been focused upon the protein chemistry and molecular biology of AD-type amyloid. It should be borne in mind that neuritic plaques are a quantitative rather than qualitative feature of AD and occur to some degree in normal aging. Recent advances in understanding the role of amyloid in AD have been reviewed by Selkoe (1990). Once Glenner and Wong (1984) identified the peptide sequence of the amyloid protein from vascular amyloid obtained from AD brain tissue, progress was rapid. It soon became clear that this fragment was part of a 695-residue polypeptide known as amyloid precursor protein (APP), a membrane-spanning protein containing a 40-amino-acid fragment, the amyloid beta protein (βP). βP is the major component of the amyloid deposits in the neuritic plaques and blood vessels of patients with AD. A few highlights from recent studies will illustrate attempts to understand the nature of these proteins, and elucidate their role in the pathogenesis of AD. First, there are at least three forms of APP, known as APP 695, APP 751, and APP 770. Recently, it has been demonstrated that the large extracellular amino terminal portion of APP 751 and APP 770 is identical to a protease inhibitor known as protease nexin II, a molecule that inactivates serine proteases. The protease nexin II component of APP has recently been found in relatively large amounts in the alpha granules of human platelets and is secreted during platelet activation (Van Nostrand, Schmaier, Farrow, & Cunningham, 1990). Together with the recent demonstration by Joachim, Mori, and Selkoe (1989) of βP in peripheral tissues such as skin and intestine, this finding has raised speculation that βP deposited in AD lesions may be derived from the peripheral circulation. This view is still a minority opinion (βP has not been identified in blood), and most investigators continued to believe that βP is neuronally produced. Other investigations have focused upon potential abnormal processing of APP that could result in excessive deposition of βP in the brain (Johnson, McNeill, Cordell, & Finch, 1990) within the hippocampus and entorhinal cortex, and which may be detectable in cerebrospinal fluid (CSF) in AD and in normal aging (Palmert et al. 1989).

In addition to characterizing the forms of APP and its fragments, investigators have also explored the biologic function of APP fragments. Whitson, Selkoe, and Cotman (1989) found that a peptide containing only the first 28 amino acids of βP actually promotes the survival of embryonic rat hippocampal cells in culture, suggesting growth factor–like activity of an APP fragment, at least in this *in vitro* system. In contrast, Yankner et al. (1989) found a very different result using an APP fragment that included the entire βP and another segment of the precursor. This group transfected pheochromocytoma cells with a gene coding for this fragment of APP. When the pheochromocytoma cells were induced to differentiate into neuron-like cells by nerve growth factor (NGF), they perished. It therefore appears that different fragments of APP may have very different functions. It is also not clear of course that these *in vitro* experiments are relevant to the biology of APP and βP in humans. Another important chemical feature of neuritic plaques is the presence of heparan sulfate proteoglycan, a normal constituent of the vascular basement membrane, which may be involved in the abnormal deposition of amyloid in plaques (Snow et al., 1988).

An approach to finding a basic molecular defect in AD has been pioneered by Davies and Wolozin (1987). They found an antibody (Alz 50) which recognized a 68-kDa protein that appears to accumulate fairly specifically in brain tissue from patients with AD and Down's syndrome but not in other dementing disorders. This A68 *antigen* may be related to the microtubule-associated protein tau (Ksiezak-Reding et al., 1988), which has been found to be a major constituent of intraneuronal neurofibrillary tangles in AD. A68 may appear before the formation of neurofibrillary tangles and neuritic plaques (Hyman et al., 1988), and is probably part of a larger molecule called Alzheimer's disease–associated protein (ADAP). In a recent study in which ADAP was quantified in human postmortem brain tissue utilizing an Alz 50 immunoassay, ADAP was clearly detected in 93% of 43 AD cases and all of three elderly Down's syndrome cases, but in no elderly normal controls or patients with dementia secondary to non-AD neurologic diseases (Ghanbari et al., 1990). These findings suggest that this immunoassay may be helpful in the postmortem neuropathologic diagnosis of AD. An antemortem diagnostic test using the Alz 50 immunoassay in CSF would be extremely valuable, but to this point early findings suggesting diagnostic utility in a small group of subjects (Davies, 1991) have not yet been replicated. Such diagnostic tools have become even more needed with the recent description of dementing disorders such as those associated with Lewy bodies (see below), which can be confused antemortem and even postmortem with AD.

The attempt to understand the basic chemistry of intraneuronal neurofibrillary tangles has been hampered by their extreme insolubility. Recent success in dissolving neurofibrillary tangles using formic acid has led to the demonstration of such cytoskeletal proteins as tau (which appears to be in an abnormally phosphorylated state in neurofibrillary tangles), ubiquitin, MAP2 and several neurofilament subunits (Perry, 1987).

F. Environmental Toxins

Search for possible environmental etiologies of AD have been discouraging to date, but recent studies possibly implicating a neurotoxin in the etiology of Parkinson's disease as well as the demonstration that there is a high rate of discordant expression of AD among monozygotic twin pairs (Nee *et al.* 1987) provide rationale for continued epidemiologic and other studies seeking an environmental cause.

Several studies have suggested that aluminum, the third most common element in the earth's crust, may be implicated in the pathogenesis of AD. This element has been linked to the dementia seen in chronic renal dialysis patients, and neurofibrillary-like changes can be induced in rabbits by injecting aluminum into the central nervous system. Several studies (Crapper, Krishnan, & Dalton, 1973; Trapp, Miner, Zimmerman, Mastri, & Heston, 1978) have found increased aluminum in postmortem brain tissue in AD, and Perl and Brody (1980) demonstrated by x-ray spectrometry focal intraneuronal accumulations of aluminum within neurofibrillary tangle–bearing neurons in AD. Tangle-free neurons from AD patients and from nondemented controls fail to show similar degrees of aluminum accumulation. In addition, neuritic plaques have been reported to contain aluminosilicate (Candy *et al.* 1986). Other investigators have failed to find differences in brain aluminum between AD patients and age-matched controls (Markesberry, Ehmann, Hosain, Alauddin, & Goodin, 1981; McDermott, Smith, Igbal, & Wisniewski, 1977). Yates and Mann (1986) speculate that the aluminosilicate concentrations in plaques are likely to be a secondary phenomenon. This controversy, together with suggestive findings in a recent epidemiologic study (Graves *et al.*, 1990), support the need for further studies of aluminum and AD.

Although an infectious etiology for AD is considered unlikely, the demonstrated viral etiology of Creutzfeldt-Jakob and the occasional presence of spongiform changes at neuropathologic exam in patients with otherwise classic AD neuropathology suggest the need for further investigation. Recently, Manuelidis *et al.* (1988) reported neurohistologic damage in rodents exposed to blood components from persons with familial AD. Studies attempting to replicate this finding are currently underway. One potential risk factor for AD that has been demonstrated in several epidemiologic studies is history of head trauma (Graves *et al.*, 1990; Heyman *et al.*, 1984; Mortimer, French, Hutton, & Schuman, 1985;), which has been noted to have been more prevalent in AD patients than in normal case controls. Head trauma in these studies was remote to the onset of AD symptoms and severe enough to cause loss of consciousness, but did not produce neurologic sequelae after the patient awakened. It should be noted, however, that such a history of remote head trauma was found in fewer than 25% of AD subjects.

G. Pathophysiology of AD

Even if the pathogenesis of AD remains unclear and the cause of death or dysfunction of brain tissue elements remains unknown, understanding how such damaged brain tissue disrupts brain function can have important implications for symptomatic treatment and differential diagnosis. Attempts to understand the pathophysiology of AD and to be guided by such knowledge in the design of pharmacologic treatment strategies have received impetus from the successful application of such a strategy to dopaminergic therapies in Parkinson's disease. That such a strategy might also succeed in AD became more plausible in the late 1970s with the discovery of an apparently specific deficit in the brain cholinergic system in postmortem tissue from AD patients (Davies & Maloney, 1976; Perry, Tomlinson, Blessed, & Perry, 1978), which was manifested by substantial decreases in the synthetic enzyme for acetylcholine, choline acetyltransferase (ChAT) in hippocampal and cortical tissue from AD patients compared with nondemented age-matched normal controls. Furthermore, in 1982, Whitehouse *et al.* demonstrated extensive neuronal damage in the nucleus basalis of Meynert, the major source of cholinergic neurons projecting to neocortex and hippocampus, in postmortem AD brain tissue. In living AD patients, brain biopsy tissue showed reduced cortical ChAT activity, which was significantly correlated with the density of neuritic plaques (Neary *et al.*, 1986). In another demonstration of the AD cholinergic deficit in living patients, Raskind (1989) documented in AD patients a decreased neuroendocrine response to physostigmine of beta-endorphin and arginine vasopressin (AVP), hormones which are under stimulatory regulation by brain cholinergic systems.

Although there is debate as to whether the presynaptic cholinergic lesion in AD is a primary event or secondary to AD lesions in cortical and hippocampal cholinergic projection areas, this cholinergic deficit has generated an intense amount of research directed at ameliorating cognitive dysfunction by enhancing brain cholinergic activity. Unfortunately, these attempts have not been nearly so successful as has been enhancement of dopaminergic systems in Parkinson's disease. Administration of the acetylcholine precursors choline or lecithin (phosphatidyl choline) have been ineffective (Thal, Rosen, Sharpless, & Crystal, 1981; Brinkman *et al.*, 1982). Because the brain muscarinic receptors on postsynaptic neurons remain intact in AD, several investigators have administered muscarinic cholinergic agonists believed to be active at these receptor sites. Christie, Shering, Ferguson, and Glen, (1981) demonstrated slight cognitive improvement following intravenous arecoline. Harbaugh, Roberts, Coombs, Saunders, and Reeder, (1984) administered bethanechol continuously into AD patients' cerebral ventricles by an implantable infusion system. Unfortunately, this fairly invasive treatment did not result in reproducible cognitive improvement. Somewhat more successful have been attempts to use centrally active cholinesterase inhibitor drugs to prolong the synaptic activity of acetyl choline released from presynaptic cholinergic neurons. Intravenous administration of physostigmine produced modest improvement in cognitive function in mildly demented AD patients (Davis, Mohs, & Tinklenberg, 1979). Treatment with oral physostigmine, a more convenient dosage form with longer duration of activity, has produced modest cognitive improvement in several studies (Harrell *et al.*, 1989; Mohs *et al.*, 1985; Stern, Sano, & Mayeux, 1988; Thal, Masur, & Sharpless, 1983) but has not been consistently replicated (Jenike, Albert, Heller, Gunther & Goff, 1990; Schmechel *et al.*, 1984). An ongoing trial of an oral physostigmine preparation with enhanced bioavailability is currently in progress at multiple centers. An encouraging therapeutic trial using the cholinesterase inhibitor tetrahydroaminoacridine (THA) reported by Summers, Majorski, Marsh, Tachiki, and Kling in 1986 prompted a large multicenter clinical trial that has attempted to replicate these positive findings as well as to assess the risk:benefit ratio of THA. Although this trial is still in progress, an interim analysis was encouraging enough to continue the trial to completion. It is clear, however, that if THA is demonstrated effective and approved by the FDA for clinical use, its effect on memory will be modest, and the reversible liver toxicity produced by the drug in some patients will be problematic. A recent Canadian trial of THA failed to demonstrate efficacy (Gauthier et al., 1990). The lack of a straightforward response to enhancement of cholinergic activity in AD may be related to the recent demonstration in postmortem AD brain tissue that remaining presynaptic cholinergic neurons appear to be already working at increased capacity (Slotkin et al., 1990). It is possible that attempting to increase further the activity of already activated presynaptic cholinergic neurons in AD may be of limited utility.

Another potential problem with the cholinergic enhancement strategy is the existence of multiple neurotransmitter and neuromodulator abnormalities in AD. Prominent among these is an abnormality in the brain noradrenergic system. In postmortem AD brain tissue, cell counts in the locus ceruleus are reduced (Bondareff et al., 1987) and norepinephrine content is decreased in several areas (Mann, Yates, & Hawkes, 1982). The data are not straightforward, however, in that the concentration of the primary brain metabolite of norepinephrine, 3-methoxy-4-hydroxyphenylglycol (MHPG) is elevated in several brain areas in which norepinephrine content is decreased (Winblad, Adolfsson, Carlsson, & Gottfries, 1982). In cortical biopsy tissue from the temporal lobe of AD patients, MHPG is increased in early-onset patients (Francis et al., 1985) and, in CSF, concentrations of both norepinephrine and MHPG are elevated in early-onset AD patients with advanced disease (Raskind, Peskind, Halter, & Jimerson, 1984). The finding of decreased norepinephrine concentration in brain tissue, but increased concentration of its metabolite in brain tissue and CSF, are compatible with increased release of norepinephrine. The apparent contradiction between dramatic cell loss in the locus ceruleus and possibly increased norepinephrine release in the central nervous system in early-onset AD patients with advanced disease may represent increased activity of remaining neurons in the locus ceruleus (Hollander, Mohs, & Davis, 1986). More speculatively, the noradrenergic neuronal ingrowth from perivascular sympathetic nervous system fibers into cholinergically denervated hippocampus in the rat (Booze, Laforet, and Davis, 1986) may also be present in the cholinergically denervated hippocampus in patients with AD. If demonstrated, such noradrenergic sprouting into brain tissue in AD could have important implications for such AD symptoms as agitation and sleep disturbance.

Several neuropeptides are also decreased in AD brain tissue and CSF. Somatostatin, a neuropeptide primarily located in intrinsic cortical neurons, is reduced in AD neocortex and hippocampus (Davies, Katzman, & Perry, 1980). CSF concentrations of somatostatin are also decreased (Wood et al., 1982; Raskind et al., 1986). AVP, a neuropeptide that enhances learning in animal models, is widely distributed in extrahypothalamic brain areas. AVP concentrations in CSF in AD have consistently been demonstrated to be reduced (Sorensen, Hammer, Vorstrup, & Gjerrig, 1983; Sundquist, Forsling, Olsson, & Akerlund, 1983; Mazurek, Growden, Beal, & Martin, 1986; Raskind et al., 1986) Corticotropin-releasing factor (CRF) is decreased in brain tissue in AD (Bissette, Reynolds, Kilts, Widerlov, & Nemeroff, 1985; DeSouza, Whitehouse, Kuhar, Price, & Vale 1986), and increases in CRF-receptor concentrations have been demonstrated in cortical areas in which the concentrations of the peptide itself were reduced. This apparent up-regulation of CRF receptors in AD brain tissue suggests a meaningful neurotransmitter role for CRF. Receptor up-regulation has not been demonstrated for other neuropeptides found to be decreased in AD, although careful studies remain to be done to rule out this possibility for AVP. Taken together, these and other abnormalities in brain neuropeptides and other neurotransmitters highlight the complexity of the multiple neurochemical lesions in AD and suggest that combined replacement strategies may be necessary to compensate for the pathophysiologic abnormalities.

An exciting new area of brain research with potential relevance to prevention or restoration of cholinergic or perhaps other deficits in AD is the area of neurotrophic factors. These factors, which are usually polypeptides, affect the survival and differentiation of neurons in both the peripheral and central nervous systems (Levi-Montalcini, 1987). Growth factors are synthesized in the target areas innervated by the neurons they regulate, and bind to specific receptors on these neurons to promote neuronal growth and survival. NGF is the best characterized of these neurotrophic factors. NGF sustains viability of noradrenergic neurons in the peripheral sympathetic nervous system and cholinergic neurons in the brain. These latter cholinergic neurons are the magnocellular neurons in the nucleus basalis of Meynert and other basal forebrain areas deficient in AD. In two animal model systems relevant to AD, NGF has been demonstrated to improve cholinergic function. NGF administered to rats following fimbria fornix lesions, which separate septal cholinergic neurons from their hippocampal target-organ supply of endogenous NGF, prevents degeneration and induces axonal regrowth of these cholinergic neurons (Gage, Armstrong, Williams, & Varon, 1988; Kromer, 1987). Also, infusion of NGF into the ventricles of cognitively impaired aged rats improves retention of a spatial-learning task and increases the size of basal forebrain cholinergic neurons (Fischer *et al.*, 1987). The major problems in studying NGF in humans are its inability to cross the blood–brain barrier, lack of information concerning potential toxicity, and the lack of a reliable source of well-characterized human NGF in sufficient quantity for comprehensive research studies (Phelps *et al.*, 1989). This last problem appears to have been overcome by genetically engineered NGF production.

III. Dementia in Parkinson's Disease and the Spectrum of Lewy Body Diseases

The high prevalence of dementia in Parkinson's disease (PD) was not fully appreciated until the functional life of Parkinson's patients was extended by use of L-dopa and other specific dopaminergic-enhancing therapies. Dementia in Parkinson's disease usually presents as memory impairment and slowness of thinking with preserved language function, although aphasia and apraxia may also occur (Perry *et al.*, 1985). Estimates of the prevalence of dementia in PD have ranged from 14 to 40%. Brown and Marsden (1984) have reviewed 17 studies reported over the past 60 years including a total of 2530 patients. Some degree of dementia was present in approximately 35%. They suggest that various methodologic problems such as nonstandardized diagnostic criteria for PD and dementia and sampling variability may have resulted in an overestimation of the prevalence of dementia; they offer a more conservative estimate of approximately 20%. Mayeux *et al.* (1988a), in a study of 339 patients with idiopathic PD using standardized research criteria for dementia and idiopathic PD, found an overall prevalence of 10.9%. Demented patients were older, had a later onset of motor manifestations, a more rapid progression of physical disability, and tended to respond poorly and have more adverse effects to L-dopa than did PD patients without dementia. The incidence of dementia in PD is approximately four times higher compared to that in similarly aged adults (Rajput, Offord, Beard, & Kurland, 1987).

It has been proposed that the dementia seen in Parkinson's disease could be attributed to the concurrent presence of AD in these patients (Hakim and Mathieson, 1979; Boller *et al.*, 1980). Several other studies have suggested that the dementia of PD is not usually secondary to concomitant AD. Chui, Mortimer, and Slager (1984) reported careful histopathologic studies of cerebral cortex, hippocampus, substantia nigra, locus ceruleus, and nucleus basalis of Meynert in four PD patients with carefully documented dementia antemortem. Dementia in these patients was associated with severe neuronal loss in subcortical nuclei. Significant numbers of neuritic plaques and neurofibrillary tangles were not found in the hippocampus or cerebral cortex. Studies by Perry *et al.*, (1985) and Ball (1984) have confirmed that the dementia of PD usually occurs in the absence of substantial AD-type changes in the cortex. Perry *et al.* (1985) measured cortical ChAT levels in brains of six demented and three nondemented PD patients; none of these patients had histopathologic evidence of AD. Reductions in temporal neocortical ChAT levels correlated with the degree of mental impairment. Substantial cell loss in the noradrenergic locus ceruleus also occurs in PD. Cash *et al.* (1987) found decreased norepinephrine and MHPG (the major metabolite of norepinephrine) in the locus ceruleus of seven demented PD patients compared with 13 age-matched controls. Eight nondemented PD patients had similar norepinephrine and MHPG levels to those of the controls. Brain and tissue levels of somatostatin have been reported to be reduced in PD patients with dementia (Beal *et al.*, 1986; Epelbaum *et al.*, 1983; Jolkkonen *et al.*, 1986), and Whitehouse *et al.* (1987) have reported reductions in brain CRF in PD. Some of these PD neurochemical changes also occur in AD.

Conversely, neuropathologic changes of PD have been found in the brains of patients with the clinical and neuropathologic diagnosis of AD. Brainstem Lewy bodies have been reported in 10 to 16% (Forno, 1982; Jellinger & Grisold, 1982; Woodard, 1962) of AD cases. Ditter and Mirra (1987) studied 20 consecutive cases of pathologically confirmed AD. Neuropathologic examination revealed numerous substantia nigra Lewy bodies in 11 cases (55%); marked nigral degeneration was seen in three cases. Three of the 11 cases also had cortical Lewy bodies. Rigidity was the most common extrapyramidal sign, occurring in 80% of the cases with PD pathology. Bradykinesia occurred less often and was always seen in association with rigidity in the group with PD pathology. Tremor was not observed in any patient. Rigidity was also seen in two and bradykinesia and masked facies in a another of the nine cases without PD pathology. Rigidity and bradykinesia had been previously reported in 28 to 67% of AD patients (Molsa, Martilla, & Rinne, 1984; Pearce, 1974; Sulkava, 1982). Leverenz and Sumi (1986) found nigral pathology in 18 of

40 AD cases; retrospective review of their records revealed rigidity in 61% and tremor in 33% of the 18 cases with PD pathology.

Diffuse Lewy body disease (DLBD) is a recently described disorder (Kosaka, Tsuchiya, & Yoshimura, 1980) which may be a common cause of dementia in later life. Lewy bodies are the classic neurohistologic stigmata of PD and are located in the substantia nigra in PD. The literature on the relationship between Lewy bodies and dementing disorders is discussed in some detail because of its recent prominence and potentially great importance. In 1961, Okazaki, Lipin, and Åronsen reported two cases of progressive dementia followed by rigidity and immobility of the limbs within 14 months. Neuropathologic exam revealed Lewy bodies in substantia nigra, locus ceruleus, and hypothalamus, and widespread Lewy bodies in the cerebral cortex. Gibb, Esiri, and Lees (1985) and Burkhardt et al. (1988) review 34 similar cases reported since that time. Age at onset with few exceptions was between 50 and 80 years, and the ratio of male:female cases was approximately 2:1. The most common presentation was a neurobehavioral syndrome; memory impairment and other cognitive deficits were typical, and confusional states, paranoid delusions, and visual and auditory hallucinations were frequently reported. All but one patient eventually became demented. Rigidity was the most commonly reported parkinsonian sign; bradykinesia and tremor were less common, and the tremor was often described as *transient* or mild. Among other movement disorders were myoclonus, seen in five patients, dystonia and chorea; orthostatic hypotension and dysphagia were also reported. Duration of illness ranged from less than 1 year to 20 years with progression to severe dementia, ridigity, mutism, quadriparesis, and emaciation; pneumonia was the most frequently reported cause of death. Neuropathologic exam of these cases revealed widespread Lewy body degeneration throughout the neocortex, limbic structures, and subcortical nuclei.

Lennox, Lowe, Godwin-Austen, Landon, & Mayer (1989) and Lennox et al. (1989) reported a recent neuropathologic correlational study of 15 patients with DLBD using anti-ubiquitin neurochemistry. Conventional hematoxylin and eosin (H & E) stains provide poor contrast between cortical Lewy bodies and the surrounding cytoplasm and are unreliable in identifying cortical Lewy bodies; ubiquitin provides intense staining of cortical Lewy bodies, allowing identification of even small or tangentially cut cortical Lewy bodies and pale bodies (Lennox et al., 1989c). Ubiquitin is a small protein produced in cells. It appears to have a housekeeping role in cells by conjugating with (*ubiquinating*) abnormal proteins and targeting them for degradation (Reichsteiner, 1987). Lennox et al. (1989a, 1989b) present 15 cases characterized clinically by dementia (severe in 14 cases) and varying severity of extrapyramidal signs; typical neuropathological findings are described and correlated with dementia severity. DLBD is chracterized by widespread Lewy bodies in the cortex in addition to loss of pigmented cells in the substantia nigra with gliosis and classic Lewy body formation similar to the findings in idiopathic PD. Similar changes were also found in other subcortical nuclei: locus ceruleus, dorsal vagal nucleus, and nucleus basalis of Meynert. No significant difference was found in substantia nigra cell counts between DLBD and PD, although in DLBD, a greater proportion of the remaining substantia nigra neurons contained Lewy bodies. Cortical Lewy bodies were not detected in normal controls and very rarely in nondemented PD cases. In DLBD cases,

Lewy bodies were found most abundantly in the entorhinal, inferior temporal, insular, and anterior cingulate cortex, mainly in small-and medium-sized pyramidal neurons of the deeper cortical layers; up to 4% of anterior cingulate gyrus neurons were affected by Lewy bodies. Mean cortical Lewy body density in six cortical regions studied correlated highly with severity of dementia.

Perry *et al.* (1990) have recently described a dementing syndrome in a group of 18 patients aged 71–90 initially presenting with an acute or subacute confusional state often associated with visual hallucinations and other behavioral disturbances. These cases did not meet clinical criteria for the diagnosis of AD; compared to AD, the atypical patients were more cognitively intact at time of referral, had a shorter history, and a shorter survival time. A number of cases had mild extrapyramidal symptoms, but the typical parkinsonian triad of tremor, rigidity, and bradykinesia was not present. Detailed neuropathological exam revealed Lewy bodies in the substantia nigra and other subcortical nuclei, the limbic system, and neocortex. Numerous senile plaques were present, but neurofibrillary tangles were minimal or absent. Perry *et al.* termed this syndrome senile dementia of the Lewy body type (SDLT).

In summary, it has been suggested that the Lewy body diseases represent a spectrum ranging from age-related or subclinical pathologic changes through a primarily movement disorder with or without dementia (PD) to primarily dementing disorders with prominent psychiatric symptoms and mild extrapyramidal symptoms or rigidity (SDLT and DLBD). In addition, there is marked biochemical and morphological overlap with AD. Although dementia in Lewy body diseases may occur in the absence of AD neuropathologic changes or with plaques only, a subgroup of PD patients have typical neuropathologic findings of AD as well and, in addition, PD changes occur in the brains of a proportion of AD cases. Lewy bodies, unlike plaques and tangles, are not a common feature of normal aging; Lewy bodies were found in only 2.3% of 131 normal control brains studied over a 50-year period (Perry *et al.*, 1990). This raises interesting questions about the pathological significance of Lewy body formation and its relationship to other neurodegenerative disorders.

IV. Multi-Infarct Dementia

The erroneous notion that dementia in most elderly patients is a consequence of cerebrovascular disease was dispelled by the landmark study of Blessed, Tomlinson, and Roth (1968). In this classic clinicopathologic correlational study, AD and not cerebrovascular dementia was the principal cause of the dementia syndrome even in the eighth and ninth decades of life. However, they also demonstrated that cerebrovascular disease still contributed to a substantial minority of dementia cases in the elderly (Tomlinson, Blessed & Roth, 1970). Using greater than 50 ml of infarcted tissue as their criterion for sufficient infarcted tissue to have produced dementia, they estimated that 17% of their elderly demented population had vascular dementias and an additional 18% had a combination of vascular dementia and AD. On the basis of this carefully studied small sample, subsequent investigators have accepted multiple cerebral infarctions in sufficient quantity as a basis of dementia in late life [multi-infarct dementia (MID)], if such infarctions can be demonstrated radiologically antemortem or at postmortem pathologic examination

(Hachinski, Larson, & Marshall, 1974). There are those who argue that MID continues to be overdiagnosed in elderly demented patients (Brust, 1983).

The DSM-III-R has established diagnostic criteria for MID. The four criteria are the presence of the dementia syndrome, a step-wise deteriorating course with patchy distribution of deficits early in the course, focal neurologic signs and symptoms, and evidence from history, physical examination, or laboratory tests of significant cerebrovascular disease that is judged to be etiologically related to the disturbance. These criteria for MID have not yet been validated by careful clinicopathologic correlational studies. Zubenko (1990) has questioned the usefulness of *step-wise deteriorating course* to differentiate MID dementia from AD. He evaluated 115 patients who met DSM-III-R criteria for primary degenerative dementia of the Alzheimer type and 46 patients who met DSM-III-R criteria for multi-infarct dementia (with the exclusion of the necessary presence of a step-wise deteriorating course). Criteria were further operationalized by requiring evidence of at least two independent cerebrovascular accidents as determined by both neurologic examination and brain imaging. They found a history of step-wise deterioration in 9 (11%) of AD patients and 6 (15%) of putative MID patients. These rates of occurrence of step-wise progression did not differ statistically. At least in this population, step-wise deterioration did not differentiate AD and MID.

There is also increasing controversy concerning the utility of the most common laboratory test helpful in determining cerebrovascular diseases, that is, brain neuroimaging by computer-assisted tomography (CT) or magnetic resonance imaging (MRI). On CT scans and even more commonly with the better resolution provided by MRI scans, deep or periventricular white matter changes are commonly described in patients with dementia meeting either criteria for AD or MID, as well as in cognitively intact older individuals. Although the radiologic appearance of these periventricular white matter changes has been read as compatible with ischemic changes by some neuroradiologists, neuropathologic documentation of actual ischemic lesions correlating with these antemortem neuroradiologic findings has been scanty. Whether or not these periventricular white matter changes seen on CT or MRI contribute to cognitive dysfunction is currently unclear. George *et al.* (1986a) reviewed the CT scans of 275 normal and demented subjects. The incidence and severity of white matter changes increased significantly with age but did not differ significantly between patients and normal subjects. Within dementia subjects the severity of white matter changes did not correlate with severity of cognitive impairment. At neuropathologic examination in five AD patients, areas of white matter rarefaction were present in all brains, and there was microscopic evidence of arteriolar hyalinization. In an MRI study (George *et al.*, 1986b), this same group of investigators found that the MRI was a more sensitive instrument for demonstrating periventricular white matter changes, which were equally common in AD subjects and age-matched control subjects. However, the extent of white matter involvement was greater in the Alzheimer group, although the configuration of the patches of increased signal intensity was similar for both normal elderly and AD subjects. Periventricular white matter changes have been reported to correlate with severity of dementia in AD (Bondareff, Raval, Coletti, & Hauser, 1988; Steingart *et al.*, 1987), but whether such changes are an indication of increased water content in the brain (Bondareff *et al.*, 1988) or a more specifically ischemic lesion (Brun & Englund, 1986; Braffman *et al.*, 1988) remains to be determined. Periventricular white matter changes on MRI and CT were more common in subjects meeting DSM-III-R criteria for primary degenerative dementia (presumed AD) than in patients meeting DSM-III-R criteria for vascular dementia in a recent Scandinavian study (Erkinjuntti *et al.*, 1987). It is possible, however, that the white matter lesions seen on MRI are benign. Fein *et al.* (1990) recently reported that the presence of extensive deep white matter brain lesions on MRI for up to 7 years was not associated with impairment in cognitive, behavioral, and neurologic functioning in two elderly normal subjects. They concluded that such deep white matter brain lesions do not necessarily indicate a clinically significant CNS disease process. The diagnostic and pathophysiologic significance of white matter lesions in persons meeting criteria for AD must await further careful clinicopathologic studies in which MRI scans are performed both antemortem and postmortem with concomitant neuropathologic examination.

Despite the controversies concerning MID and the field of vascular dementia, it is reasonably clear that ischemic sequelae of cerebrovascular insufficiency produce or contribute to dementia in some elderly persons. It is probable that multiple vascular mechanisms can be involved in different individuals. Some patients have multiple infarcts involving the cerebral cortex, whereas other patients have lesions involving the perforating arteries with production of small *lacunes* in subcortical structures such as the basal ganglia, internal capsule, thalamus, brain stem, and other deep structures. These patients with multiple lacunes classically present with gait disturbance, rigidity, pseudobulbar palsy, emotional incontinence, and paucity of speech and motor activity. A third entity, presumably secondary to ischemia of subcortical white matter, has been termed Binswanger's disease. That Binswanger's disease is in fact a different entity from multiple lacunar infarctions is debatable (Roman, 1985), and as noted above, the relationship of deep white matter lesions seen on CT or MRI to Binswanger's disease is unclear.

Hachinski *et al.* (1975) proposed a diagnostic rating scale for MID, which has gained wide use. The Hachinski scale derives an *ischemic score* from 13 items based on clinical observation and history This scale has been partially validated by Rosen, Terry, Fuld, Katzman, & Peck (1980) in a retrospective chart review study of 14 neuropathologically examined patients who had been documented on neuropsychologic testing antemortem to have been moderately or severely demented. A diagnosis of MID has potential treatment implications. Meyer, Judd, Tawakina, Rogers and Mortel (1986) prospectively studied 52 MID patients for a period of 22 months. Hypertensive patients among this group improved cognitively with adequate control of systolic blood pressure within the upper limits of the normal range (135–150 mm Hg). However, systolic blood pressure reduction below this level was associated with deterioration. Furthermore, normotensive MID patients showed improved cognitive function with cessation of cigarette smoking.

V. Pick's Disease

Pick's disease is a progressive dementing disorder of middle and late life, which is clinically difficult to differentiate from AD. Although generally considered rare, one Scandinavian series found Pick's disease to be relatively common (Sjogren, Sjogren & Lindgren, 1952), and in a Minnesota series, Pick's disease accounted for 5% of progressive dementing disorders (Heston, White & Mastri, 1987). Despite its clinical similarity, the neurochemistry and neuropathology of Pick's disease differ markedly from AD. The cholinergic and somatostatinergic deficits found in AD do not occur in Pick's disease (Wood *et al.*, 1983). Frontotemporal atrophy is apparent on gross pathology and accompanying microscopic changes include neuronal cell loss and gliosis and the presence of intraneuronal Pick's bodies (massed cytoskeletal elements). However, Pick's disease and AD appear to share specific antigens in degenerating neurons (Rasool & Selkoe, 1985). Clinical similarity has been noted between the affective disturbances and excessive eating of Pick's disease and aspects of Klüver-Bucy syndrome (Cummings & Duchen 1981; Constantinidis *et al.* 1974). Heston *et al.* (1987) confirmed that excessive eating may be associated with Pick's disease; however, their patients did not have striking affective changes, and most were clinically indistinguishable from AD. Some evidence of a genetic component to Pick's disease was also found by these investigators. A recent positron emission tomography (PET) study in a Pick's disease patient demonstrated markedly decreased glucose metabolism in frontal cortex, which corresponded with extensive frontal lobe neuronal loss and gliosis postmortem (Kamo *et al.*, 1987). The PET pattern was sufficiently distinctive to suggest that PET scanning may be diagnostically useful in distinguishing Pick's from AD antemortem.

VI. Normal-Pressure Hydrocephalus

Normal-pressure hydrocephalus is probably the most important disorder producing a truly reversible dementia. Described by Adams *et al.* in 1965, the classic clinical presentation of this syndrome consists of the triad of dementia, gait disturbance, and urinary incontinence associated with ventricular dilatation without evidence of persistently elevated intracranial pressure. Although in most cases the etiology of normal-pressure hydrocephalus remains unclear, a sizable minority result from previous subarachnoid hemorrhage, meningitis, or other neurologic insults. The occasional reversal of some or all aspects of the syndrome following cerebroventricular shunting created widespread enthusiasm for surgical treatment, and this procedure was performed on large numbers of dementia patients (many of whom did not have normal-pressure hydrocephalus but AD with ventricular dilation secondary to cortical atrophy). More careful patient selection seems to have improved outcomes in recently reported series. Thomasen, Borgesen, Bruhn, and Gjerris (1986) neuropsychologically evaluated 40 patients with normal-pressure hydrocephalus before and 12 months following ventriculoatrial shunt placement. Cognitive function improved in 16 patients, was unchanged in 19, and worsened in 5. Among factors associated with good postoperative outcome were short history, absence of gyral atrophy and known cause.

   The relative severity of ventricular dilatation compared to degree of sulcal enlargement on head CT or MRI aids in differentiating normal-pressure hydrocephalus from cerebral atrophy caused by AD or other primary degenerative dementing disorders. Isotope cisternography may be helpful if abnormal CSF dynamics are demonstrated but is not absolutely diagnostic. It has been suggested (Wikkelso, Andersson, Blomstrand, & Lindqvist 1982) that drainage of 20 to 40 ml of CSF by lumbar puncture followed by temporary clinical improvement may indicate those patients most likely to benefit from shunt placement. While of interest, this finding requires a controlled evaluation before it can be accepted. Indeed it must be kept in mind when evaluating the literature on surgical treatment of normal-pressure hydrocephalus, that none of the reports is of controlled trials. Although understandable given the difficulty of adequately controlling for an invasive surgical procedure, lack of appropriate controls limits the interpretation of therapeutic efficacy.

VII. Metabolic Dementing Disorders

Metabolic disorders most commonly produce delirium; however, if persistent, they may cause dementia. Vitamin B_{12} deficiency can present with dementia even in the absence of megaloblastic anemia (Strachan & Henderson 1965). Several anecdotal reports (Wieland, 1986; Gross, Weintraub, Neufeld, & Libow, 1986) suggest some modest efficacy of B_{12} replacement in dementia presumably secondary to B_{12} deficiency. A recent large combined retrospective study in a predominantly African-American population (Lindenbaum et al., 1988) raises the possibility that neuropsychiatric problems secondary to B_{12} deficiency in the absence of macrocytic anemia may be common and reversible. Although this uncontrolled study must be interpreted cautiously, these investigators documented frequent improvement following B_{12} administration of cognitive impairment and other neurologic and behavioral problems in patients with low plasma B_{12} concentrations.

Hypothyroidism can also produce a dementia often accompanied by irritability, paranoid ideation, and depression. There is some anecdotal evidence that dementia due to hypothyroidism is reversible (Whybrow, Prange, & Treadway, 1969). However, in a more recent study, four thyroid-deficient patients diagnosed in an outpatient dementia clinic were carefully followed (Larson, Reifler, Featherstone, & English, 1984). None of these four patients had a complete reversal of their dementia and over 2 years, three developed the progressive cognitive deterioration typical of AD. In the fourth hypothyroid patient, the dementia did not progress.

Repeated episodes of hypoglycemia secondary to hypoglycemic medications in diabetic patients are a metabolic cause of dementia that merits emphasis. The possible advantages of tight control of blood glucose in elderly diabetic patients must be weighed against the risk of brain damage due to hypoglycemia, particularly in the unsupervised patient who may not maintain an adequate and regular diet.

VIII. Infectious Dementing Disorders

A. AIDS

The virus (HIV-1) that causes acquired immune deficiency syndrome (AIDS) attacks neuronal cells of the brain as well as lymphoid cells of the immune system. Dementia and other organic mental disorders caused by HIV have been recently reviewed by Perry (1990); HIV in the geriatric patient population has been reviewed by Kendig and Adler

(1990). HIV enters the brain shortly following initial infection when macrophages containing the virus cross the blood–brain barrier (Resnick, Berger, Shapstak, & Tourtellotte 1988; Janssen, Stehr-Green, & Starcher, 1989; Price, Brew & Rosenblum, 1990). The virus is released and causes an acute clinical or subclinical meningoencephalitis. Recovery from the initial infection of the brain usually occurs because the patient's immune system is not yet compromised and is able to contain the virus. However, as the patient becomes progressively more immunosuppressed, virus replication within the CNS occurs, and a progressive multifocal leukoencephalopathy can result. Postmortem neuropathological findings are most prominent in the central white matter, basal ganglia, thalamus, and brainstem; there is relative sparing of the cortex (Gray et al., 1988; Petito, 1988). Neuronal loss is not characteristic and suggests that neurotoxic effects may be due to an autoimmune process or interaction with other pathogens or from release of toxic substances from viral genes or adjacent infected cells.

It is estimated that by 1992, 100,000 Americans older than 40 will be diagnosed with AIDS; 10,000 of these will be older than 60 (Centers for Disease Control, 1989). Approximately two thirds of all AIDS patients develop clinical evidence of a neurodegenerative disorder termed AIDS dementia complex (Price et al., 1988). However, most HIV-infected patients do not have a clinically overt dementia as their primary diagnosis. Clinical studies have found that 6–14% of HIV-infected patients initially present to a medical clinic with symptoms of dementia (Navia & Price, 1987; Abos, Graus, & Alom, 1989); however, the CDC reported that only 3% of 38,666 adults had HIV encephalopathy as their only early manifestations of AIDS (Janssen et al., 1989). Early signs and symptoms of the AIDS dementia complex include changes in attention span, concentration, and personality with a slowing of information processing. The patient may appear apathetic, withdrawn, or depressed. Cognitive dysfunction may be accompanied by motor signs such as weakness, bradykinesia, and ataxia. Patients eventually progress to a picture of severe dementia, mutism, incontinence, and paraplegia (Navia, Jordan, & Price, 1986). Although the clinical expression of AIDS in older patients does not appear to differ from that in younger AIDS patients, increasing age is associated with more rapid disease progression and shorter survival time (Bacchetti et al., 1988; Rothenberg et al., 1987).

Most elderly patients with HIV infection have a history of male homosexual activity or were infected via contaminated blood products. Intravenous drug abuse is rare in the older population. HIV must be considered in the differential diagnosis of dementia and taking an adequate history includes inquiring about risk factors from the patient and spouse or partner. The presence of risk factors for HIV should prompt serologic testing as part of the dementia work-up.

Pharmacotherapy for AIDS dementia complex consists of antiviral therapy and psychotropic medications to treat associated behavioral symptoms. Zidovudine (AZT) and other antiviral drugs penetrate the CSF and may be effective in delaying progression of the AIDS dementia complex (Yarchoan et al., 1987; Brunetti et al., 1989). The neuropsychological indications for early administration of AZT are not yet known; however, for these therapies to be evaluated adequately, early recognition of HIV-induced neurologic disease is essential. The use of psychotropic medications for secondary behavioral and mood disturbances is under study. Psychostimulants may be effective for treating apathy, lethargy, and withdrawal in AIDS patients (Fernandez *et al.*, 1988; Holmes, Fernandez & Levy, 1989). The use of high-potency neuroleptics for AIDS-related delirium and psychotic symptoms has been associated with an increased frequency of severe dystonic reactions and neuroleptic malignant syndrome (Edelstein & Knight, 1987; Breitbart, Marotta, & Call, 1988; Swenson, Erman, Labell, & Dimsdale 1989). The use of benzodiazepines for agitated behaviors may be more prudent in this patient population.

B. Creutzfeldt-Jakob Disease

Several other infectious dementing disorders, while rare in the elderly population, should be considered in the differential diagnosis of dementia. Creutzfeldt-Jakob disease is a rapidly fatal neurodegenerative disease usually afflicting persons in middle to late-middle life; it presents as a rapidly progressive dementia accompanied by myoclonic jerks, seizures, ataxia, rigidity, and other signs of widespread CNS involvement. Death within 2 years of onset is the rule, and this rapid course helps differentiate Creutzfeldt-Jakob disease patients from AD patients, who may also have myoclonic jerks (Mayeux, Stern, & Spanton, 1985; Risse *et al.*, 1990). Abnormal proteins in CSF of patients with Creutzfeldt-Jakob disease may prove to be helpful in the differential diagnosis of this disorder (Harrington *et al.*, 1986). Neuropathologic exam reveals spongiform changes, neuronal loss, and gliosis. The disease is caused by a *slow virus* with a prolonged latency from exposure to expression of the disease. Human-to-human transmission has occurred via corneal transplants, use of contaminated stereotactic electroencephalogram electrodes and through parenteral administration of growth hormone prepared from pooled human pituitary glands.

C. Neurosyphilis

Neurosyphilis was previously a common cause of dementia. In this age of widespread antibiotic administration, it is now rare. However, the prolonged latency for development of general paresis (up to 20 years) raises the possibility of late diagnosis. Because the Venereal Disease Research Laboratory test (VDRL) is negative in nearly one third of patients with late syphilis, the more sensitive fluorescent treponemal antibody absorption test should be obtained if late syphilis is suspected. Treatment with high doses of penicillin may be effective, but the disease may progress despite adequate antibiotic therapy (Wilner & Brody, 1968).

IX. Alcoholic Dementia

The cognitive disorders associated with alcoholism have recently been reviewed by Lishman (1981), who argues convincingly for the existence of a true dementia secondary to chronic alcoholism. A brief discussion of the DSM-III-R criteria for amnestic syndrome and their relevance to the cognitive syndromes secondary to alcoholism is useful at this point. DSM-III-R criteria for amnestic syndrome include demonstrable evidence of impairment in both short- and long-term memory, not occurring exclusively during the course of delirium and not meeting the criteria for dementia (i.e., no impairment in abstract thinking, judgment, or nonmemory higher cortical functions, or personality change), and evidence of a specific organic factor judged to be etiologically related to the disturbance. Although Korsakoff's syndrome is usually considered a disorder producing the amnestic syndrome, most chronic alcoholic patients with severe memory impairment also demonstrate impairment of at least some higher cortical functions when tested neuropsychologically (Lishman, 1981), and thus more appropriately meet criteria for the diagnosis of dementia. In fact, neuropsychological testing even in sober alcoholics without obvious dementia consistently reveals impairment in new learning, abstract thinking, and visuospatial functions (Tarter, 1980). Also, Brewer and Perett (1971) demonstrated cortical atrophy or ventricular enlargement in a high percentage of alcoholic patients, and such cortical changes correlated significantly with cognitive impairment.

Korsakoff's syndrome is classically attributed to repeated episodes of acute Wernicke's encephalopathy, a thiamine-deficiency disorder. The acute encephalopathy presents with confusion, nystagmus, lateral gaze palsy, and ataxia reflecting damage to brain areas adjacent to the third and fourth ventricles and the medial temporal lobes. Thiamine is specifically therapeutic and a transketolase deficiency may predispose toward development of the syndrome in the absence of adequate dietary thiamine (Blass & Gibson, 1977). This treatable cause of delirium and eventual dementia may be under-recognized. Harper (1979) reported that only 7 of 51 cases of Wernicke's encephalopathy diagnosed at autopsy had been suspected antemortem, despite the fact that the great majority of patients had been known alcoholics. Alcohol may damage brain tissue beyond the classic lesions of Wernicke's encephalopathy (Riley & Walker, 1978). The importance of recognizing Wernicke's encephalopathy and Korsakoff's or chronic alcoholic dementia should be emphasized. In addition to the effective acute treatment of Wernicke's encephalopathy with thiamine, cessation of alcohol ingestion is associated with improved cognitive function in the majority of patients with alcoholic dementia. Victor et al. (1971) followed up 104 cases of Korsakoff's "psychosis." Complete recovery occurred in 21%, and some degree of recovery occurred in 53% of the remaining patients. In 19 of the 22 patients in whom recovery was judged to have been complete, the amnestic syndrome had been severe. Therefore, recovery of memory function was not simply a reflection of mildness of the clinical disorder.

X. Treatment of Secondary Behavioral Problems in Dementia _____

Behavioral problems such as depression, agitation, and psychotic symptoms including hallucinations and delusions frequently complicate the course of dementing illnesses (Reisberg et al., 1987). These secondary behavioral problems offer treatment opportunities that, if effective, can improve the quality of life of both the patient and care providers as well as postpone institutionalization. The term agitated behaviors will be used to describe such problems as pacing, violent outbursts, delusions, hallucinations, and irritability. Although antipsychotic drugs are widely prescribed to dementia patients in long-term care facilities (Prien & Caffe, 1977), their efficacy in this population has not lived up to early expectations. Open uncontrolled studies were often interpreted as markedly positive (Salzman, 1987), but the small number of placebo-controlled trials of antipsychotic drugs in this population suggest that efficacy is limited, and adverse effects often complicate treatment. These studies have recently been reviewed by Raskind, Risse, and Lampe (1987), and several will be briefly described to illustrate some of the important issues in antipsychotic drug therapy in dementia. Petrie *et al.* (1982), compared haloperidol (4–6 mg/day), loxapine (mean dose, 22 mg/day), and placebo in 64 demented inpatients (mean age, 73 years) in a large state psychiatric hospital. Although active antipsychotic drug was significantly more effective than placebo for suspiciousness, hallucinatory behavior, excitement, hostility, and uncooperativeness, only one third of antipsychotic drug–treated patients were globally rated as moderately or markedly improved. Barnes, Veith, Okimoto, Raskind, and Gumbrecht (1982) found similar results in predominantly AD patients in a nursing home. They compared thioridazine (mean dose, 63 mg/day), loxapine (mean dose, 11 mg/day), and placebo in 53 patients whose mean age was 83 years. Active medication was superior for anxiety, excitement, and uncooperativeness, but suspiciousness and hostility improved as much over time with placebo as with active drug. Again, only one third of patients in this study manifested either marked or moderate global improvement. In a small placebo-controlled study of haloperidol for behaviorally disturbed AD patients, Devanand, Sackheim, Brown, and Mayeux (1989) found that target symptoms improved modestly but that cognitive function deteriorated. The practice of maintaining elderly dementia patients on chronic antipsychotic drugs has not been prospectively evaluated. However, several studies (Barton & Hurst, 1966, and Risse, Cubberley, Lampe, Zemmers, & Raskind, 1987) have demonstrated that the majority of patients maintained on antipsychotic drugs will not significantly deteriorate if placebo is substituted over periods of 3 to 6 weeks, and in fact a subgroup of patients will improve. On balance, the few well-designed studies of antipsychotic drugs in elderly dementia patients suggest a definite but limited efficacy for such disturbed behaviors as agitation, irritability, and classic psychotic symptoms (delusions and hallucinations).

The limited role of antipsychotic drugs in the behaviorally disturbed dementia patient makes careful assessment of interpersonal and environmental therapies imperative. A central concern is providing support for the care provider, especially while the dementia patient is still residing at home. Ongoing contact with an empathic health care professional can be extremely useful to help with long-term planning, crisis intervention, education, and provision of psychotherapy to the care provider. Self-help groups that have been fostered by the national Alzheimer's Association can be of great therapeutic benefit to family members and other care providers.

Many nonpharmacologic therapies for agitated behaviors in dementia have been attempted, but the mainstay of therapy continues to be provision of a safe, secure, and consistent environment, designed to compensate for the deficits of the individual dementia patient. Pacing and wandering are a particularly difficult problem both in the home and in the long-term care setting. Pharmacologic management of wandering is generally ineffective, and such adverse effects as akathisia (motor restlessness from antipsychotic drugs) and postural instability (from benzodiazepines) can aggravate the situation. Provision of a secure area in which the dementia patients can wander at any hour without harming themselves or causing disruption to others is one of the few workable solutions. However, such environments are not always available, and wandering is one of the behavioral problems that prompts institutionalization. Other more formal approaches to both cognitive and secondary behavioral problems in dementia patients, such as reality orientation and classic behavioral techniques, have not been evaluated well enough to define specific indications or establish efficacy (Raskind, 1989).

XI. Dementia and Depression

The problem of depression either complicating or mimicking a dementing disorder has received extensive attention in the literature. Because antemortem biologic markers are not available for either dementia or depression, and because signs and symptoms in the two disorders overlap, the interaction between depression and dementia continues to produce both diagnostic and clinical management uncertainty. A pure depressive disorder presenting with severe enough cognitive disturbance to mimic the dementia syndrome [so-called depressive pseudodementia (Kiloh, 1961)], is relatively uncommon compared to a depressive disorder superimposed upon AD or another dementing disorder. However, depressive pseudodementia [a term that has been justly criticized by Reifler (1982)] will be retained in this discussion for its widespread acceptance among practicing clinicians (Wells, 1979). Depressive pseudodementia is usually distinguishable from AD or other dementing disorders by a careful history and clinical examination (Post, 1975). It is unusual for cognitive changes to occur in depressive pseudodementia before the other signs and symptoms of depression have become obvious. In contrast, the true dementia patient's problems begin with memory and other cognitive deficits, and depressive signs and symptoms appear later in the clinical course. On examination, the depressive pseudodementia patient is likely to give "don't know" answers rather than to demonstrate clear memory deficits, and if the depressed patient can overcome motivational deficits, performance improves. In addition, aphasia and apraxia are not present in the pseudodementia patient. Persistently confusing diagnostic problems are best resolved by inpatient hospitalization.

It is generally accepted that depressive signs and symptoms are common in AD. The study of Reifler, Larson, and Hanley (1982), which found a 23% prevalence of depression in AD patients in an outpatient clinic, has been supported by a number of other investigators. Depression in AD patients is associated with greater functional impairment for a given level of cognitive impairment (Pearson, Teri, Reifler, & Raskind, 1989) and therefore offers potential treatment opportunities both to improve function and mood and potentially to improve the components of cognitive dysfunction that may be secondary to depression. Although uncontrolled studies have suggested that standard tricyclic antidepressant therapy is effective in the treatment of depression complicating AD (Reifler, Larson, Teri & Poulsen 1986), a recent double-blind placebo-controlled study testing this hypothesis has produced less optimistic results. In this study (Reifler et al., 1989), the efficacy of imipramine was compared to placebo in patients with AD who were concurrently diagnosed as suffering from major depressive disorder by DSM-III criteria. Substantial improvement was documented in both placebo and active medication groups, but there was no difference in outcome between groups. Another unexpected finding of this study was that the anticholinergic antidepressant imipramine at plasma concentrations of approximately 120 ng/ml had no clinically significant adverse effect on cognitive function (Teri *et al.*, in press). Although imipramine plasma concentrations in this study were somewhat lower than those suggested as therapeutic in younger, nondemented depressed patients (Glassman, Perel, Shostak, Kantor, Fleiss, 1977), imipramine concentrations were similar to those associated with efficacy as compared to placebo in a study of elderly depressed patients with ischemic heart disease (Veith *et al.*, 1982; Raskind, Veith, Barnes & Gumbrecht, 1982b). It appears that mild to moderate depressive signs and symptoms in AD outpatients improve with participation of the patient and caregiver in a study, but that the tricyclic antidepressant drug was not the specific therapeutic agent. That tricyclic antidepressants or other antidepressant agents may be specifically effective in AD patients with more severe depression or depressions with prominent endogenous features has not yet been addressed by controlled treatment evaluations.

Neuroendocrine approaches have been used experimentally to help differentiate depression from dementia and help diagnose depression complicating dementia. Early anecdotal studies suggested that the dexamethasone-suppression test (DST) might be useful in the differential diagnosis of depression in dementia. That is, a positive DST (early escape of plasma cortisol from dexamethasone suppression) would support the diagnosis of either primary depression or depression complicating AD or other dementing disorders in the cognitively impaired patient. However, a series of studies have demonstrated that AD and multi-infarct dementia are associated with a positive DST, whether or not a concomitant depressive syndrome is present (Raskind *et al.*, 1982a; Spar & Gerner, 1982; Balldin *et al.*, 1983; Abou-Saleh, 1987). The resistance to dexamethasone suppression together with increased cortisol secretion in AD raise interesting questions about the basic neuroendocrinology of AD. In fact, Sapolsky, Armamini, Packan, & Tombaugh (1987) have demonstrated that corticosteroids can be toxic to hippocampal neurons. However, the DST does not appear to have clinical value in the differential diagnosis of depression and AD or other dementing disorders. The blunted response of thyroid-stimulating hormone (TSH) to its hypothalamic releasing factor, thyrotropin-releasing hormone (TRH), which has been associated with depression in studies of nondemented individuals (Loosen & Prange, 1982), has also been evaluated in AD. The TSH response to TRH appears normal in nondepressed AD subjects (Dysken *et. al.*, 1990; El Sobky *et al.*, 1986; Lampe *et al.*, 1988; Peabody *et al.*, 1986), although Sunderland *et al.* (1985), found a blunted TSH response in AD compared to normal elderly control subjects. Further studies of the TRH stimulation test comparing dementia patients with coexistent depression to dementia patients without depression are needed.

That the depressive disorder complicating AD is related to major depressive disorder in nondemented individuals has received recent support from a study of Pearlson *et al.* (1990). They demonstrated that depressed AD patients had significantly more first- and second-degree relatives with depression than did nondepressed AD patients, and that the lifetime risk of depression was greater in first-degree relatives of AD patients with depression. They interpreted their data as supporting a genetic relationship of depression in AD to primary major depressive disorder. If this is true, then recent neuropathologic findings

(Zweig *et al.*, 1988) comparing the histology of the noradrenergic locus ceruleus, the major source of brain noradrenergic neurons, in AD patients with and without concomitant depression is of potential significance both for depression complicating AD and for primary major depressive disorder. In this study, locus ceruleus cell counts were significantly more reduced in AD patients with a history of depression than in AD patients who had not had a depression complicating their clinical course. This type of clinical pathologic correlational study in AD patients with secondary psychiatric symptomatology offers a unique opportunity to explore the neuropathology of psychiatric syndromes at the basic level.

The clinical observation that memory complaints are at least as common in depressed nondemented patients as they are in patients suffering from a dementing disorder has received support from a recent British epidemiologic study that examined memory complaints as well as objective cognitive impairment in normal, depressed, and demented elderly persons in the community (O'Connor, Pollitt, Roth, Brook, & Reiss, 1990). They found that depressed elderly persons reported memory problems more often than did normal elderly subjects; although memory complaints *per se* were no more common in the depressed group than in the demented elderly patients, the depressed subjects reported indecisiveness, impaired concentration, and mental slowing more frequently than did the demented subjects. As would be predicted, subjective memory complaints and objective memory performance correlated poorly in both the normal elderly subjects and the depressed elderly subjects.

XII. The Relationship of Depression in Parkinson's Disease to Dementia in Parkinson's Disease

Depression appears to be a common complicating psychiatric syndrome in Parkinson's disease. Rabins (1982) diagnosed a depressive syndrome in 46% of parkinsonian patients, and Mayeux *et al.* (1986) found major depressive disorder or dysthymic disorder in 40% of 49 consecutive patients with PD. Two recent studies suggest that there may be an interaction between the depressive syndrome that complicates PD and the dementia that PD patients may develop during their illness. In a consecutive series of 105 patients with PD, Starkstein, Preziosi, Bolduc, and Robinson (1990) evaluated depression and neuropsychological deficits. Severity of depression was found to be the single most important factor associated with severity of cognitive impairment. Sano *et al.* (1989) found a prevalence of 10.9% for dementia, 51% for depression, and 5.4% for coexistent depression and dementia in their population of parkinsonian patients. Based on previous studies demonstrating decreased CSF concentrations of the serotonin metabolite 5-hydroxyindolacetic acid (5HIAA) in depressed PD patients (Mayeux, Stern, Sano, Williams, & Cote, (1988b), they examined CSF 5HIAA concentrations in their subjects. PD patients who were either depressed or demented had lower concentrations of this serotonin metabolite than did PD patients without psychiatric morbidity. Patients who were both depressed and demented had the lowest 5HIAA levels in CSF. They interpreted their findings as suggesting that CNS serotonergic systems may be involved in both depression and dementia complicating PD. In a small, open pilot study, these investigators demonstrated improvement in depression with the serotonin precursor 5-hydroxy tryptophan. With the current availability of antidepressant drugs that appear to act on brain serotonergic systems, trials of these agents in depressed and/or demented PD patients appear warranted.

XIII. Delirium

The greatest potential for improvement in cognitive function in the dementia patient lies in the detection and reversal of a superimposed delirium. Delirium is a syndrome of diverse organic etiologies that disrupt brain physiology. The most prominent feature is a disorder of attention. DSM-III-R criteria for delirium include

1. reduced ability to maintain attention to external stimuli;
2. disorganized thinking as indicated by rambling, irrelevant, or incoherent speech;
3. at least two of the following: reduced level of consciousness; perceptual disturbances such as misinterpretations, illusions, or hallucinations; disturbance of sleep-wake cycle; increased or decreased psychomotor activity; disorientation as to time, place, or person; or memory impairment;
4. clinical features develop over a short period (usually hours or days) and tend to fluctuate over the course of a day; and
5. either evidence of a specific organic factor, or in the absence of such evidence, an organic factor can be presumed if the disturbance cannot be accounted for by any non-organic mental disorder.

It should be noted that for elderly patients, criterion 4, "clinical features develop over a short period of time," may be misleading. Elderly persons who develop delirium from the gradual accumulation of long-acting benzodiazepines may present with an insidious onset and gradual progression of their cognitive impairment, which may mimic AD. Such patients highlight the need to discontinue, if at all possible, any potentially cognitive-active medications in a patient who presents with cognitive dysfunction. It should also be noted that the presence of the delirium syndrome usually reflects disrupted brain physiology, whereas the dementia syndrome usually reflects structural damage to brain tissue. Of course, many patiens have a delirium superimposed on an underlying dementia. Etiologic factors for the delirium syndrome are numerous and include systemic medical illnesses, toxic CNS effects of both prescribed and non-prescribed medications, metabolic disorders, neurologic disorders, and such often hospital-based problems as the postoperative state and the intensive-care-unit syndrome. Withdrawal from addiction to alcohol and sedative hypnotic drugs can occur both in the community and in the hospital setting, particularly if the patient denies this form of substance abuse.

Treatment should be directed toward the underlying disorder. Frequently, however, an underlying disorder is either not discernible or not completely correctable, and symptomatic treatment becomes necessary if agitation, anxiety, delusions, hallucinations, or other behavioral symptoms interfere with patient management or threaten the safety of the patient or others in the environment. Mild symptoms may respond to reassurance from a family member, a trusted nurse, or a physician whose role is clear to the patient. An environment in which stimulation is provided at a moderately low and constant level can be helpful. A night light may be useful for patients whose delirium is exacerbated during the night (sundown syndrome). Although it is ideal to avoid adding medications to the delirious patient's regimen, pharmacologic intervention may be necessary. If delirium is secondary to withdrawal from a CNS-depressant drug such as ethanol or benzodiazepines, treatment with a cross-tolerant sedative hypnotic drug such as a medium-duration half-life barbiturate or benzodiazepine is indicated. In other types of delirium in which agitated behaviors demand attention, low doses of neuroleptic medication can be helpful. It should be kept in mind that neuroleptics may produce problematic hypotension or lower seizure threshold in the fragile, elderly delirious patient. The goal in using medication to control disruptive symptoms of delirium is to improve function while minimizing sedative or anticholinergic drug effects.

XIV. Conclusion

AD and other dementing illnesses are the most important neuropsychiatric disorders of the elderly, devastating millions of patients and their caregivers and costing the country and patients' families tens of billions of dollars for care at home and in institutional settings. During the past two decades, however, substantial progress has been made in understanding AD and related disorders, and effective treatments based on new knowledge are on the horizon. Although we still can not prevent or reverse the primary cognitive deficits of AD, we are increasingly aware of the need to treat superimposed delirium and noncognitive problems such as depression, agitated behaviors, and psychotic symptoms and to support the needs of caregivers with respite care programs and community services. Managing the elderly patient with dementia is a rewarding experience, and will become even more so as effective treatment modalities become available.

References

Abos, J., Graus, F., & Alom, J., (1989). Incidence of the AIDS dementia complex as the first manifestation of AIDS: a prospective study. In *Abstracts of the Fifth International Conference on AIDS*. Montreal: International Development Research Centre.

Abou-Saleh, M. T., Spalding, E. M., Kellet, J. M., & Coppen, A. (1987). Dexamethasone suppression test in dementia. *Journal of American Geriatrics Society, 35*, 271.

Adams, R. D., Fisher, C. M., Hakim, S., (1965). Symptomatic occult hydrocephalus with normal cerebrospinal-fluid pressure: A treatable syndrome. *New England Journal of Medicine, 273*, 117–126.

American Psychiatric Association. (1987). *Diagnostic and Statistical Manual of Mental Disorders* (3rd ed., rev.). Washington, DC: American Psychiatric Association.

Bacchetti, P., Osmond, I., Chaisson, R. E., Dritz, S., Rutherford, G. W., & Swig, L. (1988). Survival patterns of the first 500 patients with AIDS in San Francisco. *Journal of Infectious Diseases, 157*, 1044–1047.

Ball, M. J. (1984). The morphological basis of dementia in Parkinson's disease. *Canadian Journal of Neurological Sciences, 11*, 180–184.

Balldin, J., Goufries, C. G., Karlsson, I., Lingstedt, G.,Långström, G., & Wålinder, J. (1983). DST and serum prolactin in dementia. *British Journal of Psychiatry, 143*, 277–281.

Barnes, R., Veith, R., Okimoto, J., Raskind, M. & Gumbrecht, G. (1982). Efficacy of antipsychotic medications in behaviorally disturbed dementia patients. *American Journal of Psychiatry, 139*, 1170–1174.

Beal, M. F., Uhl, G., Mazurek, M. F., Kowall, N., Martin, J. B. (1986). Somatostatin alterations in the central nervous system in neurologic diseases. *Research Publications of the Association for Research in Nervous Mental Disease, 64*, 215–257.

Barton, R., & Hurst, L. (1966). Unnecessary use of tranquilizers in elderly patients. *British Journal of Psychiatry, 112*, 989–990.

Bissette, G., Reynolds, G., Kilts, C. D., Widerlov, E., & Nemeroff, C. B. (1985). Corticotropin-releasing factor–like immunoreactivity in senile dementia of the Alzheimer type. *Journal of the American Medical Association, 254*, 3067–3069.

Blass, J. P., & Gibson, G. E. (1977). Abnormality of a thiamine-requiring enzyme in patients with Wernicke–Korsakoff syndrome. *New England Journal of Medicine, 297*, 1367–1370.

Blessed, G., Tomlinson, B. E., & Roth, M. (1968). The association between quantitative measures of dementia and of senile change in the cerebral grey matter of elderly subjects. *British Journal of Psychiatry, 114*, 796–811.

Boller, F., Mizutani, T., Roessmann, U., & Gambetti, P. (1980). Parkinson's disease, dementia, and Alzheimer's disease: Clinicopathological correlations. *Annals of Neurology, 7*, 329-335.

Bondareff, W., Mountjoy, C. Q., Roth, M., Rossor, M. N., Iverson, L. L., Reynolds, G. P., & Hauser, D. C. (1987). Age and histopathologic heterogeneity in Alzheimer's disease. *Archives of General Psychiatry, 44*, 412–417.

Bondareff, W., Raval, J., Colletti, P. M., & Hauser, D. L. (1988). Quantitative magnetic resonance imaging and the severity of dementia in Alzheimer's disease. *American Journal of Psychiatry, 145*, 853–856.

Booze, R. M., Laforet, G., & Davis, J. M. (1986). Hippocampal sympathetic ingrowth in rats and guinea pigs. *Brain Research, 375*, 251–258.

Braffman, B. H., Zimmerman, R. A., Trojanowski, J. Q., Gonatas, N. K., Hickey, W. F., & Jchlaepfer, W. W. (1988). Brain MR: Pathologic correlation with gross and histopathology. 1. Lacunar infarction and Virchow–Robin spaces. *American Society of Neuroradiology, 9*, 621–628.

Braffman, B. H., Zimmerman, R. A., Trojanowski, J. Q., Gonatas, N. K., Hickey, W. F., Schlaepfer, W. W. (1988) Brain MR: pathologic correlation with gross and histopathology. 2. Hyperintense white-matter foci in the elderly. *American Journal of Radiology, 151*, 559–566.

Breitbart, M., Marotta, R. F., & Call, P. (1988). AIDS and neuroleptic malignant syndrome. *Lancet, 2*, 1488–1489.

Breitner, J. C. S., & Folstein, M. F. (1984). Familial Alzheimer dementia: Prevalent disorder with specific clinical features. *Psychological Medicine, 14*, 63–80.

Brewer, C., & Perrett, L. (1971). Brain damage due to alcohol consumption: An air-encephalographic, psychometric, and electroencephalographic study. *British Journal of Addiction, 66* 170–182.

Brinkman, S. D., Smith, R. C., Meyer, J. S., Vroulis, G., Shaw, T., Gordon, J. R., & Allen, R. H. (1982) Lecithin and memory training in suspected Alzheimer's disease. *Journal of Gerontology, 37*, 4–9.

Brown, R. G., & Marsden, C. D. (1984). How common is dementia in Parkinson's disease? *Lancet, 2*, 1262–1265.

Brun, A., & Englund, E. (1986). A white matter disorder in dementia of the Alzheimer type: A pathoanatomic study. *Annals of Neurology, 19*, 253–262.

Brunetti, A., Berg, G., Bi Chiro, G., Cohen, R. M., Yarchoan, R., Pizzo, P. A., Broder, S., Eddy, J., Fulham, M. J., Finn, R. O. *et al.* (1989). Reversal of brain metabolic abnormalities following treatment of AIDS dementia complex with 3'-azido-2', 3'-dideoxythymidine (AZT, zidovudine): A PET-FDG study. *Journal of Nuclear Medicine, 30*, 581–590.

Brust, J. C. M. (1983). Vascular dementia—still overdiagnosed. *Stroke, 14*, 298–300.

Burkhardt, C. R., Filley, C. M., Kleinschmidt-DeMasters, B. K., de la Monte, S., Norenberg, M. D., & Schneck, S. A. (1988). Diffuse Lewy body disease and progressive dementia. *Neurology, 38*, 1520–1528.

Candy, J. M., Klinowski, J., Perry, R. H., Oakley, A. E., Carpenter, T. A., Atack, J. R., Perry, E. K. Blessed, G., Fairbairn, A., & Edwardson, J. A. (1986). Aluminosilicates and senile plaque formation in Alzheimer's disease. *Lancet, 1*, 354–356.

Cash, R., Dennis, T., L'Heureux, A., (1987). Parkinson's disease and dementia: Norepinephrine and dopamine in locus ceruleus. *Neurology, 37*, 42–46.

Centers for Disease Control. (1989). HIV/AIDS Surveillance (Vol. 11). Atlanta, Georgia: U. S. Department of Health and Human Services, Centers for Disease Control.

Christie, J. E., Shering, A., Ferguson, J., & Glen, A. I. (1981). Physostigmine and arecoline: Effects of intravenous infusions in Alzheimer's presenile dementia. *British Journal of Psychiatry, 138,* 46–50.

Chul, H. C., Mortimer, J. A., Slager, U., Oakley, A. E., Carpenter, T. A., Atack, J. R., Perry, E. K., Blessed, G., Fairbairn, A., & Edwardson, J. A. (1984). *Pathological correlates of dementia in Parkinson's disease.* Presented at the annual scientific meeting of the Gerontological Society, San Francisco, November.

Constantinidis, J., Richard, J., & Tissot, R. (1974). Pick's disease, histological and clinical corelations. *European Neurology, 11,* 207–218.

Crapper, D. R., Krishnan, S. S., & Dalton, A. J. (1973). Brain aluminum distribution in Alzheimer's disease and in experimental neurofibrillary degeneration. *Science, 180,* 511–513.

Cummings, J. L., & Duchen, L. W. (1981). Kluver-Bucy syndrome in Pick's disease: Clinical and pathologic correlations. *Neurology, 31,* 1415–1422.

Davies, P. (1991). Alzheimer's disease: progress toward diagnosis in vivo. *Geriatrics, 46,* 79–81.

Davies, P., & Maloney, A. J. F. (1976). Selective loss of central cholinergic neurons in Alzheimer's disease. *Lancet, 2,* 1403.

Davies, P., & Wolozin, B. L. (1987). Recent advances in the neurochemistry of Alzheimer's disease. *Journal of Clinical Psychiatry, 48(5),* 23–30.

Davies, P., Katzman, R., & Perry, R. D. (1980). Reduced somatostatin-like immunoreactivity in cerebral cortex from cases of Alzheimer's disease and Alzheimer's senile dementia. *Nature, 288,* 279–280.

Davis, K. L., Mohs, R. C., & Tinklenberg, J. R. (1979). Enhancement of memory by physostigmine. *New England Journal of Medicine, 301,* 946.

DeSouza, E. B., Whitehouse, P. J., Kuhar, M. J., Price, D. L., and Vale, W. W. (1986). Reciprocal changes in corticotropin-releasing factor (CR)–like immunoreactivity and CRF receptors in cerebral cortex of Alzheimer's disease. *Nature, 319,* 593–595.

Devanand, D. P., Sackheim, H. A., Brown, R. P., & Mayeux, R. (1989). A pilot study of haloperidol treatment of psychosis and behavioral disturbance in Alzheimer's disease. *Archives of Neurology, 46,* 854–857.

Ditter, S. M., & Mirra, S. S. (1987). Neuropathologic and clinical features of Parkinson's disease in Alzheimer's disease patients. *Neurology, 37,* 754–760.

Dysken, M. W., Faek, A., Perr, B., Kuskowski, M., Krahn, D. D. (1990). Gender differences in TRH-stimulated TSH and prolactin in primary degenerative dementia and elderly controls. *Biological Psychiatry, 15,* 144–150.

Edelstein, H., & Knight, R. T. (1987). Severe parkinsonism in two AIDS patients taking prochlorperazine (letter). *Lancet, 2,* 341–342.

El Sobky, A., Shazly, M., Darwish, A. K., Davies, T., Griffin, K., & Keshaven, M. S. (1986). Anterior pituitary response to thyrotropin-releasing hormone in senile dementia (Alzheimer type) and elderly normals. *Acta Psychiatrica Scandinavica, 74,* 13–17.

Epelbaum, J., Ruberg, M., Mayse, E., Javoy-Agid, F., Dubois, B., Agid, Y. (1983). Somatostatin and dementia in Parkinson's disease. *Brain Research, 278,* 376–379.

Erkinjuntti, T., Ketonen, L., Sulkava, R., Sipponen, J., Vuorialho, M., & Iivanainen, M. (1987). Do white matter changes on MRI and CT differentiate vascular dementia from Alzheimer's disease? *Journal of Neurology, Neurosurgery, and Psychiatry, 50,* 37–42.

Evans, I. A., Funkenstein, H., Albert, M. S., Scherr, P. A., Cook, N. R., Chown, M. J., Hebert, L. E., Hennekens, C. H., & Taylor, J. O. (1989). Prevalence of Alzheimer's disease in a community population of older persons. Higher than previously reported. *Journal of the American Medical Association, 262,* 2551–2556.

Fein, G., Van Dyke, C., Davenport, L., Turetsky, B., Brant-Zawadzki, M., Zata, L., Dillon, W., & Valk, P. (1990). Preservation of normal cognitive functioning in elderly subjects with extensive white-matter lesions of long duration. *Archives of General Psychiatry, 47,* 220–223.

Fernandez, F., Adams, F., Levy, J. K., Holmes, V. F., Neidhart, M., Mansell, P. W. (1988). Cognitive impairment due to AIDS-related complex and its response to psychostimulants. *Psychosomatics, 29,* 38–46.

Fischer, W., Wictorin, K., Bjorklund, A., Williams, L. R., Varon, S., & Gage, F. H. (1987). Amelioration of cholinergic neuron atrophy and spatial memory impairment in aged rats by nerve growth factor. *Nature, 329,* 65–68.

Forno, L. S. (1982). Pathology of Parkinson's disease. In C. D. Marsden & S. Fahn (Eds.), *Movement disorders* (pp. 25–40). London: Butterworth Scientific.

Francis, P. T., Palmer, A. M., Sims, N. R., Bowen, D. M., Davidson, A. N., Esiri, M. M., Neary, D., Snowden, J. S., & Wilcock, G. K. (1985). Neurochemical studies of early-onset Alzheimer's disease. *New England Journal of Medicine, 313*, 7–11.

Gage, F. H., Armstrong, D. M., Williams, L. R., & Varon, S. (1988). Morphological response of axotomized septal neurons to nerve growth factor. *Journal of Comparative Neurology, 289*, 147–155.

Gauthier, S., Bouchard, R., Lamontagne, A., Bailey, P., Bergman, H., Ratner, J., Tesfaye, Y., Saint-Martin, M., Bacher, Y., Carrier, L., Charbonneau, R., Clarfield, A. M., Collier, B., Dastoor, D., Gauthier, L., Germain, M., Kissel, C., Krieger, M., Kushnir, S., Masson, H., Morin, J., Nair, V., Neirinck, L., & Suissa, S. (1990). Tetrahydroaminoacridine–lecithin combination treatment in patients with intermediate-stage Alzheimer's disease. *New England Journal of Medicine, 322*, 1272–1276.

George, A. E., De Leon, M. J., Gentes, C. I., Miller, J., London, E., Berdzilovich, G. N., Ferris, S., Chase, N. (1986a). Leukoencephalopathy in normal and pathologic aging: 1. CT of brain lucencies. *American Journal of Neuroradiology, 7*, 561–566.

George, A. E., de Leon, M. J., Kalnin, A., Rosner, L., Goodgold, A., & Chase, N. (1986b). Leukoencephalopathy in normal and pathologic aging: 2. MRI of brain lucencies. *American Journal of Neuroradiology, 7*, 567–570.

Ghanbari, H. A., Miller, B. E., Haigler, H. J., Arato, M., Bissette, G., Davies, P., Nemeroff, C. B., Perry, E. K., Perry, R., Ravid, R. (1990). Biochemical assay of Alzheimer's disease—associated protein(s) in human brain tissue. A clinical Study. *Journal of the American Medical Association, 6:263*, 2907–2910.

Gibb, W. R. G., Esiri, M. M., & Lees, A. J. (1985). Clinical and pathological features of diffuse cortical Lewy body disease (Lewy body dementia). *Brain, 110*, 1131–1153.

Glassman, A. H., Perel, J. M., Shostak, M., Kantor, S. J., & Fleiss, J. L. (1977). Clinical implications of imipramine plasma levels for depressive illness. *Archives of General Psychiatry, 34*, 197–204.

Glenner, G. G., & Wong, C. W. (1984). Alzheimer disease: Initial report of the purification and characterization of a novel cerebrovascular amyloid protein. *Biochemical and Biophysical Research Communications, 120*, 885–890.

Goate, A. M., Haynes, A. R., Owen, M. J., Farrall, M., James, L.A., Lai, L. Y. C., Mullan, M. J., Roques, P., Rossor, M. N., Williamson, R., & Hardy, J. A. (1989). Predisposing locus for Alzheimer's disease on chromosome 21. *Lancet, 1*, 352–355.

Graves, A. B., White, E., Koepsell, T. D., Reifler, B. V., van Belle, G., & Larson, E. V. (1990). The association between aluminum-containing products and Alzheimer's disease. *Journal of Clinical Epidemiology, 43*, 35–44.

Gray, F., Gherardi, R., Keohane, C., Farolini, M., Sobel, A., & Poirier, J. (1988). Pathology of the central nervous system in 40 cases of acquired immune deficiency syndrome (AIDS). *Neuropathological Applied Neurobiology, 14*, 3645–3680.

Gross, J. S., Weintraub, N. T., Neufeld, R. R., & Libow, L. S. (1986). Pernicious anemia in the demented patient without anemia or macrocytosis: A case for early recognition. *Journal of American Geriatric Society, 34*, 612–614.

Hachinski, V. C., Larson, N. A., & Marshall, J. (1974). Multi-infarct dementia. *Lancet, 2*, 207–210.

Hachinski, V. C., Iliff, L. D.,Zilhka, E., Barclay, G. H., McAllister, V. L., Marshall, J., Russell, R. W. & Symon, L. (1975). Cerebral blood flow in dementia. *Archives of Neurology, 32*, 632–637.

Hakim, A.M. & Mathieson, I. (1979).Dementia in Parkinson's disease: A neuropathologic study. *Neurology, 29*, 1209–1214.

Harbaugh, R. E., Roberts, D. W., Coombs, D. W., Saunders, R. L., & Reeder, T. M. (1984). Preliminary report: Intracranial cholinergic drug infusion in patients with Alzheimer's disease. *Neurosurgery, 15*, 514–518.

Harper, C. (1979). Wernicke's encephalopathy: A more common disease than realized. *Journal of Neurology, Neurosurgery, and Psychiatry, 42*, 226–231.

Harrell, L. E., Jope, R. S., Falgout, J., Callaway, R., Avery, C., Spiers, M., Leli, D., Morere, D., Halsey, J. H., Jr. (1990). Biological and neuropsychological characterization of physostigmine responders and non-responders in Alzheimer's disease. *Journal of the American Geriatrics Society, 38*, 113–112.

Harrington, M. G., Merril, C. R., Asher, D.M., Gadjusek, D. C., (1986). Abnormal proteins in the cerebro spinal fluid of patients with Creutzfeldt-Jakob disease. *New England Journal of Medicine, 315*, 279–283.

Heston, L. L., White, J. A., & Mastri, A. R. (1987). Pick's disease: Clinical genetics and natural history. *Archives of General Psychiatry, 44*, 409–411.

Heyman, A., Wilkinson, W. E., Stafford, J. A., Helms, M. J., Sigmon, A. H., & Weinberg, T. (1984). Alzheimer's disease: A study of epidemiologic aspects. *Annals of Neurology, 15*, 335–341.

Hollander, E. R., Mohs, R. L., & Davis, K. L. (1986). Antemortem markers of Alzheimer's disease. *Neurobiology of Aging, 7*, 367–386.

Holmes, V. F., Fernandez, F., & Levy, J. K. (1989). Psychostimulant response in AIDS-related complex patients. *Journal of Clinical Psychiatry, 50*, 5–8.

Hyman, B. T., Van Hoesen, G. W., Wolozin, B. L., Davies, P., Kromer, L. J., Damasie, A. R. (1988). Alz-50 antibody recognized Alzheimer-related neuronal changes. *Annals of Neurology, 23*, 371–379.

Janssen, R. S., Cornblath, D. R., Epstein, L. G., McArthur, J., and Price, R. W. (1989). Human immunodeficiency virus (HIV) infection and the nervous system: Report from the American Academy of Neurology AIDS Task Force. *Neurology, 39*, 119–122.

Jansen, R., Stehr-Green, J., & Starcher, T. (1989). Epidemiology of HIV encephalopathy in the United States. In *Abstracts of the Fifth International Conference on AIDS*. Montreal: International Development Research Centre.

Jellinger, K., & Grisold, W. (1982). Cerebral atrophy in Parkinson's syndrome. *Experimental Brain Research, 5*, 26–35.

Jenike, M. A., Albert, M. S., Heller, H., Gunther, J., & Goff, D. (1990). Oral physostigmine treatment for patients with presenile and senile dementia of the Alzheimer's type: A double-blind placebo-controlled trial. *Journal of Clinical Psychiatry, 51*, 3–7.

Joachim, C. L., Mori, H., & Selkoe, D. J. (1989). Amyloid βP deposition in tissues other than brain in Alzheimer's disease. *Nature, 341*, 226–230.

Johnson, S. A., McNeill, T., Cordell, B., & Finch, C. E. (1990). Relation of neuronal APP-751/APP-695 mRNA ratio and neuritic plaque density in Alzheimer's disease. *Science, 248*, 854–857.

Jolkkonin, J, Soininen, H., Halonen, T., Ylinen, A., Laulumaa, V., Laakso, M., Riekkinen, P. (1986). Somatostatin-like immunoreactivity in the cerebrospinal fluid of patients with Parkinson's disease and it's relation to dementia. *Journal of Neurology and Neurosurgery, 49*, 1374–1377.

Kamo, H., McGeer, P. L., Harrop, R., McGeer, E. G., Calne, D. B., Martin, W. R., Pate, B. D. (1987). Positron emission tomography and histopathology in Pick's disease. *Neurology, 37*, 439–445.

Kendig, N. E., & Adler, W. H. (1990). The implications of the acquired immunodeficiency syndrome for gerontology research and geriatric medicine. *Journal of Gerontology: Medical Sciences, 45(3)*, M77–881.

Kiloh, L. G. (1961). Pseudo-dementia. *Acta Psychiatrica Scandinavica, 37*, 336–351.

Kosaka, K., Tsuchiya, K., & Yoshimura, M. (1988). Lewy body disease with and without dementia: A clinicopathological study of 35 cases. *Clinical Neuropathology, 7*, 299–305.

Kromer, L. F. (1987). Nerve growth factor treatment after brain injury prevents neuronal death. *Science 235*, 214–217.

Ksiezak-Reding, H., Binder, L. I., Yen, S. H. (1988). Immunochemical and biochemical characterization of tau proteins in normal and Alzheimer's disease brains with Alz-50 and Tau-1. *Journal of Biological Chemistry, 263*, 7948–7953.

Lai, F., & Williams, R. S. (1989). A prospective study of Alzheimer's disease in Down's syndrome. *Archives of Neurology, 46*, 849–853.

Lampe, T. H., Playmate, S. R., Risse, S. C., Kopeikan, H., Cubberley, L., & Raskind, M. A. (1988). TSH responses to two TRH doses in men with Alzheimer's disease. *Psychoneuroendocrinology, 13*, 245–254.

Larson, E. B., Reifler, B. V., Featherstone, H. J., English, D. R. (1984). Dementia in elderly outpatients: A prospective study. *Annals of Internal Medicine, 100*, 417–423.

Lennox, G., Lowe, J. Í., Godwin-Austen, R. B., Landon, M., & Mayer, R. J. (1989). Diffuse Lewy body disease: An important differential diagnosis in dementia with extrapyramidal features. *Progress in Clinical and Biological Research, 317*, 121–130.

Lennox, G., Lowe, J., Landon, M., Byrne, E. J., Mayer, R. J., & Godwin-Austen, R. B. (1989). Diffuse Lewy body disease: Correlative neuropathology using antiubiquitin immunocytochemistry. *Journal of Neurology, Neurosurgery, and Psychiatry, 52,* 1236–1247.

Lennox, G., Lowe, J., Morrell, K., Landon, M., & Mayer, R. J. (1989). Anti-ubiquitin immunocytochemistry is more sensitive than conventional techniques in the detection of diffuse Lewy body disease. *Journal of Neurology, Neurosurgery, and Psychiatry, 52,* 67–71.

Leverenz, J., & Sumi, S. M. (1986). Parkinson's disease in patients with Alzheimer's disease. *Archives of Neurology, 43,* 662–664.

Levi-Montalcini, R. (1987). The nerve growth factor 35 years later. *Science, 237,* 1154–1162.

Lindenbaum, J., Healton, E. B., Savage, D. G., Briest, J. C., Garrett, T. J., Podell, E. R., Marcell, P. D., Stabler, S. P., Allen, R. H. (1988). Neuropsychiatric disorders caused by cobalamin deficiency in the absence of anemia or macrocytosis. *New England Journal of Medicine, 318,* 1720–1728.

Lishman, W. A. (1981). Cerebral disorder in alcoholism: Syndromes of impairment. *Brain, 104,* 1–20.

Loosen, P. T., & Prange, A. J. (1982). Serum thyrotropin response to thyrotropin-releasing hormone in psychiatric patients: A review. *American Journal of Psychiatry, 139,* 405–416.

Mann, D. A., Yates, P. O., & Hawkes, J. (1982). The noradrenergic system in Alzheimer's and multi-infarct dementias. *Journal of Neurology, Neurosurgery and Psychiatry, 45,* 113–119.

Manuelidis, E. E., De Figueiredo, J. M., Kim, J. H., Fritch, W. W., Manuelidis, L. (1988). Transmission studies from blood of Alzheimers's disease patients and healthy relatives. *Proceedings of National Academy of Science. 85,* 4898–4901.

Markesbery, W. R., Ehmann, W. D., Hossain, T. I., Alauddin, M., & Goodin, D. T. (1981). Instrumental neutron activation analysis of brain aluminum in Alzheimer disease and aging. *Annals of Neurology, 10,* 511–516.

Mayeux, R., Stern, Y., Rosenstein, R., Marder, K., Hauser, A., Cote, L., & Kahn, S. (1988). An estimate of the prevalence of dementia in idiopathic Parkinson disease. *Archives of Neurology, 45,* 260–262.

Mayeux, R., Stern, Y., Sano, M., Williams, J. B.W., & Cote, L. J. (1988b). The relationship of serotonin to depression in Parkinson's disease. *Movement Disorders, 3,* 237–244.

Mayeux, R., Stern, Y., & Spanton, S. (1985). Heterogeneity in dementia of the Alzheimer type: Evidence of subgroups. *Neurology, 35,* 453–461.

Mayeux, R., Stern, Y., Williams, J. B. W., Cote, L., Frantz, & A., Dyrenfurth, I. (1986). Clinical and biochemical features of depression in Parkinson's disease. *American Journal of Psychiatry, 143,* 756–759.

Mazurek, M. F., Growden, J. H., Beal, M. F., Martin, J. B. (1986). CSF vasopressin concentration is reduced in Alzheimer's disease. *Neurology, 36,* 1133–1137.

McDermott, J. R., Smith, A. I., Iqbal, K., & Wisniewski, H. M. (1977). Aluminum and Alzheimer's disease. *Lancet, 1,* 710–711.

McKhann, G., Drachman, D., Folstein, M., Katzman, R., Price, D., & Stadian, E. M. (1984). Clinical diagnosis of Alzheimer's disease: Report of the NINCDS-ADRDA work group under the auspices of Department of Health and Human Services Task Force on Alzheimer's disease. *Neurology, 34,* 939–944.

Meyer, J. S., Judd, B. W., Tawakina, T., Rogers, R. L., & Mortel, K. F. (1986). Improved cognition after control of risk factors for multi-infarct dementia. *Journal of the American Medical Association, 256,* 2203–2209.

Mohs, R. C., Davis, B. M., Johns, C. A., Mathie, A. A., Greenwald, B. S., Horvath, T. B., & Davis, K. L. (1985). Oral physostigmine treatment of patients with Alzheimer's disease. *American Journal of Psychiatry, 142,* 28–33.

Mohs, R. C., Breitner, J. C. S., Silverman, J. M., & Davis, K. L. (1987). Alzheimer's disease: Morbid risk among first-degree relatives. *Archives of General Psychiatry, 44,* 405–408.

Molsa, P. K., Marttila, R. J., & Rinne, U. K. (1984). Extrapyramidal signs in Alzheimer's disease. *Neurology, 34,* 1114–1116.

Mortimer, J. A. (1983). Alzheimer's disease and senile dementia: Prevalence and incidence. In B. Reisberg (Ed.), *Alzheimer's disease: The standard reference.* New York: Free Press.

Mortimer, J. A., French, I. R., Hutton, J. T., & Schuman, L. M. (1985). Head injury as a risk factor for Alzheimer's disease. *Neurology* (NY), *35,* 264–267.

Navia, B. A., & Price, R. W. (1987). The acquired immunodeficiency syndrome dementia complex as the presenting or sole manifestation of human immunodeficiency virus infection. *Archives of Neurology, 44,* 65–69.

Navia, B. A., Jordan, B. D., & Price, R. W. (1986). The AIDS dementia complex: 1. Clinical features. *Annals of Neurology, 19,* 517–524.

Neary, D., Snowden, J. S., Mann, D. M. A., Bowen, D. M., Sims, N. R., Northern, B., Yates, P. O. & Davidson, A. N. (1986). Alzheimer's disease: A correlative study. *Journal of Neurology, Neurosurgery, and Psychiatry, 49,* 229–237.

Nee, L. E., Eldridge, R., Sunderland, T., Thomas, C. B., Katz, D., Thompson, K. E., Weingartner, H., Weiss, H., Julian, C. E., Cohen, R. (1987). Dementia of the Alzheimer type: Clinical and family study of 22 twin pairs. *Neurology, 37,* 359–363.

O'Connor, D. W., Pollitt, P. A., Roth, M., Brook, P. B., & Reiss, B. B. (1990). Memory complaints and impairment in normal, depressed, and demented elderly persons identified in a community survey. *Archives of General Psychiatry, 47,* 224–227.

Okazaki, H., Lipin, L. E., & Åronson, S. M. (1961). Diffuse intracytoplasmic ganglionic inclusions (Lewy type) associated with progressive dementia and quadriparesis in flexion. *Journal of Neuropathology and Experimental Neurology, 20,* 237–244.

Palmert, M. R., Podlisny, M. B., Witker, D. S., Oltersdorf, T., Younkin, L. H., Selkoe, D. J., & Younkin, S. C. (1989). The β-amyloid protein precursor of Alzheimer's disease has soluble derivatives found in human brain and cerebrospinal fluid. *Proceedings of the National Academy of Sciences of the United States of America, 86,* 6338–6342.

Peabody, C. A., Minkoft, J. R., Davies, H. D., Winograd, C. H., Yesavage, J., & Tinklenberg, J. R. (1986). Thyrotropin–releasing hormone stimulation test and Alzheimer's disease. *Biological Psychiatry, 21,* 553–556.

Pearce, J. (1974). The extrapyramidal disorder of Alzheimer's disease. *European Neurology, 12,* 94–103.

Pearlson, G. D., Ross, C. A., Lohr, W. D., Rovner, B. W., Chase, G. A., & Folstein, M. F. (1990). Association between family history of affective disorder and the depressive syndrome of Alzheimer's disease. *American Journal of Psychiatry, 147,* 452–456.

Pearson, J. L., Teri, L., Reifler, B. V., & Raskind, M. A. (1989). Functional status and cognitive impairment in Alzheimer's patients with and without depression. *Journal of the American Geriatric Society, 37,* 1117–1121.

Pericak-Vance, M. A., Yamaoka, L. H., Haynes, C. S., Speer, M. C., Haines, J. L., Gaskell, P. C., Hung, W. Y., Clark, C. M., Heyman, A. L., & Trofatter, J. A. (1988). Genetic linkage studies in Alzheimer's diseases families. *Experimental Neurology, 102,* 271–279.

Perl, D., & Brody, A. (1980). Alzheimer's disease: Spectrometric evidence of aluminum accumulation in neurofibrillary tangle–bearing neurons. *Science, 208,* 297–299.

Perry, E., K., Curtis, M., Dick, D. J., Candy, J. M., Atack, J. R., Bloxham, C. A., Blessed, G., Fairbairn, A., Tomlinson, B. E., & Perry, R. H. (1985). Cholinergic correlates of cognitive impairment in Parkinson's disease: Comparisons with Alzheimer's disease. *Journal of Neurology, Neurosurgery, and Psychiatry, 48,* 413–421.

Perry, E. K., Marshall, E., Perry, R. H., Irving, D., Smith, C. J., Blessed, G., & Fairbairn, A. F. (1990). Cholinergic and dopaminergic activities in senile dementia of Lewy body type. *Alzheimer Disease and Associated Disorders, 4,* 87–95.

Perry, E. K., Tomlinson, B. E., Blessed, G., & Perry, R. H. (1978). Correlation of cholinergic abnormalities with senile plaques and mental test scores in senile dementia. *British Medical Journal, 2,* 1457–1459.

Perry, G. (Ed.). (1987). *Advances in behavioral biology;* (Vol. 34). *Alterations in the neuronal cytoskeleton in Alzheimer disease.* New York Plenum Press.

Perry, R. H., Irving, D., Blessed, G., Fairbairn, A., & Perry, E. K. (1990). Senile dementia of Lewy body type. A clinically and neuropathologically distinct form of Lewy body dementia in the elderly. *Journal of the Neurological Sciences, 95,* 119–139.

Perry, S. W. (1990). Organic mental disorders caused by HIV: Update on early diagnosis and treatment. *American Journal of Psychiatry, 147,* 696–710.

Petito, C. K. (1988). Review of central nervous system pathology in human immunodeficiency virus infection. *Annals of Neurology (suppl.), 23,* 554–557.

Petrie, W. M., Ban, T. A., Berney, S., Fujimoro, M., Guy, W., Raghab, M., Wilson, W. H., & Schaffer, J. D. (1982). Loxapine in psychogeriatrics: A placebo- and standard-controlled clinical investigation. *Journal of Clinical Psychopharmacology, 2,* 122–126.

Phelps, C. H., Gage, F. H., Growdon, J. H., Hefti, F., Harbaugh, R., Johnston, M. V., Khachaturian, Z. S., Mobley, W. C., Price, D. L., Raskind, M., *et al.* (1989). Potential use of nerve growth factor to treat Alzheimer's disease. *Neurobiology of Aging, 10,* 205–207.

Post, F. (1975). Dementia, depression, and pseudodementia. In D. F. Benson & D. Blumer (Eds.), *Psychiatric aspects of neurologic disease* (pp. 99–120). New York: Grune & Stratton.

Price, R. W., Brew, B., & Rosenblum, M. (1990). The AIDS dementia complex and HIV-1 brain infection: A pathogenic model of virus-immune interaction. In B. H. Waksman (Ed.), *Immunological mechanisms in neurological and psychiatric disease* New York, Raven Press.

Price, R. W., Brew, B., Sidtis, J., Rosenblum, M., Scheck, A. C., & Cleary, P. (1988). The brain in AIDS: Central nervous system HIV-1 infection and AIDS dementia complex. *Science, 239,* 586–592.

Prien, F., & Caffe, E. M. (1977). Pharmacologic treatment of elderly patients with organic brain syndrome: A survey of twelve Veterans Administration hospitals. *Comprehensive Psychiatry, 18,* 551–560.

Rabins, P. (1982). The psychopathology of Parkinson's disease. *Comprehensive Psychiatry, 12,* 421–428.

Rajput, A. H., Offord, K. P., Beard, C. M., Kurland, L. T. (1987). A case-control study of smoking habits, dementia, and other illnesses in idiopathic Parkinson's disease. *Neurology, 37,* 266–232.

Raskind, M. A. (1989). Organic mental disorders. In E. W. Busse & D. G. Blazer (Eds.), *Geriatric psychiatry* (pp. 313–368). Washington DC: American Psychiatric Press.

Raskind, M. A., Peskind, E. R., Halter, J. B., Jimerson, D. C. (1984). Norepinephrine and MHPG levels in CSF and plasma in Alzheimer's disease. *Archives of General Psychiatry, 41,* 343–346.

Raskind, M. A., Peskind, E. R., Lampe, T. H., Risse, S. C., Taborsky, G. J., & Dorsa, D. (1986). Cerebrospinal fluid vasopressin, oxytocin, somatostatin, and beta-endorphin in Alzheimer's disease. *Archives of General Psychiatry, 43,* 382–388.

Raskind, M. A., Peskind, E., Rivard, M. F., Veith, R., Barnes, R. (1982). Dexamethasone suppression test and cortisol circadian rhythm in primary degenerative dementia. *American Journal of Psychiatry, 139,* 1468–1471.

Raskind, M. A., Peskind, E. R., Veith, R. C., Risse, S. C., Lampe, T. H., Borson, S., Gumbrecht, G., & Dorsa, D. M. (1989). Neuroendocrine response to physostigmine in Alzheimer's disease. *Archives of General Psychiatry, 46,* 535–540.

Raskind, M. A., Risse, S. C., & Lampe, T. H. (1987). Dementia and antipsychotic drugs. *Journal of Clinical Psychiatry, 48,* 16–18.

Raskind, M. A., Veith, R., Barnes, R., Gumbrecht, G. M. (1982b). Cardiovascular and anti-depressant effects of imipramine in the treatment of secondary depression in patients with ischemic heart disease. *American Journal of Psychiatry, 139,* 1114–1117.

Rasool, C. G., & Selkoe, D. J. (1985). Sharing of specific antigens by degenerating neurons in Pick's disease and Alzheimer's disease. *New England Journal of Medicine, 312,* 700–705.

Rechsteiner, M. (1987). Ubiquitin-mediated pathways for intracellular proteolysis. *Annual Review of Cellular Biology, 3,* 1–30.

Reifler, B. V. (1982). Arguments for abandoning the term pseudodementia. *Journal of the American Geriatric Society, 30,* 665–668.

Reifler, B. V., Larson, E., & Hanley, R. (1982). Coexistence of cognitive impairment and depression in geriatric outpatients. *American Journal of Psychiatry, 139,* 623–629.

Reifler, B. V., Larson, E., Teri, L., & Poulsen, M. (1986). Dementia of the Alzheimer's type and depression. *Journal of the American Geriatric Society, 34,* 855–859.

Reifler, B. V., Teri, L., Raskind, M., Veith, R., Barnes, R., White, E., & McLean, P. (1989). Double-blind trial of imipramine in Alzheimer's disease patients with and without depression. *American Journal of Psychiatry, 146,* 45–49.

Reisberg, B., Borenstein, J., Salob, S. P., Ferris, S. H., Franssen, E., & Georgotas, A., (1987). Behavioral symptoms in Alzheimer's disease: Phenomenology and treatment. *Journal of Clinical Psychiatry, 48(5),* 9–15.

Resnick, L., Berger, J. R., Shapshak, P., & Tourtellotte, W. W. (1988). Early penetration of the blood–brain barrier by HIV. *Neurology, 38,* 9–14.

Riley, J. N., & Walker, D. W. (1978). Morphological alterations in hippocampus after long-term alcohol consumption in mice. *Science, 201,* 646–648.

Risse, S. C., Cubberley, L., Lampe, T. H., Zemmers, R., & Raskind, M. A. (1987). Acute effects of neuroleptic withdrawal in elderly dementia patients. *Journal of Geriatric Drug Therapy, 2,* 65–77.

Risse, S. C., Lampe, T. H., Bird, T. D., Nochlin, D., Sumi, S. M., Keenan, T., Cubberley, L., Peskind, E., & Raskind, M. A. (1990). Myoclonus, seizures and rigidity in Alzheimer's disease. *Alzheimer's Disease and Associated Disorders, 4,* 217–225.

Roman, G. C. (1985). The identify of lacunar dementia and Binswanger disease. *Medical Hypotheses, 16,* 389–391.

Rosen, W. G., Terry, R. D., Fuld, P. A., Katzman, R., & Peck, A. (1980). Pathological verification of ischemic score in differentiation of dementia. *Annals of Neurology, 7,* 486–488.

Roses, A. D., Belbout, J., Yamaoka, L., Gaskell, P. C., Hung, W-Y., Walker, A. P., Alberts, M. J., Clark, C., Welch, K., Earl, N., Hayman, A., & Paricak-Vance, M. A. (1990). Linkage of late-onset familial Alzheimer's disease on Chromosome 19. *Society for Neuroscience Abstracts, 16,* 149.

Rothenbert, R., Woelfel, M., Stoneburner, R., Milberg, J., Parker, R., & Truman, B. (1987). Survival with the acquired immunodeficiency syndrome. Experience with 5833 cases in New York City. *New England Journal of Medicine, 317,* 1297–1302.

Salzman, C. (1987). Treatment of the elderly agitated patient. *Journal of Clinical Psychiatry, 48(Suppl.),* 19–22.

Sano, M., Stern, Y., Williams, J., Cote, L., Rosenstein, R., & Mayeux, R. (1989). Coexisting dementia and depression in Parkinson's disease. *Archives of Neurology, 46,* 1284–1286.

Sapolsky, R., Armanini, M., Packan, D., & Tombaugh, G. (1987). Stress and glucocorticoids in aging. *Endocrinology Metabolism Clinic, 16,* 965–980.

Schellenberg, G. D., Bird, T. D., Wijsman, E. M., Moore, D. K., Boehnke, M., Bryant, E. M. Lampe, T. H., Nochlin, D., Sumi, S. M., Deweb, S. S., Beyreuther, K., & Martin, G. M. (1988). Absence of linkage of chromosome 21q21 markers to familial Alzheimer's disease. *Science, 241,* 1507–1510.

Schmechel, D. R., Schmitt, I., Horner, J., Wilkinson, W. E., Hurwitz, B. J., Heyman, A., & Durham, N. C. (1984). Lack of effect of oral physostigmine and lecithin in patients with Alzheimer's disease. *Neurology, 34,* 280.

Selkoe, D. J. (1990). Deciphering Alzheimer's disease: The amyloid precursor protein yields new clues. *Science, 248,* 1058–1062.

Selkoe, D. J., Abraham, C. R., Podlishny, M. B., & Duffy, L. K. (1986). Isolation of low-molecular-weight proteins from amyloid plaque fibers in Alzheimer's disease. *Journal of Neurochemistry, 146,* 1820–1834.

Sisodia, S. S., Koo, E. H., Beyreuther, K., Unterbeck, A., & Price, D. L. (1990). Evidence that β-amyloid protein in Alzheimer's disease is not derived by normal processing. *Science, 248,* 492–495.

Sjogren, T., Sjogren, H., & Lindgren, A. G. H. (1952). Morbus Alzheimer and morbus Pick. *Acta Psychiatrica Scandinavica, 82(Suppl. 82),* 1–66.

Slotkin, T. A., Seidler, F. J., Crain, B. J., Bell, J. M., Bissette, G., & Nemeroff, C. B. (1990). Regulatory changes in presynaptic cholinergic function assessed in rapid autopsy material from patients with Alzheimer disease: Implications for etiology and therapy. *Proceedings of the National Academy of Sciences of the United States of America, 87,* 1–4.

Small, G. W., Kuhl, D. E., Riege, W. H., Fujikawa, D. G., Ashford, J. W., Metter, E. J., & Mazziotta, J. C. (1989). Cerebral glucose metabolic patterns in Alzheimer's disease: Effect of gender and age at dementia onset. *Archives of General Psychiatry, 46,* 527–534.

Snow, A. D., Mar, H., Nochlin, D., Kimata, K., Sato, M., Suzuki, S., Hassell, J., & Wight, N. (1988). The presence of heparan sulfate proteoglycans in the neuritic plaques and congophilic angiopathy in Alzheimer's disease. *American Journal of Pathology, 133,* 456–463.

Sorensen, P. S., Hammer, M., Vorstrup, S. & Gjerris, F. (1983). CSF and plasma vasopressin concentrations in dementia. *Journal of Neurology, Neurosurgery, and Psychiatry, 46,* 911–916.

Spar, J., & Gerner, R. (1982). Does the dexamethasone suppression test distinguish dementia from depression? *American Journal of Psychiatry, 139,* 238–240.

Starkstein, S. E., Preziosi, T. J., Bolduc, P. L., & Robinson, R. G. (1990). Depression in Parkinson's disease. *Journal of Nervous and Mental Disease, 178,* 27–31.

Steingart, A., Hachinski, V. C., Lau, C., Fox, A. J., Fox, H., Lee, D., Inzitari, E., & Marskey, H. (1987).

Cognitive and neurologic findings in demented patients with diffuse white matter lucencies on computed tomographic scan (leuko-araoisis). *Archives of Neurology, 44,* 36–39.

Stern, Y., Sano, M., & Mayeux, R. (1988). Long-term administration of oral physostigmine in Alzheimer's disease. *Neurology, 38,* 1837–1841.

St. George-Hyslop, P. H., Tanzi, R. E., Polinsky, J. L., Haines, J. L., Nee, L., Watkins, P. C., Myers, R. H., Feldman, R. G., Poiten, D., Drachman, D., *et al.,* (1987). The genetic defect causing familial Alzheimer's disease maps on chromosome 21. *Science, 235,* 885–889.

Strachan, R. W., & Henderson, J. G. (1965). Psychiatric syndromes due to avitaminosis B_{12} with normal blood and bone marrow. *Quarterly Journal of Medicine, 34,* 303–309.

Sulkava, R. (1982). Alzheimer's disease and senile dementia of Alzheimer type: A comparative study. *Acta Neurologica Scandinavica, 65,* 636–650.

Summers, W. K., Machovski, L. V., Marsh, G. M., Tachiki, K., & Kling, A. (1986). Oral tetrahydro-aminoacridine in long-term treatment of senile dementia, Alzheimer type. *New England Journal of Medicine, 315,* 1241–1245.

Sunderland, T., Tarlot, P. N., Mueller, E. A., Newhouse, P. A., Murphy, D. L., & Cohen, R. M. (1985). THR stimulation test in dementia of the Alzheimer type and elderly controls. *Psychiatry Research, 16,* 269–275.

Sundquist, J., Forsling, M. L., Olsson, J. E., & Akerlund, M. (1983). Cerebrospinal fluid arginine vasopressin in degenerative disorders and other neurological diseases. *Journal of Neurology, Neurosurgery, and Psychiatry, 46,* 14–17.

Swenson, J. R., Erman, M., Labell, J., & Dimsdale, J. E. (1989). Extrapyramidal reactions: Neuropsychiatric mimics in patients with AIDS. *General Hospital Psychiatry, 11,* 248–253.

Tanzi, R. E., Gusella, J. I. Watkins, P. C., Burns, G. A., St. George-Hyslop, P., VanKleuren, M. L., Patterson, D., Pagan, S., Kurnit, D. M., Neve, R. L. (1987). Amyloid β protein gene: cDNA, mRNA distribution and genetic linkage near the Alzheimer locus. *Science, 235,* 880–884.

Tarter, R. E. (1980). Brain damage in chronic alcoholics: A review of the psychological evidence. In D. Richter (Ed.), *Addiction and Brain Damage.* (pp. 267–297), London: Croom Helm.

Teri, L., Reifler, B. V., Raskind, M., Veith, R. C., Barnes, R., White, E., & McLean, P. (in press). Imipramine in the treatment of depressed Alzheimer's patients: impact on cognition. *Journal of Gerontology.*

Thal, I. J., Rosen, W., & Sharpless, N. S., (1981). Choline chloride fails to improve cognition in Alzheimer's disease. *Neurology of Aging, 2,* 205–208.

Thal, I. J., Fuld, P. A., Masur, D. M., & Sharpless, N. S. (1983). Oral physostigmine and lecithin improve memory in Alzheimer's disease. *Annals of Neurology, 13,* 491–496.

Thomasen, A. M., Borgesen, S. E., Bruhn, P., & Gjerris, F. (1986). Prognosis of dementia in normal-pressure hydrocephalus after a shunt operation. *Annals of Neurology, 20,* 304–310.

Thomlinson, B. E., Blessed, G., & Roth, M. (1970). Observations on the brains of demented old people. *Journal of the Neurological Science, 11,* 205–242.

Trapp, G. A., Miner, G. D., Zimmerman, R. L., Mastri, A. R., & Heston, L. L. (1978). Aluminum levels in brain in Alzheimer's disease. *Biological Psychiatry, 13,* 709–718.

Van Nostrand, W. E., Schmaier, A. H., Farrow, J. S., & Cunningham, D. S. (1990). Protease nexin-II (amyloid β-protein precursor): A platelet δ-granule protein. *Science, 248,* 745–748.

Veith, R. C., Raskind, M. A., Caldwell, J. H., Barnes, R. F., Gumbrecht, G., & Ritchie, J. L. (1982). Cardiovascular effects of the tricyclic antidepressants in depressed patients with chronic heart disease. *New England Journal of Medicine, 306,* 954–959.

Victor, M., & Adams, R. D. (1971). *The Wernicke–Korsakoff syndrome.* Philadelphia: F. A. Davis.

Wells, C. E. (1979). Pseudodementia. *American Journal of Psychiatry, 136,* 895–890.

Whitehouse, P. J., Price, I. L., Struble, R. G., Clark, A. W., Coyle, J. T., & Dilon, M. R. (1982). Alzheimer's disease and senile dementia: Loss of neurons in the basal forebrain. *Science, 215,* 1237–1239.

Whitehouse, P. J., Vale, W. W., Zweig, R. M., Singer, H. S., Mayeux, R., Kuhar, M. J., Price, D. L., & DeSouza, L. B. (1987). Reductions in corticotropin-releasing factor–like immunoreactivity in cerebral cortex in Alzheimer's disease, Parkinson's disease, and progressive supranuclear palsy. *Neurology, 37,* 905–909.

Whitson, J. S., Selkoe, D. J., & Cotman, C. W. (1989). Amyloid β-protein enhances the survival of hippocampal neurons *in vitro, Science, 243,* 1488–1490.

Whybrow, P. C., Prange, A. J., Jr., & Treadway, C. A. (1969). Mental changes accompanying thyroid gland dysfunction. A reappraisal using objective psychological measurement. *Archives of General Psychiatry, 20,* 48–53.

Wieland, R. G. (1986). Vitamin B_{12} deficiency in the nonanemic elderly. *Journal of the American Geriatric Society, 34,* 618–619.

Wikkelso, C., Andersson, H. Blomstrand, C., & Lindqvist, G. (1982). The clinical effect of lumbar puncture in normal pressure hydrocephalus. *Journal of Neurology, Neurosurgery, and Psychiatry, 45,* 64–69.

Wilner, E., & Brody, J. A. (1968). Prognosis of general paresis after treatment. *Lancet, 2,* 1370–1371.

Winblad, B., Adolfsson, R., Carlsson, A., & Gottfries, C. G. (1982). Biogenic amines in hairs of patients with Alzheimer's disease. In S. Corkin, K. L. Davis, J. H. Growden, E. Usdin & R. J. Wurtman (Eds.), *Alzheimer's disease: A report of progress in research* (pp. 25–33). New York: Raven Press.

Wood, P. L. Etienne, P., Lal, S., Gauthier, S., Cajal, S., & Nair, N. P. (1982). Reduced lumbar CSF somatostatin levels in Alzheimer's disease. *Life Sciences, 31,* 2073–2079.

Wood, P. L., Nair, N. P., Etienne, P., Lal, S., Gauthier, S., Robitaille, Y., Bird, E. D., Pals, J., Haltin, M., & Paetau, A. (1983). Lack of cholinergic deficit in the neocortex in Pick's disease. *Progress in Neuropsychopharmacology, Biology, and Psychiatry, 7,* 725–727.

Woodard, J. H. S. (1962). Concentric hyaline inclusion body formation in mental disease analysis of 27 cases. *Journal of Neuropathology and Experimental Neurology, 21,* 442–449.

Yankner, B. A., Dawes, L. R., Fisher, S., Villa-Komaroff, L., Oster-Granite, M. L., & Neve, R. L. (1989). Neurotoxicity of a fragment of the amyloid precursor associated with Alzheimer's disease. *Science, 245,* 417–420.

Yarchoan, R., Berg, G., Brouwers, P., Fishchel, M. A., Spitzer, A. R., Wichman, A., Grafman, J., Thomas, R. V., Safai, B., & Brunetti, A. (1987). Response of human immunodeficiency virus–associated neurological disease to 3'azido-3'deoxythymidine. *Lancet, 1,* 132–135.

Yates, P. O., & Mann, D. M. A. (1986). Aluminosilicates and Alzheimer's disease. *Lancet, 1,* 681–682.

Zubenko, G. S. (1990). Progression of illness in the differential diagnosis of primary dementia. *American Journal of Psychiatry, 147,* 435–438.

Zubenko, G. S. (1988). Familial risk of dementia associated with a biologic subtype of Alzheimer's disease. *Archives of General Psychiatry, 45,* 889–900.

Zweig, R. M., Ross, C. A., Hedreen, J. C., Steele, C., Gardillo, J. L., Whitehouse, P. J., Folstein, M., & Price, D. L. (1988). The neuropathology of aminergic nuclei in Alzheimer's disease. *Annals of Neurology, 24,* 232–242.

19

Alcohol and Substance-Use Disorders in the Elderly

Roland M. Atkinson, Linda Ganzini, and Michael J. Bernstein

I. Introduction
II. Epidemiology
    A. Risk Factors for Substance-Use Disorders
    B. Under-Recognition of Substance-Use Disorders in Later Life
    C. Comparative Prevalence of Substance-Use Disorders
III. Principles of Assessment and Management
    A. Assessment of Substance-Use Disorders
    B. Management and Treatment
IV. Alcohol-Use Disorders
    A. Epidemiology
    B. Patterns of Alcohol Use and Abuse
    C. Clinical Features of Alcohol-Use Disorders
    D. Course
    E. Management and Treatment
V. Prescription Psychoactive Drug-Use Disorders
    A. Epidemiology of Sedative–Hypnotic Drug Use and Problems
    B. Clinical Features and Complications of Benzodiazepine Dependence
    C. Assessment and Management of Benzodiazepine-Use Disorders
    D. Prescription Analgesic Drug Use and Abuse
VI. Other Substances
    A. Illegal Drugs
    B. Over-the-Counter Drugs
    C. Tobacco (Nicotine) Dependence
    D. Polysubstance-Use Disorders
VII. Looking Ahead
    A. Predicting Future Case Volume
    B. Research Directions
    C. Planning Services
    D. Prevention
    References

Handbook of Mental Health and Aging, Second Edition
Copyright © 1992 by Academic Press, Inc. All rights of reproduction in any form reserved.

I. Introduction

Gerontologists and addiction experts have been slow to acknowledge that significant substance abuse occurs in later life. Recent evidence, however, indicates that persons in their 60s and beyond do experience significant alcohol and drug problems (Atkinson, 1984, 1990; Atkinson & Kofoed, 1982; J. H. Atkinson & Schuckit, 1984; Schuckit, 1977). In this chapter we will present a general review of substance abuse in the elderly, followed by special sections on alcohol, prescription drugs, and other substances: illicit, over-the-counter, and tobacco products. The chapter closes with comments on future prospects, including planning for services and prevention.

We view aging as a complex process, with important cellular–genetic, organismic, psychosocial, and cultural dimensions. The interaction of these processes produces great diversity among individuals: older adults are a highly heterogeneous population. Vulnerability to disease is a function of aging. The actual occurrence and manifestations of illness, however, as well as responses to disease, are variable (*secondary aging*) (Busse, 1989). In affected individuals, substance abuse interacts with, and complicates, all features of aging, illness, and dysfunction.

In Table I, several terms are defined as they will be used in this chapter. A general model of substance abuse, embracing alcohol, licit, and illicit psychoactive drugs, is supported by recent research suggesting common biobehavioral bases for these disorders (Donovan, 1988; Maloff & Levinson, 1980; National Academy of Sciences, 1977). Interest in recent years has broadened from an exclusive focus on the pharmacology of abused substances to the perspective of substance-use behavior, which also considers the characteristics of the user and the social context of use. Explicit criteria for diagnosis of substance-use disorders, available since 1980, have aided epidemiologic and clinical research. Two currently used sets of criteria for substance dependence, the fundamental behavioral disorder underlying most drug problems, are listed in Table II. For further information, the reader may consult general sources. We have referenced some representative works on clinical disorders (Lowinson & Ruiz, 1981; Schuckit, 1989) and research on substance abuse (Donovan & Marlatt, 1988; Kissin & Begleiter, 1983a, 1983b). The reader unfamiliar with the drug classes discussed in this chapter may wish to consult a standard pharmacology text (for example, Goodman, Goodman, Rall, & Furad, 1985).

II. Epidemiology

A. Risk Factors for Substance-Use Disorders

1. Cohort and Period Effects

Cohort and period effects must be considered apart from aging effects to understand risks for substance abuse in the elderly (Mandolini, 1981). Cohort effects are especially important, as substance-use habits and attitudes typically are established by early adulthood and

Table I

Definitions

- **Psychoactive**—any chemical (alcohol, therapeutic agent, industrial compound, or illicit drug) with important effects on the central nervous system.

- **Substance**—a psychoactive that typically is associated with a substance-use disorder. The term includes alcohol, opioids, sedative–hypnotics, and antianxiety agents of the barbiturate and benzodiazepine types, psychomotor stimulants, especially amphetamines and cocaine, tobacco products, and certain over-the-counter psychoactives. The terms **chemical** and **drug** in this context are synonymous with substance (e.g., *chemical dependence, drug abuse*).

- **Use**—appropriate medical or social consumption of a psychoactive in a manner that minimizes the potential for dependence or abuse.

- **Heavy use**—use of a substance in greater quantity than the usual norms, but without obvious negative social, behavioral, or health consequences. Heavy alcohol or tobacco users may be dependent upon the substance.

- **Misuse**—use of a prescribed drug in a manner other than directed. The term can mean overuse, underuse, improper dose sequencing, lending or borrowing another's medication, with or without harmful consequences (Strategy Council on Drug Abuse, 1979).

- **Problem use**—use of a substance in a manner that induces negative social, behavioral, or health consequences. A *problem* user may or may not meet criteria for substance dependence or abuse, although most do. Alcohol "problems" or drug "problems" are categories that often have been used by epidemiologists in community prevalence surveys.

- **Abuse**—substance abuse is defined by three criteria: (1) a maladaptive pattern of use manifest by (a) continued use despite knowledge of prior harmful consequences, or (b) recurrent use in hazardous situations (as in driving while intoxicated); (2) signs of the disorder have persisted for longer than a month; and (3) person has never met the criteria for dependence upon the substance in question (American Psychiatric Association, 1987). *Harmful use* (World Health Organization, 1988) approximates abuse in definition.

- **Dependence**—substance dependence is defined by nine criteria, any three of which must be met to justify the diagnosis. Table II lists two recently established criteria sets for dependence. These approaches set aside the older distinction between **physical dependence** and **psychological dependence,** which are now viewed as differing manifestations of similar disorders. The terms *alcoholism* and *addiction* are usually used as synonyms for dependence on alcohol and other drugs, respectively.

- **Substance-use disorder**—a clinical condition in which substance abuse or substance dependence can be diagnosed (American Psychiatric Association, 1987).

- **Substance abuse, chemical dependence,** and **addictions**—these terms are often used to refer to the entire professional–scientific field.

---

depend on prevailing but ever-changing social norms. The Prohibition Era (1920–1933) inculcated negative values about alcohol use that have biased the practices and views of elders currently in their late 70s and older (Malin, Coakley, & Laelber, 1982). During World War II (1941–1945) social sanctions against the use of alcohol and tobacco by women were relaxed, and the gender gap for use of these substances has steadily narrowed since then (Cloninger, Reich, Sigvardsson, von Knorring, & Bohman, 1987; Reich, Cloninger, Van Eerdewegh, Rice, & Mullaney, 1988). Period effects include developments in clinical practice and biomedical research. For example, emerging awareness that substance-use disorders exist in older persons will be likely to increase their reported

Table II

DSM-III-R versus ICD-10 (provisional) Criteria for Substance Dependence

DSM-III-R Criteria[a]	ICD-10 Criteria[a]
1. Substance taken in larger amounts or over longer time than person intended	1. Strong desire or sense of compulsion to take the substance
2. Persistent desire or one or more unsuccessful efforts to cut down or control use of the substance	2. Subjective awareness of an impaired capacity to control substance-taking behavior in terms of onset, termination, or levels of use
3. Great deal of time spent in activities necessary to get or use substance, or recovering from its effects	3. Substance used with the intention of relieving withdrawal symptoms and with awareness that this strategy is effective
4. Frequent intoxication or withdrawal symptoms when expected to fulfill major role obligations at work, school, or home, or when substance use is physically hazardous, e.g., when driving	4. Physiological withdrawal state
	5. Evidence of tolerance such that an increased amount is required to achieve effects originally produced by lesser amounts
5. Important social, occupational, or recreational activities given up or reduced because of substance use	6. Narrowing of personal repertoire of patterns of substance use (e.g., a tendency to use in the same way on weekdays and weekends, whatever social constraints there may be regarding appropriate or safe use)
6. Continued substance use despite knowledge of having a persistent or recurrent social, psychological, or physical problem that is caused or exacerbated by use of substance	7. Progressive neglect of alternative pleasures or interests in favor of substance use
7. Marked tolerance: need for increased amounts of substance in order to achieve intoxication or desired effect, or diminished effect with continued use of the same amount	8. Persisting with use despite clear evidence of overtly harmful consequences (medical, social, psychological)
8. Characteristic withdrawal symptoms	9. Evidence that return to substance use after a period of abstinence leads to more rapid reappearance of other features of dependence than occurs with nondependent individuals
9. Substance often taken to relieve or avoid withdrawal symptoms	

[a]DSM-III-R, Diagnostic and Statistical Manual of Mental Disorders, 3rd ed., rev. (American Psychiatric Association, 1987). ICD-10, International Classification of Diseases, 10th ed., provisional version (World Health Organization, 1988). For either system, at least three of the nine listed criteria must be met in order to make the diagnosis of dependence on a substance.

incidence and prevalence, quite apart from any true change in the rate of their occurrence. The synthesis of benzodiazepine drugs created new opportunities for the occurrence of sedative dependence after 1960.

2. Biological Risk Factors

The elderly show increased sensitivity to the effects of most psychoactives. Pharmacokinetic processes (mechanisms of drug deactivation and elimination—or *what the body does to drugs*) and pharmacodynamic processes (mechanisms of drug action upon the central nervous system and other organs—or *what drugs do to the body*) determine drug sensitivity. Changes with age in several pharmacokinetic systems, affecting absorption, distribution, protein binding, and metabolism and excretion of drugs, have been recently reviewed (Jenike, 1989; Robertson, 1984), as have age-related changes in systems affecting tissue responsiveness to drugs (Freund, 1984a, 1984b; Salzman, 1984; Timiras, 1988). Findings to date support a multivariate model: modified drug sensitivity is based on age-related change in several biological systems, contributions from each of which vary with the drug in question (see Chapters 7 and 27 for further discussion).

Psychoactives can also increase the symptoms of certain medical disorders that are more common in the elderly, especially cognitive dysfunction, and cardiovascular and pulmonary disorders. Furthermore, there can be clinical complications from the adverse interaction of psychoactive substances and other prescribed medications (drug–drug interactions). Alterations in biological sensitivity to drugs can influence the potential for substance abuse in several ways: larger effects from smaller doses can discourage consumption, or lead to problems at consumption rates that caused no problems earlier in life.

3. Psychosocial and Psychiatric Risk Factors

Although gerontologists have often attributed late substance-use problems to major loss and other life stress, this relationship is complex. Life stressors are ubiquitous among the elderly, while only a minority develop substance abuse. Persons who abuse alcohol and drugs are more prone to create crises in their lives. A narrow conception of *stress* is evident in most studies of the question (Finney & Moos, 1984). Major losses and other dramatic life events, long-term strains, and the ordinary tribulations of daily life constitute distinctive forms of life stressors, but their relative contributions to substance-use disorders have not been defined. Mediating processes (e.g., prior substance dependence, availability of the substance) and moderating processes (e.g., social support network, alternative coping means) are also rarely incorporated in studies of individual susceptibility to substance-use problems under stress. Similar stress factors—for example, physical debility, decreased drive, and lack of money—have been invoked to explain spontaneous recovery from long-standing alcohol and opioid dependence in old age (Atkinson & Kofoed, 1982).

Subjective symptoms of chronic illness, such as pain, insomnia, anxiety, and depression, may increase the likelihood of some elderly persons to abuse various substances in self-medication efforts. Permissive or fatalistic attitudes of relatives or caregivers also sometimes abet substance abuse (Atkinson & Kofoed, 1982). Relatives may supply substances (surreptitiously at times) to an elderly person; family members may become drinking partners; or family may support ill-advised prescribing by the physician. Caregivers may also become overcontrolling, using *as needed* sedatives excessively to suppress "inappropriate" behavior. These and other risk factors are summarized in Table III.

B. Under-Recognition of Substance-Use Disorders in Later Life

Special clinical features, social factors, and professional biases contribute to under-recognition of these problems in the elderly. Signs and symptoms of substance-use disorders in old age can be subtle, atypical, or can mimic symptoms of other geriatric illness, making

Table III
Risk Factors for Substance Abuse in the Elderly

Demographic factors	***Iatrogenic factors***
Male gender (alcohol, illicit substances)	Prescription-drug dependence
Female gender (sedative–hypnotics)	Drug–drug and alcohol–drug interactions
Substance-related factors	Caregiver overuse of *as needed* medication
Prior substance abuse	Physician advice or permission to use alcohol
Family history (alcohol)	***Psychosocial factors***
Increased biological sensitivity	Loss and other major life stress
Drug sensitivity	Discretionary time, money
Pharmacokinetic factors	Social isolation
Pharmacodynamic factors	Family collusion
Medical illnesses associated with aging	***Psychiatric factors***
Cognitive loss	Depression
Cardiovascular disease	Dementia
Metabolic disorders	Subjective symptoms of chronic illness
	Cohort and period effects

diagnosis difficult (Atkinson, 1990; Atkinson & Kofoed, 1982). Substance abuse can produce delirium or dementia (Freund, 1987), which the clinician may falsely attribute to other causes. Nonspecific presenting signs and symptoms, for example, poor grooming, malnutrition, bladder and bowel incontinence, muscle weakness, gait disorders, recurring falls, burns, head trauma, or accidental hypothermia, may be caused by unsuspected alcohol or drug abuse.

Younger abusers often are first identified by others: employer, spouse, arresting officer, or judge. Older persons who are retired and living in isolation may not have sufficient contact with others, so that opportunities for detection are missed. Family members may also cover up the abuse because of embarrassment or a misguided wish to preserve the dignity or indulge the "final pleasures" of their elder relative. Caregivers may gradually assume functional roles of the impaired elderly abuser, further masking the substance abuse to outside view.

Health and social services providers often fail to consider the possibility of substance abuse in geriatric patients. One reason is that many older abusers are middle class and do not conform to the public stereotype of the substance abuser as down-and-out or anti-social. Influential early studies of alcohol (Drew, 1968) and opioid (Winick, 1962) dependence have perpetuated the myth that, because of high early mortality and spontaneous recovery in survivors, these disorders are uncommon after middle age. Failure to diagnose substance abuse may stem from a fatalistic view about the quality of life of elderly patients, or pessimism about treatment prospects. Under-recognition, under-reporting, and under-referral were substantial in several hospital studies (Beresford, Blow, Brower, K. M. Adams, & Hall, 1988; Curtis, Geller, Stokes, Levine, & Moore, 1989; Shuckit & P. L. Miller, 1976; Stinson, Dufour, & Bertolucci, 1989).

C. Comparative Prevalence of Substance-Use Disorders

Despite differing methods and study populations, all reports comparing the prevalence of heavy use or abuse of different substances in older persons agree that alcohol problems are more common than drug problems, and that licit drug problems are far more common than illicit drug problems. In community surveys of the elderly, for example, daily or nearly daily alcohol users exceed tranquilizer and sedative users by ratios of 1.4:1 (Guttman, 1978) to 5.5:1 (Smart & Adlaf, 1988). In a large urban community, elderly-mental-health outreach setting, primary alcohol abuse cases exceeded primary drug abuse cases by 5:1 (Reifler, Raskind, & Kethley, 1982b). In a large, hospitalized series, alcohol-dependence cases exceeded drug-dependence cases by 11:1 (Finlayson, 1984). Tobacco dependence, however, is more common than all other elder substance dependence combined.

III. Principles of Assessment and Management

A. Assessment of Substance-Use Disorders

Denial of substance abuse is common in affected persons of all ages. Reasons for this include substance-induced amnesia for many intoxication episodes, shame about reliance on alcohol or drugs, pessimism about recovery, and, of course, the desire to continue use. For these reasons, careful rapport building through repeated contacts, inquiry with relatives, caregivers, and others in the social network, reviews of medical and pharmacy records, and home visitation are especially useful case-assessment methods. There is no good general screening instrument, covering all substances, that is validated for use with elderly persons. The DSM-III-R and ICD-10 dependence criteria (Table II) offer a reasonable guide for acquiring information in order to establish a diagnosis, but no study of item-response frequencies for these criteria in age-stratified samples has yet confirmed their validity in the elderly. Toxicological examinations of urine, blood, and breath samples for suspected substances are the most useful medical test findings to corroborate the history. Neuropsychological and neurological evaluation may identify complicating brain disorders.

B. Management and Treatment

The goals of substance-abuse treatment in the elderly are threefold: stabilization and reduction of substance consumption, treatment of coexisting problems, and arrangement of appropriate social interventions. Reducing consumption may be a simple and straightforward matter of providing education and advice in mild dependence cases, especially if the older person is highly cooperative; or it may be very complicated and hazardous, requiring hospital care or a protracted outpatient course, in cases of long-standing, high-dose dependence. Treatment of coexisting problems can be a crucial step, especially when chronic pain, chronic insomnia, or a mood disorder has been a major factor sustaining the substance dependence, or when serious complications of substance abuse are present. Social interventions range from informal plans, such as arranging for increased visitation by loved ones or enrollment in a senior activity center, to major formal interventions (e.g., admission to a senior substance-abuse program, or to a nursing home). Persuading the elderly substance abuser and family to accept treatment often requires carefully arranged counseling (Atkinson, 1985). The geriatric healthcare team—with representatives from the medical, mental health, social and rehabilitative disciplines—is ideally constituted to evaluate needs, plan, and provide services in typically complex cases of severe substance abuse in the elderly, if the team is adequately trained for such cases (see Section VI,C). Inclusion of a geriatric substance-abuse specialist on the team may be the best approach in some settings.

IV. Alcohol-Use Disorders

A. Epidemiology

1. Use, Heavy Use, and Problem Use in the Elderly

A majority of persons older than 60 to 65 continue to drink beverage alcohol (reviewed in Atkinson, 1990). The best-available prevalence studies on heavy and problematic alcohol use are summarized in Table IV. There are few data available on ethnic or racial differences in elderly alcohol abuse, but two clinical studies suggest that rates of active alcoholism may be higher in older African-Americans (Blum & Rosner, 1983; McCusker, Cherubin, & Zimberg, 1971). With regard to gender, men in present elderly cohorts are two to six times more likely than women to have documented alcohol problems. Indeed, prevalence data support the conclusion that alcohol problems now constitute a public health problem of moderate proportion in young-old men.

2. Age versus Cohort Effects on Prevalence

Cross-sectional studies show declining prevalence of alcohol use and abuse with age (studies summarized in Atkinson, 1990). These findings may be partly accounted for by premature deaths of early-onset alcoholics, and by moderation or cessation of drinking with age by surviving alcoholics and others (W. L. Adams, Garry, Rhyne, Hunt, & Goodwin, 1990; Hermos, LoCastro, Glynn, Bouchard, & DeLabry, 1988; Nordstrom & Berglund, 1987; Vaillant, 1983, p. 153–155). Cross-sectional surveys, however, cannot separate cohort effects from age effects. Moreover, in such surveys there tends to be undersampling of elderly persons in general, and of elderly heavy drinkers in particular (Clark & Midanik, 1982). To further complicate matters, the elderly are less candid and less likely to recall accurately when reporting their alcohol consumption, especially when asked retrospectively to estimate their *usual* alcohol intake (Graham, 1986; Werch, 1989).

Data from two large longitudinal studies (Dufour, Colliver, Stinson, & Grigson, 1988; Glynn, Bouchard, LoCastro, & Laird, 1985) suggest that apparent decline in drinking prevalence may be a cohort, rather than an age, effect. In the Boston Normative Aging Study, a mail survey of alcohol use by 1700 men was conducted at two points in time

Table IV

Surveys of Drinking Behavior in the Elderly

Study (cohort age ≥ 60 unless stated)	Footnote	Men	Men and women	Women
Heavy drinking—community surveys				
Clark & Midanik (1982) U.S. 1979; age ≥65	a	8		2
Cahalan et al. (1969) U.S. 1964–65; age ≥65	b	7		1
Room (1972) U.S. late 1960s	b	12		1
Smart & Adlaf (1988) Ontario 1976–77	c		10	
Smart & Adlaf (1988) Ontario 1982–84	c		14	
Meyers et al. (1982) Boston 1977	d		6	
Glynn et al. (1983) Boston 1973	e	17		
Barnes (1979) NY State 1975; age 60–69	b	24		0
Barnes (1979) NY State 1975; age 70–96	b	6		2
Busby et al. (1988) rural New Zealand; age ≥70	f	24		10
Problem drinking—community surveys				
Saunders et al. (1989) Liverpool; age ≥65	g	1.5		0.6
Holzer et al. (1984) ECA—3 U.S. cities 1980–82	h	1.9–4.6		0.1–0.7
Glynn et al. (1983) Boston 1973	i	2		
Borgatta et al. (1982) U.S. 1978, 80; age ≥65	k		7	
Meyers et al. (1982) Boston 1977	j		4	
Cahalan (1970) U.S. 1964–65, 67; age 60–69	j	12		1
Cahalan (1970) U.S. 1964–65, 67; age ≥70	j	1		≤0.5
Currently active alcoholism: clinical samples				
General hospital medical wards				
Schuckit et al. (1980) U.S.—VA medical wards	l	6		
Cheah et al. (1979) U.S.—VA geri. med. eval. unit	m	8		
Outpatient/outreach settings				
Malcolm (1984) Liverpool, psychiat. home eval.	n	21	9	5
Reifler et al. (1982a) Seattle; age ≥60	o		10	
Reifler et al. (1982b) Seattle; age 60–69	o		17	
Bridgewater et al. (1987) Newcastle gen. prac.	p	23	17	11

[a] ≥1 oz ethanol/day.
[b] 2–3 drinks, ≥3 times/week.
[c] Nearly daily use.
[d] ≥2 drinks/day; mail survey.
[e] ≥2 drinks/day.
[f] Daily drinking; general practice rolls; ? date.
[g] Geriatric Mental State Examination; general practice rolls, 1982–83.
[h] DSM-III alcohol dependence or alcohol abuse, past 6 months.
[i] Problem drinking variously defined; mail survey.
[j] Problem drinking variously defined.
[k] Intemperate drinking otherwise undefined.
[l] Alcohol-related major life problem(s) without preexisting psychiatric disorders; age ≥65.
[m] Alcohol abuse (undefined but pre–DSM-III); 88% age ≥65; others younger.
[n] Alcohol problem (undefined); age ≥65.
[o] Alcohol abuse (undefined but pre–DSM-III); geri. mental health outreach team.
[p] CAGE questionnaire: affirmative answers ≥2 of 4.

(Glynn *et al.*, 1985). Older cohorts reported less alcohol consumption on the initial survey, but each age cohort reported unchanged consumption levels nine years later. Estimates of prevalence reconstructed from retrospective reports collected in cross-sectional community surveys (Cloninger *et al.*, 1987; Holzer *et al.*, 1984; Reich, *et al.*, 1988), show that the prevalence of alcohol-use disorders by age period has tended to increase steadily in successive birth cohorts during this century.

Individuals reaching age 21 during prohibition (1920–1933) attained age 65 between 1964 and 1977, and survivors are now in their 80s. It is of interest that the most recently reported national community household surveys of alcohol use and problems were conducted in the years 1964 to 1982 (see Table IV). Thus the very cross-sectional studies that represent the prevalence "gold standard" at this time—studies that show lower prevalence rates for persons older than 60 to 65—were conducted with an older cohort that would have been most influenced by prohibition values. To summarize, several lines of epidemiological evidence suggest that cohort effects account for a substantial portion of the apparently lower prevalence of alcohol-use disorders reported in today's elderly. Relatively higher levels of alcohol consumption and problems in old age might be expected in birth cohorts entering their 60s in the 1980s and beyond.

B. Patterns of Alcohol Use and Abuse

1. Motives for Nonpathological Drinking

Some old people may drink more than they did when they were younger because they now have more time and money to do so (Barnes, 1979; Busby, Campbell, Borrie, & Spears, 1988), and alcohol may be used medicinally by some older persons (Hartford & Samorajski, 1982). Conventional motives of enhancing social experience and relaxation, however, probably are the most common reasons that older people drink alcohol (Alexander & Duff, 1988; Christopherson, Escher, & Bainton, 1984). Social expectations may influence alcohol use in retirement communities (Alexander & Duff, 1988).

2. Therapeutic Use and Health Maintenance Value of Alcohol

Several careful studies (reviewed in Atkinson & Kofoed, 1984) have demonstrated that modest amounts of alcohol can enhance patient socialization and morale in residential-care settings. Residents who have cardiovascular or cognitive disorders, or are prescribed psychiatric medications, however, should not use alcohol. For outpatients, controls are absent that, in the residential studies, assured limits in quantity consumed and use within a positive social context. Similar cautions apply to advising older patients to use alcohol for appetite enhancement or sleep induction (Hartford & Samorajski, 1982).

An intriguing epidemiological finding is the association of regular but moderate alcohol use (up to two drinks/day) with lower morbidity and mortality from coronary heart disease in men, when compared to heavy users and abstainers, suggesting that moderate consumption of alcohol has an apparent protective value against coronary heart disease (Colsher & Wallace, 1989; Gordon & Doyle, 1987; Hegsted & Ausman, 1988; Klatsky, Friedman, & Siegelaub, 1981; Marmot, 1984). Although biochemical hypotheses have been proposed that could explain the findings, another interpretation is that the abstainer group is predisposed to cardiac disease. In a recent large British study of male non-alcoholics, abstainers, who had higher mortality than moderate drinkers, often had serious medical illnesses that predated (and were the probable motive for) drinking cessation (Shaper, Wannamethee, & Walker, 1988). These considerations raise doubts about the validity of the alcohol-protective hypothesis (Lancet editorial, 1988; Shaper *et al.*, 1988).

3. Heavy Drinking

Because of increasing alcohol sensitivity with age, it is not surprising that in some carefully studied elderly clinical cohorts, alcohol consumption levels are lower than is typical of younger alcoholics (Schuckit, Atkinson, Miller, & Berman, 1980). However, there are studies in which amounts consumed by elderly alcoholics are impressively high. For example, Dupree, Broskowski, & Schonfeld (1984) reported that their patients averaged 23 drinking days/month, 15 intoxicated days/month, and consumed the mean equivalent of 12.2 ounces of 100-proof alcohol on a typical drinking day. Elderly heavy drinkers in one study (Nakamura *et al.*, 1990), compared to others, had used more alcohol before age 40, smoked more cigarettes after age 40, and were more likely to report a cohabiting residence, lower educational achievement, and better health as measured by lack of use of prescribed medicines and unimpaired ratings on a scale of daily living activities.

4. Reactive Drinking

Despite its popularity, the stress-reactive hypothesis for problem drinking in old age has been difficult to validate (Atkinson, 1990; Finney & Moos, 1984; Gomberg, 1985; Schuckit, 1977). In community surveys, *coping* reasons are not commonly endorsed by elderly drinkers (Christopherson *et al.*, 1984; Huffine, Folkman, & Lazarus, 1989), and retirement was found to have little impact on alcohol consumption in a large urban sample of men (Ekerdt, DeLabry, Glynn, & Davis, 1989). On the other hand, a recent study by Moos and his associates has confirmed links between stress and problem drinking in older persons. Compared with nonproblem drinkers of similar age, community-dwelling problem drinkers aged 55 to 65 reported more negative life events, chronic stressors, and social resource deficits (Brennan & Moos, 1990). They were also more likely to cope with life stressors by making avoidant responses (Moos, Brennan, Fondacaro, & Moos, 1990). Older persons who demonstrate increasing alcohol problems in association with major losses are also commonly encountered in clinical practice (Finlayson, Hurt, Davis, & Morse, 1988; Atkinson, 1990), although often in such cases it is difficult to determine the causal links between drinking and life events (Graham, Zeidman, Flower, Saunders, & White-Campbell, 1989). Persons with prior alcohol-use disorders (in remission for several years) may be especially vulnerable to recurrent late-life alcohol problems with stress. Persons suffering from major depression (Atkinson & Kofoed, 1982) or dementia (King, 1986) may abuse alcohol.

5. Alcohol Use and Cognition

The neurotoxicity of alcohol increases with age (Freund, 1984a, 1984b). A nonalcoholic man in his 60s may have a peak blood alcohol level 20% higher than a man in his 30s after a standard alcohol load, because of altered volume of distribution with age (Vestal *et al.*, 1977). Even when one controls for blood-alcohol level, cognitive and cerebellar functions are more impaired with age after a standard alcohol load, indicating an increasing neuropharmacodynamic effect of alcohol with age, as well (Vogel-Sprott & Barrett, 1984). While unreplicated, this finding is consistent with similar findings in studies of aging rodents (Wood, Armbrecht, & Wise, 1982; York, 1983).

Neuropsychological deficits in chronic alcoholics are magnified with age. This relationship appears to be a function of age-related increase in central nervous system susceptibility to alcohol toxicity rather than duration of alcoholism (Parsons & Leber, 1982; Ryan & Butters, 1984). Alcohol impairs memory, abstract reasoning, and cognitive adaptation to novel stimuli in alcohol abusers. Neuropsychological evidence does not support a *premature aging* effect of alcohol. Similar but more subtle effects have been reported in older moderate to heavy social drinkers tested when sober (reviewed in Atkinson & Kofoed, 1982). These findings, however, could be explained by differences between light and heavy social drinkers in their innate cognitive abilities or anxiety levels during testing (reviewed in Waugh, Jackson, Fox, Hawke, & Tuck, 1989).

6. Early versus Late-Onset Alcohol Problems

Although gerontologists often have doubted the existence of late-onset alcoholism, reports in the last decade clearly confirm this phenomenon. Several retrospective studies of community samples have noted subsets among the elderly who report increasing their alcohol consumption in later life, either for the first time or following a fluctuating pattern established earlier (Busby *et al.*, 1988; Dunham, 1981; Giordano & Beckham, 1985). Data from elderly clinical samples demonstrate that onset of initial drinking problems at or after age 60 is common, occurring in 29 to 68% of cases in three recent series (Atkinson, 1990; Atkinson, Tolson, & Turner, 1990b; Finlayson *et al.*, 1988; Wiens, Menustik, Miller, & Schmitz, 1982–1983). Later onset appears to be related to higher socioeconomic status (Atkinson, 1984) and gender, having been found to be more common among elderly women alcoholics than among men (Holzer *et al.*, 1984). Late-onset alcohol problems are often milder and more circumscribed than those beginning earlier in life (Atkinson *et al.*, 1990b). The assertion in DSM-III-R (American Psychiatric Association, 1987, p. 174), that later-onset alcohol dependence typically occurs secondary to mood or organic mental disorder, was not upheld by findings from two large datasets (Atkinson, 1990; Atkinson *et al.*, 1990b; Finlayson *et al.*, 1988).

7. Family Patterns

Familial and *nonfamilial* forms of alcohol-use disorders are seen in the elderly, but older alcoholics in treatment tend to report lower rates of family alcoholism, later onset of alcohol problems, and milder alcohol problems (Atkinson, 1990; Atkinson *et al.*, 1990b; Atkinson, Turner, Kofoed, & Tolson, 1985). In occasional late-onset cases with strong family loading for alcoholism, a genetic influence could be a contributing cause. Conversely, as Volicer and associates have observed (Volicer, Volicer, & D'Angelo, 1983), a negative family history may predict freedom from alcoholism in early adulthood, but may have far less predictive value for lifetime risk.

C. Clinical Features of Alcohol-Use Disorders

1. Essential and Associated Features

Graham (1986) has observed that there are problems in applying to the elderly the measures commonly used for characterizing alcoholism in younger persons: consumption level, alcohol-related social and legal problems, alcohol-related health problems, symptoms of drunkenness or dependence, and self-recognition of an alcohol problem. With these limitations in mind, it can be said that there is no evidence that the primary symptoms of alcohol dependence or abuse in the elderly are different from those seen in younger adults. One study (Willenbring, Christensen, Spring, & Rasmussen, 1987) employing factor analysis of responses of hospitalized elderly male alcoholics on the Michigan Alcoholism Screening Test (MAST), a self-report questionnaire on alcoholism-related symptoms, found that the symptom constellation in these men was not distinctly different from that of younger alcoholics. In a much larger hospital survey, however, many items on the MAST were demonstrated to correlate poorly with alcohol problems in older patients. A new geriatric version (MAST-G) is being developed (F. C. Blow, personal communication, October, 1990). Circumscribed abuse (for example, complication of a preexisting medical disorder, or drinking and driving, without evidence of other problems) is common in late-onset cases (Atkinson *et al.,* 1990b).

Intoxication may occur at lower dose levels in older persons, because of increased biological sensitivity. Several characteristic laboratory abnormalities also accompany many cases of alcohol dependence (Hurt, Finlayson, Morse, & Davis, 1988). Self-reported depressive symptoms occur in more than half of older alcoholics entering treatment, as is also true for younger patients. Such findings generally are interpreted as correlates or consequences of recent heavy drinking in alcoholics rather than as evidence of primary mood disorders, since scores on depression self-report measures usually fall to normal levels without specific antidepressant treatment after two to four weeks' sobriety. Mood disorders are diagnosed much less often than simple depressed mood. Finlayson and colleagues (1988) found that 12% of patients hospitalized for alcoholism had currently coexisting affective disorders, typically major depression. Dementias are more common, occurring in 25% of Finlayson's cases. Clinical features and screening tests for alcoholism in the elderly have been reviewed more extensively elsewhere (Atkinson, 1990).

2. Complications

Alcohol-withdrawal disorders include the tremulous syndrome, hallucinosis, seizures, and delirium tremens. While there is no evidence that these disorders occur at different rates in the elderly (Atkinson, 1988), there is evidence in animal studies of increasing alcohol-dependence liability with age (Ritzmann & Melchior, 1984). In older persons, alcohol-withdrawal disorders are more difficult to treat (Liskow, Rinck, Campbell, & DeSouza, 1989), and may be associated with greater mortality (Feuerlein & Reiser, 1986). Organic central nervous system complications include prolonged reversible cognitive impairment (Grant, K. M. Adams, & Reed, 1984), dementia associated with alcoholism (Pfefferbaum, Rosenbloom, Crusan, & Jernigan, 1988; Ron, 1983), deterioration of another form of dementia, such as Alzheimer's (King, 1986), and amnestic (Korsakoff) disorder. Accurate diagnosis among these disorders may at times be difficult (Atkinson, 1988).

Alcohol problems are implicated in a high proportion of elderly suicide cases in some series (Blazer, 1982; Martin & Streissguth, 1982), but not in others (Conwell, Rotenberg, & Caine, 1990). Social impairment ranges from mild to very severe—presenting in extreme cases as *senile squalor* or *Diogenes syndrome,* in which a chaotic, disorganized living pattern not attributable to dementia or depression improves in supervised residential care (Droller, 1964; Kafetz & Cox, 1981; MacMillan & Shaw, 1966; Wattis, 1981). In some cases family discord can be prominent, especially if there are family drinking partners.

Diseases of other organ systems caused or exacerbated by alcohol excess include those of concern at all ages. In severe cases, alcohol excess can intensify multiple geriatric illness (Atkinson & Kofoed, 1982). Hypoglycemia, unstable diabetes mellitus, hyperuricemia, hypertriglyceridemia, osteoporosis, anemias, hypertension, congestive heart failure, aspiration pneumonia, and parkinsonism all can be caused or aggravated by alcohol dependence. Unexpected response to prescribed medication may also be the first clue to undisclosed alcohol abuse.

D. Course

No adequate longitudinal studies of alcoholics spanning the later years have been reported; available studies offer only fragmentary glimpses of the course of alcohol-use disorders beyond age 65. Shuckit and colleagues (1980) studied prospectively, over 3 years, two very small cohorts of active ($N = 9$) and remitted ($N = 9$) older alcoholics in their late 60s and early 70s, along with a control group of 113 medical patients. They found relapses and remissions in several cases, as well as onset of new problem drinking in 5% of controls. Cross-sectional surveys of problem drinking that are further stratified for age after 60 show steadily declining prevalence with age, receding to negligible levels after 85, but it is unclear to what extent such differences represent age versus cohort effects.

There is no information about rates of spontaneous remission in older alcoholics. Schuckit and associates have marshaled some evidence to suggest that the course of chronic alcoholism runs about 20 to 25 years, irrespective of onset age, but this observation lacks confirmation (reviewed in Atkinson & Kofoed, 1982). Among older outpatient male-war-veteran problem drinkers, the span from first alcohol problem to date of entry into current treatment can be as long as 50 years (Atkinson, 1990). Over this course, drinking may have been steady, progressive, or variable; in some cases, there had been sober periods of 10 years or more between problem-drinking episodes. Mortality rates are very high when active drinking continues in the face of frank dementia (Simon, Epstein, & L. Reynolds, 1968) or active alcohol-related liver disease (Hurt *et al.,* 1988; Woodhouse & James, 1985). Those with liver disease who stop drinking have a better outcome (Woodhouse & James, 1985).

E. Management and Treatment

Older alcoholics have tended to fare as well as or better than younger persons in a variety of alcohol-treatment settings (Atkinson, 1984; Atkinson & Kofoed, 1982; Janik & Dunham, 1983; Schuckit 1977). In the largest outpatient compliance study reported to date, Atkinson, Tolson, and Turner (1990a) followed 205 problem-drinking male veterans, aged 55–76, during a one-year, age-specific treatment program. Fifty-seven percent completed the program, versus only 27% of younger patients in a comparable treatment condition.

Various treatment approaches have been described, including outpatient social support groups (Atkinson *et al.*, 1990a; Dunlop, Skorney, & Hamilton, 1982; Kofoed, Tolson, Atkinson, Turner, & Toth, 1984; Zimberg, 1978), family therapy (Dunlop *et al.*, 1982), behavioral–educational groups (Dupree *et al.*, 1984), home-based outreach interventions (Graham *et al.*, 1989), and hospital treatment (Finlayson *et al.*, 1988; Wiens *et al.*, 1982–1983). None of the studies, however, employed controls, randomized assignments, or comparison treatments. Using a *historical controls* approach, one small study (Kofoed, Tolson, Atkinson, Toth, & Turner, 1987) demonstrated enhanced compliance with social group treatment when older alcoholics were placed in elder-specific groups rather than mixed-age groups. In a large study of factors affecting outpatient elder-specific group treatment compliance (Atkinson *et al.*, 1990a) court supervision (of drinking drivers) and concurrent spouse counseling independently increased one-year outpatient program completion. Management of persons with coexisting major mental disorders is discussed in Section VI,C.

V. Prescription Psychoactive Drug-Use Disorders _____

A. Epidemiology of Sedative–Hypnotic Drug Use and Problems

1. Introduction

The elderly receive far more prescribed drugs than do younger people (Basen, 1977; Vestal, 1982), although younger persons use and abuse a wider variety of prescribed psychoactive agents. Aging persons primarily develop problems from sedative–hypnotic agents, especially benzodiazepines, while opioid analgesics are a distant second, and psychostimulant abuse is virtually unknown (Finlayson, 1984; Raffoul, Cooper, & Love, 1981; Smart & Adlaf, 1988; Stephens, Haney, & Underwood, 1981). The abuse potential of other commonly prescribed psychoactives, for example, antidepressants and neuroleptics, is too low in the elderly for them to be considered in the context of substance abuse.

2. Benzodiazepine Use by the Community Elderly

This class of sedative–hypnotics has achieved dominance over the past 30 years because of the relative safety and efficacy of these agents in the treatment of insomnia and anxiety. (See Chapter 27 for a list of benzodiazepines.) Barbiturates, in contrast, now account for only a small proportion of anxiolytic prescriptions for the elderly in the United States

(Mellinger, Balter, & Uhlenhuth, 1984) and United Kingdom (Morgan, Dallosso, Ebrahim, Arie, & Fentem, 1988). Although the number of benzodiazepine prescriptions peaked in the mid-1970s and has since been in decline worldwide (Balter, Manheimer, Mellinger, & Uhlenhuth, 1984), use of these drugs in the elderly has not changed appreciably in recent years (Smart & Adlaf, 1988; Sullivan *et al.*, 1988). Surveys of community-dwelling elderly suggest that about 5 to 15% have on hand currently prescribed benzodiazepines (Cadigan, Magaziner, & Fedder, 1989; Sullivan *et al.*, 1988). Women may be more likely than men to receive benzodiazepine prescriptions (Mellinger *et al.*, 1984; Smart & Adlaf, 1988), although not all studies find such gender distinctions (Mant *et al.*, 1988). No information is available on ethnic, racial, or socioeconomic factors in sedative use or abuse.

Similar surveys also suggest that most older persons in the community use these agents as directed (American Psychiatric Association, 1990). When misuse occurs, it tends to be in the direction of underuse (Abrams & Alexopoulos, 1987; Pinsker & Suljaga-Petchel, 1984; Quinn, Applegate, Roberts, Collins, & Vanderzwaag, 1983). Recreational use (taking the drug to get "high") is rare except among prior substance abusers. Still, many healthcare professionals believe that the rate of benzodiazepine use in all age groups is excessive (Higgitt, 1988).

3. Institutional Benzodiazepine Use

Wide concern has been expressed that, in nursing homes and residential care facilities, older patients may be particularly likely to be dosed with excessive sedatives to control behavior. Several surveys indicate that a relatively high proportion of residents receive sedative–hypnotic (20–28%) and antianxiety (8–21%) drugs, mainly benzodiazepines, typically on a regular, daily basis (Avorn, Dreyer, Connelly, & Soumerai, 1989; Beardsley, Larson, Burns, Thompson, & Kamerow, 1989; Beers *et al.*, 1988; DeLeo & Stella, 1989). Information critical for determining the extent of dependence liability or overdose, such as drug dose and duration, unfortunately are not reported in these studies (see Chapter 27 for further information).

4. Long-Term Benzodiazepine Use and the Development of Dependence

It is now well established that regular, daily therapeutic doses of any benzodiazepine, if prolonged beyond 6 to 12 months, can result in the development of dependence, even without dose escalation (APA, 1990; Higgitt, 1988). There is little tolerance to the antianxiety effects of diazepam, alprazolam, or other drugs in this class (Ashton, 1984; Pinsker & Suljaga-Petchel, 1984; Rodrigo, King, & Williams, 1988). Thus persons with anxiety disorders may continue to enjoy symptom relief for prolonged periods without needing to increase drug doses. Tolerance to their hypnotic (sleep-inducing) effects, on the other hand, is well documented, so that addiction to increasingly high doses is also possible, especially in persons who take a benzodiazepine over a protracted period for chronic insomnia.

Community surveys indicate that the elderly are more likely to receive benzodiazepines for prolonged periods than are younger persons (Mant *et al.*, 1988; Mellinger *et al.*, 1984). A U.S. national survey of noninstitutionalized adults concluded that long-term benzodiazepine users were more likely to be older, have more psychological distress, and suffer from chronic somatic illnesses, especially cardiovascular disease and arthritis (Uhlenhuth, Dewit, Balter, Johanson, & Mellinger, 1988). In two recent British studies, over 60% of elderly benzodiazepine users had received their prescriptions for more than a year (Morgan, 1988; Sullivan *et al.*, 1988). Although receipt of a prescription does not necessarily mean that the patient uses the drug every day, these findings demonstrate that many elderly patients are placed at risk for developing benzodiazepine dependence by the manner in which these drugs are prescribed.

The community prevalence of drug dependence of all types in persons aged 65 and older is very low—well under 1% (Myers *et al.*, 1984). These data, however, almost certainly underestimate, or quite possibly ignore entirely, low-dose benzodiazepine dependence, which may be unrecognized by the patient and poorly measured by the dependence criteria (Table II).

5. Other Risk Factors for Benzodiazepine Dependence

Besides duration of treatment, other pharmacological variables influencing the likelihood of dependence are higher drug dose, shorter duration of action, and higher milligram potency of the agent (APA, 1990). Patient factors include prior or concurrent alcoholism, prior sedative drug dependence, chronic insomnia (rather than anxiety) as the target symptom for which the drug is prescribed, and coexisting chronic painful physical illness or personality disorder (APA, 1990). The most common reasons elderly patients give for long-term benzodiazepine use are pain and insomnia (Finlayson, 1984; Higgitt, 1988). Insomnia is a common complaint among old people and stems in part from changes with age in brain physiology during sleep (see Chapter 20). Of all treatment strategies available for insomnia, a hypnotic prescription requires the least effort by both patient and clinician and provides rapid, if not long-lasting, relief. Coexistent somatic illnesses and pain may also disrupt sleep. The presence of chronic, undiagnosed depression may also predispose to long-term benzodiazepine use and dependence in older patients. In one group of elderly patients (F. Miller, Whitcup, Sacks, & Lynch, 1985), a pattern was noted of benzodiazepines prescribed for symptoms of depression misdiagnosed as anxiety by one or more primary care physicians. The longer depression went undiagnosed, the more likely the patient was to receive additional benzodiazepine prescriptions.

6. Limitations of the Epidemiologic Data

Data gathered by self-report questionnaire may underestimate actual drug use. In the Liverpool Study, Sullivan and colleagues (1988) concluded that the elderly benzodiazepine-use prevalence figure of 14% was low compared to national prescription audits and may have represented under-reporting. In another British survey, a structured questionnaire was given to elderly people living at home. *Occasional* use for sleep was reported by 16%. However, 89% of those people said they had taken a dose the night before the interview (Morgan, *et al.*, 1988). Mellinger and associates (1984) addressed the issue of under-reporting by verifying self-reports of medication use with examination of prescription bottles provided by the patients. They concluded that some under-reporting did occur, but found an 83% correlation between reported and actual consumption.

Most epidemiologic studies of benzodiazepine use do not properly make the distinction between their use to treat anxiety versus insomnia, the definition of which seems to rest more on the time of day the medication is taken rather than on clinical indication or pharmacologic grounds. Morgan and colleagues (1988) argue that while this distinction is irrelevant in terms of the general effects and toxicity of benzodiazepines, failure to distinguish between these two uses of the agents obscures possible important differences in both the etiology of misuse and proposals of alternative treatment strategies.

B. Clinical Features and Complications of Benzodiazepine Dependence

1. Low-Dose Dependence

Low-dose dependence may cause few if any adverse signs or symptoms, until abrupt cessation leads to withdrawal symptoms. Persistence of the patient in assuring a steady supply of the agent is perhaps the most noteworthy behavioral feature. Dependence may develop within as little as four to six weeks of continuous treatment (Murphy, Owen, & Tyrer, 1984; Power, Jerrom, Simpson, & Mitchell, 1985), at doses as low as 6 to 10 mg diazepam equivalent (Ashton, 1987). Not everyone receiving long-term treatment, however, will develop dependence. The proportion of long-term users who experience withdrawal symptoms upon sudden discontinuation is estimated as 15 to 44% (Higgitt, Lader, & Fonagy, 1985).

2. High-Dose Dependence

A person believed to be taking only low doses of a benzodiazepine drug as prescribed may be receiving the same or similar medications from other sources simultaneously. This phenomenon is not uncommon in the elderly (Abrams & Alexopoulos, 1987; F. Miller *et al.*, 1985). This information may be withheld by the patient out of confusion or ignorance that two drugs from different sources are of the same class, or purposefully to conceal a high-dose dependence problem (Raffoul *et al.*, 1981). Sometimes healthcare providers simply fail to inquire about medications from other sources.

High-dose dependence is most likely to occur when these drugs are prescribed for many months for the treatment of insomnia, especially in persons with prior addiction to alcohol or sedatives. Tolerance to sleep-inducing effects of these agents is very rapid, some studies showing loss of effects on sleep after as little as one week's nightly dosing (APA, 1990).

3. Acute Side-Effects and Toxicity

When initiating benzodiazepine treatment or stepping up the dose, there is a transitional period until a new plasma steady-state drug level is achieved, during which toxic effects may occur transitorily, typically consisting of one or more of the following symptoms: sedation, cerebellar ataxia, or increased reaction time (APA, 1990). Age-related pharmacokinetic and pharmacodynamic changes render the elderly especially vulnerable to these effects, and the duration until steady state is more protracted with age, as well (Cook, 1986; Cook, Huggett, Graham-Pole, Savage, & James, 1983). The sensitivity of the aging brain to these agents is well illustrated by a study comparing psychomotor performance between young and old volunteers after a single dose of nitrazepam, in which significantly more deficits occurred among the elderly despite similar serum levels of the drug (Castleden, George, Marcer, & Hallett, 1977).

4. Chronic Toxicity

Persistent toxicity is most likely to occur when dose escalation follows the development of tolerance. In older persons, toxicity may be manifest by persistent ataxia leading to falls and fractures (Ancill, Embury, MacEwan, & Kennedy, 1987); depressed mood, which can be mistaken for an affective disorder; oversedation; and memory impairment and other cognitive dysfunction, which can be mistaken for progressive dementia. Memory impairment typically is the consequence of drug disruption of memory consolidation (transfer of information from short- to long-term memory) (APA, 1990). Benzodiazepines can also induce anterograde amnesia. This action occurs when these agents are used intravenously in preanaethesia, but oral doses of short-acting, high-potency agents such as alprazolam can also induce anterograde amnesia. In a study of elderly demented patients, 5% had clinically significant cognitive improvement after discontinuation of their benzodiazepine medication (Larson, Reifler, Featherstone, & English, 1984) (See Chapter 27 for further discussion of benzodiazepine toxicity).

5. Complications Associated with Other Disorders

Benzodiazepines may contribute to respiratory insufficiency in persons with pulmonary disorders, or deteriorating status of demented or depressed patients. These agents potentiate the effects of alcohol and opioids. Cimetidine and propranolol interfere with the metabolism of benzodiazepines and can raise their blood levels (F. Miller *et al.*, 1985), but the clinical importance of these effects appears to be small.

6. Discontinuance Symptoms

Following abrupt termination of benzodiazepines after long-term use, distressing and sometimes very serious symptoms can occur, only some of which are true withdrawal phenomena (defined as new or novel symptoms for that patient, with early or late onset, but typically lasting only 2 to 4 weeks) (APA, 1990). *Rebound* symptoms are identical to those for which the drug was originally prescribed, for example, anxiety, but they reoccur rapidly, are more severe or intense than in the past, and resolve in a few days. *Reoccurrence* symptoms are also identical to the original symptoms, but are of the same intensity, and they persist. They represent a return to the chronic symptom pattern that had been suppressed by drug therapy. Some symptoms, like restlessness or irritability, are common and can represent any of the three types of discontinuance phenomena, depending upon the history, intensity, and time course. Other symptoms, like psychosis, seizures, or delirium, are uncommon and almost always represent true withdrawal phenomena.

C. *Assessment and Management of Benzodiazepine-Use Disorders*

1. Assessment of Dependence and Withdrawal

Many cases of dependence on benzodiazepines are evident when one simply considers the low-dose dependence phenomenon. Professional bias that drug dependence only occurs in the young can block timely recognition in the elderly (Whitcup & F. Miller, 1987). Benzodiazepine toxicity and dependence should be considered whenever an elderly person who receives these drugs suffers from poorly explained sedation, incoordination, depression, or deteriorating cognitive status. Acute confusional states are a common manifestation of benzodiazepine withdrawal in the elderly (Foy, Drinkwater, March, & Mearrick, 1986). Cases in which benzodiazepine withdrawal produced autonomic hyperactivity or fever have been misdiagnosed as hypertension, myocardial infarction, or acute infection (F. Miller *et al.*, 1985; F. Miller & Whitcup, 1986). A search for undisclosed prescription bottles should be conducted, with the aid of relatives and home visitation, when there is strong suspicion of benzodiazepine overuse.

2. Drug Discontinuation and Rehabilitation of the Dependent Patient

Gradual discontinuation of the drug is indicated, at least in those drug-dependent persons who suffer from chronic toxicity or other complications, or who have developed tolerance with dose escalation above the therapeutic range (APA, 1990; Higgitt *et al.*, 1985). One's goal is to proceed slowly enough in decremental dose reductions to avoid major withdrawal and minimize other discontinuance symptoms. Although many patients experience no major withdrawal symptoms even after abrupt termination of benzodiazepines, some, especially those who have developed lengthy, high-dose habits, may require many months' tapering to avert serious discontinuance symptoms. As the dose reaches lower levels, the size and frequency of decrements may have to be reduced even further, especially for high-potency, short-acting drugs like alprazolam. One must, in the end, tailor the reduction schedule to meet individual needs, although a period of 1 to 4 months is often sufficient. It is no small feat to persuade some elderly persons to give up benzodiazepines, and various intervention strategies may be needed (Atkinson, 1985). Several drug substitutes have been tried to ease withdrawal, but none clearly merits widespread use (APA, 1990).

Recovery following withdrawal is problematic. Although most patients will complete gradual-withdrawal regimens, many will experience symptoms of depression or anxiety, which may take up to a year to resolve (Ashton, 1984). A social–emotional support group for older persons withdrawing from benzodiazepines may aid the process (A. MacDonald, personal communication, December, 1987). Relapse rates have not been well studied in the general population, and objective information on elderly relapse rates and risk factors for relapse is needed. In a followup survey of mixed age patients 10 months to 3.5 years after withdrawal, 48% were considered fully recovered, while the remainder showed some degree of psychiatric difficulty or had relapsed on benzodiazepines (Ashton, 1987). Age was inversely correlated with positive outcome, but other factors such as duration of dependence, psychological profile, dose, and severity of symptoms showed no correlation. Comprehensive study of rehabilitation of older, sedative-dependent persons is limited by the small number of cases in any given healthcare program or geographic area.

3. Preventing Misuse and Dependence

There is considerable controversy over the indications for long-term prescribing of benzodiazepines in the elderly (Rickels, Case, Winokur, & Swenson, 1984). Higgitt (1988) advocates against any long-term use in geriatric patients, while Uhlenhuth and associates (1988) provide evidence that long-term risk is often exaggerated, and that certain patients with chronic anxiety benefit from continuing therapy. This is a view supported by the recent American Psychiatric Association task force on benzodiazepine dependence (APA, 1990), which advocated the long-term use of these drugs for generalized anxiety symptoms associated with chronic physical illness in older patients, even though dependence can be expected to occur in a substantial number of such patients. In contrast to the treatment of anxiety, most investigators agree that the use of long-term benzodiazepines in the treatment of chronic insomnia exposes the elderly patient to increased risks, while providing rapidly diminishing therapeutic effect (Reynolds, Kupfer, Hoch, & Sewich, 1985).

Higgitt and her associates (1985) have proposed several ways to reduce the risk of benzodiazepine dependence. Clinicians should prescribe in low doses and for short durations, avoid automatic refills, and educate patients about side-effects and risks of dependence. The high prevalence of undiagnosed depression in long-term users (F. Miller *et al.*, 1985), and the results of a survey by Mellinger and colleagues (1984) showing that most long-term benzodiazepine users had not sought psychiatric help, indicate that earlier and more frequent involvement of mental health practitioners in geriatric cases might reduce inappropriate benzodiazepine prescribing.

D. Prescription Analgesic Drug Use and Abuse

Little information is available concerning elderly use of prescribed analgesics. One reason may be the rapid rise in consumption of benzodiazepines and the overshadowing controversies and fears related to their use. Another obstacle to understanding geriatric analgesic use is that most surveys of drug consumption do not differentiate among the various types of analgesics. Thus data on the two most common types, opioids and nonsteroidal antiinflammatory drugs, are often combined in reports. One study divided analgesics simply into *strong* and *mild* without further definition (Cadigan *et al.*, 1989). This obscures important information on abuse and dependence, since chronic opioid use is attended by some risk of dependence, while nonsteroidal analgesics have virtually no dependence liability. Reports from two hospitalized elderly case series indicate that opioid analgesic dependence was less common than dependence on antianxiety and sedative–hypnotic agents (Finlayson, 1984; Whitcup & F. Miller, 1987). Opioid use often began before old age but gradually escalated, typically for treatment of chronic pain.

VI. Other Substances _____

A. *Illegal Drugs*

1. Varieties of Drugs and Disorders

Common illegal drugs include marijuana, opioids, hallucinogens, and psychostimulants such as amphetamines and cocaine. Use of illegal drugs may impair social functioning and promote excessive risk taking. Clinical disorders caused by illegal drugs vary by drug class, and include intoxication, withdrawal, delirium, dementia, and delusional, mood, and amnestic disorders. Space does not permit a description of disorders for each drug class; for this, readers may consult general sources (APA, 1987; Lowinson & Ruiz, 1981; Schuckit, 1989). Little is known about age-related changes in the pattern or manifestations of these disorders, or about the special treatment needs of elderly drug abusers.

2. Prevalence of Disorders

Illegal drug use by present elderly cohorts is very uncommon, a conclusion uniformly supported by community surveys (Myers *et al.*, 1984), surveys of the homeless (Koegel, Burnam, & Farr, 1988), reports of adverse drug reactions (Klein-Schwartz, Oderda, & Booze, 1983; Petersen & Thomas, 1975), and drug arrests (Jamieson & Flanagan, 1988; P. J. Taylor & Parrott, 1988). Illicit drug use occurs mainly among aging criminals and long-term heroin addicts. A recent, sporadically occurring phenomenon, however, is abuse of illicit substances by middle-class elderly susceptible to influence by younger persons who themselves are drug abusers. The authors have observed such cases involving marijuana and cocaine abuse.

3. Opioid Dependence

The most well studied of elderly illicit drug abusers are opioid addicts. Addicts older than 60 constituted less than .005% of all methadone maintenance clients in New York City in 1974, but their numbers increased to 2% by 1985 (Pascarelli, 1985). Low incidence of new opioid abuse after age 25 years, high mortality associated with illegal drug use, imprisonment, and increasing abstinence associated with age, are all factors that contribute to the low prevalence of aged addicts (Des Jarlais, Joseph, & Courtwright, 1985; Ghodse, Sheehan, C. Taylor, & Edwards, 1985; Harrington & Cox, 1979; Maddux & Desmond, 1980; Vaillant, 1973). Continued addiction into old age may be reinforced in part by one's identity as an addict, social ties in the drug subculture, and associated crime and drug dealing (Anglin, Brecht, Woodward, & Bonett, 1986; Capel, Goldsmith, Waddell, & Stewart, 1972; Pottieger & Inciardi, 1981; Wilbanks & Kim, 1984).

Those opiate addicts who do survive into old age typically bring a history of several decades of opiate use, although in one survey old addicts were often found who began their addiction in middle age (Capel *et al.*, 1972; Shuckit, 1977). In studies of urban American whites, blacks and Chinese, aged addicts tend to lead socially isolated lives and are often secretive regarding their drug use (Capel *et al.*, 1972; Deely, Kaufman, Yen, Jue, & Brown, 1979; Des Jarlais *et al.*, 1985; Pascarelli, 1985). They may reduce their daily drug dose because of lack of money or difficulty competing in the drug subculture, but their use tends to be steady, without periods of abstinence or binges. Typically they manage to avoid the attention of law enforcement agencies and often support their drug habit through legal employment. Survival of elderly addicts may be related to their tendency to practice scrupulous hygiene regarding needles and syringes, and their ability to obtain a steady supply of relatively pure drug, often substituting cleaner synthetic opioids such as hydromorphone (Dilaudid) for heroin (Capel *et al.*, 1972; Des Jarlais *et al.*, 1985; Pascarelli & Fischer, 1974). Many enter methadone maintenance as they become too old to "hustle," though it has been suggested that elderly addicts tolerate methadone poorly (Capel & Peppers, 1978; Pascarelli, 1979). For those who are without family and have outlived their contemporaries, the methadone maintenance clinic may be their only source of social support. Despite increased social stability, these elderly addicts usually tolerate detoxification from methadone maintenance poorly.

The consequences of intravenous (IV) opioid abuse are of concern in the elderly. Of all elderly with acquired immunodeficiency syndrome (AIDS), 3% contracted the disease through IV drug use (Moss & Miles, 1987). Long-term heroin addicts develop neuro-psychologic and neuroimaging abnormalities and are at high risk for medical problems, which consequently impair their function in the community (Schuckit, 1977; Strang & Gurling, 1989). As these addicts age and develop impairments in functioning, they face considerable discrimination by healthcare professionals and social service agencies. Alcohol abuse in aging opioid-dependent persons becomes an increasing source of comorbidity. Ironically, those who manage to avoid alcohol dependence and survive to their seventh or eighth decade usually die of the consequences of tobacco dependence (Des Jarlais *et al.*, 1985).

Historically opioid use was associated with aging. In China prior to the 1930s, opium smoking was primarily a habit of older men (Deely *et al.*, 1979). In Britain prior to 1960, 60% of known addicts were older than 50 (Bean, 1974). Opium use was predominantly associated with increasing age and debility in the United States before the passage of the Harrison Narcotic Act in 1914 (Anglin *et al.*, 1986; Capel & Peppers, 1978). This suggests that the present low prevalence of illegal opioid use in the elderly is mediated more by factors of low availability, cost, stigma, sanctions against use, and cohort effects, than by physiologic aversion.

4. Other Drugs

Little information is available regarding the use of other illegal drugs by the elderly. The 1-year prevalence of marijuana use in people older than 50 years was 1% in 1982 (J. D. Miller *et al.*, 1983). With the rising incidence of cocaine use, there are now sporadic case reports of abuse in the elderly but no systematic studies (Abrams & Alexopoulos, 1988). There is some speculation that amphetamines may be less euphorogenic in the elderly, and early clinical studies of amphetamines showed lower sympathomimetic response after standard doses with age (reviewed in Atkinson & Kofoed, 1982).

B. Over-the-Counter Drugs

1. Prevalence of Use

More than 300,000 over-the-counter (OTC) preparations (those medications that can be purchased without a prescription) are marketed, containing over 700 active ingredients (Gilbertson, 1986). In general, the use of OTC medications increases with age (Kofoed, 1985). However, psychoactive OTC use in the elderly is uncommon (Darnell, Murray, Martz, & Weinberger, 1986; Helling *et al.*, 1987; May, Stewart, Hale, & Marks, 1982). Hypnotic use rates are reported in the range of 1.5 to 2.5% (Guttman, 1978; Vener, Krupka, & Climo, 1979), with comparable or lower rates for stimulant use (Parry, Balter, Mellinger, Cisin, & Manheimer, 1973; Stephens *et al.*, 1981). The use of psychoactive OTC medications is less common among community elderly than is use of prescribed medications with similar effects (Guttman, 1978; Vener *et al.*, 1979). In a national age-stratified sample, decrease in use of psychoactive OTC sedatives, stimulants, and tranquilizers was seen with increasing age, especially among women (Parry *et al.*, 1973).

2. Factors Affecting Use and Misuse of OTCs

It has been proposed that OTC use is promoted by such diverse factors as lack of access to medical care, poverty, reluctance to admit illness, and reinforcement of self-sufficiency (Abrams & Alexopoulos, 1988; Kofoed, 1985). OTC use has also been associated with more frequent physician visits and lower prescription drug use (Stoller, 1988). Users of psychoactive OTCs were found to have higher educational achievement and social class than others (Parry *et al.*, 1973). Stoller (1988) found that elderly people living in the community usually used OTC treatments as their initial response for mild, self-limiting illness. Users are modest in their expectations about the usefulness of these drugs, regard them as only marginally effective, and rarely describe them as necessary for their daily functioning (Guttman, 1978; Parry *et al.*, 1973).

Untoward effects of OTC medications often are not recognized by the elderly person or the healthcare provider. Many persons conceal their OTC drug use or do not consider them drugs (Gardner & Hall, 1982; Ostrom, Hammarlund, Christensen, Plein, & Kethley, 1985). Consumers believe these drugs are safe and often do not read the instructions. Only about one sixth of patients tell their physicians about their OTC use (Ellor & Kurz, 1982; Guttman, 1978). Persons with cognitive impairment may be especially vulnerable to OTC drug misuse (Abrams & Alexopoulos, 1988).

3. OTC Hypnotics

OTC sedative–hypnotics are predominantly antihistamines, and the most common is diphenhydramine (Benadryl). Scopolamine–methapyrilene combinations and bromides, which were included in most OTC hypnotics before recent years, have been eliminated (Caro & Walker, 1986). In frail elderly persons, diphenhydramine causes a variety of side-effects of concern at the usual recommended doses because of its anticholinergic effects. Paradoxical excitement may occur at therapeutic doses, and elderly persons are more prone to exhibit this effect. Anticholinergic agents impair memory and new learning, and elevated serum anticholinergic levels in nursing home patients have been found to be related to decreased cognition and capacity for self-care (McEvoy *et al.*, 1987; P. S. Miller *et al.*, 1988; Potamianos & Kellett, 1982; Rovner *et al.*, 1988). Patients with Alzheimer's disease may be especially vulnerable to central anticholinergic effects because the primary neurotransmitter deficit in Alzheimer's is in the cholinergic system (Peters, 1989). These drugs also cause constipation, urinary retention, dry mouth, blurred vision, and impaired heat dissipation. Side-effects, even when mild, can result in falls, functional decline, and failure to thrive (Peters, 1989). There are case reports of abuse of diphenhydramine for its psychoactive effects, and fatalities have resulted from overdose (Feldman & Behar, 1986; Koppel, Ibe, & Tenczer, 1987). Elders also may be exposed unknowingly to diphenhydramine and other anticholinergic drugs contained in OTC cold remedies.

4. OTC Stimulants

Caffeine is the only active ingredient in OTCs marketed as stimulants. Each dose of OTC stimulant contains 100–200 milligrams of caffeine, similar to that found in 1–2 cups of coffee (Caro & Walker, 1986). Caffeine improves alertness and decreases fatigue, but in higher doses can cause insomnia, tremor, headache, and rarely, a mild form of delirium. Withdrawal symptoms include headache and fatigue. Elderly people are more sensitive to the physical effects of caffeine but report fewer psychological effects than do younger subjects (Swift & Tiplady, 1988). Other preparations with prominent stimulant effects include phenylpropanolamine and, less commonly, ephedrine and pseudoephedrine. Phenylpropanolamine, chemically similar to amphetamine, is often an active ingredient in OTC cold remedies and appetite suppressants. In older persons this drug has been associated with hypertension (especially in subjects with autonomic insufficiency or those prescribed monoamine oxidase–inhibiting medications), stroke, cerebral hemorrhage, and cardiac arrhythmias (Appelt, 1986; Biaggioni, Onrot, Stewart, & Robertson, 1987; Kase, Foster, Reed, Spatz, & Girgis, 1987; Pentel, 1984). Toxic psychiatric effects of phenylpropanolamine are also recognized, but fortunately these are uncommon in the elderly (Lake, Alagna, Quirk, Moriarty, & Reid, 1985). Phenylpropanolamine is often combined with antihistamines in OTC preparations, which may increase the risk of toxicity (Pental, 1984).

5. Other Drugs

Although not marketed primarily for their psychoactive properties, some OTCs have significant psychoactive effects when overused or combined with other medications (Glantz, 1981; Lamy, 1982). The most common OTC medications used by the elderly are vitamins, laxatives, antacids, and analgesics (Helling *et al.*, 1987; May *et al.*, 1982; Ostrom *et al.*, 1985; Stoller, 1988; Vener *et al.*, 1979).

Older adults have been the target of misinformation and fraud regarding the benefits of megadoses of vitamins, minerals, and other supplements. Supplements promoted as anti-aging and sex rejuvenating include Vitamin E (used by 5–13% of community elders), selenium, zinc, bee pollen, and RNA pills. Vitamins C and B have been promoted as preventing cancer (Herbert, 1988; May *et al.*, 1982; Schneider & Nordlund, 1983). These claims are not supported by scientific evidence, and toxicity syndromes (with mental status changes) have been reported for most of these preparations at large doses (Aflin-Slater, 1988). Laxatives, despite their lack of psychoactive effects, are frequently misused, especially by elderly women. Overuse of laxatives may be promoted by age-related increases in constipation but also by the mistaken belief that a daily bowel movement is necessary for good health. Compulsive laxative use can assume addictive proportions.

OTC analgesics, including aspirin products, acetaminophen, and the newer ibuprofen, are commonly used by the elderly because of the age-related increase in arthritis (Lamy, 1982). The risk of salicylate toxicity increases with age even though the elderly use lower average doses of salicylates (Grigor, Spitz, & Furst, 1987). Toxic manifestations include a dementia-like picture with tinnitus and irritability. In one series of 20 patients with chronic salicylate toxicity, the median age was 77 years. Eighty percent showed abnormal mental status, and 85% had some functional dependence when first evaluated (Bailey & S. R. Jones, 1989). Aspirin and ibuprofen are common causes of adverse drug reactions (primarily gastritis and gastric bleeds) requiring hospital admission of elderly persons (Colt & Shapiro, 1989; Griffin, Ray, & Schaffner, 1988). Analgesic preparations may contain alcohol or caffeine, and dependence and abuse of the psychoactive ingredient may result in toxicity from the analgesic (Murray, 1980).

C. Tobacco (Nicotine) Dependence

1. Dependence and Its Prevalence

Tobacco dependence is the most common of all substance-use disorders, is entirely obvious, thus taking no special effort to establish the diagnosis, and arguably accounts for far more medical disability and mortality in the elderly than abuse of all other substances combined. Because of its low behavioral toxicity, however, tobacco dependence has held little interest for mental health professionals. Nicotine is the psychoactive agent in tobacco, and regular, daily tobacco use produces a nicotine-dependence disorder. The pharmacologic and behavioral processes that determine nicotine dependence are similar to processes that determine addiction to drugs such as heroin and cocaine. They include pleasurable effects, regular and compulsive patterns of use, withdrawal syndromes, tolerance to effects with compensatory increased intake, and relapse with abstinence (Hughes, Gust, & Pechacek, 1987; U.S. Department of Health and Human Services, 1988a).

Cigarette smoker prevalence among adults has declined steadily over the past 25 years. Rates are lower after age 64, because of mortality among smokers (U.S. Department of Health and Human Services, 1988b) and smoking cessation. In 1987, the following smoking prevalence rates were determined for the United States: age 45–64: men 33.5%, women 28.6%; age 65–74: men 20.2%, women 18%; age 75 or older; men 11.3%, women 7.5% (U.S. Department of Health and Human Services, 1989b).

2. Adverse Health Consequences of Tobacco Dependence

Smoking is the leading preventable cause of death in adults, and tobacco use continues to be a critical public health concern in the elderly. Smoking causes cancer—including lung, larynx, oral cavity, kidney, bladder, and pancreatic cancers, heart disease, peripheral vascular disease, cerebrovascular disease, chronic obstructive lung disease, peptic ulcer disease, and osteoporosis (Agner, 1985; Mellstrom, Rundgren, Jagenburg, Steen, & Svanborg, 1982; Rundgren & Mellstrom, 1984). Elderly smokers weigh less than their nonsmoking contemporaries and have impaired sense of taste and smell (Rimer, 1988). Smoking also interferes with the metabolism of many drugs in the elderly (Dawson & Vestal, 1984). Fatal burns are the fifth leading injury cause of death in the elderly, and 30% of fatal burns in elderly older than 60 are smoking related (Gulaid, Sacks, & Sattin, 1989; Parks, Noguchi, & Klatt 1989).

3. Smoking Cessation and Its Effects on Health in the Elderly

In the current cohort of living elderly, 60% of women and 70% of men who have at any time been tobacco dependent are now abstinent (U.S. Department of Health and Human Services, 1988a). Of these former smokers, one in five have ceased smoking in the last five years, and among those elderly who continue to smoke, half have attempted to quit in the preceding year (Pierce, Giovino, Hatziandreu, & Shopland, 1989). Older smokers, both those who have never attempted to quit and those who have failed to quit, may have stronger nicotine dependence than do younger smokers (Bosse, Garvey, & Glynn, 1980). Studies of the effect of age on the success of quitting provide conflicting results (Garvey, 1984), but the most extensive and recent U.S. survey indicates that age is correlated with success (Fiore *et al.*, 1990). Increased dependence may be balanced by other factors that promote quitting, such as the presence of a smoking-related illness, or death of a loved one who smoked (Garvey, 1984).

Significant beneficial health effects follow smoking cessation. Elders who quit smoking at age 65 will live an average of 2 to 4 years longer than age-matched smokers who continue the habit (Sachs, 1986). Morbidity and mortality from heart disease is significantly decreased in elderly who quit smoking. (Aronow, 1990; Hermanson, Omenn, Kronmal, & Gersch, 1988). The risk of a fatal cardiac event in smokers aged 65–74 begins to decrease in the first year of abstinence, and within 5 years decreases to the level of persons who never smoked (Jajich, Ostfeld, & Freeman, 1984). Examined 13 years after the first episode of unstable angina or myocardial infarction, men who continued to smoke had a mortality rate of 82.1% compared to 36.9% among quitters (Daly, Mulcahy, Graham & Hickey, 1983). Compared to aged nonsmokers, old smokers have a significant decrease in cerebral blood flow, and substantial improvement in cerebral blood circulation occurs steadily over the first year of abstinence among elderly who have smoked for 3 to 4 decades (Rogers, Meyer, Judd & Mortel, 1985; Yamashita, Kobayashi, Yamaguchi, Kitani, & Tsunematsu, 1988). Decreases in pulmonary function are diminished in quitters during the first 5 years of abstinence (Bosse, Sparrow, Rose, & Weiss, 1981). The alleged effect of smoking in possibly preventing Alzheimer's disease has not been confirmed (Jones, Reith, Philpot, & Sahakian, 1987).

4. Smoking-Cessation Methods and Outcomes

Ninety percent of all adult smokers who quit do so without a specialized treatment program, typically by stopping abruptly (Fiore *et al.*, 1990). In addition to age, among predictors of success, more men than women, more white than blacks, and more college-educated persons than persons without college training, succeed in quitting smoking. Most quitters, independent of methods used, say they stopped smoking because of health concerns, and a physician's advice to quit is often a significant motivator (Garvey, 1984). Persons who choose a formal smoking-cessation program tend to be heavier smokers and at greater risk for tobacco-related illness (Fiore *et al.*, 1990). Specialized smoking-cessation strategies include behavioral techniques such as aversion therapies (rapid smoking, satiation), cognitive therapies, relaxation training, social support, coping-skills training, hypnosis, acupuncture, group and individualized counseling, and, more recently, nicotine polacrilex gum to decrease craving and diminish withdrawal symptoms (Heinold, 1984; Rimer, 1988; U.S. Department of Health and Human Services, 1988a). Multicomponent trials combining two or more of these techniques have the best outcomes with up to 50% abstinence at 1 year (U.S. Department of Health and Human Services, 1988a).

Effective interventions for the elderly may not differ substantially from those generally available, but little investigation has been done comparing efficacy of different methods by age group (Sachs, 1986). The elderly are less likely than younger groups to choose such strategies as candy–coffee–tea substitutes, bets with friends, or use of hypnosis. They are less responsive to mass media campaigns such as the Great American Smokeout and are more likely to choose and respond to counseling-type programs (Heinold, 1984; Vetter & Ford, 1990). One study showed that male smokers older than 75 years did not believe that smoking was harmful to their health but did agree that children's health is affected by others' cigarette smoke, and that people have a right to breathe smoke-free air (Vetter, Charny, Farrow, & Lewis, 1988). Thus strategies based on altruism and appeal to pride as a role model may improve motivation.

Rapid smoking and nicotine polacrilex gum may be contraindicated because of increased health risks in some older patients with heart disease, hypertension, diabetes, or peptic ulcer disease. Some physicians continue to believe that there is little justification for advising healthy elders to give up smoking, as older patients may find it traumatic to give up one of their few remaining pleasures (Ebrahim *et al.*, 1988). Others point out that competent elderly, on balance, will be able to weigh the risks and benefits of quitting when given the most accurate information available (Abramson, 1977).

D. Polysubstance-Use Disorders

The potential risk for mixed disorders in the elderly is suggested by Guttman's (1978) findings in a household survey of OTC drug use: 55% were regular users of concurrent OTCs (typically analgesics), prescription drugs (most often cardiovascular or sedative–tranquilizer compounds), and/or alcohol. Over 17% used all three types of drugs concurrently. In a study of random urine drug screens conducted in an alcohol-treatment clinic (Kania & Kofoed, 1984), about 5% of specimen from older patients were positive for benzodiazepines, although the treatment program explicitly forbade their use. Finlayson and colleagues (1988), assessing 216 elderly inpatients with primary alcohol-use disorders, found that 52% were also dependent upon tobacco, 9% were dependent upon legally prescribed psychoactives, and another 5% were abusing them. Finlayson (1984) also reported on 34 patients hospitalized for primary dependence on prescription psychoactives: in this group there were 21 instances of dependence on opioid analgesics; 15, on antianxiety agents; and 14, on sedative–hypnotics, indicating multiple coexisting drug addictions in a number of the patients. In addition, 15 (44%) were also dependent on alcohol. Illicit polysubstance disorders in elderly cohorts are seen only among aging criminals and long-standing heroin addicts.

VII. Looking Ahead

A. Predicting Future Case Volume

Based on earlier experience with meprobamate (Miltown) and propoxyphene (Darvon), it is likely that physicians will moderate their prescribing of benzodiazepines as they become educated about dependence and toxicity hazards in the elderly. It is equally probable, however, that new classes of prescription drugs with dependence liability will emerge. Future psychoactive OTC-, tobacco-, and illicit drug–dependence rates are impossible to predict. For alcohol-use disorders, on the other hand, one can expect perhaps a threefold to fourfold increase in elderly cases in the United States over the next 40 years. Numbers could run higher, but certainly even this conservative estimate justifies further efforts to understand, identify, treat, and prevent these disorders in old age.

B. Research Directions

There is a general need for information on distinctive gender, ethnic, and socioeconomic patterns of geriatric substance use and abuse. Three of the nine areas established in the research agenda of the U.S. Surgeon General's 1988 Workshop on Health Promotion and Aging concerned substance abuse: alcohol, mental health consequences of prescribed and OTC drugs, and smoking cessation (Walker, 1989). An especially ambitious research agenda, covering epidemiology, clinical problems, and health promotion has been suggested by the Health Promotion and Aging Alcohol Working Group (U.S. Department of Health and Human Services, 1989a). Other alcoholism-related themes deserving special emphasis include (1) development of improved methods for determining elder alcohol consumption (Werch, 1989) and for early identification of cases by clinicians; (2) clarification of the relationship of late-onset and relapsing varieties of alcoholism to life stress and to coexisting mental disorders; and (3) studies of the prevalence, management, and prevention of problem alcohol and prescription psychoactive use in nursing homes and other long-term care facilities.

C. Planning Services

To understand and treat older adults who have alcohol or drug dependence, what is called for within the geriatric healthcare team or other treatment staff is a synthesis of the perspectives of clinical gerontology, chemical-dependence counseling, and mental health assessment and treatment (Merrill, Kraft, Gordon, Holmes, & Walker, 1990). At this time few professional degree programs or certificate programs in either chemical-dependence counseling or gerontology offer this combined emphasis. Services discussed in prior sections and below will be effective to the extent that properly trained staff are available to meet the unique needs of alcohol- and drug-dependent elders.

Acute inpatient care for these problems can usually be accomplished satisfactorily within existing settings, for example, in age-heterogeneous medical or psychiatric wards, substance-abuse residential programs, or geriatric medical or psychiatric evaluation units. Longer-term recovery–rehabilitation typically requires an elder-specific group program of education, social support, and active counseling, including provision for counseling relatives and home visitation. An effective program can be sustained for as few as four or five clients with the part-time services of one professional leader (who may have other roles and clientele, as well). Such a program can be located in a medical geriatrics or substance-abuse clinic, nursing home, or other residential facility. Access to medical and psychiatric consultation is essential.

New models of care are currently being tested. For example, alcohol–drug free foster care coupled with enrollment in an intensive outpatient treatment program can stabilize clients for whom more routine outpatient care alone would not suffice at first (J. Dunlop, personal communication, September, 1990). Adjunctive models of supervised peer volunteer counseling, outreach, and home visitation are also being attempted for homebound community elderly recovering from alcoholism (J. Annand, personal communication, September, 1990). When available, age-specific chapters of Alcoholics Anonymous (AA) may offer excellent adjunctive or definitive support for sustained recovery of the elderly. The original tenets of AA, however, discouraged segregated groups based on demographic, social, or other special criteria, with the result that elder-specific chapters are not fostered in all communities. Most elders are offended by younger members' disclosure of illicit drug use and antisocial or promiscuous behavior, and by their profanity, in mixed-age AA groups.

For chemically dependent elderly with coexisting dementia or other major mental disorders, treatment within a psychiatric or neurobehavioral clinic or day hospital is often the best arrangement. In intractable cases, where life-threatening drinking or drug use persists despite treatment efforts, guardianship may be necessary, permitting temporary or more long-term placement of the patient in a controlled, alcohol- and drug-free residential setting.

D. Prevention

Alcohol and drug dependence in the elderly can be reduced. Prevention should begin with public and private institutions sponsoring better preretirement planning for employees' future roles and constructive uses of time, including substance-use education (Brody, 1982). Retirement communities, and senior organizations and periodicals, can promote smoking cessation and moderation of alcohol use. Health caregivers and social case-workers can provide advice and education on the adverse health and behavioral effects of alcohol and tobacco, and programs for smoking cessation and alcohol-use reduction can be made more easily accessible. Medical practitioners need continuing education on conservative prescribing of psychoactives and on screening for early recognition of alcohol and benzodiazepine dependence. Neurobehavioral and dementia clinics need to closely monitor alcohol use by their clients (King, 1986). Improved institutional milieus for the aging must address alcohol use and alternatives to sedation for behavioral control.

References

Abrams, R. C., & Alexopoulos, G. S. (1987). Substance abuse in the elderly: Alcohol and prescription drugs. *Hospital and Community Psychiatry, 38,* 1285–1287.

Abrams, R. C., & Alexopoulos, G. S. (1988). Substance abuse in the elderly: Over-the-counter and illegal drugs. *Hospital and Community Psychiatry, 39,* 822–823, 829.

Abramson, J. H. (1977). The hazard of persistent cigarette smoking in later life. *American Journal of the Medical Sciences, 274,* 35–43.

Adams, W. L., Garry, P. J., Rhyne, R., Hunt, W. C., & Goodwin, J. S. (1990). Alcohol intake in the healthy elderly: Changes with age in a cross-sectional and longitudinal study. *Journal of the American Geriatrics Society, 38,* 211–216.

Aflin-Slater, R. B. (1988). Vitamin use and abuse in elderly persons. In J. E. Morley (moderator). Nutrition in the elderly. *Annals of Internal Medicine, 109,* 890–904.

Agner, E. (1985). Smoking and health in old age: A ten-year follow-up study. *Acta Medica Scandinavica, 218,* 311–316.

Alexander, F., & Duff, R. W. (1988). Social interaction and alcohol use in retirement communities. *The Gerontologist, 28,* 632–638.

American Psychiatric Association (1987). *Diagnostic and Statistical Manual of Mental Disorders,* (Third ed., rev.) Washington, DC: American Psychiatric Press.

American Psychiatric Association (1990). *Benzodiazepine dependence, toxicity and abuse.* Washington, DC: American Psychiatric Press.

Ancill, R. J., Embury, G. D., MacEwan, G. W., & Kennedy, J. S. (1987). Lorazepam in the elderly—A retrospective study of the side-effects in 20 patients. *Journal of Psychopharamacology, 2,* 126–127.

Anglin, M. D., Brecht, M. L., Woodward, J. A., & Bonett, D. G. (1986).. An empirical study of maturing out: Conditional factors. *The International Journal of the Addictions, 21,* 233–246.

Appelt, G. D. (1986). Weight-control products. In American Pharmacy Association (Ed.), *Handbook of nonprescription drugs* (8th ed., pp. 343–358). Washington, DC: American Pharmacy Association.

Aronow, W. S. (1990). Cardiac risk factors: Still important in the elderly. *Geriatrics, 45,* 71–80.

Ashton, H. (1984). Benzodiazepine withdrawal: An unfinished story. *British Medical Journal, 288,* 1135–1140.

Ashton, H. (1987). Benzodiazepine withdrawal: Outcome in 50 patients. *British Journal of Addiction, 82,* 665–671.

Atkinson, J. H., & Schuckit, M. A. (1984). Geriatric alcohol and drug misuse and abuse. *Advances in Substance Abuse, 3,* 195–237.

Atkinson, R. M. (1984). Substance use and abuse in late life. In R. M. Atkinson (Ed.), *Alcohol and drug abuse in old age* (pp. 1–21). Washington, DC: American Psychiatric Press.

Atkinson, R. M. (1985). Persuading alcoholic patients to seek treatment. *Comprehensive Therapy, 11* (11),16–24.

Atkinson, R. M. (1988). Alcoholism in the elderly population. (Editorial). *Mayo Clinic Proceedings, 63,* 825–829.

Atkinson, R. M. (1990). Aging and alcohol use disorders: Diagnostic issues in the elderly. *International Psychogeriatrics, 2,* 55–72.

Atkinson, R. M., & Kofoed, L. L. (1982). Alcohol and drug abuse in old age: A clinical perspective. *Substance and Alcohol Actions/Misuse, 3,* 353–368.

Atkinson, R. M., & Kofoed, L. L. (1984). Alcohol and drug abuse. In C. K. Cassell & J. R. Walsh (Eds.),

Geriatric Medicine. Volume II. Fundamentals of Geriatric Care (pp. 219–235). New York: Springer-Verlag.

Atkinson, R. M., Tolson, R. L., & Turner, J. A. (1990a). Factors affecting outpatient treatment compliance of older male problem drinkers. Revised manuscript submitted for publication.

Atkinson, R. M., Tolson, R. L., & Turner, J. A. (1990b). Late- versus early-onset problem drinking in older men. *Alcoholism (New York), 14,* 574–579.

Atkinson, R. M., Turner, J. A., Kofoed, L. L., & Tolson, R. L. (1985). Early- versus late-onset alcoholism in older persons: Preliminary findings. *Alcoholism (New York), 9,* 513–515.

Avorn, J., Dreyer, P., Connelly, K., & Soumerai, S. B. (1989). Use of psychoactive medication and the quality of care in rest homes. *The New England Journal of Medicine, 320,* 227–232.

Bailey, R. B., & Jones, S. R. (1989). Chronic salicylate intoxication: A common cause of morbidity in the elderly. *Journal of the American Geriatrics Society, 37,* 556–561.

Balter, M. B., Manheimer, D. I., Mellinger, G. D., & Uhlenhuth, E. H. (1984). A cross-national comparison of anti-anxiety–sedative drug use. *Current Medical Research and Opinion, 8* (Suppl. 4), 5–20.

Barnes, G. M. (1979). Alcohol use among older persons: Findings from a western New York State general population survey. *Journal of the American Geriatrics Society, 27,* 244–250.

Basen, M. M. (1977). The elderly and drugs—Problem overview and program strategy. *Public Health Reports, 92,* 43–48.

Bean, P. (1974). *The social control of drugs.* London: Martin Robertson.

Beardsley, R. S., Larson, D. B., Burns, B. J., Thompson, J. W., & Kamerow, D. B. (1989). Prescribing of psychotropics in elderly nursing home patients. *Journal of the American Geriatrics Society, 37,* 327–330.

Beers, M., Avorn, J., Soumerai, S. B., Everitt, D. E., Sherman, D. S., & Salem, S. (1988). Psychoactive medication use in intermediate-care facility residents. *Journal of the American Medical Association, 260,* 3016–3020.

Beresford, T. P., Blow, F. C., Brower, K. J., Adams, K. M., & Hall, R. C. W. (1988). Alcoholism and aging in the general hospital. *Psychosomatics, 29,* 61–72.

Biaggioni, I., Onrot, J., Stewart, C. K., & Robertson, D. (1987). The potent pressor effect of phenylpropanolamine in patients with autonomic impairment. *Journal of the American Medical Association, 258,* 236–239.

Blazer, D. G. (1982). *Depression in late life* (p. 37). St. Louis, MO: C. V. Mosby.

Blum, L., & Rosner, F. (1983). Alcoholism in the elderly: An analysis of 50 patients. *Journal of the National Medical Association, 75,* 489–495.

Borgatta, E. F., Montgomery, R. J. V., & Borgatta, M. L. (1982). Alcohol use and abuse, life crisis events, and the elderly. *Research on Aging, 4,* 378–408.

Bosse, R., Garvey, A. J., & Glynn, R. J. (1980). Age and addiction to smoking. *Addictive Behavior, 5,* 341–351.

Bosse, R., Sparrow, D., Rose C. L., & Weiss, S. T. (1981). Longitudinal effect of age and smoking cessation on pulmonary function. *American Review of Respiratory Diseases 123,* 378–381.

Brennan, P. L., & Moos, R. H. (1990). Life stressors, social resources, and late-life problem drinking. *Psychology and Aging. 5,* 491–501.

Bridgewater, R., Leigh, S., James, O. F. W., & Potter, J. F. (1987). Alcohol consumption and dependence in elderly patients in an urban community. *British Medical Journal, 295,* 884–885.

Brody, J. A. (1982). Aging and alcohol abuse. *Journal of the American Geriatrics Society, 30,* 123–126.

Busby, W. J., Campbell, A. J., Borrie, M. J., & Spears, G. F. S. (1988). Alcohol use in a community-based sample of subjects aged 70 years and older. *Journal of the American Geriatrics Society, 36,* 301–305.

Busse, E. W. (1989). The myth, history, and science of aging. In E. W. Busse & D. G. Blazer (Eds.), *Geriatric Psychiatry* (pp. 3–34). Washington, DC: American Psychiatric Press.

Cadigan, D. A., Magaziner, J., & Fedder, D. O. (1989). Polymedicine use among community older women: How much of a problem? *American Journal of Public Health, 79,* 1537–1540.

Cahalan, D. (1970). *Problem drinkers: A national survey.* San Francisco: Jossey-Bass.

Cahalan, D., Cisin, I. H., & Crossley, H. M. (1969). *American drinking practices: A national study of drinking behavior and attitudes.* Monograph No. 6. New Brunswick, NJ: Rutgers Center of Alcohol Studies.

Capel, W. C., & Peppers, L. G. (1978). The aging addict: A longitudinal study of known abusers. *Addictive Diseases, 3,* 389–403.

Capel, W. C., Goldsmith, B. M., Waddell, K. J., & Stewart, G. T. (1972). The aging narcotic addict: An increasing problem for the next decades. *Journal of Gerontology, 27,* 102–106.

Caro, J. P., & Walker, C. A. (1986). Sleep aid and stimulant products. In American Pharmacy Association (Ed.), *Handbook of non-prescription drugs* (8th ed., pp. 359–370). Washington, DC: American Pharmacy Association.

Castleden, C. M., George, C. F., Marcer, D., & Hallett, C. (1977). Increased sensitivity to nitrazepam in old age. *British Medical Journal, 1,* 10–12.

Cheah, K.-C., Baldridge, J. A., & Beard, O. W. (1979). Geriatric evaluation unit of a medical service: Role of a geropsychiatrist. *Journal of Gerontology, 34,* 41–45.

Christopherson, V. A., Escher, M. C., & Bainton, B. R. (1984). Reasons for drinking among the elderly in rural Arizona. *Journal of Studies on Alcohol, 45,* 417–423.

Clark, W. B., & Midanik, L. (1981). Alcohol use and alcohol problems among U.S. adults. In N.I.A.A.A.: *Alcohol consumption and related problems.* Alcohol and Health Monograph No. 1. (pp 3–52). DHHS Pub. No. (ADM) 82–1190. Washington, D.C., Supt. of Documents, U.S. Govt. Printing Office.

Cloninger, C. R., Reich, T., Sigvardsson, S., von Knorring, A.-L., & Bohman, M. (1987). The effects of changes in alcohol use between generations on the inheritance of alcohol abuse. In R. M. Rose & J. E. Barrett (Eds.), *Alcoholism: Origins & outcome* (pp. 49–74). New York: Raven Press.

Colsher, P. L., & Wallace, R. B. (1989). Is modest alcohol consumption better than none at all? An epidemiologic assessment. *Annual Review of Public Health, 10,* 203–219.

Colt, H. G., & Shapiro, A. P. (1989). Drug-induced illness as a cause for admission to a community hospital. *Journal of the American Geriatrics Society, 37,* 323–326.

Conwell, Y., Rotenberg, M., & Caine, E. D. (1990). Completed suicide at age 50 and over. *Journal of the American Geriatrics Society, 38,* 640–644.

Cook, P. J., (1986). Benzodiazepine hypnotics in the elderly. *Acta Psychiatrica Scandinavica, 74* (suppl. 332), 149–158.

Cook, P. J., Huggett, A., Graham-Pole, R., Savage, I. T., & James, I. M. (1983). Hypnotic accumulation and hangover in elderly inpatients: A controlled double-blind study of temazepam and nitrazepam. *British Medical Journal, 286,* 100–102.

Curtis, J. R., Geller, G., Stokes, E. J., Levine, D. M., & Moore, R. D. (1989). Characteristics, diagnosis, and treatment of alcoholism in elderly patients. *Journal of the American Geriatrics Society, 37,* 310–316.

Daly, L. E., Mulcahy, R., Graham, I. M., & Hickey, N. (1983). Long-term effect on mortality of stopping smoking after unstable angina and myocardial infarction. *British Medical Journal, 287,* 324–326.

Darnell, J. C., Murray, M. D., Martz, B. L., & Weinberger, M. (1986). Medication use by ambulatory elderly: An in-home survey. *Journal of the American Geriatrics Society, 34,* 1–4.

Dawson, G. W., & Vestal, R. E. (1984). Smoking, age, and drug metabolism. In R. Bosse & C. L. Rose (Eds.), *Smoking and aging* (pp. 131–156). Lexington, MA: Lexington Books.

Deely, P. J., Kaufman, E., Yen, M. S., Jue, B. A., & Brown, E. (1979). The special problems and treatment of a group of elderly Chinese opiate addicts in New York City. *British Journal of Addiction, 74,* 403–409.

DeLeo, D., & Stella, A. G. (1989). Prescription of psychotropic drugs in geriatric institutions. *International Journal of Geriatric Psychiatry, 4,* 11–16.

Des Jarlais, D. C., Joseph, H., & Courtwright, D. T. (1985). Old age and addiction: A study of elderly patients in methadone maintenance treatment. In E. Gottheil, K. A. Druley, T. E. Skoloda, & H. M. Waxman (Eds.), *The combined problems of alcoholism, drug addiction, and aging* (pp. 201–209). Springfield, IL: Charles C Thomas.

Donovan, D. M. (1988). Assessment of addictive behaviors: Implications of an emerging biopsychosocial mode. In D. M. Donovan & G. A. Marlatt (Eds.), *Assessment of addictive behaviors* (pp. 3–48). New York: Guilford.

Donovan, D. M., & Marlatt, G. A. (Eds.) (1988). *Assessment of addictive behaviors.* New York: Guilford.

Drew, L. R. H. (1968). Alcoholism as a self-limiting disease. *Quarterly Journal of Studies on Alcohol, 29,* 956–967.

Droller, H. (1964). Some aspects of alcoholism in the elderly. *Lancet, 2,* 137–139.

Dufour, M., Colliver, J., Stinson, F., & Grigson, B. (1988, November). *Changes in alcohol consumption with age: NHANES I Epidemiologic Followup.* Paper presented at the 116th Annual Meeting of the American Public Health Association, Boston, November 13–17.

Dunham, R. G. (1981). Aging and changing patterns of alcohol use. *Journal of Psychoactive Drugs, 13,* 143–151.

Dunlop, J., Skorney, B., & Hamilton, J. (1982). Group treatment for elderly alcoholics and their families. *Social Work in Groups, 5,* 87–92.

Dupree, L. W., Broskowski, H., & Schonfeld, L. (1984). The Gerontology Alcohol Project: A behavioral treatment program for elderly alcohol abusers. *The Gerontologist, 24,* 510–516.

Ebrahim, S., Dallosso, H., Morgan, K., Bassey, J., Fentem, P., & Arie, T. (1988). Causes of ill health among a random sample of old and very old people: Possibilities for prevention. *Journal of the Royal College of Physicians of London, 22,* 105–107.

Ekerdt, D. J., DeLabry, L. O., Glynn, R. J., & Davis, R. W. (1989). Change in drinking behaviors with retirement: Findings from the Normative Aging Study. *Journal of Studies on Alcohol, 50,* 347–353.

Ellor, J. R., & Kurz, D. J. (1982). Misuse and abuse of prescription and nonprescription drugs by the elderly. *Nursing Clinics of North America, 17,* 319–330.

Feldman, M. D., & Behar, M. (1986). A case of massive diphenhydramine abuse and withdrawal from the drug. *Journal of the American Medical Association, 255,* 3119–3120.

Feuerlein, W., & Reiser, E. (1986). Parameters affecting the course and results of delirium tremens treatment. *Acta Psychiatrica Scandinavica,* (suppl.) *329,* 120–123.

Finlayson, R. E. (1984). Prescription drug abuse in older persons. In R. M. Atkinson (Ed.), *Alcohol and drug abuse in old age* (pp. 61–70). Washington, DC: American Psychiatric Press.

Finlayson, R. E., Hurt, R. D., Davis, L. J., & Morse, R. M. (1988). Alcoholism in elderly persons: A study of the psychiatric and psychosocial features of 216 inpatients. *Mayo Clinic Proceedings, 63,* 761–768.

Finney, J. W., & Moos, R. H. (1984). Life stressors and problem drinking among older persons. In M. Galanter (Ed.), *Recent developments in alcoholism* (Vol. 2, pp. 267–288). New York: Plenum Press.

Fiore, M. C., Novotny, T. E., Pierce, J. P., Giovino, G. A., Hatziandreu, E. J., Newcomb, P. A., Surawicz, T. S., & Davis, R. M. (1990). Methods used to quit smoking in the United States. *Journal of the American Medical Association, 263,* 2760–2765.

Foy, A., Drinkwater, V., March, S., & Mearrick, P. (1986). Confusion after admission to hospital in elderly patients using benzodiazepines. *British Medical Journal, 293,* 1072.

Freund, G. (1984a). Neurobiologic relationships between aging and alcohol abuse. In M. Galanter (Ed.), *Recent developments in alcoholism* (Vol. 2, pp. 203–221). New York: Plenum Press.

Freund, G. (1984b). Neurotransmitter function in relation to aging and alcoholism. In J. T. Hartford & T. Samorajski (Eds.), *Alcoholism in the elderly. Social and biomedical issues* (pp. 65–83). New York: Raven.

Freund, G. (1987). Drug- and alcohol-induced dementias. In W. G. Wood & R. Strong (Eds.), *Geriatric clinical pharmacology* (pp. 95–105). New York: Raven.

Gardner, E. R., & Hall, R. C. W. (1982). Psychiatric symptoms produced by over-the-counter drugs. *Psychosomatics, 23,* 186–190.

Garvey, A. J. (1984). Age, health status, and other factors in smoking cessation. In R. Bosse & C. L. Rose (Eds.), *Smoking and aging* (pp. 187–202). Lexington, MA: Lexington Books.

Ghodse, A. H., Sheehan, M., Taylor, C., & Edwards, G. (1985). Deaths of drug addicts in the United Kingdom, 1967–1981. *British Medical Journal, 290,* 425–428.

Gilbertson, W. E. (1986). The FDA's OTC drug review. In American Pharmacy Association (Ed.), *Handbook of non-prescription drugs* (8th ed., pp. 1–8). Washington, DC: American Pharmacy Association.

Giordano, J. A., & Beckham, K. (1985). Alcohol use and abuse in old age: An examination of Type II alcoholism. *Journal of Gerontological Social Work, 9,* 65–83.

Glantz, M. (1981). Predictions of elderly drug abuse. *Journal of Psychoactive Drugs, 13,* 117–126.

Glynn, R. J., Bouchard, G. R., LoCastro, J. S., & Laird, N. M. (1985). Aging and generational effects on drinking behaviors in men: Results from the Normative Aging Study. *American Journal of Public Health, 75,* 1413–1419.

Glynn, R. J., LoCastro, J. S., Hermos, J. A., & Bosse, R. (1983). Social contexts and motives for drinking in men. *Journal of Studies on Alcohol, 44,* 1011–1025.

Gomberg, E. L. (1985). Gerontology and alcohol studies. In E. Gottheil, K. A. Druley, T. E. Skoloda, & H. M. Waxman (Eds.), *The combined problems of alcoholism, drug addiction and aging* (pp. 51–73). Springfield, IL: Charles C Thomas .

Goodman, A. G., Goodman, L. S., Rall, T. W., & Furad, F. (1985). *Goodman and Gilman's the pharmacological basis of therapeutics* (7th ed.) New York: Macmillan.

Gordon, T., & Doyle, J. T. (1987). Drinking and mortality: the Albany study. *American Journal of Epidemiology, 125*, 263–270.

Graham, K. (1986). Identifying and measuring alcohol abuse among the elderly: Serious problems with existing instrumentation. *Journal of Studies on Alcohol, 47*, 322–326.

Graham, K., Zeidman, A., Flower, M. C., Saunders, S. J., & White-Campbell, M. (1989). *Case study analyses of elderly persons who have alcohol problems.* Final report to the Canadian National Health Research and Development Program, Project No. 6606-3414-43DA, 1987–1989.

Grant, I., Adams, K. M., & Reed, R. (1984). Aging, abstinence, and medical risk factors in the prediction of neuropsychologic deficit among long-term alcoholics. *Archives of General Psychiatry, 41*, 710–718.

Griffin, M. R., Ray, W. A., & Schaffner, W. (1988). Nonsteroidal anti-inflammatory drug use and death from peptic ulcer in elderly persons. *Annals of Internal Medicine, 109*, 359–363.

Grigor, R. R., Spitz, P. W., & Furst, D. E. (1987). Salicylate toxicity in elderly patients with rheumatoid arthritis. *The Journal of Rheumatology, 14*, 60–66.

Gulaid, J. A., Sacks, J. J., & Sattin, R. W. (1989). Deaths from residential fires among older people, United States, 1984. *Journal of the American Geriatrics Society, 27*, 331–334.

Guttman, D. (1978). Patterns of legal drug use by older Americans. *Addictive Diseases, 3*, 337–356.

Harrington, P., & Cox, T. J. (1979). A twenty-year followup of narcotic addicts in Tucson, Arizona. *American Journal of Drug and Alcohol Abuse, 6*, 25–37.

Hartford, J. T., & Samorajski, T. (1982). Alcoholism in the geriatric population. *Journal of the American Geriatrics Society, 30*, 18–24.

Hegsted, D. M., & Ausman, L. M. (1988). Diet, alcohol, and coronary heart disease in men. *Journal of Nutrition, 118*, 1184–1189.

Heinold, J. W. (1984). The efficacy of smoking-cessation strategies: Does it vary with age? In R. Bosse & C. L. Rose (Eds.), *Smoking and aging* (pp. 203–220). Lexington, MA: Lexington Books.

Helling, D. K., Lemke, J. H., Semla, T. P., Wallace, R. B., Lipson, D. P., & Cornoni-Huntley, J. (1987). Medication-use characteristics in the elderly: The Iowa 65+ rural health study. *Journal of the American Geriatrics Society, 35*, 4–12.

Herbert, V. (1988). Megavitamins, food fads, and quack nutrition in health promotion: Risks and myths. In R. Chernoff & D. A. Lipschitz (Eds.), *Health promotion and disease prevention in the elderly* (pp. 45–66). New York: Raven Press.

Hermanson, B., Omenn, G. S., Kronmal, R. A., & Gersch, B. J. (1988). The beneficial six-year outcome of smoking cessation in older men and women with coronary artery disease—Results from the CASS registry. *The New England Journal of Medicine, 319*, 1365–1369.

Hermos, J. A., LoCastro, J. S., Glynn, R. J., Bouchard, G. R., & DeLabry, L. O. (1988). Predictors of reduction and cessation of drinking in community-dwelling men: Results from the Normative Aging Study. *Journal of Studies on Alcohol, 49*, 363–368.

Higgitt, A. C. (1988). Indications for benzodiazepine prescriptions in the elderly. *International Journal of Geriatric Psychiatry, 3*, 239–243.

Higgitt, A. C., Lader, M. H., & Fonagy, P. (1985). Clinical management of benzodiazepine dependence. *British Medical Journal, 291*, 688–690.

Holzer, C. E., III, Robins, L. N., Myers, J. K., Weissman, M. M., Tischler, G. L., Leaf, P. J., Anthony, J., & Bednarski, P. B. (1984). Antecedents and correlates of alcohol abuse and dependence in the elderly. In G. Maddox, L. N. Robins, & N. Rosenberg (Eds.), *Nature and extent of alcohol problems among the elderly* (pp. 217–244). Research Monograph No. 14. Rockville, MD: National Institute on Drug Abuse, DHHS, U.S. Government Printing Office.

Huffine, C. L., Folkman, S., & Lazarus, R. S. (1989). Psychoactive drugs, alcohol, and stress and coping processes in older adults. *American Journal of Drug and Alcohol Abuse, 15*, 101–113.

Hughes, J. R., Gust, S. W., & Pachacek, T. F. (1987). Prevalence of tobacco dependence and withdrawal. *American Journal of Psychiatry, 144*, 205–208.

Hurt, R. D., Finlayson, R. E., Morse, R. M., & Davis, L. J. (1988). Alcoholism in elderly persons: Medical aspects and prognosis of 216 inpatients. *Mayo Clinic Proceedings, 63*, 753–760.

Jajich, C. L., Ostfeld, A. M., & Freeman, D. H. (1984). Smoking and coronary artery disease mortality in the elderly. *Journal of the American Medical Association, 252,* 2831–2834.

Jamieson, C., & Flanagan, T. J. (Eds.) (1988). *Sourcebook of criminal justice statistics - 1988.* Office of Justice Programs, Bureau of Justice Statistics, Washington, DC: U.S. Government Printing Office.

Janik, S. W., & Dunham, R. G. (1983). A nationwide examination of the need for specific alcoholism treatment programs for the elderly. *Journal of Studies on Alcohol, 44,* 307–317.

Jenike, M. A. (1989). Metabolic changes with aging. In *Geriatric psychiatry and psychopharmacology: A clinical approach* (pp. 25–32). Chicago: Year Book Medical Publishers.

Jones, G. M. M., Reith, M., Philpot, M. P., & Sahakian, B. J. (1987). Smoking and dementia of the Alzheimer type. *Journal of Neurology, Neurosurgery, and Psychiatry, 50,* 1383.

Kafetz, K., & Cox, M. (1982). Alcohol excess and the senile squalor syndrome. *Journal of the American Geriatrics Society, 30,* 706.

Kania, J., & Kofoed, L. (1984). Drug use by alcoholics in outpatient treatment. *American Journal of Drug and Alcohol Abuse, 10,* 529–534.

Kase, C. S., Foster, T. E., Reed, J. E., Spatz, E. L., & Girgis, G. N. (1987). Intracerebral hemorrhage and phenylpropanolamine use. *Neurology, 37,* 399–404.

King, M. B. (1986). Alcohol abuse and dementia. *International Journal of Geriatric Psychiatry, 1,* 31–36.

Kissin, B., & Begleiter, H. (Eds.) (1983a). *The pathogenesis of alcoholism: Biological factors.* New York: Plenum.

Kissin, B., & Begleiter, H. (Eds.) (1983b). *The pathogenesis of alcoholism: Psychosocial factors.* New York: Plenum.

Klatsky, A. L., Friedman, G. D., & Siegelaub, A. B. (1981). Alcohol and mortality: A 10-year Kaiser–Permanente experience. *Annals of Internal Medicine, 95,* 139–145.

Klein-Schwartz, W., Oderda, G. M., & Booze, L. (1983). Poisoning in the elderly. *Journal of the American Geriatrics Society, 31,* 195–199.

Koegel, P., Burnam, A., & Farr, R. K. (1988). The prevalence of specific psychiatric disorders among homeless individuals in the inner city of Los Angeles. *Archives of General Psychiatry, 45,* 1085–1092.

Kofoed, L. L. (1985). OTC drug overuse in the elderly: What to watch for. *Geriatrics, 55,* 55–60.

Kofoed, L. L., Tolson, R. L., Atkinson, R. M., Turner, J. A., & Toth, R. F. (1984). Elderly groups in an alcoholism clinic. In R. M. Atkinson (Ed.), *Alcohol and drug abuse in old age* (pp. 35–48). Washington, DC: American Psychiatric Press.

Kofoed, L. L., Tolson, R. L., Atkinson, R. M., Toth, R. L., & Turner, J. A. (1987). Treatment compliance of older alcoholics: An elder-specific approach is superior to "mainstreaming." *Journal of Studies on Alcohol, 48,* 47–51; correction *48,* 183.

Koppel, C., Ibe, K., & Tenczer, J. (1987). The clinical symptomatology in diphenhydramine overdose: An evaluation of 136 cases in 1982 to 1985. *Clinical Toxicology, 25,* 53–70.

Lake, R. C., Alagna, S. W., Quirk, R. S., Moriarty, K. M., & Reid, A. A. (1985). Does phenylpropanolamine cause psychiatric disorders? In J. P. Morgan, D. V. Kagan, & J. S. Brody (Eds.), *Phenylpropanolamine: Risks, benefits and controversies* (pp. 285–314). New York: Praeger.

Lamy, P. P. (1982). Over-the-counter medication: The drug interactions we overlook. *Journal of the American Geriatrics Society, 30* (Suppl.), S69–S75.

Lancet editorial (1988). Alcohol and mortality: The myth of the U-shaped curve. *Lancet, 2,* 1292–1293.

Larson, E. B., Reifler, B. V., Featherstone, H. J., & English, D. R. (1984). Dementia in elderly outpatients: A prospective study. *Annals of Internal Medicine, 100,* 417–423.

Liskow, B. I., Rinck, C., Campbell, J., & DeSouza, C. (1989). Alcohol withdrawal in the elderly. *Journal of Studies on Alcohol, 50,* 414–421.

Lowinson, J. H., & Ruiz, P. (Eds.) (1981). *Substance abuse: Clinical problems and perspectives.* Baltimore: Williams & Wilkins.

MacMillan, D., & Shaw, P. (1966). Senile breakdown in standards of personal and environmental cleanliness. *British Medical Journal, 2,* 1032–1037.

Maddux, J. F., & Desmond, D. P. (1980). New light on the maturing-out hypothesis in opioid dependence. *Bulletin on Narcotics, 32,* 15–25.

Malcolm, M. T. (1984). Alcohol and drug use in the elderly visited at home. *The International Journal of the Addictions, 19,* 411–418.

Malin, H., Coakley, J., & Laelber, C. (1982). An epidemiologic perspective on alcohol use and abuse in the

United States. In NIAAA, *Alcohol and health monograph no. 1: Alcohol consumption and related problems.* DHHS Publ. no. (ADM) 82-1190. Washington, DC: Superintendent of Documents, U.S. Government Printing Office.

Maloff, D. R., & Levinson, P. K. (Eds.) (1980). *Issues in controlled substance use: Papers and commentary.* Washington, DC: National Academy of Sciences.

Mandolini, A. (1981). The social contexts of aging and drug use: Theoretical and methodological insights. *Journal of Psychoactive Drugs, 13,* 135–142.

Mant, A., Duncan-Jones, P., Saltman, D., Bridges-Webb, C., Kehoe, L., Lansbury, G., & Chancellor, A. H. B. (1988). Development of long-term use of psychotropic drugs by general practice patients. *British Medical Journal, 296,* 251–254.

Marmot, M. G. (1984). Alcohol and coronary heart disease. *International Journal of Epidemiology, 13,* 160–166.

Martin, J. C., & Streissguth, A. P. (1982). Alcoholism and the elderly: An overview. In C. Eisdorfer & W. E. Fann (Eds.), *Treatment of psychopathology in the aging* (pp. 242–280). New York: Springer.

May, F. E., Stewart, R. B., Hale, W. E., & Marks, R. G. (1982). Prescribed and nonprescribed drug use in an ambulatory elderly population. *Southern Medical Journal, 75,* 522–528.

McCusker, J., Cherubin, C. E., & Zimberg, S. (1971). Prevalence of alcoholism in a general municipal hospital population. *New York State Journal of Medicine, 71,* 751–754.

McEvoy, J. P., McCue, M., Spring, B., Mohs, R. C., Lavori, P. W., & Farr, R. M. (1987). Effects of amantadine and trihexyphenidyl on memory in the elderly normal volunteers. *American Journal of Psychiatry, 144,* 573–577.

Mellinger, D. G., Balter, M. B., & Uhlenhuth, E. H., (1984). Prevalence and correlates of the long-term regular use of anxiolytics. *Journal of the American Medical Association, 251,* 375–379.

Mellstrom, D., Rundgren, A., Jagenburg, R., Steen, B., & Svanborg, A. (1982). Tobacco smoking, aging and health among the elderly: A longitudinal population study of 70-year-old men and an age cohort comparison. *Age and Ageing, 11,* 45–58.

Merrill, M., Kraft, P. G., Gordon, M., Holmes, M. M., & Walker, B. (1990). *Chemically dependent older adults. How do we treat them?* Minneapolis: Hazelden.

Meyers, A. R., Hingson, R., Mucatel, M., & Goldman, E. (1982). Social and psychological correlates of problem drinking in old age. *Journal of the American Geriatrics Society, 30,* 452–456.

Miller, F., & Whitcup, S. (1986). Benzodiazepine use in psychiatrically hospitalized elderly patients. *Journal of Clinical Psychopharmacology, 6,* 384–385.

Miller, F., Whitcup, S., Sacks, M., & Lynch, P. E. (1985). Unrecognized drug dependence and withdrawal in the elderly. *Drug and Alcohol Dependence, 15,* 177–179.

Miller, J. D., Cisin, I. H., Gardner-Keaton, H., Harrell, A. V., Wirtz, P. W., Abelson, H. I., & Fishburne, P. M. (1983). *National survey on drug abuse: Main findings, 1982.* (DHHS Publication No. [ADM] 83-1263). Washington, DC: U.S. Govt. Printing Office.

Miller, P. S., Richardson, J. S., Jyu, C. A., Lemay, J. S., Hiscock, M., & Keegan, D. L. (1988). Association of low serum anticholinergic levels and cognitive impairment in elderly presurgical patients. *American Journal of Psychiatry, 145,* 342–345.

Moos, R. H., Brennan, P. L., Fondacaro, M. R., & Moos, B. S. (1990). Approach and avoidance coping responses among older problem and nonproblem drinkers. *Psychology and Aging, 5,* 31–40.

Morgan, K. (1988). Hypnotic drug use for the elderly. *British Medical Journal, 296,* 930.

Morgan, K., Dallosso, H., Ebrahim, S., Arie, T., & Fentem, P. H. (1988). Prevalence, frequency, and duration of hypnotic drug use among the elderly living at home. *British Medical Journal, 296,* 601–602.

Moss, R. J., & Miles, S. H. (1987). AIDS and the geriatrician. *Journal of the American Geriatrics Society, 35,* 460–464.

Murphy, S. M., Owen, R., & Tyrer, P. (1984). Withdrawal symptoms after six weeks' treatment with diazepam. *Lancet, 2,* 1389.

Murray, R. M. (1980). Minor analgesic abuse: The slow recognition of a public health problem. *British Journal of Addiction, 75,* 9–17.

Myers, J. K., Weissman, M. M., Tischler, G. L., Holzer, C. E., Leaf, P. J., Orvaschel, H., Anthony, J. C., Boyd, J. H., Burke, J. D., Kramer, M., & Stoltzman R. (1984). Six-month prevalence of psychiatric disorder in three communities, 1980–1982. *Archives of General Psychiatry, 41,* 959–967.

Nakamura, C. M., Molgaard, C. A., Stanford, E. P., Peddecord, K. M., Morton, D. J., Lockery, S. A.,

Zuniga, M., & Gardner, L. D. (1990). A discriminant analysis of severe alcohol consumption among older persons. *Alcohol and Alcoholism, 25,* 75–80.

National Academy of Sciences (1977). *Common processes in habitual substance use: A research agenda.* Washington, DC: National Academy of Sciences.

Nordstrom, G., & Berglund, M. (1987). Ageing and recovery from alcoholism. *British Journal of Psychiatry, 151,* 382–388.

Ostrom, J. R., Hammarlund, E. R., Christensen, D. B., Plein, J. B., & Kethley, A. J. (1985). Medication usage in an elderly population. *Medical Care, 23,* 157–164.

Parks, J. G., Noguchi, T. T., & Klatt, E. C. (1989). The epidemiology of fatal burn injuries. *Journal of Forensic Sciences, 34,* 339–406.

Parry, H. J., Balter, M. B., Mellinger, G. D., Cisin, I. H., & Manheimer, D. I. (1973). National patterns of psychotropic drug use. *Archives of General Psychiatry, 28,* 769–783.

Parsons, O. A., & Leber, W. R. (1982). Premature aging, alcoholism, and recovery. In W. G. Wood & M. F. Elias (Eds.), *Alcoholism and aging: Advances in research* (pp. 79–96). Boca Raton, FL: CRC Press.

Pascarelli, E. F. (1979). An update on drug dependence in the elderly. *Journal of Drug Issues, 9,* 47–54.

Pascarelli, E. F. (1985). The elderly in methadone maintenance. In E. Gottheil, K. A. Druley, T. E. Skoloda, & H. M. Waxman (Eds.), *The combined problems of alcoholism, drug addiction, and aging* (pp. 210–214). Springfield, IL: Charles C Thomas.

Pascarelli, E. F., & Fischer, W. (1974). Drug dependence in the elderly. *International Journal of Aging and Human Development, 5,* 347–356.

Pentel, P. (1984). Toxicity of over-the-counter stimulants. *Journal of the American Medical Association, 252,* 1898–1903.

Peters, N. L. (1989). Snipping the thread of life: Antimuscarinic side-effects of medications in the elderly. *Archives of Internal Medicine, 149,* 2414–2420.

Petersen, D. M., & Thomas, C. W. (1975). Acute drug reactions among the elderly. *Journal of Gerontology, 30,* 552–556.

Pfefferbaum, A., Rosenbloom, M., Crusan, K., & Jernigan, T. L. (1988). Brain CT changes in alcoholics: Effects of age and alcohol consumption. *Alcoholism (New York), 12,* 81–87.

Pierce, J., Giovino, G., Hatziandreu, E., & Shopland, D. (1989). National age and sex differences in quitting smoking. *Journal of Psychoactive Drugs, 21,* 293–298.

Pinsker, H., & Suljaga-Petchel, K. (1984). Use of benzodiazepines in primary care geriatric patients. *Journal of the American Geriatrics Society, 32,* 595–597.

Potamianos, G., & Kellett, J. M. (1982). Anticholinergic drugs and memory: The effects of benzhexol on memory in a group of geriatric patients. *British Journal of Psychiatry, 140,* 470–472.

Pottieger, A. E., & Inciardi, J. A. (1981). Aging on the street: Drug use and crime among older men. *Journal of Psychoactive Drugs, 13,* 199–210.

Power, K. G., Jerrom, G. W. A., Simpson, R. J., & Mitchell, M. (1985). Controlled study of withdrawal symptoms and rebound anxiety after six-week course of diazepam for generalised anxiety. *British Medical Journal, 290,* 1246–1248.

Quinn, B. P., Applegate, W. B., Roberts, K., Collins, T., & Vanderzwaag, R. (1983). Knowledge and use of medications in a group of elderly individuals. *Journal of the Tennessee Medical Association, 76,* 647–649.

Raffoul, P. R., Cooper, J. K., & Love, D. W. (1981). Drug misuse in older people. *The Gerontologist, 21,* 146–150.

Reich, T., Cloninger, C. R., Van Eerdewegh, P., Rice, J. P., & Mullaney, J. (1988). Secular trends in the familial transmission of alcoholism. *Alcoholism (New York), 12,* 458–464.

Reifler, B. V., Kethley, A., O'Neill, P., Hanley, R., Lewis, S., & Stenchever, D. (1982a). Five-year experience of a community outreach program for the elderly. *American Journal of Psychiatry, 139,* 220–223.

Reifler, B., Raskind, M., & Kethley, A. (1982b). Psychiatric diagnoses among geriatric patients seen in an outreach program. *Journal of the American Geriatrics Society, 30,* 530–533.

Reynolds, C. F., Kupfer, D. J., Hoch, C. C., & Sewich, D. E. (1985). Sleeping pills for the elderly: Are they ever justified? *Journal of Clinical Psychiatry, 46,* 9–12.

Rickels, K., Case, G. W., Winokur, A., & Swenson, C. (1984). Long-term benzodiazepine therapy: Benefits and risks. *Psychopharmacology Bulletin, 20,* 608–615.

Rimer, B. (1988). Smoking among older adults: The problem, consequences and possible solutions. In *Surgeon General's report on health promotion for older adults*. Washington, DC: U.S. Department of Health and Human Services.

Ritzmann, R. F., & Melchior, C. L. (1984). Age and development of tolerance to and physical dependence on alcohol. In J. T. Hartford & T. Samorajski (Eds.), *Alcoholism in the elderly. Social and biomedical issues* (pp. 117–138). New York: Raven.

Robertson, D. (1984). Drug handling in old age. In J. C. Brocklehurst, (Ed.), *Geriatric pharmacology and therapeutics* (pp. 41–59). Oxford: Blackwell Scientific Publications.

Rodrigo, E. K., King, M. B., & Williams, P. (1988). Health of long-term benzodiazepine users. *British Medical Journal, 296,* 603–606.

Rogers, R. L., Meyer, J. S., Judd, B. W., & Mortel, K. F. (1985). Abstention from cigarette smoking improves cerebral perfusion among elderly chronic smokers. *Journal of the American Medical Association, 253,* 2970–2974.

Ron, M. A. (1983). The alcoholic brain: CT scan and psychological findings. *Psychological Medicine* (Monograph suppl.), *3,* 1–33.

Room, R. (1972). Drinking patterns in large U.S. cities: A comparison of San Francisco and national samples. *Quarterly Journal of Studies on Alcohol* (Suppl.), *6,* 28–57.

Rovner, B. W., David, A., Lucas-Blaustein, M. J., Conklin, B., Filipp, L., & Tune, L. (1988). Self-care capacity and anticholinergic drug levels in nursing home patients. *American Journal of Psychiatry, 145,* 107–109.

Rundgren, A., & Mellstrom, D. (1984). The effect of tobacco smoking on the bone mineral content of the ageing skeleton. *Mechanisms of Ageing and Development, 28,* 273–277.

Ryan, C., & Butters, N. (1984). Alcohol consumption and premature aging: A critical review. In M. Galanter (Ed.), *Recent developments in alcoholism* (Vol. 2, pp. 223–250). New York: Plenum.

Sachs, D. P. L. (1986). Cigarette smoking: Health effects and cessation strategies. *Clinics in Geriatric Medicine, 2,* 337–362.

Salzman, C. (1984). Neurotransmission in the aging central nervous system. In *Clinical geriatric psychopharmacology* (pp. 18–31). New York: McGraw-Hill.

Saunders, P. A., Copeland, J. R. M., Dewey, M. E., Davidson, I. A., McWilliam, C., Sharma, V. K., Sullivan, C., & Voruganti, L. N. P. (1989). Alcohol use and abuse in the elderly: Findings from the Liverpool longitudinal study of continuing health in the community. *International Journal of Geriatric Psychiatry, 4,* 103–108.

Schneider, C. L., & Nordlund, D. J. (1983). Prevalence of vitamin and mineral supplementation in the elderly. *Journal of Family Practice, 17,* 243–247.

Schuckit, M. A. (1977). Geriatric alcoholism and drug abuse. *The Gerontologist, 17,* 168–174.

Schuckit, M. A. (1989). *Drug and Alcohol Abuse* (3rd ed.). New York: Plenum.

Schuckit, M. A., & Miller, P. L. (1976). Alcoholism in elderly men: A survey of a general medical ward. *Annals of the New York Academy of Sciences, 273,* 558–571.

Schuckit, M. A., Atkinson, J. H., Miller, P. L., & Berman, J. (1980). A three year followup of elderly alcoholics. *Journal of Clinical Psychiatry, 41,* 412–416.

Shaper, A. G., Wannamethee, G., & Walker, M. (1988). Alcohol and mortality in British men: Explaining the U-shaped curve. *Lancet, 2,* 1267–1273.

Simon, A., Epstein, L. J., & Reynolds, L. (1968). Alcoholism in the geriatric mentally ill. *Geriatrics, 23,* 125–131.

Smart, R. G., & Adlaf, E. M. (1988). Alcohol and drug use among the elderly: Trends in use and charcteristics of users. *Canadian Journal of Public Health, 79,* 236–242.

Stephens, R. C., Haney, C. A., & Underwood, S. (1981). Psychoactive drug use and potential misuse among persons aged 55 years and older. *Journal of Psychoactive Drugs, 13,* 185–193.

Stinson, F. S., Dufour, M. C., & Bertolucci, D. (1989). Alcohol-related morbidity in the aging population. *Alcohol Health and Research World, 13,* 80–87.

Stoller, E. P. (1988). Prescribed and over-the-counter medicine use by ambulatory elderly. *Medical Care, 26,* 1149–1157.

Strang, J., & Gurling, H. (1989). Computerized tomography and neuropsychological assessment in long-term high-dose heroin addicts. *British Journal of Addiction, 84,* 1011–1019.

Strategy Council on Drug Abuse (1979). *Federal strategy for drug abuse and drug traffic prevention, 1979.* Washington, DC: Strategy Council on Drug Abuse.

Sullivan, C. F., Copeland, J. R. M., Dewey, M. E., Davidson, I. A., McWilliam, C., Saunders, P., Sharma, V. K., & Voruganti, L. N. P. (1988). Benzodiazepine usage among the elderly: Findings of the Liverpool community survey. *International Journal of Geriatric Psychiatry, 3,* 289–292.

Swift, C. G., & Tiplady, B. (1988). The effects of age on the response to caffeine. *Psychopharmacology, 94,* 29–31.

Taylor, P. J., & Parrott, J. M. (1988). Elderly offenders: A study of age-related factors among custodially remanded prisoners. *British Journal of Psychiatry, 152,* 340–346.

Timiras, P. S. (1988). Aging of the nervous system: Structural and biochemical changes. In *Physiological basis of geriatrics* (pp. 123–143). New York: Macmillan.

Uhlenhuth, E. H., DeWit, H., Balter, M. B., Johanson, C. E., & Mellinger, G. D. (1988). Risks and benefits of long-term benzodiazepine use. *Journal of Clinical Psychopharmacology, 8,* 161–167.

U.S. Department of Health and Human Services (1988a). *The health consequences of smoking: Nicotine addiction—A report of the Surgeon General.* (DHSS Pub # [CDC] 88-8406). Washington, DC: U.S. Government Printing Office.

U.S. Department of Health and Human Services (1988b). State-specific estimates of smoking-attributable mortality and years of potential life lost—United States, 1985. *Morbidity and Mortality Weekly Review, 37,* 689–693.

U.S. Department of Health and Human Services (1989a). Surgeon General's workshop on health promotion and aging: Summary recommendations of the Alcohol Working Group. *Morbidity and Mortality Weekly Report, 38,* 385–388.

U.S. Department of Health and Human Services (1989b). Tobacco use by adults—United States, 1987. *Morbidity and Mortality Weekly Report, 38,* 685–687.

Vaillant, G. E. (1973). A 20-year followup of New York narcotics addicts. *Archives of General Psychiatry, 29,* 237–241.

Vaillant, G. E. (1983). *The Natural History of Alcoholism.* Cambridge, MA: Harvard University Press.

Vener, A. M., Krupka, L. R., & Climo, J. J. (1979). Drug usage and health characteristics in noninstitutionalized retired persons. *Journal of the American Geriatrics Society, 27,* 83–90.

Vestal, R. E. (1982). Pharmacology and aging. *Journal of the American Geriatrics Society, 30,* 191–200.

Vestal, R. E., McGuire, E. A., Tobin, J. D., Andres, R., Norris, A. H., & Mezey, R. (1977). Aging and ethanol metabolism in man. *Clinical Pharmacology and Therapeutics, 21,* 343–354.

Vetter, N. J., & Ford, D. (1990). Smoking prevention among people aged 60 and over: A randomized controlled trial. *Age and Ageing, 19,* 164–168.

Vetter, N. J., Charny, M., Farrow, S., & Lewis, P. A. (1988). The Cardiff health survey. The relationship between smoking habits and beliefs in the elderly. *Public Health, 102,* 359–364.

Vogel-Sprott, M., & Barrett, P. (1984). Age, drinking habits, and the effects of alcohol. *Journal of Studies on Alcohol, 45,* 517–521.

Volicer, B. J., Volicer, L., & D'Angelo, N. (1983). Variation in length of time to development of alcoholism by family history of problem drinking. *Drug and Alcohol Dependence, 12,* 69–83.

Walker, S. N. (1989). Health promotion for older adults: Directions for research. *American Journal of Health Promotion, 3,* 47–52.

Wattis, J. P. (1981). Alcohol problems in the elderly. *Journal of the American Geriatrics Society, 29,* 131–134.

Waugh, M., Jackson, M., Fox, G. A., Hawke, S. H., & Tuck, R. R. (1989). Effect of social drinking on neuropsychological performance. *British Journal of Addiction, 84,* 659–667.

Werch, C. E. (1989). Quantity-frequency and diary measures of alcohol consumption for elderly drinkers. *International Journal of the Addictions, 24,* 859–865.

Whitcup, S. M., & Miller, F. (1987). Unrecognized drug dependence in psychiatrically hospitalized elderly patients. *Journal of the American Geriatrics Society, 35,* 297–301.

Wiens, A. N., Menustik, C. E., Miller, S. I., & Schmitz, R. E. (1982–1983). Medical–behavioral treatment of the older alcoholic patient. *American Journal of Drug and Alcohol Abuse, 9,* 461–475.

Wilbanks, W., & Kim, P. K. H. (Eds.). (1984). *Elderly Criminals* (pp. 1–31; 41–53). Lanham, MD: University Press.

Willenbring, M. L., Christensen, K. J., Spring, Jr., W. D., & Rasmussen, R. (1987). Alcoholism screening in the elderly. *Journal of the American Geriatrics Society, 35,* 864–869.

Winick, C. (1962). Maturing out of narcotic addiction. *United Nations Bulletin on Narcotics, 14,* 1–7.

Wood, W. G., Armbrecht, H. J., & Wise, R. W. (1982). Ethanol intoxication and withdrawal among three age groups of C57BL/6NNIA mice. *Pharmacology and Biochemistry of Behavior, 17,* 1037–1041.

Woodhouse, K. W., & James, O. F. W. (1985). Alcoholic liver disease in the elderly: Presentation and outcome. *Age and Ageing, 14,* 113–118.

World Health Organization (1988). Mental, behavioural and developmental disorders. Clinical descriptions and diagnostic guidelines: Chapter V, Categories F00-F99. *International classification of diseases* (10th ed. 1988 draft). Geneva: World Health Organization, Division of Mental Health.

Yamashita, K., Kobayashi, S., Yamaguchi, S., Kitani, M., & Tsunematsu, T. (1988). Effects of smoking on regional cerebral blood flow in the normal aged volunteers. *Gerontology, 34,* 199–204.

York, J. L. (1983). Increased responsiveness to ethanol with advancing age in rats. *Pharmacology and Biochemistry of Behavior, 19,* 687–691.

Zimberg, S. (1978). Psychosocial treatment of elderly alcoholics. In S. Zimberg, J. Wallace, & S. B. Blume (Eds.), *Practical approaches to alcoholism psychotherapy* (pp. 237–251). New York: Plenum.

Sleep Disorders and Aging

Carolyn C. Hoch, Daniel J. Buysse, Timothy H. Monk, and Charles F. Reynolds III

I. Introduction
II. Sleep and Aging
III. Sleep Disturbances
    A. Sleep-Disordered Breathing
    B. Nocturnal Myoclonus
    C. Insomnia
    D. Excessive Daytime Sleepiness
    E. Circadian System
    F. Physical Illness
    G. Depression
    H. Dementia
    I. Pseudodementia
    J. Mortality
IV. Clinical and Laboratory Assessment
V. Pharmacologic Treatment Approaches
VI. Nonpharmacologic Treatment Approaches
VII. Conclusions
    References

I. Introduction

Research in sleep and aging over the past 15 years has yielded many exciting and promising discoveries. It has become clear that sleep is affected by the aging process, with complex interactions occurring between aging, sleep, and illness (mental and physical). The 1990 National Institutes of Health (NIH) Consensus Development Conference on the Treatment of Sleep Disorders of Older People agreed that sleep disturbances in general, as well as those associated with late-life depression and dementia, represent a major public health problem among elderly individuals, with up to 35% of persons older than 65 having sleep-related problems (NIH, 1990). The elderly are the age group most severely affected by disorders of initiating and maintaining sleep and tend to consume disproportionate quantities of sedative hypnotics (NIH, 1990). Frequently, nighttime sleep disturbances and/or the medication used to treat them lead to marked deterioration in daytime alertness and functioning, causing significant distress for the elderly and their families (Carskadon & Dement, 1981; Carskadon, Brown, & Dement, 1982). Sleep-related behavioral disturbances such as wandering, confusion, and agitation also occur and are often the factors that precipitate a family's decision to institutionalize the elderly individual (Rabins, Mace, & Lucas, 1982; Sanford, 1975).

The purpose of this chapter is to address (1) sleep and aging; (2) sleep disturbances and their etiologies; (3) clinical and laboratory assessment of sleep disturbances; (4) pharmacological treatment approaches; and (5) nonpharmacological treatment approaches; and (6) conclusions.

II. Sleep and Aging

Sleep is a set of complex physiological processes involving a predictable sequence of operating states within the central nervous system. These states are identified by electroencephalographic (EEG) patterns and by specific behaviors. During sleep two different operating states occur in the central nervous system: *rapid eye movement* (REM) sleep, representing an activated brain; and *non–rapid eye movement* (NREM) sleep with a quiescent brain. NREM sleep is divided into four stages numbered from 1 (drowsy or transitional) to 4 (deep or slow-wave sleep). NREM sleep is characterized by a general slowing of physiological processes, such as respiration and heart rate, relative to wakefulness. The EEG shows progressive slowing and synchronization with the deeper NREM sleep stages, and subjective mental activity decreases as well. During REM sleep the heart rate, respiratory rate, and blood pressure increase relative to NREM sleep, and show great variability. The ventilatory response to increased concentrations of inhaled CO_2 is decreased compared to that of NREM sleep. Most characteristics of REM sleep are the tonic suppression of skeletal muscle tone; the mixed-frequency, low-voltage EEG; and the phasic bursts of rapid eye movements. REM is also associated with substantial mental activity, i.e., dreaming. The onset of REM sleep is mediated by the firing of cholinergic cells in the pontine tegmentum, while NREM sleep depends on neuronal activity of the basal forebrain area and the midbrain raphe. REM sleep is regulated to a large degree by circadian factors, occurring near the nadir or lowpoint of the circadian temperature rhythm. Slow-wave sleep, on the other hand, is regulated by homeostatic factors (Kryger, Roth, & Dement, 1989).

EEG sleep processes are summarized and quantified using measures of sleep continuity, sleep architecture, and REM sleep (Table I). Sleep-continuity measures describe the overall pattern of sleep and wakefulness and include total recording period, sleep latency, awake time after sleep onset, time spent asleep, arousal sleep efficiency, sleep maintenance. Sleep architecture describes the amount and percentage of the different sleep stages. More specific measures of REM sleep include REM latency, REM activity, REM density, and REM intensity. Other physiologic events during sleep, including apnea, hypopnea, oxygen

Table I

EEG Measures of Selected Sleep Processes

Sleep continuity measures

Total recording period (TRP)	Total number of minutes from initial plug-in to the end of the recording.
Sleep latency (SL)	Time from lights out until the appearance of 10 min of stage 2 sleep interrupted by not more than two min of wakefulness or stage 1.
Awake (WASO)	Time spent awake after sleep onset and before the final morning awakening.
Time spent asleep (TSA)	Time spent asleep, less any awake time during the night after sleep onset.
Arousal	Period of wakefulness lasting thirty sec or longer.
Sleep efficiency (SE)	Ratio of time spent asleep to total recording period.
Sleep maintenance (SM)	Ratio of time spent asleep to total recording period after sleep onset.

Sleep architecture

Stage 1	NREM sleep with low-voltage activity waves three to seven cycles per sec; a transition between wakefulness and sleep.
Stage 2	NREM sleep marked by the appearance of sleep spindles and/or K-complexes.
Stage 3	NREM sleep with delta waves occupying 20 to 50% of EEG activity.
Stage 4	Deepest NREM sleep, with delta waves occupying more than 50% of EEG activity.

REM sleep measures

REM latency	Number of minutes of sleep until the first REM period.
REM time	Total number of minutes of REM sleep.
REM activity	Rapid eye movements throughout the night.
REM density	Ratio of total REM activity to total REM time.
REM intensity	Ratio of REM activity to time spent asleep.
REM period	Occurrence of at least 3 consecutive min of REM sleep separated by no less than 30 min of NREM sleep from the next occurence of REM sleep.

Sleep-disordered breathing

Apnea	Cessation of airflow during sleep lasting 10 sec or longer.
Hypopnea	Decreased air flow and respiratory movement during sleep to one third of baseline for 10 sec or longer.
Oxygen desaturation	Decrease in oxyhemoglobin level during sleep to less than baseline.

desaturation, and periodic leg movements can also be recorded during nocturnal polysomnography.

Age-dependent changes in sleep structure and patterns in 60-, 70-, and 80-year-olds have been documented (Figure 1) (Brendel, *et al.*, 1990; Feinberg, 1974; Hayashi & Endo, 1982; Kahn & Fischer, 1969; Kahn, Fischer, & Lieberman, 1970; Kales, Wilson, & Kales, 1967; Prinz, 1977; Reynolds, Kupfer, Taska, Hoch, Sewitch, & Spiker, 1985a; Webb & Swinbrune, 1982). The most important of these age-related changes are decreased sleep continuity, characterized in particular by numerous transient microarousals

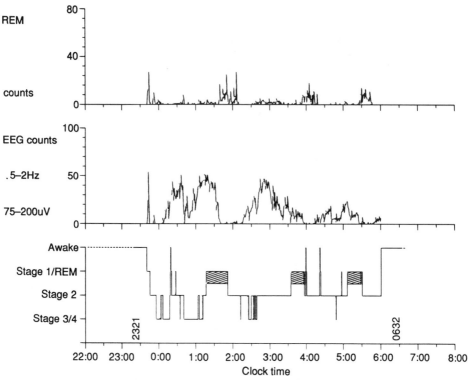

Figure 1 The sleep histogram of a healthy elderly (73-year-old) woman (bottom panel) displays the progression of sleep stages across the night. This subject shows good sleep continuity with few awakenings and robust Stage 3/4 NREM sleep. In contrast to younger subjects, the first REM period (hatched bar) is long in comparison to subsequent REM periods. Computer measurements of rapid eye movements (top panel) and EEG counts in the delta frequency range (middle panel) provide more detailed quantitative information about physiological events during various sleep stages.

(3–15 sec in duration); decreased NREM stages 3 and 4 slow-wave sleep with increased NREM stages 1 and 2 sleep; decreased absolute amounts of REM sleep; and a tendency for REM sleep to occur earlier in the night (NIH, 1990; Webb, 1989). These characteristics demonstrate the increased fragility of sleep in the elderly.

In addition, older individuals may show a redistribution of sleep across the 24-hr day, reflecting circadian rhythm disturbances. Many people report retiring earlier at night and rising earlier in the morning as they become older, reflecting a phase advance of their major sleep period relative to the 24-hr clock. Elders also develop a polyphasic sleep–wake cycle consisting of multiple, short sleep–wake periods over the 24-hr day (Reynolds, Hoch, & Monk, 1989).

Some authors have suggested that these sleep–wake pattern changes may reflect age-related changes in endogenous circadian rhythms, such as lowering of amplitude or a phase advancement relative to the 24-hour clock (Vitiello, Smallwood, Avery, 1986; Weitzman, Moline, Czeisler, & Zimmerman, 1982; Zepelin, 1983). However, the issue is far from resolved, since the elderly may also have less activity, more illness, more medication use, and a variety of other factors that influence their circadian rhythms and sleep.

Other age-associated changes in sleep include a decrement in growth-hormone secretion (which typically is maximal during the first 2 hr of sleep, in association with NREM states 3 and 4 sleep), decreases in a sleep-associated prolactin and testosterone, increase in plasma norepinephrine levels, and increases in cortisol secretion, particularly in depressed elderly (For review, see Kryger, Roth, & Dement, 1989).

Another important characteristic of the sleep of elders is daytime napping. Evidence exists that daytime sleepiness among the elders may be a compensatory response to fragmented nocturnal sleep (Carskadon, Brown, & Dement, 1982; Carskadon, van der Hoed, & Dement, 1980). Lifestyle changes and social factors such as boredom, loneliness, and custom may also play contributory roles in napping behavior.

The ability to sleep versus need for sleep is another issue in sleep and healthy aging (Dement, 1990). Age-related EEG sleep patterns support the view that the elderly have less ability to sleep rather than less need for sleep, since the ability to have slow-wave sleep and long interrupted sleep periods declines with age. Therefore, the occurrence of daytime sleepiness in many elderly may be a manifestation of unmet sleep need. Recent research also, however, suggests that some aspects of age-related sleep alterations may be reversible. For example, following a period of a sleep deprivation or a sleep-restriction pattern of progressively and systematically spending less time in bed, the elderly responded with recovery sleep, having increased amounts of delta (slow-wave) sleep and improved sleep continuity (Reynolds et al., 1986; Spielman, Raskin, & Thorpy, 1983).

Gender-related differences have also been reported in the sleep of the healthy elderly, with men showing more impaired sleep maintenance and less delta sleep than women (Hoch, Reynolds, Kupfer, & Berman, 1988; Reynolds, Kupfer, Taska, et al., 1985a; Williams, Karacan, & Hursch, 1974). It is interesting to note, however, that older women complain more frequently of sleep disturbance and receive sleeping pills more often than older men (Miles & Dement, 1980a). A possible explanation may be the gender-related differences in sleep perception and effects of sleep disruption on mood. Elderly women show higher and more stable correlations between estimates of sleep quality and objective laboratory measures of sleep (Hoch, Reynolds, Kupfer, Berman, Houck, & Stack, 1987), and elderly women find sleep deprivation to be a more mood-disturbing experience than do elderly men (Reynolds et al., 1986). Thus it is possible that elderly women may be more sensitive to sleep quality and sleep loss than are elderly men.

In order to determine if advancing age continues to affect the stability of sleep structure and subjective reports of sleep quality, longitudinal studies of sleep in healthy elders have been initiated. Hoch and colleagues (1988) examined EEG sleep characteristics and perceptions of sleep quality among healthy elders over a 2-year interval. Most EEG sleep variables and subjective perceptions of sleep quality were stable at 2 yr. Elderly men and women showed significantly more awakenings during the second recording series; gender-dependent sleep changes were noted only in phasic REM measures; and REM activity, density, and intensity increased in men over time and decreased in the women. Finally, subjective estimates of sleep quality, although stable over time, showed gender-dependent differences, with women reporting a lower sleep quality than men.

With respect to other behaviors observed during sleep in late life, snoring has received considerable attention. Koskenvuo *et al.* (1985, 1987), in a large-scale study, found habitual snoring in 9% of men (n = 3847) and 3.6% of women (n = 3664) aged 40 to 69. Snoring was more prevalent in men and women with hypertension (relative risk, 1.94 and 3.19, respectively), and in men (n = 4388) with ischemic heart disease (relative risk, 1.91) or stroke (relative risk, 2.38). Lugaresi and colleagues (1975, 1978, 1983) have also found that heavy snoring may have a negative association with cardiac and circulatory functioning. In their epidemiological study of snoring in all ages (*n* = 5713), 16.8% of men and 14.1% of women reported occasional snoring. Nineteen percent of the participants reported habitual snoring (24.1% men, 13.8% women). The prevalence of snoring also increased with age with more than 60% of men and 40% of women older than 60 reporting habitual snoring. Clinically, it is believed that more severe snoring is likely to reflect sleep apnea (i.e., occlusion of the airway during sleep) (Reynolds, 1990).

III. Sleep Disturbances

In addition to the sleep changes associated with the normal aging process, several *intrinsic* sleep disorders have been studied in relation to advancing age: sleep-disordered breathing, nocturnal myoclonus, insomnia, excessive daytime sleepiness, and circadian dysrhythmias. Sleep disturbances related to specific pathological factors such as physical illness, depression, dementia (including *sundowning* and nursing home residents), pseudodementia, and mortality have also been examined.

A. Sleep-Disordered Breathing

Sleep-disordered breathing and its relation to advancing age is detected during nocturnal polysomnographic recordings with oral and nasal thermistors to measure air flow and bellows to monitor respiratory effort. Sleep apnea occurs when at least five apneas or hypopneas occur per hour of sleep, with each apnea or hypopnea event lasting a minimum of 10 sec (Figure 2). Apnea index (AI) is the number of apneas per hour of sleep; apnea-hypopnea index (AHI), also known as respiratory disturbance index (RDI), is the number of apneas and hypopneas per hour of sleep. Apneic events are usually followed by an awakening or arousal, and can be associated with many symptoms including decreased blood oxygen levels, cardiac arrhythmias, hypertension, nighttime confusion, and daytime neuropsychiatric impairment.

The prevalence of sleep-disordered breathing has been examined in healthy elders as well as in randomly selected, community-resident elders. Results consistently demonstrate age-related increases of sleep-disordered breathing. Estimates of AI and/or AHI of five or greater have been reported in one fourth to one third of the elderly studied (Ancoli-Israel & Kripke, in press; Berry & Phillips, 1988; Hoch *et al.*, 1986; Mosko *et al.*, 1988; Reynolds, Kupfer, Taska, Hoch, Sewitch, Restifo, *et al.*, 1985b). Gender differences have also been noted with increased prevalence of sleep apnea in elderly men versus elderly women (Ancoli-Israel, Kripke, & Mason, 1984; Hoch *et al.*, 1986; Mosko *et al.*, 1988;

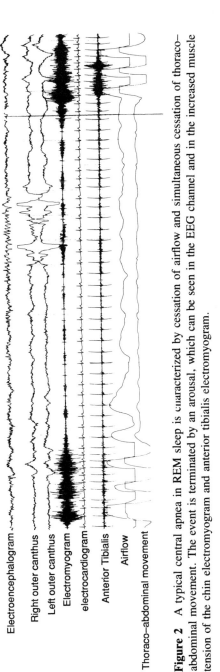

Electroencephalogram

Right outer canthus

Left outer canthus

Electromyogram

electrocardiogram

Anterior Tibialis

Airflow

Thoraco–abdominal movement

Figure 2 A typical central apnea in REM sleep is characterized by cessation of thoraco–abdominal movement. The event is terminated by an arousal, which can be seen in the EEG channel and in the increased muscle tension of the chin electromyogram and anterior tibialis electromyogram.

Reynolds *et al.*, 1985b). However, the significance of sleep-disordered breathing at mild levels without clinical symptoms is not clear, nor is the indication for intervention (NIH, 1990).

The impact of sleep-disordered breathing may be greater in medically and neuropsychiatrically compromised elders. Higher rates of sleep apneas have been found among randomly selected elderly medical-ward patients and nursing-home residents than in community-dwelling elderly (Ancoli-Israel, 1989b; Ancoli-Israel & Kripke, 1988; Ancoli-Israel, Parker, Sinall, Mason, & Kripke, 1989). The higher rates of sleep apnea in the medical ward patients were attributed to congestive heart failure (Ancoli-Israel, 1989b). Other studies have also reported significant associations between sleep-disordered breathing and substantial pulmonary and cardiovascular disease (Guilleminault, Connolly, & Winkle, 1983; Kales, Bixler, & Cadieux, 1984; Lavie, Rachamin, & Rubin, 1984).

The rate of sleep-disordered breathing in depressed elderly patients does not appear to be significantly greater than that of age- and sex-matched controls. Reynolds *et al.* (1985) and Hoch *et al.* (1986) have reported a 16 to 18% occurrence rate of sleep apnea (AHI ≥ 5) in depressed elderly versus 4 to 6% in healthy controls. A significantly higher prevalence of sleep-disordered breathing has been documented in elderly patients with probable Alzheimer's disease than in elderly controls by some investigators (Hoch *et al.*, 1986; Moldofsky *et al.*, 1983; Reynolds, *et al.*, 1985b; Smirne *et al.*, 1981) but not by all (Smallwood, Vitiello, Giblin, & Prinz, 1983). The functional significance of sleep-disordered breathing in Alzheimer's disease has also been examined. For instance severity of dementia was significantly correlated with severity of sleep apnea (and with percentage of indeterminate NREM sleep) (Hoch *et al.*, 1986; Reynolds *et al.*, 1985). Data also suggest that sleep-disordered breathing in nonmedicated Alzheimer's patients is relatively mild and is not a predictor of overnight changes in respiration, nocturnal oxyhemoglobin desaturation, overnight mental status changes, and nocturnal behavior (Hoch *et al.*, 1989a). Finally, in elderly patients with mixed symptoms of depression and cognitive impairment who had died by 2-yr followup, apnea–hypopnea indices (and REM latency) correctly predicted 77% of survivors. Patients with REM latency of more than 40 min and an apnea–hypopnea index of more than 3 were assigned a relative mortality risk of 3.7 ($p < .05$). (Hoch, Reynolds, Houck, *et al.* 1989).

B. Nocturnal Myoclonus

Nocturnal myoclonus or periodic leg movements in sleep is a sleep disturbance characterized by brief (.5–5.0 sec), repetitive jerking movement in the extremities having a periodicity of 20 to 40 sec, which may lead to transient arousals. The movements are measured by polysomnographic recordings of anterior tibialis muscle activity (Figure 3). Myoclonus arousal index (MAI) is the ratio of periodic leg movements associated with arousals and microarousals to total sleep time in hours (Coleman, 1982). While there is no absolute consensus, a MAI ≥ 5 is generally considered abnormal. Among elderly with sleep complaints, the rates of nocturnal myoclonus range (MAI ≥ 5) from 4 to 31% (Ancoli-Israel, Kripke, Mason, & Messin, 1981; Reynolds *et al.*, 1980). However, in studies with healthy elderly people, rates of myoclonus range from 25 to 60%. (Dickel,

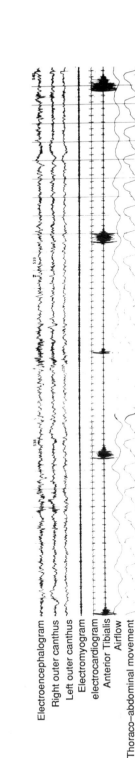

Figure 3 Periodic leg movements during Stage 2 NREM sleep are indicated by rhythmic *bursts* of increased muscle tension in the anterior tibialis electromyogram. The first and third movements are associated with transient arousal in the EEG tracing.

Sassin, & Mosko, 1986; Okudaira *et al.*, 1983). The 1990 NIH Consensus Conference on the "Treatment of Sleep Disorders of Older People" highlighted the controversy surrounding the diagnosis and symptomatic consequences of periodic leg movements in sleep (Kripke, 1990). Some experts believe that periodic leg movements in sleep can cause insomnia, as expressed in difficulties with initiating and maintaining sleep or daytime sleepiness, resulting from disrupted nocturnal sleep. Others, however, argue that periodic leg movements in sleep are no more common among insomniacs than in noncomplaining subjects, and, therefore, are not an etiologic factor in insomnia (Kales *et al.*, 1982; Kripke, 1990).

C. Insomnia

1. Insomnia and Psychiatric Disorders

Insomnia is the subjective complaint that sleep is inadequate or abnormal. Generally included are nocturnal symptoms of difficulty initiating sleep, frequent awakenings from sleep, a short sleep time, and *nonrestorative* sleep; and daytime symptoms, resulting from the poor sleep, of fatigue, sleepiness, depression, anxiety, and other mood changes. These symptoms are similar to those complaints most frequently offered by elders about their sleep. Studies confirm that the elderly are the largest age group affected by insomnia complaints and disorders (Carskadon & Dement, 1981; Dement, Miles, & Carskadon, 1982; Miles & Dement, 1980a).

Insomnia in the elderly (as in younger age groups) is a *symptom* with many possible causes, rather than a unitary *disorder* (Buysse & Reynolds, 1990). Medical illness, psychiatric illness, medication use or withdrawal, substance abuse, and sleep–wake schedule changes can all lead to complaints of insomnia. Very often, multiple causes for sleep disturbance can be identified. Furthermore, an insomnia complaint may originate from one source (such as an acute medical problem or psychosocial stress), but may be perpetuated by maladaptive conditioning that arises in response to the original stress. A similar scenario may arise with medications: drugs initially used to treat the symptom of insomnia may, through tolerance and withdrawal phenomena, actually perpetuate the problem. Since insomnia in the elderly can arise from so many sources, it is critical that the evaluation of insomnia include a detailed history examining each of the possible factors mentioned above.

2. Insomnia and Bereavement

The recent NIMH epidemiologic catchment area survey of individuals provides supporting data regarding the potential links of insomnia and hypersomnia to the development of psychiatric disorders (Ford & Kamerow, 1989). Between 1981 and 1985, 7954 respondents were questioned at a baseline interview and then again 1 year later about sleep complaints and psychiatric symptoms using the Diagnostic Interview Schedule. This community resident sample reported rates of 10.2% for persistent insomnia and 3.2% for hypersomnia on first interview. Rates of prevalent and incident insomnia complaints were highest among the 1801 respondents aged 65 and older: 12% and 7.3% respectively. By contrast, only 1.6% of those aged 65 and older had persistent hypersomnia at initial interview, with an additional 1.8% at followup interview. Of all respondents with insomnia, 40% had a psychiatric disorder as compared with 16% of the sample without sleep complaints. Furthermore, the risk of development of new major depression was higher in those respondents (of any age) who had insomnia at both baseline and followup interviews compared with those without insomnia (odds ratio, 39:8) or among those individuals whose insomnia had resolved by the second interview (odds ratio, 1:6). Ford and Kamerow suggested that early recognition and treatment of sleep disturbances can prevent future psychiatric disorders.

Longitudinal epidemiologic study by Rodin and colleagues (1988) examined relationships among aging, insomnia, and depression in 264 community-residing elderly aged 62 and older. The focus was on how the frequency of depressed affect over time relates to poor sleep. Results showed that frequency of depressed affect over a 3-yr period was "related positively to sleep disturbance, even when subjects' age, gender, and health status were considered simultaneously (p. 47)." Further, the authors noted that "early morning awakening was the sleep symptom most consistently related to depressed mood over the course of the study (p. 51)." Poor health and female gender showed positive but less consistent relationships to the sleep complaints than depression.

Insomnia is also a persistent and debilitating symptom in late-life spousal bereavement. Clayton and colleagues (1972) studied 149 bereaved persons at 1 month from the loss event and found that 76% of subjects reported sleep disturbances; at 13 months, 48% had evidence of persistent sleep disturbance. The frequency of spousal loss through death has been estimated at 1.6 and 3% yearly for older adult males and females, respectively (Murrell & Himmelfarb, 1989; Murrell, Norris & Hutchins, 1984). Given the large number of spousally bereaved elderly, the strong likelihood of concurrent sleep disturbances, and the risk for developing major depression posed by persistent sleep disturbance, the public-health importance of sleep disturbance in late-life bereavement is evident. It also seems plausible to suggest that sleep loss in bereavement may contribute not only to bereavement-related depression but also to bereavement-related self-medication with alcohol and sleeping pills.

3. Summary

Complaints of persistent insomnia (lasting longer than one month) are clinically and epidemiologically important in late life. A strong association of persistent insomnia with depressed mood (Rodin et al., 1988), with risk for the development of major depression (Ford & Kamerow, 1989), and with bereavement (where it is a persistent and debilitating symptom) (Clayton et al., 1972) is supported by the data.

D. Excessive Daytime Sleepiness

Excessive daytime sleepiness can be the final result of several different processes including (1) disorders marked by an increase in sleep propensity, such as narcolepsy; (2) a reduction of or disturbance during nighttime sleep such as night apnea or myoclonus; or

(3) medication effects. Excessive daytime sleepiness in the elderly may, therefore, be indicative of underlying health states. In addition, changes in circadian rhythms of temperature, alertness–sleepiness, and social time cues are also important. Finally, the presence of degenerative central nervous system disorders, such as dementias of the Alzheimer's type, lead to polyphasic sleep–wake patterns, that is, the loss of consolidation of sleep at night and its redistribution during the day (Vitiello & Prinz, 1989). Investigations have also shown that the elderly take more naps than younger people (Carskadon, Brown, & Dement, 1982; Tune, 1968; Webb & Swinburne, 1971). Daytime sleepiness is measured objectively by the multiple sleep latency test (MSLT) using polysomnography during four or five daytime naps lasting 20 min each. The MSLT measures how long it takes an individual to fall asleep during and whether REM sleep occurs. Research has demonstrated that elderly consistently fall asleep in less than 15 min, more quickly than other comparative age groups (Richardson, Carskadon, & Flagg, 1978). When elders are asked to subjectively describe their sleep and daytime functioning, most report that their sleep is satisfactory, but they also report daytime sleepiness (Ancoli-Israel, Kripke, & Mason, 1984).

E. Circadian System

From both animal and human studies (Brock, 1985), there is evidence of a reduction in circadian rhythm amplitude with advancing age. Moreover, sleep-diary studies have confirmed the conventional wisdom that older people tend to retire to bed earlier, and get up earlier than their younger counterparts (Tune, 1968). This increased tendency toward *morningness* may be explained by a shortening with age of the *natural* (free-running) period of the endogenous circadian pacemaker (Weitzman, Moline, Czeisler, & Zimmerman, 1982).

Studies of circadian temperature rhythms in the elderly have shown that the reduction in amplitude appears to result from an increase in the nadir temperature level (Vitiello *et al.*, 1986; Weitman, Moline, Czeisler, & Zimmerman, 1982). In normal diurnal situations, this results in a smaller nighttime drop in temperature in the old than in the young (Zepelin, 1983). The circadian temperature rhythm exerts powerful effects on the regulation of sleep. Sleep disturbances such as insomnia are associated with diminished amplitude in the body-temperature rhythm. The body-temperature cycle is the generally accepted marker of the circadian clock that drives the daily cycles in REM sleep propensity, alertness, and vigilance (Weitzman, Moline, Czeisler, & Zimmerman, 1982). REM sleep is most abundant near the nadir or low point of the daily temperature rhythm.

There are several explanations why circadian amplitudes may be reduced in the elderly. First, perhaps the circadian oscillator is generating a weaker signal resulting in a desynchronized temperature rhythm. Although it is appealing to hypothesize that the age-related decreases in circadian amplitude merely result from a weakening of the signal coming from the endogenous circadian pacemaker, this may not always be the case. Other explanations are that Zeitgeber (time cue) impoverishment (particularly in *shut-ins*) and/or weaker entrainment mechanisms may result in a failure to properly entrain the circadian system.

F. Physical Illness

It has been estimated that two thirds of the individuals older than 65 have one or more chronic medical illness (Miles & Dement, 1980a). It is commonplace in clinical geriatric practice that elderly report disrupted sleep in relation to physical discomfort, though there has been little systematic study of this area. Physical illness can cause sleep problems in several ways. First, symptoms of medical illness such as pain or breathing problems can interrupt nighttime sleep. Second, physical illness such as dementia and strokes may directly affect brain structures responsible for sleep and wakefulness. Third, medications used to treat physical illness can disrupt sleep or lead to daytime sleepiness.

One hundred participants at the Pittsburgh site of the National Heart, Lung, and Blood Institute (NHLBI)-funded Cardiovascular Health Study (CHS; Reynolds, 1990) recently completed the Pittsburgh Sleep Quality Inventory (Buysse, Reynolds, Monk, Berman, & Kupfer, 1989). Participants in the multisite CHS are required to be aged 65 and older, well enough to come to the University, and able to climb onto an examining table. Of the 100 respondents, 59% reported that nocturia had disturbed their nighttime sleep three or more times a week during the past month. Other symptoms leading to sleep disruption were the following: leg cramps (6%), pain (12%), coughing or difficulty breathing (16%), feeling cold (10%), feeling hot (8%), and dreams (3%). Nocturia, which is extremely common in old people, is related to different factors (e.g., diabetes, use of diuretics, decreased bladder capacity, and decrease in renal concentrating ability).

G. Depression

Electroencephalographic sleep changes associated with late-life depressive illness include high REM sleep percentage, long first REM periods, greater density of phasic rapid-eye movements, shorter REM latency, and extreme sleep maintenance difficulty (Hoch, Buysse, & Reynolds, 1989). Several of the sleep changes that occur in late-life depression also occur, although to a lesser extent, during the course of normal aging (Table II and Figure 4). An age-dependent increase in wakefulness after sleep onset and decrease in slow-wave sleep occur in both normal aging and depression. REM-sleep latency shortens considerably in depression and may also be a component of normal aging (Kupfer, Frank, & Ehlers, 1989). The capacity to sustain REM-sleep inhibition during the first half of the night is diminished by advancing age as well as by depressive illness. Additionally, the shortening of REM-sleep latency and alteration of intranight temporal distribution of REM sleep with greater early REM-sleep density specifically characterizes the sleep of elders with major depressive disorders. Sleep-maintenance difficulties of depressed elders also correlate significantly with the severity of depression, as measured by Hamilton depression ratings (Reynolds, Kupfer, Hoch, & Sewitch, 1985c). Finally, the sleep characteristics of depressed and healthy individuals are consistently different across a range of ages (Gillin et al., 1981; Ulrich, Shaw, & Kupfer, 1980), and elderly depressed, demented, and healthy subjects can be reliably distinguished on the basis of sleep EEG findings (Reynolds et al., 1988).

An interactive relationship between sleep regulation and depression has also been

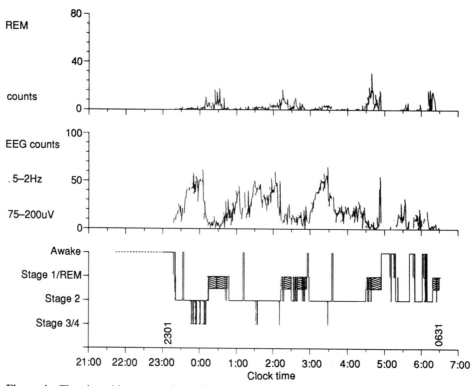

Figure 4 The sleep histogram of an elderly (70-year-old) depressed woman shows decreased slow-wave sleep, an increased amount of wakefulness after sleep onset, and a large amount of early-morning wakefulness. This particular patient does not have a short REM-sleep latency. The pattern of computer REM and delta-frequency EEG counts can further discriminate depressed patients from healthy controls and patients with dementia.

supported through self-report measures of sleep disturbances and depressed feelings in community-resident elders (Rodin, McAvay, & Timko, 1988). Frequency of depressed mood has been associated with reports of difficulty falling asleep, waking up frequently in the night, early morning awakening, and not feeling rested in the morning. This finding is consistent with EEG sleep studies, which have suggested the importance of early-morning awakening as a significant finding among depressed elders (Kupfer *et al.*, 1989).

H. Dementia

Elderly individuals with probable Alzheimer's disease frequently have disturbances in nocturnal sleep and sleep–wake cycles and disruptive nocturnal behaviors such as insomnia, wandering, and sundowning. These sleep-related disturbances may result from degenerative changes in the Alzheimer's disease process such as loss of or damage to the neuronal pathways that initiate and maintain sleep and that control respiration (Hirano & Zimmerman, 1962; Smallwood, Vitiello, Giblin, & Prinz, 1983).

The sleep of elderly individuals with probable Alzheimer's dementia, compared with that of healthy elderly controls, has been characterized by greater disruption of sleep continuity, decreased REM sleep time and activity, *indeterminate* NREM sleep, (i.e., NREM stage 2 without characteristic wave forms), and decreased or absent slow-wave sleep (Table II). Frequent daytime naps with periods of wakefulness also occur (Hoch *et al.*, 1986; Prinz *et al.*, 1982; Reynolds *et al.*, 1985b; Vitiello & Prinz, 1989). Concurrent with advancing dementia, Alzheimer's patients show a gradual but progressive loss of phasic activity, both of rapid eye movements in REM sleep and of spindles and K-complexes in NREM sleep. Finally, Alzheimer's patients have significantly more sleep-disordered breathing (Ancoli-Israel, Parker, & Butters, 1985; Frommlet, Prinz, & Vitiello, Ries, & Williams, 1986; Hoch, 1989; Hoch *et al.*, 1986; Reynolds, *et al.*, 1985; Vitiello *et al.*, 1984). These sleep variables have been explored as potential biological markers for Alzheimer's disease. However, definitive markers in early or mild dementia have not yet been isolated (Vitiello & Prinz, 1989).

The disruptive sleep disturbances and behaviors of demented elderly often precipitate their admission to nursing homes. Sleep patterns among nursing home residents have been observed around the clock. Increasing amounts of sleep in a 24-hr period usually result

Table II

Selected EEG Sleep Changes Associated
with Normal and Pathologic Aging

Normative aging changes
  Decreased sleep continuity
  Sleep fragmentation
  Decreased NREM stages 3 and 4
  Increased NREM stages 1 and 2
  Decreased amount of REM
  Tendency for REM to occur earlier in the night
  Phase advancement of major sleep period
  Presence of sleep-disordered breathing

Changes in depressed elders
  High REM sleep percentage
  Long first REM period
  Greater density of phasic rapid eye movement
  Shorter REM latency
  Extreme sleep maintenance difficulty

Changes in dementia
  Disruption of sleep continuity
  Decreased REM sleep time and activity
  Indeterminate NREM sleep
  Loss of phasic activity
  Significantly more sleep-disordered breathing than among
    healthy elders

from increased daytime sleep rather than an increase in nocturnal sleep (Regestein & Morris, 1987). Investigations have also demonstrated large amounts of individual variability in the sleep patterns of the nursing-home residents (Bliwise, Bevier, & Bliwise, 1987; Jacobs, Ancoli-Israel, & Parker, in press).

Portable nocturnal polysomnography was utilized in a randomly selected group of elderly nursing-home patients (mean age, 81.9 years). These patients averaged only 39.5 min of sleep per hour in any hour of the night, and 50% woke up at least two times per hour (Jacobs, Ancoli-Israel, & Parker, in press). When a subgroup of these nursing home residents were recorded for a full 24 hr, patients spent some portion of every hour asleep. In addition, their sleep was so fragmented that they rarely experienced even a single hour of consolidated sleep (Ancoli-Israel, Parker, Sinall, Mason, & Kripke, 1989). Sleep-disordered breathing is also more prevalent among nursing home residents than among community-residing elders (Ancoli-Israel & Kripke, in press).

Sundowning is agitated behavior manifested either verbally or physically, which occurs in the evening and night hours. This phenomena has been empirically studied by Evans (1987) and associated with a diagnosis of dementia and/or fluid and electrolyte imbalances. Symptoms occurred more frequently in patients recently admitted to a nursing care facility, in patients whose rooms had been changed within the past month, and in patients who participated in fewer daytime activities. Sundowning has also been linked to sensory deprivation, loneliness, diminished social and physical time cues (lighting, visitors), partial arousal from REM sleep (Feinberg, Koresko, & Heller, 1967), and with sleep apnea (Hoch *et al.*, 1989). The phenomenon of sundowning may be the final expression of several mechanisms, some related to changes in sleep–wake rhythmicity and some to the physical and psychosocial time cues that impinge upon internal circadian systems.

I. Pseudodementia

Sleep physiological measures have also been examined for diagnostic clarification of patients with depressive pseudodementia versus primary degenerative dementia with secondary depression. Reynolds and associates (1988) performed discriminant function analyses of sleep alteration in diagnostically *pure* (nondemented) depressed and (nondepressed) demented patient groups. Overall, 80% of the diagnostically *pure* patients were correctly identified. The four measures that contributed most to the successful separation of depressed and demented patients were REM latency (lower in depressives), REM percentage (higher in depressives), *indeterminate* NREM sleep percentage (higher in demented patients, reflecting greater loss of spindles and K-complexes), and early-morning awakening (more marked in depressives). This discriminant function classification was successfully cross-validated in independent subsamples of pure depressed and pure demented patients.

In order to further clarify the utility of sleep electrophysiologic measures for diagnosis in patients with mixed symptoms of depression and cognitive impairment, Buysse *et al.* 1988) examined several clinical ratings and sleep EEG measures before and after one night of sleep deprivation. Subjects had three undisturbed nights of baseline sleep, one night of sleep deprivation (36 to 40 hr total), and two recovery nights. Patients with depressive pseudodementia had less-severe cognitive impairment at baseline and showed significant improvement in Hamilton depression ratings after sleep deprivation. By contrast, those patients having dementia with secondary depression showed no changes or worsening in Hamilton depression ratings. Further, baseline sleep measures demonstrated significantly higher REM percentage and phasic REM activity–intensity in the pseudodemented versus demented patients. While both groups had increases in sleep efficiency, sleep maintenance, and slow-wave sleep after sleep deprivation, the second recovery night was characterized by greater first-REM-period duration in depressive pseudodementia than in dementia with secondary depression. These differences in REM-sleep duration and density (using a first-REM-period duration of $\geq$ 25 min) permitted correct identification of 88.5% of the patients.

J. Mortality

Mortality rates during various times at night have been studied. Mortality rate from all causes is estimated to increase 30% during sleep (Smolensky, Halberg, & Sargent, 1972). Above-average frequencies of death between 2 AM and 8 AM have been found, with the peak being relatively specific to ischemic heart disease in persons older than 65 years (Mitler, Hajukovic, & Shafor, 1987). Studies have also shown that people who report either sleeping less than 7 hr or more than 8 hr have a higher mortality rate, with 86% of these deaths occurring among individuals older than 60 yr (Belloc, 1973; Kripke, Simons, & Garfinkel, 1979).

IV. Clinical and Laboratory Assessment

Sleep disturbances in the elderly reflect numerous factors:

1. age-dependent changes in sleep;
2. increased prevalence of sleep-disordered breathing and nocturnal myoclonus;
3. sleep-phase alterations;
4. neuropsychiatric disorders such as depression and dementia;
5. medical disorders and physical symptoms such as nocturia, pain limitation of mobility, and gastroesophageal reflux;
6. medications;
7. poor sleep hygiene practices and/or negative conditioning;
8. adverse environmental factors such as excessive heat or noise, or inadequate lighting that may encourage sleeping at times other than the major sleep period; and
9. psychosocial factors such as loneliness, inactivity, and boredom (Reynolds, in press; Reynolds, Kupfer, Hoch, & Sewitch, 1985c).

The primary aims of clinical assessment are to determine the duration of the patient's sleep-related complaint and the probable contributing factors. For example, transient sleep disturbances such as insomnia are usually situationally determined and last less than 3 weeks. More persistent disturbances, however, last longer than a month and are usually indicative of a more serious underlying medical or neuropsychiatric problem. The 1983 NIH Consensus Conference on Drugs and Insomnia emphasized that long-term insomnia of 1 month or longer requires special medical, physiological, and psychiatric evaluation (NIH, 1984).

Sources of diagnostic information should include interviews with both the elderly individual and bed partner. A sleep–wake log, kept daily over a minimum of a 2-week period should be completed in order to establish the distribution and quality of the individual's sleep during the 24-hr day. The log should also include daily information about naps, alcohol use, medications, and the timing of meals, exercise, social activities, and other indicators of social rhythms. A physical examination and portable screening (monitoring for cardiac arrhythmia, cassette tape of the patient's breathing during sleep, or body-temperature measurements to document circadian rhythm abnormalities) may also be indicated.

Sleep laboratory evaluation, polysomnography, can be useful for the elderly individual with a sleep disorder and is definitely indicated if one suspects sleep apnea, nocturnal myoclonus, or sleep-phase disturbance of irregularity. Laboratory evaluation should also be considered if routine treatment for persistent insomnia have not been effective.

V. Pharmacologic Treatment Approaches

An accurate diagnosis of the specific disorder and identification of its causes are the most important prerequisites for any type of medication treatment. For example, the treatment of insomnias secondary to arthritis pain, sleep apnea, depression, or transient situational disturbance are all quite different. Often, the most effective pharmacotherapy involves the *discontinuation* of a medication, or changing to medications that have less effect on sleeping and waking, rather than adding a new medication.

Insomnia secondary to medical problems is best addressed by optimizing treatment of the medical disorder. This may involve changing the timing of medications to maximize the patient's sleeping and waking function. For instance, L-dopa given at night to a patient with parkinsonism may worsen sleep continuity, while the same dose during the day would pose no problem. Adequate treatment of painful conditions can improve nighttime sleep continuity, but narcotic analgesics should be minimized, since they can disrupt sleep and cognitive function at higher doses.

Insomnia associated with depression can be effectively treated with antidepressant medications. Clinical trials have demonstrated the efficacy of drugs such as nortriptyline, imipramine, doxepin, trazodone, fluoxetine, and phenelzine in the treatment of late-life depression (Feighner & Cohn, 1985; Georgotas, McCue, & Cooper, 1989; Gerner, Estabrook, Sterner, & Jarvik, 1980; Reynolds *et al.*, 1989). Obviously, these drugs are associated with different sedative potential. In one study, approximately 45% of patients complained of daytime sedation with doxepin, while approximately 15% had insomnia with fluoxetine (Feighner & Cohn, 1985). Differences in daytime performance have also been demonstrated with different antidepressants in the elderly. For instance, daytime administration of 100 mg trazadone caused less impairment of vigilance and tracking performance than did 50 mg amitriptyline (Burns, Moskowitz, & Jaffe, 1986).

Medication treatment of insomnia associated with transient or situational disturbances is often appropriate, but caution is warranted in using benzodiazepine hypnotics for this purpose. Specific concerns relate to (1) the prolonged duration of action of hypnotics in the elderly; (2) the possibility of exacerbating sleep apnea; (3) effects on daytime alertness and performance; and (4) interactions with other medications that might potentiate the sedative effects of sleeping pills (Reynolds, Hoch, & Monk, 1989).

The duration of action and elimination half-lives of many drugs—including benzodiazepines and antidepressants—are prolonged in the elderly, and benzodiazepines may have half-lives well over 100 hr (Salzman, 1982). In part because of lower baseline scores, and in part because of altered pharmacokinetics, elderly subjects have significantly greater performance impairments than do younger subjects after ingestion of benzodiazepines (Heinrichs & Ghoneim, 1987; Pomara, Stanley, Block, Berchou, & Stanley, 1985). Healthy elderly subjects may also show worsening of sleep apnea with benzodiazepines (Guilleminault, Silvestri, Mondine, & Coburn, 1984).

In older patients who have *chronic* insomnia without specific medical or psychiatric causes, and who cannot function without maintenance sleep-promoting medication, the use of a low-dose sedating antidepressant, such as 25–50 mg trazodone or trimipramine, may be preferable to using a benzodiazepine on a long-term basis.

Antidepressants may retain their sedating effects longer than benzodiazepines, but with less tolerance. However, it is essential that orthostatic blood pressure changes during therapy be monitored. Such elderly patients often have minor affective disorders and/or low-grade sleep apnea that might be diminished by a tricyclic antidepressant (Reynolds, in press). Specific contraindications to benzodiazepine use in elders include heavy snoring, systemic illnesses that decrease the ability to eliminate the medication, the use of other medication with potentially dangerous interactions and alcohol, jobs requiring alertness, and suicidal risk. If a physician determines that a benzodiazepine is indicated for an elderly patient, then the smallest effective dose (one third to one half that prescribed in younger adults) should be established. The patient should be instructed to take the medication about 30 min before bedtime. Daytime consequences should be monitored. The patient should be followed regularly with an effort to limit the use of benzodiazepines to fewer than 20 doses per month over a period not exceeding 3 months. The patient and significant others should be encouraged to increase use of nonpharmacologic approaches to sleep disturbances (Reynolds, in press; Reynolds, Hoch, & Monk, 1989).

There is a paucity of literature regarding controlled pharmacotherapeutic trials on well-diagnosed samples of elderly patients with dementia or organic brain syndromes (Reynolds, Hoch, & Monk, 1989); of the available studies, none used sleep laboratory or objective methods for assessment of drug effects (Linnoila & Viukari, 1976; Linnoila, Viukari, Lamminsivu, 1980; Linnolia, Viukari, Numminen, 1980a; Schubert, 1984; Strotsky, Cole, Tang, 1971; Viukari, Linnoila, & Aalto, 1978), using nursing observations of sleep-onset time, sleep duration, and number and duration of arousals during the night as the dependent measures. The studies investigated the effects of several different psychoactive agents on sleep including butabarbital, nitrazepam, thioridazine, flurazepam, chloral hydrate, lorazepam, oxazepam, temazepam, and hydroxyzine. With the exception of thioridazine, all compounds were associated with significant and negative side-effects, such as increased daytime sleepiness, drug-withdrawal insomnia, and diminished capability for performing activities of daily living.

If clinical evaluation confirms that periodic leg jerks during sleep are a major factor in the elderly patient's insomnia, then the use of a short-acting benzodiazepine may well be helpful for the patient. Benzodiazepine therapy does not suppress myoclonus activity; it overrides the arousal effects of the periodic leg jerks, allowing maintenance of sleep continuity (Reynolds, in press).

In cases of sleep disturbance related to sleep apnea, the decision whether to treat and, if so, how to intervene is complex and depends on the severity and type of apnea as well as the physiological and behavioral sequelae. Interventions include behavioral (weight loss, training for the patient to sleep on the side), prosthetic (continuous positive airway pressure), pharmacologic (acetazolamide), and surgical (uvulopalatopharyngoplasty or tracheotomy) (Reynolds, in press).

VI. Nonpharmacologic Treatment Approaches

One of the most important interventions is to teach elderly individuals and their families that some sleep disturbances may be an unavoidable consequence of aging. That is, their ability to sleep diminishes with age. Reinforcement of a regular sleep–wake rhythm is essential in order to combat the age-related tendency to lose the consolidation of sleep and to develop a polyphasic sleep–wake cycle. In practical terms, the elderly person should be encouraged to maintain temporal control by going to bed only when sleepy, by getting up at the same time each morning, by reducing naps to no more than 30 min daily, and by limiting nightly time in bed to 7 hr. Hoch and colleagues (1987) noted that elderly persons who habitually restrict themselves to $6\frac{1}{2}$ to 7 hr in bed at night tend to have sleep continuity superior to that observed in persons who remain in bed 8 or more hr and whose lives are generally less active and less structured. The elderly patient should also be taught to maintain stimulus control by avoidance of the bedroom for activities not conducive to sleep. The use of such stimulus control will serve to keep the bed as a powerful stimulus to sleep. Alcohol and caffeine should be avoided in the evening hours. In practice, strengthening temporal and stimulus control, together with education and reassurance, help to give the elderly individual a sense of increased control and diminish the need for sedating nighttime medications.

VII. Conclusions

Late-life sleep disturbances are chronic and intermittent problems probably associated with medical and psychiatric conditions. It is an essential challenge to develop and test effective nonpharmacologic interventions such as the use of bright light to affect the human circadian pacemaker (Czeisler *et al.*, 1986). It is also necessary to conduct controlled pharmacological studies to find safe and effective hypnotic drugs for elderly.

References

Ancoli-Israel, S. (1989). Epidemiology of sleep disorders. *Clinics in Geriatric Medicine, 5*, 347–362.

Ancoli-Israel, S., & Kripke, D. F. (in press). Epidemiology of sleep apnea in the elderly. *Sleep.*

Ancoli-Israel, S., & Kripke, D. F. (1988). Epidemiology of sleep apnea in three populations of elderly. *9th European Congress Sleep Research Program Abstracts, 162.*

Ancoli-Israel, S., Kripke, D. F., & Mason, W. J. (1984). Obstructive sleep apnea in a senior population. *Sleep Research, 13,* 130.

Ancoli-Israel, S., Kripke, D. F., & Mason, W. (1987). Characteristics of obstructive and central sleep apnea in the elderly: An interim report. *Biological Psychiatry, 22,* 741–750.

Ancoli-Israel, S., Parker, L., & Butters, N. (1985). Respiratory disturbances during sleep and mental status: Preliminary results from a TNH. *The Gerontologist, 25,* 6.

Ancoli-Israel, S., Kripke, D. F., Mason, W., & Messin, S. (1981). Sleep apnea and nocturnal myoclonus in a senior population. *Sleep, 4,* 349–358.

Ancoli-Israel, S., Parker, L., Sinall, R., Mason, W., & Kripke, D. F. (1989). Sleep fragmentation in patients from a nursing home. *Journal of Gerontology, 44,* M18–21.

Berry, D. T. R., & Phillips, B. A. (1988). Sleep-disordered breathing in the elderly: Review and methodological comment. *Clinical Psychological Review, 8,* 101–120.

Bliwise, D. L., Beveer, W. C., Bliwise, N. G., & Dement, W. C. (1987). Systematic behavioral observation of sleep–wakefulness in skilled care nursing home. *Sleep Research, 16,* 170.

Belloc, N. B. (1973). Relationship of health practices and mortality. *Preventive Medicine, 2,* 67–81.

Brendel, D. H., Reynolds, C. F., Jennings, J. R., Hoch, C. C., Monk, T. H., Berman, S. R., Hall, F. T., Buysse, D. J., Kupfer, D. J. (1990). Sleep stage physiology, mood, and vigilance responses to total sleep deprivation in healthy eighty-year-olds and twenty-year-olds *Psychophysiology, 27,* 677–686.

Brock, M. A. (1985). Biological clocks and aging. *Review of Biological Research in Aging, 2,* 445–462.

Bureau of the Census. (1986). *Age structure of the U.S. population in the 21st century,* (SB-1-86). Washington, DC: U.S. Government Printing Office.

Burns, M., Moskowitz, H., & Jaffe, J. (1986). A comparison of the effects of trazodone and amitriptyline on skills performance by geriatric subjects. *Journal of Clinical Psychiatry, 47,* 252–254.

Buysse, D. J., & Reynolds, C. F. (1990). Insomnia. In M. J. Thorpy (Ed.), *Handbook of Sleep Disorders* (pp. 373–431). New York: Marcel Dekker.

Buysse, D. J., Reynolds, C. F., Kupfer, D. J., Houck, P. R., Hoch, C. C., Stack, J. A., and Berman, S. R. (1988). EEG sleep in depressive pseudodementia. *Archives of General Psychiatry, 45,* 568–575.

Buysse, D. J., Reynolds, C. F., Monk, T. H., Berman, S. R., & Kupfer, D. J. (1989). The Pittsburgh sleep quality index: A new instrument for psychiatric practice and research. *Psychiatry Research, 28,* 193–213.

Carskadon, M. A., & Dement, W. C. (1981). Cumulative effects of sleep restriction on daytime sleepiness. *Psychophysiology, 18,* 107–122.

Carskadon, M. A., Brown, E. D., & Dement, W. C. (1982). Sleep fragmentation in the elderly: Relationship to daytime sleep tendency. *Neurobiology of Aging, 3,* 321–327.

Carskadon, M. A., van den Hoed, J., & Dement, W. C. (1980). Sleep and daytime sleepiness in the elderly. *Journal of Geriatric Psychiatry, 13,* 135–151.

Clayton, P. J., Halikas, J. A., & Mauria, W. L. (1972). The depression of widowhood. *British Journal of Psychiatry, 120,* 71–78.

Coleman, R. M. (1982). Periodic movements in sleep (nocturnal myoclonus) and restless legs syndrome. In C. Guilleminault & W. C. Dement (Eds.), *Sleeping and waking disorders: Indications and techniques* (pp. 155–182). Menlo Park, CA: Addison-Wesley.

Czeisler, C. A., Allan, J. S., Strogatz, S. H., Ronda, J. M., Sanchez, R., Rios, D., Freitag, W. Q., Richardson, G. S., & Kronauer, R. E. (1986). Bright light resets the human circadian pacemaker independent of the timing of the sleep–wake cycle. *Science, 233,* 667–671.

Dement, W. C., Miles, L. E., & Carskadon, M. A. (1982). "White paper" on sleep and aging. *Journal of the American Geriatrics Society, 8,* 20–29.

Dickel, M. J., Sassin, J., & Mosko, S. (1986). Sleep disorders in an aged population: Preliminary findings of a longitudinal study. *Sleep Research, 15,* 116.

Evans, L. K. (1987). Sundown syndrome in institutionalized elderly. *Journal of the American Geriatric Society, 35,* 101–108.

Feighner, J. P., & Cohn, J. B. (1985). Double-blind comparative trials of fluoxetine and doxepin in geriatric patients with major depressive disorder. *Journal of Clinical Psychiatry, 46,* 20–25.

Feinberg, I. (1974). Changes in sleep-cycle pattern with age. *Journal of Psychiatric Research, 10,* 283–306.

Feinberg, I., Koresko, R. L., & Heller, N. (1974). EEG sleep patterns as a function of normal and pathologic aging in men. *Journal of Psychiatric Research, 10,* 283–306.

Ford, D. E., & Kamerow, D. B. (1989). Epidemiological studies of sleep disturbances and psychiatric disorders: An opportunity for prevention? *Journal of the American Medical Association, 262,* 1479–1484.

Frommlet, M., Prinz, P., Vitiello, M. V., Ries, R., & Williams, D. (1986). Sleep hypoxemia and apnea are elevated in females with mild Alzheimer's disease. *Sleep Research, 15,* 189.

Georgotas, A., McCue, R. E., & Cooper,. T. B. (1989). A placebo-controlled comparison of nortriptyline and phenelzine in maintenance therapy of elderly depressed patients. *Archives of General Psychiatry, 46,* 783–786.

Gerner, T., Estabrook, W., Steven, J., & Jarvik, L. (1980). Treatment of geriatric depression with trazodone, imipramine, and placebo: A double-blind study. *Journal of Clinical Psychiatry, 41.* 216–220.

Gillin, J. C., Duncan, W. C., Murphy, D. L., Post, R. M., Wehr, T. A., Goodwin, F. K., Wyatt, R. J., & Bunney, W. E. (1981). Age-related changes in sleep in depressed and normal subjects. *Psychiatry Research, 4,* 73–78.

Guilleminault, C., Connolly, S. J., & Winkle, R. A. (1983). Cardiac arrhythmia and conduction disturbances during sleep in 400 patients with sleep apnea syndrome. *American Journal of Cardiology, 52,* 490–494.

Guilleminault, C., Silvestri, R., Mondini, S., & Coburn, S. (1984). Aging and sleep apnea: Action of benzodiazepine, acetazolamide, alcohol, and sleep deprivation in a healthy elderly group. *Journal of Gerontology, 39,* 655–661.

Hayashi, Y., & Endo, S. (1982). All-night sleep polygraphic recording of healthy aged persons: Rem and slow-wave sleep. *Sleep, 5,* 277–283.

Hildebrandt, G., & Stratmann, I. (1979). Circadian system response to night work in relation to the individual circadian phase position. *International Archives of Occupational and Environmental Health, 43,* 73–83.

Hinrichs, J. V., & Ghoneim, M. M. (1987). Diazepam, behavior, and aging: Increased sensitivity or lower baseline performance? *Psychopharmacology, 92,* 100–105.

Hirano, A., & Zimmerman, H. M. (1962). Alzheimer's neurofibrillary changes. *Archives of Neurology, 7,* 227–242.

Hoch, C. C., Buysse, D. J., & Reynolds, C. F. (1989). Cleep and depression in late life. *Clinics in Geriatric Medicine, 5,* 259–274.

Hoch, C. C., Reynolds, C. F., Kupfer, D. J., & Berman, S. R. (1988). Laboratory note: Stability of EEG sleep and sleep quality in healthy seniors. *Sleep, 11,* 521–527.

Hoch, C. C., Reynolds, C. F., Houck, P. R., Hall, F., Berman, S. R., Buysse, D. J., Dahl, R. E., & Kupfer, D. J. (1989). Predicting mortality in mixed depression and dementia using EEG sleep variables. *The Journal of Neuropsychiatry and Clincial Neurosciences, 1,* 366–371.

Hoch, C. C., Reynolds, C. F., Kupfer, D. J., Berman, S. R., Houck, P. R., & Stack, J. A. (1987). Empirical note: Self-report versus recorded sleep in healthy seniors. *Psychophysiology, 24,* 293–299.

Hoch, C. C., Reynolds, C. F., Kupfer, D. J., Houck, P. R., Berman, S. R., & Stack, J. A. (1986). Sleep-disordered breathing in normal and pathologic aging. *Journal of Clinical Psychiatry, 47,* 499–503.

Hoch, C. C., Reynolds, C. F., Kupfer, D. J., Houck, P. R., Berman, S. R., & Stack, J. A. (1987). The superior sleep of healthy elderly nuns. *International Journal of Aging and Human Development, 25,* 1–8.

Hoch, C. C., Reynolds, C. F., Nebes, R. D., Kupfer, D. J., Berman, S. R., & Campbell, D. W. (1989). Clinical significance of sleep-disordered breathing in Alzheimer's disease: Preliminary data. *Journal of the American Geriatrics Society, 37,* 138–144.

Jacobs, D., Ancoli-Israel, S., & Parker, L. (in press). Twenty-four-hour sleep–wake patterns in a nursing home population. *Psychological Aging.*

Kahn, E., & Fischer, C. (1969). The sleep characteristics of the normal aged male. *Journal of Nervous and Mental Disorders, 148,* 477–494.

Kahn, E., Fischer, C., & Lieberman, L. (1970). Sleep characteristics of the normal aged female. *Comprehensive Psychiatry, 11,* 274–278.

Kales, A., Bixler, E. O., & Cadieux, D. W. (1984). Sleep apnea in a hypertensive population. *Lancet, ii,* 1005–1008.

Kales, A., Wilson, T., & Kales, J. D. (1967). Measurement of all-night sleep in normal elderly persons: Effects of aging. *Journal of the American Geriatric Association, 15,* 405–410.

Kales, A., Bixler, E. O., Soldatos, C. R., Vela-Bueno, A., Caldwell, A. B., & Cadieux, R. J. (1982). Role of sleep apnea and nocturnal myoclonus. *Psychosomatics, 23,* 589–600.

Koskenvuo, M., Kaprio, J., Partinen, M., Langinvainio, H., Sarna, S., & Heikkila, K. (1985). Snoring as a risk factor for hypertension and angina pectoris. *Lancet, 1,* 893–896.

Koskenvuo, M., Kaprio, J., Telaviki, T., Partinen, M., Heikkila, K., & Sarina, S. (1987). Snoring as a risk factor for ischemic heart disease and stroke in men. *British Medical Journal, 294,* 16–19.

Kryger, M. H., Roth, T., & Dement, W. C. (1989). *Principles and practice of sleep medicine.* Philadelphia: Saunders.

Kupfer, D. J., Frank, E., & Ehlers, C. L. (1989). EEG sleep in young depressions: First and second night effects. *Biological Psychiatry, 25,* 87–97.

Kupfer, D. J., Reynolds, C. F., Ulrich, R. F., Shaw, D. H., & Coble, P. A. (1982). Sleep, depression, and aging. *Neurobiology of Aging: Experimental and Clinical Research, 3,* 351–360.

Kripke, D. F. (1990). Periodic movements in sleep: Clinical consequences and treatment. In National Institute of Health (Ed.) *The treatment of sleep disorders of older people* (pp. 69–71). Washington, D.C.: U.S. Government Printing Office.

Kripke, D. F., & Ancoli-Israel, S. (1983). Epidemiology of sleep apnea among the aged: Is sleep apnea a fatal disorder? In C. Guilleminault & E. Lugaresi (Eds.), *Sleep/wake disorders: Natural history, epidemiology and long-term evolution* (pp. 137–142). New York: Raven Press.

Kripke, D. F., Ancoli-Israel, S., & Mason, W. (1983). Sleep-related mortality and morbidity in the aged. In M. H. Chase & E. D. Weitzman (Eds.), *Sleep disorders: Basic and Clinical Research* (pp. 415–429). New York: Spectrum Publications.

Kripke, D. F., Ancoli-Israel, S., & Mason, W. J. (1986). Sleep apnea, long and short sleep. *Sleep Research, 15,* 139.

Kripke, D. F., Simons, R. N., Garfinkel, L., & Hammond, E. D. (1979). Short and long sleep and sleeping pills: Is increased mortality associated? *Archives of General Psychiatry, 36,* 103–106.

Lavie, P., Rachamin, B., & Rubin, A. E. (1984). Prevalence of sleep apnea syndrome among patients with essential hypertension. *American Heart Journal, 108,* 373–376.

Linnoila, M., & Viukari, M. (1976). Efficacy and side-effects of nitrazepam and thioridazine as sleeping aids in psychogeriatric inpatients. *British Journal of Psychiatry, 128,* 566–569.

Linnoila, M., Viukari, M., Lamminsevu, U., & Auvinen, J. (1980). Efficacy and side-effects of lorazepam, oxazepam, and temazepam as sleeping aids in psychogeriatric inpatients. *International Pharmacopsychiatry, 15,* 129–135.

Linnoila, M., Viukari, M., Numminen, A., & Auvinen, J. (1980). Efficacy and side-effects of chloralhydrate and tryptophan as sleeping aids in psychogeriatric patients. *International Pharmacopsychiatry, 15,* 124–128.

Lugaresi, E., Coccagna, G., & Cirignotta, F. (1978). Snoring and its clinical implications. In C. Guilleminault & W. C. Dement (Eds.), *Sleep apnea syndromes* (pp. 13–22). New York: Alan R. Liss.

Lugaresi, E., Coccagna, G., Farneti, P., Mantobani, M., & Cirignotta, F. (1975). Snoring. *Electroencephalography and Clinical Neurophysiology, 39,* 59–64.

Mahler, B. (1981). The meaning of health for all by the year 2000. *World Health Forum, 2*(1), 5–22.

Miles, L. E., & Dement, W. C. (1980a). Sleep–wake complaints of elderly men and women. *Sleep, 3,* 121–129.

Miles, L. E., & Dement, W. C. (1980b). Sleep and aging. *Sleep, 3,* 119–120.

Mitler, M. M., Hajdukovic, R. M., & Shafer, R. (1987). When people die; cause of death versus time of death. *American Journal of Medicine, 82,* 266–274.

Moldolsky, H., Goldstein, R., McNicholas, W. T., Lue, F., Zamel, N., & Phillipson, E. A. (1983). Disordered breathing during sleep and overnight intellectual deterioration in patients with pathological aging. In C. Guilleminualt & E. Lugaresi (Eds.), *Sleep/Wake Disorders: Natural History, Epidemiology, and Long-Term Evolution* (pp 143–150). New York: Raven Press.

Mondini, S., Zucconi, M., Cirignotto, F., Umberto, A., Lenzi, L., Zauli, C., & Lugaresi, E. (1983). Snoring as a risk factor for cardiac and circulatory problems: An epidemiologic study. In C. Guilleminault & E. Lugaresi (Eds.), *Sleep/Wake Disorders: Natural History, Epidemiology, and Long-Term Evolution* (pp. 96–106). New York: Raven Press.

Monk, T. H. (1989). Circadian rhythm. In T. Roth & T. A. Roehrs (Eds.), *Clinics in Geriatric Medicine, 5,* 331–346.

Mosko, S. S., Deckel, M. J., Paul, T., Dhillon, S., Ghanim, A., & Sassin, J. F. (1988). Sleep apnea and sleep-related periodic leg movements in community resident seniors. *Journal of the American Geriatrics Society, 36,* 502–508.

Murrell, S. A., & Himmelfarb, S. (1989). Effects of attachment bereavement and pre-event condition on subsequent depressive symptoms in older adults. *Psychology of Aging, 4,* 166–172.

Murrell, S. A., Norris, F., & Hutchins, G. (1984). Distribution and desirability of life events in older adults: Population and policy implications. *Journal of Community Psychology, 12,* 301–311.

National Institutes of Health (1984). Consensus development conference: Drugs and insomnia—the use of medications to promote sleep. *Journal of American Medical Association, 251,* 2410–2414.

National Institutes of Health. (1990). *The treatment of sleep disorders of older people.* Washington, DC: U.S. Government Printing Office.

Okudaira, N., Fukuda, H., Nishihara, K., Ohtani, K., Endo, S., & Torii, S. (1983). Sleep apnea and nocturnal myoclonus in elderly persons in Vilcabamba, Ecuador. *Journal of Gerontology, 38,* 436–438.

Pomara, N., Stanley, B., Block, R., Berchou, R. C., Greenblatt, I. J., Newton, R. E., & Gerson, S. (1985). Increased sensitivity of the elderly to the central depressant effects of diazepam. *Journal of Clinical Psychiatry, 46,* 185–187.

Prinz, P. (1977). Sleep patterns in the healthy aged: Relationships with intellectual functions. *Journal of Gerontology, 32,* 179–180.

Prinz, P. N., Peskund, E. R., Vitaliano, P. P., Raskind, M. A., Eisdorfer, C., Zemuznikov, N., & Gerber, C. J. (1982). Changes in the sleeping and waking EEGs of nondemented and demented elderly subjects. *Journal of the American Geriatrics Society, 30,* 86–93.

Rabin, D. I. (1985). *Waxing of the gray, waning of the green, in American aging–health in an older society.* Washington, D.C.: National Acdemy Press.

Rabins, P. V., Mace, N. L., & Lucas, M. J. (1982). The impact of dementia on the family. *Journal of the American Medical Association, 248,* 333–335.

Regestein, Q. R., & Morris, J. (1987). Daily sleep patterns observed among institutionalized elderly. *Journal of the American Geriatrics Society, 35,* 767–772.

Reynolds, C. F. (in press). Sleep disorders of late life. In J. Sadavoy, L. Lazarus, & L. Jarvik (Eds.), *Comprehensive review of geriatric psychiatry.* New York: American Psychiatric Press.

Reynolds, C. F. (1990). Subjective and objective sleep complaints in late life. In National Institutes of Health (Ed.), *The treatment of sleep disorders of older people.* Washington, DC: U.S. Government Printing Office.

Reynolds, C. F., Coble, P. A., Black, R. S., Holzer, B., Carroll, R., & Kupfer, D. J. (1982). Sleep disturbances in a series of elderly patients: Polysomnographic findings. *Journal of the American Geriatrics Society, 23,* 164–170.

Reynolds, C. F., Hoch, C. C., & Monk, T. H. (1989). Sleep and chronobiologic disturbances in late life. In E. W. Busse & D. G. Blazer (Eds.), *Geriatric psychiatry* (pp. 475–488). Washington, DC: American Psychiatric Press.

Reynolds, C. F., Kupfer, D. J., Hoch, C. C., & Sewitch, D. E. (1985c). Sleeping pills for the elderly: Are they ever justified? *Journal of Clinical Psychiatry, 46,* 9–12.

Reynolds, C. F., Kupfer, D. J., Hoch, C. C., Stack, J. A., Houck, P. R., Berman, S. R. (1986). Sleep deprivation in healthy elderly men and women: Effects on mood and on sleep during recovery. *Sleep, 9,* 492–501.

Reynolds, C. F., Kupfer, D. J., Houck, P. R., Hoch, C. C., Stack, J. A., Berman, S. R., & Zimmer, B. (1988). Reliable discrimination of elderly depressed and demented patients by EEG sleep data. *Archives of General Psychiatry, 45,* 258–264.

Reynolds, C. F., Kupfer, D. J., Taska, L. S., Hoch, C. C., Sewitch, D. E., & Spiker, D. G. (1985a). The sleep of healthy seniors: A revisit. *Sleep, 1,* 20–29.

Reynolds, C. F., Kupfer, D. J., Taska, L. S., Hoch, C. C., Sewitch, D. E., Restifo, K., Spiker, D. G., Zimmer,

B., Marin, R. S., Nelson, J., Martin, D., & Morcyz, R. (1985b). Sleep apnea in Alzheimer's dementia: Correlation with mental deterioration. *Journal of Clinical Psychiatry, 46,* 257–261.

Reynolds, C. F., Perel, J. M., Frank, E., Imber, S., Thornton, J., Morycz, R. K., Cornes, C., & Kupfer, D. J. (1989). Open-trial maintenance pharmacotherapy in late-life depression: Survival analysis. *Psychiatry Research, 27,* 225–231.

Richardson, G. S., Carskadon, M. A., & Flagg, W. (1978). Excessive daytime sleepiness in man: Multiple sleep latency measurement in narcoleptic and control subjects. *Electroencephalography and Clinical Neurophysiology, 45,* 621–627.

Rodin, J., McAvay, G., & Timko, C. (1988). A longitudinal study of depressed mood and sleep disturbances in elderly adults. *Journal of Psychological Science, 43,* 45–52.

Salzman, C. (1982). Key concepts in geriatric psychopharmacology. *Psychiatric Clinics of North America, 5,* 181–191.

Sanford, J. R. A. (1975). Tolerance of debility in elderly dependents by supporter at home: Its significance for hospital practice. *British Medical Journal, 3,* 471–473.

Schubert, D. S. P. (1984). Hydroxyzine for acute treatment of agitation and insomnia in organic mental disorder. *Psychiatric Journal of the University of Ottawa, 9,* 59–60.

Smallwood, R. G., Vitiello, M. V., Giblin, E. C., & Prinz, P. (1983). Sleep apnea: Relationship to age, sex, and Alzheimer's dementia. *Sleep, 6,* 16–22.

Smirne, S., Franceschi, M., Bareggi, S. R., Comi, G., Mariani, E., & Mastrangelo, M. (1981). Sleep apneas in Alzheimer's disease. In W. P. Koella (Ed.), *1980 European Congress sleep research* (pp. 422–444). Basel: Karger.

Smolensky, M., Halberg, F., & Sargent, F. I. (1972). Chronobiology of the late-life sequence. In I. S. Tokyo (Ed.), *Advances in Climatic Physiology* (pp. 281–318). New York: Springer Verlag.

Speilman, A., Saskin, P., & Thorpy, M. (1983). Sleep restriction treatment for insomnia. *Sleep Research, 12,* 286.

Stotsky, B. A., Cole, J. O., Tang, Y. T. & Gahm, I. G. (1971). Sodium butabarbital as a hypnotic agent for age to psychiatric patients with sleep disorders. *Journal of the American Geriatrics Society, 19,* 860–870.

Tune, G. S. (1968). Sleep and wakefulness in normal adults. *British Medical Journal, 2,* 269–271.

Ulrich, R. F., Shaw, D. H., & Kupfer, D. J. (1980). Effects of aging on EEG sleep in depression. *Sleep, 3,* 31–40.

Vitiello, M. V., & Prinz, P. N. (1989). Alzheimer's disease: Sleep and sleep–wake patterns. *Clinics in Geriatric Medicine, 5,* 289–299.

Vitiello, M. V., Bokan, J. A., Kukull, W. A., Muniz, R. L., Smallwood, R. G., & Prinz, P. N. (1984). Rapid-eye-movement sleep measures of Alzheimer's dementia patients and optimally healthy individuals. *Biological Psychiatry, 19,* 721–734.

Vitiello, M. V., Smallwood, R. G., Avery, D. H., Pascualy, R. A., Martin, D. C., & Prinz, P. N. (1986). Circadian temperature rhythms in young adult and aged men. *Neurobiology of Aging, 7,* 97–100.

Viukari, M., Linnoila, M., & Aalto, U. (1978). Efficacy and side-efects of flurazepam, fosazepam, and nitrazepam as sleeping aids, in psychogeriatric patients. *Acta Psychiatrica Scandinavica, 57,* 27–35.

Webb, W. B. (1989). Age-related changes in sleep. *Clinics in Geriatric Medicine, 5,* 275–287.

Webb, W. B., & Swinburne, H. (1971). An observational study of sleep in the aged. *Perceptive Motor Skills, 32,* 895–898.

Weitzman, E. D., Moline, M. L., Czeisler, C. A., & Zimmerman, J. C. (1982). Chronobiology of aging: Temperature, sleep–wake rhythms, and entrainment. *Neurobiology of Aging, 3,* 299–309.

Williams, R. L., Karacan, I., & Hursch, C. J. (1974). *EEG of human sleep: Clinical applications,* New York: Wiley and Sons.

Zepelin, H. (1983). Normal age-related change in sleep. In M. Chase & E. Weitzman (Eds.), *Sleep disorders: Basic and clinical research* (pp. 431–444). New York: Spectrum.

Aging in Persons with Developmental Disabilities ___

Marsha Mailick Seltzer

I. Introduction
II. Population Characteristics and Demographic Trends
    A. Population Size
    B. Life Expectancy
    C. The Aging of Cohorts
III. Age-Related Changes
    A. Cognitive Abilities
    B. Functional Abilities
    C. Health and Mental Health Status
IV. Formal and Informal Supports
    A. Formal Supports
    B. Family and Informal Supports
V. Summary
VI. The Need for Future Research: The Mental Health
    of Older Persons with Developmental Disabilities
    References

I. Introduction ___

At the present time, a considerably larger number of persons with developmental disabilities live to old age than was the case in the past. As a result, researchers and policy analysts have become increasingly interested in how the aging process is manifested in persons with developmental disabilities. A body of knowledge about this population has only recently begun to coalesce. It is clear, however, that persons with developmental disabilities will become a growing proportion of the general aging population (Janicki & Wisniewski, 1985). Therefore, it is necessary for gerontologists to develop an understanding of the characteristics of this subgroup of the aging population, their patterns of mortality and morbidity, and their needs for formal and informal support.

The purpose of this chapter is to review the literature about aging in persons with developmental disabilities in order to set the stage for future research. First, consideration will be given to the demographic trends that characterize this group, including its size, life expectancy data, and future population projections. Second, a description will be presented of age-related changes characteristic of older persons with developmental disabilities, including changes in functional and cognitive abilities, and health and mental health status. Third, this group's need for support will be examined, with discussion of formal service-utilization patterns and family and other informal supports. Last, the chapter will present recommendations for future research. Throughout, special attention will be focused on older persons with Down syndrome, as these individuals have an increased risk for, and earlier onset of, Alzheimer's disease. Before dealing with these issues, however, it is necessary to define the basic terms that will be used throughout this chapter, including developmental disabilities and aging.

A developmental disability, as defined by PL 95-602 (the Rehabilitation, Comprehensive Services, and Developmental Disabilities Amendments of 1978), is a severe chronic disability of a person, that

1. is attributable to a mental or physical impairment or combination of mental and physical impairments;
2. is manifested before the person attains age 22;
3. is likely to continue indefinitely;
4. results in substantial functional limitations in three or more of the following areas of major life activity: (a) self-care, (b) receptive and expressive language, (c) learning, (d) mobility, (e) self-direction, (f) capacity for independent living, and (g) economic self-sufficiency; and
5. reflects the person's need for a combination and sequence of special, interdisciplinary, or generic care, treatment, or other services that are of lifelong or extended duration and are individually planned and coordinated.

Developmental disabilities are thus defined on the basis of the functional characteristics of the affected individual rather than on the basis of the individual's categorical diagnosis. Nevertheless, the most commonly included categories of developmental disability are mental retardation, cerebral palsy, epilepsy, and autism.

The largest subgroup of the population with developmental disabilities consists of persons with mental retardation. Most available knowledge about older persons with developmental disabilities was generated from research on older persons with mental retardation. According to the American Association on Mental Retardation, mental retardation is defined as significantly subaverage general intellectual functioning (an IQ score of approximately 70 or below), existing concurrently with deficits in adaptive behavior, and manifested during the developmental period (before age 18) (Grossman, 1983). The most prevalent known cause of mental retardation is Down syndrome, a chromosomal anomaly in which there is an extra 21st chromosome.

The definition of *old age* in the general population has posed conceptual and methodological challenges for gerontologists for several decades. While it is generally the case that old age is defined in years (Siegel, 1980), there is variation in the specific age used to define the onset of this stage of life—age 60, 62, or 65. The *young-old* have been differentiated from the *old-old* (Streib, 1983), although the age that separates these two groups has not been consistent from study to study. Some gerontologists have developed non-age–based functional definitions for old age (Birren, 1959; Eisdorfer, 1983), stressing the different trajectories of biological, psychological, and social aging.

The application of these various definitions of old age to the population with developmental disabilities has been even more challenging than their application to the general population. Definitions based on age alone are problematic because, as will be described below, some subgroups of the population with developmental disabilities, notably those with Down's syndrome, age prematurely, with age-related declines observable by age 40 or 50 (Evenhuis, 1990; Zigman, Schupf, Lubin, & Silverman, 1987). Functional definitions of aging are especially problematic for this population, because the definition of developmental disabilities includes functional limitations, which would make a functional approach to defining the onset of old age in this group redundant with the group's basic definition. Most studies of older persons with developmental disabilities have used age 55 as the lower age boundary in an attempt to include at least some of those of those who age prematurely (see Seltzer & Krauss, 1987, for a review of literature about this issue).

The definition of old age in persons with developmental disabilities remains an unresolved issue. From a policy perspective, it has been argued that age 60 should be used in order to be consistent with the Older Americans Act (Rose & Janicki, 1986). From a clinical perspective, it has been argued that a single chronological age cut-off is not useful, in that there is so much heterogeneity in the point of onset of old age in this population (Cotten & Spirrison, 1986). From a research perspective, there is a need to measure age-related changes in cognitive, functional, and health characteristics for each subgroup of the population with developmental disabilities in order to reach an empirically sound understanding of the process of aging in this group (Seltzer & Krauss, 1987).

II. Population Characteristics and Demographic Trends

A. Population Size

At the present time, the true size of the older population with development disabilities is not known. Several factors make this population difficult to count. First, there is the unresolved problem of defining the lower age boundary of this population, as described above. Second, all counts of this population are based on those older persons with developmental disabilities who are known to the formal mental retardation–developmental disabilities (MR–DD) service system in each state (Janicki, Knox, & Jacobson, 1985). These individuals (age 55+) total about 200,000 persons nationally (Jacobson, Sutton, & Janicki, 1985). However, individuals who have not been recipients of formal MR–DD services in adulthood or who receive generic (non-MR–DD) services are generally not identified in population enumerations of this group (Krauss, 1988). A third problem in determining the size of this population is that individuals with developmental disabilities other than mental retardation (e.g., cerebral palsy or epilepsy) are less consistently counted in some states than are those with mental retardation.

Some efforts have been made to estimate (rather than to count) the size of the older population with developmental disabilities on the basis of prevalence rates. However, age-adjusted prevalence rates are not available for either the population with developmental disabilities as a whole or for the various diagnostic groups included within the population with developmental disabilities. To illustrate with the example of mental retardation, in childhood about 3% of the population is diagnosed as having mental retardation, while in adulthood, the prevalence is believed to be only about 1% (Seltzer, 1989). This decrease is believed to occur because there are fewer intellectual challenges encountered in adulthood than during school years. Many adults with mild mental retardation do not have a continual need for formal services (Edgerton, 1988). In old age, some persons who were classified as having mental retardation during their childhood, but who were not labeled in adulthood may reenter the formal service-delivery system, if they become frail or socially isolated.

Two additional factors have an effect on the size of the older population with developmental disabilities. The first of these factors is the life expectancy of the population, while the other pertains to the aging of cohorts of different sizes.

B. Life Expectancy

As noted earlier, there has been a marked increase in the life expectancy of persons with developmental disabilities (Janicki, 1988). This increase is owing, in part, to new medical technology and the improved health care provided to this population. For example, fully one third of all children born with Down syndrome have congenital heart defects (Pueschel, 1987). In the past, these children generally died at a young age. However, because of improved surgical procedures and changed social attitudes toward medical intervention with persons with disabilities, the length of life of these individuals has been extended considerably.

Very little current data are available about the life expectancy of persons with each of the various causes of developmental disabilities. It is believed that individuals with an organic basis of their disability and severe to profound retardation have a shorter life expectancy than does the general population, but the differences in life expectancy among the specific disorders (e.g., chromosomal anomalies versus metabolic disorders versus teratogenic effects, etc.) have not been adequately described. However, those who have no organic basis for their disability and mild or moderate retardation are believed to have a life expectancy that is close or equal to that of the general population (Lubin & Kiely, 1985).

Eyman, Call, and White (1989) have studied the life expectancy of persons with mental retardation in California. They report that the death rate in this population is curvilinear, with the highest death rates occurring before age 5 and after age 55. Those with severe or profound retardation have a higher death rate at all ages than those with mild or moderate retardation.

Persons with Down syndrome have a reduced life expectancy as compared with those with other causes for their retardation. Those with this diagnosis can be divided into two groups with respect to their life expectancy (Eyman, Call, & White, 1991). Those who have no ambulation or feeding skills have a short life expectancy—usually less than 30 years. However, most persons with Down syndrome are ambulatory and can feed themselves; these individuals have a life expectancy of about 50 or 55 years. A primary reason that the latter group has a shorter lifespan than the general population is their increased risk for Alzheimer's disease (Wisniewski & Merz, 1985). Nearly 100% of persons with Down syndrome who survive to the age of 35 manifest the neuropathology of Alzheimer's (detected upon autopsy) (Lott & Lai, 1982), although only about 45% manifest the behavioral symptoms (Thase, 1982). Among middle-aged adults with Down syndrome, the risk of the behavioral symptoms of Alzheimer's appears to increase with advancing age.

C. The Aging of Cohorts

In addition to the effects of increased longevity, the increase in the size of the older population with developmental disabilities is attributed to the aging of larger cohorts than in the past. In particular, the members of the baby-boom generation with developmental disabilities are currently approaching midlife and will reach old age during the beginning of the next century (Baird & Sadovnick, 1985). Owing to the large size of this cohort, the population of older persons with developmental disabilities will increase. In addition, because the most dramatic reductions in mortality that have been made during the past two decades have been reductions in infant mortality (Lubin & Kiely, 1985), another large increase in the size of the older population with developmental disabilities can be expected when this cohort reaches old age.

To summarize, while the size of the population of older persons with developmental disabilities is difficult to estimate precisely, we do know that two interrelated trends have a continuing and dynamic effect on it: (1) changes in the life expectancy of various subgroups of the population with developmental disabilities, and (2) changes in the size of successive cohorts with developmental disabilities. There is a great need to develop an understanding of age-specific prevalence rates for the major subgroups of the population with developmental disabilities, both for planning purposes and to clarify our understanding of the processes of development and aging in this group.

III. Age-Related Changes

Life span development is characterized by both stability and change. This is true for older persons with developmental disabilities, although the paucity of longitudinal research on this group makes it difficult to characterize their trajectories of stability and change in various psychological, behavioral, and social domains. The confounds of cohort effects and true age effects have been described for the general population (Schaie, 1988) and for those with developmental disabilities (Seltzer, 1985a; in press). In that aging and cohort effects have not been disentangled in much of the literature on older persons with developmental disabilities, some descriptions of age-related changes in this population are confounded.

A. Cognitive Abilities

Of particular interest are changes in cognitive abilities. As in the general population, most persons with developmental disabilities maintain their cognitive abilities and even show evidence of intellectual development throughout their adult years (Eyman & Widaman, 1987; Hewitt, Fenner, & Torpy, 1986; Janicki & Jacobson, 1986), with declines manifested only after age 60 or 70. However, as noted earlier, persons with Down syndrome are at increased risk for Alzheimer's disease, and those who manifest the behavioral symptoms of the disease show a pattern of cognitive decline starting at age 40 or 50. Dalton (1982) reported that the average age of onset of memory loss in persons with Down syndrome was 49. However, he noted that the heterogeneity of this group with respect to memory loss was great, and that there are persons with Down syndrome in their 60s who do not show evidence of cognitive decline. Thase (1982) compared older persons with Down syndrome with age- and IQ-matched controls. The subjects with Down syndrome had significantly greater impairment than did the controls on measures of orientation, attention span, digit-span recall, visual memory, and object identification.

B. Functional Abilities

The pattern of age-related changes in functional abilities parallels the trajectories for cognitive abilities. Persons with retardation continue to develop new functional abilities throughout their adult years, but the acquisition of new skills levels off and begins to decline in older age. In persons with mild and moderate retardation who do not have Down syndrome, declines in activities of daily living are not routinely observed until the mid-70s, but motoric skills tend to begin to decline two decades earlier (Bell & Zubek, 1960; Janicki & Jacobson, 1986). In persons with severe and profound retardation who survive to old age, the declines in functional abilities are not so marked as in those who are less impaired, perhaps because of their more limited initial abilities (Janicki & Jacobson, 1986). Persons with Down syndrome who manifest the symptoms of Alzheimer's disease begin to decline in their functional abilities by age 40 or 50 (Evenhuis, 1990; Zigman et al., 1987). At all levels of retardation, regression in self-care skills and mobility is a significant predictor of morality (Eyman et al., 1989).

Several studies have compared the patterns of functional decline as manifested by persons with mental retardation and those of other older at-risk or disabled groups. For example, Sherwood and Morris (1983) studied persons with mental retardation, mental illness, and elderly nondisabled persons, all of whom were participants in the Pennsylvania Domiciliary Care Program. The three groups were found to respond similarly over time to placement in the domiciliary care program. However, those with mental retardation declined in functional abilities, while the other two groups did not. Callison, et al., (1971) compared elderly persons with mental retardation, elderly schizophrenics, and elderly persons who were not disabled with respect to changes in their visual ability, hearing, and grip strength. While all three groups were found to decline, those with mental retardation declined the most in hearing and vision. While these studies suggest that persons with mental retardation manifest more pronounced age-related declines than other diagnostic groups and than the general population, their results should be cautiously generalized. These studies were conducted on local samples, which may not be representative of the population with developmental disabilities, and who undoubtedly received poorer services in their childhood and adulthood than would be the case today. Therefore, it is difficult to separate the true differences in aging patterns between the general older population and persons with developmental disabilities from artifactual differences associated with poor services and poor health care.

Interestingly, even though older persons with developmental disabilities manifest age-related declines in functional and cognitive abilities, cross-sectional comparisons of younger and older adults with developmental disabilities reveal unexpected patterns. Krauss and Seltzer (1986) compared adults with mental retardation between the ages of 18 and 54 with those age 55 and older in both institutional and community-based settings. They found that the younger individuals were significantly more impaired cognitively and functionally than were the older group. The explanation for these unexpected findings was that the younger and older cohorts were composed of a different mix of persons. These differences were the result of changes in diagnostic practices, placement patterns, and mortality that have occurred during the last century. The members of the younger cohort included a higher proportion of persons with severe and profound retardation, who in the past were less likely to survive beyond childhood, while the older cohort included a higher proportion of persons having *borderline* mental retardation, who would not be included in the younger cohort as a result of contemporary diagnostic practices. This example illustrates the distinction between true aging influences and cohort effects, which are particularly marked in the population with developmental disabilities.

C. Health and Mental Health Status

With selected exceptions, older persons with developmental disabilities have similar health status and health care needs to those of their age peers without disabilities (Anderson, Lakin, Bruininks, & Hill, 1987). Older persons with developmental disabilities manifest the expected age-related increases in chronic diseases and medical problems (Janicki & Jacobson, 1986), as well as increases in the extent to which they utilize health care services (Janicki & MacEachron, 1984). However, access to health care services tends to be a function of living arrangement, with older persons who live in community-based group homes having more frequent contact with physicians than do those who live with their families (Janicki, Jacobson, & Ackerman, 1985). A history of institutionalization is associated with more medical problems and a shorter life span (Krauss & Seltzer, 1986; Lubin & Kiely, 1985; Tait, 1983), but these studies do not separate the effects of the possible differential characteristics of the individuals placed in institutions from the negative impact of the institutional setting on health and longevity.

Older persons with Down syndrome have a number of medical problems in addition to

Alzheimer's disease and sequelae of congenital heart disease. They have a higher-than-average incidence of acquired cataracts, leukemia, hypothyroidism, and skeletal abnormalities (Pueschel, 1987). In addition, a number of investigators have reported that persons with Down syndrome manifest a marked pattern of impaired auditory abilities associated with advancing age (Brooks, Wooley, & Kanjilal, 1972; Kaiser, Montague, Wold, Maune, & Pattison, 1981).

Another important domain of age-related stability and change pertains to the mental health of older persons with developmental disabilities. While it has been well documented that there is an increased prevalence of mental health problems among persons with developmental disabilities (Cohen & Bregman, 1988; Menolascino & Potter, 1989; Reiss, 1990), it is not known whether there are age-related patterns in the manifestation of such problems.

In sum, most persons with developmental disabilities manifest the patterns of declines in cognitive and functional abilities and health status that are characteristic of the general aging population. There is some evidence that the declines may begin somewhat earlier or are somewhat steeper in persons with developmental disabilities, but for the most part there are more similarities than differences. The exceptions include those whose developmental disabilities are due to specific disorders, notably those with Down syndrome. These individuals manifest accelerated and atypical patterns of aging.

IV. Formal and Informal Supports

As compared with the general older population, older persons with developmental disabilities have a relatively high need for formal and informal supports. There are a number of reasons for this higher need for support. First, these individuals, by definition, have impairments in their ability to function, and need compensatory supports in order to manage their daily activities, maintain their health, and enjoy a reasonable quality of life. Second, since most older persons with developmental disabilities do not marry or have children, they lack the most basic supports that are provided to most older persons by members of the nuclear family. Instead, they must depend for family support on their aging parents or on siblings. Third, their disabilities and their advancing age may interfere with their ability to develop meaningful relationships with friends who could provide support to them (Berkson & Romer, 1980; Krauss, 1989; Landesman-Dwyer, Sackett, & Kleinman, 1980). For all of these reasons, older persons with developmental disabilities may be especially vulnerable and lonely, and therefore have a high need for formal support, as well as continued informal support from their family of origin and from friends.

A. Formal Supports

Older persons with developmental disabilities receive services from three formal service sectors (Seltzer & Krauss, 1987):

1. the age-integrated developmental disabilities service sector;
2. the age-specialized developmental disabilities service sector; and
3. the generic aging service sector.

The dominant approach to providing services to older persons with developmental disabilities in the United States is the age-integrated developmental disabilities service sector. Age-integrated developmental disabilities services include older clients in residential and day programs without making age-based eligibility criteria or modifications in the programs. In one study that examined the patterns of service utilization of older persons with retardation in Massachusetts, it was found that about two thirds of the services received by these older persons were provided by the age-integrated developmental disabilities service sector (Seltzer, 1988).

There are advantages and disadvantages associated with utilization of age-integrated developmental disabilities services by older persons with developmental disabilities. As regards the advantages, this option avoids making chronological age *the* issue in service delivery. In addition, individuals have continuity in their activities and friendship groups, and the opportunity to participate in active treatment programs that are stimulating and challenging. However, there are disadvantages with this service model, including the inability of many programs to be responsive to age-related needs as they emerge, the absence of retirement options in most employment-oriented day programs, and the limited number of age-peers.

The second service sector utilized by older persons with developmental disabilities is the age-specialized developmental disabilities service sector. In the Massachusetts analysis of patterns of service utilization (Seltzer, 1988), it was found that only 5% of the services utilized by the population of older persons with mental retardation were classified as age-specialized services. In this sector, special services are developed for older persons with developmental disabilities in order to respond specifically to their age-related needs. Programmatic features of these day and residential services include a slower pace, more room for personal choice, a greater emphasis on recreational and leisure-time activities, and an increased attention to health care services. In 1985, Seltzer and Krauss conducted a national survey of age-specialized services for older persons with mental retardation (Seltzer & Krauss, 1987). In total, 529 programs in 43 states and the District of Columbia were identified. About 60% of these programs were located in community-based settings, while 40% were institution-based. Combining institution and community programs, about 65% were residential programs and 35% were day programs. About half began as age-integrated mental retardation programs that became age-specialized as their clients aged, while the other half were developed specifically to serve the needs of older persons with mental retardation.

As with age-integrated services, age-specialized services have both advantages and disadvantages. Advantages include the potential to create flexible, individualized, and age-appropriate services. Retirement options are most likely to be included in this service sector. Also, such programs appear to be particularly effective at creating the context in which peer relationships will flourish, as participants interact with others similar to them in age and skill level. Weaknesses of the age-integrated service sector include the possibility that programs might be isolated or segregated by age and disability. Participants might be separated from their past friends and placements, which may be particularly problematic at a time in life when new relationships are often difficult to establish.

The third service sector providing services to older persons with developmental disabilities is the generic aging service sector. Utilization of these services involves the inclusion of older persons with developmental disabilities in services that were designed for the general elderly population. These include all of the services in the aging network: home-health services, day-health services, senior centers, congregate housing, home-delivered meals, nutrition sites, etc. There actually is rather widespread participation of older persons with developmental disabilities in such services, usually in conjunction with, rather than as a substitution for, services sponsored by the developmental disabilities services system (Seltzer, Krauss, Litchfield, & Modlish, 1989). It is generally the less severely disabled individuals among the population of older persons with developmental disabilities who participate in generic aging programs.

Advantages of generic aging programs include the high level of social integration of such programs. Participation in such programs is believed to be normalizing and beneficial for developing relationships with age peers. However, the disadvantages include a lack of staff with expertise in serving individuals with disabilities and attitudinal barriers on the part of both staff and other participants, who might not welcome the participation of older persons with developmental disabilities. There is also a problem with the level of task demands made of participants, which might involve intellectual or motoric capacities beyond all but the most mildly handicapped.

During the next decade, three trends will affect the patterns of service utilization of older persons with developmental disabilities. First, as noted earlier, there will be an increase in the absolute size of this population, necessitating an increase in the service options available to them. Second, it can be expected that as the population of older persons with developmental disabilities continues to age, these individuals will become more frail, resulting in an increase in the intensity of services that are needed. Third, there will be an increased familiarity by aging network service providers with the needs of older persons with developmental disabilities. It is to be hoped that this will result in an increase in the appropriateness of the services that are delivered to these individuals.

B. Family and Informal Supports

It is very common for persons with developmental disabilities to live with their families, in many cases for their entire lives (Fujiura, Garza, & Braddock, 1989; Lakin, 1985). There is currently a great deal of attention focused on aging parents who have provided long-term care to their adult children with developmental disabilities (Engelhardt, Brubaker & Lutzer, 1988; Heller & Factor, 1988; Seltzer, 1985b). This interest is the result of several factors. First, researchers, policy makers, and service providers are all concerned about the impacts on parents of the increased longevity of persons with developmental disabilities. The demographic shifts described earlier in this chapter pose new challenges to family caregivers, the impacts of which are not yet well understood.

Second, gerontologists are interested in the capacity of older persons to be family resources. While in much past research, elderly persons were viewed as family burdens, this perspective is now changing (Greenberg & Becker, 1988; Rowe & Kahn, 1987). It is now recognized that intergenerational relationships are often reciprocal, with the older generation providing assistance to, as well as receiving assistance from, the younger generation. However, it is necessary to develop an understanding of how the aging process affects parental caregiving capacity. This is particularly true when the parents are in their 70s and 80s and continue to have caregiving responsibilities for the younger generation.

While family caregiving is not an unusual role, especially for women, several factors set apart the experiences of aging parents who care for an adult child with developmental disabilities. First, whereas the provision of care by a parent for a child is normative when the child is young, this arrangement is not normative when the mother is approaching or has reached old age, and the son or daughter has reached adulthood. The family life cycle for these families is *off cycle* (Farber, 1959; Turnbull, Summers, & Brotherson, 1986). It is often assumed that the effects on parents of off-cycle caregiving responsibilities are negative, but this assumption has not yet been tested. It is possible that there are positive as well as negative effects of long-term family caregiving, especially in those instances in which the adult with developmental disabilities provides assistance to a physically impaired or infirm parent, or when the parent derives a continued purpose in life from caregiving.

Another unique aspect of the caregiving experiences of aging parents who care for their adult son or daughter with developmental disabilities is the duration of the caregiving responsibility. National data indicate that the period of family caregiving for an elderly relative averages about 5 years (Stone, Cafferta, & Sangl, 1987). In contrast, the period of care for an aging son or daughter with developmental disabilities can span 5 or 6 decades, or even longer.

Seltzer and Krauss (1989), in a longitudinal study of 450 mothers (aged 55 to 85) who provide care to their son or daughter with mental retardation (aged 15 to 66), are examining a number of the issues discussed above. The overall purpose of the study is to investigate the correlates of well-being in the sample of older caregiving mothers, to identify the predictors of continuing in-home versus out-of-home placement for their adult children with retardation, and to describe the patterns of stability and change in the adults with retardation.

The preliminary findings of this study suggest that the older women in the sample are coping surprisingly well with their continuing caregiving responsibilities. Although it was hypothesized that they would be at risk for poor physical and mental health owing to their long years of caregiving, it was found that they, in fact, compare favorably with samples of age peers and samples of other caregivers. Specifically, the aging mothers in the Seltzer and Krauss study were substantially healthier and had better morale than did other samples of caregivers for the elderly. Furthermore, they reported no more burden or stress than did other caregivers. Thus, despite the long duration of their caregiving roles, and despite the unique characteristics of their children, many of these mothers appear to be resilient, optimistic, and able to function well in multiple roles.

A second hypothesis of the Seltzer and Krauss study that was tested in preliminary analyses pertained to the mothers of the sons and daughters with Down syndrome (37% of the total sample). It was hypothesized that these mothers would have poorer physical and mental health than the other mothers in the sample because adults with Down syndrome have a higher rate of chronic health problems and are at risk for premature aging. Comparison between the mothers of the adults with Down syndrome and those whose retardation was due to other factors revealed that, contrary to expectations, the mothers of the adults with Down syndrome manifested better overall well-being (Seltzer, 1990). Even when between-group differences on socioeconomic and disability factors were controlled, the mothers of the adults with Down syndrome perceived their families to be more cohesive and less conflictual, were more satisfied with their social supports and with the services provided to their adult children, and were less stressed and less burdened by their caregiving responsibilities than were the other mothers in the sample.

These differences mirror patterns that have been reported regarding young families with a child with Down syndrome as compared with other groups with developmental disabilities (Holroyd & McArthur, 1976; Krauss, 1989; Mink, Nihira, & Meyers, 1983). Although it was not expected that the mothers of the adults with Down syndrome would have superior well-being in older age, these differences may be persistent sequelae to the diagnosis. Possible reasons include the greater level of scientific knowledge about Down syndrome as compared with other diagnostic groups, the greater prevalence of Down syndrome than other diagnoses and therefore possibly greater public familiarity with it, and temperamental differences between children with Down syndrome and comparison groups of children with other causes of their mental retardation. It is possible that these *protective factors* buffer some of the stresses associated with having a child with retardation that are manifested more negatively by families of children with other diagnoses.

V. Summary

This chapter has provided an overview of the currently available knowledge about aging in persons with developmental disabilities. The challenges of defining old age in this population are substantial, as a result of the atypical aging manifested by some members of this group and because of their early-life onset of functional limitations. There appears to be an emerging consensus that age 55 should be used to define the onset of old age in persons with developmental disabilities.

The size of this group is difficult to ascertain, not only as a result of definitional problems but also because many older persons with developmental disabilities are not known to the formal service-delivery system. Nevertheless, it is known that there has been an increase in life expectancy among persons with developmental disabilities which, in conjunction with the aging of the baby-boom generation, has resulted in an increase in the size of the adult and older segment of this population.

Some information is now available about the trajectory of change in cognitive and functional abilities across the life span in persons with developmental disabilities, with declines reported only by age 60 or 70. Persons with Down syndrome age atypically, manifesting declines by age 40 or 50. Changes in health status appear to be similar to those manifested by the general population, although certain factors (e.g., of history of institutional placement) increase the risk of poor health in old age. No information is currently available about mental health changes characteristic of this group in old age.

Older persons with developmental disabilities have a particularly high need for formal and informal support. Formal support is provided by three service sectors: the age-integrated developmental disabilities service sector, the age-specialized developmental disabilities service sector, and the generic aging service sector. Each has advantages and disadvantages. Informal support is provided by parents and, after they are no longer able to provide care, by siblings of the older person with developmental disabilities. New patterns of family caregiving are emerging in this context, including previously unidentified caregiving capacities (e.g., aging persons serving as family resources rather than being viewed as family burdens) and consequences (e.g., caregiving responsibilities lasting as long as 6 decades of a parent's life). Families of adults with Down syndrome do not appear to be so negatively affected as other families in the long-term caregiving role, probably as a result of protective mechanisms characteristic of this subgroup.

VI. The Need for Future Research: The Mental Health of Older Persons with Developmental Disabilities _____

Knowledge about aging in persons with developmental disabilities has only recently begun to accumulate. As compared with just one decade ago, a great deal is now understood about the characteristics of this population and the extent to which they are similar to and different from the larger population of older Americans. However, most research that has been conducted on this population to date is descriptive. In order for substantial progress to be made in our understanding of the aging patterns of this population, it is necessary for future research to be more theory driven and analytic. Further, and of particular relevance to this chapter, little information exists about the manifestation of specific mental health problems in older persons with developmental disabilities.

Many issues regarding aging in the population with developmental disabilities warrant additional investigation. Four stand out as particularly important. First, there is great interest in the link between Down syndrome and Alzheimer's disease. Among the important questions that should be examined are the elucidation of the genetic relationship between these two disorders and an understanding of why the neuropathology of Alzheimer's is accompanied by behavioral pathology in fewer than 45% of the cases with Down syndrome, whereas neuropathology and behavioral pathology are more strongly associated in the general population. In addition, there is interest in the extent to which there is a greater risk of Alzheimer's in relatives of persons affected with Down syndrome. This problem has particular significance because Alzheimer's disease places a substantial burden on the mental health system, both with respect to the treatment of Alzheimer's patients and the provision of mental health services to their family caregivers.

A second problem that warrants attention in future research pertains to the mental health characteristics and needs of older persons with developmental disabilities. As reviewed in this chapter, there is a preliminary understanding of the age-related changes in cognitive, functional, and health status in older persons with developmental disabilities.

However, there has been no systematic investigation of the mental health status of this population. Some have hypothesized that there is an increased risk of depression in this group because of their social isolation, but this hypothesis remains to be tested. A particular challenge will be the development of measures of mental health and psychopathology that can be reliably and validly used with this population.

A third important issue pertains to the extent to which there is reciprocity in caregiving between aging parents and their middle-aged children with developmental disabilities. Gerontological interest in the capacity of older persons to be family resources, rather than family burdens, would be addressed by an analysis of caregiving patterns in two-generation aging families. However, it is also necessary to examine the consequences of parental responsibility in old age and of dependent adults outliving their parents. In that adults with developmental disabilities tend not to have a spouse or their own children on whom to depend after care by a parent is no longer an option, there is a need for either formal or informal support to replace parental care. These substitute types of support may be derived either from family members (primarily siblings, who may be ambivalent about assuming this responsibility), or from the developmental disabilities or mental health service delivery system.

Finally, there is a need to investigate the heterogeneity of the population of older persons with developmental disabilities. While there has been some attention to the atypical aging manifested by persons with Down syndrome, other subgroups that have distinct developmental patterns have not been studied. For example there is good reason to believe that persons with cerebral palsy, autism, and epilepsy, among others, will age atypically. This may also be true of those dually diagnosed as having mental retardation and mental illness. However, at the present time, all of these subgroups, as well as many others, are included in the heterogeneous grouping of developmental disabilities. While diagnostic distinctions might not be relevant for purposes of service delivery, for research purposes it is necessary to understand the complex relationships among etiology, life experience, and patterns of aging.

References

Anderson, D. J., Lakin, K. C., Bruininks, R. H., & Hill, B. K. (1987). *A national study of residential and support services for elderly persons with mental retardation.* (Report No. 22). Minneapolis: University of Minnesota, Department of Educational Psychology.

Baird, P. A., & Sadovnick, A. D. (1985). Mental retardation in over half-a-million consecutive livebirths: An epidemiological study. *American Journal of Mental Deficiency, 89,* 323–330.

Berkson, G., & Romer, D. (1980). Social ecology of supervised communal facilities for mentally disabled adults: I. Introduction. *American Journal of Mental Deficiency, 85,* 219–228.

Bell, A., & Zubek, J. P. (1960). The effect of age on the intellectual performance of mental defectives. *Journal of Gerontology, 15,* 285–295.

Birren, J. E. (1959). Principles of research on aging. In J. E. Birren (Ed.), *Handbook of aging in the individual* (p. 3–42). Chicago: University of Chicago Press.

Brookes, D. N., Wooley, A., & Kanjilal, G. C. (1972). Hearing loss and middle-ear disorders in patients with Down's (Mongolism). *Journal of Mental Deficiency Research, 16,* 21–29.

Callison, D. A., Armstrong, H. F., Elam, C., Cannon, R. L., Paisley, C. M., & Himwich, H. (1971). The effects of aging on schizophrenic and mentally defective patients: Visual, auditory, and grip-strength measurements. *Journal of Gerontology, 26,* 137–145.

Cohen, D. J., & Bregman, J. D. (1988). Mental disorders and psychopharmacology of retarded persons. In J. F.

Kavanaugh (Ed.), *Understanding mental retardation: Research accomplishments and new frontiers.* Baltimore, MD: Brookes.

Cotton, P. D., & Spirrison, C. L. (1986). The elderly mentally retarded (developmentally disabled) population: A challenge for the service-delivery system. In J. S. Brody & G. E. Ruff, (Eds.), *Aging and rehabilitation: Advances in the state of the art.* New York: Springer.

Dalton, A. J. (1982). *A prospective study of Alzheimer's disease in Down syndrome.* Paper presented at the Sixth Meeting of the International Association for the Scientific Study of Mental Deficiency, Toronto.

Edgerton, R. (1988). Aging in the community—A matter of choice. *American Journal of Mental Retardation, 92,* 331–335.

Eisdorfer, C. (1983). Conceptual models of aging: The challenge of a new frontier. *American Psychologist, 38,* 197–202.

Engelhardt, J. L., Brubaker, T. H., & Lutzer, V. D. (1988). Older caregivers of adults with mental retardation: Service utilization. *Mental Retardation, 26,* 191–195.

Evenhuis, J. M. (1990). The natural history of dementia in Down's syndrome. *Archives of Neurology, 47,* 263–267.

Eyman, R. K., Call, T. L., & White, J. F. (1989). Mortality of elderly mentally retarded persons in California. *Journal of Applied Gerontology, 8,* 203–215.

Eyman, R. K., Call, T., & White, J. F. (1991). Life expectancy of persons with Down syndrome. *American Journal of Mental Retardation, 95,* 603–612.

Eyman, R. K., & Widaman, K. F. (1987). Lifespan development of institutionalized and community-based mentally retarded persons revisited. *American Journal of Mental Deficiency, 91,* 559–569.

Farber, B. (1959). Effects of a severely mentally retarded child on family integration. *Monographs of the Society for Research in Child Development, 24* (2 Serial No. 71).

Fujiura, G. T., Garza, J., & Braddock, D. (1989). *National survey of family support services in developmental disabilities.* Chicago, IL: University of Illinois, Chicago.

Greenberg, J., & Becker, M. (1988). Aging parents as family resources. *The Gerontologist, 28,* 786–791.

Grossman, H. J. (Ed.) (1983). *Classification in mental retardation.* Washington, DC: American Association on Mental Deficiency.

Heller, T., & Factor, A. (1988). Permanency planning among black and white family caregivers of older adults with mental retardation. *Mental Retardation, 26,* 203–208.

Hewitt, K. E., Fenner, M. E., & Torpy, D. (1986). Cognitive and behavioral profiles of the elderly mentally handicapped. *Journal of Mental Deficiency Research, 30,* 217–225.

Holroyd, J., & McArthur, D. (1976). Mental retardation and stress on the parents: A contrast between Down's syndrome and childhood autism. *American Journal of Mental Deficiency, 80,* 431–436.

Jacobson, J. W., Sutton, M. S., & Janicki, M. P. (1985). Demography and characteristics of aging and aged mentally retarded persons. In M. P. Janicki & H. M. Wisniewski (Eds.), *Aging and developmental disabilities: Issues and approaches.* Baltimore: MD Brookes.

Janicki, M. P. (1988). Aging: The new challenge. *Mental Retardation, 26,* 177–180.

Janicki, M. P., & Jacobson, J. W. (1986). Generational trends in sensory, physical, and behavioral abilities among older mentally retarded persons. *American Journal of Mental Deficiency, 90,* 490–500.

Janicki, M. P., Jacobson, J. W., & Ackerman, L. J. (1985). *Patterns of health and support services among elderly mentally retarded persons living in community group home settings.* Paper presented at the XIII International Congress of Gerontology, New York.

Janicki, M. P., Knox, L. A., & Jacobson, J. W. (1985). Planning for an older developmentally disabled population. In M. P. Janicki & H. M. Wisniewski (Eds.), *Aging and developmental disabilities: Issues and approaches.* Baltimore, MD: Brookes.

Janicki, M. P., & MacEachron, A. E. (1984). Residential, health, and social service needs of elderly developmentally disabled persons. *The Gerontologist, 24,* 128–137.

Janicki, M. P., Seltzer, M. M., & Krauss, M. W. (1987). *Contemporary issues in the aging of persons with mental retardation and other developmental disabilities.* Washington, DC: NARIC.

Janicki, M. P., & Wisniewski, H. M. (Eds.) (1985). *Aging and developmental disabilities: Issues and approaches.* Baltimore, MD: Brookes.

Kaiser, H., Montague, J., Wold, D., Maune, S., & Pattison, D. (1981). Hearing of Down's syndrome adults. *American Journal of Mental Deficiency, 85,* 467–472.

Krauss, M. W. (1988). Long-term care issues in mental retardation. In J. Kavanagh (Ed.), *Understanding mental retardation: Research accomplishments and new frontiers.* Baltimore, MD: Brookes.

Krauss, M. W. (1989). *Parenting a young child with disabilities: Differences between mothers and fathers.* Paper presented at the 22nd Annual Gatlinburg Conference on Research and Theory in Mental Retardation and Developmental Disabilities, Gatlinburg, TN.

Krauss, M. W., & Seltzer, M. M. (1986). Comparison of elderly and adult mentally retarded persons in community and institutional settings. *American Journal of Mental Deficiency, 75,* 354–360.

Lakin, K. C. (1985). Service system and settings for mentally retarded people. In K. C. Lakin, B. Hill, & R. Bruininks (Eds.), *An analysis of Medicaid's ICF-MR program.* Minneapolis: University of Minnesota.

Landesman-Dwyer, S., Sackett, G. P., & Kleinman, J. S. (1980). Relationship of size to resident and staff behavior in small community residences. *American Journal of Mental Deficiency, 85,* 6–17.

Lott, I. T., & Lai, F. (1982). Dementia in Down's Syndrome: Observations from a neurology clinic. *Applied Research in Mental Retardation, 3,* 233–239.

Lubin, R. A., & Kiely, M. (1985). Epidemiology of aging in developmental disabilities. In M. P. Janicki & H. M. Wisniewski (Eds.), *Aging and developmental disabilities: Issues and approaches.* Baltimore, MD: Brookes.

Menaloscino, F. J., & Potter, J. F. (1989). Mental illness in the elderly mentally retarded. *Journal of Applied Gerontology, 8,* 192–202.

Mink, I. T., Nihira, K., & Meyers, C. E. (1983). Taxonomy of family life styles: I. Homes with TMR children. *American Journal of Mental Deficiency, 87,* 484–497.

Pueschel, S. M. (1987). Health concerns in persons with Down syndrome. In S. M. Pueschel, C. Tingey, J. E. Rynders, A. C. Crocker, & D. M. Crutcher (Eds.), *New perspectives on Down syndrome* (pp. 113–134). Baltimore: Brookes.

Rehabilitation, Comprehensive Services, and Developmental Disabilities Amendments of 1978, PL 85-602,92 Stat. 2955 (1978).

Reiss, S. (1990). Prevalence of dual diagnosis in community-based day programs in the Chicago metropolitan area. *American Journal of Mental Retardation, 94,* 578–585.

Rose, T., & Janicki, M. P. (1986). Older mentally retarded adults: A forgotten population. *Aging Network News, 3,* 17–19.

Rowe, J. W., & Kahn, R. L. (1987). Human aging: Usual and successful. *Science, 237,* 143–149.

Schaie, K. W. (1988). The impact of research methodology on theory building in the developmental sciences. In J. E. Birren & V. L. Bengston (Eds.), *Emergent theories of aging.* New York: Springer.

Seltzer, M. M. (1985a). Research in social aspects of aging and developmental disabilities. In M. P. Janicki & H. M. Wisniewski (Eds.), *Aging and developmental disabilities: Issues and Approaches* (p. 161–173). Baltimore, MD: Brookes.

Seltzer, M. M. (1985b). Informal supports for aging mentally retarded persons. *American Journal of Mental Deficiency, 90,* 259–265.

Seltzer, M. M. (1988). Structure and patterns of service utilization by elderly persons with mental retardation. *Mental Retardation, 26,* 181–185.

Seltzer, M. M. (1989). Introduction to aging and lifelong disabilities: Context for decision making. In E. F. Ansello & T. Rose (Eds.), *Aging and lifelong disabilities: Partnership for the 21st century.* College Park, MD: University of Maryland Center on Aging.

Seltzer, M. M. (1990). *Continuing effects of etiology in adulthood: Down syndrome vs. other diagnostic groups.* Paper presented at the 23rd Annual Gatlinburg Conference on Research and Theory in Mental Retardation, Brainerd, Minnesota, March, 1990.

Seltzer, M. M. (in press). Family caregiving across the full lifespan. In L. Rowitz (Ed.), *Mental retardation in the year 2000.* New York: Springer.

Seltzer, M. M., & Krauss, M. W. (1987). *Aging and mental retardation: Extending the continuum.* Washington, DC: American Association on Mental Retardation.

Seltzer, M. M., & Krauss, M. W. (1989). Aging parents with mentally retarded children: Family risk factors and sources of support. *American Journal on Mental Retardation, 94,* 303–312.

Seltzer, M. M., Krauss, M. W., Litchfield, L. C., & Modlish, N. J. K. (1989). Utilization of aging network services by elderly persons with mental retardation. *The Gerontologist, 29,* 234–238.

Siegel, J. S. (1980). On the demography of aging. *Demography, 17*, 245–364.

Sherwood, S., & Morris, J. N., (1983). The Pennsylvania domiciliary care experiment: I. Impact on quality of life. *American Journal of Public Health, 73*, 646–653.

Stone, R., Cafferta, G. L., & Sangl, J. (1987). Caregivers of frail elderly: A national profile. *The Gerontologist, 27*, 616–626.

Streib, G. (1983). The frail elderly: Research dilemmas and research opportunities. *The Gerontologist, 23*, 40–44.

Tait, D. (1983). Mortality and aging among mental defectives. *Journal of Mental Deficiency Research, 27*, 133–142.

Thase, M. E. (1982). Longevity and mortality in Down's syndrome. *Journal of Mental Deficiency Research, 26*, 117–192.

Turnbull, A. P., Summers, J. A., & Brotherson, M. J. (1986). Family life cycle: Theoretical and empirical implications and future directions for families with mentally retarded members. In J. J. Gallagher & P. M. Vietze (Eds.), *Families of handicapped persons: Research, programs, and policy issues* (p. 45–65). Baltimore, MD: Brookes.

Wisniewski, H. M., & Merz, G. S. (1985). Aging, Alzheimer's disease, and developmental disabilities. In M. P. Janicki & H. M. Wisniewski (Eds.), *Aging and developmental disabilities: Issues and approaches.* Baltimore, MD: Brookes.

Zigman, W. B., Schupf, N., Lubin, R. A., & Silverman, W. P. (1987). Premature regression of adults with Down syndrome. *American Journal of Mental Deficiency, 92*, 161–168.

Assessment, Treatment, and Prevention

Neuropsychiatric Assessment ___

Eric D. Caine and Hillel Grossman

I. Introduction
II. Framework for Assessment
    A. Approaches to Case Reasoning
    B. Aims of Assessment
III. Data Acquisition
    A. History and Present Illness
    B. Mental-Status Assessment
    C. Standardized Assessment Procedures
    D. Medical and Neurological Examination
    E. Laboratory Procedures
IV. Differential Diagnosis
    A. Delirium
    B. Dementia and Other Disturbances of Intellect
    C. Affective Disorder
    D. Psychotic Disorders
    E. Other Psychiatric Disturbances
V. Conclusion of Assessment
    References

I. Introduction ___

Neuropsychiatric assessment is fundamentally a process of integration. It requires the use of disparate, but historically distinctive case reasoning approaches in the evaluation of a patient. The exercise of clinical skill and experience, the *art* of medicine rather than its technology, comes into play when deciding which of these approaches is most useful for dealing with complementary aspects of a patient's illness. Art also implies understanding how to mix these separate elements into a cohesive treatment plan that is suited for the unique circumstances of each patient.

Neuropsychiatry shares with neurology the view that behavior reflects brain function, and that neurobiology provides the basis for all that is observed clinically (Caine & Joynt, 1986). From psychiatry it draws its emphasis on mental disorders. The neuropsychiatrist strives to understand the content of behavior, in addition to describing its form, and appreciates the multiple influences that shape behavior, including family and environment, nurture and nature both. As we will discuss, these assumptions require that the clinician utilizes parallel, at times diverging, methods of data gathering and clinical reasoning. The clinician is faced with the daunting task of weaving these separate views into a single conception, one that fits the particular needs of the patient at hand. Fundamental to this approach is the implicit understanding that determining what is *functional* and what is *organic* may not be possible (indeed, for us the terms have little practical meaning); often the clinician must choose among empirically defined therapies, those that have been tested through trial and error, rather than having been derived from scientific understanding.

Assessing the patient's *functional integrity* is the focal point for integrating the distinctive clinical approaches that are used by the neuropsychiatrist. Attention to function underscores the utilitarian aim of assessment. One may choose to espouse biological (homeostatic) or psychosocial viewpoints, but evaluating the functional significance of constructs such as *symptoms, psychological meaning, diseases,* or *illnesses,* forces the clinician to employ a variety of assessment methods, even though some may have little common ground with others. Ultimately, treatment evaluation is based on measuring the impact of our interventions on function.

Engel coined the biopsychosocial model to contrast with a more technologically oriented biomedical model (Engel, 1977). He advocated a *systems approach* for understanding human illness, rather than a strictly defined disease model. In this chapter, we will distinguish, at times, between the expression of disease or disorder (defined pathobiologically) and illness (defined psychologically, socially, and culturally). Assessment of functional integrity will be the point of integration of factors that lead to both disease and illness. The biopsychosocial perspective calls for integrating these factors for a complete understanding; but first, the neuropsychiatric assessment requires that they be pulled apart in order to collect data useful for a complete evaluation. We will emphasize scrutiny of three separate, but overlapping perspectives, including examination of (1) brain–behavior relationships, (2) symptomatic and syndromic features that lead to diagnosis, and (3) personal and developmental attributes that uniquely affect each patient throughout the life course.

Nonspecificity of symptoms is the bane of the clinician. There are few final common behavioral pathways for the expression of disordered behavior, no matter what the origin (Caine & Joynt, 1986). These include

1. arousal, attention, and concentration;
2. affective state, including both the expression of emotion and the feeling of mood;
3. perception, including ideational and physical, internal and external;
4. intellectual function (e.g., memory, language, or the organization of thought processes);
5. personality (e.g., "He's not the same as he used to be," or "He's always been that way."); and
6. motor function.

Disturbances along these dimensions may present distinctive patterns of failure. However, behavioral abnormalities tend to be nonspecific: More than one pathophysiologically distinct medical or cerebral disorder can cause the same phenomenological abnormality (e.g., Davison & Bagley, 1969); or, secondary mental disorders due to medical conditions can mimic primary psychiatric disturbances (Caine, in press).

No patient can be evaluated effectively without appreciating the influence of age on the expression of illness. Aging represents an evolving biological, psychological, and social process. The art of clinical assessment entails an appreciation of how the shifting background of age influences or defines the pathological meaning of clinical symptoms and signs. A consideration of age-related effects cannot be segregated into a separate section in a chapter on assessment. It must be interwoven. The examiner does not come to the end of the clinical evaluation and then consider the age-related meanings of the findings. The evaluative process requires blending serially ordered assessments with intuitive, gestalt-oriented reasoning. One must understand the potential meaning of findings as one proceeds, especially if one seeks to develop an inquisitive, hypothesis-testing method of neuropsychiatric appraisal.

Indeed, the evaluative process is dynamic rather than static. That is, the clinician must view symptoms as evolving, and place current findings in a time-oriented context. Interviewing and the gathering of pertinent historical data might be considered to be an effort in sequential mental status examination, where one seeks to elicit evidence of a developing mental disorder that can be most fully defined during the current encounter. The clinician seeks to understand form and course, as well as content and meaning. Moreover, one struggles to discern the overall pattern of illness and *predict* its future evolution. This is an essential component of planning treatment, and perhaps most importantly, evaluating the correctness of initial conclusions or formulations. Therapeutic intervention should lead to a predictable response; a predictable negative outcome can also prove revealing, but the clinician should be most concerned when confronted by unanticipated clinical alterations. In essence, the clinical process inserts the evaluator in the midst of an imaginary time line, where the clinician measures its force and direction, with the aim of altering the process of illness toward a beneficial outcome.

II. Framework for Assessment

A. Approaches to Case Reasoning

Neuropsychiatrists can draw upon three complementary approaches to case reasoning when considering the problems presented by new patients. The first method relies upon clinical–pathological correlation. The neuropsychiatrist considers brain function as the foundation of behavior, understanding that neuroanatomy, neurophysiology, and neurochemistry underlie all that is considered clinically, both abnormal and normal. When focusing on disease processes, one seeks to define the *site of the lesion,* based on thorough symptom-oriented history and careful examination for definable signs. Knowing where the lesion lies in the central nervous system allows probabilistic determination of its pathology, which leads to a consideration of pathophysiology and pathogenesis. From these, the clinician develops a differential diagnostic array from most to least probable, and in turn initiates *rational treatment*. This method presupposes predictable, lawful relationships in central nervous system functioning, where all nervous systems are created equal: Each behaves in an identical fashion, given the same set of provocative conditions. Traditional clinical–pathological correlation is complicated, however, by our current understanding that major neuropsychiatric disorders (e.g., degenerative diseases, affective disturbances) are a reflection of disordered neurochemical systems that are difficult to localize discretely in the brain. In the past, advances in clinical–pathological correlation were based on postmortem study of lesions related to vascular anatomy or missile wounds. These cut across neurochemical systems' boundaries or functional zones. Although great strides were made during the past century, with such focal disorders providing our primary research models, they have generally proven less illuminating for studying primary and secondary behavioral disturbances such as depression, psychosis, dementia, agitation, or violence.

The strength of the clinical–pathological correlative method is also its weakness. It focuses exclusively on diseases, while failing to consider nonphysiological factors that contribute to illness and dysfunction. Ultimately, consideration of brain–behavior relationships is a highly abstracting process that requires no consideration of the patient as a person. In the extreme, the clinician attempts to put right the physiological imbalance that has been detected. Alone, this strategy is often insufficient for developing an effective therapeutic plan.

A second method of clinical reasoning emphasizes rigorous syndromic diagnosis. This approach has regained adherents during the past two decades, stimulated both by a desire for psychiatry to become more scientific, as well as the needs of psychopharmacologists to have more clearly defined target symptoms for their pharmacotherapeutic agents. For some psychiatrists, this was also a reaction to the post-World War II movement toward a psychodynamic psychiatry, in which attention to psychological theory was emphasized and concern about specific psychopathological abnormalities waned. Modern psychopharmacology has been built empirically through trial and error. Using criteria based diagnoses, one is able to generalize from case to case, learn from mistakes, and in time, apply therapeutic tools with greater precision. "Cases" are defined by both content and form, and attention to disease course has been paramount. With the inception of the third edition of the Diagnostic and Statistical Manual (DSM-III) in 1980 (American Psychiatric Association, 1980), psychiatrists sought to enhance the inter-rater reliability of clinicians by explicitly defining diagnostic features. As well, the aim was to assist clinicians when gathering the historical and clinical data necessary for effectively assessing the presence of cardinal symptoms and signs, thus reducing tendencies toward idiosyncratic data collection or highly varied use of diagnostic labels.

Most neuropsychiatric diagnostic entities are syndromes, not anatomically or etiologically defined diseases. No methods are available for externally establishing the validity of these disorders. That is, there are no specific tests that use alternative classification methods, beyond psychopathology itself, to define the presence of particular diseases. One must apply empiric and probabilistic, rather than specific treatments. By its very nature, descriptive diagnosis is stereotyping and leads to the loss of recognition of the individual, in a fashion akin to neurological case reasoning. However, it offers the ability to generalize one's success, thus providing a powerful tool clinically.

The final method that we employ involves the attempt to discern the patient as a unique person, a dynamic and interactive product of his life experiences, his personal psychological makeup, and his current life circumstances. The ultimate goal is to reveal the individual. Formal diagnosis is less important, while understanding the meaning of the patient's apparent pathology (in the unique terms of his own experience) becomes the essential key for developing a caring, therapeutic intervention. This methodology grew, to a great extent, from a dissatisfaction with the abilities of neurologically oriented case reasoning and descriptive psychopathology to fully encompass the problems that patients presented to their clinicians, as they typically brought themselves and their connected psychological and social worlds, rather than their diseases (Havens, 1973). When taken to the extreme, however, formal diagnosis becomes an afterthought when using this method. Generalization from case to case is impossible. Nonetheless, most of us wish to be seen as uniquely ourselves rather than stereotypic clinical conceptions. This method also offers the opportunity to form a powerful working collaboration around jointly defined problems that the patient comprehends as well as (or better than) the clinician. It is a rare patient who thinks of himself in terms of a diagnosis or a brain–behavior relationship, although understanding such issues may be reassuring.

Historically, these methods of clinical reasoning have been kept quite separate, and have been practiced most often by clinicians who spoke to one another rarely. There has been no tradition in medicine for integrating these approaches, and efforts in that direction often make clinicians uncomfortable, as they most readily identify with one or two, but not all three, methods. Although Engel called for a biopsychosocial model (Engel, 1977), one that describes many of the same features, he provided little direction on how one might develop that model in a practical fashion. The point of juncture for us involves the clinician's attention to function, through defining a patient's functional strengths and deficits, and seeking to understand the contributions of various factors to any evident impairment. For example, one attempts to appreciate the nature of the disease process and its specifically debilitating effects, while delineating specific symptoms and signs that may be responsive to therapeutic intervention. In addition to discovering the special meaning that these symptoms may hold for the patient, the clinician attends as well to those social factors that contribute to the illness.

B. Aims of Assessment

The objectives or aims of clinical evaluation grow directly from understanding the methods of case reasoning employed. As noted, the overall goal ultimately involves defining those factors that interfere with functional integrity. The clinician utilizes history taking, mental-status assessment, and laboratory procedures to establish whether any definable central nervous system disruption can account for the observed behavioral disturbances. At the same time, there must be constant attention to detecting noncerebral, primary medical disorders that have a causal or contributing effect. Maintaining a high *index of suspicion* is essential, both during the beginning of an evaluative process as well as later during the course of treatment, especially when one confronts symptomatic changes that were not anticipated.

Developing the clinical description necessary for considering brain–behavior relationships also provides the opportunity for refining a psychopathological diagnosis. The search for etiological or anatomical causes does not preclude careful definition of target symptoms that may be amenable to treatment. Indeed, as response to psychotropic agents has been defined empirically, it is not surprising that secondary (i.e., symptomatic) disorders also improve in a fashion similar to those primary psychiatric disturbances to which they are related phenomenologically. (Secondary syndromes, such as the behavioral disturbances that may follow traumatic brain injury or those that are associated with Alzheimer's disease, often respond robustly to treatment, even when no specific cure is available.) However, one must remember that descriptive psychopathological boundaries are arbitrary, and there are no clear-cut points of rarity or demarcation separating one disease cluster from another, despite commonly accepted clinical assumptions (Kendell, 1975).

While evaluating aspects of the patient's disease process, the clinician is also learning more about his illness. This entails establishing where the patient is in his life course, evaluating personal strengths and social supports, and defining resources for future treatment. As well, it entails clarification regarding long-term patterns of dealing with illness and assessment of how the patient sees himself working in collaboration with the clinician.

Thus, the major objective during initial assessment is the establishment of the foundations for treatment. The time for evaluation is also the time when the therapeutic relationship begins to form. Ideally, it provides the opportunity for the patient to demonstrate a commitment to taking part in his own care, while the clinician takes the opportunity to demonstrate expertise and begins infusing hope.

III. Data Acquisition

A. History and Present Illness

Neuropsychiatric assessment follows closely on standard medical examination, and includes attention to present illness, psychiatric history, medical history, family history, social and developmental history, personal habits, review of systems, mental-status examination, physical examination, and laboratory assessment. Central to the process is the determination of when the patient functioned autonomously and effectively—if ever—and illumination of those factors or events that contributed to the patient's decline. As well, the clinician must identify those personal strengths and social supports that have tended to mitigate the illness. The clinical history provides the means for describing the evolution of symptoms and signs, in the fashion of sequential mental-status assessment, and establishes the framework for specifying those target symptoms that will be amenable to therapeutic intervention. The examiner should develop, whenever possible, a full understanding of what the illness may mean to the patient, both in psychodynamic terms and with respect to the patient's perception of its effects on future life.

Clinical data should be gathered from all available sources, even when the patient can cooperate effectively with the evaluation. Spouse, children, co-workers, neighbors, and previous care providers may provide useful insights. Frequently they may have distinctive or disparate views of the patient's illness (e.g., MacKenzie, Robiner, & Knopman, 1989). Depending on the patient alone is often insufficient, especially when evaluating questions of dementia, affective disturbance, or late-life paranoia. The clinician may benefit from using DSM-III-R as a type of inventory for assessment. Indeed, a variety of structured interviews have been developed, which can facilitate the work of both the clinician and the researcher (e.g., Spitzer, Williams, & Gibbon, 1987). Even when these are not used in practice, the clinician must actively assess whether patients have suffered symptoms from particular domains (e.g., reflecting affective, psychotic, or anxiety disorders) and not depend solely on the patient's providing information spontaneously. One may say to the patient, "Please tell me about your difficulties," but this often proves inadequate. Once the patient has responded with complaints and the *story,* the clinician must backtrack to the time when the patient most recently functioned at *normal* level and begin to assist with the development of an organized, time-tagged rendition of the development of the illness. Once cardinal or lead symptoms have been elicited, the clinician must generate specific hypotheses regarding contributing disorders, and also inquire whether other associated phenomena are present. It becomes possible in this fashion to begin to shape a better understanding of the symptom cluster(s) suffered by the patient. This is an essential step toward developing a syndromic diagnosis. Quite apparently, syndromic definition requires a culturally shared recognition of complaints and subjective experiences (Kleinman, 1988), enabling patient and clinician to form a common view of the illness. Lack of cultural congruity can interfere significantly, and the clinician may need assistance from another who has a greater cultural understanding of the patient, especially as the same symptoms may connote widely different meanings (Kleinman, 1986).

While collecting the patient's history, the examiner actively describes what we term the functional anatomy of the illness. We focus on the patient's day-to-day activity, and attempt to understand how the illness has affected personal routine. For example, attention is paid to sleep patterns, self-care, meal preparation, shopping and personal support, interaction with friends, hobbies, personal interests, clubs and outside recreational events, work or structured retirement activities, ability to take care of personal finances, attention to current events, and interest in activities such as sporting events. The examiner should identify particular pursuits in which the patient had been most involved, and then determine how the illness has affected the patient's ability to participate or function effectively. In essence, the most important illustrations of the impact from the illness must be drawn in a personalized fashion; illuminating these areas during evaluation provides the clinician with the framework for later assessing the efficacy of treatment, as it is within the same arena that one will assess whether the patient has improved.

Definition of social and developmental history, medical history, family history, personal habits, and review of systems is undertaken to clarify what other factors may have contributed to the illness. Detection of comorbid medical conditions is critical for establishing whether the neuropsychiatric disturbance is primary or secondary, or coincidentally contributing to functional decline. Principal areas of assessment are outlined in Table I. Of particular import, one must inquire about current medications, their recognized side-effects, and symptoms that may indicate possible central nervous system actions (e.g., sleepiness, dizziness, agitation, fluctuating awareness). Detailing allergic reactions and reactions to medications or radiological contrast agents is also valuable. Although the

Table I

Topics for Medical History, Family History, Developmental
and Social History, and Assessment of Personal Habits

Medical history
  Major illnesses
  Surgical procedures
  Hospitalizations
  Pregnancies
  Current medications and side-effects
  Prior medications and side-effects
  Allergies and allergic reactions
  Worries–misconceptions regarding physical disorders

Family history
  Psychiatric disorders (suicide)
  Neurological disorders (movement disorders)
  Dementing disorders
  Institutionalizations
  General medical disorders (e.g., cardiac diseases, diabetes, cancer)

Developmental and social history
  Birth–early family life–relations with parents and siblings
  Major early-life trauma, if any
  Peer relations
  School–educational attainment
  Chronological occupational history (including possible toxic occupa-
    tional exposures)
  Adult social relations
  Sexual history
  Marital history–family formation
  Adult transitions–maturation
  Retirement
  Death of parents, peers, spouse

Personal habits
  Smoking
  Drinking–substance use (including over-the-counter preparations)
  Reading, current events
  Hobbies–recreation
  Family events
  Structured nonvocational activities

patient may deny having had a formal psychiatric diagnosis in the past, questions regarding the use of specific psychotropics (e.g., antidepressants) may prove revealing, as these are frequently prescribed by family physicians and internists: Establishing past therapeutic responses will provide the clinician with an indication of possibly effective future agents. Though not typically considered part of the medical history, the clinician should elicit from the patient any worries, concerns, or misconceptions regarding physical disorders. This may bring out unreasonable or exaggerated somatic complaints. We and our colleagues have noted the association between fears of cancer and completed suicide (Conwell, Caine, & Olsen, in press).

Documenting family history of psychiatric and neurological disorders may help with differential diagnostic consideration, as well as providing a lead to potential therapeutic interventions. Although great effort has been made to educate professionals regarding the inappropriate usage of the term senility, patients and their families continue to apply it indiscriminately. It is not uncommon to encounter an individual or relative who states unequivocally that there is no history of neuropsychiatric disturbance, dementia, or Alzheimer's disease, but then readily describes senility in parents and grandparents. Similarly, questions about long-term institutionalization may prove rewarding.

When collecting an elaborate developmental and social history, the clinician works to define the patient's prior experiences and coping abilities, as well as clarifying the social supports that may have diminished the adverse effects of the illness. Developmental and social history establish the context for understanding further the patient's personal habits and current symptoms.

B. Mental-Status Assessment

The mental-status evaluation provides the formal structure used by the clinician to examine thoughts and cognitive abilities. It constitutes an essential element in neuropsychiatric diagnosis, a process that intertwines a detailed appreciation of the patient's present state of mind and a broadly viewed clinical history. The examination fulfills several, complementary functions; it (1) provides an initial assessment of a patient's mental strengths, deficiencies, and abnormalities; (2) establishes the basis for future comparison, enabling a clinician to document improvement or decline; (3) enhances communication between clinicians by defining a common structure for evaluation; and (4) improves the ability to compare descriptions developed for different patients.

Formal mental-status examination has been a part of neuropsychiatric diagnosis for perhaps 100 years, at most. Pinel (1806), Rush (1812), and Esquirol (1845) had no sections in their books on the method of patient examination. It is clear that Esquirol, in particular, placed great importance on the productions of patients, but he presented no systematized approach for documenting them. Bucknell and Tuke (1858) described the value of noting the patient's appearance and motor behavior, but they were less concerned about the form and content of his thoughts. Initially it was the German neuropsychiatrists of the mid-1800s, particularly Griesinger (1867), who began attending to intellectual functions in a systematic manner.

For Kraepelin, the individual most identified with modern diagnostic classification, the form of patient's thought processes provided a principal pillar in the structure of syndromic analysis. The opening sections of his *Textbook of Psychiatry* (1919) were devoted to what was, in effect, an outline and definition of the major abnormalities of mental functioning. Textbooks in the United States immediately following Kraepelin's work also showed the mental status examination as the first major topic for discussion. After the ascendance of psychoanalytic and personality theory in this country, however, the systematic evaluation of intellectual functions received less attention.

Although numerous mental examinations now exist that focus on specific diagnostic entities, the approaches psychiatrists utilize in testing mental status often fail to exploit potential contributions from neuropsychology, neurology, and memory–learning theory. In the last 20 to 30 years, careful clinical correlations between cognitive deficits and cortical lesions have clarified the nature of functional localization in man. Studies of patients with unilateral temporal lobectomy, commissurotomy, and focal cerebral lesions have documented distinct hemispheric cognitive strategies and capabilities. Techniques and theories developed in college learning laboratories are being applied to clarify disorders of neuropsychiatric patients. Strub and Black (1985) provide a detailed introduction to these areas.

Psychiatric diagnosis comprises more than the formal evaluation of mental state. However, the perfunctory style with which the mental-status examination was taught for many years to students of psychiatry suggested that it had little to add to history taking and symptom description. With increased attention to aging, dementia, and behavior disorders due to cerebral diseases, the mental status examination has emerged again as a source of potentially valuable diagnostic information.

A comprehensive mental-status examination requires an evaluation of all major mental functions that might be affected by neuropsychiatric disorders. It affords a means of surveying problems and determining those dysfunctions needing more detailed evaluation and description. It stresses the consideration of an individual's disabilities and relative strengths. We shall discuss briefly each major category of function needing examination.

1. General Description

Among the purposes of mental assessment, two involve the composition of a clear picture describing a newly encountered patient, and the effective communication of this picture to another professional. Beginning with a depiction of the patient's appearance and behavior, the examination is developed in a manner that encourages the formulation of a detailed verbal representation of the patient, with a consideration of both broad psychological processes and specific intellectual functions. The clinician must observe the patient's self-care, motoric behavior, and interactive style. It is always useful to record where the patient looked during the examination (e.g., Did he make eye contact?). Typically we note in this section whether the patient manifests any grossly evident sensory impairments, and indicate what sensory aids (e.g., glasses, hearing assist) are used.

2. Level of Consciousness

The examiner can detect many subtle gradations of consciousness between the fully alert, responsive state and unresponsive coma. Such designations are often arbitrary; the major requirement is that each clinician maintain an internal consistency, with his colleagues being aware of what is meant by all descriptive terms. In some published outlines of mental status examination, *sensorium* is included as one of the last items for reporting. It should be one of the first! If mental function is impaired grossly, owing to an altered level of consciousness, it is essential to communicate this immediately. When evaluating delirium, the clinician must see the patient on multiple occasions, to document the fluctuation of arousal that often characterizes the condition. (In cases of mild delirium, changes in arousal level may be difficult to detect, and the examiner may note only changes in attention and organization of thought.)

3. Attention

Attention, along with comprehension, forms the foundation on which the remainder of the mental-status examination is built. A deficit in attention may be subtle, but it can lead to impaired intellectual functioning on a number of tasks. Patients often present with a spontaneously varying level of attention, with fluctuations due to disorders of neurophysiological arousal, environmental distractions, or preoccupying internal thoughts. It is essential to assess patients on a number of structured and unstructured procedures in order to establish their ability to shift and focus attention, as well as their ability to sustain it. It may also be necessary to observe them in informal settings (e.g., when they are talking with other individuals) to gain the fullest appreciation of their attentional skills.

4. Language

Language function is judged by evaluating an individual's comprehension, verbal output, and repetition skills. Comprehension must be effectively assessed before other intellectual functions can be evaluated meaningfully. Verbal output is described in terms of fluency (phrase length), prosody (melody or intonation), syntactic structure, word content (e.g., telegraphic, fluent but empty), word-finding difficulties (e.g., paraphasic errors, circumlocutions), and a qualitative description (e.g., soft or loud, circumstantial, pedantic). Repetition is tested for simple sounds, and multisyllabic words and phrases. Naming to confrontation is also evaluated routinely. In special cases, color naming and body part naming–recognition will need to be examined. Language function also provides a convenient, though potentially biased, means of defining a patient's level of general intelligence. The clinician should always attempt to establish an estimate of intellectual abilities (beyond screening for dementia) as part of planning an overall treatment approach. By knowing the patient's educational level, and assessing the use of vocabulary, one can make a rough estimate. However, this method requires caution, as low education, a cultural background different from that of the examiner, or English as a second language can contribute to apparently diminished verbal and intellectual facility.

5. Thought

A consideration of language logically leads next to the description of a patient's thought processes, both in form and content. Someone may have normal language function (e.g., adequate variety of words, with proper intonation and grammar) but disordered connection of ideas (a disturbance in form). Similarly, an individual might articulately and coherently describe an organized persecutory system (a disturbance in content). In evaluating thought disorder, clarity of definition is crucial (Andreasen, 1979); verbatim examples of the patient's disturbance avoid ambiguity or misunderstanding. The examiner must note somatic complaints, and encourage the patient to discuss any fears and preconceptions. In addition to also noting preoccupations and concerns, the clinician must always assess suicidal ideation. This involves eliciting responses regarding passive (e.g., "better off dead" or "wished I was no longer alive") as well as active ideas. Specific questions must deal with plans regarding implementation, and the examiner should discover contemplated means, location, time of day, and thoughts regarding contact with possible rescuers. For all patients, the examiner should inquire about their view of the future, their sense of self-worth, and their sense of personal effectiveness.

6. Affective State

The examiner evaluates the overt manifestation of emotion (affect), the expressed internal feeling state (mood), and the congruence of affect and mood. One must note spontaneously manifested emotions; facial, vocal, and body expressions; and responses to specific (probing) questions. It is essential to remember that, in the elderly, sadness or despair may not be the presenting features of an affective disorder. Rather, they may describe reduced interest, energy, and joy, increased pessimism, and diminished self-worth, while communicating discouragement or bewilderment about their functional decline. We routinely attempt to engage the patient in some humorous conversation, both to assess the ability to appreciate humor, as well as the ability to sustain a positive affect. Occasionally we encounter patients with *pseudobulbar* affect, or *affective incontinence*. These signs reflect cerebral lesions, and are characterized most often by an *affective overshoot* or *disconnected affect*. In the former, the patient responds to an appropriate stimulus, but the expression is exaggerated. The latter denotes a severing of internal mood state from affective expression; the patient responds to an emotion stimulus with a bizarrely inappropriate emotion (e.g., a sad statement followed by giddy laughter). The patient may acknowledge that the emotional outburst does not match the felt internal state. These affective abnormalities often coexist, and careful observation should provide the examiner with sufficiently consistent findings to determine that these manifestations are not within the range of behaviors typically seen in patients with primary psychiatric disorders (e.g., the inappropriate smiling seen in some schizophrenic patients).

7. Judgment, Abstraction, and Insight

These functions are the most difficult to define; they often defy adequate assessment. In the past, the standard questions (e.g., "What do you do when you find a stamped, sealed letter on the ground?") provided little indication about an individual's judgment; often they were an invitation to lighthearted, joking answers. Questions that require individuals to consider how they would behave in a difficult social situation can prove more revealing (e.g., "What would you do if someone came up to you on the street and became angry with you, thinking that you were someone else?" or "What would you say to someone who broke something of yours that meant a lot to you?"). As well, we ask patients to judge the nature of their important social relationships.

Proverb interpretation may prove useful for assessing abstraction abilities, despite its lack of specificity. Noting the qualitative nature of someone's deficit is essential, as failure to adequately interpret proverbs can reflect a multitude of causes, including low intelligence, poor education, and unfamiliarity with the concept of proverbs, as well as focal brain disease, schizophrenia, depression, etc. Proverbs often provide a fruitful means of inviting people to share their inner thoughts, a short-hand projective test.

Insight is evaluated most effectively by determining the patient's understanding of his or her present state and the reasons for hospitalization. An individual's insight may also be noted when an examiner presents specific questions concerning affective state.

8. Focal Cognitive Functions

Although commonly assumed to be intact in many psychiatric patients, focal cognitive functions tests must be performed for the complete evaluation of cerebral functioning. They may prove useful in separating dementia from depression, detecting subtle focal cortical lesions, evaluating toxic states, or assessing the side-effects of electroconvulsive therapy (in conjunction with memory tests). Constructional skills (particularly copying) must be assessed on all patients. Other *higher cortical functions* include mathematics, reading, writing, finer sensory function (stereognosis, graphesthesia, two-point discrimination), right–left orientation, motor praxis, and finger gnosis. It is essential to realize that all neuropsychological functions do not uniformly localize to the same specific regions in all people. Apparent localization may be affected by cerebral dominance, individual variation, minor developmental deficits, the speed with which a lesion develops (i.e., gradual versus acute), or other undetermined factors. All deficits must be interpreted *by the company they keep*.

9. Memory

Evaluating memory is dealt with at greater length, given its central role in geriatric neuropsychiatry. Disordered memory is found in a wide variety of diseases. It may be the unique manifestation of dysfunction or one of several intellectual impairments. The former disorders might be termed specific (e.g., Korsakoff syndrome, transient global amnesia), the latter *multifunctional* (e.g., dementia of the Alzheimer type). Impairments may be *persistent* or *transient*. Onset may be acute, or insidious and gradual.

When examining a patient with memory dysfunction, there are two major domains which require assessment: (1) Recall of previously well-remembered information, and (2) the ability to learn new material. The first can be done by questioning the patient about life events and major current events that took place early in the patient's life (before the onset of any disease process). It proves helpful to have a spouse or family member present to verify the accuracy of the patient's statements. Too often, inexperienced examiners ask overly general questions, which can be answered by patients with severe retrograde amnesia (i.e., the inability to remember previously learned material). For example, a question about the name of the town where one grew up might be answered easily, while a request to describe in detail the house where one lived as a child might elicit a deficit. Emotionally laden events are usually recalled vividly by normal individuals (e.g., "What were you doing when you heard that Pearl Harbor was bombed?" or "Tell me about your wedding day," or "Where were you when you heard that John Kennedy was shot?"). If it is not possible to verify a patient's responses to highly personal queries, detailed questions about historical persons or events may prove more reliable (e.g., "What was the name of Roosevelt's dog?"—for those examiners and patients who were either alive at that time or know historical trivia—or, "What was the name of the man who shot John Kennedy?" or "Can you tell me about Watergate?").

When questioning patients concerning their recall of previously learned material, an examiner may find a pattern—or combination of patterns—of memory deficit. Patients with alcoholic Korsakoff's syndrome often show their most marked impairment for recall of events or persons from the years immediately preceding the onset of their disorder.

Questions aimed at eliciting information from the more distant past typically yield more accurate answers.

It is often evident that a major element of retrograde amnesia is the disruption of temporal ordering, in which an event may be remembered but its time relationship to other events is forgotten. This is seen dramatically in patients with traumatic amnesia and other kinds of acquired memory disorders (Whitty & Zangwill, 1977). Retrograde amnesia is not an all-or-none phenomenon in the great majority of cases.

Generally, the inability to learn and remember new information is also not an all-or-none phenomenon. Most of what we know about disorders with anterograde amnesia relates to verbal materials; it is not possible to generalize to visual, acoustic, or olfactory stimuli. Deficits can occur in memory acquisition, retention, or retrieval. These can be separated by systematically varying the kinds of stimuli employed, the delay between exposure and recall testing, and the nature of the recall tests utilized. All clinical testing must be conducted on the basis of a patient's output; inferences about the mechanisms of memory failure are of necessity indirect.

A variety of memory tasks can be used. These can be divided into incidental learning procedures, where the individual is not told that he or she is expected to recall the material later, and instructed learning tests, where the patient is told about the need for later recall. In normal individuals, incidental learning is as effective as instructed recall, but for purposes of initial evaluation, the latter is more desirable. If the patient fails when consciously expending effort, it is most likely that a memory impairment is present. Tasks may vary from formally developed batteries [e.g., the Wechsler Memory Scale, Revised (Wechsler, 1987)] to recall tests of digits, word lists of varying lengths, or reading a paragraph and remembering its details.

For a very brief evaluation, a short list of words can prove useful. The examiner might present stimulus words after presenting these instructions—"I am going to tell you a list of words that I want you to remember. I will say them all to you at first, and I want you to repeat them to me when I finish. Later I will ask you to recall them again." Thereupon the examiner presents the word list, spoken at a one word per 2–3 sec rate: For example, "daisy, cat, seventeen, friend, church, sad." The patient's ability to repeat immediately and accurately points to intact initial acquisition skills. A list of six items is close to or within most normal individuals' memory span or "chunk size." This is then rehearsed for 3 to 5 trials, with the examiner repeating the entire list on each occasion and asking the patient to recall. It is discontinued after the fifth trial or when the patient has repeated the list correctly two times in a row (whichever comes sooner). Then, the patient is engaged for 10 min in other tasks such as history taking or physical examination. Recall is elicited by saying, "Please tell me the words I asked you to remember before." The patient's output is recorded, giving a measure of delayed recall. If this is deficient, the examiner presents a categorical *cue,* which is employed to improve recall of those items that were not remembered spontaneously. "A flower" would be the categorical cue for daisy. If the patient did not produce the target item after the cuing procedure, he or she would be presented with a multiple-choice task: "Was it rose, violet, daisy, or lily?" These last two procedures are intended to determine whether the subject remembers the stimulus item under any circumstances; the ultimate test presents the stimulus itself in the multiple-choice (recognition) paradigm. When the patient does not spontaneously recall the to-be-remembered item, but produces it in either cued or recognition formats, he or she is said to have a retrieval failure. The item is in memory, but is not retrieved without prompting.

C. Standardized Assessment Procedures

We shall briefly review several standardized procedures that can be used by the clinician to readily augment mental status examination and functional evaluation. These include both self-report and examiner-rated forms. Two useful compendiums of such instruments have been published in recent years (Crook, Ferris, & Bartus, 1983; Raskin & Niederhe, 1988), and we shall only highlight several measures that we have found to be particularly helpful.

There are a variety of tools available to aid in overall psychopathological assessment, as well as in the quantitation of symptoms related specifically to mood disorders. The Sandoz Clinical Assessment-Geriatric (SCAG) Scale was developed for psychopharmacological research (Shader, Harmatz, & Salzman, 1974). As a general-purpose rating scale, it is particularly helpful when using the guidelines developed by Venn (1983) for reliably scoring the eighteen items on the scale, which then fall into five factor clusters, including cognitive dysfunction, interpersonal relationships, affective disorders, apathy, and somatic functioning. In a similar vein, the Brief Psychiatric Rating Scale (Overall & Beller, 1984; Overall & Gorham, 1962) has been shown to have substantial utility with geriatric populations. Though developed in nongeriatric settings, it has been widely used in pharmacotherapeutic trials on patients of all ages, and is readily used with both outpatients and inpatients. The Hamilton Depression Rating Scale (Hamilton, 1967) is another instrument that was not developed for the geriatric population, but has been used frequently in pharmacotherapeutic studies. The Hamilton must be applied cautiously with the elderly, however, as unrelated but coexisting medical disorders can contribute substantially to items on the scale (Caine, in press). Self-rating scales of depression may also add to the rigor of the clinical assessment, and are easily utilized in both inpatient and outpatient settings. In our experience, the Geriatric Depression Scale (GDS) (Yesavage *et al.*, 1983) and the Beck Depression Inventory (BDI) (Beck, Ward, Mendelson, Mock, & Erbaugh, 1961) are less heavily contaminated by comorbid medical illnesses. The GDS has an acceptably high specificity and sensitivity for detecting major depression in both inpatients and outpatients (Koenig, Meador, Cohen, & Blazer, 1988), although it does not demonstrate validity in populations of cognitively impaired individuals (Burke, Houston, Bonst, & Roccaforte, 1989). The Beck Depression Inventory has been used with neurologically impaired patients, such as those with Parkinson's disease (Mayeux, Stern, Rosen, & Leventhal, 1981; Levin, Llabre, & Weiner, 1988), and the effects of depression can be separated from those of the disease process itself. We have used the short form of the BDI (Beck & Beck, 1972), which correlates highly with the original version, and is particularly suited for the elderly given its brevity.

Cognitive assessment can be aided by using structured, brief tests of intellectual function. The most widely employed procedure during the past decade has been the Mini Mental State Examination (MMSE) developed by Folstein and colleagues (Folstein, Folstein, & McHugh, 1975). Its convergent validity with other procedures has been documented (Folstein, *et al.*, 1975; Thal, Grundman, & Golden, 1986), as has its sensitivity and specificity (Anthony, LeResche, Niaz, vonKorff, & Folstein, 1982). It correlates robustly with overall intellectual functioning, as measured with the Wechsler Adult Intelligence Scale (Farber, Schmitt, & Logue, 1988), and has been used extensively during the epidemiological catchment area studies performed by the National Institute of Mental Health. It is now also included in the geriatric evaluation procedure developed by Roth and colleagues, the CAMDEX (Cambridge Mental Disorders of the Elderly Examination) (1986). Confounding errors on the MMSE that might lead to a false positive designation of impairment have been related to older age, lower educational level, ethnicity, and language background (Anthony *et al.*, 1982; Escobar *et al.*, 1986). Our own experience, as well as those of Folstein and colleagues (personal communication, November 1985), indicate that it has a false-negative rate of about 10%, failing to detect outpatients suffering dementia of the Alzheimer type. This has been related to the examination of patients early in their disease course; annual reassessment has consistently demonstrated functional decline and developing deficits on the MMSE. It is notable that the protocol is not satisfactory for defining focal versus diffuse hemisphere disease (Dick *et al.*, 1984), and we have observed that patients with circumscribed impairments (e.g., mild to moderate amnestic disorders) may have stable significant deficits on detailed neuropsychological assessment procedures that are not manifest significantly on the MMSE.

There are a variety of instruments available for functional evaluation of older patients. These have recently been reviewed by Applegate, Blass, and Williams (1990). Functional capacity has been assessed typically by measuring self-maintenance activities (e.g., activities of daily living) such as dressing, toileting, feeding, etc., or instrumental self-care activities that require a higher level of personal competence (e.g., shopping, using money, driving, etc.). The scales of Lawton and Brody (Lawton & Brody, 1969), the Instrumental Activities of Daily Living and the Physical Self-Maintenance Scale are time tested, reliable, and valid, and have been employed in a number of settings. They are especially sensitive to the effects of developing dementia, and often reflect abnormalities evidenced by elderly patients with major depression or psychosis. However, many subjects may eventually surpass the *ceiling* of these scales as they recover. Unfortunately, instruments for assessing the function of more competent psychiatric patients are not available.

D. Medical and Neurological Examination

It is beyond the scope of this chapter to consider the general physical and neurological examinations in detail. However, these are essential components of a comprehensive neuropsychiatric assessment, and compose a major element in deciding whether behavioral disturbances are primary, due to idiopathic psychiatric disorders, or secondary syndromes, symptomatic manifestations of disordered cerebral functioning or systemic medical disease. Medical disorders may be etiologically related (leading to secondary behavioral syndromes), or comorbid conditions. The latter may contribute to primary psychiatric disturbances, confound them by adding to overall functional decline, or merely be incidental factors that the knowledgeable clinician should appreciate at the time of treatment planning.

Thorough physical examination and medical assessment often require consultation with internists and other medical specialists. The neuropsychiatric clinician must articulate specific questions to consultants, as their advice is most helpful in the differential diagnostic process when it is focused and addresses defined medical issues. Neurological examination is necessary to establish the integrity of the cranial nerves, the motor system as it relates to strength, complex and general sensory function, muscle-stretch reflexes, and motoric behavior (including posture and gait). The clinician searches for any findings indicative of subtle pathology, especially sensory impairments, asymmetrical alterations in reflexes, and abnormalities of movement. These and other evaluations are described amply in Albert's *Clinical Neurology of Aging* (1984). Similar to medical consultation, questions to the neurological consultant must be focused and thoughtful. Inquiries about such vague concerns as *organic pathology* frequently prove unrewarding, as the neurologist must often depend on the behaviorally oriented clinician to identify which behaviors are uncharacteristic of primary psychiatric disorders. Careful case reasoning requires that a clinical syndrome must have positive features to include it as a possible primary psychiatric disturbance. Failing to find a primary cerebral or systemic medical cause does not automatically denote a disorder as *psychiatric,* nor does discerning the presence of a physical abnormality automatically lead one to decide that a behavioral disturbance is secondary or symptomatic. The clinician must weigh factors such as the time course of the behavioral disturbance, the evolution of the medical disorder, and apparent laboratory abnormalities, with an understanding of which behavioral disturbances are related to specific physical derangements. However, even the most experienced clinician may confront situations in which he is uncertain regarding the etiologic tie between definable physical disruptions and psychopathological syndromes that need treatment.

E. Laboratory Procedures

The neuropsychiatric assessment has as its goal the description, definition, and explanation for a disturbance in mental life. Laboratory evaluations provide a means for further defining cerebral and systemic medical disturbances. They take their lead from the clinical history, mental-status and physical examinations, following the path of clinical intuition toward a suspected etiological cause. A secondary function of the laboratory evaluation is to screen for incidental medical illness unrelated to the neuropsychiatric disturbance, but previously undetected.

1. Clinical Laboratory Assessment

Psychiatric patients suffer increased rates of medical illness and are less likely than others to seek treatment or comply with therapeutic recommendations. They suffer higher rates of morbidity and mortality from medical illness (Brugha, Wing, & Smith, 1989). While there is some controversy regarding the yield and cost–benefit ratio of extensive screening examinations, there is a consensus that patients older than 50 years and those with suspected primary medical pathology should be studied more exhaustively (Brugha *et al.,* 1989; Ferguson & Dudleston, 1986; Koran *et al.,* 1989). The onset of a major psychiatric disturbance after ages 45–50 years is an indication for a maximally vigorous assessment.

Table II presents a simple, preliminary laboratory examination. These procedures screen for abnormalities in organ systems (e.g., blood, kidney, liver) in which dysfunction can impair mental life, and provide a relatively inexpensive health maintenance evaluation as well. Table II also lists tests that can be added to a patient's initial battery if he has not received regular or recent medical care.

Beyond this screening laboratory evaluation, specific testing must be tailored to the patient's individual presentation. *Informed clinical suspicion* must lead the examiner when selecting which tests confirm or disconfirm initial leads. A lower threshold is used when ordering less intrusive or inexpensive procedures. Table III presents some additional tests helpful in defining the etiology of neuropsychiatric disturbances.

Blood tests are the least invasive and least expensive ancillary tests, and as such, the threshold for ordering them is lower. Neuroimaging can be integral to the diagnostic process, though it is costly and may be uncomfortable for the patient. The technologies available and their indications are discussed shortly. Lumbar puncture may involve considerable discomfort to the patient. It is indicated when the cause for neuropsychiatric disturbance remains unclear after appropriate blood testing and imaging studies, or if there is a suspicion of an intracranial infection. It is contraindicated when there is evidence of raised intracranial pressure. When possible, imaging should be obtained before lumbar puncture to ascertain that there is no structural lesion that might cause elevated intracranial pressure. One must also rely on the clinical examination, specifically noting the absence of papilledema or other signs of raised pressure.

The electroencephalogram (EEG) is a noninvasive and easily accessible test of brain function. It measures, through the skull, the electrical activity over the cerebral hemispheres. Disturbances in the proportion of the various electrical-wave rhythms (alpha, delta, beta, and theta) are detected and recorded. The EEG is fairly sensitive to cortical

Table II

General Screening Laboratory Evaluation

Complete blood count (CBC)
Erythrocyte sedimentation rate (ESR)
Electrolytes
Glucose
Blood urea nitrogen (BUN)/serum creatinine
Liver function tests
Serum calcium and phosphorous
Thyroid function tests
Serum protein
Levels of all drugs
Urinanalysis
Pregnancy test for women of childbearing age
Electrocardiogram (EKG)

For Patients without Regular Medical Care
Chest X-ray
Stool for occult blood
Mammogram
PAP smear

Table III

Ancillary Tests Useful in Neuropsychiatric Assessment

Blood	*Cerebrospinal Fluid*
Blood cultures	Glucose, protein
Rapid plasma reagin (RPR)	Cell count
Arterial blood gas (ABG)	Cultures (bacterial, viral, fungal)
Serum heavy metals	Cryptococcal antigen
Serum copper	Veneral Disease Research Laboratory (VDRL)
Ceruloplasmin	*Radiography*
Serum B_{12}, RBC folate	Computerized tomography (CT)
Urine	Magnetic resonance imaging (MRI)
Culture	Positron emission tomography (PET)
Toxicology	Single photon emission computed tomography (SPECT)
Heavy metal screen	
Electrography	
Electroencephalography (EEG)	
Evoked potentials	
Polysomnography	
Nocturnal penile tumescence (NPT)	

dysfunction, but quite nonspecific. There are few disturbances that can be attributed to a specific disease process (Lishman, 1987, p. 110). Beyond its use in epilepsy, the EEG's greatest utility in neuropsychiatry is in the detection of mild encephalopathy or delirium, space-occupying lesions, and complex partial seizures where the patient continues to remain conscious, though behaviorally impaired. It is highly sensitive to metabolic disturbances and toxic states, displays a diffuse slowing of rhythm in such cases, and may be extremely useful when verifying a clinical suspicion of delirium. It cannot distinguish, however, between different etiologies. The EEG can display focal slowing in the presence of space-occupying cranial lesions, cerebral abscesses, or subdural hematomas. Localization, however, is far from infallible, as the lesion may not result in an electrical disruption or may also disturb rhythm in other cerebral locations (Lishman, 1987, p. 112). The EEG changes with age, with a general reduction in the alpha rhythm, and increase in the amount of theta and delta waves. In dementia, these same changes are accentuated (Soininen, Partanen, Helkala, & Riekkinen, 1982). The EEG has been useful in distinguishing demented from nondemented patients, but patients with severe dementia can present with a normal EEG, and normal elderly individuals may have mild abnormalities (Soininen *et al.*, 1982). The EEG changes in dementia are nonspecific; in dementia of the Alzheimer's type (DAT), these changes manifest earlier and to a greater extent than in multi-infarct dementia (MID) or mixed presentations (Ettlin *et al.*, 1989). Brenner, Reynolds, and Ulrich (1989) utilized EEG abnormalities to distinguish demented patients with depressive features from patients with depressive pseudodementia.

2. Neuroimaging

Imaging merits a detailed discussion, as it provides the clinician a means to study directly the organ of neuropsychiatric function and pathology, the brain. Not since the discovery of the electroencephalogram by Hans Berger in 1929 has there been such an explosion in the available technologies for investigating the brain. Long-standing techniques for study of neuropsychiatric conditions, such as pneumoencephalography, ventriculography, and isotope cisternography, have been displaced by computerized tomographic (CT) scanning and magnetic resonance imaging (MRI). These technologies have become readily available and are now an integral part of the assessment. The newness of these technologies, however, remains evident in the ambiguities that surround the interpretation of many detected *abnormalities*. For example, there is no fully comprehensive or standardized, normative baseline across the age spectrum for comparative MRI interpretation. We will review five imaging techniques currently available for neuropsychiatric assessment.

a. X-ray radiography.   X-ray films of the skull have been part of the diagnostic armamentarium for nearly a century. They are able to visualize only bony structures and have been used to infer underlying brain abnormalities. They were, at one point, considered a standard part of psychiatric assessment. With the advent of CT and MRI, utility of skull films has become limited to those instances in which a bony abnormality is specifically suspected, as myeloma, Paget's disease, or old skull fractures.

b. Computerized tomographic (CT) scanning.   CT, the first technology for studying brain tissue in a live patient, came into widespread use during the mid-1970s. The technique involves a computerized image reconstruction of brain tissues, based on their relative densities and absorption values when exposed to a beam of x-rays. The technique is 100 times more sensitive than standard x-rays, yet produces no greater radiation exposure. The CT scan can describe both the extent and type of focal abnormalities (such as primary cerebral neoplasms, extracerebral tumors, nonmalignant abscesses and calcifications, subdural and epidural hematomas, and cerebral infarctions), as well as generalized structural alterations such as cerebral edema and hydrocephalus. It has proven inestimably valuable for delineating the type, location, age, and size of lesions—tasks previously dependent on clinical guesswork.

Clinical and research use with the degenerative dementias, such as DAT, display both the promise and limits of CT imaging. DAT is diagnosed on presumptive clinical grounds after all other possible etiologies have been eliminated. The CT is most useful for excluding other causes for the dementia, but it has not provided a *rule in* or identifying factor for DAT. CT scanning cannot image those brain structures that are pathologically affected by the disease process (e.g., the hippocampus). Thus, indices of developing brain atrophy must depend on indirect measurements of expanding fluid-filled spaces (e.g., lateral ventricles, temporal horns), rather than gathering direct evidence of specific shrunken brain sites. While there is a group correlation between the prevalence and severity of dementia with the extent of cortical atrophy, the correlation is imperfect; there are severely demented patients with little atrophy and normal elderly patients with prominent atrophy. Atrophy usually does not become apparent until the dementing process is well underway and is easily recognized by the clinician (Kido *et al.*, 1989). Cortical atrophy remains a nonspecific finding on CT, generally more prominent in the cognitively impaired, but also present in normal elderly patients, schizophrenics, and those with bipolar disorder (Weinberger, 1984; Pearlson & Veroff, 1981). CT cannot provide diagnostic markers or preclinical indicators of risk, or prognostic signs for the degenerative dementias.

Though the head CT scan can provide rich information, both its expense and its radiation exposure have prompted a search for clinical guidelines for its use. McClellan, Eisenberg, & Giyanani (1988) reviewed the records of 261 patients who had received routine head CT scans as part of an admission evaluation. After excluding patients with known neurologic disease, focal neurological findings, seizures, or complaints of head-ache, they found no CT abnormalities that were felt to be clinically related to the patient's condition. They concluded that head CT scanning should be utilized only if the physical examination and history detect focal neurologic deficits or other findings such as pa-pilledema, seizures, or headache. Weinberger (1984) reviewed the literature regarding the yield of the head CT in general psychiatric patients and concluded that the studies are inadequate and contradictory. He emphasized that, while the yield of positive results is low, the potential for uncovering occult primary neurological disease was high. He pro-posed the following guidelines for obtaining a head CT:

1. confusion or dementia of unknown etiology;
2. first episode of psychosis of unknown etiology;
3. movement disorder of unknown etiology;
4. anorexia nervosa;
5. prolonged catatonia; or
6. first episode of an affective disorder or personality change occurring after the age of fifty years.

While these guidelines again underscore the need to investigate focal neurological find-ings with a head CT scan, they also include changes in personality, affect, and cognition as indications for study. Perhaps a single condensation of these guidelines is that any patient, previously functioning adequately or independently who presents with an ac-quired neurological deficit or mental impairment should have a brain imaging study, either CT scan or MRI, depending on the specific questions being studied.

c. Magnetic resonance imaging (MRI). MRI has become available for clinical application during the past decade, though the technology of nuclear magnetic resonance has been used for the greater part of this century. Images are obtained by computer analysis of the tissue distribution of hydrogen ions as their polarity is altered by radio frequency pulses through a magnetic field (Conlon & Trimble, 1987). The patient is not exposed to x-ray radiation. Recent reviews of the technology and its applications to psychiatry are available (Conlon & Trimble, 1987; Gordon, Kraiuhin, & Meares, 1986). The MRI expands the potential for evaluation of the brain. It provides greater mor-phological detail than CT scanning, and allows direct measurement of structures such as the thalamus, basal ganglia, hippocampus, and amygdala (Conlon & Trimble, 1987; Johnson et al., 1987). The MRI is insensitive to bone and its therefore of great utility in looking at those structures obscured by bone on the head CT scan, such as the temporal and apical areas of the brain, as well as the posterior fossa structures. MRI also provides for greater discrimination of the interface between gray matter and white matter. It has been validated against autopsy findings for accuracy regarding brain volume, sulcal and ventricular cerebrospinal fluid (CSF) distribution, and gray matter volume (Jernigan, Press, & Hesselink, 1990). In comparison with head CT, MRI has been found to detect more lesions with greater delineation of the extent of the lesion (Garber, Weilbury, Buonanno, Manschreck, & New, 1988; Tanridag & Kirschner, 1987). In particular, the MRI has been shown to be far more sensitive than the CT in detecting white-matter lesions. MRI is superior for detecting lesions in the periventricular and subcortical white matter (Harrel, Callaway, & Sekar, 1987; Johnson *et al.*, 1987; Erkinjuntti *et al.*, 1987). The meaning of findings such as periventricular *rims* and *caps* and *unidentified bright objects* is still uncertain. Autopsy correlations generally show that these findings represent true anatomical structures and are not artifacts (Jernigan *et al.*, 1990; Leifer, Buonanno, & Richardson, 1990), but their pathophysiological contribution remains to be clarified. They are detected, for example, in younger patients with multiple sclerosis or HIV infection, but are also found in older subjects having no known diseases or clinical correlates. While it was hoped that the increased sensitivity of MRI would provide the means for definitive diagnosis of neuropsychiatric conditions until now dependent solely on clinical description, this promise has not been realized. White-matter hyperintensities (WMH) provide an example. Erkinjuntti *et al.* (1987) found that all 28 patients with MID in their study had WMH, as compared to only eight of 22 patients with DAT. They concluded that WMH on MRI was a distinguishing factor for the diagnosis of MID. However, others have compared demented and nondemented elderly patients and found that WMH did not distinguish the two groups (Duara, Barker, Lowenstein, Pascal, & Bowen, 1989; Hershey, Modic, Greenough, & Jaffee, 1987; Leys *et al.*, 1990). Ebmeier *et al.* (1987) were unable to separate DAT from MID based on WMH, though they and others have found a descending frequency of WMH, highest in MID, intermediate in DAT, lower in unimpaired elderly, and extremely rare in young normals (Aharon-Peretz, Cummings, & Hill, 1988; Kertesz, Polk, & Carr, 1990; Kobari, Meyer, & Ichijo, 1990). WMH has been shown to correlate with age (Hunt *et al.*, 1989; Jernigan *et al.*, 1990; Kobari *et al.*, 1990), but not cognitive, behavioral, or motor dysfunction (Fein *et al.*, 1990; Hunt *et al.*, 1990; Leys *et al.*, 1990). In summary, WMH on the MRI can probably be viewed in the same light as cortical atrophy on the CT, a highly sensitive but nonspecific finding. WMH is more extensive and frequent in demented patients (and more common in MID than DAT), but too variable to contribute to individual diagnosis and/or prognosis. At this time, the MRI remains useful only in conjunction with the clinical examination. Like CT, its greatest utility in the evaluation of dementia arises from what it might exclude, namely a reversible lesion, as opposed to its ability to specifically determine the disease process.

Indications for MRI are similar for those for head CT. MRI is preferred over head CT when studying those areas of the brain for which it has greater resolution. MRI is warranted when the clinical picture is not adequately explained by the known pathology, when multiple pathologies (e.g., combined MID and DAT) are suspected, or when a CT (or IV contrast) is contraindicated (Sachdev, 1990). MRI requires a patient to enter a narrow tube, remain there for approximately 45–90 min, and to be exposed to an electromagnet. It is contraindicated in patients with metal implants or surgical clips, as these may move in response to the magnetic field. Patients with pacemakers are at risk for desynchronization (Garber *et al.*, 1988). Patients with claustrophobia or agitation do not tolerate MRI well. In these instances, CT is preferable. CT is also the instrument of choice when examining bony structures or expected calcified lesions, such as meningiomas, as MRI is insensitive to calcium or bone.

d. Physiological imaging techniques. In addition to the progress in imaging anatomical structures, two new technologies have been developed for direct imaging of brain function. Single photon emission-computed tomography (SPECT) involves the injection of a radiopharmaceutical that follows the cerebral blood flow. Recent studies have demonstrated perfusion deficits in patients with DAT, when compared with age-matched normals (Johnson *et al.*, 1990), and regional-flow distinctions between patients with DAT and those with MID (Ebmeier *et al.*, 1987; Gemmel *et al.*, 1987). Positron emission tomography (PET) allows the injection of naturally occurring substances, such as oxygen or glucose tagged with radioisotopes, that can be followed through their metabolic pathways. Drugs can also be tagged and followed to determine their sites of receptor binding. Thus, PET scanning illuminates the physiological and biochemical basis of cerebral activity. PET, like SPECT, is now being applied to the study of a variety of neuropsychiatric disorders. While neither of these techniques has been found exact enough, as yet, to serve as diagnostic tools, they hold promise for further delineating the brain basis of psychopathology.

3. Neuropsychological Testing

During the past two decades, neuropsychological and cognitive tests have become a critically important adjunct to the evaluation process. They provide a standardized, quantitative, and reproducible method for initial assessment and periodic reevaluation. Neuropsychological test protocols go far beyond the bedside mental-status assessment in characterizing a patient's intellectual strengths and deficiencies, and often provide valuable information for establishing a successful treatment plan, as they aid the clinician in exploiting or promoting the patient's resources while downplaying his weaknesses. In addition, many neuropsychological tests have been subjected to repeated study to define possible clinical–pathological correlates (Kertesz, 1983; Lezak, 1983), thus providing a means for guiding study of underlying cerebral dysfunction.

There are presently a variety of distinctive, competing neuropsychological schools of thought (Grant & Adams, 1986). When obtaining consultation, the clinician is well advised to learn more about his consultant's background, theoretical frame of reference, and particular outlook on how neuropsychological assessment should be undertaken. Different methods have distinctive strengths, as often occurs in relatively young fields of study, thus arguing for a maximally interactive process where, before the evaluation, the clinician and the consultant discuss the patient's history, clinical and laboratory findings, and the questions for assessment. The clinician should strive to develop a greater understanding of the tests that are utilized, and invite the consultant to assist in the treatment-planning process, where results from specific test situations can be applied to the practical tasks of enhancing functional integrity.

IV. Differential Diagnosis _____

Differential diagnosis of a neuropsychiatric disturbance can be a daunting challenge. Nearly every disease or toxic state with systemic potential can influence behavior, emotion, or cognition. The neuropsychiatric assessment must organize data in a sequential, probabilistic fashion that ranks and limits differential diagnostic possibilities. It is accomplished by establishing at the outset a firm sense of the patient's premorbid functioning and personality, and defining the onset and course of the current changes. This always requires input from family or friends who knew the patient before and after the start of the current condition. This is followed by a rigorous physical examination and mental-status examination. Laboratory tests are then used to prove or disprove the clinical suspicions.

For purposes of initial assessment, neuropsychiatric disorders may be divided into four major descriptive categories: delirium, dementia, and other disturbances of intellect, affective disorders, and psychotic disorders. When establishing a differential diagnosis, one must ask whether the patient's condition falls into one of these broad classes. The clinician seeks to exclude first those disorders that are symptomatic of cerebral or systemic medical diseases. He then evaluates primary affective and psychotic disturbances. During this process, the clinician considers the variety of diseases that may lead to behavior disruptions, included in the mnemonic, $(TIC)^2P^2M^2D^3$: trauma, tumor, infection, immune and autoimmune disorders, cardiovascular diseases, congenital–hereditary disorders, (primary) psychopathology, physiological disruptions, metabolic diseases, malingering, degenerative and demyelinating disorders, and drug-toxic states.

A. Delirium

Delirium can mimic any and every possible psychiatric disorder; apathy, anergia, anorexia, depressed mood, mania, irritability, delusions, hallucinations—all are possible in a delirious patient and can be mistaken for primary psychiatric illness. The cardinal features of delirium are a disturbance of consciousness. The mode of onset is usually acute or subacute, presenting with a fluctuating course or on occasion a chronic, stable course. The disturbance of consciousness may be manifest during the clinical interview, with the patient becoming drowsy, hyperalert, or vacillating between different levels of arousal. However, disturbance of consciousness can also be manifest only in a daily waxing and waning pattern. The clinician who observes the patient once daily may see him only when he appears to be fully conscious. A careful history from family or nursing staff will reveal the instability in the patient's level of arousal. Associated features of delirium are a disturbance of the sleep–wake cycle, and at times, incontinence. Other features are listed on Table IV. Clinical examination can usually detect a disturbance of consciousness if it is moderate or severe. If mild, it may not become obvious until the patient is asked to perform a task requiring sustained concentration or attention, such as counting backward by 7s or digit span. Personality, mood, and behavioral changes often accompany delirium, but the hallmark is the disturbance of consciousness. The neurologic examination can be entirely normal or may demonstrate nonfocal abnormalities, such as asterixis, clonus, or hyperreflexia. The EEG may demonstrate diffuse slowing and verify the clinical impression. Once the clinician has determined that a disturbance of consciousness is present, aggressive efforts are warranted to find the etiological agent. Delirium is a final common pathway for most structural, infectious, metabolic, and toxic insults. Table V presents common causes of delirium in the elderly.

Table IV

Clinical Features of Delirium[a]

Arousal	Psychomotor Activity	Personality	Mood
Waxing–waning	Restlessness	Apathy	Lability
Nighttime confusion	Somnolence	Irritability	Depression
("sundowning")	Agitation	Disinhibition	Euphoria
Drowsy	Posturing	Bizarre behaviors	**EEG**
Vigilant	Reversal of sleep–wake	**Neurological**	Mild delirium:
Stupor & coma when	cycle	Tremor	Mild slowing, low
severe	**Cognitive**	Nystagmus	voltage
Abnormal Beliefs	Perplexity	Asterixis	Severe delirium:
Suspiciousness	Disorientation	Myoclonus	Diffuse severe slow-
Paranoia	Distractibilty	Hyperactive reflexes	ing; progressive
Misperceptions	Perseveration		disorganization
Illusions	Poor memory		
Hallucinations			
(especially visual &			
tactile)			

[a]All are present in fluctuating course.

The elderly are particularly prone to develop delirium. Both local (affecting the brain) and systemic factors can cause delirium. Local factors include space-occupying lesions, such as tumors, subdural hematomas, and abscesses. These can cause an acute or subacute delirium depending on the location, extent, and pace of the space occupying process. More often, space-occupying lesions result in a chronic dementing process. Systemic febrile illnesses are common causes of delirium. For example, minimal elevations in temperature caused by urinary tract or respiratory infections may be accompanied by confusion and disorientation. Partial seizures due to infarctions, tumors, or metabolic imbalance are often difficult to detect. Infarctions are the most common underlying cause of seizures in the elderly, in contrast to tumors among the middle-aged. Metabolic and endocrine disorders can also produce both delirium and dementia, but more commonly produce acute or subacute delirium. Any reduction of oxygen to the brain can compromise arousal, either through pulmonary or hematologic processes, or through a direct compromise of vascular flow (e.g., progressive carotid stenosis or cerebral embolism). Chronic nutritional deficiency has occasionally led to mild delirium. Minor elevations in the levels of therapeutic agents, even within the *normal* laboratory range, can also be etiologic in the elderly. Withdrawal deliria are often misdiagnosed on medical and surgical services. The unsuspecting clinician does not recognize the cause of the delirium that emerges 24–72 hr following admission, when the alcohol-or (usually prescribed) tranquilizer-dependent elderly patient suddenly suffers a change in mental status following surgery or an emergency admission to the hospital.

Some psychiatrists describe a *manic delirium,* or *catatonic excitement* as delirium. However, these are uncommon among the elderly, and they are diagnoses that must be consistent with psychiatric histories. When antipsychotic medications have been prescribed, a delirium associated with muscle rigidity and fever may herald neuroleptic

Table V

Common Causes of Delirium in the Elderly

Tumor
  Space occupying (cerebral tumors)
  Remote effects
    Secreting tumors (bronchocarcinoma)
    Paraneoplastic syndromes

Trauma

Infection
  Local (encephalitis, meningitis)
  Systemic (pneumonia, urinary tract infection, sepsis, cellulitis)

Infarction
  Acute cerebral vascular accident

Cardiovascular
  Myocardial infarction
  Cardiac arrhythmia
  Congestive heart failure
  Hypertensive encephalopathy
  Transient ischemic attack
  Cerebral embolism

Physiological
  Epilepsy (psychomotor seizures; postictal state)

Primary Psychiatric
  "Manic delirium"
  "Catatonic excitement"

Metabolic
  Renal, pancreatic, hepatic compromise
  Anoxia
    Anemic ('silent' bleed)
    Anoxic (pneumonia, chronic obstructive pulmonary disease, acute carbon monoxide poisoning)
  Endocrinopathies (hyper and hypothyroidism; hyper and hypoglycemia; hyper and hypoparathyroid states;
    Addisonian crisis)
  Vitamin deficiences (Wernicke's encephalopathy)

Drugs (toxic)
  Prescription medications
    Anticholinergics
    Psychotropics (tricyclic antidepressants, lithium carbonate, neuroleptics)
    Anticonvulsants
    Sedative–hypnotics (intoxication; withdrawal)
    Digitalis
    Histamine antagonists
    Analgesics (opiates)
  Over-the-counter medications
    Antihistamines

Postanesthesia

Alcohol (intoxication; withdrawal)

---

malignant syndrome. When considering differential clinical description, one should not exclude delirium until convinced that the level of the patient's consciousness has been stable, and that the clinical-symptom picture has been persistent and consistent. Only then should one proceed to considering other syndromic patterns.

B. Dementia and Other Disturbances of Intellect

Dementia is characterized by a *persistent* diminution in cognition in the presence of a stable level of consciousness. Dementia denotes a decrement in two or more intellectual functions, in contrast to focal or specific impairments, such as amnestic disorder or aphasia. The persistent and stable nature of the impairment distinguishes dementia from delirium, with its fluctuating deficits and altered consciousness. Dementia must also be distinguished from long-standing mental subnormality, as the former represents an acquired loss of prior capacities. Dementia can also be associated with noncognitive symptoms, such as a change in personality, depression, or paranoia. The most common causes of dementia are noted in Table VI.

Dementia syndromes can be distinguished from each other clinically by the relative impairment and sparing of various neuropsychological functions. Two basic patterns of dementia have been characterized clinically: *Cortical* and *subcortical* (Cummings & Benson, 1984). These terms are *pseudoanatomical* diagnoses, and are imperfect as strict designations of anatomical loci for the degenerative disease process. They were intended to define clinical presentations that had specific cerebral localizations. However, cortical degenerative disorders that cause dementia tend to spread and involve subcortical structures, and subcortical diseases affect regions beyond the subcortex, especially the frontal lobes, given the brain's robust frontal–subcortical connections. Nonetheless, these clinical labels usefully define distinctive patterns of behavioral and cognitive impairment, especially during the early stages of the disease process when correct diagnosis is most crucial.

Cortical dementias are characterized by impairments in memory and gnostic–practic abilities, primarily involving language, visuospatial processing, calculation, motor praxis, and *executive functions* such as organization, judgment, abstraction, and insight. General motor function (e.g., gait) is usually intact until late in the disease. Affect and personality are often spared, with the patient frequently displaying an indifference to cognitive deficits. Despite these generalizations, it is important to recognize that DAT patients commonly develop depression, and show concern about their intellectual decline, especially in the early stages of decline.

Subcortical dementias are characterized by a generalized slowing of mental processes; we have described them as primarily involving modulatory or psychomotor functions (Caine, Bamford, Schiffer, Shoulson, & Levy, 1986). Specific skills such as calculation, naming, or copying can be spared initially. Planning and organizational skills are quite disrupted. Abnormal movements are common, typically associated with obvious disturbances in gait, posture, and speech (e.g., chorea in Huntington's disease; bradykinesia, tremor, and rigidity in Parkinson's disease; oculomotor paralysis and a toppling gait in progressive supranuclear palsy). Language is less affected, despite the abnormal produc-

Table VI

Etiologies for Dementia

Tumor[a]
  Primary cerebral
  Metastatic

Trauma
  Hematomas[a]
  Post-traumatic dementia[a]

Infection (chronic)
  Syphilis[a]
  Jakob-Creutzfeldt disease[b]
  AIDS dementia complex[c]

Cardiovascular (infarction)
  Single[a]
  Multi-infarct dementia
    Lacunar state[c]
    Subcortical arteriosclerotic encephalopathies (Binswanger's disease)[c]

Congenital–Hereditary
  Huntington's disease[c]

Primary psychiatric
  Pseudodementia[c]

Physiological
  Epilepsy[a]
  Normal-pressure hydrocephalus (NPH)[a]

Metabolic
  Vitamin deficiencies[a]
  Chronic metabolic disturbances[a]
  Chronic anoxic states[a]
  Chronic endocrinopathies[a]

Degenerative dementias
  Alzheimer's disease[b]
  Pick's disease[b]
  Huntington's disease[c]
  Parkinson's disease[a]
  Progressive supranuclear palsy (PSP)[c]
  Idiopathic cerebral ferrocalcinosis (Fahr's disease)[c]

Demyelinating
  Multiple sclerosis (MS)[c]

Drug (toxic)
  Alcohol[a]
  Heavy metals[a]
  Carbon monoxide poisoning[a]
  Medications[a]

[a]variable or mixed pattern.
[b]cortical.
[c]subcortical.

tion of speech. Personality change is marked, with patterns of apathy, inertia, and diminished spontaneity. Affective disorders are more common. Of note, the presentations of cortical and subcortical dementias become nearly indistinguishable from one another as the basic cerebral degenerative processes progress.

The first task in differential diagnosis of dementia is to distinguish clinically between a subcortical and cortical process. Once the pattern has been established, the clinician seeks identifying characteristics for diseases within the category of subcortical or cortical dementias. Among the cortical dementias, DAT may be distinguished from Pick's disease early in the degenerative process by the tendency for the latter to affect personality more than intellectual ability. DAT is distinguished from MID by its time course, the former being insidious in onset with gradual progression. MID may begin more suddenly, but often progresses slowly as well. It can, at times, be characterized by a step-wise deterioration, and is typically associated with hypertension and clinical stigmata of cerebrovascular disease (e.g., resolving ischemic episodes, reflex asymmetry, or motor dysfunction noted on physical examination). The pattern of dementia associated with infarction depends on the size and location of the lesion or lesions. Large single infarctions may result in a discrete loss of one particular function, such as language, though not a formal dementia. MID usually has an earlier age of onset than DAT. Lacunar infarctions are small, deep lesions caused by disease of the small arteries, usually involving the basal ganglia, thalamus, and internal capsule. The neurologic and cognitive deficits may resolve quickly after each of these small strokes. However, deficits gradually accumulate, leading to persisting functional and intellectual decline. Pseudobulbar palsy characterized by dysarthria, dysphasia, and emotional incontinence is common in MID.

Binswanger's disease, or subcortical arteriosclerotic encephalopathy, is characterized by microinfarctions of the white matter with sparing of the cortex. Unlike MID, this produces a subcortical pattern of dementia, and again must be considered when there is a history of long-standing hypertension and a subacute progression of subcortical dementia and neurological deficits. Binswanger's encephalopathy was previously considered a rare condition, diagnosed by autopsy alone. Its prevalence is now being reexamined, in light of the frequency of white-matter lesions being detected with the new imaging technologies.

Infectious processes usually produce a fulminant deterioration with acute delirium. Chronic infectious processes, however, can have a more insidious and subtle course. Syphilis, the classic example of a treatable neuropsychiatric condition, must be considered because it is a potentially reversible condition. It is likely to be resurgent during the coming years. Central nervous system syphilis can manifest as late as 25 years after initial infection. It can present as almost any form of psychiatric disturbance or dementia syndrome. The classical grandiose presentation of general paresis has become rare, while depressive or cognitive presentations have become more frequent (Lishman, 1987, p. 282). Neurologic examination can be most informative with evidence of oculomotor dysfunction, reflex abnormalities, or the sensory and proprioceptive loss of tabes dorsalis. The clinician must be attuned to a history of previous venereal disease and be suspicious for the presence of a chronic syphilitic condition.

Cognitive impairment due to human immunodeficiency virus (HIV) infection must be suspected in any patient from appropriate high-risk categories, regardless of age. In North

America, these risk categories include homosexuals, blood-product recipients, Haitians, and IV-drug users. Anyone who has had sexual contact with a high-risk subject is also susceptible to HIV disease. HIV can produce dementia either by direct cerebral viral infection or by secondary suprainfection from an opportunistic organism. Primary HIV infection of the brain causes a subcortical-pattern dementia (Marotta & Perry, 1989; Navia, Jordan, & Price, 1986), which may be the only presenting abnormality (Navia & Price, 1987). Opportunistic infections commonly include the herpes simplex encephalitis and cryptococcal cerebral abscesses.

Jakob-Creutzfeldt disease is a rapidly progressive cortical-pattern dementia that is accompanied frequently by myoclonus. It is caused by a slow virus, one that incubates for years before the development of clinical symptoms.

Tumors and hematomas, like other space-occupying lesions, can cause dementia, depending on their location and the extent of cerebral involvement. Systemic cancer can also have remote effects on cerebral function through brain metastases, supraimposed infection, metabolic disturbances, or *paraneoplastic syndrome.*

Vitamin deficiencies can be found often in elderly patients, associated with chronic illnesses that interfere with feeding or gastrointestinal absorption, or with a chronically deficient diet. Vitamin B_{12} (cyanocobalamin) deficiency can cause anergia, slowing, and memory impairment that may resolve partially or completely with replenishment of the deficiency. Macrocytic anemia is a nearly invariant concomitant and should raise suspicion for the disorder in a patient presenting with dementia. Vitamin B_1 (thiamine) deficiency can cause an acute Wernicke's encephalopathy characterized by ophthalmoplegia, ataxia, and delirium. Even as this clears, a persisting Korsakoff's syndrome supervenes, characterized by severe memory and new-learning impairment, with relative preservation of other cognitive functions. Both conditions, together called the Wernicke-Korsakoff syndrome, are far more common in patients with a history of chronic alcohol abuse. It remains to be established whether alcohol amnestic disorder is actually due to the vitamin deficiency or to the toxic effects of alcohol (Lishman, 1987, p. 497). Iron depletion may also result from poor dietary intake, and can contribute to a progressive dementing condition, associated with a characteristic microcytic anemia.

Metabolic disturbances, like those found in renal, hepatic, or pancreatic compromise, are more common in the elderly. Acute onset causes delirium, but a slow and insidious exposure to the insulting agent leads to a chronic dementia. The characteristics are those of a subcortical dementia, with slowing, memory impairment, and motor abnormalities, without frank aphasia or agnosia (Cummings & Benson, 1983, p. 169). Anoxia due to cardiovascular, pulmonary, or hematologic etiologies can cause such dementia as well.

Normal pressure hydrocephalus (NPH) predominantly affects patients in their 60s and 70s. It is caused by partial obstruction of the flow of cerebrospinal fluid into the subarachnoid space. The classical triad of symptoms—dementia, incontinence, and gait disturbance—is not uniformly present in all patients with hydrocephalus, especially early in the course, but it nearly always emerges if NPH goes unrecognized or untreated. The dementia syndrome is variable and can include features of both cortical and subcortical patterns. Diagnostic assessment has utilized, in the past, pneumoencephalography and isotope cisternography, but these have been replaced by MRI. The presence of significant ventricular dilatation, in the absence of prominent sulcal widening, is a telltale sign.

Of the demyelinating disorders, multiple sclerosis is the most common. It is an idiopathic disorder characterized by the development of demyelinating lesions throughout the nervous system. Its clinical course is variable, with frequent relapses and remissions. The presence and type of cognitive impairments can vary between patients, or even within the same patient, owning to the variable nature of the development of lesions. Affective symptoms are common. MRI has been demonstrated to be of great value in detecting the multiple sclerosis plaques, though one group of investigators found no correlation between the number or distribution of lesions with degree of dementia (Huber *et al.*, 1987). Multiple sclerosis should be suspected in any patient with concomitant cognitive and motor (especially ocular) impairments associated with a remitting and relapsing course.

Among toxic causes, alcohol is the most common. As noted above, there is some controversy as to whether alcohol can cause a dementia directly, or only indirectly through nutritional deficiencies. Cummings and Benson (1983) review the literature regarding alcohol dementia and note that a mild dementia is reported, characterized by forgetfulness, psychomotor retardation, circumstantiality, perseveration, and poor attention. More focal, gnostic, or practic deficits may be observed. As well, there is no specific boundary clinically between persisting alcohol amnestic disorder and alcohol dementia. While the former is defined as a specific disorder, and the latter, as multifunctional, severely memory-disordered patients often show mild decrements in other cognitive abilities. A history of alcohol use must be obtained in every patient, and must be considered in a differential diagnosis for dementia whenever it is elicited. Alcohol-induced cognitive deficits may improve during the months following cessation of drinking; thus, it is a potentially treatable cause of intellectual impairment that warrants careful assessment. Heavy metals, such as lead, mercury, manganese, and arsenic are also associated with dementing processes, and must be considered in those patients who have had occupational or environmental exposures. Carbon monoxide poisoning can cause basal ganglia calcification or necrosis, as well as other cerebral lesions, and may lead to a chronic dementing process, even after the exposure has been removed.

In summary, the etiologies for dementia are numerous. A clinician must progress in an orderly fashion, utilizing clues from the history, physical examination, mental-status examination, and laboratory evaluation.

C. Affective Disorder

Affective disorder, particularly depression, is common in the elderly (Blazer & Williams, 1980). Delirium, which can present with a mood disturbance, may be mistaken for a primary affective disorder, but disturbance of consciousness and fluctuations in mood characterize delirium. Affective disorders may be distinguished by *sustained* and *pervasive* disturbances in mood in the presence of clear consciousness. They can be superimposed on a dementia, though the evaluation and diagnosis of depression becomes much more difficult in a patient with communication and memory limitations. Affective disorders may, in themselves, present with a cognitive impairment, described by terms such as pseudodementia or dementia of depression. Here the impairments are primarily in attention, mental processing speed, memory retrieval, and paucity of verbal elaboration

(Caine, 1981). These patients may be quick to put off the examiner, or respond "I don't know," but at times they may be coaxed into a more accurate or sustained task performance. They have great difficulty with spontaneous recall, but are often better able to recognize material when presented with cues. Recently, several investigators have described a mild anomia in elderly depressives (King, Caine, Conwell, & Cox, in press; Speedie, Rabins, Pearlson, & Moberg, 1990), but the pathobiological significance of these findings is undetermined. The onset of cognitive impairment coincident with mood symptoms can alert the clinician to a recognition of primary depression. Anxiety, chronic pain, and hypochondriasis are other "masks" depression can wear in the elderly.

Affective disorders can be primary (idiopathic) or occurring secondarily in the context of a medical or neurological disorder. The idiopathic disorders more commonly have onset earlier in life. A secondary depressive disorder must always be considered when an elderly patient experiences a new onset of symptoms. Subcortical dementia, characterized by apathy, inertia, and anergia, can simulate depressive symptoms. The diminished range of facial expression and the bradykinesia of subcortical disease can be mistaken for a depressive affect and psychomotor retardation. Here the patient's self-reported mood is essential for developing a correct diagnosis.

Depression has been demonstrated to be a frequent concomitant of stroke. Poststroke depression can resemble idiopathic major depression of dysthymic disorder in almost all their clinical aspects (Robinson, Morris, & Federoff, 1990). Thirty to 60% of inpatient and outpatient populations developed an affective disorder over a 6–24 month period after stroke (Lipsey & Parikh, 1989). The occurrence and severity of depression is independent of the degree of functional or cognitive impairment (Robinson & Starkstein, 1990). Left frontal and basal ganglia lesions have been found to be associated more commonly with poststroke depression than with right-hemisphere lesions; the latter may be related to poststroke mania (Robinson & Starkstein, 1990). Patients with poststroke affective disorders have been shown to be less likely to have personal or family histories of a previous affective disorder (Robinson et al., 1990). Taken together, these results suggest that poststroke affective syndromes arise specifically from focal injury to identifiable brain regions. The clinician must be highly vigilant for evidence of a stroke in a patient over 50 years who presents with a new onset of depression or mania.

Hypothyroidism can present frequently with depression, with apathy and lethargy being the most prominent symptoms. It is recognized by its clinical symptoms and signs, most obviously dry skin; puffy and edematous facial appearance; coarse, stiff, and thinning hair; and a hoarsened voice. Hypothyroidism should be suspected in any patient with a depressive syndrome that remains unresponsive to standard antidepressant treatment. Hypothyroid-induced depression is highly amenable to treatment of the primary thyroid disease. Both elevated and depressed calcium, related to parathyroid dysfunction, have been associated with changes in mood and behavior.

Therapeutic medications for systemic diseases have often been implicated as causative agents of depression, particularly in the elderly. Pascualy and Veith (1989) reviewed the literature and found depression associated with a number of drug classes, including steroids, antihypertensives, and histamine receptor antagonists. A thorough drug history is always indicated. Withdrawal of the medication alone can sometimes be adequate treatment.

As discussed previously, the subcortical dementias are associated with affective disorders. Mayeux (1990) found that 53% of a population of Parkinson's patients had a history of depression at some point during their illness. Affective disorder, particularly depression, is a well-known component of Huntington's disease (Caine & Shoulson, 1983). Depression has been found to be more common in patients with multiple sclerosis than in control patients with other neurologic disease (Rabins, 1989). Depression is also common in both Cushing's and Addison's diseases, and responds well to treatment of the underlying pathology.

Mania can also present in the context of a primary medical or neurological disorder. Krauthammer and Klerman (1978) reviewed the reported cases of secondary mania, while disregarding those associated with confusion or delirium. They identified multiple causes, including a variety of therapeutic compounds, encephalitides, and specific tumors. They detected a later age of onset and a lack of family history of affective disorder among the patients with secondary mania. Stone (1989), in his review, found a later age of onset for primary mania than reported by previous investigators. He noted too that patients with cerebral impairment had a significantly later age of onset and rarely had a family history of affective disorder. Robinson and co-workers identified a cohort of patients who developed mania after stroke. These patients had a high frequency of right-hemispheric lesions, particularly in the basitemporal cortex (Robinson & Starkstein, 1990).

Manic symptomatology, like depression, is only presumed to be primary in nature when a stable level of consciousness is present. New onset of mania after the age of 50 years must be evaluated exhaustively to rule out another primary etiology. Frontal-lobe pathology can mimic depression or mania; the abulia and lack of initiative of dorsolateral lesions can seem depressive in origin. The disinhibition and euphoria of orbitomedial lesions can appear as mania. Here the clinician must be as attentive to the presenting cognitive deficits and neurologic abnormalities as to the affective symptoms. Mania, like depression, may mimic a dementing process. Inattention and distractibility of the manic patient can impair intellectual performance. The clinician must review the patient's psychiatric history, the evolution of the current disturbance, and the affective coloration of its presentation.

D. Psychotic Disorders

The clinician must first presume the existence of a primary cerebral lesion or systemic disease in any person older than 50 years with the new onset of delusions, hallucinations, ideas of reference, or other first-rank symptoms. Delirium must be excluded, as it may manifest with florid psychotic symptoms. Visual hallucinations are often associated with *organic* hallucinosis (Lishman, 1987, p. 127), particularly with the delirium of alcohol withdrawal (delirium tremens). Dementia must also be excluded; all forms of distortions, misinterpretations, and frank psychotic symptoms are possible during a dementing illness. Affective disorders in the elderly commonly present with prominent psychotic features. These are usually mood congruent; for example, delusions of poverty and guilt, or depreciatory auditory hallucinations in depression. Olfactory hallucinations can actually be seizures originating from the uncus.

Primary psychotic disorders do exist in the elderly. They are discussed in detail elsewhere in this book. As with schizophrenia, these are diagnoses of exclusion. A patient must have clear consciousness, without significant cognitive impairment, and with a stable euthymic mood before a psychotic disorder can be considered.

E. Other Psychiatric Disturbances

In this section on differential diagnosis, we have discussed disorders that involve five of the six *behavioral pathways* for expressing psychopathology, including disorders that are manifest through disruptions of arousal–consciousness, affective expression, perception, intellectual function, and motoric behavior. Change of personality may also serve as an initial complaint. In our experience, it is more commonly expressed by family members than by patients themselves. As we have emphasized when considering differential diagnostic approaches, the clinician must first exclude cerebral or systemic medical disorders, and recognize that altered personality may be the first manifestation of degenerative disease or chronic delirium. It may also be the primary presenting symptomatology for an affective disturbance, in which the patient may deny dysphoria, but display reduced initiative, diminished energy and interest, and increased dependency and social withdrawal. Alternatively, the apparent emergence of disturbed personality functioning may reflect a life-long pattern of diminished coping or adaptive abilities, in which the patient benefited previously from the support of other caring individuals (e.g., a spouse). In the face of reduced social resources, functionally significant disordered personality emerges. It is critically important to remember that the expression of personality disturbances is particularly dependent on the setting in which they are expressed; syndrome description does not suffice when attempting to fully capture the quality of the dysfunction. In sum, differential diagnostic evaluation of disordered personality requires especially careful consideration of brain–behavior, description psychopathologic, and psychosocial factors.

V. Conclusion of Assessment _____

We have emphasized the evaluation of person, diagnosis, and disease process. We have alluded to brain–behavior correlations, standardized criteria-based diagnoses that enhance reliability, and consideration of the patient in the context of his unique life setting. These efforts subserve the process of thoughtfully establishing a comprehensive treatment plan. Improved functional integrity is the ultimate measure of therapeutic success. Symptom resolution by itself is insufficient. Using this standard, one recognizes that conitions such as DAT, which are not presently curable or reversible, may be ameliorated with treatment, as the depressive, psychotic, or other behavioral complications, which may be part of the overall clinical picture, can be reduced significantly with appropriate therapeutic intervention. Function may then improve substantially, although the primary disease process has been unaffected.

Treatment planning and evaluation is as dynamic a process as is initial assessment. We have emphasized the need to *think over time*. That applies for considering future therapeutic response, akin to judging the prior evolution of the patient's illness. The clinician should anticipate in an active fashion the desired positive outcomes from his planned interventions, as well as any undesirable side-effects. Moreover, it proves helpful to consider how the patient will appear if the proposed treatment fails. That is, one should contemplate how the illness might progress further in the absence of an effective therapy. In this way, the clinician is prepared to evaluate his efforts to steer the course of the illness toward a new direction. When the patient responds in a fashion that has not been anticipated, the clinician will be alerted to the possibility that the basic nature of the illness was not fully or correctly understood. This provides a stimulus for further reviewing and refining one's evaluation, and establishes the framework for considering the relative benefits and dangers of more invasive or vigorous diagnostic and therapeutic procedures.

There is no simple formula for undertaking the integrative processes that form the basis of neuropsychiatric assessment. The clinician is often faced with making definitive therapeutic decisions when data are incomplete or unavailable. Vigilant evaluation of the patient's progress becomes both the yardstick for monitoring the effectiveness of the initial evaluation, and the alarm system for warning that further scrutiny is warranted.

Acknowledgment

This work was supported, in part, by grants from the National Institute of Mental Health (UR-NIMH CRC/PE #MH40381, and NRSA #MH18911). Janet Werkheiser and Helen Bennett assisted with manuscript preparation.

References

Aharon-Peretz, J., Cummings, J. L., & Hill, M. A. (1988). Vascular dementia and dementia of the Alzheimer type: Cognition, ventricular size, and leuko-araiosis. *Archives of Neurology, 45,* 719–721.

Albert, M. L. (Ed.). (1984). *Clinical neurology of aging.* New York: Oxford University Press.

Andreasen, N. C. (1979). Thought, language, and communication disorders: I. Clinical assessment, definition of terms, and evaluation of their reliability. *Archives of General Psychiatry, 36,* 1315–1321.

Anthony, J. C., LeResche, L., Niaz, U., vonKorff, M. R., & Folstein, M. F. (1982). Limits of the "Mini-Mental State" as a screening test for dementia and delerium among hospital patients. *Psychological Medicine, 12,* 397–408.

Applegate, W. B., Blass, J. B., & Williams, T. F. (1990). Instruments for the functional assessment of older patients. *New England Journal of Medicine, 322,* 1207–1214.

Beck, A. T., & Beck, R. W. (1972). Screening depressed patients in family practice. *PostGraduate Medicine, 52,* 81–85.

Beck, A. T., Ward, C. H., Mendelson, M., Mock, J. E., & Erbaugh, J. (1961). An inventory measuring depression. *Archives of General Psychiatry, 4,* 561–571.

Blazer, D., & Williams, C. D. (1980). Epidemiology of dysphoria and depression in an elderly population. *American Journal of Psychiatry, 137* (4), 439–444.

Brenner, R. P., Reynolds, C. F., & Ulrich, R. F. (1989). EEG findings in depressive pseudodementia and dementia with secondary depression. *Electroencephalography and Clinical Neurophysiology, 72,* 298–304.

Brugha, T. S., Wing, J. K., & Smith, B. L. (1989). Physical health of the long-term mentally ill in the community: Is there unmet need? *British Journal of Psychiatry, 155,* 777–781.

Bucknell, J. C., & Tuke, D. H. (1858). *A manual of psychological medicine* (Facs. ed., 1965). New York: Hefner.

Burke, W. J., Houston, M. J., Boust, S. J., & Roccaforte, W. H. (1989). Use of the geriatric depression scale in dementia of the Alzheimer type. *Journal of the American Geriatric Society, 37,* 856–860.

Caine, E. D. (1981). Pseudodementia: Current concepts and future directions. *Archives of General Psychiatry, 38,* 1359–1364.

Caine, E. D. (in press). Standing at the mental health–physical health interface: Is current caregiver research valid? In E. Light, B. D. Lebowitz, & G. T. Niederehe (Eds.), Untitled volume. New York: Springer.

Caine, E. D., Bamford, K. A., Schiffer, R. B., Shoulson, I., & Levy, S. (1986). A controlled neuropsychological comparison of Huntington's disease and multiple sclerosis. *Archives of Neurology, 43,* 249–254.

Caine, E. D., & Joynt, R. J. (1986). Neuropsychiatry . . . again. *Archives of Neurology, 43,* 325–327.

Caine, E. D., & Shoulson, I. (1983). Psychiatric syndromes in Huntington's disease. *American Journal of Psychiatry, 140* (6), 728–733.

Conlon, P., & Trimble, M. R. (1987). Magnetic resonance imaging in psychiatry. *Canadian Journal of Psychiatry, 32,* 702–711.

Conwell, Y., Caine, E. D., & Olsen K. (in press). Suicide and cancer in late life. *Hospital and Community Psychiatry.*

Crook, T., Ferris, S., & Bartus, R. (1983). Assessment in geriatric psychopharmacology. New Canaan, CT: Mark Powley.

Cummings, J. L., & Benson, D. F. (1983). Dementia: A clinical approach. Boston, MA: Butterworths.

Cummings, J. L., & Benson, D. F. (1984). Subcortical dementia: Review of an emerging concept. *Archives of Neurology, 41,* 874–878.

Davison, K., & Bagley, C. R. (1969). Schizophrenic-like psychoses associated with organic disorders of the central nervous system: A review of the literature. *British Journal of Psychiatry, Special Publication #4,* 113–184.

Diagnostic and Statistical Manual of Mental Disorders (3rd ed.). (1980). Washington, DC: American Psychiatric Association.

Dick, J. P. R., Guiloff, R. J., Stewart, A., Blackstock, J., Bielawska, C., Paul, E. A., & Marsden, C. D. (1984). Mini-Mental State Examination in neurological patients. *Journal of Neurology, Neurosurgery, and Psychiatry, 47,* 496–499.

Duara, R., Barker, W., Loewenstein, D., Pascal, S., & Bowen, B. (1989). Sensitivity and specificity of positron emission tomography and magnetic resonance imaging studies in Alzheimer's disease and multi-infarct dementia. *European Journal of Neurology, 29* (suppl. 3), 9–15.

Ebmeier, K. P., Besson, J. A. O., Crawford, J. R., Palin, A. N., Gemmel, H. G., Sharp, P. F., Cherryman, G. R., & Smith F. W. (1987). Nuclear magnetic resonance imaging and single photon emission tomography with radioiodine-labeled compounds in the diagnosis of dementia. *Acta Psychiatrica Scandinavica, 75,* 549–556.

Engel, G. L. (1977). The need for a new medical model. *Science, 196,* 129–136.

Erkinjuntti, T., Ketonen, L., Sulkava, R., Sipponen, J., Vuorialho, M., & Iivanainen, M. (1987). Do white matter changes on MRI and CT differentiate vascular dementia from Alzheimer's disease. *Journal of Neurology, Neurosurgery, and Psychiatry, 50,* 37–42.

Escobar, J. I., Burnam, A., Karno, M., Forsythe, A., Landsverk, J., & Golding, J. M. (1986). Use of the Mini-Mental State Examination (MMSE) in a community population of mixed ethnicity: Cultural and linguistic artifacts. *Journal of Nervous and Mental Disease, 174,* 607–614.

Esquirol, J. E. D. (1845). *Mental maladies: A treatise on insanity* (Facs. ed., 1963). New York: Hefner.

Ettlin, T. M., Staehelin, H. B., Kishka, U., Ulrich, J., Scollo-Lavizzari, G., Wiggli, U., & Seiler, W. O. (1989). Computed tomography, electroencephalography, and clinical features in the differential diagnosis of senile dementia. *Archives of Neurology, 46,* 1217–1220.

Farber, J. F., Schmitt, F. A., & Logue, P. E. (1988). Predicting intellectual level from the Mini-Mental State Examination. *Journal of the American Geriatric Society, 36,* 509–510.

Fein, G., VanDyke, C., Davenport, L., Turetsky, B., Brant-Zawadzki, M., Zatz, L., Dillon, W., & Valk, P. (1990). Preservation of normal cognitive functioning in elderly subjects with extensive white-matter lesions of long duration. *Archives of General Psychiatry, 47,* 220–223.

Ferguson, B., & Dudleston, K. (1986). Detection of physical disorder in newly admitted psychiatric patients. *Acta Psychiatrica Scandinavica, 74,* 485–489.

Folstein, M. F., Folstein, S. E., & McHugh, P. R. (1975). "Mini-Mental State": A practical method for grading the cognitive state of patients for the clinician. *Journal of Psychiatric Research, 12,* 189–198.

Garber, H. J., Weilburg, J. B., Buonanno, F. S., Manschreck, T. C., & New, P. F. J. (1988). Use of magnetic resonance imaging in psychiatry. *American Journal of Psychiatry, 145*, 164–171.

Gemmell, H. G., Sharp, P. F., Besson, J. A. O., Crawford, J. R., Ebmeier, K. P., Davidson, J., & Smith F. W. (1987). Differential diagnosis in dementia using the cerebral blood flow agent ^{99m}Tc HM-PAO: A SPECT study. *Journal of Computer-Assisted Tomography, 11* (3), 398–402.

Gordon, E., Kraiuhin, C., & Meares, R. A. (1986). Review images of the brain in psychiatry. *Australian and New Zealand Journal of Psychiatry, 20*, 122–133.

Grant, I., & Adams, K. M. (Eds.). (1986). *Neuropsychological assessment of neuropsychiatric disorders.* New York: Oxford University Press.

Griesinger, W. (1867). *Mental pathology and therapeutics* (Facs. ed., 1967). New York: Hefner.

Hamilton, M. (1967). Development of a rating scale for primary depressive illness. *British Journal of Social & Clinical Psychology, 6*, 278–296.

Harrell, L. E., Callaway, R., & Sekar, B. C. (1987). Magnetic resonance imaging and the diagnosis of dementia. *Neurology, 37*, 540–543.

Havens, L. L. (1973). *Approaches to the mind: Movement of the psychiatric schools from sects toward science.* Boston, MA: Little, Brown.

Hershey, L. A., Modic, M. T., Greenough, P. G., & Jaffe, D. F. (1987). Magnetic resonance imaging in vascular dementia. *Neurology, 37*, 29–36.

Huber, S. J., Paulson, G. W., Shuttleworth, E. C., Chakeres, D., Clapp, L. E., Pakalnis, A., Weiss, K., & Rammohan, K. (1987). Magnetic resonance imaging correlates of dementia in multiple sclerosis. *Archives of Neurology, 44*, 732–736.

Hunt, A. L., Orrison, W. W., Yeo, R. A., Haaland, K. Y., Rhyne, R. L., Garry, P. J., & Rosenberg, G. A. (1989). Clinical significance of MRI white-matter lesions in the elderly. *Neurology, 39*, 1470–1474.

Jernigan, T. L., Press, G. A., Hesselink, J. R. (1990). Methods for measuring brain morphologic features on magnetic resonance images. *Archives of Neurology, 47*, 27–32.

Johnson, K. A., Davis, K. R., Buonanno, F. S., Brady, T. J., Rosen, T. J., & Growdon, J. H. (1987). Comparison of magnetic resonance and roentgen-ray computed tomography in dementia. *Archives of Neurology, 44*, 1075–1080.

Johnson, K. A., Holman, L., Rosen, T. J., Nagel, J. S., English, R. J., & Growdon, J. H. (1990). Iofetamine I^{123} single photon emission computed tomography is accurate in the diagnosis of Alzheimer's disease. *Archives of Internal Medicine, 150*, 752–756.

Kendell, R. E. (1975). *The role of diagnosis in psychiatry.* Oxford: Blackwell Scientific Publication.

Kertesz, A. (Ed.). (1983). *Localization in neuropsychology.* New York: Academic Press.

Kertesz, A., Polk, M., & Carr, T. (1990). Cognition and white-matter changes on magnetic resonance imaging in dementia. *Archives of Neurology, 47*, 387–391.

Kido, D. K., Caine, E. D., LeMay, M., Ekholm, S., Booth, H., & Panzer, R. (1989). Temporal lobe atrophy in patients with Alzheimer's disease: A CT study. *American Journal of Neuroradiology, 10*, 551–555.

King, D. A., Caine, E. D., Conwell, Y., & Cox, C. (in press). The neuropsychology of depression in the elderly: A comparative study with normal aging and Alzheimer's disease. *Journal of Neuropsychiatry.*

Kleinman, A. (1986). *Social origins of distress and disease: Depression, neurasthenia, and pain in modern China.* New Haven: Yale University Press.

Kleinman, A. (1988). *Rethinking psychiatry: From cultural category to personal experience.* New York: Free Press.

Kobari, M., Meyer, J. S., & Ichijo, M. (1990). Leuko-araiosis, cerebral atrophy, and cerebral perfusion in normal aging. *Archives of Neurology, 47*, 161–165.

Koenig, H. G., Meador, K. G., Cohen, H. J., & Blazer, D. G. (1988). Self-rated depression scales and screening for major depression in older hospitalized patient with medical illness. *Journal of American Geriatrics Society, 36*, 699–706.

Kolman, P. B. R. (1985). Predicting the results of routine laboratory tests in elderly psychiatric patients admitted to hospital. *Journal of Clinical Psychiatry, 46*, 532–534.

Koran, L. W., Sox, H. C., Martron, K. I., Moltzen, S., Sox, C. H., Kraemer, H. C., Imai, K., Kelsey, T. G., Rose, T. G., Jr., Levin, L. C., & Chandra, S. (1989). Medical evaluation of psychiatric patients. *Archives of General Psychiatry, 46*, 733–740.

Kraepelin, E. (1919). *Dementia praecox and paraphrenia.* (R. M. Barclay, Trans.) from 8th German ed., *"Textbook of Psychiatry,"* Vol. iii, Part ii) (Facs. ed., 1971). New York: Krieger.

Krauthammer, C., & Klerman, G. L. (1978). Secondary mania. *Archives of General Psychiatry, 35,* 133–1339.

Lawton, M. P., & Brody, E. M. (1969). Assessment of older people: Self-maintaining and instrumental activities of daily living. *Gerontologist, 9,* 179–186.

Leifer, D., Buonanno, F. S., & Richardson, E. P. (1990). Clinicopathologic correlations of cranial magnetic resonance imaging of periventricular white matter. *Neurology, 40,* 911–918.

Levin, B. E., Llabre, M. M., & Weiner, W. J.(1988). Parkinson's disease and depression: Psychometric properties of the Beck Depression Inventory. *Journal of Neurology, Neurosurgery, and Psychiatry, 51,* 1401–1404.

Levin, H. S., Amparo, E., Eisenberg, H. M., Williams, D. H., High, W. M., McArdle, C. B., & Weiner, R. L. (1987). Magnetic resonance imaging and computerized tomography in relation to the neurobehavioral sequelae of mild and moderate head injuries. *Journal of Neurosurgery, 66,* 706–713.

Leys, D., Soetaert, G., Petit, H., Fauquette A., Pruvo, J. P., & Steinling, M. (1990). Periventricular and white-matter magnetic resonance imaging hyperintensities do not differ between Alzheimer's disease and normal aging. *Archives of Neurology, 47,* 524–527.

Lezak, M. D. (1983). *Neuropsychological assessment* (2nd ed.). New York: Oxford University Press.

Lipsey, J. R., & Parikh, R. M. (1989). Depression and stroke. In R. G. Robinson & P. V. Rabins (Eds.), *Aging and clinical practice: Depression and coexisting disease* (pp. 186–201). New York: Igaku-Shoin.

Lishman, W. A. (1987). *Organic psychiatry. The psychological consequences of cerebral disorder* (2nd ed.). Oxford: Blackwell Scientific Publications.

Mackenzie, T. B., Robiner, W. N., & Knopman, D. S. (1989). Differences between patient and family assessments of depression in Alzheimer's disease. *American Journal of Psychiatry, 146,* 1174–1178.

Marotta, R., & Perry, S. (1988). Early neuropsychological dysfunction caused by human immunodeficiency virus. *Journal of Neuropsychiatry, 1* (3) 225–235.

Mayeux, R. (1990). Parkinson's disease. A review of cognitive and psychiatric disorders. *Neuropsychiatry, Neuropsychology, and Behavioral Neurology, 3* (1), 3–14.

Mayeux, R., Stern, Y., Rosan, J., & Leventhal, J. (1981). Depression, intellectual impairment, and Parkinson's disease. *Neurology, 31,* 645–650.

McClellan, R. L., Eisenberg, R. L., & Giyanani, V. L. (1988). Routine CT screening of psychiatry inpatients. *Radiology, 169,* 99–100.

Navia, B. A., Jordan, B. D., & Price R. W. (1986). The AIDS dementia complex: I. Clinical features. *Annals of Neurology, 19,* 517–524.

Navia, B. A., & Price, R. W. (1987). The acquired immunodeficiency syndrome dementia complex as the presenting or sole manifestation of human immunodeficiency virus infection. *Archives of Neurology, 44,* 65–67.

Overall, J. E., & Beller, S. A. (1984). The brief psychiatric rating scale (BPRS). In Geropsychiatric Research: I. Factor structure on an inpatient unit. *Journal of Gerontology, 39,* 187–193.

Overall, J. E., & Gorham, D. R. (1962). The brief psychiatric rating scale. *Psychological Reports, 10,* 799–812.

Pascualy, M., & Veith, R. C. (1989). Depression as an adverse drug reaction. In R. G. Robinson & P. V. Rabins (Eds.), *Aging and clinical practice: Depression and coexisting disease* (pp. 132–151). New York: Igaku-Shoin.

Pearlson, G. D., & Veroff, A. E. (1981). Computerized tomographic scan changes in manic-depressive illness. *The Lancet, 12* (8244), 470.

Pinel, R. (1806). *A treatise on insanity* (Facs. ed., 1962). New York: Hefner.

Rabins, P. V. (1989). Depression and multiple sclerosis. In R. G. Robinson & P. V. Rabins (Eds.), *Aging and clinical practice: Depression on coexisting disease* (pp. 226–233). New York: Igaku-Shoin.

Raskin, A., & Niederehe, G. (Eds.). (1988). Assessment in diagnosis and treatment of geriatric psychiatry patients. *Psychopharmacology Bulletin, 24,* 509–810.

Robinson, R. G., Morris, P. L. P., & Fedoroff, J. P. (1990). Depression and cerebrovascular disease. *Journal of Clinical Psychiatry, 51* (7), 26–31.

Robinson, R. G., & Starkstein, S. E. (1990). Current research in affective disorders following stroke. *Journal of Neuropsychiatry, 2,* 1–14.

Roth, M., Tym, E., Mountjoy, C. Q., Huppert, F. A., Hendrie, H., Verma, S., & Goddard, D. (1986). CAMDEX: A standardized instrument for the diagnosis of mental disorder in the elderly with special reference to the early detection of dementia. *British Journal of Psychiatry, 149,* 698–709.

Rush, B. (1812). *Medical inquiries and observations upon the diseases of the mind* (Facs. ed., 1962). New York: Hefner.

Sachdev, P. (1990). Magnetic resonance imaging in clinical psychiatry. *Acta Psychiatrica Scandinavica, 81,* 378–385.

Shader, R. I., Harmatz, J. S., & Salzman, C. (1974). A new scale for clinical assessment (SCAG). *Journal of the American Geriatrics Society, 22,* 107–113.

Soininem, H., Partanen, V. J., Helkala, E. L., & Riekkinen, P. J. (1982). EEG findings in senile dementia and normal aging. *Acta Neurologica Scandinavica, 65,* 59–70.

Speedie, L., Rabins, P., Pearlson, G., & Moberg, P. (1990). Confrontation naming deficit in dementia of depression. *Journal of Neuropsychiatry, 2,* 59–63.

Spitzer, R. L., Williams, J. B. W., & Gibbon, M. (1987). *Structured clinical interview for DSM-III-R patient version (SCID-P).* New York: Biometrics Research Department, New York State Psychiatric Institute.

Stone, K. (1989). Mania in the elderly. *British Journal of Psychiatry, 155,* 220–224.

Strub, R. L., & Black, F. W. (1985). *The mental status examination in neurology* (2nd ed.). Philadelphia: F. A. Davis.

Tanridag, O., & Kirshner, H. S. (1987). Magnetic resonance imaging and CT scanning in neurobehavioral syndromes. *Psychosomatics, 28,* 517–528.

Thal, L. J., Grundman, M., & Golden, R. (1986). Alzheimer's disease: A correlational analysis of the Blessed information–memory–concentration test and the Mini-Mental State Exam. *Neurology, 36,* 262–264.

Venn, R. D. (1983). The Sandoz clinical assessment–geriatric (SCAG) scale. *Gerontology, 29,* 185–198.

Wechsler, D. (1987). *Wechsler Memory Scale - Revised.* San Antonio: The Psychological Corporation.

Weinberger, D. R. (1984). Brain disease and psychiatric illness: When should a psychiatrist order a CAT scan? *American Journal of Psychiatry, 141* (12), 1521–1527.

Whitty, C. W. M., & Zangwill, O. L. (1977). Amnesia (2nd ed.). London: Butterworths.

Yesavage, J., Brink, T., Rose, T., Lum, O., Huang, O., Adey, V., & Leirer, V. (1983). Development and validation of a geriatric screening scale: A preliminary report. *Journal of Psychiatric Research, 17,* 37–49.

Neuropsychological Assessment

Asenath La Rue, Janet Yang, and Sheryl Osato

I. Introduction
II. Trends in Research and Practice
  A. Understanding Brain–Behavior Relations
  B. Neuropsychological Testing Procedures
III. Diagnostic Applications
  A. Dementia versus Normal Aging
  B. Dementia versus Depression
  C. Distinguishing Different Types of Dementia
IV. Treatment Planning and Evaluation
V. Summary and Conclusions
  References

I. Introduction

Expansion of the older population, public awareness of Alzheimer's disease, and growing interest in neuropsychology as a profession have increased the demand for neuropsychological assessment of elderly patients. The general aims of this type of evaluation are threefold: to document strengths and weaknesses in cognitive function and emotional status; to interpret test outcomes diagnostically, using normative data for older adults and various pathological groups; and to make recommendations for treatment and management of problem behaviors, taking into account the constraints imposed by brain impairment.

Most older patients who come to the attention of a neuropsychologist have been referred by physicians or other professionals because of indications of failing memory or other cognitive problems. Some have clear brain impairment, but there is an interest in knowing more specifically which skills are impaired and preserved. For others, there is only a suspicion of brain disorder, and the issue is to determine whether problems are severe enough to warrant a more complete diagnostic assessment. This is particularly true for individuals with depression or other psychiatric disorders, since emotional problems can greatly exacerbate normal age-related cognitive failures. Recently, with expanded publicity about Alzheimer's disease, there has also been an increase in the number of older people who seek out a cognitive evaluation on their own because of concerns about diminished abilities.

This chapter examines the current state of geriatric neuropsychology, describing advances that have taken place in the past 10 years and highlighting areas in which additional research is needed. The first section reviews recent trends in research and clinical practice. The second section summarizes findings that bear upon common diagnostic questions (e.g., distinguishing dementia from normal aging), and the third discusses applications of neuropsychological assessment in treatment planning and monitoring.

II. Trends in Research and Practice

A. Understanding Brain–Behavior Relations

Neuropsychology is the study of interrelations between brain function and behavior. In human neuropsychology, the aim is to understand the role of brain processes in such complex activities as learning, communicating, and thinking, in both normal individuals and those with neuropsychiatric disorders.

1. Neuroimaging Research

Technical advances of the past 10 to 15 years have facilitated this endeavor by making it possible to monitor brain structure and function in relatively safe and noninvasive ways. Computerized axial tomography (CT), magnetic resonance imaging (MRI), positron emission tomography (PET), and single photon emission tomography (SPECT) complement earlier procedures such as pneumoencephalography, cerebral blood-flow studies, and electroencephalography (EEG), producing increasingly precise information on brain structure and metabolism. EEG methodology has been expanded to include analysis of spectral densities and a variety of evoked responses. Cerebral blood-flow measurement has also become more precise and regionally specific. For neuropsychological researchers, these techniques offer an additional means of validating behavioral tests (for reviews, see Poon, 1986) and an opportunity to address more fundamental questions about the organization of brain and behavior.

Detailed discussion of neuroimaging procedures and their applications to geriatrics and gerontology can be found in Albert and Moss (1988) and in the chapter by Rapoport and Grady in this book. Here, only a few general points can be made.

With respect to normal aging, it has become increasingly apparent that the extent of brain change varies with general health status. In optimally healthy research subjects, those with no identified illnesses and no medications, the evidence for decline in brain function is equivocal or modest in extent, at least through the seventh decade (for discussions and reviews, see Albert & Stafford, 1988; Duffy & McAnulty, 1988; Metter, 1988).

In less carefully screened samples, or in those with identified chronic medical illness, there is often greater evidence for declining brain function compared to young adults. In effect, two normal-aging literatures are emerging—one for exceptionally healthy old people and the other for individuals who exhibit some of the chronic health problems common among older cohorts. Which of these two pictures represents the most useful baseline for understanding normal aging or for comparing normal aging with pathology is unclear at this time.

A second issue concerns associations that have been reported between brain measures and cognitive performance. When recent studies are compared with those of a decade or so ago, there is a trend toward stronger and more consistent correlations in recent research (Albert & Stafford, 1988; Duffy & McAnulty, 1988; La Rue & Jarvik, 1982); this presumably reflects the increased sensitivity of improved neuroimaging procedures. However, the pattern of associations varies across studies and is often hard to interpret. Simple models that relate a particular behavior to a single, focal brain region find relatively little support, particularly when complex behaviors—such as those tapped by clinical neuropsychological tests—are investigated (e.g., Duffy, Albert, McAnulty, & Garvey, 1984; Riege, Harker, & Metter, 1986). Therefore, newer technologies have only served to reinforce the need for a systems approach to brain–behavior correlations (Parks *et al.*, 1989).

Neuroimaging techniques have been more extensively used in research on dementing disorders than in studies of normal aging, and there is somewhat greater consistency in outcomes reported to date. On the average, patients who meet research diagnostic criteria for dementia of the Alzheimer type (DAT; American Psychiatric Association, 1987) or probable Alzheimer's disease (pAD; McKhann *et al.*, 1984) differ significantly from healthy older controls on a host of brain indices, including quantitative CT measures (Albert & Stafford, 1988), cerebral blood flow, PET, and SPECT (Metter, 1988), EEG, and late components of the evoked response (Duffy & McAnulty, 1988). These techniques have also shown promise for helping to distinguish pAD from multi-infarct dementia (MID). For example, in MID, a *patchiness* in the distribution of brain dysfunction can often be noted in blood-flow patterns (Metter, 1988), glucose metabolic rates (Riege & Metter, 1988), and on quantitative EEG (Leuchter, Spar, Walter, & Weiner, 1987).

Whether any of the existing procedures will prove capable of detecting very early or incipient dementia remains an open question. There have been several reports in which patients with mild or questionable DAT (generally with memory deficits only) have shown declines in parietal glucose metabolism on PET before demonstrating clear impairments on tests on intelligence, language, or visuospatial function (Cutler *et al.*, 1985; Grady *et al.*, 1988; Kuhl *et al.*, 1987). This is different, however, from detecting dementia before its manifestation in the form of memory loss. In general, researchers who are interested in beginning signs of dementia face the same problems as those who study normal aging; that is, since the magnitude of changes in both brain processes and behavior is small, the precision of measurement may not be sufficient to detect distinctive associations.

2. Implications for Neuropsychological Practitioners

For the clinical neuropsychologist, questions arise about the integration of behavioral test outcomes with the results of various neurodiagnostic measures. For example, older patients may show signs of atrophy on CT or mild slowing on EEG, but still score within normal limits on neuropsychological tests. Enough is known about these findings to indicate that neither atrophy nor slowing, if mild, is sufficient to call the normalcy of behavioral performance into doubt. However, the significance of some other neuroimaging results is currently less clear. For example, although changes in the white matter surrounding the ventricles on MRI are noted with a high prevalence in patients diagnosed with MID (Meyer, McClintic, Rogers, Sims, & Mortel, 1988; Mirsen & Hachinski, 1988), these findings are also quite common in mentally normal older adults (especially those with hypertension) and in patients with DAT (Mirsen & Hachinski, 1988; Rezek, Morris, Fulling, & Gado, 1987). At present, such an MRI pattern cannot be used to confirm a vascular origin for observed behavioral impairments, nor should it be used in diagnosing MID when deficits in memory or other cognitive functions are lacking (Berg, 1988).

In general, therefore, although the sensitivity of brain-imaging measures is improving, only a partial consensus should be expected between neuropsychological findings and such measures, particularly when the diagnosis under question is one of the diffuse or multi-focal brain disorders so common in older adults.

B. Neuropsychological Testing Procedures

In the late 1970s and early 1980s, the inadequacy of the normative data base for older adults on neuropsychological tests, and the questionable appropriateness of these tests for later life, were viewed as serious impediments to clinical evaluation (e.g., Albert, 1981; Schaie & Schaie, 1977). In the past decade, considerable progress has been made in addressing these concerns; for example, many studies have validated standard tests for various aged populations, and several new clinical tools have been developed specifically for older adults.

1. Renorming Standard Tests

The clinical literature now includes old-age normative data for several of the standard neuropsychological tests that have proved useful in assessment of younger brain-injured adults (for a summary of normative data, see D'Elia & Boone, in press). A few of the more noteworthy normative investigations include published findings for old-old adults on several of Benton's neuropsychological measures (Benton, Eslinger, & Damasio, 1981), including the Visual Retention Test (Benton, 1974), Controlled Oral Word Associations (Benton & Hamsher, 1976), and the Test of Line Orientation (Benton, Varney, & Hamsher, 1978); further descriptive studies conducted with the original version of the Wechsler Memory Scale (WMS; Wechsler, 1945; see review by D'Elia, Satz, & Schretlen, 1989); the development of old-age norms for the Selective Reminding Test (Buschke & Fuld, 1974; Banks, Dickson, & Plasay, 1987; Masur, Fuld, Blau, Levin, & Aronson, 1989; Ruff, Light, & Quayhagen, 1988), a multi-trial verbal free recall task that has been popular in research on aging; and new findings on the Halstead-Reitan Neuropsychological Battery for normal adults with different ages and educational backgrounds (Heaton, Grant, & Matthews, 1986).

Other properties of standard tests (e.g., test–retest reliability and stability) have also been examined for older populations. For example, one-year test–retest findings for normal older adults have now been reported for the Wechsler Adult Intelligence Scale-Revised (WAIS-R; Wechsler, 1981), in complete form (Snow, Tierney, Zorzitto, Fisher, & Reid, 1989) and a short-form administration (Mitrushina & Satz, in press). Since older patients are commonly referred for repeat evaluation after a few months or a year, findings such as these are critical for interpreting whether rate of change exceeds expectations for age.

2. Revising and Adapting Standard Measures

Revisions of standard tests reflect an increased sensitivity to the value of including older adults during standardization than was true a few decades ago. The WAIS-R and the revised Wechsler Memory Scale (WMS-R; Wechsler, 1987) both included individuals as old as 74 years in their national standardization samples. For some other well-known tests, scoring manuals have been revised to incorporate methods for making age adjustments (e.g., for the Color-Word Interference Test, see Golden, 1978; for the Hooper Test of Visual Organization, see the Western Psychological Services, 1983).

3. New Tests

The past decade has also witnessed the development of many new tests that include old-age normative data. For example, the Luria Nebraska Neuropsychological Battery (Golden, Hammeke, & Purisch, 1980; Purisch & Sbordone, 1986), which attempts to standardize some of the assessment techniques used by Luria in his clinical work (e.g., Luria, 1974, 1980), includes an age- and education-adjusted baseline for determining the presence of impairment; a short form has been devised that is specifically recommended for geriatric applications (McCue, Shelly, & Goldstein, 1985). In the area of learning and memory, the California Verbal Learning Test (Delis, Kramer, Kaplan, & Ober, 1987), which adapts and extends the Rey Auditory Verbal Learning Test (Rey, 1964), and the Continuous Visual Memory Test (Trahan & Larrabee, 1988), a nonverbal recognition test, have also been normed for a broad age span (17 to 80 years and 18 to 91 years, respectively).

A few new measures have made specific accommodations to the characteristics of older adults. Larrabee and Crook (1989) have developed a computerized memory battery that uses realistic stimuli to assess traditional memory functions (e.g., face-name pairs for associative learning); this battery is not presently available for clinical use, but pencil and paper versions of several of the measures are described in the literature (e.g., Crook, Ferris, & McCarthy, 1979; McCarthy, Ferris, Clark, & Crook, 1981). This approach addresses one of the common criticisms of standard tests for older adults—that is, questionable relevance for the task of everyday life. Another example is Fuld's (1981) Object Memory Evaluation. Developed for persons aged 70 and older, this test uses a short list of familiar objects that can be identified in several ways (e.g., by touch as well as by sight). This serves to increase motivation and helps to counteract the effects of limited education and stamina, both of which are commonly observed in geriatric clinical populations.

Other investigators have applied findings from the literature on normal aging to develop clinical tests. For example, the Delayed Word Recall Test (Knopman & Ryberg, 1989) is predicated on the ability of normal older adults to benefit from encoding enhancement (Craik, 1977; Perlmutter & Mitchell, 1982). Initially, the patient makes up sentences about each of 10 words; after a brief delay, free recall of the words is elicited. The sentence generation procedure presumably promotes more effective encoding than might occur spontaneously, and in fact, normal older adults perform quite well on this task, whereas those with DAT recall very little. The Controlled Learning and Cued Recall procedure (Grober & Buschke, 1987; Grober, Buschke, Crystal, Bang, & Dresner, 1988) examines the effects of both encoding and retrieval enhancement. A set of 16 items, each accompanied with a category cue, is initially presented in sets of four to assure that they are adequately learned. Both free recall and cued recall (using the cue words presented during learning) are then examined. Normal elderly individuals perform near ceiling under these optimized conditions, but patients with even very early dementia appear to have substantial reductions with this task.

These measures are potentially valuable additions to the field. Tests such as the California Verbal Learning Test, while not specifically designed for the elderly, at least provide normative standards for age interpretation. *Familiarized* tests such as those of Crook and Larrabee may be helpful in the testing process; that is, they may promote rapport and help a patient to feel that his or her problems are being directly and realistically addressed. Tasks such as the Controlled Learning and Cued Recall procedure, which incorporate knowledge of normal aging *processes,* may ultimately prove more sensitive to early pathology than measures that have not been designed with the elderly in mind. As with all new tests, however, replication and validation studies are needed before the clinical value of these measures can be estimated.

4. Brief, Focused Batteries

A final popular area of psychometric research pertains to the search for brief assessment batteries that can address specific diagnostic questions. For example, several dementia-screening batteries, comprising small sets of standard neuropsychological measures, have been identified. The best known are the Washington University battery (Storandt, Botwinick, Danziger, Berg, & Hughes, 1984), which includes Logical Memory and Mental Control from the WMS, a verbal fluency test, and Trails A (Reitan, 1955), and the Iowa Dementia Battery (Eslinger, Damasio, Benton, & Van Allen, 1985), comprising the Visual Retention Test, Controlled Oral Word Associations, and a temporal orientation measure. In initial validation studies, both of these batteries were highly effective in distinguishing patients with mild dementia (DAT and/or mixed dementia cases) from healthy older controls. However, subsequent studies suggest that the value of these batteries is more limited. For example, while Tierney, Snow, Reid, Zorzitto, and Fisher (1987) confirmed the sensitivity of the Washington battery in distinguishing dementia patients and controls, they did not find it to be useful in distinguishing among types of dementia (e.g., DAT versus multi-infarct versus Parkinson's dementia). Ryan, Paolo, and Oehlert (1989), who used both batteries with an unselected sample of neuropsychological referrals, found hit rates of only about 78 and 66% for the Washington and Iowa batteries, respectively, for detecting dementia compared to other forms of brain disorder. Effectively, therefore, these batteries merely screen for the presence of cognitive impairment and cannot be used to identify a particular type of dementia. Whether they are any better for this purpose than a standardized mental status examination such as the Mini-Mental State (MMSE; Folstein, Folstein, & McHugh, 1975) or geriatric screening batteries developed in previous years (e.g., Kendrick, 1965; cf. Miller, 1980) is currently unclear.

III. Diagnostic Applications

Testing for diagnostic purposes continues to be the bread-and-butter task of clinical neuropsychologists. On geriatric services, a majority of referrals revolve around one of three issues: distinguishing dementia from normal aging changes; distinguishing *pseudodementias* caused by psychiatric conditions from *organic* dementia; and distinguishing among different types of dementia.

A. Dementia versus Normal Aging

For the first of these issues—differentiating between dementia and normal aging—the lion's share of the literature pertains to DAT. In the past 10 years, the number of investigations of various cognitive and behavioral functions in DAT has increased at such a rapid rate that it is difficult to keep abreast of new results. For example, a recent compilation of biological and behavioral studies on DAT cited 1200 such papers published from 1983 to 1988, compared to fewer than 100 from 1974 to 1982 (Costa, Whitfield, & Stewart, 1989).

A majority of neuropsychological investigations of DAT have compared the performance of individuals with obvious, clinically significant dementia (DAT or pAD) with carefully screened healthy normal adults. Several generalizations can be drawn from the results of these studies (for a summary, see Table I).

For patients with pAD or DAT of mild to moderate severity, multiple areas of impairment can usually be expected on cognitive testing. In one investigation, 83% of persons who met criteria for pAD had deficits (≥ 2 *standard deviations* [SDs] below the means for matched controls) in at least two areas on a battery of neuropsychological tests, and 68% were impaired in three or more areas (Huff *et al.*, 1987). Other studies also show deficits in a wide range of cognitive functions (e.g., Bayles, Boone, Tomoeda, Slauson, & Kaszniak, 1989; Storandt & Hill, 1989). In most cases, deficits in memory are the most consistent and most severe type of cognitive impairment. The memory loss of DAT is characterized by a striking reduction in the ability to learn new facts and details, impairments in accessing semantic memory, and difficulties in retaining newly learned information over time. Memory deficits are most readily detected on effortful memory tasks (e.g., free recall), but in contrast to either normal aging or certain other pathologies (see Section III, B and C, below), impairments are also likely to be noted on recognition and cued recall tasks. Other common areas of neuropsychological impairment include reductions in cognitive flexibility and executive functions as measured by tasks such as the Trail-

Table I

Summary of Neuropsychological Test Findings in DAT

Typical presentation
Disproportionate loss of memory, accompanied by
Deficits in cognitive flexibility and speeded perceptual–motor integration
Deficits in language production and comprehension, and/or
Visuospatial impairments

Variations in presentation (present in some cases)
Moderate deficits in attention and short-term memory
Depression, psychosis, anxiety, or agitation
Differential severity of language versus visuospatial impairments

Most informative tests
Secondary memory measures
Quantitative deficit relative to age and education norms on all such tests
Qualitative features present in many cases
Paragraph recall—intrusions, confabulation; ≥50% decline on delayed recall
Associative learning—intrusions; additional decline on delayed recall
List learning and recall—impairment in storage as well as retrieval; impaired recognition relative to
norms
Reproduction of designs—omission of complete figure; gross distortions; perseveration from one design
to the next
Semantic memory and language processes
Quantitative deficit relative to age and education norms
Qualitative features present in many cases
Object naming—marked circumlocution; remote semantic associations; perseverations
Verbal fluency—perseveration; loss of set
Picture description—fluent, but many vague terms; word-finding problems

Findings that raise doubt about the diagnosis
Any of the following in early stages of illness
Focal neurological signs and symptoms
Motor impairments (e.g., gait disturbance, tremor)
Speech problems
Severe attention deficits

Cautions
Very early DAT cannot be reliably distinguished from normal aging by cognitive tests
Autopsy is required to confirm AD pathology

Making Test or Digit Symbol; language problems, including impaired word finding, decreased word fluency, impaired language comprehension and written expression, and the presence of paraphasic errors; and visuospatial difficulties, including perceptual inaccuracies and construction deficits. Most patients with pAD have problems in each of these areas, although a few have much more pronounced deficits in language than visuospatial functioning or the reverse (e.g., Friedland, 1988; Martin *et al.*, 1986). For a few patients, deficits in attention and other central executive functions may precede serious secondary memory losses (Becker, 1988).

When DAT is at an early or questionable stage, many of the characteristic deficits noted above are not yet evident on testing. A recent study by Storandt and Hill (1989) illustrates this result. In a previous investigation, these researchers found that a battery of four tests

(Logical memory and Mental Control from the WMS, the Trail-Making Test, Part A, and a word-fluency task) accurately differentiated normal older adults from patients with a clear dementia of mild severity (Clinical Dementia Ratings of 1; see Hughes, Berg, Danziger, Coben, & Martin, 1982). However, in their more recent investigation (Storandt & Hill, 1989), these and other tests failed to distinguish between controls and patients whose dementia was questionable (Clinical Dementia Rating, .5). Discrimination between normals and mildly demented subjects continued to be good based on a three-test battery (Logical Memory, Digit Symbol, and the Boston Naming Test), which again implicated secondary memory, complex psychomotor integration, and language impairment as core deficits in DAT. However, the overlap in distributions for the questionable dementia patients and controls was too great to permit reliable differentiation of these groups. The investigators concluded that absolute levels of performance will probably not be useful in identifying very early dementia, but suggested that knowledge of previous level of function might be of help in making such distinctions more accurately.

In clinical practice, most examiners try to estimate baseline function and to calibrate conclusions about the severity of decline relative to this baseline. Precisely how this is done varies widely among examiners. Regression equations combining variables such as the person's age, education, occupation, and geographical region of residence have been proposed for estimating overall IQ (Barona, Reynolds, & Chastain, 1984; Wilson *et al.*, 1978). The usefulness of these equations with clinical populations has been questioned in a recent study (cf. Klesges & Troster, 1987; Sweet, Moberg, & Tovian, 1990, for a review). Since they were developed on younger samples, the formulas may not apply directly to elderly populations, given that the relationship between key variables (e.g., intellectual level and formal education) is likely to differ between older and younger cohorts. Another method for estimating premorbid ability capitalizes on the relatively good preservation of word-reading skills in dementias such as DAT; a brief test for assessing this ability has been developed (Nelson & McKenna, 1975) for which some data for North American populations are now available (Blair & Preen, 1989). Other methods, such as taking an individual's highest performance as baseline—whether estimated from history or from current test results—have also been discussed (Lezak, 1983), but the validity of this procedure is doubtful given the wide intraindividual variability in cognitive skill levels noted in normal populations (Matarazzo & Prifitera, 1989).

Because deficits in secondary memory appear to be an early-occurring feature in DAT, much effort has been directed at developing memory tests that may prove more sensitive to mild dementia than standard clinical measures. List-learning tasks such as the Selective Reminding Test (SRT; Buschke & Fuld, 1974) have been widely used in clinical research with DAT patients. These measures provide estimates of several component memory processes (e.g., storage versus retrieval) that may be differentially affected by normal aging and DAT. They also appear to be sensitive to the effects of cholinergic drugs and other cognition-enhancing medications (Flicker, 1988). Research comparing carefully screened normal volunteers and patients with either mild DAT or depression on selective reminding tasks has found DAT patients to be impaired on storage and recognition as well as on measures of retrieval, in contrast to patients with depression, whose deficits were primarily limited to retrieval processes (Hart, Kwentus, Hamer, & Taylor, 1987; La Rue, D'Elia, Clark, Spar, & Jarvik, 1986a). When old-old patients in "very early stages" of

DAT (mean error score on the Blessed Dementia Scale, 12.9) were compared with normal subjects on the SRT, demented patients performed more poorly on all memory indices, with scores on recall, delayed recall, recognition, and retrieval from long-term storage distinguishing DAT and normal aging with 80% sensitivity and 95% specificity (Masur *et al.*, 1989). Deficits in storage had a specificity of 100% for DAT, but low sensitivity. These findings suggest that the SRT and related tests may be quite useful in clinical geriatric assessment; however, there are several limitations of this procedure. As noted by Loring and Papanicolaou (1987) and others, empirical support is lacking for the contention that different subtest scores (e.g., retrieval from short-term versus long-term storage) are tapping different memory processes. Also, for some of the populations in which diagnostic discriminations are particularly difficult (old-old adults or psychiatric inpatients), neither the sensitivity (Masur *et al.*, 1989) nor specificity (La Rue, 1989) of selective reminding measures is as high as one might hope.

Tests that evaluate an individual's ability to benefit from encoding or retrieval support may prove to be more useful than unsupported learning tasks in these difficult clinical situations. In a series of two investigations with samples of advanced age (mean age, 78 to 79 years), the Controlled Learning and Cued Recall procedure (Grober & Buschke, 1987; Grober *et al.*, 1988), described above, correctly distinguished 98% of normal older adults and 99% of patients with fairly mild DAT (mean prorated verbal IQ, 99.9; mean Blessed Mental Status score, 12.2 errors). This level of discrimination, based on results for enhanced cued recall, was considerably higher than that observed for either standard free recall or recognition testing.

Paying attention to the types of errors made during learning and recall may also increase the confidence that can be placed in a diagnostic impression in certain situations. For example, Loewenstein, Wilkie, Eisdorfer, Guterman, and Berkowitz (1989) found some support for the hypothesis (Fuld, Katzman, Davies, & Terry, 1982) that monitoring of intrusion errors may be helpful in identifying DAT. Fifty percent of patients with mild DAT (scoring ≥ 21 on the MMSE) made at least one unrelated intrusion during testing with the Object Memory Evaluation. In addition, the ratio of the number of intrusions to the overall number of responses was considerably higher for patients with moderate dementia than either the mild DAT or normal groups (cf. Butters, Granholm, Salmon, Grant, & Wolfe, 1987). Several studies report a considerably higher rate of intrusions in DAT than in certain other disorders that are common in old age, including depression (La Rue *et al.*, 1986a; Loewenstein *et al.*, 1989; Whitehead, 1973) and MID (Fuld *et al.*, 1982; Loewenstein *et al.*, 1989; Reed, Jagust, & Seab, 1988). These outcomes suggest that when errors of intrusion occur, the diagnosis of DAT should be given careful consideration. However, the absence of such errors cannot be used to exclude DAT. In general, lengthy test batteries appear more likely to elicit intrusions than briefer testing (Ober, Koss, Friedland, & Delis, 1985), and delayed or cued recall may also increase intrusion rate relative to immediate memory testing (Kramer *et al.*, 1988).

Other investigations have focused on erosion of language processes in DAT (e.g., Bayles & Kaszniak, 1987; Bayles *et al.*, 1989). A decrease in the number of ideas expressed in spontaneous speech and problems with complex language comprehension may be helpful in distinguishing DAT from some other dementing disorders in which fluency may be reduced without a loss of comprehension or ideational content (Bayles &

Kaszniak, 1987; Cummings, Darkins, Mendez, Hill, & Benson, 1988; Hier, Hagen-locker, & Schindler, 1985; Powell, Cummings, Hill, & Benson, 1988). Verbal fluency and confrontation naming tests, which provide a structured assessment of the ability to access semantic memory, are also relatively sensitive to mild DAT (e.g., Eslinger *et al.*, 1985; Huff, Corkin, & Growdin, 1986; Storandt *et al.*, 1984; Storandt & Hill, 1989).

While there is good agreement on the general types of neuropsychological impairment that are likely to observed in DAT (e.g., see Table I), there is no consensus regarding a diagnostic test profile for DAT. Fuld (1984) proposed an algorithm based on WAIS scores that might be helpful in identifying DAT, but the sensitivity of this formula appears to be low (see section on distinguishing DAT and MID, below). More recently, Christensen and colleagues (Christensen, Multhaup, Nordstrom, & Voss, 1990) have suggested a method for categorizing profiles derived from a broader battery of tests assessing word knowl-edge, memory, reasoning, and executive function. In an initial study of 31 patients with pAD and an equal number of matched controls, the profile similarity index, which is independent of level of performance, produced a perfect separation of groups. However, replication studies and investigations with other brain-damaged groups are clearly needed before the clinical value of this profile approach can be ascertained.

B. Dementia versus Depression

A second popular topic of neuropsychological research in the past decade pertains to distinctions—or the lack thereof—between cognitive deficits which result from depres-sion versus those produced by DAT or other organic dementias. The roots of this research can be found in case descriptions of patients, many of whom were elderly, who had severe cognitive deficits during depressive episodes that remitted, in whole or in part, with treatment or the passage of time (e.g., Kiloh, 1961). Terms such as depressive pseudode-mentia (Wells, 1979) or dementia syndrome of depression (DSD; Folstein & McHugh, 1978) have been coined to denote these cognitive impairments, and a substantial literature has developed, aimed at identification and treatment of this condition.

This discussion will use the term DSD in referring to severe depression-related cog-nitive impairments. The organic dementias with which DSD is compared include condi-tions such as DAT, in which there is substantial, currently irreversible, structural brain impairment. Neurobiological correlates have been postulated for DSD as well (e.g., catecholamine changes, see Weingartner & Silberman, 1982), but at present, these are believed to represent a more transient, metabolic disturbance that does not qualify for the label of brain damage in the sense that the term is usually used.

Findings of the past 10 years have clarified a few of the issues related to DSD. It now seems clear, for example, that a majority of older depressed patients do *not* show severe or generalized cognitive problems when they become depressed (for a discussion, see Niederehe, 1986). Subjective complaints of poor concentration and memory problems are very common in depressives at all ages (e.g., Kahn, Zarit, Hilbert, & Niederehe, 1975; Popkin, Gallagher, Thompson, & Moore, 1982), but on objective testing, many studies report either no measurable deficit compared to controls or relatively mild impairments that are restricted to certain areas (e.g., effortful cognitive processing such as free recall;

see Blau & Ober, 1988; Niederehe & Yoder, 1989; Reisberg, Ferris, Gerogatas, de Leon, & Schneck, 1982; Weingartner, Cohen, Murphy, Martello, & Gerdt, 1981). It is only among severely depressed individuals, most of whom are inpatients, that DSD is relatively common; among older inpatients, some 10–20% are likely to score in the organic range of commonly used cognitive tests (McAllister, 1983; Rabins, 1983).

What distinguishes patients with this level of cognitive deficit from other depressed patients? This question is only beginning to be addressed. DSD seems most likely to occur in patients whose global functional level is compromised (La Rue, Spar, & Hill, 1986b) and who have prolonged episodes of depression (La Rue & Goodman, 1989); low levels of education or general intelligence also seem to account for some of the poor performances observed (La Rue *et al.*, 1986b; Post, 1966). In some studies, delusional depressives or those with unusually high levels of anxiety or agitation are also disproportionately likely to exhibit DSD (La Rue *et al.*, 1986b; Post, 1966; Rabins, Merchant, & Nestadt, 1984). In all of these investigations, however, sample sizes have been small, and the reliability of identified "risk factors" for DSD is not well established.

The prognosis for patients with DSD is also an open question. Some studies report that DSD patients show a good response to standard antidepressant therapies and have a favorable prognosis, at least for a year or two after treatment (La Rue *et al.*, 1986b; Rabins *et al.*, 1984). However, other studies suggest that a large proportion of patients with DSD will progress to a frank dementia within a few years (e.g., Kral & Emery, 1989; Reding, Haycox, & Blass, 1985). DSD patients are undoubtedly a heterogeneous group, with some having cognitive problems that are solely related to depression, and others having the beginnings of structural brain impairment. Interestingly, studies that have shown a less-favorable course appear to have focused on patients who were first brought to clinical attention because of failing cognitive abilities, and only later judged to have depression instead of dementia (e.g., Kral & Emery, 1989; Reding *et al*, 1985). Those in whom depression was the first or most prominent clinical concern appear more likely to be the *true* DSD patients. Therefore, as suggested by Wells (1979), clinical history remains important for clinical diagnosis in these difficult cases. Also, as other reviewers have pointed out (e.g., Caine, 1986; Marcopulos, 1989; Stoudemire *et al.*, 1988), there are many cases in which depression and dementia coexist, and in which treatment may lead to only partial improvement in functional cognitive ability.

On neuropsychological testing, there are several fairly distinctive features of performance that are commonly observed in patients with depression (see Table II for a summary). For example, memory problems are most pronounced on tasks that require substantial spontaneous effort on the patient's part, either in organizing information during learning or in retrieving it at a later time (Hart, Kwentus, Hamer, & Taylor, 1987; Weingartner *et al.*, 1981); on tasks in which the organization of information is more readily apparent or retrieval is enhanced (e.g., as in multiple-choice recognition) deficits are often not detectable on standard clinical tests. Similarly, incidental learning and rate of forgetting are usually not impaired compared to normals in older depressed patients (Hart, Kwentus, Taylor, & Harkins, 1987; Hart, Kwentus, Wade, & Hamer, 1987; Kopelman, 1986). Problems are noted quite often on tests of cognitive flexibility, which require shifting of attention or thought (Caine, 1981, 1986; Raskin, 1986), and tests of abstract reasoning (e.g., Savard, Rey, & Post, 1980; Silberman, Weingartner, & Post, 1983). These tasks

Table II

Summary of Neuropsychological Findings in Geriatric Depression

---

Typical presentation
   Depressed mood or pervasive loss of interest, accompanied by
      Mild memory deficit
      Mild to moderate visuospatial impairment
      Reduced abstraction and cognitive flexibility
Behavior during testing
   Self-critical of performance; may underestimate ability or reject positive comments from the examiner; global
      as opposed to circumscribed cognitive complaints
   Complaints of fatigue or physical distress, often accompanied by an objective loss of stamina
   Complaints of poor concentration, but usually can attend to tasks if encouraged
Most informative tests
   List-learning tests
      Storage, recognition, and rate of forgetting close to normal
      Mild-to-moderate impairments in recall
      Low rate of intrusion errors
      Benefit from cueing and encoding enhancement
   Intelligence testing
      Verbal IQ close to normal levels
      Digit Span ≤ other verbal subtests
      Mild-to-moderate impairment on performance subtests, due primarily to slowing, carelessness, or refusal to
         complete the task
Findings that raise doubt about the diagnosis
   Depressive symptoms mild or questionable
   Problems in language comprehension
   Severe memory deficit
Cautions
   Cognitive loss may be linked more closely to global dysfunction than to severity of depression *per se.*
   Depression often coexists with organic brain disorder.
   10–20% of patients have diffuse cognitive problems that are hard to distinguish from DAT or other organic
      dementias.

---

also require considerable effort, and in many cases are performed under conditions that place a premium on speed. Another common finding is for relatively greater deficits on visuospatial as opposed to verbal tasks (e.g., performance IQ lower than verbal IQ; e.g., Dean, Gray, & Seretny, 1987). As previously indicated, problems in these areas are absent or mild in severity for many depressed individuals, but may be discernible statistically when groups of patients are compared.

Whether this "depressive profile" can be used clinically to distinguish individual cases of DSD from DAT or other organic dementias is a question that has not been adequately researched. Caine (1981) concluded that these types of problems were characteristic of DSD patients, but did not provide quantitative data to illustrate these results. In practice, examiners often find DSD patients to be very difficult to test, since many have severely reduced motivation or ability to apply themselves. This limits the accumulation of a consistent body of findings that may be of help in characterizing a DSD profile or profiles.

C. Distinguishing Different Types of Dementia

Different systems have been proposed in classifying organic dementias. The DSM-III-R (American Psychiatric Association, 1987) presents criteria for a generic dementia syndrome, with additional criteria provided for two of the most common dementing disorders, Primary Degenerative Dementia of the Alzheimer Type (DAT) and Multi-Infarct Dementia (MID). Others (e.g., Albert, 1978; Cummings & Benson, 1983, 1988) have proposed a broader, more inclusive classification based on the primary site of neuropathological involvement. Specifically, a distinction is drawn between *cortical* dementias (including DAT and Pick's disease) and *subcortical* dementias [including Huntington's disease and Parkinson's disease (PD)].

Both of these systems have been the subject of considerable criticism. The feasibility of making valid antemortem diagnostic distinctions between DAT and MID, using criteria such as those in DSM-III-R, has been questioned by several reviewers (e.g., Brust, 1988; Liston & La Rue, 1983a,b). The cortical–subcortical distinction has been criticized because disorders in either category often entail a combination of cortical and subcortical pathology (e.g., nucleus basalis involvement in DAT, frontal systems deficits in PD; see Whitehouse, 1986) and because clinically, within-group differences (e.g., between various cortical disorders) are often as striking as between-group distinctions (i.e., between cortical and subcortical conditions; see Chui, 1989). Nonetheless, it is apparent that there are important differences in behavioral impairments among dementia patients, and the need for criteria to organize these distinctions continues to be felt.

1. DAT versus PD

The most striking features differentiating PD from DAT are the behavioral manifestations associated with motor functioning. For individuals with PD, motor impairment is evident at the first stages of disease, and generally involves one or more of the following: resting tremor, bradykinesia (motor retardation), ataxic gait, dystonia, cogwheel rigidity, hypophonia (reduced speech volume), and dysarthria (poorly articulated speech). In DAT, by contrast, motor functioning generally remains intact until the late stages of disease.

Differences on neuropsychological testing are less clear, although several differentiating trends have been reported (see Table III). Studies comparing groups of patients with PD with those with DAT have reported greater global cognitive impairment (as evidenced by lower mental status exam scores) in DAT than in PD (e.g., Huber, Freidenberg, Shuttleworth, Paulson, & Christy, 1989). Also, while visuospatial deficits are common in both disorders (Boller *et al.*, 1984; Huber, Shuttleworth, Paulson, Bellchambers, & Clapp, 1986), language deficits (especially comprehension problems) are more pronounced in DAT than in PD, whereas speech problems (reduced phrase length, articulatory deficits) are often more noticeable in PD (e.g., Cummings *et al.*, 1988). Memory deficits and frontal systems impairments are noted in both diseases; however, their relative prominence in early stages of disease may differ. In DAT, secondary memory loss tends to be the most striking area of impairment, whereas in PD, frontal lobe dysfunction (e.g., as evidenced by impaired shifting on tasks such as the Wisconsin Card Sort or a lack of spontaneity in everyday interactions) are comparatively more prominent (e.g., Hietanen

Table III

Summary of Neuropsychological Test Findings in PD

Typical presentation
  Motor slowing and/or tremor, accompanied by
    Disproportionate loss of cognitive flexibility
    Visuospatial impairment
    Speech problems
    Mild memory deficit

Most informative tests
  Cognitive flexibility and attentional switching
    Reduced speed of performance relative to age and education norms
    Qualitative features present in many cases
      Sorting or categorization—Perseveration; difficulty in inferring or switching categories
      Complex sequencing—Difficulty comprehending task; loss of set
  List-learning tests
    Storage, recognition, and rate of forgetting within normal limits
    Impaired consistency of retrieval
    Impaired recall of serial position
    Low rate of intrusion errors

Findings that raise doubt about the diagnosis
  Any of the following in early stages of illness:
    Severe memory impairment
    Severe attentional deficit
    Deficits in language comprehension
    Loss of verbal intellectual ability

Cautions
  Only a rough parallel should be expected between the severity of motor symptoms and extent of cognitive loss
  Depression is commonly observed and may exacerbate cognitive problems
  10–20% of patients have diffuse cognitive problems that are hard to distinguish from DAT

& Teravainen, 1986; Lees & Smith, 1983; Pillon, Dubois, Lhermitte, & Agid, 1986). In mild PD, memory problems tend to be confined to effortful tasks (Weingartner, Burns, Diebel, & LeWitt, 1984), and even then, there are many patients with no clear evidence of impairment (El-Awar, Becker, Hammond, Nebes, & Boller, 1987; Lees & Smith, 1983). Research also suggests that depression may be more common or more severe in PD than in DAT (Gainotti, Caltagirone, Masullo, & Micelli, 1980; Huber *et al.*, 1986).

Awareness of these differentiating trends can be helpful in testing PD patients. Generally, these patients are referred to a neuropsychologist when there are questions about the severity of cognitive impairment or about whether the pattern of impairments is consistent with PD alone. However, methodological problems in this area reduce the degree of confidence that can be placed in the generalizations noted above (for recent critical reviews, see Bayles, 1990; Levin, 1990). In many investigations, PD and DAT groups have not been matched for global dementia severity; therefore, the more severe memory loss of DAT may simply reflect the relatively greater global dementia. Questions also arise about *how* to match for dementia severity, since tests like the MMSE primarily tap cortically based functions and may not be a valid indication of the extent of subcortical dementia. Another issue concerns the effects of motor dysfunction on neuropsychological measures. Many visuospatial tests, language tests, and nonverbal memory measures contain a constructive component or require a speedy response. When such tests are used with a PD patient, they may lead to an underestimation of cognitive abilities which, in fact, might be intact if motor-minimizing tests were given. In clinical settings, therefore, it may be best to use conservative criteria in applying the label of dementia with PD patients.

2. DAT versus MID

MID is generally considered to be the second most common form of dementia in older adults, exceeded only by DAT. However, prevalence estimates vary widely, since the antemortem diagnosis of MID continues to be difficult (for contrasting viewpoints, see Brust, 1988; O'Brien, 1988).

Currently, many research and clinical settings rely on one version or another of the Ischemia Score (Hachinski et al., 1975; Loeb, 1988; Rosen, Terry, Fuld, Katzman, & Peck, 1980) to identify patients whose dementia might be due to vascular disorder, and in particular, to multiple small or large infarcts. This checklist of historical and clinical features includes items that are sensitive to stroke, other indications of cardio- or cerebrovascular disease, and several psychiatric and behavioral features (e.g., presence or absence of depression or emotional incontinence). A high score is generally taken as support for a cerebrovascular etiology of dementia; a low score suggests the absence of significant cerebrovascular disease, and thus increases confidence that the dementia is of a primary degenerative type (e.g., DAT). However, both clinical and pathological validation studies have raised doubts about the accuracy of diagnoses based on the Ischemia Score (IS) or similar scales (for details, see Liston & La Rue, 1983a,b). Many of the clinical features composing the IS are also found in substantial proportions of DAT patients (e.g., hypertension, depressive features). Other features are quite uncommon in either diagnostic group (e.g., stepwise deterioration, emotional incontinence). In general, the items that withstand the test of validation best are those that pertain most directly to a history of stroke (e.g., presence or absence of focal neurological signs and symptoms or abrupt onset of impairment).

CT or MRI findings are also commonly used to try to differentiate MID and DAT. Often, the presence of one or more distinct areas of lucency on CT or hyperintensity on MRI, suggesting small strokes, is taken as support for a clinical diagnosis of MID. However, since small strokes are often behaviorally silent, this method might lead to an overdiagnosis of MID relative to DAT (Brust, 1988). The relevance of small, deep, white-matter lesions, unless extensive, is even less clear.

These diagnostic problems have had a dampening effect on research on MID. In terms of neuropsychological studies, for example, there are far fewer investigations focusing on MID than on DAT, and considerably fewer than for PD. The few studies of MID that are available have generally included samples that are heterogeneous with respect to the site and extent of vascular lesions, thereby obscuring relationships that might exist between cerebral and behavioral impairments.

Early studies by Perez and colleagues (Perez, Gay, Taylor, & Rivera, 1975; Perez et al., 1975) came to the conclusion that the deficits observed on both the WAIS and WMS in DAT and MID were quite similar in pattern on the average, but that the severity of impairment tended to be greater in DAT than in MID. However, there was no indication that the groups were at a comparable stage of illness at the time of these comparisons. Similarly, although Powell *et al.* (1988) noted greater language impairment in DAT than in MID, the DAT patients also had somewhat greater global dementia severity (mean MMSE, 15.7 versus 18.8).

A more recent study (Loewenstein *et al.*, in press) compared matched groups of mildly impaired DAT and MID patients (mean MMSE score, 22.9 versus 23.5, respectively). No differences were observed on verbal or nonverbal intelligence subtests, language tests, or visuospatial functions. Total retrieval on the Object Memory Evaluation and the number of intrusion errors made during this test were the only measures that discriminated the groups, with the DAT patients tending to have more severe impairment on these measures. Holborn (1990) also compared DAT and MID groups, controlling for differences in dementia severity in statistical analyses. No single neuropsychological measure accurately distinguished these groups. However, a discriminant function equation based on the MMSE, Boston Naming Test, delayed recall from the Object Memory Evaluation, and WAIS-R Vocabulary correctly classified 74% of the patients (21 of 29 with MID, 28 of 35 with DAT). In general, poor performance on the MMSE, naming, and delayed-recall tasks, combined with a high score on Vocabulary, was associated with the diagnosis of DAT.

Fuld (1984) proposed that the following WAIS formula, based on age-scaled scores, may have some utility in distinguishing patients with DAT from those with MID:

$$A > B > C \le D, \text{ and } A > D,$$

where A = the mean of Information and Vocabulary, B = the mean of Similarities and Digit Span, C = the mean of Digit Symbol and Block Design, and D = Object Assembly. In Fuld's (1984) study, approximately one-half of patients with DAT and young subjects with drug-induced cholinergic deficiency displayed this subtest pattern, compared to fewer than 10% of MID patients and young adult controls.

Replication studies examining this formula have provided variable results. Brinkman and Braun (1984) also found that the profile was more common in DAT than in MID, and others have reported that it rarely occurs in normal aging (Satz, Van Gorp, Soper, & Mitrushina, 1987) or geriatric depression (Bornstein, Termeer, Longbrake, Heger, & North, 1989). However, additional studies indicate that the profile occurs with similar frequencies in DAT and other forms of dementia, including MID (Filley, Koyabashi, & Heaton, 1987; Logsdon, Teri, Williams, Vitiello, & Prinz, 1989).

In general, the neuropsychological literature on MID is too limited and inconsistent to permit a listing of characteristic test outcomes. On the average, it appears that patients with MID do not differ greatly from those with DAT on standard clinical tests when the overall level of dementia is equated (cf. Erkinjuntti, 1987).

There are a few test findings that can serve to reinforce an impression of MID. For example, patients who have multiple, large cerebral infarctions in different cortical regions would be expected to show pronounced intertest variability. However, for those with lacunar infarcts alone (see Hachinski, Lassen, & Marshall, 1974) or Binswanger's disease, intertest differences may not exceed those observed in normal aging or DAT. The presence of motor speech impairments may be more consistent with MID than DAT, as is the *absence* of intrusion errors. However, neither of these findings has been studied enough to give firm estimates of diagnostic sensitivity and specificity. Patients with Binswanger's disease or infarcts limited to subcortical regions will sometimes, but not invariably, have impairments that fit a pattern of subcortical dementia (e.g., Derix, Hijdra, & Verbeeten, 1987). For those with cortical infarcts, deficits consistent with established stroke syndromes (e.g., aphasia or apraxia) may be expected.

IV. Treatment Planning and Evaluation

In addition to aiding in diagnosis, neuropsychological tests have potential utility in treatment planning for the patient and family. For example, after noticing memory deficits in a relative, and particularly if the person has been labeled as having dementia, family members may begin to treat the patient as if he or she is impaired in all daily tasks. This in turn could lead to demoralization and *excess disability,* i.e., losses of function not inherently related to the disease. By identifying a patient's retained areas of strength, neuropsychological assessment can help in tailoring a plan for sharing everyday responsibilities between the patient and significant others. Test findings can also document deficits that suggest the need for greater assistance or supervision on an everyday level. For example, in a study of patients with pAD (Henderson, Mack, & Williams, 1989), visuoconstructive deficits combined with memory loss were identified as significant predictors of everyday spatial disorientation, as indicated by caregivers' reports of wandering, getting lost, and failing to recognize familiar surroundings. That is, patients with deficits on visuospatial tests were more likely to wander than were other patients with comparable levels of memory impairment.

Investigations like that of Henderson *et al.* are quite rare in the literature on geriatric neuropsychology. Most of the research examining the utility of neuropsychological testing for predicting everyday function has been conducted with younger adults, and the emphasis has been placed on predicting performance in educational or occupational settings (for a review, see Heaton & Pendleton, 1981). With the elderly, research has been quite limited in method and scope. Most studies have compared performance on brief mental status exams to relatives' or professionals' ratings of patients' functional ability (e.g., Breen, Larson, Reifler, Vitaliano, & Lawrence, 1984; Kahn, Goldfarb, Pollack, & Gerber, 1960; Wilson, Grant, Witney, & Kerridge, 1973; Winograd, 1984). In general, only a modest relationship has been found between such measures. One recent study (Reed, Jagust, & Seab, 1989) observed significant associations between Mini-Mental State scores and relatives' ratings of both physical and instrumental activities (rs, .68 and .51, respectively) for patients with relatively severe dementia (MMSE < 14), but not for those with milder dementia severity (MMSE > 15). The investigators suggested that particularly at early stages of disease, familiarity with tasks (i.e., degree of overlearning), motivation, and opportunity to engage in different skills might all influence functional level in ways that cannot be detected by cognitive mental status exams.

In general, the more thorough the neuropsychological assessment, the greater are the prospects of making meaningful predictions about everyday functional abilities. However, since research on external validity is so limited, treatment-planning applications are dependent on the clinical skill and experience of the examiner.

Heaton and Pendleton (1981) provide some useful clinical generalizations about areas of deficit that may impinge on specific realms of everyday function. With respect to driving, for example, they suggest that deficits in any one of several areas (attention, sequencing, right–left discrimination, nonverbal memory, visuoconstruction, and concept formation) may be sufficient to raise a question about driving safety. Ultimately, a professional assessment of driving ability would be needed to evaluate competence, but test findings might help to alert a patient or family member to potential problems in this area. Other high-risk activities, such as taking medications, might also be predicted to a degree by formal cognitive testing. There are indications that even healthy, mentally normal older adults have difficulty learning and retaining information related to medications (e.g., Morrell, Park, & Poon, 1989); therefore, if testing indicates that these skills are impaired beyond normal levels, assistance in scheduling and administering medications should be strongly recommended.

Assessment findings may also be helpful in selecting appropriate therapies or supportive activities. The literature on stroke patients suggests that cognitive test results can help to predict rehabilitation outcome beyond the information obtained from standard neurological exams (Caplan, 1982; Heaton & Pendleton, 1981; Sundet, Finset, & Reinvang, 1988), and for psychiatric patients, basic level of cognitive function appears to have a bearing on the benefit obtained from participation in psychotherapy (Heaton & Pendleton, 1981).

Older patients with focal or nonprogressive brain impairment may be candidates for neuropsychological rehabilitation programs to ameliorate cognitive and behavioral impairments, including memory loss for particular materials or activities (Wilson, 1987; Wilson & Moffat, 1984). Even among patients with DAT, there is wide variation in individuals' abilities to benefit from psychosocial interventions, including individual and group psychotherapy (Group for the Advancement of Psychiatry, 1988; Jarvik & Winograd, 1988). For these applications, baseline neuropsychological testing may provide one of the best means available for selecting interventions that are suited to the patient's abilities and personal dynamics.

Monitoring the impact of treatment is another important use of neuropsychological testing. Tests of attention, learning and memory, and psychomotor speed have played a critical role in clinical trials of psychoactive medications for older patients, including experimental drugs for memory enhancement (see Flicker, 1988, for a review). In assessing treatment outcomes, it is important to select measures that are sensitive to the specific cognitive process under investigation, that can be repeated multiple times, and that will not produce ceiling or floor effects (La Rue, 1987). With impaired older patients, brevity and high face validity are also desirable. Flicker (1988) has ranked many commonly used neuropsychological tests on these dimensions. Brief structured batteries such as the Alzheimer's Disease Assessment Scale (ADAS; Rosen, Mohs, & Davis, 1984), which provides simple tests of several cognitive domains and ratings of mood and behavior, may be preferable in some treatment studies to more extensive neuropsychological testing. For normal older adults or those with very mild impairment, computerized batteries such as the one designed by Larrabee and Crook (1989) or Branconnier (1986) are good candidates for measuring treatment effects.

V. Summary and Conclusions _____

This chapter discussed recent developments in geriatric neuropsychological practice, including research and clinical applications. One important new development is improved neuroimaging technology, which permits safer and more precise visualization of brain process involved in cognition. This provides exciting opportunities to examine brain–behavior changes in normal and pathologic aging and a means of cross-validating impressions based on clinical tests. There have also been many improvements in neuropsychological testing procedures in the past decade. Several standard tests have been revised, providing more complete and representative old-age norms than earlier versions. New tests have been developed and normed across a broad age range, and a few tests have been specifically designed for elderly patients. Despite these developments, however, some important limitations persist in assessment procedures, including a paucity of norms for very old adults and limited data on the practical significance of poor test performance.

Three common diagnostic applications of geriatric neuropsychology were examined in this chapter: distinguishing normal aging and DAT, distinguishing depression and DAT, and differentiating various dementing conditions (e.g., DAT versus MID). DAT usually results in multiple neuropsychological impairments, with deficits in learning and memory being particularly prominent; language deficits, visuospatial impairments, and declining cognitive flexibility often accompany memory changes. In very early phases of the disease, however, no test or set of tests has been identified that can reliably distinguish patients from controls. Questions of when, where, and how to draw the line between normal and abnormal decline hinge in part on the general medical and psychosocial status of the individual, since trajectories of *normal* decline appear to differ for various aging subgroups. Therefore, until a valid biological marker for DAT is discovered, or normal aging is better understood, detection of beginning dementia is likely to remain a problem.

Cognitive effects of DAT and major depression can be distinguished with acceptable accuracy for about 80% of cases, since most of the time, depression produces milder and more circumscribed impairments. Compared to patients with DAT, depressed patients are less likely to have language impairments or to make errors of intrusion or confabulation during testing; memory problems are often limited to effortful tasks (e.g., free recall as opposed to recognition). For patients in whom more severe cognitive losses coexist with depression, there is still no consensus about methods for ruling out possible early dementia as a basis for cognitive problems. Followup testing, allowing time for treatment and improvement in depressive symptoms, continues to be of value in gaining a clearer picture of cause and effect in these individuals.

Research attempting to distinguish among types of dementia that are common in old age is still in an unsatisfactory state. Neuropsychological research on MID remains too limited to permit many useful generalizations, and clinical diagnostic criteria such as patchiness of deficits or stepwise decline, as noted in the DSM-III-R, have never been operationalized. For PD, there is a larger and more detailed literature, but fundamental issues about the prevalence and causes of cognitive decline in PD remain to be resolved. In general, patients with PD tend to have relatively prominent impairments in executive functions, but less severe language and memory impairments, compared to patients with DAT. However, the degree of cognitive problems varies considerably from one PD patient to another, and interpretation of test outcomes is complicated by motor slowing, tremor, and articulation problems. To advance knowledge of neuropsychological patterns in MID and PD, greater emphasis needs to be placed on subject selection (especially on subgrouping of patients with similar brain pathology) and on following samples to obtain autopsy confirmation of disease.

A final area of discussion concerned the application of neuropsychological testing to treatment planning and evaluation. The information gained from testing about an individual's strengths and impairments can provide valuable clues to potential problems in everyday function and constitutes an objective basis for determining effects of different treatments. However, in most geriatric care settings, greater effort needs be directed at educating the patient and family about the implications of test results and in helping them to identify helpful supports and interventions when brain impairment is part of the clinical picture.

References

Albert, M. L. (1978). Subcortical dementia. In R. Katzman, R. D. Terry, & K. L. Bick (Eds.), *Alzheimer's disease: Senile dementia and related disorders* (pp. 173–180). New York: Raven.

Albert, M. S. (1981). Geriatric neuropsychology. *Journal of Consulting and Clinical Psychology, 49,* 835–850.

Albert, M. S., & Moss, M. B. (Eds.). (1988). *Geriatric neuropsychology.* New York: Guilford.

Albert, M. S., & Stafford, J. L. (1988). Computed tomography studies. In M. S. Albert & M. B. Moss (Eds.), *Geriatric Neuropsychology* (pp. 211–227). New York: Guilford.

American Psychiatric Association. (1987). *Diagnostic and statistical manual of mental disorders (DSM-III-R)* (3rd ed., rev.). Washington DC: Author.

Banks, P. G., Dickson, A. L., & Plasay, M. T. (1987). The verbal selective reminding test: Preliminary data for healthy elderly. *Experimental Aging Research, 13,* 203–206.

Barona, A., Reynolds, C., & Chastain, R. (1984). A demographically based index of premorbid intelligence for the WAIS-R. *Journal of Consulting and Clinical Psychology, 52,* 885–887.

Bayles, K. A. (1990). Language and Parkinson disease. *Alzheimer Disease and Associated Disorders, 4,* 171–180.

Bayles, K. A., & Kaszniak, A. W. (1987). *Communication and cognition in normal aging and dementia.* Boston, MA: College-Hill.

Bayles, K. A., Boone, D. R., Tomoeda, C. K., Slauson, T. J., & Kaszniak, A. W. (1989). Differentiating Alzheimer's patients from the normal elderly and stroke patients with aphasia. *Journal of Speech and Hearing Disorders, 54,* 74–87.

Becker, J. T. (1988). Working memory and secondary memory deficits in Alzheimer disease. *Journal of Clinical and Experimental Neuropsychology, 10,* 739–753.

Benton, A. L. (1974). *Revised Visual Retention Test* (4th ed.). New York: Psychological Corporation.

Benton, A. L., & Hamsher, K. de S. (1976). *Multilingual Aphasia Examination.* Iowa City: University of Iowa Press.

Benton, A. L., Eslinger, P. J., & Damasio, A. R. (1981). Normative observations on neuropsychological test performances in old age. *Journal of Clinical Neuropsychology, 3,* 33–42.

Benton, A. L., Varney, N. R., & Hamsher, K. deS. (1978). Visuospatial judgment: A clinical test. *Archives of Neurology, 35,* 364–367.

Berg, L. (1988). The aging brain. In R. Strong, W. G. Wood, & W. J. Burke (Eds.), *Central nervous disorders of aging: Clinical intervention and research* (pp. 1–16). New York: Raven.

Blair, J., & Preen, O. (1989). Predicting premorbid IQ: A revision of the National Adult Reading Test. *The Clinical Neuropsychologist, 3,* 129–136.

Blau, E., & Ober, B. A. (1988, January). *The effect of depression on verbal memory in older adults.* Paper presented at a meeting of the International Neuropsychological Society, New Orleans, LA.

Boller, F., Passafiume, D., Keefe, N. C., Rogers, K., Morrow, L., & Kim, Y. (1984). Visuospatial impairment in Parkinson's disease. *Archives of Neurology, 41*, 485–490.

Bornstein, R. A., Termeer, J., Longbrake, K., Heger, M., & North, R. (1989). WAIS-R cholinergic deficit profile in depression. *Psychological Assessment, 1*, 342–344.

Branconnier, R. J. (1986). A computerized battery for behavioral assessment in Alzheimer's disease. In L. W. Poon (Ed.), *Handbook for clinical memory assessment of older adults* (pp. 189–196). Washington, DC: American Psychological Association.

Breen, A. R., Larson, E. B., Reifler, B. V., Vitaliano, P. P., & Lawrence, G. L. (1984). Cognitive performance and functional competence in coexisting dementia and depression. *Journal of the American Geriatrics Society, 32*, 132–137.

Brinkman, S. D., & Braun, P. (1984). Classification of dementia patients by a WAIS profile related to central cholinergic deficiencies. *Journal of Clinical Neuropsychology, 6*, 393–400.

Brust, J. C. M. (1988). Vascular dementia is overdiagnosed. *Archives of Neurology, 45*, 799–801.

Buschke, H., & Fuld, P. A. (1974). Evaluating storage, retention, and retrieval in disordered memory and learning. *Neurology, 24*, 1019–1025.

Butters, N., Granholm, E., Salmon, D., Grant, I., & Wolfe, J. (1987). Episodic and semantic memory: A comparison of amnestic and demented patients. *Journal of Clinical and Experimental Neuropsychology, 9*, 479–497.

Caine, E. (1981). Pseudodementia: Current concepts and future directions. *Archives of General Psychiatry, 38*, 1359–1364.

Caine, E. D. (1986). The neuropsychology of depression: The pseudodementia syndrome. In I. Grant & K. M. Adams (Eds.), *Neuropsychological assessment of neuropsychiatric disorders* (pp. 221–243). New York: Oxford University Press.

Caplan, B. (1982). Neuropsychology in rehabilitation: Its role in evaluation and intervention. *Archives of Physical Medicine and Rehabilitation, 63*, 362–366.

Christensen, K. J., Multhaup, K. S., Nordstrom, S., & Voss, K. (1990). Cognitive test profile analysis for the identification of dementia of the Alzheimer type. *Alzheimer Disease and Associated Disorders, 4*, 96–109.

Chui, H. C. (1989). Dementia: A review emphasizing clinicopathologic correlation and brain–behavior relationships. *Archives of Neurology, 46*, 806–814.

Costa, P. T., Jr., Whitfield, J. R., & Stewart, D. (Eds.) (1989). *Alzheimer's disease: Abstracts of the psychological and behavioral literature.* Washington, DC: American Psychological Association.

Craik, F. I. M. (1977). Age differences in human memory. In J. E. Birren & K. W. Schaie (Eds.), *Handbook of the psychology of aging* (pp. 384–420). New York: Van Nostrand Reinhold.

Crook, T., Ferris, S., & McCarthy, M. (1979). The misplaced-object task: A brief test for memory dysfunction in the aged. *Journal of the American Geriatrics Society, 27*, 284–287.

Cummings, J. L., & Benson, D. F. (1983). *Dementia: A clinical approach.* Boston, MA: Butterworths.

Cummings, J. L., & Benson, D. F. (1988). Psychological dysfunction accompanying subcortical dementias. *Annual Review of Medicine, 39*, 53–61.

Cummings, J. L., Darkins, A., Mendez, M., Hill, M. A., & Benson, D. F. (1988). Alzheimer's disease and Parkinson's disease: Comparison of speech and language alterations. *Neurology, 38*, 680–684.

Cutler, N. R., Haxby, J. V., Duara, R., Grady, C. L., Moore, A. M., Parisi, J. E., White, J., Heston, L., Margolin, R. M., & Rapoport, S. I. (1985). Brain metabolism as measured with positron emission tomography: Serial assessment in a patient with familial Alzheimer's disease. *Neurology, 35*, 1556–1561.

D'Elia, L. F., & Boone, K. B. (in press). *Handbook of normative data for neuropsychological assessment.* New York: Oxford University Press.

D'Elia, L., Satz, P., & Schretlen, D. (1989). Wechsler Memory Scale: A critical appraisal of the normative studies. *Journal of Clinical and Experimental Neuropsychology, 11*, 551–568.

Dean, R. S., Gray, J. W., & Seretny, M. L. (1987). Cognitive aspects of schizophrenia and primary affective depression. *International Journal of Clinical Neuropsychology, IX*, 33–36.

Delis, D. C., Kramer, J. H., Kaplan, E., & Ober, B. A. (1987). *The California Verbal Learning Test, research edition.* New York: Psychological Corporation.

Derix, M. M. A., Hijdra, A., & Verbeeten, B. W. J., Jr. (1987). Mental changes in subcortical arteriosclerotic encephalopathy. *Clinical Neurology and Neurosurgery, 89*, 71–78.

Duffy, F. H., & McAnulty, G. (1988). Electrophysiological studies. In M. S. Albert & M. B. Moss (Eds.), *Geriatric neuropsychology* (pp. 262–289). New York: Guilford.

Duffy, F. H., Albert, M. S., McAnulty, G., & Garvey, A. J. (1984). Age-related differences in brain electrical activity of healthy subjects. *Annals of Neurology, 16*, 430–438.

El-Awar, M., Becker, J. T., Hammond, K. M., Nebes, R. D., & Boller, F. (1987). Learning deficit in Parkinson's disease. *Archives of Neurology, 44*, 180–184.

Erkinjuntti, T. (1987). Differential diagnosis between Alzheimer's disease and vascular dementia: Evaluation of common clinical methods. *Acta Neurologica Scandinavica, 76*, 433–442.

Eslinger, P. J., Damasio, A. R., Benton, A. L., & Van Allen, M. (1985). Neuropsychologic detection of abnormal mental decline in older persons. *Journal of the American Medical Association, 253*, 670–674.

Filley, C. M., Kobayashi, J., & Heaton, R. K. (1987). Wechsler Intelligence Scale profiles, the cholinergic system, and Alzheimer's disease. *Journal of Clinical and Experimental Neuropsychology, 9*, 180–186.

Flicker, C. (1988). Neuropsychological evaluation of treatment effects in the elderly: A critique of tests in current use. *Psychopharmacology Bulletin, 4*, 535–556.

Folstein, M. F., Folstein, S. E., & McHugh, P. R. (1975). Mini-Mental State: A practical method for grading the cognitive state of patients for the clinician. *Journal of Psychiatric Research, 12*, 189–198.

Folstein, M. F., & McHugh, P. R. (1978). Dementia syndrome of depression. In R. Katzman, R. D. Terry, & K. L. Bick (Eds.), *Alzheimer's disease: Senile dementia and related disorders* (pp. 87–96). New York: Raven Press.

Friedland, R. P. (1988). Alzheimer disease: Clinical and biological heterogeneity. *Annals of Internal Medicine, 109*, 298–311.

Fuld, P. A. (1981). *The Fuld Object-Memory Evaluation*. Chicago: Stoelting Instrument Company.

Fuld, P. A. (1984). Test profile of cholinergic dysfunction and of Alzheimer-type dementia. *Journal of Clinical Neuropsychology, 6*, 380–392.

Fuld, P. A., Katzman, R., Davies, P., & Terry, R. O. (1982). Intrusions as a sign of Alzheimer dementia: Chemical and pathological verification. *Annals of Neurology, 11*, 155–159.

Gainotti, G., Caltagirone, C., Massullo, C., & Micelli, G. (1980). Patterns of neuropsychologic impairment in various diagnostic groups of dementia. In A. Amaducci, A. Davison, & P. Antuono (Eds.), *Aging of the brain and dementia* (pp. 245–250). New York: Raven Press.

Golden, C. J. (1978). *Stroop color and word test: A manual for clinical and experimental uses*. Chicago: Stoelting.

Golden, C. J., Hammeke, T. A., & Purisch, A. D. (1980). *The Luria-Nebraska Neuropsychological Battery Manual*. Los Angeles: Western Psychological Services.

Grady, C. L., Haxby, J. V., Howitz, B., Sundaram, M., Berg, G., Schapiro, M., Friedland, R. P., & Rapoport, S. I. (1988). Longitudinal study of the early neuropsychological and cerebral metabolic changes in dementia of the Alzheimer type. *Journal of Clinical and Experimental Neuropsychology, 10*, 576–596.

Grober, E., & Buschke, H. (1987). Genuine memory deficits in dementia. *Developmental Neuropsychology, 3*, 13–36.

Grober, E., Buschke, H., Crystal H., Bang, S., & Dresner, R. (1988). Screening for dementia by memory testing. *Neurology, 38*, 900–903.

Group for the Advancement of Psychiatry (1988). *The psychiatric treatment of Alzheimer's disease*. New York: Brunner/Mazel.

Hachinski, V. C., Iliff, L. D., Zilhka, E., Du Boulay, G. H., McAllister, V. L., Marshall, J., Russell, R. W., & Symon, L. (1975). Cerebral blood flow in dementia. *Archives of Neurology, 32*, 632–637.

Hachinski, V. C., Lassen, N. A., & Marshall, J. (1974). Multi-infarct dementia: A cause of mental deterioration in the elderly. *Lancet, 2*, 207–209.

Hart, R. P., Kwentus, J. A., Hamer, R. M., & Taylor, J. R. (1987). Selective reminding procedure in depression and dementia. *Psychology and Aging, 2*, 111–115.

Hart, R. P., Kwentus, J. A., Taylor, J. R., & Harkins, S. W. (1987). Rate of forgetting in dementia and depression. *Journal of Consulting and Clinical Psychology, 55*, 101–105.

Hart, R. P., Kwentus, J. A., Wade, J. B., & Hamer, R. M. (1987). Digit Symbol performance in mild dementia and depression. *Journal of Consulting and Clinical Psychology, 55*, 236–238.

Heaton, R. K., & Pendleton, M. G. (1981). Use of neuropsychological tests to predict adult patients' everyday functioning. *Journal of Consulting and Clinical Psychology, 49*, 807–821.

Heaton, R. K., Grant, I., & Matthews, C. G. (1986). Differences in neuropsychological test performance associated with age, education, and sex. In I. Grant & K. M. Adams (Eds.), *Neuropsychological assessment of neuropsychiatric disorders* (pp. 100–120). New York: Oxford University Press.

Henderson, V. W., Mack, W., & Williams, B. W. (1989). Spatial disorientation in Alzheimer's disease. *Archives of Neurology, 46,* 391–394.

Hier, D. B., Hagenlocker, K., & Shindler, A. G. (1985). Language disintegration in dementia: Effects of etiology and severity. *Brain and Language, 25,* 117–133.

Hietanen, M. & Teravainen, H. (1986). Cognitive performance in early Parkinson's disease. *Acta Neurologica Scandinavica, 73,* 151–159.

Holborn, P. J. (1990). *Differentiating multi-infarct dementia from dementia of the Alzheimer type.* Unpublished doctoral dissertation, University of Manitoba, Winnipeg, Canada.

Huber, S. J., Freidenberg, D. O., Shuttleworth, E. C., Paulson, G. W., & Christy, J. A. (1989). Neuropsychological impairments associated with severity of Parkinson's disease. *Journal of Neuropsychiatry, 1,* 155–158.

Huber, S. J., Shuttleworth, E. C., Paulson, G. W., Bellchambers, M. J. G., & Clapp, L. E. (1986). Cortical vs. subcortical dementia. *Archives of Neurology, 43,* 392–394.

Huff, F. J., Becker, J. T., Belle, S. H., Nebes, R. D., Holland, A. L., & Boller, F. (1987). Cognitive deficits and clinical diagnosis of Alzheimer's disease. *Neurology, 37,* 1119–1124.

Huff, F. J., Corkin, S., & Growdon, J. H. (1986). Semantic impairment and anomia in Alzheimer's disease. *Brain and Language, 28,* 235–249.

Hughes, C. P., Berg, L., Danziger, W. L., Coben, L. A., & Martin, R. L. (1982). A new clinical scale for the staging of dementia. *British Journal of Psychiatry, 140,* 566–572.

Jarvik, L. F., & Winograd, C. H. (Eds.). (1988). *Treatments for the Alzheimer patient: The long haul.* New York: Springer.

Kahn, R. L., Goldfarb, A. I., Pollack, M., & Gerber, I. E. (1960). The relationship of mental and physical status in institutionalized aged persons. *American Journal of Psychiatry, 117,* 120–124.

Kahn, R. L., Zarit, S. H., Hilbert, N. M., & Niederehe, G. (1975). Memory complaint and impairment in the aged. *Archives of General Psychiatry, 32,* 1569–1573.

Kendrick, D. C. (1965). Speed and learning in the diagnosis of diffuse brain damage in elderly subjects: A Bayesian statistical approach. *British Journal of the Society for Clinical Psychology, 4,* 141–148.

Kiloh, L. G. (1961). Pseudo-dementia. *Acta Psychiatrica Scandinavica, 37,* 336–351.

Klesges, R. C. & Troster, A. I. (1987). A review of premorbid indices of intellectual and neuropsychological functioning: What have we learned in the past five years? *International Journal of Clinical Neuropsychology, 9,* 1–11.

Knopman, D. S., & Ryberg, S. (1989). A verbal memory test with high predictive accuracy for dementia of the Alzheimer type. *Archives of Neurology, 46,* 141–145.

Kopelman, M. D. (1986). Clinical tests of memory. *British Journal of Psychiatry, 148,* 517–525.

Kral, V. A., & Emery, O. B. (1989). Long-term follow-up of depressive pseudodementia of the aged. *Canadian Journal of Psychiatry, 34,* 445–446.

Kramer, J. H., Delis, D. C., Blusewicz, M. J., Brandt, J., Ober, H. A., & Strauss, M. (1988). Verbal memory errors in Alzheimer's and Huntington's dementias. *Developmental Neuropsychology, 4,* 1–15.

Kuhl, D. E., Small, G. W., Riege, W. H., Fujikawa, D. G., Metter, E. J., Benson, D. F., Ashford, J. W., Mazziotta, J. C., Maltese, A., & Dorsey, D. A. (1987). Cerebral metabolic patterns before the diagnosis of probable Alzheimer's disease. *Journal of Cerebral Blood Flow Metabolism, 7* (Suppl. 1), S-406.

La Rue, A. (1987). Methodological concerns: Longitudinal studies of dementia. *Alzheimer Disease and Associated Disorders, 1,* 180–192.

La Rue, A. (1989). Patterns of performance on the Fuld Object Memory Evaluation in elderly inpatients. *Journal of Clinical and Experimental Neuropsychology, 11,* 409–422.

La Rue, A. & Goodman, S. (1989). *Clinical correlates of impaired memory in geriatric depression.* Paper presented at a meeting of the Gerontological Society of America, Minneapolis, November, 1989.

La Rue, A., & Jarvik, L. F. (1982). Old age and biobehavioral changes. In B. Wolman (Ed.), *Handbook of developmental psychology* (pp. 791–806). New York: Prentice-Hall.

La Rue, A., D'Elia, L. F., Clark, E. O., Spar, J. E., & Jarvik, L. F. (1986a). Clinical tests of memory in dementia, depression, and healthy aging. *Psychology and Aging, 1,* 69–77.

La Rue, A., Spar, J., & Hill, C. (1986b). Cognitive impairment in late-life depression: Clinical correlates and treatment implications. *Journal of Affective Disorders, 11,* 179–184.

Larrabee, G. J., & Crook, T. H. (1989). Dimensions of everyday memory in age-associated memory impairment. *Psychological Assessment: A Journal of Consulting and Clinical Psychology, 1,* 92–97.

Less, A. J., & Smith, E. (1983). Cognitive deficits in the early stages of Parkinson's disease. *Brain, 106,* 257–270.

Leuchter, A., Spar, J. E., Walter, D. O., & Weiner, H. (1987). Electroencepthalographic spectra and coherence in the diagnosis of Alzheimer's type and multi-infarct dementia. *Archives of General Psychiatry, 44,* 993–998.

Levin, B. E. (1990). Spatial cognition in Parkinson disease. *Alzheimer Disease and Associated Disorders, 4,* 161–170.

Lezak, M. D. (1983). *Neuropsychological assessment* (2nd ed.). New York: Oxford University Press.

Liston, E. H., & La Rue, A. (1983a). Clinical differentiation of primary degenerative and multi-infarct dementia: A critical review of the evidence. Part I: Clinical studies. *Biological Psychiatry, 18,* 1451–1465.

Liston, E. H., & La Rue, A. (1983b). Clinical differentiation of primary degenerative and multi-infarct dementia: A critical review of the evidence. Part II: Pathological studies. *Biological Psychiatry, 18,* 1467–1484.

Loeb, C. (1988). Clinical criteria for diagnosis and classification of vascular and multi-infarct dementia. In J. S. Meyer, J. Marshall, H. Lechner, & J. F. Toole (Eds.), *Vascular and multi-infarct dementia* (pp. 13–22). Mount Kisco, NY: Futura.

Loewenstein, D. A., D'Elia, L., Guterman, A., Eisdorfer, C., Wilkie, F., La Rue, A., Mintzer, J., & Duara, R. (in press). The occurrence of different intrusive errors in patients with Alzheimer disease, multiple cerebral infarctions and major depression. *Brain and Cognition.*

Loewenstein, D. A., Wilkie, F., Eisdorfer, C., Guterman, A., & Berkowitz, N. (1989). An analysis of intrusive error types in Alzheimer's disease and related disorders. *Development Neuropsychology, 5,* 115–126.

Logsdon, R. G., Teri, L., Williams, D. E., Vitiello, M. V., & Prinz, P. N. (1989). The WAIS-R profile: A diagnostic tool for Alzheimer's disease? *Journal of Clinical and Experimental Neuropsychology, 11,* 892–898.

Loring, D. W., & Papanicolaou, A. C. (1987). Memory assessment in neuropsychology: Theoretical considerations and practical utility. *Journal of Clinical and Experimental Neuropsychology, 9,* 340–358.

Luria, A. (1974). *The working brain.* London: Penguin.

Luria, A. (1980). *Higher cortical functions in man* (2nd ed.). New York: Basic Books.

Marcopulos, B. A. (1989). Pseudodementia, dementia, and depression: Test differentiation. In T. Hunt & C. J. Lindley (Eds.), *Testing older adults* (pp. 70–91). Austin, TX: Pro-ed.

Martin, A., Browers, P., Cox, C., Teleska, P., Fedio, P., Foster, N. L., & Chase, T. H. (1986). Towards a behavioral typology of Alzheimer's patients. *Journal of Clinical and Experimental Neuropsychology, 8,* 594–610.

Masur, D. M., Fuld, P. A., Blau, A., Levin, H. S., & Aronson, M. K. (1989). Distinguishing normal and demented elderly with the selective reminding test. *Journal of Clinical and Experimental Neuropsychology, 11,* 615–630.

Matarazzo, J. D., & Prifitera, A. (1989). Subtest scatter and premorbid intelligence: Lessons from the WAIS-R standardization sample. *Psychological Assessment: A Journal of Consulting and Clinical Psychology, 1,* 186–191.

McAllister, T. W. (1983). Overview: Pseudodementia. *American Journal of Psychiatry, 140,* 528–533.

McCarthy, M., Ferris, S. H., Clark, E., & Crook T. (1981). Acquisition and retention of categorized material in normal aging and senile dementia. *Experimental Aging Research, 7,* 127–135.

McCue, M., Shelley, C., & Goldstein, G. (1985). A proposed short form of the Luria-Nebraska Neuropsychological Battery oriented toward assessment of the elderly. *International Journal of Clinical Neuropsychology, 7,* 96–101.

McKhann, G., Drachman, D., Folstein, M., Katzman, R., Price, D., & Stadlan, E. M. (1984). Clinical diagnosis of Alzheimer's disease: Report of the NINCDS-ADRDA Work Group. *Neurology, 34,* 939–944.

Metter, E. J. (1988). Postron tomography and cerebral blood flow studies. In M. S. Albert & M. B. Moss (Eds.), *Geriatric neuropsychology* (pp. 228–261). New York: Guilford.

Meyer, J. S., McClintic, K. L., Rogers, R. L., Sims, P., & Mortel, K. F. (1988). Aetiological considerations and risk factors for multi-infarct dementia. *Journal of Neurology, Neurosurgery, and Psychiatry, 51,* 1489–1497.

Miller, E. (1980). Cognitive assessment of the older adult. In J. E. Birren & R. B. Sloane (Eds.), *Handbook of mental health and aging* (pp. 520–536). Englewood Cliffs, NJ: Prentice-Hall.

Mirsen, T., & Hachinski, V. (1988). Epidemiology and classification of vascular and multi-infarct dementia. In

J. S. Meyer, J. Marshall, H. Lechner, & J. F. Toole (Eds.), *Vascular and multi-infarct dementia* (pp. 61–76). Mount Kisco, NY: Futura.

Mitrushina, M., & Satz, P. (in press). Test–retest reliability of WAIS-R Satz-Mogel short form in a normal elderly sample. *International Journal of Clinical Neuropsychology.*

Morrell, R. W., Park, D. C., & Poon, L. W. (1989). Quality of instructions on prescription drug labels: Effects on memory and comprehension in young and old adults. *The Gerontologist, 29,* 345–354.

Nelson, H. E., & McKenna, P. (1975). The use of current reading ability in the assessment of dementia. *British Journal of Social and Clinical Psychology, 14,* 259–267.

Niederehe, G. (1986). Depression and memory impairment in the aged. In L. W. Poon (Ed.), *Handbook for clinical memory assessment of older adults* (pp. 226–237). Washington, DC: American Psychological Association.

Niederehe, G., & Yoder, C. (1989). Metamemory perceptions in depressions of young and older adults. *Journal of Nervous and Mental Disease, 177,* 4–14.

O'Brien, M. D. (1988). Vascular dementia is underdiagnosed. *Archives of Neurology, 45,* 797–798.

Ober, B. A., Koss, E., Friedland, R. P., & Delis, D. C. (1985). Processes of verbal memory failure in Alzheimer type dementia. *Brain and Cognition, 4,* 90–103.

Parks, R. W., Crockett, D. J., Tuokko, H., Beattie, B. L., Ashford, J. W., Coburn, K. L., Zec, R. F., Becker, R. E., McGeer, P. L., & McGeer, E. G. (1989). Neuropsychological "system efficiency" and positron emission tomography. *Journal of Neuropsychiatry, 1,* 269–282.

Perez, F. I., Gay, J. R. A., Taylor, R. L., & Rivera, V. M. (1975). Patterns of memory performance in the neurologically impaired aged. *Canadian Journal of Neurological Sciences, 2,* 347–355.

Perez, F. I., Rivera, V. M., Meyer, J. S., Gay, J. R. A., Taylor, R. L., & Mathew, N. T. (1975). Analysis of intellectual and cognitive performance in patients with multi-infarct dementia, vertebrobasilar insufficiency with dementia, and Alzheimer's disease. *Journal of Neurological and Neurosurgical Psychiatry, 38,* 533–540.

Perlmutter, M., & Mitchell, D. B. (1982). The appearance and disappearance of age differences in adult memory. In F. I. M. Craik & S. Trehub (Eds.), *Aging and cognitive processes* (pp. 127–143). New York: Plenum.

Pillon, B., Dubois, B., Lhermitte, F., & Agid, Y. (1986). Heterogeneity of cognitive impairment in progressive supranuclear palsy, Parkinson's disease, and Alzheimer's disease. *Neurology, 36,* 1179–1185.

Poon, L. W. (Ed.). (1986). *Handbook for clinical memory assessment of older adults.* Washington, DC: American Psychological Association.

Popkin, S. J., Gallagher, D., Thompson, L. W., & Moore, M. (1982). Memory complaint and performance in normal and depressed older adults. *Experimental Aging Research, 8,* 141–145.

Post, F. (1966). Somatic and psychic factors in the treatment of elderly psychiatric patients. *Journal of Psychosomatic Research, 10,* 13–19.

Powell, A. L., Cummings, J. L., Hill, M. A., Benson, F. (1988). Speech and language alterations in multi-infarct dementia. *Neurology, 38,* 717–719.

Purisch, A. D., & Sbordone, R. J. (1986). The Luria-Nebraska Neuropsychological Battery. In G. Goldstein & R. E. Tarter (Eds.), *Advances in clinical neuropsychology* (pp. 291–316). New York: Plenum.

Rabins, P. V. (1983). Reversible dementia and the misdiagnosis of dementia: A review. *Hospital and Community Psychiatry, 34,* 830–835.

Rabins, P. V., Merchant, A., & Nestadt, G. (1984). Criteria for diagnosing reversible dementia caused by depression: Validation by 2-year follow-up. *British Journal of Psychiatry, 144,* 488–492.

Raskin, A. (1986). Partialing out the effects of depression and age on cognitive functions: Experimental data and methodologic issues. In L. W. Poon (Ed.), *Handbook for clinical memory assessment of older adults* (pp. 244–256). Washington, DC: American Psychological Association.

Reding, M., Haycox, J., & Blass, J. (1985). Depression in patients referred to a dementia clinic. A three-year prospective study. *Archives of Neurology, 42,* 894–896.

Reed, B. R., Jagust, W. J., & Seab, J. P. (1989). Mental status as a predictor of daily function in progressive dementia. *The Gerontologist, 29,* 804–807.

Reed, B. R., Jagust, W. J., & Seab, J. P. (1988, February). *Differences in rates of confabulatory intrusions in Alzheimer's disease and multiinfarct dementia.* Paper presented at a meeting of the International Neuropsychological Society, New Orleans, LA.

Reisberg, B., Ferris, S. H., Georgotas, A., de Leon, M. J., & Schneck, M. K. (1982). Relationship between cognition and mood in geriatric depression. *Psychopharmacology Bulletin, 18*, 191–193.

Reitan, R. M. (1955). The distribution according to age of a psychologic measure dependent upon organic brain functions. *Journal of Gerontology, 10*, 338–340.

Rey, A. (1941). L'examen psychologique dans les cas d'encephalopathie traumatique. *Archives de Psychologie, 28*, 286–340.

Rezek, D. L., Morris, J. C., Fulling, K. H., & Gado, M. H. (1987). Periventricular white-matter lucencies in senile dementia of the Alzheimer type and in normal aging. *Neurology, 37*, 1365–1368.

Riege, W. H., & Metter, E. J. (1988). Cognitive and brain imaging measures of Alzheimer's disease. *Neurobiology of Aging, 9*, 69–86.

Riege, W. H., Harker, J. O., & Metter, E. J. (1986). Clinical validators: Brain lesions and brain imaging. In L. W. Poon (Ed.), *Handbook for clinical memory assessment of older adults* (pp. 314–336). Washington, DC: American Psychological Association.

Rosen, W. G., Mohs, R. C., & Davis, K. L. (1984). A new rating scale for Alzheimer's disease. *American Journal of Psychiatry, 141*, 1356–1364.

Rosen, W. G., Terry, R. D., Fuld, P. A., Katzman, R. & Peck, A. (1980). Pathological verification of ischemic score in differentiation of dementias. *Annals of Neurology, 7*, 486–488.

Ruff, R. M., Light, R. H., & Quayhagen, M. (1988). Selective reminding tests: A normative study of verbal learning in adults. *Journal of Clinical and Experimental Neuropsychology, 11*, 539–550.

Ryan, J. J., Paolo, A. M., & Oehlert, M. E. (1989, June). Dementia screening: A tale of two tests. *VA Practitioner*, 51–54.

Satz, P., Van Gorp, W. G., Soper, H. V., & Mitrushina, M. (1987). A WAIS-R marker for dementia for the Alzheimer type? An empirical and statistical induction test. *Journal of Clinical and Experimental Neuropsychology, 9*, 767–774.

Savard, R. J., Rey, A. C., & Post, R. M. (1980). Halstead-Reitan Category Test in bipolar and unipolar affective disorders. *Journal of Nervous and Mental Disease, 168*, 297–303.

Schaie, K. W., & Schaie, J. P. (1977). Clinical assessment and aging. In J. E. Birren & K. W. Schaie (Eds.), *Handbook of the psychology of aging* (pp. 692–723). New York: Van Nostrand Reinhold.

Silberman, E. K., Weingartner, H., & Post, R. M. (1983). Thinking disorder in depression. *Archives of General Psychiatry, 40*, 775–780.

Snow, W. G., Tierney, M. C., Zorzitto, M. L., Fisher, R. H., & Reid, D. W. (1989). WAIS-R Test–retest reliability in a normal elderly sample. *Journal of Clinical and Experimental Neuropsychology, 11*, 423–428.

Storandt, M., & Hill, R. D. (1989). Very mild senile dementia of the Alzheimer type: II. Psychometric test performance. *Archives of Neurology, 46*, 383–386.

Storandt, M., Botwinick, J., Danziger, W. L., Berg, L., & Hughes, C. P. (1984). Psychometric differentiation of mild senile dementia of the Alzheimer type. *Archives of Neurology, 41*, 497–499.

Stoudemire, A., Hill, C. D., Kaplan, W., Hill, D., Morris, R., Coen-Cole, S., & Houpt, J. L. (1988). Clinical issues in the assessment of dementia and depression in the elderly. *Psychiatric Medicine, 6*, 40–49.

Sundet, K., Finset, A., & Reinvang, I. (1988). Neuropsychological predictors in stroke rehabilitation. *Journal of Clinical and Experimental Neuropsychology, 10*, 363–379.

Sweet, J. J., Moberg, P. J., & Tovian, S. M. (1990). Evaluation of Wechsler Adult Intelligence Scale—Revised premorbid IQ formulas in clinical populations. *Psychological Assessment: A Journal of Consulting and Clinical Psychology, 2*, 41–44.

Tierney, M. C., Snow, G., Reid, D. W., Zorzitto, M. L., & Fisher, R. H. (1987). Replication and extension of the findings of Storandt and co-workers. *Archives of Neurology, 44*, 720–722.

Trahan, D. E., & Larrabee, G. J. (1988). *Continuous visual memory test: Professional manual*. Odessa, FL: Psychological Assessment Resources.

Wechsler, D. (1945). A standardized memory scale for clinical use. *Journal of Psychology, 19*, 87–95.

Wechsler, D. (1981). *Wechsler Adult Intelligence Scale—Revised*. New York: The Psychological Corporation.

Wechsler, D. (1987). *Wechsler Memory Scale—Revised*. New York: The Psychological Corporation.

Weingartner, H., & Silberman, E. (1982). Models of cognitive impairment: Cognitive changes in depression. *Psychopharmacology Bulletin, 18*, 27–42.

Weingartner, H., Burns, S., Diebel, R., & Le Witt, P. A. (1984). Cognitive impairments in Parkinson's disease:

Distinguishing between effort-demanding and automatic cognitive processes. *Psychiatry Research, 11,* 223–235.

Weingartner, H., Cohen, R. M., Murphy, D. L., Martello, J., & Gerdt, C. (1981). Cognitive processes in depression. *Archives of General Psychiatry, 38,* 42–47.

Wells, C. E. (1979). Pseudodementia. *American Journal of Psychiatry, 136,* 895–900.

Western Psychological Services (1983). *Hooper Visual Organization Test (VOT) manual* (1983 ed.). Los Angeles, CA: Author.

Whitehead, A. (1973). Verbal learning and memory in elderly depressives. *British Journal of Psychiatry, 123,* 203–208.

Whitehouse, P. J. (1986). The concept of subcortical and cortical dementia: Another look. *Annals of Neurology, 19,* 1–6.

Wilson, B. A. & Moffat, N. (Eds.) (1984). *Clinical management of memory problems.* London: Croom Helm.

Wilson, B. A. (Ed.) (1987). *Rehabilitation of memory.* New York: Guilford.

Wilson, L. A., Grant, K. Witney, P. M., & Kerridge, D. F. (1973). Mental status of elderly hospital patients related to occupational therapist's assessment of activities of daily living. *Gerontologica Clinica, 15,* 197–202.

Wilson, R. S., Rosenbaum, G., Brown, G., Rourke, D., Whitman, D., & Gisell, J. (1978). An index of premorbid intelligence. *Journal of Consulting and Clinical Psychology, 46,* 1554–1555.

Winograd, C. H. (1984). Mental status tests and the capacity for self-care. *Journal of the American Geriatrics Society, 32,* 49–55.

Functional Assessment in Geriatric Mental Health

Bryan J. Kemp and Judith M. Mitchell

I. The Conceptual Basis of Functional Assessment
   A. Definitions of Function
   B. Kinds of Functional Ability
   C. Determinants of Function
   D. The Importance of a Functional Assessment
   E. The Concept of Psychiatric Rehabilitation
   F. A Hierarchical Model of Functional Assessment
II. The Effect of Mental Illness on Function
   A. Diagnosis
   B. Kind of Function
   C. Chronic versus Acute
   D. Presence of Other Problems
III. Functional Assessment Principles
   A. Purpose of Assessment
   B. Clinical versus Research Use
   C. Screening versus Assessment
   D. General versus Disorder Specific
   E. Reliability
   F. Validity
IV. Survey of Functional-Assessment Instruments
   A. Unidimensional Scales
   B. Functional Assessment of Dementia Patients
   C. Multidimensional Scales
V. Discussion and Summary
   References

I. The Conceptual Basis of Functional Assessment _____

Thorough assessment of an older person with a psychiatric problem is a necessary starting point of treatment. In fact, proper and thorough assessment constitutes the basis for any rational, systematic, and effective treatment program. But, assessment of what? A human being is a complex biological, psychological and social animal; the array of things that could be assessed is almost limitless. The answer to the question of what to assess is determined by the purposes of the assessment.

In geriatric mental health, any assessment is done for one or more of the following reasons: (1) to establish a diagnosis; (2) to determine the personal, social, and environmental dynamics that maintain, control and influence the behavior; (3) to establish a baseline measure from which to assess the effects of treatment or natural changes in one disorder; and (4) to assess the person's ability to look after himself or herself and to function in various environments. The latter purpose is the main topic of this chapter: namely, to review and discuss the rationale and methods of functional assessment of older persons with psychiatric problems.

A. Definitions of Function

Historically, the concept of function in psychiatry has had three distinct meanings. First that of a nonorganic cause of psychiatric disturbance. In the early history of modern psychiatry, an important breakthrough was to discover and demonstrate that psychiatric disorder could and did have a cause outside a purely organic–biological basis (Alexander & Selanick, 1966). Freud, trained as a neurologist, recognized the role of unconscious, wish-fulfilling, and ego-defensive mechanisms as a cause of psychiatric illness. The suspected source of functional psychiatric disorders varies from theorist to theorist, but each recognizes that functional, i.e., purposeful, albeit maladaptive, psychological processes can underlie psychiatric disorder. This opened avenues of investigation and clinical interventions in addition to biological treatment. This approach stresses the question, "What is the function of this symptom?"

The second idea of function is the approach based largely upon learning theory. This approach to psychiatric disorders is based upon principles such as reinforcement, stimulus control, shaping, and modeling. This approach stresses specific behaviors ranging from verbal self-descriptions to social interaction. In this approach, the diagnosis of the patient is largely irrelevant. The focus of analysis and treatment is on discrete behaviors and the environmental (as opposed to internal) factors that control and regulate the behavior. This approach stresses the question, "What environmental variables function to maintain and alter this behavior?"

The third definition of function examines what people are capable of doing in their own environment, that is, the factors that allow the person to function with the most independence and in the least restrictive environment possible. Function in this sense, and in this chapter, refers to a set of performance capabilities that allow the person to look after himself or herself and to survive in the community.

B. Kinds of Functional Ability

In this chapter, functional assessment will focus primarily on areas that have come to be known as activities of daily living (ADLs) and instrumental activities of daily living

(IADLs). In addition, it will touch upon the physiological substrates of functional performance, skilled performance, and social-role performance. For a discussion of other functional assessment domains, the reader should see Lawton (1986) or Patterson (1990).

ADLs are generally divided into seven tasks:

1. eating;
2. dressing;
3. grooming;
4. toileting;
5. bathing;
6. transferring; and
7. mobility.

These seven abilities constitute the skills of self-maintenance or those needed to care for one's body within a limited space, such as at home. Disruptions of these abilities represent major risks to independent living at home for the older person (Fulton & Katz, 1986; Patterson, 1990; Rogers, 1990). Dysfunction of ADL abilities places a large burden for caregiving on the formal (e.g., organized and funded) and informal care systems, (e.g., the family) (Brody, 1985). Assessment of these functional abilities is paramount to any comprehensive and independence-oriented geriatric mental health care program.

IADLs refers to the skills and behaviors needed to survive in the community. Lawton and Brody (1969) originally coined this exact term for these abilities, and the term is now widely used in health care programs, although other terms, such as community skills and independent-living skills have been used. IADL skills have the following components:

1. money management;
2. household chores;
3. use of transportation;
4. shopping;
5. health maintenance;
6. communication; and
7. safety preparedness.

People who cannot perform IADLs may be able to live at home alone if they can perform ADLs, but they need outside assistance or supervision. Patterns of dysfunction on ADLs and IADLs often relate to underlying disorders. For example, people with dementia lose the ability to perform IADLs before they lose the ability to perform ADLs, largely because IADLs require more cognitive skill, and ADLs require more physical skills. People with severe depression may simultaneously lose the ability (or, more correctly, the desire) to perform either ADLs or IADLs.

Social-role performance is still another area of functional ability. This area consists of highly skilled performance and interpersonal functioning. Factors in this area include (but are not limited to) the following:

• job performance
• friendships

- intimacy
- parenthood/grandparenthood
- recreation
- helping others

At the other end of the continuum of functional abilities lie the physiological substrates necessary for basic ADL performance. These include the following:

- endurance
- strength
- range of motion (flexibility)
- coordination.

Without these abilities, very little of a physical nature can be done. Different ADL skills require different degrees of each of these components. For example, bathing is heavily dependent upon strength, while eating requires range of motion in the upper extremities.

Skilled performance is yet another area of function, lying between IADLs and social-role performance in terms of complexity and level of skill. These skills involve intellectual, motor, and personality skills.

C. Determinants of Function

All functioning, from being able to dress oneself to performing a job, has multiple determinants. These determinants are generally divided into biological, psychosocial, and environmental components. The relationship among these components are described in Figure 1. As can be seen, functioning is a product of the interaction of all of these

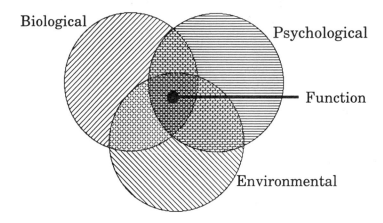

Figure 1 Functional abilities are a product of biological, psychological, and environmental factors.

components. No aspect of functioning is attributable to only one component. Biological factors include the presence of illnesses, sufficient strength, endurance, speed of behavior, range of motion, and ability to move. Psychosocial factors include desire to perform the activity, a reason for doing it, knowledge of how to do it, and help or support from others. Environmental factors can facilitate or impede functioning. For example, stairs would prevent a person who has limited mobility from leaving the home, whereas a ramp might facilitate leaving the home and doing things in the community. Since environmental factors can play such a big role in the functioning of older persons, it is important to make sure that assessments are conducted under the most favorable of environmental conditions and that the older person's home environment is carefully assessed.

This perspective also leads to the practical position that impairment in functioning requires that all of the potential biological, psychosocial and environmental factors be examined.

Psychiatric disorders can and do affect social-role performance, skilled-performance IADLs, and ADLs, and eventually even the physiological substrates of performance. Symptoms of all psychiatric disorders fall into affective, cognitive, physiological, and behavioral categories. If the disorder is severe enough, all areas are affected, regardless of the nature of the disorder. Since functional performance, both skilled and nonskilled, has biological, psychosocial, and environmental components, psychiatric disorders cause tremendous functional impairments as well as specific symptomatology.

D. The Importance of a Functional Assessment

Assessment of function plays an important role in psychiatric care of the older persons for three distinct reasons. First, assessment of function is a part of any psychiatric diagnosis. The Diagnostic and Statistical Manual (DSM) III-R (American Psychiatric Association, 1987) as well as most texts on psychiatric diagnosis stress the need to determine whether and how much the functional abilities of the older (or younger) person are affected before making a diagnosis. For example, in order to meet a diagnostic criterion for dementia, a person must have at least three characteristics: (1) a decrement in memory, (2) a decrement in at least one other area of cognition, and (3) a decrement in personal, social, or vocational functioning. Without the functional component, the person doesn't meet criteria. He or she may have no disorder at all or may have a different disorder. Similarly, a diagnosis of depression is not made until a person shows (1) an altered mood, (2) other symptoms of depression (sleep, lowered self-esteem, thinking disturbance, etc.), and (3) decrements in functioning of a personal, social, or vocational nature. Thus it is recognized that assessment of function is necessary to establish diagnosis.

Secondly, it is important to assess function because diagnosis alone does not predict outcome or the ability to live independently. This is a critical point in both the psychiatric literature as reviewed by Anthony and Liberman (1986), Liberman and Foy (1983), and Hursh and Anthony (1983), and in medical literature as reviewed by Granger (1984), Katz, Ford, Maskowitz, Jackson, and Jaffe (1963), and Brummel-Smith (1990). Knowledge of the patient's diagnosis (either psychiatric or physical) predicts symptomatology but does not predict performance, daily functioning, or ultimate outcome in terms of living situation, work capacity or even relapse.

Therefore, whatever goes into assessment, a functional assessment needs to be done to determine what the person can and cannot do. Knowledge of the person's condition (diagnosis) tells little about how that person can perform. Two people with the same diagnosis (e.g., dementia) can perform quite differently. Two people with different diagnoses may perform quite the same. Since treatment is aimed at *both* ameliorating the distress symptoms of psychiatric disorder *and* improving function, and since diagnosis is unrelated to functional performance, it follows that a separate and thorough assessment of function must occur and must be followed by treatment to improve it.

The third reason a functional assessment is important in geriatric psychiatry is to help support and educate others as to the person's/patient's performance capacities and support needs. Family members provide over 80% of the day-to-day care of older persons (Brody, 1985). Providing only a diagnosis is of limited value in terms of understanding what the family will need to help the older individual. Also, the psychiatric disorder itself appears to play a lesser role in the stress and burden of caregivers than the need for help with functional activities and behavioral disturbances. In dementia research, for example, the cognitive impairment is less a factor in measured family burden than are the behavioral deficiencies and excesses (Teri, Boorsun, Kiyak, & Yamagishi, 1989; Zarit & Zarit, 1984). Similarly, professional staff need to know the patient's performance capabilities in order to avoid excessive pessimism about treating patients with dementia (Dawson, Kline, Wiancko, & Wells, 1986) and thereby overrestricting individuals.

E. The Concept of Psychiatric Rehabilitation

Several models relating psychiatric illness to functional ability and to treatment have been proposed. Liberman and Evans (1985), and Anthony, Cohen, and Cohen, (1983) propose a psychiatric rehabilitation concept. This model states that (1) the functional consequences of severe or chronic psychiatric illness cannot be predicted by diagnosis; (2) amelioration or reduction of psychiatric symptoms does not correlate with improvements in functional status; (3) functional abilities are largely learned skills and require specific programs of treatment geared toward relearning of impaired skills over and above primary psychiatric intervention; and (4) functional assessment is an essential part of psychiatric care for older persons.

A number of general principles of assessment can be derived from the rehabilitation viewpoint.

1. A functional assessment should be a part of any comprehensive psychiatric assessment of an older person.
2. The content of the functional assessment should be guided by the purpose of the assessment, the nature of the disorder, and the chronicity of the problems.
3. Social role, IADLs, ADLs, and physiological substrates of performance encompass the range of functional abilities.
4. Changes in performance across these levels of function measure severity of the disorder and the degree of support the older person needs.
5. Improvements in functional ability through treatment programs are the best indicator of treatment success.

F. A Hierarchical Model of Functional Assessment

An examination of the relationship among various kinds of functional abilities may help illustrate the factors that are involved in each, as well as their underlying requirements. The relationship among different kinds of functional abilities can be described in many ways. Lawton (1986) took a similar view in diagraming the relationship between levels of *behavioral competence* and well-being among older persons. Spector, Katz, Murphy, and Fulton (1987) also used a hierarchical model in studies of community-dwelling older persons.

Each level of functional ability requires, in varying proportions, certain physical, psychological, and social skills. As the demands for performance change from daily-survival types of ability to social interaction, the proportion of each of these factors likewise changes. However, even social performance has inherent physical capacities that must be satisfied; therefore, no level of functional ability is completely devoid of combined physical, psychological, and social components.

As can be seen from Figure 2, when the level of functional ability increases from the more physically determined to the more socially determined, the kinds of performance change. The prerequisite abilities increase to encompass those at a lower level, and new skills and attributes at successive new levels are added. Assessment of functional abilities can include physical substrates, ADLs, IADLs, skilled performance, and social roles, depending on the particular needs of the clinician or investigator. Assessments may be made either by clinical observation or by formal assessment. Health care specialists may be called on to make an assessment. A physical therapist may assess physical substrates and ADLs; an occupational therapist may assess ADLs and IADLs; and a social worker or other professional may assess IADLs and social roles.

1. Physical Substrates

The area of physical substrates has been reviewed very well by Jones (1984). Various measures are available for assessing endurance, range of motion, strength, and coordination. In and of themselves most psychiatric disorders do not affect these factors. However, these abilities are highly subject to deterioration due to disuse, hospitalization, or bed rest (Corcoran, 1981). Depression probably affects these physiological parameters most due to its impact on motivation, desire, and perseverance. Decrements in these substrates put further strain on organ-system integrity. This may help to account for high rates of subsequent, as well as concurrent medical illnesses in older persons with psychiatric disorders (e.g., Cohen, 1989).

2. ADLs

Rogers (1990) has recently reviewed the literature on ADLs in geriatric rehabilitation. Manton (1988) has related adequacy of ADLs performance to the ability to live independently in the community. The loss of ability to perform any four of the seven basic ADLs dramatically increases the risks of institutionalization and death. Psychiatric disorders can and do directly affect ADL performance. Depressive disorders, anxiety disorders, cognitive impairment, substance abuse, and psychotic disorders all are likely to cause ADL impairment. Depression may affect all ADLs; dementia affects the subtle aspects of ADL performance, such as forgetting the social context, and standards for eating or toileting.

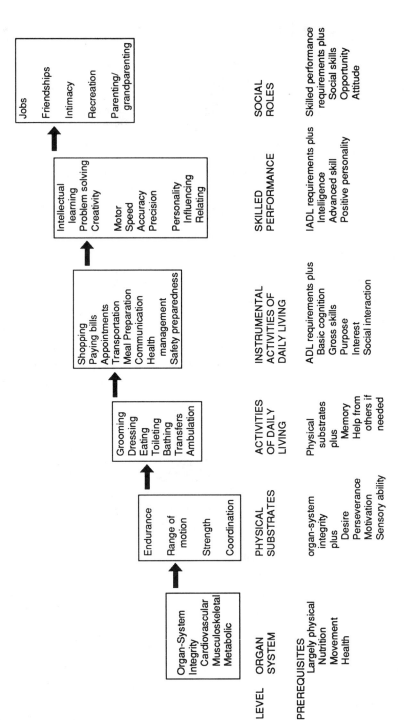

Figure 2 A hierarchical model of functional abilities.

3. IADLs

Lawton and Brody (1969) coined this term to apply to community functioning. In order to be performed independently, these skills require the abilities from previous levels and more cognition, especially judgment, and some ability to interact with others. This level of ability is easily disrupted by psychiatric and/or neurological impairments. Dementia, by the time it is diagnosed, almost always causes decrements in IADLs, though not yet severely affecting ADLs. Usually, people who cannot perform IADLs are not at high risk of institutionalization as long as there is sufficient formal or informal support to supplement the person's inability (Brody, 1985).

4. Skilled Performance

This level of ability includes driving, operating equipment, solving new everyday problems, relating well to others, learning new tasks and procedures, and high levels of expression. These abilities require advanced intellectual skill, positive personality attributes, and intact motor skills. Abilities at this level are disrupted by psychiatric disorders and show up early in the progress of the disorder. A person with the beginnings of dementia may become lost while driving or change personality before losing the ability to shop.

5. Social Roles

These are the most complex and demanding of functional abilities and therefore the most susceptible to psychiatric illness. The ability to relate to friends and others in a sensitive, rational, and mature manner, the ability to perform most paid jobs, and the ability to maintain an intimate relationship are disrupted by even mild forms of most psychiatric disorders that affect older persons, including mood disorders, substance abuse, anxiety disorders, cognitive impairment, and psychoses (Patterson *et al.*, 1982; Patterson, 1990). Instruments to assess social-role performance have been difficult to establish (Lawton, 1986) owing to the multiple behavioral areas that could be assessed and the complexity of distinguishing performance from capacity and from opportunity for social interaction with older persons. As Figure 2 implies, impairment of social-role performance may be followed by disruption of skilled performance, IADLs, ADLs, etc., as the disorder worsens.

II. The Effect of Mental Illness on Function ⎯⎯⎯⎯⎯⎯⎯⎯⎯⎯⎯⎯

Mental illnesses affect function in the reverse order of their complexity, i.e., from social roles to physiological substrates as the condition worsens. Several variables affect the relationship between mental illness and functional performance. These include (1) the specific underlying disorder; (2) the kind of function under consideration; (3) the chronicity of the psychiatric disorder; and (4) the presence of other, coexisting, problems. These issues should be kept in mind when deciding what functional measures to assess.

A. Diagnosis

Not all psychiatric disorders affect functioning in the same way or to the same extent. Very few data actually compare this effect. However, from different studies one can see that dementing illnesses cause a great deal of functional impairment, first at the highest level and then progressively impairing lower levels (Chui & Smith, 1990; Warren *et al.*, 1989; Wilson, Grant, Witney, & Kerrige, 1973; Winograd, 1986). Bipolar and psychotic disturbances are correlated with substantial functional loss (Dion, Tohen, Anthony, & Waternavx, 1988; Klein & Phillip, 1980; Ross, Kedward, & Henry, 1978). Depressive disorders other than bipolar disorders cause relatively lesser functional decrements, everything else considered (Berkman, *et al.*, 1986). This difference seems to imply a severity difference among disorders, at least as far as daily functioning is involved, the disorders with more cognitive involvement causing the greatest functional impairment.

B. Kind of Function

The nature of the function assessed influences the relationship between psychiatric disorder and performance. Using the gradient of social role, skilled performance, IADLs, ADLs, and physiological substrates of performance as a rough scale, it appears that the "higher" or more skilled the activity, the more easily it is disrupted. Thus job performance is affected by nearly all psychiatric disorders to some extent, as is social interaction, but ADLs are impaired more often by advanced dementing illnesses and long-standing psychotic disorders (Patterson, 1990). Depressive disorders affect ADLs more by lack of interest and motivation than by inability to perform them (e.g., Blazer, 1982).

C. Chronic versus Acute

One of the most important determinants of functional disruption is duration of the problem. People affected by the acute onset of a psychiatric disorder may sustain temporary and/or minor disruptions to their daily living abilities. If properly treated, they usually can return to their previous activities as their symptoms are controlled without additional services. However, as the duration of the psychiatric disorder continues, especially past 2 years, and becomes chronic, the person's ability to function may not spontaneously return, even if symptoms are controlled. This appears to be independent of the symptoms themselves (Liberman & Evans, 1985; Anthony & Liberman, 1986) and is attributable to loss of skill, the development of negative self-attitudes, institutionalization, and low social support. Older individuals with early-life psychiatric disorder, a growing population in the United States, have the greatest degree of functional disability (Patterson, 1990).

D. Presence of Other Problems

As individuals age, the likelihood of their having *only* a psychiatric disorder decreases (Cohen, 1989). The presence of other coexisting problems increases, especially medical illnesses. Older persons are often undercounted in terms of mental health problems because their psychiatric disorders are seen as medically related (Blazer & Williams, 1980; Spitzer *et al.*, 1978). Thus the prevalence of psychiatric disorder may be underrepresented in late life. When medical and psychiatric disorders coexist, a common occurrence in late life, there is a much greater impact on functioning than with either separately (Berkman *et al.*, 1986). For research purposes, controlling for these other conditions is essential. Vital data as to the nature and consequences of these dual diagnoses in mental health problems are often overlooked.

III. Functional Assessment Principles

A number of principles guide the selection of assessment procedures and specific tools or methods.

A. Purpose of Assessment

Functional assessment instruments serve several major purposes. From the clinical perspective, assessment assists in diagnosis, planning for therapy, and assuring appropriate use of services. It operates as a useful tool in supplementing the medical history and physical exam by the physician. In rehabilitation settings, periodic assessment provides monitoring of improvement or deterioration. Geriatric assessment programs rely upon formal assessment to provide measurable and objective information in the domains of physical health, psychological health, functional ability, and social parameters. This information is a valuable adjunct when a medical team needs to make decisions regarding community or institutional placement and use of available community-support services. In research, formal functional assessment is used for epidemiological studies, exploring group differences, and following standardized change scores over time. Clinical scales often need to be shorter to fit the patient's capabilities. Research scales are more concerned with reliability issues and other technical parameters.

B. Clinical versus Research Use

Functional assessment instruments can be used for a variety of purposes including clinical assessment, research studies, program evaluation and policy decisions. Practitioners and researchers/evaluators have different needs and may use existing instruments in different ways. Kane and Kane (1981) provide an in-depth list of clinical and research needs in the functional-assessment field.

The primary clinical usefulness of an instrument is its ability to determine a patient's present functional status and reflect subsequent change over time. Instruments chosen need to provide useful information for diagnosis, treatment plans, and discharge status. Issues when choosing a clinical measure are ease of scoring and interpretation of results, ease of administration, and relevance of the content measured to clinical focus and decision making. A major concern is the user-friendliness of the scale for both the medical personnel and the patient. Scales that are long, complicated, or confusing are not appropriate for clinical settings. Multidimensional scales, while providing a rich amount of information, will probably require staff training. Applegate (1987) recommends using several short scales to measure different aspects of functioning, rather than one long multidimensional scale. High levels of inter-rater reliability become crucial when a chosen instrument will be used by many different staff members. An important concern for the physician and rehabilitation staff is a scale's capability to detect small increments of change over time. The scoring systems of many formal functional instruments are not sensitive enough to detect these small changes, even though the patient achieved a great deal of improvement in function.

Use of assessment instruments in research and program evaluation emphasizes objective data-collection procedures, a consistent approach to each patient, and minimal use of subjective judgement when scoring the items. The purpose of research is comparison of population differences in assessment scores or longitudinal studies of population changes over time. Assessment scales appropriate for research require psychometric properties of adequate validity and reliability, clear definition of the construct being measured, and production of a final score that can be compared to existing norms.

C. Screening versus Assessment

Screening is a preliminary assessment based upon quick and often observational measures, and is used to identify people who need a more thorough assessment. In clinical settings, screening procedures are used for case finding and to determine eligibility for services. Screening devices need to be very sensitive or allow cutoff criteria for identifying cases. In clinical practice, it is important not to overlook individuals who may have a problem, even if later assessment eventually indicates a false alarm. Formal assessment is a lengthier process, done with an identified at-risk patient to help make a diagnosis, to map out the full range of deficits, and to monitor progress. Assessment implies a more in-depth set of items that will thoroughly identify the type and severity of functional problems (Kane & Kane, 1981).

Screening is appropriate for use in office settings and with suspected high-risk populations, such as persons coming to a hospital clinic. Some elderly adults may ignore symptoms of functional decline or not volunteer this information to the physician. Quick screening for any loss of function by the physician will help target overlooked problems early (Pace, 1989). At-risk populations for functional decline can also include those who are recently bereaved, socially isolated, or suffering mild cognitive impairment (Kennie, 1984).

Scales best suited for screening are inexpensive, quick to administer, and easy to score and interpret. Functional scales used for screening include the five-item ADL subscale on the Older American Resources and Services Scale (OARS), the PULSES, (see p. 689, for explanation), and a five-item IADL tool developed by Fillenbaum (1985). Instruments more appropriate for assessment are multidimensional scales, ADL scales that require observation of performance such as the Performance Test of ADL (PADL), and scales that require professional judgement in scoring of the items.

D. General versus Disorder Specific

The majority of functional-assessment instruments were designed to be used across a variety of disorders. They tend to be broad, eclectic, and not fundamentally disorder specific in their focus. Since older adults are more likely to present with several illnesses and chronic disorders, a general and broad functional approach has proven to be of better utility than a disorder-specific focus. However, some disorders require special consideration.

Dementia patients suffer from cognitive and behavioral impairments, thereby making a self-report functional assessment more difficult. Assessment of these patients must rely on informant or caregiver reports, or an observation of performance. When direct observation is done, an instrument designed for that purpose is used. If the intent is to relate cognitive functioning with daily functioning, many clinicians prefer to use one instrument that includes both. The most widely used instrument for this purpose is the Blessed-Roth Dementia Scale, which combines functional assessment items with memory items that influence IADLs.

A few scales have been developed with a specific disorder in mind. The Barthel Index was developed and normed on stroke patients, and is most often used in stroke-rehabilitation settings. The Range of Motion Scale was developed for patients with rheumatoid arthritis and measures the motions in different joints rather than capacity to perform ADLs.

E. Reliability

Reliability is the degree to which an instrument's scores are consistent over time, reproducible, and free from errors of measurement. The problem in using a scale with no demonstrated reliability is that scale scores may fluctuate unpredictably or represent measurement error. Three different methods of testing reliability exist—internal consistency, test—retest reliability, and inter-rater reliability. Internal consistency measures whether the instrument items hold together as one scale and represent one construct. Scales lacking internal consistency will produce scattered results that lack interpretation. Test–retest reliability looks at an instrument's stability over time and whether it produces similar scores in the absence of any actual change. Functional-assessment instruments used to monitor increments of change in improvement or deterioration must demonstrate good test–retest reliability for actual change to be accurately assessed. Inter-rater reliability tests whether a scale produces the same results when used by different clinicians. This type of reliability is particularly important in clinical settings where different medical personnel may use the instruments. Inter-rater reliability is improved with staff training and standardized procedures.

F. Validity

Validity is the degree to which an instrument truly reflects the construct it is intended to measure. Four major types of validity exist: face, concurrent, predictive, and construct.

Face validity exists when the items in the scale appear to measure the identified construct and cover the appropriate content. Face validity of most functional assessment scales is high, since there is general agreement about what items constitute relevant ADLs and IADLs.

Concurrent validity determines the effectiveness of a scale by comparing the results against existing and alternate criteria. In functional assessment, new instruments are typically compared to clinician assessments, or correlated with results from older and more established scales.

Predictive validity explores whether scales are capable of predicting expected outcomes or ongoing progress as defined by the construct, and accurately identifying and classifying groups of people.

Construct validity is concerned with the construct being tested by the instrument. In order to accurately measure a construct, the scale should be embedded in a conceptual framework that emphasizes what characteristics significantly represent that construct. The construct guides the development of the test items and suggests what types of relationships should exist between test results and other clinical variables. When choosing an instrument, a clinician needs to be aware of the actual construct measured by the scale and to evaluate whether this is also the construct intended by the clinician.

Lastly, instruments used for diagnostic purposes should provide information on the sensitivity or specificity of the scale. Sensitivity is the scale's capability to accurately classify patients with a characteristic, and specificity is the scale's capability to accurately classify patients without a characteristic.

IV. Survey of Functional-Assessment Instruments

This section provides an overview of many of the frequently used instruments as well as some recently developed instruments that show promise. The section is divided into unidimensional scales, scales especially developed for cognitive impairment, and multidimensional scales. Table I provides an outline that can be used as a quick reference on scale content, clinical and research use, and reliability and validity for each of the scales. Other surveys of functional assessment scales can be found in Kane and Kane (1981), Branch and Meyers (1987), and Law and Letts (1989).

Table I

Characteristics of Selected Measures of Functional Assessment[a]

Scale	Functional content		Psychosocial content	Clinical use	Research use	Reliability	Validity
Katz ADL Index (Katz *et al.*, 1963)	Bathing Feeding Transfer	Continence Toileting Feeding		Institutions Rehabilitation Psychiatric	Epidemiological studies General research studies	Simultaneous observations, differences in fewer than 1 of 20	Correlates with mobility & home confinement after discharge
Pulses (Granger & Greer, 1976)	Physical condition Self-care Mobility Sensory Excretory		Mental & emotional status	Hospital settings	Rehab outcomes	Not reported	Correlates with Barthel & patient outcomes
Barthel Index (Mahoney & Barthel, 1965)	Feeding Grooming Toilet Transfers	Ambulation Continence Bathing Use of Stairs		Rehabilitation Stroke patients	Rehab outcomes	Not reported	Correlates with clinical judgement scores, predicts mortality
Kenny Self-Care Evaluation (Schoening & Iverson, 1968)	Transfers Dressing Hygiene	Locomotion Feeding Continence		Rehabilitation Community settings	Rehab outcomes	Not reported	Face & content validity
Rapid Disability Rating Scale (Linn & Linn, 1982)	Eating Walking Mobility Bathing Dressing	Toileting Grooming Adaptive tasks	Mental confusion Depression Cooperation	Hospital settings	Program evaluation	Inter-rater, .91	Correlates with physician prognosis, number of previous hospitalizations, 6-month mortality

(*continued*)

Table I (*Continued*)

Scale	Functional content	Psychosocial content	Clinical use	Research use	Reliability	Validity
Health Assessment Scale (Fries *et al.*, 1980)	Dressing Arising Eating Mobility Hygiene Reach Grip Outside activities Sex activities		Arthritis patients	None mentioned	Test–retest, .85	Compared self-report with actual performance
PADL (Kuriansky *et al.*, 1976)	16 items related to: Eating Grooming Dressing Telephone Ambulation		Community settings Hospital settings Psychiatric patients	None mentioned	Inter-rater, .90	Predictive validity with mortality
PSMS (Lawton & Brody, 1969; Lawton, 1972)	Toilet Bathing Dressing Feeding Grooming Ambulation		Community settings Hospital settings Psychiatric patients	General research	Inter-rater: Nurse, .87 Research, .91	Correlates with clinician judgement & other rating scales
IADL (Lawton & Brody, 1969; Lawton, 1972)	Telephone Shopping Food prep Housekeeping Laundry Transportation Medication Finances		Community settings Hospital settings Psychiatric patients	General research	Inter-rater, .85	
Blessed-Roth Dementia Rating Scale (Blessed *et al.*, 1968)	Performance of everyday activities Eating Dressing Continence	Changes in personality	Patients with dementia	General research	Not reported	Correlates with mental function & measures of post-mortem neuropathological & neurochemical findings

(*continued*)

Table I (*Continued*)

Scale	Functional content		Psychosocial content	Clinical use	Research use	Reliability	Validity
Direct Assess of Functional Status (Loewenstein et al., 1989)	Time orientation Communication Transportation Financial skills	Shopping Eating Dressing Grooming		Patients with dementia	None mentioned	Test–retest, .87–.92	Correlates with Blessed dementia scale
Functional Activities Questionnaire (Pfeffer et al., 1982)	10 items related to: Finances Shopping Cooking	Memory and attention Travel		Community settings Patients with dementia	None mentioned	Inter-rater .80–.97	Correlates with IADL Scale. Predictive of neurological ratings & cognitive scores
OARS (George & Fillenbaum, 1985; Fillenbaum & Smyer, 1981)	Dressing Feeding Grooming Walking Transfers Continence Medication	Telephone Travel Shopping Cooking Housework Finances	Social contacts, loneliness, availability and source of help	Community Psychiatric Institutions	Epidemiological studies Community-based research	Inter-rater, per subscale ADL, .86 Social, .82	Correlates with clinical ratings by medical personnel, distinguishes between community, clinic & institutional patients
Functional Assessment Inventory (Cairl et al., 1983)	Shortened version of OARS		Shortened version of OARS	Community Psychiatric Institutions	Community-based research	Test–retest, .71	Correlates with the full OARS; distinguishes between 4 groups of placement sites for older adults
MAI (Lawton et al., 1982)	Uses PSMS and IADL Scales		Leisure activities, social interaction	Community Setting Residential homes	Epidemiological studies	Internal consistency "usable" test–retest is high	Correlates with different residential populations

(*continued*)

687

Table I (*Continued*)

Scale	Functional content	Psychosocial content	Clinical use	Research use	Reliability	Validity
CARE (Gurland *et al.*, 1977)	Basic ADLs & IADLs	Social issues of isolation, background, activities and problems	Community settings	Longitudinal research General research	Inter-rater per subscale: Psychiatric, .88–.92 ADL, .48–.61 Social, .72–.79	Several studies validating subscales, correlates with medical personnel, predictive of mortality after 1 yr.

[a]Information derived in part from Kane and Kane (1981); Branch and Meyers (1987); Law and Letts (1989); Israel, Kozarevic, and Sartorius (1984).

A. Unidimensional Scales

1. Katz Index of ADL

The Katz Index (Katz *et al.*, 1963) is one of the more well-known, widely used and carefully studied of the ADL instruments (Kane & Kane, 1981). It has been used as a prototype and guide for many of the scales developed after it. The Index evaluates individuals on a three point level of independence–dependence for six ADL areas and produces a final rank ordered score representing the combined independent/dependent pattern for all the ADLs. Branch *et al.* (1984) modified the Index by including ambulation and personal grooming.

2. PULSES

The PULSES, developed by Moskowitz, Vernon, and McCann (1957) and modified by Granger and Greer (1976), was modeled after a systemic functional classification developed by the Canadian army. The name PULSES is an acronym with each letter referring to a different area of assessment (P = physical condition; U = upper extremities/self care; L = lower extremities/mobility; S = sensory perception; E = excretory functions; S = mental and emotional state). The instrument operates as a global screening tool rather than a detailed assessment instrument. The physician identifies the degree to which the patient has abnormalities (i.e., none, minor, moderate, or severe) in each of the six domains using information from the physical examination and medical history. This information provides a brief profile of patient functioning (or the lack thereof) in these six areas and can quickly highlight areas of functional limitations. However, minimal information on the specificity of limitations is given. Validity studies of the PULSES have been done with stroke patients (Granger & Greer, 1976).

3. Barthel Index and Barthel Self-Care Ratings

The Barthel Index is one of the more well-developed scales with acceptable reliability and validity testing (Mahoney & Barthel, 1965). The scale produces a score for each of the eight ADL areas, with weighted score values ranging from 0 to 15 and indicating different levels of independence. The modified Barthel, called the Barthel Self-Care Ratings (Sherwood, Morris, Morr, & Gutkin, 1977) increased the number of items to 15 and divided the items into two components of self-care (representing ADLs) and mobility. Items are scored on a four-point scale from intact, limited, helper required, and null. The Barthel, along with the Kenny scale, is one of the more sensitive scales used to monitor change among stroke-rehabilitation inpatients (Donaldson, Wagner, & Gresham, 1973). It has been used to predict gain through rehabilitation and discharge placement for stroke patients.

4. Kenny Self-Care Evaluation

This scale (Schoening & Iverson, 1968) was designed to measure self-care in the home or other similar environments. It measures 17 specific activities in six ADL categories on a five-point scale from 0 (complete dependence) to 4 (complete independence). This scale has been used to identify different learning curves in functional rehabilitation for right versus left hemiplegic patients (Schoening & Iverson, 1968). According to the authors, the learning curves can be used to predict expected learning patterns of different stroke patients as well as the time required to learn certain functional skills.

5. Rapid Disability Rating Scale (RDRS)

This scale (Linn & Linn, 1982) was developed for older chronically ill patients in nursing homes or hospital settings. The scale has 18 items in three categories: ADLs, Degree of Disability, and Degree of Special Problems. The ADL category includes basic ADLS and one item on adaptive tasks, which refers to all components of IADLs. The Degree-of-Disability category addresses communication, hearing, sight, diet, in bed during the day, continence, and medication. The category on special problems has three global items of mental confusion, uncooperativeness, and depression. The adaptive tasks and degree of specific problems are global categories and are to be used for screening purposes only.

6. Health Assessment Questionnaire

The Health Assessment Questionnaire (Fries, Spitz, Kraines, & Holman, 1980) was developed as a disability-outcome scale, particularly for patients with rheumatoid arthritis. This scale assesses general ADL tasks in five areas, and additional tasks of reach, grip, outside activity, and sexual activities. Reach and grip are not typically found in ADL scales, but are included in this scale because they represent the physiological substrates likely to be affected by arthritis and thereby also affecting ADL performance. Each category is made up of one to three items representing functional capability in that category for a total of 19 items. This is a recently developed scale and requires more testing in reliability and validity.

7. Performance Test of Activities of Daily Living (PADL)

The PADL (Kuriansky & Gurland, 1976) is a structured performance test of ADLs based on actual observation of a patient's performance. It is specifically designed to be used with geriatric psychiatric patients. The patient is asked to demonstrate his or her ability to perform 16 detailed tasks that measure basic ADL functions. Scale scores have been found to correlate with patient physical health, mental status, and prediction of mortality 3 months after hospitalization (Kuriansky & Gurland, 1976). The PADL appears to be a better predictor of patient functional status than either patient or informant self-report (Kuriansky, Gurland & Fleiss, 1976). When assessing psychiatric geriatric patients, using a performance scale is particularly helpful, since affective states can easily influence self-report and accurate recall of ADL and IADL activities. Additionally, observing a patient's performance and reaction to various tasks can provide the assessor with information on how the patient's mental status is affecting his or her ADL activity.

8. Physical Self-Maintenance Scale (PSMS) and Instrumental Activities of Daily Living (IADL)

Lawton and Brody (1969) have developed two scales that measure ADLs and IADLs among community and hospitalized older adults. While both scales use a dichotomous scoring system, items for each category are designed in a Guttman format with each item representing a higher level of independent functioning than those below it. The PSMS is an ADL scale similar to the Katz Index and measures the six basic ADL functions. Each function is assessed by five items representing increasing independence. The IADL measures self-report performance with five items per category in the areas of telephone use, food preparation, housekeeping, laundry, mode of transportation, handling medications, and handling finances. Scores on the IADL are higher for women than for men, because the tasks measured overemphasize skills typically performed by women (Lawton, 1972).

B. Functional Assessment of Dementia Patients

The three scales listed below were designed to measure ADL and IADL status for patients with cognitive impairments, in particular Alzheimer's disease and other forms of dementia. To accurately determine the functional capacity of patients with dementia, these scales include items on memory tasks relevant to various IADLs, and rely heavily on information from a caregiver, relative, or other informant in close and continual contact with the patient. The scales are best interpreted when used in conjunction with measures of cognitive status that assess long-term and recent memory, concentration, and attention.

1. Blessed-Roth Dementia Rating Scale

The Blessed-Roth Dementia Rating Scale (Blessed, Tomlinson & Roth, 1968) is a well-established scale of general functional status and has been used in a variety of research and clinical settings. It was developed on the basis of neuropathological studies. The scale has three categories: changes in performance of everyday activities, changes in habits, and changes in personality, with the first two covering items of IADLs and ADLs respectively. In some clinical settings, the changes-in-habits category has been expanded to include walking, alertness, and talking. Change in performance of everyday activities is a combination of basic IADL items such as performing household tasks and managing small sums of money, and dementia-related items. These latter items include ability to recall recent events, to interpret surroundings, and to find ones way around familiar indoor and outdoor surroundings. Changes in personality measures a variety of possible personality changes associated with dementia, for example, increased rigidity and/or egocentricity, and diminished emotional response.

2. Direct Assessment of Functional Status (DAFS)

This scale (Loewenstein, *et al.*, 1989) was developed by the authors to provide a measure sensitive to subtle changes in specific subskills that can occur in different phases of Alzheimer's disease and other dementias. Similar to the PADL, the DAFS measures actual patient performance and relies on direct observation, making it less susceptible to informant-report bias. The scale assesses seven functional domains of time orientation, communication abilities, transportation, financial skills, shopping skills, eating skills, and dressing–grooming skills. Each of the categories has 5 to 17 items asking the patient to perform specific related tasks. This scale has promise based on its use of actual observation and its inclusion of many detailed tasks to measure each domain. Since it was recently developed, additional studies are needed to demonstrate its overall validity as a functional assessment tool for dementia patients.

3. Functional Activities Questionnaire (FAQ)

This questionnaire (Pfeffer, Kurosaki, Harrah, Chance, & Filos, 1982) was developed as an assessment tool for dementia in conjunction with neurological and psychological evaluations. According to Pfeffer *et al.* (1981), previous scales have not always been sensitive enough to detect persons at the mildly demented level and have items that are difficult only for severely affected individuals. The FAQ assesses ten activities of IADLs on a four-point scale. The FAQ scale is a good predictor of cognitive and social function, and has been found to be a slightly better predictor than the IADL scale by Lawton and Brody (Pfeffer *et al.*, 1982). Pfeffer *et al.* (1982) report the scale to have better sensitivity than the IADL scale when classifying a patient as dysfunctional, and it can operate as a screening tool when used alone.

C. Multidimensional Scales

1. Older Americans Resources and Services (OARS)

This instrument (Fillenbaum & Smyer, 1981; George & Fillenbaum, 1985) was developed for the purpose of program evaluation, needs assessment, and resource-allocation decisions. It is intended to be used for clinical, research, and policy needs. The OARS is divided into two parts: Section A, which assesses individual functioning, and Section B, which assesses services used. The combination of multidimensional assessment along with use of services fits the biological–psychological–social model of older adults seeking medical care (Kemp, Brummel-Smith, & Ramsdell, 1990) and the fact that many older adults will require some kind of community-service assistance. The OARS questionnaire provides functional information in the five domains of social resources, economic resources, mental health, physical health, and ADL status. The activities of daily living section combines both ADL and IADL activities, covering the typical activities in those areas with a list of 15 items. The social-resources section assesses social competence in the areas of availability of help from family and kin, perception of loneliness, and frequency and satisfaction of contact with others. The mental health section covers cognitive function, psychiatric status, and self-evaluation. Validity has been based on comparisons with clinical judgments and ability to discriminate between different populations of community residents, clinic patients, and people living in institutions.

2. Functional Assessment Inventory (FAI)

This assessment inventory (Cairl, Pfeiffer, Keller, Burke, & Samis, 1983) is a 30-min abbreviated version of the OARS. It covers the same components and provides information on the same five domains. Pfeiffer, Johnson, and Chiofolo (1981) report that the FAI successfully distinguished between older adults at four different sites of nursing homes, day care centers, adult congregate living facilities, and senior centers. Correlations between the FAI and OARS were highest for the scales of mental health, physical health, and ADLs. The social-resource and economic-resource scales had lower correlations and were somewhat unstable in test–retest reliability (Cairl *et al.*, 1983). While the need for a shortened version of the OARS may exist, the FAI may require further study before it becomes an accepted replacement for the OARS.

3. Multilevel Assessment Instrument (MAI)

The Multilevel Assessment Instrument was developed by Lawton and associates at the Philadelphia Geriatric Center (Lawton, Moss, Fulcomer, & Kleban, 1982). It is based on a conceptual model of the well-being of older people and the use of the OARS as an example of comprehensive assessment. The MAI contains seven scales of physical health, cognition, ADLs, time use, social interaction, personal adjustment, and perceived environment. The ADL measure is composed of the PSMS and IADL scales by Lawton and Brody (1969). Social competency is assessed by the two scales of Time Use and Social Interaction. The Time Use scale is a 19-item checklist of various different leisure activities. The Social Interaction scale measures the frequency and quality of contacts with others, with two final scores representing separate factors of interaction with friends and interaction with family. Test–retest reliability by Lawton *et al.* (1982) is reported as acceptable. Validity is tested by expected differences in three criterion groups.

4. Comprehensive Assessment and Referral Evaluation (CARE)

This scale is a lengthy questionnaire of 1500 items designed to be administered in a semistructured format. It was developed to provide extensive and reliable information on older people in urban communities, and was initially used to gather cross-national comparative data on residents in New York and London (Gurland *et al.*, 1977). Information is provided on psychiatric, medical, nutritional, economic, and social problems. The Social Segment component of the scale covers both the functional and social-competence topics. Functional information assesses basic ADLs and IADLs. Social-competence information covers social background, retirement activities, social problems, and a Social Isolation Index. Efforts to reduce the CARE and produce a shorter version have led to several useful CARE derivatives (Gurland & Wilder, 1984). Two of these are the CORE-CARE, which has 314 items and retains the conceptual framework of the original CARE, and the SHORT-CARE, which assesses three major areas of depression, dementia, and disability. The SHORT-CARE could be potentially relevant for older patients with psychiatric concerns.

V. Discussion and Summary _____

Functional assessment is a vital part of psychiatric intervention with older persons. Psychiatric impairments produce more than distressing emotional, cognitive, and physiological symptoms for the older person. Psychiatric impairments also produce functional deficits in terms of affecting what the person does and can do for himself or herself. These *functional abilities* range from being able to relate to other people effectively to being able to provide for basic necessities of food, clothing, and shelter at home.

In this chapter, a case was made for a hierarchical arrangement of functional abilities. By targeting functional assessments to these areas, the effect of psychiatric disorders can be determined, interventions can be designed to compensate for the older person's functional deficits, proper living arrangements can be defined, and improvements resulting from psychiatric care can be measured. Without a functional assessment, only the person's degree of distress and suffering can really be known.

This chapter also reviewed many of the measures of functional performance available today. Many are easily adopted into a battery. At a minimum, an older person with a psychiatric disorder should receive a measure of ADL functioning and IADL functioning. These are the most essential for living adequately in the community. Care must be taken with self-report measures because older persons usually believe that health professionals are questioning their ability to live at home. Therefore self-report is often a report of "how it was," but not necessarily how it is.

Finally, care must be taken to remember that how well a person can function depends on his or her abilities and the environment in which he or she lives. The degree of disability can be changed either by altering the person's abilities (increasing function) or by decreasing the demands of the environment. A truly comprehensive approach to geriatric psychiatry should also take a functional view of the environment and determine what aspects of it are impairing functioning and what could be altered to help make the older person function better.

References

Alexander, F. G., & Selesnick, S. T. (1966). *The history of psychiatry*. New York: Harper & Row.

American Psychiatric Association. (1987). *Diagnostic and statistical manual* III-Revised, Washington, DC: APA.

Anthony, W., & Liberman, R. (1986). The practice of psychiatric rehabilitation: Historical, conceptual, and research base. *Schizophrenia Bulletin, 12*, 542–559.

Anthony, W. A., Cohen, M. R., & Cohen, B. F. (1983). Philosophy, treatment process, and principles of the psychiatric rehabilitation approach. In L. Packrach (Ed.), *New directions for mental health services: Deinstitutionalization*. San Francisco: Jossey-Bass.

Applegate, W., (1987). Use of assessment instruments in clinical settings. *Journal of the American Geriatric Society, 35*, 45–50.

Berkman, L., Berkman, C. S., Kasl, S., Freeman, D., Leon, L., Ostfeld, A., Cornoni-Huntley, J. & Brody, J. (1986). Depressive symptoms in relation to physical health and functioning in the elderly. *American Journal of Epidemiology, 124*, 372–388.

Blazer, D. G. (1982). *Depressions in late life*. New York: Mosby.

Blazer, D. & Williams, G. (1980). The epidemiology of depression and dysphoria in an elderly population. *American Journal of Psychiatry, 137*, 439–444.

Blessed, G., Tomlinson, B., & Roth, M. (1968). The association between quantitative measures of dementia and senile change in the cerebral gray matter of elderly. *British Journal of Psychiatry, 114*, 797–811.

Branch, L., Katz, S., Kniepmann, K., & Papsidero, J. (1984). A prospective study of functional status among community elderly. *American Journal of Public Health, 74*, 266–268.

Branch, L. G., & Meyers, A. R. (1987). Assessing physical function in the elderly. *Geriatric Assessment, 3(1)*, 29–51.

Brody, E. (1985). Parent care as a normative family stress. *Gerontologist, 25*, 19–29.

Brummel-Smith, K. (1990). Introduction. In B. J. Kemp, K. Brummel-Smith, & J. Ramsdell (Eds.), *Geriatric rehabilitation*. (pp. 3–22). Boston: College Hill Press.

Cairl, R., Pfeiffer, E., Keller, D. M., Burke, H., & Samis, H. V. (1983). An evaluation of the reliability and validity of the Functional Assessment Inventory. *Journal of the American Geriatrics Society, 31,* 607–612.

Chui, H. & Smith, B. (1990). Rehabilitation and Alzheimer's disease. In B. J. Kemp, K. Brummel-Smith & J. Ramsdell (Eds.), *Geriatric rehabilitation* (pp. 389–404). Boston: College Hill Press.

Cohen, G. D. (1989). The interface of mental and physical health phenomena in later life: New directions in geriatric psychiatry. *Gerontology and Geriatric Education, 9,* 27–38.

Corcoran, P. (1981). Disability consequences of bed rest. In W. C. Stolov and M. P. Clowers (Eds.). *Handbook of severe disabilities.* (pp. 55–63). Washington, D.C.: U.S. Department of Education.

Dawson, P., Kline, K., Wiancko, D. & Wells, D. (1986). Nurses must learn to distinguish between excess and actual disability to prolong the patient's competence. *Geriatric Nursing, 7,* 298–301.

Dion, G., Tohen, M., Anthony, W. & Waternavx, C. (1988). Symptoms and functioning of patients with bipolar disorder six months after hospitalization. *Hospital and Community Psychiatry, 39,* 652–657.

Donaldson, S., Wagner, C., & Gresham, G. (1973). A unified ADL evaluation form. *Archives of Physical Medicine & Rehabilitation, 54,* 175–179.

Fiebel, J. H., & Springer, C. J. (1982). Depression and failure to resume social activities after stroke. *Archives of Physical Medicine and Rehabilitation, 63,* 276–281.

Fillenbaum, G. (1985). Screening the elderly: A brief instrumental activities of daily living measure. *Journal of the American Geriatrics Society, 33,* 698–705.

Fillenbaum, G., & Smyer, M. (1981). The development, validity and reliability of the OARS multidimensional functional assessment questionnaire. *Journal of Gerontology, 36,* 428–434.

Fries, J., Spitz, P., Kraines, R., & Holman, H. (1980). Measurement of patient outcome in arthritis. *Arthritis & Rheumatism, 23,* 137–145.

Fulton, J. P., & Katz, S. (1986). Characteristics of the disabled elderly and implications for rehabilitation. In S. J. Brody & G. E. Ruff (Eds.), *Aging and rehabilitation: Advances in the state of the art.* (pp. 36–46). New York: Springer.

George, K., & Fillenbaum, G. (1985). OARS methodology: A decade of experience in geriatric assessment. *Journal of the American Geriatrics Society, 33,* 607–615.

Granger, C. (1984). Goals of rehabilitation of the disabled elderly in a conceptual approach. In S. Brody & G. Ruff (Eds.), *Aging and rehabilitation: Advances in the state of the art.* (pp. 27–35). New York: Springer.

Granger, C., & Greer, D. (1976). Functional status measurement and medical rehabilitation outcomes. *Archives of Physical Medicine & Rehabilitation, 57,* 103–109.

Gurland, B., Kuriansky, J., Sharpe, L., Simon, R., Stiller, P., & Birkett, P. (1977). The Comprehensive Assessment and Referral Evaluation (CARE)—Rationale, development and reliability. *International Journal of Aging and Human Development, 8,* 9–42.

Gurland, B., & Wilder, D. (1984). The CARE interview revisited: Development of an efficient, systematic clinical assessment. *Journal of Gerontology, 39,* 129–137.

Hurst, N. C. & Anthony, W. A. (1983). The vocational preparation of the chronic psychiatric patient in the community. In I. Barofsky & R. Budson (Eds.), *The chronic psychiatric patient in the community.* San Francisco: Medical and Scientific Books.

Israel, L., Kozarevic, D., & Sartorius, N. (1984). *Sourcebook of geriatric assessment.* New York: World Health Organization.

Jones, R. (1984). Deconditioning. In T. F. Williams (Ed.) *Rehabilitation in the aging.* New York: Raven Press.

Kane, R. A., & Kane, R. L. (1981). *Assessing the Elderly: A Practical Guide to Measurement,* Massachusetts: Lexington Books.

Katz, S., Ford, A., Maskowitz, R., Jackson, B., & Jaffe, M. (1963). Studies of illness in the aged. The index of ADL: A standardized measure of biological and psychosocial function. *Journal of the American Medical Association, 185,* 914–919.

Kemp, B., Brummel-Smith, K., & Ramsdell, J. (1990). *Geriatric Rehabilitation.* Boston: College-Hill Press.

Kennie, D. V., (1984). Health maintenance of the elderly. *Journal of the American Geriatrics Society, 32,* 316–323.

Klein, S., & Phillip, F. (1980). Token economy program for developing independent living skills in geriatric patients. *Psychological Rehabilitation Journal, 4,* 1–11.

Kuriansky, J., Gurland, B., & Fleiss, J. L. (1976). The assessment of self-care capacity in geriatric psychiatric patients by objective and subjective methods. *Journal of Clinical Psychology, 32,* 95–102.

Kurinasky, J., & Gurland, B. (1976). The performance test of activities of daily living. *International Journal of Aging and Human Development, 7(4),* 343–352.

Law, M. & Letto, L. (1989). A critical review of scales of activities of daily living. *American Journal of Occupational Therapy, 43,* 522–528.

Lawton, M. (1972). Assessing the competence of older people. In D. Kent, R. Kastenbuam, & S. Sherwood (Eds.), *Research, planning and action for the elderly.* New York: Behavioral Publications.

Lawton, M., Moss, M., Fulcomer, M., & Kleban, M. (1982). Research and service-oriented multilevel assessment instrument. *Journal of Gerontology, 37,* 91–99.

Lawton, P., & Brody, E. (1969). Assessment of older people: Self-maintaining and instrumental activities of daily living. *Gerontologist, 9,* 179–186.

Lawton, M. P. (1986). Functional assessment. In L. Teri & P. M. Lewinsoh (Eds.), *Geropsychological assessment and treatment: Selected topics.* (pp. 39–84). New York: Springer.

Liberman, R., & Evans, C. C. (1985). Behavioral rehabilitation for chronic mental patients. *Journal of Clinical Psychopharmocology, 5,* 85–145.

Liberman, R., & Foy, D. (1983). Psychiatric rehabilitation for chronic mental patients. *Psychiatric Annals, 13,* 539–545.

Linn, M., & Linn, B. (1982). The Rapid Disability Rating Scale. *Journal of The American Geriatrics Society, 30,* 378–382.

Loewenstein, D., Amigo, E., Duara, R., Guterman, A., Hurwitz, D., Berkowitz, N., Wilke, F., Weinberg, G., Black, B., Gittleman, B., & Eisdorfer, C. (1989). A new scale for the assessment of functional status in Alzheimer's disease and related disorders. *Journal of Gerontology, 44(4),* 114–121.

Mahoney, F., & Barthel, D. (1965). Functional evaluation: The Barthel index. *Maryland State Medical Journal, 14,* 61–65.

Manton, K. G. (1988). Activities of daily living, death and institutionalization in older persons. *Annual Review of Geriatrics and Gerontology, 8,* 217–255.

Moskowitz, E., Vernon, M., & McCann, C. (1957). Classification of disability in the chronically ill and aging. *Journal of Chronic Disease, 5,* 342–346.

Pace. W. (1989). Geriatric assessment in the office setting. *Geriatrics, 44,* 29–35.

Patterson, R. L., Dupree, L. W., Eberly, D. A., Jackson, G., O'Sullivan, M., Penner, L., & Kelly, C. D. (1982). *Overcoming deficits of aging: A behavioral approach.* New York: Plenum.

Patterson, R. L. (1990). Psychogeriatric Rehabilitation. In R. P. Liberman (Ed.), *Rehabilitation of the psychiatrically disabled.* (pp. 191–207). New York: Springer.

Pfeffer, R., Kurosaki, T., Harrah, C., Chance, J., Bates, D., Detels, R., Filos, S., & Butzke, C. (1981). A survey diagnostic tools for senile dementia. *American Journal of Epidemiology, 114(4),* 515–527.

Pfeffer, R., Kurosaki, T., Harrah, C., Chance, J., & Filos, S. (1982). A survey diagnostic tool for senile dementia. *American Journal of Epidemiology, 114,* 515–527.

Pfeiffer, E., Johnson, T., & Chiofolo, R. (1981). Functional assessment of elderly subjects in four service settings. *Journal of the American Geriatrics Society, 10,* 433–437.

Rogers, J. C. (1990). Improving the ability to perform daily tasks. In B. J. Kemp, K. Brummel-Smith, & J. R. Ramsdell (Eds.), *Geriatric rehabilitation.* (pp. 137–156). Boston: College Hill.

Ross, H. E., Kedward, H. B., & Henry, B. (1978). Social functioning and self-care in hospitalized psychogeriatric patients. *Journal of Nervous and Mental Disease, 166,* 25–33.

Schoening, H., & Iverson, I. (1968). Numerical scoring of self-care status: A study of the Kenny Self-Care Evaluation. *Archives of Physical Medicine and Rehabilitation, 49,* 221–229.

Sherwood, S., Morris, V., Morr, & Gutkin, C. (1977). *Compendium of measures for describing and assessing longterm care populations.* Boston: Hebrew Rehab Center for Aged.

Spector, W. D., Katz, S., Murphy, J. B., & Fulton, J. P. (1987). The hierarchical relationship between activities of daily living and instrumental activities of daily living. *Journal of Chronic Disease, 40,* 481–489.

Spitzer, R., Endicott, J., & Robins, E. (1978). Research diagnostic criteria: Rationale and rehabilitation. *Archives of General Psychiatry, 35,* 773–782.

Teri, L., Borson, S., Kiyak, H. A., & Yamagishi, M. (1989). Behavioral disturbance, cognitive dysfunction, and functional skill. *Journal of the American Geriatrics Society, 37,* 109–116.

Warren, E., & Grek, A. (1989). A correlation between cognition, performance, and daily functioning in elderly people. *Journal Geriatric Psychiatry and Neurology. 2,* 96–100.

Wilson, C. A., Grant, K., Witney, P. M., & Kerrige, D. F. (1973). Mental status of elderly hospital patients related to occupational therapists' assessment of activities of daily living. *Gerontological Clinics, 15* 197–202.

Winograd, C. (1986). Mental status tests and the capacity for self-care. *Gerontologist, 32,* 49–55.

Zarit, S., & Zarit, J. M. (1984). Psychological approaches to families of the elderly. In M. Eisenberg, L. Sutkin, & M. Janson (Eds.), *Chronic illness and disability through the life span.* New York: Springer.

25

Behavioral and Psychotherapeutic Interventions

Nancy A. Newton and Lawrence W. Lazarus

I. Introduction
II. Establishing the Therapeutic Relationship
III. Individual Psychotherapy: Psychodynamic Approaches
IV. Individual Psychotherapy: Behavioral Interventions
V. Individual Psychotherapy: Empirical Investigations
VI. Group Psychotherapy
VII. Marital Therapy
VIII. Multigenerational Family Therapy
IX. Conclusions
References

I. Introduction

Interest in psychotherapy with the elderly from theoretical, research, and service-delivery perspectives is a relatively recent phenomenon. Within the psychodynamic tradition, pessimism about the usefulness of psychotherapy with older adults has a long history, dating back to 1905 with Freud's early dictum that individuals over the age of 55 are unanalyzable (Freud, 1957). In their 1982 survey of primary journals devoted to behavior research and therapy, Wisocki and Mosher (1982) found that only .6% of articles dealt with elderly subjects. From 1964 to 1980, a total of only 107 articles focusing on behavioral psychotherapy with the elderly was uncovered. Similar lack of attention to the elderly has historically been present in marital and family therapy as well.

In contrast, the last decade has witnessed significant interest in the application of a variety of treatment models to older adults. This interest is exemplified by the publication of numerous books devoted specifically to this topic (Gallagher & Thompson, 1981;

Hussian, 1981; Hussian & Davis, 1985; Lewinsohn & Terri, 1983; Myers, 1984; Nemiroff & Colarusso, 1985, 1990; Sadovoy & Leszcz, 1987; Storandt, 1983) and the inauguration of journals such as *Clinical Gerontologist, Psychology and Aging, International Journal of Behavioral Geriatrics,* and *International Psychogeriatrics.*

Acknowledging the diversity within the elderly population, this literature has addressed the application of a variety of therapy techniques to specific treatment goals rather than searching for therapeutic generalizations applicable to the *elderly.* This increased specificity has allowed for reconsideration of earlier generalizations; for example, the usefulness of psychoanalysis in treating older adults. It has led to application of techniques found useful with younger adults, such as behavioral, cognitive, multigenerational family, and marital therapy to an older adult population. In providing an overview of recent developments, this chapter will reflect this diversity. Within psychodynamic psychotherapy, increased focus on insight-oriented treatment and the use of developmental and self-psychology perspectives in understanding the older adult will be discussed. Behavioral interventions that have been developed to address a variety of specific late life problems will be reviewed. Recent developments in group psychotherapy, marital, and multi-generational family therapy will also be described.

II. Establishing the Therapeutic Relationship

Engaging the patient in treatment and establishing an effective therapeutic relationship is crucial to all forms of psychotherapy. The development of such a relationship with the elderly patient presents particular challenges. These issues can be seen from two perspectives—facilitating the patient's access to the mental health professional and then actively engaging the patient in a therapeutic relationship.

The underutilization of mental health services by older adults is well documented (Botwinick, 1981). This phenomenon reflects a number of complex patient- and therapist-related factors, including cohort and/or age-related discomfort with acknowledging psychological problems and the need for treatment (Butler & Lewis, 1982). Other barriers to treatment include limited financial resources (Gottlieb, this volume), and biases among mental health professionals against treating the elderly (Butler & Lewis, 1982). Greater understanding of the issues that contribute to negative countertransference among potential service providers and recent increases in Medicare funding of outpatient psychotherapy (Gottlieb, this volume) have helped to overcome some of these health care-related barriers.

Aggressively marketing services and providing treatment in nontraditional settings are also promising means of increasing the accessibility of treatment to the elderly. Reaching out to older adults may involve going beyond traditional referral source networks. For example, Gallagher and Thompson (1982) and Steuer *et al.,* (1984) recruited patients for their outpatient cognitive–behavioral psychotherapy programs through local newspapers, radio programs, and senior-citizen organizations.

Providing interventions in a variety of settings is another way of reaching potential older adult patients. The usefulness of group psychotherapy and behavior-management programs (Hussian, 1981) within nursing home and retirement residences is well established. Behavioral treatment programs have also been developed within the patient's home (Hussian & Davis, 1985; Patterson, 1987; Pinkston & Linsk, 1984b). In these programs, family members and the patient are involved in establishing treatment goals and implementing treatment interventions. Wasson *et al.*, (1984) effectively used an outreach team consisting of a psychiatrist, a social worker, and a nurse to conduct in-home assessments and to develop community-based interventions for elderly patients who were unable or unwilling to come to a health care center for treatment. Thompson & Gallagher (1984) treated subclinical depression in older adults through a 6-week behaviorally oriented psychoeducational course at community sites such as senior centers and residential facilities. This *coping class* project enabled older adults to learn techniques for coping with stress in a more casual environment, thus avoiding the stigma frequently associated with more traditional mental health settings.

Once the older patient has demonstrated an initial willingness to enter treatment, particular attention to relationship-building strategies is essential to engage his or her active participation in therapy. Crucial to these strategies is the therapist's attitude. Elderly clients can arouse strong negative countertransference feelings in therapists that reflect ageist cultural biases and stereotypes as well as unconscious remnants of the therapist's early parental interactions (Grotjahn, 1955; Zinberg, 1964). Working through the elderly patient's own potentially negative attitudes about psychotherapy and transference reactions toward the generally younger therapist is often another crucial aspect of establishing the therapeutic relationship (Newton, Brauer, Gutmann, & Grunes, 1986).

Many modifications in psychotherapeutic technique are directed at building the therapeutic alliance, such as maintaining a less-formal relationship with the patient (Knight, 1979) and assuming a more-active stance in providing direction to the treatment and identifying and exploring areas of conflict (Weinberg, 1975; Yesavage & Karasu, 1982). Steur and Hammen (1983) and Gallagher and Thompson (1982) believe that the structured nature of cognitive–behavioral interventions have particular advantages in engaging the elderly depressed patient. Learning behavioral skills and cognitive techniques directly counters the passivity and helplessness that characterize depression in late life, challenges negative beliefs and stereotypes about aging, and allows the client to gain a sense of competence and control.

Although it may require considerable effort to establish a treatment relationship with resistant elderly patients, the impact of such a relationship, once established, can be very powerful. The therapist's role as an empathic, trustworthy listener can, in and of itself, provide a stabilizing influence. Viewing the patient as a worthwhile and effective person can help reestablish his or her personal sense of self-worth and self-esteem, compensating for the negative impact of age-related assaults. If the therapist serves to neutralize nihilistic thoughts and feelings about aging, patients may use the therapist for emotional refueling to restore psychic equilibrium (Cath, 1967). In their study of the process and outcome of brief psychodynamic psychotherapy with elderly outpatients, Lazarus *et al.* (1984) found that patients identified with their therapist's respectful, empathic, and understanding attitude, and tended to experience what their therapists said as reaffirming their views of themselves as competent.

The therapist may also be required to be more flexible in dealing with termination. For many elderly patients, continued contact with the therapist on a limited, infrequent basis may be more appropriate than a final termination, particularly for patients expected to experience further losses or medical problems, who have few other relationships, or who require ongoing support to maintain treatment gains.

III. Individual Psychotherapy: Psychodynamic Approaches ⎯⎯⎯⎯

Many psychodynamic and psychoanalytically-oriented therapists have long advocated the use of supportive treatment approaches with the elderly, particularly the frail elderly patient. Published case material exemplifies the effectiveness of these techniques (Alexander, 1944; Grotjahn, 1955; Kaufman, 1940; Meerloo, 1953; Pfeiffer & Busse, 1973; Wayne, 1953; Weinberg, 1975). Using supportive psychotherapy, the therapist can help the older frail patient maintain his or her current level of functioning or reestablish his or her premorbid level of functioning by compensating for failing ego functions and shoring up stressed defense mechanisms. By reconfirming the patient's strengths in the face of losses and physical impairments, the therapist can enable the patient to reestablish a sense of self-continuity and self-esteem. The therapist may also be called upon to serve as a less-critical superego for the overly self-demeaning and critical patient (Meerloo, 1961).

Although the value of supportive psychotherapeutic techniques with depleted, psychologically regressed elderly patients has long been accepted, recent case reports illustrate the effectiveness of insight-oriented psychotherapy with psychologically healthier aging persons (DaSilva, 1967; Kahana, 1983; Myers, 1984, 1989; Sandler, 1978; Segal, 1958). Psychodynamic treatment has been used successfully to treat patients with even long-held, apparently intractable psychiatric symptoms (Myers, 1984).

There is generally very little difference in insight-oriented psychotherapy approaches and treatment objectives between younger and older adults. Criteria for selecting insight-oriented therapy for the younger adult are applicable to the older patient (Cath, 1982) and include factors such as the patient's diagnosis, personality structure, cognitive resources, psychological-mindedness, capacity for introspection, and ability to establish a therapeutic alliance. Treatment objectives, including achievement of insight, modification of personality structure, and development of more mature defense mechanisms, are equally applicable to older and younger adults in insight-oriented psychotherapy.

Increasing attention is being given to the treatment of elderly patients with personality disorders. These patients may present for treatment with increasing helplessness and anxiety, escalating demands on family members for assistance, or depressive withdrawal (Lazarus, Sadavoy, & Langsley, 1991). Sadavoy (1987) describes a treatment approach for these patients in a long-term care setting that incorporates understanding of the personality issues that underlie the problematic behavior, behavioral techniques, and the assistance of the patient's social-support system in setting limits for the patient's behavior.

Brief psychodynamic approaches have been applied to elderly patients experiencing circumscribed problems that can be expected to resolve within a limited time (Kirshner, 1988; Lazarus *et al.*, 1984). Examples of problems amenable to brief psychotherapy include adjustment disorder, grief reaction, and traumatic stress disorder that has not become chronic. Setting a time limit on therapy reinforces the patient's confidence in his or her ability to resolve the problem, focuses and accelerates the therapeutic process, diminishes the patient's fear of protracted dependency on the therapist, and considers the patient's limited finances. In a study of the effectiveness of 15 sessions of brief psychotherapy, Lazarus *et al.* (1984) found that seven of the eight patients treated demonstrated significant lessening of their presenting symptoms and some resolution of underlying focal conflict.

A primary contribution of psychodynamic theory has been development of frameworks for understanding the psychological issues that confront the older adult, and the relationship of these issues to personality structure and earlier life development. It is assumed that late-life presentation of psychological symptoms in reaction to age-related stressors such as retirement, widowhood, and physical illness must be understood within the context of the psychological meaning of the stressor for the individual, his or her personality structure, lifelong psychological development, and the impact of aging on ego structure and defense mechanisms. In more psychologically vulnerable elderly, stressors such as loss of significant others and retirement can undermine long-standing life structures that served to compensate for deficits and shore up functioning (Jacobowitz & Newton, 1990).

Psychodynamic developmental models propose that throughout life each person is involved in an ongoing process of confronting both age or stage-expectable challenges and idiosyncratic crises (Erikson, Erickson, & Kivnick, 1986; Gutmann, 1987). At each period the individual can master the challenge, adapt to new demands, integrate the self-awareness gained, and thus experience further psychological maturation. At the opposite extreme, inability to master the challenge can so strain defensive-coping mechanisms that internal conflict and psychological regression results.

Late life presents its own particularly salient psychological issues. Hildebrand (1982) suggests that age-related changes challenge narcissistic investment in one's sense of identity; diminished differentiation within marital roles highlights difficulties in object relations; and physiological changes require renegotiation of feelings about one's own sexuality. Successful aging also necessitates reworking of earlier life issues, such as autonomy and trust, as well as resolving issues related to ego integrity (Erikson *et al.*, 1986).

Gutmann (1987) believes that late life may be accompanied by the emergence of other aspects of the self, including long-dormant inner potentials. In their mid to late 50s, older men who were formerly preoccupied with production and competition during the achievement, career-oriented period of adulthood are confronted with previously repressed and thus newly emerging needs to nurture and desires for intimacy. During this same developmental phase, women become more aware of previously submerged strivings to be assertive and to live out their own more instrumental, sometimes career-oriented, needs (Cooper & Gutmann, 1988). Adults who are threatened by the occurrence of these normal psychological changes and/or whose marriage cannot sustain these changes, may be more vulnerable to developing emotional problems for the first time in later life (Gutmann, Griffin, & Grunes, 1982).

Psychotherapy from a developmental perspective takes into account the individual's lifelong developmental history and the impact of age-related psychological tasks (Colarusso & Nemiroff, 1987; Nemiroff & Colarusso, 1985, 1990). Transference issues are viewed from the perspective of the individual's entire history of significant relationships with peers, children, and spouse, as well as unconscious ties to significant parental figures of childhood (Nemiroff & Colarusso, 1985). Published case studies illustrate specific aspects of psychotherapy from this perspective (Hildebrand, 1982, 1985, 1987; Levinson, 1985).

The application of the psychology of the self to aging focuses on the impact of aging on the individual's core sense of self (Kohut, 1972; Lazarus, 1980; Meissner, 1976). The self may be defined as an experienced constancy formed in early childhood that constitutes a coherent, vital core of the personality. It is a developmental psychological structure responsible for maintenance of one's self-image, self-esteem, feelings, and affects associated with bodily and psychological cohesiveness and relative need for others to idealize and to help sustain self-esteem. Persons vary in their sense of cohesiveness and integration, from sustained feelings of vitality and spontaneity to feelings of enfeeblement, depletion, and, where functioning is seriously disrupted, a sense of inner fragmentation (Kohut & Wolf, 1978).

Even for people whose investment in the self is healthy and whose self-image is realistic, age-correlated experiences, such as decline in physical and mental effectiveness, restrictions in economic resources and social roles, and diminished genital sexuality and physical attractiveness can attack the essential sense of self and undermine self-esteem–regulating systems. For the individual whose sense of self is fragile, with self-esteem based on illusions of omnipotence and on roles and relationships that served to gratify narcissistic needs, assaults of aging present even greater challenges. When loss of roles and shifts in interpersonal relationships undermine these illusions and disrupt need gratification, alienation from self and others can result.

Conceptualizing self-esteem maintenance from a sociological perspective, sociologist Atcheley (1982) believes that persons who lose self-esteem in later life tend to do so because of self-esteem problems earlier in life, because profound physical changes force one to accept a less-desirable self-image; because self-esteem was previously too dependent on work or social roles; and because of loss of control over their lives and environment. In these elderly people, narcissistic loss can result in compensatory reactions, such as pronounced jealousy, envy of the young, rigid adherence to no longer gratifying but previously effective behavior patterns, excessive entitlement, and adherence to an illusion of self-sufficiency (Kernberg, 1977; Levin, 1977). Other manifestations of problems in self-esteem include sensitivity to minor slights or disappointments, propensity to shame, rage, and depression, overdependence on others for approval, vacillations in mood and self-esteem, and hypochondriasis. Since maintaining self-esteem and sense of personal dignity is a pivotal issue for many elderly patients, therapists often observe the ebb and flow of self-esteem balance and imbalance. Discussing brief psychotherapy of adult patients with stress-response syndromes, Horowitz (1976) noted: "Narcissistic considerations are present in every character type, not just the narcissistic personality, and some nuances of treatment (of the narcissistic personality) might be pertinent at any time" (p. 184).

Elderly patients with disorders of the self often enter therapy following a narcissistic loss and are therefore sensitive and responsive to the therapist's empathic approach. Experiencing the need for therapy as a narcissistic insult, some patients feel ashamed about entering a therapeutic relationship and may resist engaging the therapist by appearing aloof or arrogant, and devaluing the therapist. These behaviors may, however, serve as a defense against the establishment of an idealizing transference.

Since one of the major goals of therapy with these patients is restoration of self-esteem, the therapist functions as an empathic self-object by empathizing with the patient's understandable reactions to narcissistic injury, initial resistances to therapy, and reactions to the therapist's inevitable empathic failures (e.g., when the patient feels misunderstood). The patient may reminisce about past accomplishments, recount innumerable past narcissistic injuries and blame others for his or her problems to bolster a diminished sense of self. The relationship with the empathic therapist may serve as a bridge to encourage the patient to reestablish old, or develop new, sustaining relationships.

The therapist may experience boredom and annoyance with the patient's continual need for approval. Stolorow (1975) suggests recognizing that "their narcissism is literally in the service of the psychic survival of the self" (p. 184). The therapist may feel uncomfortable with the patient's defensive devaluation or idealization and misidentify the latter as a defense against hostility. An appropriate therapeutic response in the initial phases of treatment of elderly patients with disorders of the self is to accept the idealization.

The psychodynamic tradition provides a variety of perspectives for understanding the older adult, particularly the relationship between early childhood and adult development and psychological issues that emerge in late life and the psychological significance of external age-related stresses (loss, physical illness, retirement). While published case material illustrates specific aspects of applying these treatment approaches, empirical studies need to be undertaken to validate their effectiveness.

IV. Individual Psychotherapy: Behavioral Interventions _____

With its emphasis on the interrelationship between the individual and the environment, behavioral models provide a promising approach to understanding and treating many of the psychiatric, behavioral, and physiological problems experienced by the elderly. Problems amenable to behavior therapy include psychiatric disorders such as depression and paranoia, disorders with a physiological component such as pain, incontinence, and insomnia, and other behavioral problems, such as wandering and socially inappropriate behavior (Carstensen & Edelstein, 1987; Lewinsohn & Terri, 1983). These are commonly occuring problems that can directly affect the quality of the older adult's life, frustrate the efforts of caregivers, and affect decisions about institutional placement. For example, urinary incontinence can result in long-term placement (Ouslander, 1983) as well as exclusion from social activities and loss of self-esteem. Use of medication in the treatment of pain and insomnia, while common with the elderly (Bootzin & Engle-Friedman, 1987; Sturgis, Dolcle, & Dickerson, 1987), can cause troublesome side-effects and requires careful monitoring. Thus, the availability of specific behavioral interventions as an alternative or supplement to the judicious use of medications can be an important component of the total treatment plan.

An operant learning model provides the foundation for these behavioral interventions. This model emphasizes the functional relationship between the patient's behavior and the environment within which it occurs. Modifiability of the behavior is assumed to be possible through the manipulation of environmental cues that prompt it (stimulus-control techniques) or the environmental consequences that reinforce the behavior's occurrence. Essential to treatment success is a clear definition of the target behavior and analysis of the behavior's normally occuring antecedents and consequences. In addition to functional analysis of the immediate situation, Eyde and Rich (1982) suggest that knowledge of past reinforcement history and awareness of potential future reinforcements beyond the specific situation may be important in developing effective treatment interventions for older adults. Based on this information, interventions are designed to (1) increase the occurrence of desired behaviors (for example, social interaction); (2) diminish the frequency of inappropriate behaviors (for example, wandering); and (3) shape new behaviors (i.e., coping strategies for sleep disturbance) (Eyde & Rich, 1982).

One type of operant-learning approach focuses on the modification of the behavior's antecedents, that is, the stimulus cues that prompt it. For example, enhanced social interaction among institutionalized elderly patients has been achieved through modifications in the environment, including rearrangement of furniture, reminders of social activities, and refreshments (Carstensen, 1987). These interventions make the institutional environment more like social situations outside the institution in which the individual has likely been reinforced for social interaction in the past.

Dementia can impair the older adult's ability to accurately process normal environmental cues, thus disrupting normal stimulus control of behavior (Hussian, 1987). For example, Hussian found that some types of wandering reflect this disruption—the client may appear to be wandering because he or she is following other ambulatory people. This process is further exacerbated when available cues are limited. Even when processing deficits have an organic basis, such as in dementia, enhancement of environmental cues (using signs, colored symbols) may increase the effectiveness of those cues. Specific training programs that increase stimulus saliency can further strengthen the relationship between the environmental cues and the desired behavior. For example, using colored symbols that have been paired with noxious noises to mark areas in the institution that patients are not to enter discourages wandering into those areas (Hussian, 1982).

Operant-learning models also emphasize the modifiability of behavior through manipulation of environmental consequences that reinforce the behavior's occurrence. Maladaptive behavior may reflect absence of a relationship between behavior and environmental consequences (*learned helplessness*), insufficient reinforcement of adaptive behaviors, or inadvertent reinforcement of undesirable behaviors. Many problematic behaviors may occur in older adults when the physical environment or caregivers inadvertently reinforce and thus maintain maladaptive, rather than adaptive, behaviors. Using an operant-observational design to record resident–staff interactions in a nursing home, Baltes (1988) found that dependent self-care behaviors were followed by a supportive social response, while independent behaviors were ignored. For example, patients who did not eat independently received staff attention while no social interaction was provided to self-feeding patients. Modifying the behavior-reinforcement contingencies by training staff to increase independence-supportive behaviors and to minimize dependence-supportive behaviors were found to change the patient's behavior in an independent direction (Sperbeck & Whitbourne, 1981).

In contrast to interventions that focus on treating discrete behavior problems in debilitated or demented patients whose ability to actively participate in a treatment plan may be limited, behavioral self-management approaches focus on the individual's role in shaping his or her own environment as well as on the impact of the environment on the individual (Haley, 1983). Self-management techniques require the patient's active participation in treatment, as education and collaborative problem solving play a crucial role. He or she is taught to modify maladaptive cognitions and behavior through improved coping skills and self-reinforcement strategies.

Self-management techniques provide a basis for addressing psychiatric problems, such as depression and anxiety, which have a pervasive impact on the individual's affect, cognitions, and behavior. An example is the behavioral approach used by Gallagher and Thompson (1981) to treat major depressive disorders in community-dwelling older adults. This model, based on Lewinsohn's (1974) response-contingent positive reinforcement model of depression, emphasizes interpersonal events and social skills. Lewinsohn argues that depression may result from a decrease in the rate with which one's behaviors secure positive reinforcing consequences from the environment. Daily monitoring of mood and completion of pleasant and unpleasant event schedules enable the patient to identify the relationship between mood and life events. Through acquisition of specific behavioral skills, patients learn to increase the ratio of positive to negative life events. Depending on the specific needs identified, homework assignments and structured interventions provide training in relaxation, social skills, self-control strategies, and thought-modification techniques.

While this approach is drawn from behavioral therapy for depression in younger adults, Zeiss and Lewinsohn (1986) suggest that some modification may be necessary for an older adult population. These modifications include adapting skill-training techniques to compensate for age-related changes in cognitive functioning, modifications in relaxation training to accommodate physical limitations, and increased focus on the specific pleasant and unpleasant events present in late life.

Behavioral techniques have also been used to treat problematic behavioral manifestations of severe psychiatric disorders. Haley (1983) used behavioral self-management techniques to treat agitation and aggressive verbal behavior in a 71-year-old nursing home resident with a long history of psychiatric hospitalizations for paranoid schizophrenia. The patient was taught through education, relabeling of her responses, role-playing, and progressive muscle relaxation to respond more appropriately when angered by other staff or residents. Proulx and Campbell (1986) diminished "paranoid" behavior in an elderly man with multi-infarct dementia by teaching the patient's wife to manipulate reinforcement contingencies. Carstensen and Fremouw (1981) used a combination of individual sessions and behavioral interventions in a nursing-home setting to treat paranoid verbal behavior in an elderly woman. The individual sessions provided an opportunity for the patient to ventilate her fears and to correct misinterpretations of everyday events. Staff were taught to verbally acknowledge appropriate verbalizations and to ignore inappropriate statements. The patient was also taught to maintain a chart of times she helped other residents, thus reinforcing her positive interactions.

A number of debilitating behavioral problems confronting the elderly, such as insomnia and incontinence, can have a physiological basis. A variety of cognitive–behavioral techniques are being investigated as an alternative or adjunct to the use of medication in the treatment of insomnia. In stimulus control (SC) treatments (Bootzin, Engle-Friedman, & Hazelwood, 1983), subjects are taught to regulate the circadian rhythm (i.e., eliminate daytime naps, arise at a set time each morning) and to curtail sleep-incompatible behaviors (i.e., use the bedroom only for sleep and sex; leave the bedroom when unable to sleep). Imagery training (IT) techniques attempt to modify the cognitive arousal that potentially interferes with sleep by teaching the patient to focus attention on a sequence of neutral objects (i.e., candle, hourglass, bowl of fruit) (Woolfolk & McNulty, 1983). Morin and Azrin (1988) found that both SC and IT techniques led to significant improvements in decreasing awakening duration, and that treatment gains were maintained over 3- and 12-month follow-ups. The SC procedures were, however, relatively more effective than the IT techniques, and clients viewed them as both more credible and more satisfactory.

In their review of behavioral treatment of incontinence, Burgio and Engel (1987) identify four basic approaches. In habit training, frequency of episodes of incontinence is diminished by training the staff to establish a temporal voiding schedule (for example, every 2 hours). Bladder training attempts to enable the patient to extend the interval between voiding through use of a toileting schedule, whether or not the physical sensation to void is present. Rewards (verbal approval, food, and clothing privileges) are used to reinforce appropriate voiding in contingency-management programs. Finally, biofeedback is used to increase the patient's awareness and control of the bladder and pelvic floor muscle responses that mediate continence.

Whitehead, Burgio, and Engel (1985) and Burgio, Whitehead, and Engel (1985) effectively used behavioral self-management techniques (self-monitoring, self-scheduled toileting, and biofeedback) in the outpatient treatment of fecal and urinary incontinence. Results of research on institutionalized elderly with dementia has been less-consistently positive (Pinkston, Howe, & Blackman, 1987). Pinkston *et al.* (1987), however, were successful in reducing episodes of incontinence in three wheelchair-bound, demented nursing home residents, using a combination of scheduled toileting and reinforcement (praise and cookies) for appropriate toileting.

Pinkston and Linsk (1984a,b) applied operant models to home-based family treatment of impaired elderly patients. During an extensive assessment phase, the elderly client and family caregiver are taught to objectively define behavior problems (such as aggression, withdrawal, toileting behavior, and self-care skills) and to record baseline data on the occurrence of the targeted behaviors. Patient, caregiver, and therapist jointly develop an intervention plan, and caregivers are taught to use appropriate behavioral procedures. This plan uses reinforcement and stimulus-control techniques to ensure the necessary differential cues and consequences needed to foster positive behaviors. For example, praise or food may be used to reinforce bathing or dressing while caregivers may be taught to ignore inappropriate behavior. Using single case research designs to study 66 patients, Pinkston, Linsk, and Young (1988) found improvement in 76% of the behaviors treated. While treatment gains were generally smaller than found with younger patients, they were viewed as significant in improving the quality of life for both the caregiver and patient because of the debilitating nature of the symptoms.

As suggested in this brief overview, behavior therapy can be an effective treatment for a wide variety of discrete behavioral problems, even when cognitive impairment inhibits the patient's capacity to actively engage in treatment, or physiological changes directly contribute to the behavior's occurrence. Behavior therapy has also been used to treat major depression in elderly outpatients. These techniques can be used in a variety of settings. Symptom improvement can sometimes occur quite rapidly. A particular strength of behavioral interventions is their amenability to empirical investigation and to the use of objective measurement to monitor and evaluate treatment effectiveness.

Behavioral treatment also has limitations. Although research supports the effectiveness of these interventions for specific behavioral problems in nursing-home settings, these strategies do not appear to be in widespread use (Guy & Morice, 1985). One reason for their limited use may be that implementation requires caregiver training, whether the caregivers are institutional staff or family members. In addition, maintenance of treatment gains often depends on consistent maintenance of appropriate environmental contingencies so that ongoing caregiver investment in treatment must be reinforced.

Concerns have also been raised about the generalization of treatment gains. For example, based on her review of the behavioral literature on social interactions, Carstensen (1987) concludes that while these interventions frequently increase social contact within the specific context of the intervention, evidence of generalization to behavior outside of that context or to enhanced sense of well-being has not been demonstrated. Maintenance of social contact following withdrawal of reinforcement may also be limited. Generalization may be more likely to occur when behaviors that will naturally be reinforced by the social environment are shaped or when the reinforced behavior assumes intrinsic value so that the patient continues to be invested in maintaining it once external reinforcement contingencies end (Carstensen, 1987).

V. Individual Psychotherapy: Empirical Investigations

Thompson and Gallagher (Gallagher & Thompson, 1982; Thompson & Gallagher, 1984; Thompson, Gallagher, & Breckenridge, 1987) conducted a series of studies investigating the effectiveness of short-term (16–20 sessions) outpatient psychotherapy in the treatment of elderly patients between the ages of 60 and 80 diagnosed with major depressive disorder, using Research Diagnostic Criteria (RDC). Three psychotherapy approaches were compared: behavioral (Gallagher & Thompson, 1981), cognitive, and brief psychodynamic therapy (following the approach of Horowitz & Kaltreider, 1979). Thompson and Gallagher based their cognitive therapy on Beck, Rush, Shaw, and Emery (1979), with modifications designed specifically for an older adult population (Emery, 1981). The focus of cognitive therapy is teaching patients to identify and modify the negative thoughts that contribute to the development and maintenance of depression.

These three treatment models were compared with a wait-list control group. Improvement was assessed through completion of self-report measures (Beck Depression Scale, Geriatric Depression Scale, and Brief Symptom Inventory) and therapist rating scales (Hamilton Rating Scale for Depression and Schedule for Affective Disorders and Schizophrenia) before and after treatment. Of 91 clients who completed treatment with one of the three treatment modalities, 70% demonstrated substantial improvement (Thompson et al., 1987). In contrast, patients placed in a 6-week wait-list control group did not demonstrate improvement when compared to psychotherapy patients at the 6-week point in treatment.

Followup interviews suggested a relatively low relapse rate (approximately 9%) for patients whose symptoms remained in remission for at least 2 months following termination of treatment. These results are comparable to psychotherapy outcome results with younger adults, and support the effectiveness of psychotherapy in treating major depression in elderly outpatients.

Client variables associated with positive response to treatment have also been identified. Within their sample, age was not related to treatment response nor was severity of depression before treatment (Thompson & Gallagher, 1984). Patients with nonendogenous depression (using RDC criteria) responded better and more quickly than patients with endogenous depression (Gallagher & Thompson, 1983). Presence of personality disorder [using Diagnostic & Statistical Manual, third edition (DSM-III) criteria] was associated with poorer treatment response (Thompson, Gallagher, & Czirr, 1988). Availability of social support and the nature of the patient's alliance with the therapist were also associated with treatment outcome, although the importance of these factors was related to the specific type of treatment utilized (Gaston, Marmar, Thompson, & Gallagher, 1988; Marmar, Gaston, Gallagher & Thompson, 1989). Commitment to treatment appears to be particularly important in symptom reduction in cognitive therapy, while capacity for self-exploration, self-reflection, and self-disclosure related to improvement in both cognitive and brief psychodynamic therapy.

VI. Group Psychotherapy

The use of supportive group psychotherapy with the elderly has a long history (Linden, 1953; Silver, 1950; Wolff, 1957). The group format provides an opportunity for members to build relationships with peers who have had similar experiences and are confronting similar psychological issues. Thus, group members can both learn from the perspectives of others and serve as a resource and support system for other members. This can enhance self-esteem and lessen dependency on the "expert" therapist, diminish the social isolation experienced by many older adults, and provide assistance within a structure that may be more acceptable for many elderly people.

A variety of group techniques have been developed to specifically address the needs of the institutionalized elderly who experience significant psychological and cognitive impairments. These group techniques, including reality orientation, remotivation, resocialization, and reminiscence, all share similar goals of enhancing client self-esteem, increasing social contact with peers, and increasing activity level and interest in the environment. Each technique, however, has its own particular focus.

Reality orientation is based on the assumption that awareness of basic information is essential to a reasonable level of functioning, even in the confused elderly (Baines, Saxby, & Ehlert, 1987; Liptzin, this volume). Within the group, leaders present current factual information (date, weather, current events). Ongoing presentation of the information during the day further reinforces client awareness. Although research with mildly and moderately confused elders suggests that reality orientation can lessen disorientation and increase verbal communication, evidence of generalization beyond the specific verbal information presented has not been consistently demonstrated to improve interpersonal behavior, increase activity level, and enhance self-care (Baines *et al.*, 1987; Hussian, 1987). The focus on acquisition of new information may also have deleterious consequences (Akerlund & Norberg, 1986). Reminding patients of deficits can undermine rather than enhance self-esteem. Staff may also become discouraged when the group content becomes routine or their efforts have so little generalized impact.

Other group interventions have been explored for cognitively impaired patients which can increase social contact and stimulation without highlighting the patient's cognitive deficits. These interventions include expressive group therapy (Johnson, 1985), socialization groups, and reminiscence or life-review therapy.

Life review appears to be a naturally occurring phenomenon for many older people, and many clinicians (Butler & Lewis, 1982; Kaminsky, 1984) have stressed the use and value of the reminiscence process in individual (Grunes, 1981) and family (Hughston & Cooledge, 1989) as well as group psychotherapy. Engaging in an active reminiscence process can serve many functions for the elderly person. Reinvestment in the self and experiences of the past can reestablish a sense of self-worth and self-continuity as well as compensate for the less-gratifying present. Discharge of affect associated with past painful experiences can enable the patient to master the past and thus more freely face the present and future. The process of putting one's life in order and gaining a perspective on oneself and one's life experiences helps to prepare for eventual death. An essential component of the therapeutic value of reminiscence may be attending to the here-and-now implications of the remembered event (Poulton & Strassberg, 1986).

However, reminiscence therapy is not appropriate for all older people, and it can have deleterious effects for some. For example, focus on the past may serve as a means of avoiding issues in the present. It can also serve to reinforce negative comparisons between the present and past, thus exacerbating feelings of loss and low self-esteem (Poulton & Strassberg, 1986).

Baines *et al.* (1987) found that beginning a reminiscence group with reality orientation led to enhanced cognitive and behavioral functioning in nursing-home residents, while either technique in isolation was not so effective. Christopher, Loeb, Zaretsky, & Jassani (1988) combined reminiscence and insight-oriented techniques in a psychotherapy group that prepared elderly rehabilitation patients for hospital discharge. The group served to offset the negative impact of hospitalization and to promote the qualities of self-determination and self-reliance necessary for readjustment to the community. Lesser, Lazarus, Frankel, & Havasy (1981) found that with an inpatient psychiatric population, replacement of an unstructured psychodynamic group therapy with a reminiscence format led to increased group participation and more positive outcome.

Within the last decade, there has been increasing interest in group psychotherapy with higher-functioning older adults. Using a self-psychology perspective to treat a group of 70 to 95-year-old men, Leszcz, Feigenbaum, Sadavoy, & Robinson (1985) found group psychotherapy to be a valuable modality for addressing issues of social isolation, depression, and demoralization. Steurer *et al.* (1984) compared the effectiveness of cognitive–behavioral and psychodynamic groups for 20 community-dwelling elders with significant history of major depressive disorder. Patients in the cognitive–behavioral group were taught strategies for increasing pleasurable activities in their lives and for examining and changing distorted cognitions. The psychodynamic group employed interventions such as support, corrective emotional experiences, confrontation, and interpretation. Each group participated in 46 sessions over a 9-month period. In both groups, there were significant changes in level of depression and anxiety, as measured by both observer and self-report ratings.

VII. Marital Therapy

More than 30% of older adults reside independently with a spouse (Beckham & Giordano, 1986). The majority of these couples are involved in long-term marriages, suggesting that mutually acceptable relationship patterns are well established (Wolinsky, 1986). At the same time, retirement, physical disability, relocation, and loss of friends can challenge long-maintained marital interaction patterns (Beckham & Giordano, 1986). These challenges provide developmental opportunities within the marital relationship as the couple redefines intimacy in view of the possibility for increased time together, renegotiates instrumental marital roles, develops new ways of expressing affection that accommodate physical changes, and integrates past and anticipated losses (Wolinsky, 1986). Even within healthy marriages, successful incorporation of these changes into the marital relationship can require new communication patterns (Patten & Piercy, 1989). These changes and the accompanying demands for greater fluidity, flexibility, and role equalization can be even more disruptive to tenuous relationships in which stability depends on the presence of rigid role boundaries (Crose & Duffy, 1988).

Although these issues suggest the potential usefulness of marital therapy for older couples, this approach has received little attention in the literature. Case studies suggest that marital therapy in late life is likely to include focus on age-related issues, such as preparation for the death of the spouse, by addressing symbiotic aspects of the relationship (Carni, 1989), coping with loss, and adjustment to the impact of physical disability on long-established role patterns within the relationship (Crose & Duffy, 1988).

Given the nature of the marital issues confronting older adults, the long-established interaction patterns, and the potential presence of complicating factors such as physical or cognitive decline, treatment models designed for younger adults are likely to require substantial modification for use with aging couples (Gafner, 1987). Wolinsky (1986) suggests a model for marital therapy with the elderly couple that draws on an understanding of both the individual and marital developmental tasks of late life.

VIII. Multigenerational Family Therapy

Late-life changes may also bring the older adult into a more central focus within the intergenerational family system and challenge long-standing patterns of family interaction (Greene, 1986). For many older adults, family support is an essential component in maximizing independent functioning, providing meaningful social contact, obtaining services from social-service agencies, and addressing crises. Effectively providing this assistance frequently requires negotiation of a more mature intergenerational relationship that facilitates the older adult's sense of autonomy and self-control, while also recognizing the fully adult status of the younger generation. Achieving this balance can be a psychologically challenging endeavor. Shifts in the frequency and nature of family contact can also give renewed immediacy to long-standing, unresolved conflicts that hamper the family's capacity to deal with immediate issues and to establish more mature parent–child relationships.

The midlife child and elderly parent are likely to be dealing with their own age-related psychological issues that provide a new developmental context for the relationship. For example, age-appropriate redistribution and sharing of power, examination of previously unspoken loyalties and obligations, and recognition of each member's autonomy may be inherent within the process (Williamson, 1981, 1982a). Multigenerational family therapy provides a framework for understanding and addressing these issues (Duffy, 1986).

While maintaining the focus on the importance of system issues as the context in which problems emerge and should be addressed, multigenerational family therapy broadens the definition of the relevant family network beyond the nuclear family. Inclusion of the adult child's nuclear family in the treatment of the older adult can enable family members to more appropriately respond to the needs of its elderly members by allowing them to learn more about the aging process, to develop greater insight into the needs of elderly family members, and to come to terms with their own feelings (Greene, 1989). Historical family conflicts that reemerge with increased contact and family stress can be addressed.

Several treatment models have been proposed to accomplish these goals. Eyde and Rich (1983) propose an integrated model of family management that incorporates family members as a resource throughout identification, assessment, and treatment of the older adult's presenting problems. Viney, Benjamin and Preston (1988) apply a constructivist model in assisting family members to understand, accept, and modify the constructs that guide family relationships in a way that inhibits the psychosocial functioning of elderly family members. Systemic approaches modify interaction patterns within the family that serve to undermine the healthy development and independence of elderly family members (Keller & Bromley, 1989).

Inclusion of elders within the treatment of the younger-generation nuclear family can also provide an invaluable resource in facilitating the younger generation's assumption of more functional, adult roles (Boszormenyi-Nagy & Spark, 1973; Spark, 1974). The elders' knowledge of family history provides a broader context in which issues can be understood, potentially facilitating their resolution. Williamson (1981, 1982a,b) proposes a treatment model focused on enabling both generations to work together to terminate the hierarchical boundaries, thus allowing younger adults to psychologically leave home and to assume responsibility for their own lives.

Effective inclusion of multiple generations may require modification of traditional treatment structures and flexibility in developing interventions. An essential component is the therapist's stance of *multidirectional partiality* which facilitates the presentation and discussion of issues without scapegoating of any family member (Boszormenyi-Nagy & Spark, 1973). Education may be required to enable patients to reframe issues within a family-system perspective, and treatment goals may involve addressing concrete management concerns as well as psychological issues (Greene, 1989).

Sessions in the older adult's home facilitate further diagnostic work and accommodate the needs of physically disabled family members (Duffy, 1986). Extended sessions or multiple sessions over a few days permit therapeutic work with family members when they visit from out of town (Duffy, 1986). Written or audiotaped letters, audiotaped or guided telephone calls, and audiotaped sessions allow for direct communication across geographical distance (Duffy, 1986; Williamson, 1982b). Revisions of letters within the therapy can enable the adult child to clarify and work through issues, even in the absence of direct contact with the parent.

IX. Conclusions

The last 10 years have witnessed the development of a rich resource of psychotherapy approaches for older adults. Recognition of the diversity within this population has allowed for the development of techniques that are appropriate for specific problems, whether those be functional or organic in origin. Treatment decisions for an individual patient are based on an understanding of the particular patient's needs. Awareness of background, ability and motivation to actively participate in treatment, nature of the presenting complaints, cognitive and physical status, personality structure, and available support system must also be taken into consideration in developing a potentially effective treatment. Psychotherapy needs to be individualized and provided in a flexible manner (Yesavage & Karasu, 1982). Ongoing, age-related changes in the patient may necessitate modifications in the initial treatment approach. The role of other interventions, such as medication, in conjunction with psychotherapy must also be considered (Salzman, this volume).

This review suggests areas that warrant continuing investigation and research. Within the area of psychodynamic therapy, the last 15 years have witnessed the development of a variety of frameworks, such as self-psychology and developmental models, that enrich the therapist's understanding of the psychological issues that accompany aging and their relationship to earlier stages of development. Further study using both empirical and case-study methodologies will lead to enhanced understanding of the application of these frameworks within psychotherapy. While empirical investigations demonstrate the effectiveness of various behavior therapy approaches in addressing particularly debilitating problems such as incontinence and inappropriate social behavior, strategies for increasing the use of these techniques, both within the institutional setting and in the community, need to be developed. An important aspect of this is likely to be the development of cost-effective staff and family-caregiver training programs. In contrast, use of marital and multigenerational family therapy with the elderly is relatively recent. The early promise of these approaches suggests that they deserve further study and investigation.

Acknowledgments

The authors express appreciation to Ms. Carolyn Milligan for her invaluable assistance in researching this paper and in preparing it for publication, and to Dr. Judith Dygdon for her helpful critique of the section on behavioral psychotherapies.

References

Akerlund, B. M., & Norberg, A. (1986). Group psychotherapy with demented patients. *Geriatric Nursing,* March/April, 83–84.

Alexander, F. G. (1944). The indications for psychoanalytic therapy. *Bulletin of the New York Academy of Medicine, 20,* 319–344.

Atchley, R. C. (1982). The aging self. *Psychotherapy: Theory, Research and Practice, 19,* 388–396.

Baines, S., Saxby, P., & Ehlert, K. (1987). Reality orientation and reminiscence therapy: A controlled cross-over study of elderly confused people. *British Journal of Psychiatry, 151,* 222–231.

Baltes, M. M. (1988). The etiology and maintenance of dependency in the elderly: Three phases of operant research. *Behavior Therapy, 19,* 301–319.

Beck, A. T., Rush, J. A, Shaw, B. F., & Emery, G. (1979). *Cognitive therapy of depression.* New York: Guilford Press.

Beckham, K., & Giordano, J. A. (1986). Illness and impairment in elderly couples: Implications for marital therapy. *Family Relations, 34,* 257–264.

Bootzin, R. R., Engle-Friedman, M., & Hazelwood, L. (1983). Insomnia. In P. M. Lewinsohn & L. Teri (Eds.), *Clinical geropsychology: New directions in assessment and treatment.* (pp. 81–115). Elmsford, NY: Pergamon.

Bootzin, R. R., & Engle-Friedman, M. (1987). Sleep disturbances. In L. L. Carstensen & B. A. Edelstein (Eds.), *Handbook of clinical gerontology* (pp. 238–251). New York: Pergamon Press.

Boszormenyi-Nagy, I., & Spark, G. M. (1973). *Invisible loyalties: Reciprocity in intergenerational family therapy.* New York: Harper & Row.

Botwinick, J. (1981). *Aging and behavior.* New York: Springer.

Burgio, K. L., & Engel, B. T. (1987). Urinary incontinence: Behavioral assessment and treatment. In L. L. Carstensen & B. A. Edelstein (Eds.), *Handbook of clinical gerontology* (pp. 252–266). New York: Pergamon Press.

Burgio, K. L., Whitehead, W. E., & Engel, B. T. (1985). Urinary incontinence in the elderly: Bladder-sphincter biofeedback and toileting skills training. *Annals of Internal Medicine, 103*(4), 507–515.

Butler, R. N., & Lewis, M. I. (Eds.) (1982). *Aging and mental health: Positive psychosocial and biomedical approaches.* St. Louis: C. V. Mosby.

Carni, E. (1989). To deal or not to deal with death: Family therapy with three enmeshed older couples. *Family therapy, 16*(1), 59–68.

Carstensen, L. L. (1987). Age-related changes in social activity. In L. L. Carstensen & B. A. Edelstein (Eds.), *Handbook of clinical gerontology* (pp. 222–237). New York: Pergamon.

Carstensen, L. L., & Edelstein, B. A. (Eds.) (1987). *Handbook of clinical gerontology.* New York: Pergamon Press.

Carstensen, L. L., & Fremouw, W. J. (1981). The demonstration of a behavioral intervention for late-life paranoia. *The Gerontologist, 21*(3), 329–333.

Cath, S. H. (1967). Persistence of early emotional problems in a seventy-year-old woman: Discussion. *Journal of Geriatric Psychiatry, 1,* 67–71.

Cath, S. H. (1982). Psychoanalysis and psychoanalytic psychotherapy of the older patient. *Journal of Geriatric Psychiatry, 15,* 43–53.

Christopher, F., Loeb, P., Zaretsky, H., & Jassani, A. (1988). A group psychotherapy intervention to promote the functional independence of older adults in a long-term rehabilitation hospital: A preliminary study. *Physical and Occupational Therapy in Geriatrics, 6*(2), 51–61.

Colarusso, C. A., & Nemiroff, R. A. (1987). Clinical implications of adult developmental theory. *American Journal of Psychiatry, 144*(10), 1263–1270.

Cooper, K. L., & Gutmann, D. L. (1987). Gender identity and ego mastery style in middle-aged, pre- and post-empty nest women. *The Gerontologist, 27*(3), 347–352.

Crose, R., & Duffy, M. (1988). Separation as a therapeutic strategy in marital therapy with older couples. *Clinical Gerontologist, 8*(1), 71–73.

DaSilva, G. (1967). The loneliness and death of an old man: Three years' psychotherapy of an eighty-one-year-old depressed patient. *Journal of Geriatric Psychiatry, 1,* 5–27.

Duffy, M. (1986). The techniques and contexts of multigenerational therapy. In T. L. Brink (Ed.), *Clinical gerontology: A guide to assessment and intervention* (pp. 347–362). New York: The Haworth Press.

Emery, G. (1981). Cognitive therapy with the elderly. In G. Emery, S. D. Hollon, & R. C. Bedrosian (Eds.), *New directions in cognitive therapy* (pp. 84–98). New York: Guilford.

Erikson, E. H., Erikson, J. M., & Kivnick, H. Q. (1986). *Vital involvement in old age.* New York: W. W. Norton.

Eyde, D. R., & Rich, J. A. (1982). A family-centered model for routine management of disturbing behaviors in the aged. *Clinical Gerontologist, 1*(1), 69–87.

Eyde, D. R., & Rich, J. A. (1983). *Psychological distress in aging: A family-management model.* Rockville, MD: Aspen.

Freud, S. (1957). On psycho-therapy. In J. Strachey (Ed. and Trans.), *The standard edition of the complete psychological works of Sigmund Freud* (Vol. 7, pp. 257–268). London: Hogarth Press. (Original work published 1905)

Gafner, G. (1987). Engaging the elderly couple in marital therapy. *The American Journal of Family Therapy, 15*(4), 305–315.

Gallagher, D., & Thompson, L. W. (1981). *Depression in the elderly: A behavioral treatment manual.* Los Angeles: The University of Southern California Press.

Gallagher, D. E., & Thompson, L. W. (1982). Treatment of major depressive disorders in older adult outpatients with brief psychotherapies. *Psychotherapy, Theory, Research and Practice, 19*(4), 482–490.

Gallagher, D. E., & Thompson, L. W. (1983). Effectiveness of psychotherapy for both endogenous and nonendogenous depression in older adult outpatients. *Journal of Gerontology, 38*(6), 707–712.

Gaston, L., Marmar, D. R., Thompson, L. W., & Gallagher, D. (1988). Relation of patient pretreatment characteristics to the therapeutic alliance in diverse psychotherapies. *Journal of Consulting and Clinical Psychology, 56*(4), 483–489.

Greene, R. (1986). The functional-age model of intergenerational therapy: A social casework model. In T. L. Brink (Ed.), *Clinical gerontology: A guide to assessment and intervention* (pp. 335–346). New York: Haworth.

Greene, R. (1989). A life systems approach to understanding parent–child relationships in aging families. *Journal of Psychotherapy and the Family, 5*(1–2), 57–69.

Grotjahn, M. (1955). Analytic psychotherapy with the elderly. *Psychoanalytic Review, 42,* 419–427.

Grunes, J. (1981). Reminiscences, regression and empathy—A psychotherapeutic approach to the impaired elderly. In S. I. Greenspan & G. H. Pollock (Eds.), *The course of life: Psychoanalytic contributions toward understanding personality development. Vol. III: Adulthood and the aging process.* Washington, DC: Government Printing Office.

Gutmann, D. (1987). *Reclaimed powers: Toward a new psychology of men and women in later life.* New York: Basic Books.

Gutmann, D. L., Griffin, B., & Grunes, J. (1982). Developmental contributions to the late-onset affective disorder. In O. B. Brim & P. B. Balters (Eds.), *Life-span development and behavior, Vol. 4* (pp. 243–261). New York: Academic Press.

Guy, D. W., & Morice, H. O. (1985). A comparative analysis of behavior management in the nursing home. *Clinical Gerontologist, 4*(2), 11–17.

Haley, W. E. (1983). Behavioral self-management: Application to a case of agitation in an elderly chronic psychiatric patient. *Clinical Gerontologist, 1*(3), 45–51.

Hildebrand, H. P. (1982). Psychotherapy with older patients. *British Journal of Medical Psychology, 55,* 19–28.

Hildebrand, H. P. (1985). Object loss and development in the second half of life. In R. A. Nemiroff & C. A. Colarusso (Eds.), *The race against time* (pp. 211–228). New York: Plenum.

Hildebrand, H. P. (1987). Psychoanalysis and aging. *Annual of Psychoanalysis, 15,* 113–125.

Horowitz, M. (1976). *Stress-response syndromes.* New York: Jason Aronson.

Horowitz, M., & Kaltreider, N. (1979). Brief therapy of the stress-response syndrome. *Psychiatric Clinics of North America, 2,* 365–377.

Hughston, G. A., & Cooledge, N. J. (1989). The life review: An underutilized strategy for systemic family intervention. *Journal of Psychotherapy and the Family, 5*(1–2), 47–55.

Hussian, R. A. (1981). *Geriatric psychology: A behavioral perspective.* New York: Van Nostrand Reinhold.

Hussian, R. A. (1982). Stimulus control in the modification of problematic behavior in elderly institutionalized patients. *International Journal of Behavioral Geriatrics, 1,* 33–46.

Hussian, R. A. (1987). Wandering and disorientation. In L. L. Carstensen & B. A. Edelstein (Eds.), *Handbook of Clinical Gerontology* (pp. 177–189). New York: Pergamon.

Hussian, R. A., & Davis, R. L. (1985). *Responsive care: Behavioral interventions with elderly persons.* Champaign, IL: Research.

Jacobowitz, J., & Newton, N. (1990). Time, context and character: A life-span view of psychopathology during the second half of life. In R. A. Nemiroff & C. A. Colarusso (Eds.), *Frontiers of adult development.* New York: Basic Books.

Johnson, D. R. (1985). Expressive group psychotherapy with the elderly: A drama therapy approach. *International Journal of Group Psychotherapy, 35*(1), 109–127.

Kahana, R. J. (1983). Psychotherapy of the elderly: A miserable old age—What can therapy do? *Journal of Geriatric Psychiatry, 16*(1), 33–38.

Kaminsky, M. (Ed.) (1984). *The uses of reminiscence: New ways of working with older adults.* New York: Haworth.

Kaufman, M. R. (1940). Old age and aging. The psychoanalytic point of view. *American Journal of Orthopsychiatry, 10,* 73–84.

Keller, J. F., & Bromley, M. C. (1989). Psychotherapy with the elderly: A systemic model. *Journal of Psychotherapy and the Family, 5*(1–2), 29–46.

Kernberg, O. (1977). Normal psychology of the aging process—revisited. II. Discussion. *Journal of Geriatric Psychiatry, 10,* 27–45.

Kirshner, L. A. (1988). A model of time-limited treatment for the older patient. *Journal of Geriatric Psychiatry, 21*(2), 155–168.

Knight, B. (1979). Psychotherapy and behavior change with the non-institutionalized aged. *International Journal of Aging and Human Development, 9,* 221–236.

Kohut, H. (1972). Thoughts on narcissism and narcissistic rage. *Psychoanalytic Study of the Child, 27,* 360–400.

Kohut, H., & Wolf, E. (1978). The disorders of the self and their treatment: An outline. *International Journal of Psychoanalysis, 59,* 413–425.

Lazarus, L. W. (1980). Self-psychology and psychotherapy with the elderly: Theory and practice. *Journal of Geriatric Psychiatry, 13,* 69–88.

Lazarus, L. W., Groves, L., Newton, N., Gutmann, D. L., Ripeckyj, A., Frankel, R., Grunes, J., & Havasy-Galloway, S. (1984). Brief psychotherapy with the elderly: A review and preliminary study of process and outcome. In L. W. Lazarus (Ed.), *Psychotherapy with the elderly* (pp. 15–35). Washington, DC: American Psychiatric Press.

Lazarus, L. W., Sadavoy, J., & Langsley, P. R. (1991). Individual psychotherapy. In J. Sadavoy, L. Lazarus, & L. Jarvik (Eds.), *Comprehensive Review of Geriatric Psychiatry.* Washington, DC: American Psychiatric Association Press, Inc..

Lesser, J., Lazarus, L. W., Frankel, R., & Havasy, S. (1981). Reminiscence group therapy with psychotic geriatric inpatients. *The Gerontologist, 21,* 291–296.

Leszcz, M., Feigenbaum, E., Sadavoy, J., & Robinson, A. (1985). A men's group: Psychotherapy of elderly men. *International Journal of Group Psychotherapy, 35*(2), 177–196.

Levin, S. (1977). Normal psychology of the aging process revisited—II. *Journal of Geriatric Psychiatry, 10,* 3–7.

Levinson, G. A. (1985). New beginnings at seventy: A decade of psychotherapy in late adulthood. In R. A. Nemiroff & C. A. Colarusso (Eds.), *The race against time* (pp. 171–188). New York: Plenum.

Lewinsohn, P. A. (1974). A behavioral approach to depression. In R. Friedman & M. Katz (Eds.), *The psychology of depression: Contemporary theory and research.* New York: Wiley.

Lewinsohn, P. M., & Teri, L. (Eds.) (1983). *Clinical geropsychology: New directions in assessment and treatment.* New York: Pergamon.

Linden, M. (1953). Group psychotherapy with institutionalized women: Study in gerontological relations. *International Journal of Group Psychotherapy, 3,* 150–170.

Marmar, C. R., Gaston, L., Gallagher, D., & Thompson, L. W. (1989). Alliance and outcome in late-life depression. *The Journal of Nervous and Mental Disease, 177*(8), 464–472.

Meerloo, J. A. M. (1953). Contributions of psychoanalysis to the problems of the aged. In M. Heimann (Ed.), *Psychoanalysis and social work* (pp. 321–337). New York: International Universities Press.

Meerloo, J. M. (1961). Modes of psychotherapy in the aged. *Journal of the American Geriatrics Society, 9,* 225–234.

Meissner, W. W. (1976). Normal psychology of the aging process revisited—I: Discussion. *Journal of Geriatric Psychiatry, 9,* 151–159.

Morin, C. M., & Azrin, N. H. (1988). Behavioral and cognitive treatments of geriatric insomnia. *Journal of Consulting and Clinical Psychology, 56*(5), 748–753.

Myers, W. A. (1984). *Dynamic therapy of the older patient.* New York: Jason Aronson.

Myers, W. A. (1989). I can't play ball anymore. *Journal of Geriatric Psychiatry, 23*(1), 121–144.

Nemiroff, R. A., & Colarusso, C. A. (1985). Adult development and transference. In R. A. Nemiroff & C. A. Colarusso (Eds.), *The race against time* (pp. 59–72). New York: Plenum.

Nemiroff, R. A., & Colarusso, C. A. (1990). *Frontiers of adult development.* New York: Basic Books.

Newton, N. A., Brauer, D., Gutmann, D. L., & Grunes, J. (1986). Psychodynamic therapy with the aged: A review. In T. L. Brink (Ed.), *Clinical gerontology: A guide to assessment and intervention* (pp. 205–230). New York: Haworth.

Ouslander, J. G. (1983). Incontinence and nursing homes: Epidemiology and management. *The Gerontologist, 23,* 257.

Patten, P. C., & Piercy, F. P. (1989). Dysfunctional isolation in the elderly: Increasing marital and family closeness through improved communication. *Contemporary Family Therapy, 11*(2), 131–147.

Patterson, R. (1987). Family management of the elderly. In L. L. Carstensen & B. A. Edelstein (Eds.), *Handbook of clinical gerontology* (pp. 267–276). New York: Pergamon.

Pinkston, E. M., Howe, M. W., & Blackman, D. K. (1987). Medical social work management of urinary incontinence in the elderly: A behavioral approach. *Journal of Social Service Research, 10*(2–4), 179–194.

Pinkston, E. M., & Linsk, N. L. (1984a). Behavioral intervention with the impaired elderly. *The Gerontologist, 24*(6), 576–583.

Pinkston, E. M., & Linsk, N. L. (1984b). *Care of the elderly: A family approach.* New York: Pergamon.

Pinkston, E. M., Linsk, N. L., & Young, R. N. (1988). Home-based behavioral family treatment of the impaired elderly. *Behavior Therapy, 19*(3), 331–344.

Poulton, J. L., & Strassberg, D. S. (1986). The therapeutic use of reminiscence. *International Journal of Group Psychotherapy, 36*(3), 381–398.

Proulx, G. B., & Campbell, K. B. (1986). The management of apparent "paranoid" behavior in a patient with multi-infarct dementia. *Gerontologist, 6*(2), 121–129.

Sadavoy, J. (1987). Character disorders in the elderly: An overview. In J. Sadavoy & M. Esszca (Eds.), *Treating the elderly with psychotherapy: The scope for change in later life.* Madison, CT: International Universities Press.

Sadavoy, J., & Leszcz, M. (Eds.) (1987). *Treating the elderly with psychotherapy: The scope for change in later life.* Madison, CT: International Universities Press.

Sandler, A. M. (1978). Psychoanalysis in later life. Problems in the psychoanalysis of an aging narcissistic patient. *Journal of Geriatric Psychiatry, 11,* 5–36.

Segal, H. (1958). Fear of death. Notes on the analysis of an old man. *International Journal of Psycho-Analysis, 39,* 178–181.

Silver, A. (1950). Group psychotherapy with senile psychotic patients. *Geriatrics, 5,* 147–150.

Spark, G. M. (1974). Grandparents and intergenerational family therapy. *Family process, 13,* 225–237.

Sperbeck, D. J., & Whitbourne, S. K. (1981). Dependency in the institutional setting: A behavioral training program for geriatric staff. *The Gerontologist, 21*(3), 268–275.

Steuer, J. L., & Hammen, C. L. (1983). Cognitive–behavioral group therapy for the depressed elderly: Issues and adaptations. *Cognitive Therapy and Research, 7*(4), 285–296.

Steuer, J. L., Mintz, J., Hammen, C. L., Hill, M. A., Jarvik, L. F., McCarley, T., Motoike, P., & Rosen, R. (1984). Cognitive–behavioral and psychodynamic group psychotherapy in treatment of geriatric depression. *Journal of Consulting and Clinical Psychology, 52*(2), 180–189.

Stolorow, R. (1975). Toward a functional definition of narcissism. *International Journal of Psycho-Analysis, 56,* 179–185.

Storandt, M. (1983). *Counseling and therapy with older adults.* Boston: Little, Brown.

Sturgis, E. T., Dolcle, J. J., & Dickerson, P. C. (1987). Pain management in the elderly. In L. L. Carstensen & B. A. Edelstein (Eds.), *Handbook of clinical gerontology* (pp. 190–203). New York: Pergamon.

Thompson, L. W., & Gallagher, D. (1984). Efficacy of psychotherapy in the treatment of late-life depression. *Advanced Behavioral Research Therapy, 6*, 127–139.

Thompson, L. W., Gallagher, D., & Breckenridge, J. S. (1987). Comparative effectiveness of psychotherapies for depressed elders. *Journal of Consulting and Clinical Psychology, 55*(3), 385–390.

Thompson, L. W., Gallagher, D., & Czirr, R. (1988). Personality disorder and outcome in the treatment of late-life depression. *Journal of Geriatric Psychiatry, 21*(2), 133–146.

Viney, L. L., Benjamin, Y. N., & Preston, C. (1988). Constructivist family therapy with the elderly. *Journal of Family Psychology, 2*(2), 241–258.

Wasson, W., Ripeckyj, A., Lazarus, L. W., Kupferer, S., Barry, S., & Force, F. (1984). Home evaluation of psychiatrically impaired elderly: Process and outcome. *The Gerontologist, 24*(3), 238–242.

Wayne, G. J. (1953). Modified psychoanalytic therapy in senescence. *Psychoanalytic Review, 40*, 99–116.

Weinberg, J. (1975). Geriatric psychiatry. In A. M. Freedman, H. L. Kaplan, & B. J. Sadock (Eds.), *Comprehensive textbook of psychiatry*, 2nd ed. (vol. 2, pp. 2405–2420). Baltimore, MD: Williams & Wilkins.

Whitehead, W. E., Burgio, K. L., & Engel, B. T. (1985). Biofeedback treatment of fecal incontinence in geriatric patients. *Journal of the American Geriatrics Society, 33*, 320–324.

Williamson, D. S. (1981). Personal authority via termination of the intergenerational hierarchical boundary: A "new" stage in the family life cycle. *Journal of Marital and Family Therapy, 7*, 441–452.

Williamson, D. S. (1982a). Personal authority via termination of the intergenerational hierarchical boundary: Part II—The consultation process and the therapeutic method. *Journal of Marital and Family Therapy, 8*, 23–37.

Williamson, D. S. (1982b). Personal authority in family experience via termination of the intergenerational hierarchical boundary: Part III—Personal authority defined, and the power of play in the change process. *Journal of Marital and Family Therapy, 8*, 309–323.

Williamson, P. N., & Ascione, F. R. (1983). Behavioral treatment of the elderly. *Behavior Modification, 7*(4), 583–610.

Wisocki, P. A., & Mosher, P. (1982). The elderly: An understudied population in behavioral research. *International Journal of Behavioral Geriatrics, 1*, 5–14.

Wolff, K. (1957). Group psychotherapy with geriatric patients in a mental hospital. *Journal of American Geriatrics Society, 5*, 13.

Wolinsky, M. A. (1986). Marital therapy with older couples. *The Journal of Contemporary Social Work, 67*(8), 475–483.

Woolfolk, R. L. & McNulty, T. F. (1983). Relaxation treatment for insomnia: A component analysis. *Journal of Consulting and Clinical Psychology, 51*(4), 495–503.

Yesavage, J. A., & Karasu, T. B. (1982). Psychotherapy with elderly patients. *American Journal of Psychotherapy, 36*, 41–55.

Zeiss, A. M., & Lewinsohn, P. M. (1986). Adapting behavioral treatment for depression to meet the needs of the elderly. *The Clinical Psychologist, Fall*, 98–100.

Zinberg, N. W. (1964). Psychoanalytic consideration of aging. *Journal of the American Psychoanalytic Association, 12*, 151–159.

26

Psychopharmacologic Treatment

Carl Salzman and Joyce Nevis-Olesen

I. Overview
II. Factors Complicating Prescription of Psychotropic Drugs
    A. Nonspecific Symptoms and Diagnosis
    B. Concomitant Illness
    C. Nonspecificity of Psychotropic Drug Effects
    D. Drug Interactions and Polypharmacy
    E. Prescribing Patterns
    F. Compliance Problems: Overuse, Underuse, Inappropriate Use, Nonuse
III. Age-Related Changes in Pharmacologic Drug Effect
    A. Altered Ability to Metabolize and Excrete Psychotropic Drugs (Pharmacokinetic Changes)
    B. Altered Central Nervous System and Psychotropic Drugs (Pharmacodynamic Changes)
IV. Psychotropic Treatment of Behavior Disorders, Agitation, and Psychosis
    A. Diagnostic Concerns
    B. Neuroleptics
    C. Treatment with Nonneuroleptics
    D. New Research Directions
V. Treatment of Depression
    A. Diagnostic Concerns
    B. Antidepressants
    C. Monoamine Oxidase Inhibitors
    D. Antidepressants with Atypical Structure
    E. Psychomotor Stimulants
    F. New Research Directions
VI. Treatment of Mania
VII. Treatment of Anxiety
    A. Diagnostic Considerations
    B. Benzodiazepines

C. Other Anxiolytic Drugs
D. Prescribing Guidelines for Anxiolytic Drugs for Older Patients
E. New Research Directions
VIII. Treatment of Sleep Disorders
A. Diagnostic Considerations
B. Selection of Drug
C. Prescribing Principles
IX. Treatment of Memory Loss and Cognitive Dysfunction
A. Diagnostic Considerations
B. Experimental Treatment Approaches
X. Summary and Conclusions
References

To meet the needs of increasing numbers of older patients, the field of geriatric psychopharmacology has developed from a fledgling area of inquiry into a major subspecialty within the field of general psychopharmacology during the past dozen years. Both research and clinical experience have vastly increased the knowledge database on the specific use of psychotropic drugs for older people as well as on nondrug factors that influence the effect of psychotropic drugs in this population.

I. Overview

Psychotropic drug treatment for geriatric patients requires an understanding of several age-related factors that influence the effects of these drugs. Diagnosis, variable treatment response, and increased predisposition to drug side-effects provide the essential foundation. At least four additional areas of information bear directly and indirectly upon appropriate and successful psychotropic drug use for this population:

1. High prevalence of concomitant physical illness;
2. Increased likelihood of the use of multiple drugs (polypharmacy) and the consequent potential for harmful drug interactions;
3. Increased sensitivity of the aging central nervous system (CNS) to the effects of psychotropic drugs (pharmacodynamics); and
4. Alterations in the aging body's ability to bind, distribute, and dispose of psychotropic drugs (pharmacokinetics).

All these factors affect therapeutic as well as adverse reactions.

The nonpharmacological context of drug treatment for the psychiatric problems of geriatric patients raises issues that include the relationship between patient and physician; the patient's relationships with family; prior experience with psychotropic drugs; the ability to understand the nature of the illness and the treatment being prescribed; and the degree of compliance possible. These considerations, based on the premise that psychotropic drug use requires careful evaluation and monitoring of the patient, constitute the working principles for rational psychotropic drug treatment. Taken together, they reflect the dual pharmacological–nonpharmacological focus of this chapter.

II. Factors Complicating Prescription of Psychotropic Drugs _____

One of the key advances in the field of geriatric psychopharmacology over the past decade has been recognition of the critical role of the aging process, not only in choosing the drug or drug subclass most appropriate for an individual, but also in specifying the disorder for which the drug is prescribed.

A. Nonspecific Symptoms and Diagnosis

Determining diagnosis and etiology of a psychiatric disorder is more complex with geriatric patients than it is with younger adults, to which several factors contribute:

- Presenting symptoms of older patients are often different than those of younger adults with similar illness.
- Some elderly persons cannot describe their symptoms adequately.
- Lack of reliable biological markers of psychiatric illness in older persons often raises questions as to whether symptoms are caused by physiological or psychological factors.
- Symptoms that arise from concomitant treatments can confuse the diagnostic picture.

Because these factors can blur important diagnostic distinctions, it is essential that the clinician's differential diagnosis process include evaluation of the consequences of normal aging in addition to current health status, drug regimen, and history of psychiatric disorders.

B. Concomitant Illness

1. Impact of Physical Illness on Psychiatric Symptoms

In the older patient, psychiatric symptoms may be the initial presenting symptoms of physical illness, or they may be components of the clinical picture of a particular physical illness. Pancreatic carcinoma, hypothyroid and hypoadrenal states, and chronic viral infection, for example, are known to produce affective disturbance, and injury to the brain from several sources frequently results in psychiatric dysfunction. Persons with neurologic illness, particularly stroke, often develop significant depression, either in response to the experience of physical debilitation (Robinson, 1982) or as a complication specific to brain damage (Folstein, Maiberger, & McHugh, 1977).

   The presence of physical or neurologic disorder in an older patient complicates diagnosis of psychological disorder as well as the selection of appropriate pharmacologic treatment for the disorder. Although psychotropic drugs may alleviate many psychological disturbances that accompany physical disorders, physical illness, in turn, may alter the effects of these drugs and limit their usefulness. For example, impaired hepatic function due to illness may have two results: first, diminished production of plasma proteins reduces protein binding of psychotropics, resulting in greater toxicity; and second, impaired hepatic biotransformation leads to higher plasma levels, resulting in greater toxicity and prolonged effects. Regarding the effect of illness on specific psychotropics, reduced renal clearance, for example, affects psychotropics by raising the plasma levels of lithium as well as water-soluble toxic metabolites of antidepressants. Each type of result causes increased drug toxicity in the older patient.

2. Impact of Psychotropic Side-Effects on Psychiatric Symptoms

Psychotropic drugs frequently affect the symptoms of physical illness. For example, heterocyclic antidepressants may exacerbate cardiac arrhythmias commonly found in older people; the anticholinergic side-effects of neuroleptics and antidepressants markedly increase symptoms of prostatic hypertrophy, occular accommodation, and decreased gastric motility; and the extrapyramidal side-effects of neuroleptics almost always increase the tremor and akinesia of Parkinson's disease.

C. Nonspecificity of Psychotropic Drug Effects

Psychotropic drugs have nonspecific, often unpredictable effects in older patients, due to increased central nervous system (CNS) sensitivity and age-related changes in the body's ability to metabolize and excrete them. These factors affect the therapeutic as well as the toxic effects of these drugs.

1. Lack of Predictable Drug Response

The disorders for which psychotropic drugs are commonly prescribed for elderly patients are severe behavior problems (particularly agitation) and psychosis, depression, mania, anxiety, and sleep disorders. Treatment of these disorders for older people involves the same drug classes as those used for younger adults, although dosages may be adjusted. Too often, however, psychotropic drug treatment for older persons is based on the assumption that symptoms in older and younger adults indicate the same disease process—an assumption that presents exceptions. First, symptom patterns are less well defined in older patients; treatment response may not always follow the pattern expected with younger adults. Most psychopharmacologic research on the effects of psychotropic drugs was conducted on young adults, and, thus, may not always provide an adequate guide to effective and safe drug treatment for geriatric patients.

Diagnostic specificity for psychiatric disturbance for some elderly patients may thus become blurred and interfere with therapeutic precision. When an older patient's symptoms span two or more diagnostic categories, determining which class of psychotropics is most appropriate becomes difficult. It is not surprising, therefore, that accurate prediction of therapeutic as well as adverse response to psychotropic drugs may not always be possible. In some cases where diagnosis and predictable response remain uncertain, clinicians are faced with the decision to treat symptoms without having discerned their cause. Empirical trials of psychotropic medications may offer substantial symptomatic relief, even when all criteria for clear differential diagnosis have not been met. In these circumstances, careful monitoring and periodic reevaluation, which should always accompany medication, are especially necessary.

2. Psychiatric Symptoms and Psychotropic Drug Effect

A psychotropic drug prescribed to alleviate one psychiatric disorder, or symptom pattern of that disorder, either through its therapeutic effects or side-effects, may exacerbate an allied condition. For example, the anticholinergic properties of neuroleptics given to older demented patients to control agitation may exacerbate the agitation as well as the cognitive impairment or dementia that causes it (Larson, Kukull, Buchner, & Reifler, 1987) ; the behavior and cognitive function of demented patients may worsen when benzodiazepines are given to treat anxiety (APA Task Force, 1990; Salzman, Fisher, Nobel, & Wolfson, 1990); and clinical experience suggests that increased agitation can occur when patients with dementia or Parkinson's disease receive antidepressants. A very confusing clinical picture and distinct therapeutic challenge occurs when an elderly patient has schizophrenia, Parkinson's disease, and tardive dyskinesia simultaneously: if the schizophrenia is treated with a neuroleptic, the Parkinson's symptoms worsen and the tardive dyskinesia may ultimately be exacerbated; alternatively, if the Parkinson's symptoms are treated with L-dopa, the schizophrenia and tardive dyskinesia will worsen.

3. Secondary Drug Effects and the Aging Process

Clinically adverse side-effects occur more readily and at lower doses in older people than in younger adults because multiple CNS receptor sites are usually more sensitive to psychotropic drug effect in the geriatric population. For example, while the ability of a high-potency neuroleptic drug given to an older patient to block dopamine receptors is therapeutic for psychosis and agitation, it also causes extrapyramidal symptoms by blocking dopamine receptors; further, in addition to blocking histamine receptors and thus causing sedation, neuroleptics also block alpha-1 norandrenergic receptors, which causes orthostatic hypotension.

4. Therapeutic Use of Adverse and Secondary Drug Effects

Clinically significant side-effects such as sedation, peripheral and central anticholinergic blockage, orthostatic hypotension, and extrapyramidal symptoms occur more readily and with lower doses of psychotropics in older patients. Although these effects are usually considered unwanted adverse reactions, in some cases they may prove therapeutic. For example, the sedating side-effects of neuroleptics and antidepressants can be used to decrease agitation or induce sleep. However, even though judicious use of the sedating side-effect can be therapeutic, careful monitoring is necessary in order not to compromise daytime function.

Nonpsychotropic drugs are also sometimes prescribed for older patients for their salutary secondary psychotropic effects. For example, antihistamines can be prescribed for sedating purposes; beta blockers and the anticonvulsants carbamazepine and sodium valproate are used increasingly to treat agitation in demented patients as well as in serious affective disorder; and calcium channel blockers can be useful in controlling treatment-resistant mania as well as severe agitation in demented patients.

5. Nonspecific Effects of Psychotropic Drugs

In the treatment of elderly patients with psychotropics, drugs are not always used for the specific purpose denoted by their nosologic and therapeutic categories. For example, neuroleptics usually given to treat psychosis may also reduce agitation; antidepressants, in addition to treating depression, may also reduce agitation and anxiety, promote sleep, and block panic and phobic anxiety; and anxiolytic agents promote sleep.

The use of psychotropic drugs to treat older patients is therefore less precise than therapeutic classification suggests. Psychotropic drugs (as well as other drugs) have a broad range of pharmacologic actions that may affect several different neurotransmitter systems therapeutically, adversely, or in both ways. Use, of course, depends on whether or how the chronic physical illnesses experienced by the older patient or the medications taken for these illnesses (e.g., beta blockers for hypertension) contraindicate prescription of nonpsychotropic drugs for psychiatric dysfunction.

D. Drug Interactions and Polypharmacy

As people age and are more likely to become physically ill, the drugs prescribed for treatment of their illnesses, whether acute or chronic, as well as the increased number of drugs in addition to the over-the-counter medications that many older people take—all are predictable and common sources of adverse effects. Overall incidence of adverse drug reactions is two to three times that found in young adults (Nolan & O'Malley, 1988).

1. Impact of Drug Interactions

Drug interactions, a common problem in all facets of medicine, are considerably more likely and serious in older people (Lamy, 1986). Two main forms of adverse reactions may occur: those resulting when two or more drugs with similar pharmacologic properties may combine and increase an unwanted side-effect, and those that arise when drug combinations cancel the therapeutic effect of either or both agents. The mechanisms of adverse drug interactions result from altered CNS sensitivity (pharmacodynamics) or altered metabolic disposition (pharmacokinetics).

a. Altered CNS sensitivity.   Altered CNS neurotransmitter function that leads to heightened sensitivity to psychotropic drug side-effects in older patients also increases their vulnerability to adverse drug interactions, particularly if they take more than one psychoactive drug at a time. Two types of adverse pharmacodynamic interactions occur: additive interactions, which occur when two drugs with similar pharmacological effects are taken together, or counteractive interactions, which occur when two or more drugs cancel out the therapeutic effect of one or all.

The most common effects of additive interactions experienced by older patients are increased sedation and anticholinergic reactions. Progressive decreases in energy, enthusiasm, motivation, and concentration—all symptoms that may suggest either age-related decline in CNS function or depression—can be the result of the gradual but additive sedating properties of drugs taken simultaneously over time. Progressive memory impairment, orientation, and concentration—a syndrome often assumed by the older patient (and by the patient's family) to be symptoms of age-associated decline in memory function—may be the result of the incremental interaction of anticholinergic drugs.

An example of a pharmacodynamic drug interaction that interferes with therapeutic effects is seen with a neuroleptic (which blocks dopamine) that is used to treat psychosis interacts with L-dopa (which increases dopamine) that is used to treat Parkinson's disease. The therapeutic effect of each is cancelled, worsening both psychotic and Parkinson's symptoms.

b. Altered metabolic disposition.   The second major type of adverse drug interaction occurs when two drugs alter the metabolic disposition of each, resulting in either increased or decreased blood levels and clinical effect. These pharmacokinetic interactions can have subtle as well as disabling effects in older patients, even at drug doses ordinarily nontoxic in younger patients. Examples of drugs commonly used by older patients and the effects of their interaction with psychotropics are as follows:

- Antacids: impair and delay absorption of benzodiazepines;
- Cimetidine: increases plasma levels of long half-life benzodiazepines and tricyclic antidepressants;
- Thiazide diuretics: increase the plasma levels of lithium and may cause toxicity;
- Fluoxetine: increases blood levels of other antidepressants; and
- Alcohol (and smoking): decreases plasma levels of all psychotropics except lithium.

2. Over-the-Counter Medications (OTCs)

Older people are known to take a variety of over-the-counter medications (e.g., cold, cough, sleep, and pain preparations). The substantial likelihood that an older patient is already taking some form of medication when psychotropic treatment begins markedly increases the possibility of adverse interactions.

Two categories of adverse interactions between psychotropic drugs and OTCs are common in older people. The first is additive sedation, i.e., when sedating OTCs combine with sedating psychotropic drugs such as neuroleptics, antidepressants, and benzodiazepines. Second, and considerably more serious, are the additive anticholinergic effects that result from combinations of OTC cold and allergy preparations (and some sleep medications) with tricyclic antidepressants and some neuroleptics. Since older patients are more sensitive to drug-induced anticholinergic effects because of reduced amounts of acetylcholine in the CNS, the common consequence is anticholinergic toxicity. These side-effects may appear as increased forgetfulness or greater agitation, confusion, and disorientation; in extreme cases, paranoia and delirium can develop.

E. Prescribing Patterns [Replace]

Prescribing patterns of psychotropic drugs for elders may vary by site. In hospitals, one third of older patients are prescribed psychotropic drugs. In nursing homes, psychotropic drug use is as high as 74% (Ray *et al.*, 1980). More than 20% of residents with orders for these medications do not have a documented psychiatric symptom pattern or mental disorder; more than 25% have orders for more than one psychotropic drug; 11% receive medications from two or more psychotropic drug classes; and residents receiving psychotropics take 3.3 other medications concomitantly (Beardsley *et al.*, 1989). Guidelines for what is appropriate or inappropriate medication are not always clear, and knowledge of age-related factors implicated in the effects of psychotropic medication and care goals for older patients is often poorly understood (Gurwitz *et al.*, 1990). Based partially on these factors and on recommendations by the Institute of Medicine (1986), a uniform nursing home assessment system (Morris *et al.*, 1990) was mandated nationally and implemented in 1990. One of the intentions of this system, which includes criteria for use of psychotropic drugs, is to facilitate more rational psychotropic drug-prescribing by building comprehensive evaluation, accurate documentation, and adequate monitoring into the care provision process.

F. Compliance Problems: Overuse, Underuse, Inappropriate Use, Nonuse

Noncompliance with drug prescriptions in older persons has several sources. Evidence differs regarding the noncompliance of older patients: some claim that elders are under-compliant or noncompliant in taking psychotropic drugs (Folkman, Bernstein, & Lazarus, 1987; Rowe & Besdine, 1982); others (Montamat, Cusack, & Vestal, 1989; Nolan & O'Malley, 1988; Weintraub, 1990) claim that, as a group, older people are no less compliant than are patients in other age groups. When noncompliance does occur, however, it is clear that the main reasons are greater complexity of treatment regimens as chronic diseases take hold, increased sensitivity to drugs, and the impact of poor health on the patient's entire life. All these factors contribute to forgetfulness, confusion about doses and schedules, distressing side-effects, difficulty with medication containers, and discord with lifetime beliefs.

Forgetfulness can lead to undermedication and consequent suboptimal results. It can also result in overmedication. For example, the older person who awakens in the middle of the night may take a dose of a hypnotic, forgetting that he or she took a dose before bedtime, raising the risk of accidental overdoses and inadvertent toxicity.

Because older patients often take several drugs on a regular basis, confusion over different doses and dose schedules for different drugs is also common. It is not unusual to see an older person sitting at the dinner table facing a column of pill-filled vials, trying to remember which should be taken "with food," which should be taken "before food," which is taken "once a day," and which is taken "several times a day." Physicians' instructions on labels of these containers are often too small to be read easily, and verbal instructions are often forgotten.

The side-effects of psychotropic drugs, particularly the anticholinergic effects of constipation, blurred vision, or dry mouth, may be so severe that older patients do not take their medicine at all, or take lower-than-prescribed doses. This form of noncompliance is very common, particularly with antidepressants. Tremor due to lithium and sedation from antianxiety agents are other common side-effects poorly tolerated by older persons that may result in underdosing noncompliance.

Containers commonly used for dispensing prescriptions also pose problems: they are sometimes exceedingly difficult for an older patient to open; arthritic fingers, poor vision, tremor, and muscular weakness often interfere with the ability to reach medication; "safety" tops may be nearly impossible for older people to open. Frustration, embarrassment, and anger are not unusual responses and can understandably lead to noncompliance.

Noncompliance may also result from an older patient's lifetime beliefs, family traditions, or characteristic ethnic response to illness, physicians, and medications. For example, some patients may retain the conviction that taking medication is a sign of weakness. Although seeming to accept a doctor's prescription with gratitude, such a patient may take less than the prescribed dosage or not take the medication at all. Other older patients may believe that if one pill helps, then two will help twice as much and twice as fast. Still others may or may not take drugs, depending on the symptoms for which they are prescribed: some older people may believe that depression reflects lack of strength of character, and medication is evidence of failure of that strength; for the same individual, however, memory loss may be considered a natural consequence of aging, and any medication to improve memory will be considered acceptable treatment.

III. Age-Related Changes in Pharmacologic Drug Effect

The effect of a psychotropic drug depends on its concentration and activity at CNS receptor sites. Age-related alterations in absorption, distribution, metabolism, and excretion of psychotropic drugs (pharmacokinetic changes) may have a direct impact on the receptor site. The aging process also alters the sensitivity of the receptor site to psychotropic drugs (pharmacodynamic changes). These alterations are critically implicated in psychotropic drug activity and therapeutic effect.

A. Altered Ability to Metabolize and Excrete Psychotropic Drugs (Pharmacokinetic Changes)

Evidence indicating age-related alterations in drug disposition, derived from studies of normal older volunteer research subjects, elderly patients, and aging animals suggests several changes: absorption, alterations in plasma-protein binding, increased volume of distribution, diminished hepatic metabolism, and impaired renal clearance. The mechanisms involved in these changes are comprehensively reviewed by Abernethy (in press), Greenblatt & Shader (1990), Ritschel (1988), and Friedel (1978).

1. Absorption

Age has little effect on psychotropic drug absorption; most compounds are absorbed as completely and rapidly in old age as in younger years, and reductions are usually not clinically significant. One common exception to this finding does occur, however. When an older patient takes a sleeping pill at bedtime, absorption and sleep may be delayed; while awaiting sleep, the older person may not know that delay in hypnotic effect is expectable and assumes that an insufficient dose was taken; a second dose can then result in toxicity in the form of morning hangover.

2. Protein Binding

The effect of age on protein binding is less clear. The decline in plasma albumin (the primary plasma protein involved in the binding process) that has been thought to occur with age has been correlated with increased psychotropic drug toxicity (Greenblatt, Divoll, Harmatz, McLaughlin, & Shader, 1981). However, later evidence suggests that the clinical impact of reduced amounts of plasma albumin may have less significance than previously supposed (Greenblatt, Abernethy, & Shader, 1986; Greenblatt, Sellers, & Koch-Weser, 1982). Two factors account for the diminished importance of protein binding. First, observations indicate that another binding protein (alpha-1-acid glycoprotein) does *not* decrease with age, and actually increases during states of physical illness; it is possible that increased amounts of this second plasma protein will offset any age-related decline in plasma albumin. Secondly, the equilibrium between bound and unbound drugs remains unchanged in most elderly patients. Even though the total amount of protein binding may decline, the free fraction of psychotropic drug available to produce clinical or toxic effects remains unchanged (Greenblatt & Shader, 1990; Greenblatt & Shader, 1985).

3. Metabolism and Clearance

Most psychotropic drugs undergo reduced hepatic metabolism and clearance as a result of the aging process. Only lithium among psychotropics is directly cleared through the kidney. These reductions in metabolic transformation and renal clearance decrease or delay elimination of drugs and their metabolites. Clinically, decreased drug clearance in older people, in turn, leads to accumulated drugs and metabolites, increased steady-state blood levels, and prolonged elimination half-life, compared with younger adults taking the same dosage. Tricyclic antidepressants, for example, produce steady-state blood levels nearly twice as high (or higher) in older than in younger patients on the same dosage (Salzman, 1984). Similarly, the elimination half-lives of tricyclic antidepressants and long half-life benzodiazepines are two to three times longer for older compared with younger patients taking the same dose (Abernethy, in press).

Tricyclic antidepressants metabolize to water-soluble hydroxy metabolites that are then cleared by the kidney. The most recent data suggest that this metabolite is potentially cardiotoxic (Young, Alexopoulos, Shamoian, Dhar, & Kutt, 1985). Age-related reduction in renal clearance of older patients increases the blood level of this water-soluble toxic metabolite and thus the potential for cardiotoxicity. Lithium excretion through the kidney also decreases as people age, resulting in drug accumulation and plasma levels two to three times higher than expected for a younger adult taking the same dose.

B. Altered Central Nervous System and Psychotropic Drugs (Pharmacodynamic Changes)

The most profound influence of aging upon the effects of psychotropic drugs in older people may lie in the complex set of alterations that occurs in CNS receptor-site function, either naturally in the course of aging or as a result of illnesses or their treatment—an area that is only beginning to be explored. Comprehensive reviews of the mechanisms linking age-related changes in the brain and altered psychotropic drug effect appear in Sunderland (in press) and Moran & Thompson (1988).

1. Age-Related CNS Receptor Sensitivity

The effect of psychotropic drugs depends on the sensitivity of the CNS receptor site to therapeutic drug concentrations; as a group, older people appear to be significantly more sensitive to all psychotropic drugs. For example, therapeutic effects as well as side-effects of neuroleptics, antidepressants, and lithium often occur at doses and blood levels significantly below the corresponding levels required in younger adults.

2. Neurotransmitter Function

Altered CNS receptor-site sensitivity is the primary factor responsible for increased drug sensitivity in older patients. Altered receptor sensitivity may result from either structural or functional changes in the binding site or from age-related changes in neurotransmitter supply. For example, reduced levels of acetylcholine (Creasey & Rapoport, 1985) as well as dopamine (Morgan, May, & Finch, 1987; Severson, 1984) in the CNS heighten postsynaptic sensitivity to these neurotransmitters. Of the many neurotransmitter-receptor systems in the CNS subject to age-related changes, reductions in norepinephrine, dopamine, and acetylcholine are primarily responsible for psychotropic drug side-effects commonly experienced by older people.

Regardless of mechanism, the aging CNS becomes increasingly sensitive to the therapeutic as well as the toxic effects of psychotropic drugs. Clinically, this results in increased sedation, anticholinergic toxicity, and extrapyramidal effects at doses that would not usually be toxic in younger adults.

a. Dopamine.   Diminished dopamine function predisposes the older patient to increased frequency and severity of extrapyramidal symptoms when dopamine-blocking drugs such as neuroleptics are administered. Like alpha-1-norepinephrine receptors, dopamine receptors decrease during the aging process, resulting in less ability to maintain blood pressure in an upright position. Neuroleptics and antidepressants thus pose an increased risk of orthostatic hypotension, dizziness, and falls to the older patients.

b. Acetylcholine.   Decreased acetylcholine in the aging CNS occurs normally, and is hypothesized to be associated with the typical decline in recent memory experienced during the later years of life. In Alzheimer's dementia, acetylcholine is virtually absent in certain parts of the brain. Reviews of research efforts seeking to clarify the relationship between acetylcholine and memory loss and dementia include those of Tariot (in press), Whitehouse (1987), Davies & Wolozin (1987), and Bartus, Dean, Beer & Lippa (1982). Reduced amounts of acetylcholine in the CNS (Creasey & Rapoport, 1985) result in greater sensitivity to drugs such as neuroleptics and tricyclic antidepressants, which diminish acetylcholine function in the course of their pharmacologic action. Patients taking these medications can thus experience severely impaired memory, attention, and orientation as well as extrapyramidal symptoms.

IV. Psychotropic Treatment of Behavior Disorders, Agitation, and Psychosis

Psychotic, demented, or severely ill elderly patients often manifest behavioral symptoms that can become dangerous to self or others. Prevalence rates for behavior disorders (often characterized as agitation) are particularly high in nursing homes (Cohen-Mansfield, Marx, & Rosenthal, 1989; Peabody, Warner, Whiteford, & Hollister, 1987; Rovner, Kafonek, Filipp, Lucas & Folstein, 1986; Wragg & Jeste, 1988; Zimmer, Watson & Treat, 1984). Several of these manifestations (e.g., severe agitation, screaming, assaultiveness) seen frequently in the moderate to severe stages of dementia, as well as psychotic and paranoid thinking, require psychopharmacologic intervention when behavior becomes dangerous and distress cannot be alleviated solely by other interventions.

A. Diagnostic Concerns

Severe disturbances of behavior and thinking arise from both reversible and irreversible sources. One of the clinician's prime concerns before beginning psychopharmacologic treatment is to rule out treatable conditions induced by acute physical problems or adverse drug reactions. The most common reversible causes of these symptoms as well as disordered thinking are delirium and toxic states; others are infection, dehydration, electrolyte imbalance, and affective disturbance. In contrast, the dementia of organic mental disorders, particularly Alzheimer's disease, is the most common untreatable cause of severe behavior problems, which also occur with late-life schizophrenia (though the incidence and prevalence rates of schizophrenia are much lower).

Sound assessment of symptoms and subsequent diagnosis often presents complex choices for the geriatric clinician. Agitated depression in which patients manifest motoric agitation as well as dysphoric mood is a case in point. If symptoms are diagnosed accurately as primarily depressive, antidepressant medication may be effective. If, however, the same signs are diagnosed as agitation and treated with a neuroleptic, two sets of adverse side effects are possible: (1) a low-potency agent can sedate the patient, intensifying the depressive symptoms and possibly causing orthostatic hypotension, which increases the risk of falls and possible fractures, as well as anticholinergic reactions; (2) a high-potency drug, in contrast, can intensify the psychomotor disturbance the drug was intended to reduce and create others perhaps even more troublesome. More treatment alternatives for these type of situations are available now than even a decade ago.

B. Neuroleptics

Neuroleptics, which have been used almost exclusively to treat psychotic states, are also useful to manage dangerous or severely disruptive behavior in patients of all ages. They have been the traditional psychopharmacological approach to these disturbances in elderly patients for more than 30 years.

The prescribing principles presented here are based on the results of both controlled and uncontrolled research studies involving more than 5,000 patients. Reviews of clinical findings relating neuroleptic therapy to behavior problems and psychotic symptoms include those of Schneider, Pollock, & Lyness (1990); Phillipson, Moranville, Jeste, & Harris (1990); Devenand, Sackeim, & Mayeux (1988); Small (1988); Wragg & Jeste (1988); Salzman (1987b); Risse & Barnes (1986); Helms (1985); Black, Richelson, & Richardson (1985); and Maletta (1984).

1. Prescribing Guidelines

- Neuroleptics should be used only when behavior is so severely disruptive as to endanger the safety or well-being of the patient or others. Such behavior includes severe agitation, screaming, wandering, assaultiveness, and poor compliance with emergency medical treatment (e.g., as in an intensive care unit). Nonpharmacologic interventions that facilitate the patient's maximal participation within a calm, consistent environment, retain his or her dignity, and impart affection (Mace & Rabins, 1981) should be actively pursued before beginning drug treatment, and should remain a prime part of the patient's regimen if drug treatment becomes necessary in the home or long-term setting.
- In elderly patients for whom neuroleptics are therapeutic, the effects are consistent and reliable. However, for this population, therapeutic efficacy with this class of drugs is only modest, often no better than placebo, and the condition of some patients worsens. Careful and regular monitoring are essential for optimal effect as well as safety.
- Neuroleptics should *not* be used for treatment of anxiety, dysphoria, unhappiness, *or as a routine treatment for the cognitive impairment of dementia.* The frequent use of these drugs (as well as other psychotropics) in nursing homes has caused mounting concern among residents, families, clinicians, and policymakers.
- No data currently suggest that any one neuroleptic is better at controlling agitated behavior or psychotic thinking than any other, given comparable therapeutic doses.
- Selection of any one neuroleptic, or subclass of neuroleptics, in preference to another is guided by the side-effect profile of each drug or drug class in relation to the patient's history or prior drug response (or lack of response) and the nature of concomitant chronic illness and medication.

2. Side Effects

Three types of neuroleptic side effects occur regularly and may be particularly troublesome for the older patients. These are sedation, orthostatic hypotension, and extrapyramidal symptoms (see Table I).

a. Sedation   is almost always an unwanted side-effect, since a sedated confused older person may become more confused and potentially more agitated. Patients receiving neuroleptics with sedating side-effects and sedating medications with anticholinergic properties concomitantly are at particular risk of oversedation. Daytime sedation may lead to nighttime insomnia, accompanied by increased nocturnal agitation, which in turn requires more neuroleptics. Thus, a drug-taking cycle beginning with sedation, followed by agitation, leading to more drug use may be set in motion for some older patients. Low-potency neuroleptics (e.g., chlorpromazine and thioridazine) are associated with clinically significant sedation.

b. Orthostatic hypotension   increases the likelihood of falls, fractures, and in some cases, heart attacks and stroke. Older people are more sensitive to orthostatic hypotension because of reduced CNS baroreceptors that regulate blood pressure and peripheral adrenergic receptors that regulate vasomotor tone. The use of hypotension-inducing drugs such as neuroleptics consequently predisposes the elderly patient to serious risk of falls and fractures. Like sedation, clinically significant hypotension is commonly associated with low-potency neuroleptics.

c. Extrapyramidal symptoms   are caused by blockage of CNS postsynaptic dopamine receptors. High-potency neuroleptics such as haloperidol and fluphenazine

Table I
Side Effects and Dosage of Neuroleptic Drugs

Generic name	Sedation	Hypotension	Extrapyramidal symptoms	Anticholinergic symptoms	Approximate geriatric dosage range mg/day
Chlorpromazine	Marked	Marked	Moderate	Marked	10–300
Chlorprothixene	Marked	Marked	Moderate	Marked	10–300
Thioridazine	Marked	Marked	Mild-moderate	Moderate	10–300
Acetophenazine	Moderate	Moderate	Moderate	Moderate	10–60
Perphenazine	Moderate	Moderate	Moderate	Moderate	4–32
Loxapine	Moderate	Moderate	Moderate	Moderate	5–100
Molindone	Moderate	Moderate	Moderate	Moderate	5–100
Trifluoperazine	Moderate	Moderate	Moderate-marked	Moderate-mild	4–20
Thiothixene	Moderate	Moderate	Moderate-marked	Moderate-mild	4–20
Fluphenazine	Mild	Mild	Marked	Mild	0.25–6
Haloperidol	Mild	Mild	Marked	Mild	0.25–6

strongly block postsynaptic dopamine receptors and thus are very potent inducers of these reactions. Because dopamine decreases with advancing age, extrapyramidal symptoms are more frequent and more severe in older patients. Up to 50% of those older than 60 years have been reported to develop these adverse reactions (Salzman, Shader, & Pearlman, 1970), which may be more common in patients with dementia than in those with schizophrenia or affective psychosis (Salzman, 1982; Lohr & Bracha, 1988). Extrapyramidal symptoms seen frequently in the older group are akathisia and akinesia; dystonic reactions are relatively uncommon.

Akathisia, a motor restlessness, is the most common drug-induced extrapyramidal symptom and is often confused with agitation. When this occurs, clinicians frequently increase rather than decrease the neuroleptic dose, or change to a lower-potency neuroleptic, which leads to another iatrogenic cycle: agitation requires neuroleptic treatment and causes akathisia, which is mistaken for increased agitation, which, in turn, leads to increased neuroleptic dosage. This set of events is complicated by the difficulty in diagnosing confused, demented, or aphasic patients who often cannot describe their subjective experience of muscle tension and restlessness. If akathisia and agitation coexist, diagnosis and treatment are even more difficult, since prescribing a neuroleptic could worsen the akathisia (Peabody *et al.*, 1987).

Clinicians must weight the advantages of low-potency neuroleptics, which produce sedation and orthostatic hypotension but are relatively low inducers of extrapyramidal symptoms, against those of high-potency neuroleptics, which are nonsedating and nonhypotensive but may be strong inducers of these reactions. In general, high-potency neuroleptics are preferred, and their adverse effects are controlled with lower dosage.

d. Tardive dyskinesia   is one of the most severe forms of extrapyramidal disorders, and the relationship between advanced age and increased incidence and severity of the disorder is significant. However, there is no evidence to suggest that older patients taking very low doses of neuroleptics are more likely to suffer tardive dyskinesia than are their younger counterparts. To date, no research data indicate that any one neuroleptic is associated with the development of this adverse reaction, although clinically, tardive dyskinesia is a common result of use of high-potency neuroleptics.

The characteristics of tardive dyskinesia most frequently found in older people are rhythmic movements of mouth and tongue. These symptoms may be only mildly disfiguring and incapacitating but may nonetheless cause embarrassment and increase social isolation. If neuroleptics are discontinued, symptoms often disappear or significantly diminish in severity; if, however, symptoms have been present for years, reduced neuroleptic dose may bring only modest improvement. Grossly irregular movements of the body and limbs are less common. When they do occur in older patients, they are especially burdensome because they occur at a time of life when motor coordination is decreasing and tremor is increasing.

Clinicians are sometimes faced with a severely psychotic or agitated older patient who derives therapeutic results from a neuroleptic but also develops tardive dyskinesia. In such circumstances, making the appropriate decision is difficult—continuing the drug (thereby risking more severe tardive dyskinesia) versus discontinuing the drug or lowering the dose (thereby risking increased psychosis or agitation). For the majority of older patients, nonneuroleptic management of agitation may be possible, but alternative treatment for the psychotic thinking of schizophrenia is not yet available (Salzman, 1990a). Since the most severe dyskinetic symptoms are not usually experienced by very old patients, clinicians usually favor continuing the medication, which should be accompanied by careful and frequent monitoring and reappraisal of symptom severity. Other neuroleptic side-effects are relatively uncommon in older patients, who are no more likely than younger adults to develop reactions such as obstructive jaundice, agranulocytosis, weight gain, skin rashes, or grand mal seizures.

3. Selection of Neuroleptic

In considering the range of neuroleptic side-effects that cause difficulty for the older patient, clinicians must balance the risks and benefits of one type of neuroleptic over another (see Table I). Low-potency agents, which produce sedation and orthostatic hypotension, are relatively less likely to induce extrapyramidal symptoms. Thioridazine, the most commonly selected low-potency compound, is especially useful at bedtime because of its sedating properties. Daytime sedation and orthostatic hypotension can be minimized by the use of very low doses. High-potency neuroleptics are less sedating and cause less orthostatic hypotension, but are very likely to cause extrapyramidal symptoms. Since sedation and hypotension are potentially the more serious complications, high-potency neuroleptics are often preferred; induction of extrapyramidal side-effects can be controlled by using extremely low doses to control agitation and psychosis. Haloperidol, the high-potency compound most frequently used, may be especially useful for older patients whose daytime sedation can interfere with their ability to participate in leisure activities as well as activities of daily living.

Between the very high-potency and very low-potency neuroleptics, many compounds produce moderate sedation, hypotension, and extrapyramidal symptoms. With careful dosage carefully monitored, however, these drugs may be useful for the severely agitated geriatric patient. The relative advantages of high- versus low-potency compounds are found in comparing trifluoperazine and haloperidol for managing behavioral symptoms (Lovett *et al.*, 1987).

4. Dosage

Dose recommendations for elderly patients are presented in Table I. Some older patients who receive neuroleptics in doses suitable for younger adults may experience extreme toxicity, which may be minimized by using extremely low doses. For example, doses of fluphenazine or haloperidol as low as .25 mg, given 1–4 times/day can reduce substantially the number and severity of extrapyramidal side-effects; and thioridazine, in doses of 10 to 25 mg, 2–4 times a day, can reduce the degree of severity of sedation and orthostatic hypotension. In order to achieve these low doses, liquid preparations may be dissolved in a beverage.

C. Treatment with Nonneuroleptics

Neuroleptic drugs may be therapeutically inadequate for managing the behavior of some geriatric patients; for others, they may produce severe, unwanted toxicity. A promising new area of geriatric psychopharmacology focuses on nonneuroleptic strategies to control severe agitation and psychosis. A recent systematic review of nonneuroleptic treatment concludes that very little published empirical evidence exists for the use of these medications for elderly demented patients (Salzman, in press), although a growing body of clinical experience and anecdotal reports (summarized in Salzman, 1990a) suggest that drugs such as beta blockers, trazodone, anticonvulsants, lithium, and buspirone may aid in managing a variety of agitated behaviors refractory to more conventional treatment.

1. Beta Blockers

Beta-blocking agents such as propranolol, in lose doses (10–100 mg/day) are sometimes modestly helpful in reducing agitated and assaultive behavior in some patients, particularly when produced in some patients by dementia or other organic impairments (Yudofsky, Williams, & Gorman, 1981). On the one hand, however, lack of specific information on the efficacy of propranolol in elderly demented patients points to its role as an alternative for patients who cannot tolerate or respond to other treatments (Risse & Barnes, 1986). On the other hand, reports of recent clinical cases in which traditional drug treatment failed provide evidence of efficacy with no adverse effects (Weiler, Mungao, & Bernick, 1988). These drugs can be given only to elderly patients who are free of cardiovascular disorder and chronic obstructive pulmonary disease (particularly asthma). Side-effects include sedation, orthostatic hypotension, and decreased cardiac output. Extra pyramidal symptoms do not occur because dopamine neurotransmission is unaffected by beta blockers.

2. Trazodone

The antidepressant drug trazodone has been reported as an effective treatment for agitation and severely disruptive behavior (Simpson & Foster, 1986; Tingle, 1986; Greenwald, Marin, & Silverman, 1986; Pinner & Rich, 1988). Although no double-blind studies, to date, compare this drug with placebo or with neuroleptics, rapidly increasing clinical experience suggests that it is effective in doses of 50–200 mg/day, with few side-effects other than sedation.

3. Carbamazepine and Lithium Carbonate

Both lithium carbonate and carbamazepine are used to treat mania in nongeriatric adults. In doses of 50 to 200 mg/day, carbamazepine can also control chronic disruptive behavior and agitation in older patients, particularly those suffering from dementia (Leibovici & Tariot, 1988). Other anticonvulsants have not been studied. Like carbamazepine, lithium carbonate is sometimes useful in managing disruptive behavior (Holton & George, 1985). The therapeutic range is 150–600 mg, in divided doses. Because each of these drugs may produce neurotoxicity characterized by increased agitation, confusion, and disorientation, the lowest possible therapeutic dosage of both is recommended, and each should be discontinued if behavior worsens. The agitation-reducing properties of both carbamazepine and lithium, however, are not as effective as neuroleptics, beta blockers, or trazodone.

4. Buspirone

Case reports differ regarding this nonbenzodiazepine antianxiety agent with mild dopamine-blocking properties. In one instance, it has been reported effective in controlling disruptive behavior in older patients (Colenda, 1988); in another, oral dyskinesia developed in an elderly demented patient and persisted for at least 4 months after symptom onset (Strauss, 1988). As yet, research studies have not compared its effect with that of placebo or other drugs for treating agitation. The average dose is $2\frac{1}{2}$–5 mg, 2–4 times/day; side-effects are reported to be relatively mild.

D. New Research Directions

The most promising of a new subclass of neuroleptic drugs currently being synthesized and tested in human subjects is clozapine, which became available for clinical use in the United States in February of 1990. This low-potency neuroleptic resembles thioridazine in some ways, frequently producing side-effects of sedation and orthostatic hypotension. However, its pharmacological activity on dopamine neurotransmission is distinctly different, resulting in unusual efficacy for some treatment-resistant schizophrenic patients (Green & Salzman, 1990; Tamminga & Gerlach, 1987). Although studies of clozapine to date have not focused specifically on the older psychotic or agitated patient, the unusually salutary pharmacotherapeutic effects of this neuroleptic in chronically psychotic adults may lead to the pharmacological development of useful compounds for elderly patients.

Another fruitful ongoing research area is the study of nonneuroleptic drugs in addition to beta blockers, anticonvulsants, and lithium for the treatment of severely agitated behavior. Because the use of trazodone and buspirone to decrease later-life agitation raises challenging research questions regarding the role of serotonin in decreasing disruptive behaviors, the search for new, nontoxic serotonergic drugs with antiagitation effects has accelerated. Current clinical experience suggesting that the antidepressant fluoxetine has some antiagitation properties further stimulates this line of research.

V. Treatment of Depression _____

Depression is the most common psychiatric illness found in the older population (Blazer & Williams, 1980). Prevalence rates of depressive disorders in older people reach 20% for major depression and are even higher for milder forms. Suicide rates among depressed elders are particularly high (Alexopoulos, Young, Meyers, Abrams, & Shamoian, 1988). Recent research points to the high prevalence of diagnosed major depression in nursing homes and the unusually high mortality (from causes other than suicide) of persons so diagnosed (Rovner et al., 1991).

Reviews of psychopharmacologic treatment of depression include those of Salzman (1990b); Gerson, Plotkin, & Jarvik (1988); Rockwell, Lam, & Zisook (1988); and Peabody, Whiteford, & Hollister (1986).

A. Diagnostic Concerns

Older people with depressive disorders can present with signs and symptoms similar to those in younger adults, but the types of clinical manifestations that appear with relative frequency in geriatric patients are characterized by anxious, withdrawn, apathetic, symptoms and by preoccupation with fatigue as well as somatic concerns. Depressed patients older than 50 demonstrate more agitation, insomnia, and hypochondriasis than younger cohorts, and those with late-middle to late-life onset have symptoms distinguished by bodily complaints, guilt feelings, suicidal feelings and intent, and fewer family histories of depression (Brown, Sweeney, Loutsch, Koscis, & Frances, 1984).

Although the criteria for major depression in older persons are the same as those for younger adults, patterns of symptom presentation may differ. Major depression in older people must be distinguished from dysthymia or atypical depression, which are usually less severe and do not have all the hallmarks of the more serious disorder. Atypical depression is quite common in older people (Blazer & Williams, 1980); indeed, symptoms suggesting some degree of depressive affective state are so common as to be expectable.

The frequent association of depression with physical disease in older patients may occur as a response to illness or as a part of the clinical picture itself. Some type of depressive reaction to life-threatening illness is not unusual in persons of any age; myocardial infarction or the diagnosis of cancer, for example, predictably produce symptoms of depression.

Many depressed elderly patients, regardless of the form of their disorder, experience impaired cognitive function. Signs and symptoms that mimic or even meet criteria for dementia that accompanies depression include confusion, impaired memory, decreased concentration, mild aphasia, incontinence, and agitation (McAllister, 1983). In many instances, cognitive symptoms are more prominent than signs of depressive illness. The obverse is seen in demented patients who manifest classic depressive symptoms. Indeed, many cases of dementia first present with depressive symptoms.

B. Antidepressants

Before beginning treatment, a comprehensive physical examination is essential. An electrocardiogram is mandatory because of the cardiotoxicity of heterocyclic antidepressants. Since orthostatic hypotension is one of the principal serious side-effects of these drugs, baseline blood pressure reading as well as followup readings at each dosage change are necessary. The clinician should also bear in mind that antidepressants can interact adversely with drugs taken for systemic physical condition (such as hypertension), resulting in either augmented or inhibited therapeutic effect.

1. Heterocyclic Antidepressants

The most frequently used drugs to treat depressive symptoms in all age groups, heterocyclic antidepressants are classified as *tertiary* and *secondary* amines. Secondary amines are demethylated metabolites of tertiary compounds, two of which have been synthesized, marketed, and are in wide use as therapeutic agents. To date, no convincing data suggest the therapeutic superiority of any one compound for the average, depressed older patient. As with selection of neuroleptics, choice is based on the side-effects profile in conjunction with the patient's concomitant illnesses, medications, and prior treatment response.

a. Tertiary amines.   Clinical experience suggests that, as a group, tertiary heterocyclic antidepressants produce the most frequent and intense side-effects: anticholinergic symptoms, sedation, and orthostatic hypotension are particularly severe, compared with effects of other antidepressants given at similar doses. Because occurrence of side-effects depends partially on the individual patient's sensitivity to the drug and partially on dosage, tertiary amines may be relatively nontoxic for an older patient when dosages are reduced appropriately. For example, significant antidepressant results with only mild side-effects have been achieved with doxepin, in doses of 30 to 75 mg/day (Lakshmanan, Mion, & Frengley, 1986).

b. Secondary amines.   The demethylation of tertiary amines results in an active secondary amine metabolite. Two commercially produced, demethylated compounds are now in wide clinical use: nortriptyline (the demethylated metabolite of amitryptyline) and desipramine (the demthylated metabolite of imipramine). Compared with tertiary amines and other secondary amines, nortriptyline and desipramine have the least-toxic side-effect profiles.

The therapeutic dose range for secondary amines varies in older patients. Some respond to very low doses, such as 25–75 mg/day. Others, however, may require doses comparable to those given to younger adults (e.g., 150–250 mg/day). As a general rule, starting doses should be very low (10–25 mg/day), and increments of 10–25 mg should be gradual.

2. Side-Effects

Common side-effects of heterocyclic antidepressants that cause special difficulty for older patients are sedation, orthostatic hypotension, anticholinergic effects, cardiotoxicity, and memory impairment (see Table II). As is the case with neuroleptics, sedation and orthostatic hypotension may be especially hazardous, although the sedating effect of an antidepressant may initially help the older patient fall asleep. Anticholinergic effects, prominent in all heterocyclic antidepressants, frequently cause dry mouth, constipation, blurred vision, and impaired cognition; in men, exacerbation of prostatic hypertrophy can occur.

a. Sedation.   Tertiary amines such as amitriptyline, doxepin, trimipramine, and clomipramine are extremely sedating and should not be used for older patients. Desipramine is an "activating" antidepressant with less-severe sedative side-effects than other heterocyclics and may be helpful for the apathetic, anergic, older patient whose depression is characterized by psychomotor retardation. The activating property, however, can be a liability in older patients in whom it induces insomnia or agitation.

Table II

Relative Side Effects of Cyclic Antidepressants in the Elderly Patient

Drug	Approximate geriatric dosage range mg/day	Sedation	Hypotension	Anticholinergic side effects	Altered cardiac rate and rhythm
Tertiary amines					
Imipramine	10–150	Mild	Moderate	Moderate-Strong	Moderate
Doxepin	10–150	Moderate-Strong	Moderate	Strong	Moderate
Amitriptyline	10–150	Strong	Moderate	Very strong	Strong
Trimipramine	10–150	Strong	Moderate	Strong	Strong
Clomipramine	10–150	Strong	Strong	Strong	Strong
Secondary amines					
Desipramine	10–150	Activating	Mild-Moderate	Mild	Mild
Nortriptyline	10–150	Mild	Mild	Moderate	Mild
Amoxapine	10–150	Mild	Moderate	Moderate	Moderate
Protriptyline	5–15	Activating	Moderate	Strong	Moderate
Maprotiline	10–150	Moderate-Strong	Moderate	Moderate	Mild
Atypical					
Trazodone	25–300	Moderate	Moderate	Mild (except dry mouth)	Mild-Moderate
Fluoxetine	5–20	Activating	None	None	None
Bupropion	50–200	Variable	None	None	None
MAO Inhibitors					
Phenelzine	10–60	Mild	Moderate	Mild	Mild
Tranylcypromine	5–30	Activating	Moderate	Mild	Mild
Stimulants					
Methylphenidate	5–40	Activating	None	None	Mild

b. Orthostatic hypotension.   Because tertiary amines cause orthostatic hypotension they should not be prescribed for elderly patients. The secondary amine nortriptyline produces slightly less orthostatic hypotension than does imipramine (Glassman, Walsh, & Roose, 1982) and is recommended for the older patient with a history of falls, dizziness, stroke, or those for whom a drop in orthostatic blood pressure would be particularly hazardous.

c. Anticholinergic toxicity.   Anticholinergic properties of some heterocyclics may cause side-effects so severe as to limit their therapeutic usefulness: constipation and dry mouth or problems with dentures and eating that can worsen depressive anorexia are not infrequent occurrences. Because desipramine is relatively less anticholinergic than other antidepressants, it is useful for the older patient who is also vulnerable to anticholinergic side-effects or is taking other anticholinergic drugs. (Memory impairment, another anticholinergic reaction, is discussed below.)

d. Cardiotoxicity. This particular side-effect of heterocyclic antidepressants requires constant monitoring because it can occur in elderly patients taking high doses of antidepressants. At high therapeutic plasma levels, heterocyclic antidepressants tend to prolong electrical conduction through the heart, reflected in widening of the QRS complex in the electrocardiogram (ECG). At toxic levels, the QRS exceeds 100 milliseconds, resulting in possible heart block, ventricular arrhythmias, and sudden death. The ECG is sensitive to the cardiotoxic properties of antidepressants and is thus a useful guide to dosage for elderly patients. If the QRS does not widen, the patient's doses may be increased gradually, as needed, to achieve therapeutic effect; if the QRS begins to widen, dosage increase is contraindicated (Salzman, 1985).

The metabolism of both tertiary and secondary amine heterocyclic antidepressants in the liver produces a water-soluble hydroxy metabolite, which, until recently, was assumed to be either inactive or only very slightly active. Further research, however, suggests that these metabolites are potentially cardiotoxic (Young *et al.,* 1985). Their water-soluble properties and the reduced ability of the aging renal system to excrete can lead to higher blood levels in older patients and consequent increased cardiotoxic risk. Because laboratory measures of heterocyclic antidepressant blood levels do not include this metabolite, clinicians cannot gauge the potential for toxic cardiac effect by routine blood-level studies. The ECG, however, provides a reliable guide to impending toxicity.

e. Impaired memory function, a side effect of heterocyclic antidepressants to which older patients are sensitive (Branconnier, DeVitt, Cole, & Spera, 1982; Branconnier & Coles, 1981; Mattila, Liljequist, & Seppala, 1978; Liljequist, Linnoila, & Mattilla, 1974), is presumed secondary to the drug's anticholinergic activity. Because this effect disrupts short-term memory and recent recall—impairments identical to the decline in memory function that can occur normally with age—older patients taking antidepressant drugs and their prescribing clinicians may mistake drug-related memory impairment for expectable age-related memory decline or even mild cognitive decline. In addition to interfering with memory, anticholinergic effects of heterocyclic drugs can cause other cognitive dysfunction such as disorientation, confusion, and sundowning, as well as personality change.

Depression is a recurrent illness and depressed patients are often maintained on antidepressants to prevent symptom recurrence. Impaired memory function from anticholinergic toxicity is therefore a particular hazard for older patients who take these drugs on a regular maintenance basis.

C. Monoamine Oxidase Inhibitors

For some older patients with atypical depression characterized by withdrawal, lack of motivation, apathy, and lack of energy, monoamine oxidase inhibitors (MAOIs) are both safe and effective, and patients may experience increased energy and concentration as well as mood elevation. Research findings on this class of drugs have been reported by Georgotas, Mann, & Friedman (1981); Georgotas, Friedman, & McCarthy (1983); Georgotas *et al.*, (1986); and Lazarus *et al.*, (1986). Clinical overviews of the use of MAOIs include those of Jenike (1985) and Zisook (1985). Although some clinicians assert that patients with mild dementia may experience increased energy and concentration following MAOI treatment (Jenike, 1985), others hold that patients with moderate to severe dementia may become more agitated (Salzman, 1986). The combination of an MAOI and certain foods (such as cheese containing high amounts of the pressor amine tyramine) or stimulating drugs may lead to hypertension, causing heart attack or stroke.

For most older patients, these drugs are not the first-choice antidepressant for major depression, and increased sensitivity to side-effects may require lower doses (e.g., phenelzine, 15–30 mg/day; tranylcypromine, 10–40 mg/day) than those prescribed for younger adult patients (see Table II). The most frequent side-effect experienced by older patients is severe orthostatic hypotension.

MAOIs can be given only to responsible, compliant elderly patients or to those whose medication is carefully supervised. The high risk of toxic drug interactions resulting from the large average number of drugs prescribed for the geriatric population precludes this drug from being recommended for most older outpatients.

D. Antidepressants with Atypical Structure

This third broad category of antidepressants consists of three drugs: trazodone, fluoxetine, and bupropion (see Table II).

1. Trazodone

The antidepressant effects of trazodone are unpredictable, making it a poor first choice among the various available antidepressants. It is recommended, however, for older patients who have not responded to other compounds, and sometimes can produce surprising therapeutic effects in the previously treatment-resistant older patient. Although it is sedating and can cause orthostatic hypotension (Gerner, Estabrook, Steuer, & Jarvik, 1980), trazodone has minimal anticholinergic properties and does not interfere with memory (Branconnier & Cole, 1981). For these reasons, it is especially useful for the depressed geriatric patient who requires sedation and is extremely sensitive to anticholinergic side-effects. Reduced doses are advisable.

2. Fluoxetine

At usual therapeutic doses, fluoxetine induces neither anticholinergic reactions nor cardiotoxicity (Feighner & Cohn, 1985). It would thus seem to be the ideal drug for treating the depressive symptoms of older patients, although dosage ranges for older patients have not yet been clearly established. Fluoxetine may indeed be especially useful for the older patient with dysthymic disorder characterized by extreme fatigue or lack of motivation, but its very long elimination half-life may limit its usefulness. In some patients, fluoxetine causes nausea, agitation, insomnia, or sedation, but whether older patients are particularly sensitive to these adverse reactions is not known.

3. Bupropion

Bupropion, the third recently released antidepressant with an atypical structure, is effective for elderly patients, although insufficient clinical experience prevents determining which types of late-life depressions may be most appropriately treated with it. Side-effects are moderate, and excessive motor stimulation is common. At high doses, bupropion may be associated with seizures, but no data suggest that elderly patients are more likely than others to experience this adverse effect.

E. Psychomotor Stimulants

Some older patients complain of diminished energy, fatigue, and loss of motivation, initiative, and pleasure. Since they may not have symptoms characteristic of major depression, antidepressant drugs are not always therapeutic. Furthermore, clinical experience suggests that antidepressants prescribed for these patients may produce serious side-effects. When an older person develops symptoms of apathy, anergia, and anhedonia, the judicious use of a psychomotor stimulant (such as methylphenidate) may restore interest, energy, and pleasure without inducing side-effects. The daily dosage range of methylphenidate is quite broad (from 2.5 to 30 mg).

F. New Research Directions

Recent experience with fluoxetine, a selective serotonin reuptake-blocking drug, as well as research experience with selective MAOIs, suggests that future development of antidepressants will focus on compounds with selective rather than broad ranges of activity. In addition, the role of neurohormones, such as the corticotropin-releasing factor (CRF) and thyroid hormones in depression, has come under recent scrutiny. Exploration of the relationship between age-associated neurotransmitter dysfunction and the antidepressant effects of these hormones may prove particularly useful for older patients.

VI. Treatment of Mania

Mania rarely appears for the first time in late life. With advancing years, episodes occur more frequently, become more severe, and are more difficult to treat. Lithium is the primary treatment and prophylaxis for the mania of elderly patients, as it is for younger adults. Older patients are more sensitive to its effects, however, and the side-effect profile differs from that of younger patients. Reviews of lithium effects in older patients include those of Liptzin (in press), Stone (1989), Jefferson, Griest, Ackerman, & Carroll (1987), and Glasser & Rabins (1984).

Reduced renal clearance leads to accumulation of lithium and increased plasma levels in elders more readily than in younger adults taking the same dosage. In addition, because the CNS of many older patients seems to be more sensitive to the effects of this drug, therapeutic as well as toxic effects develop at lower doses and lower plasma levels. For these pharmacodynamic and pharmacokinetic reasons, therapeutic plasma levels for older manic patients may be as low as .2–.6 MEq/liter, in contrast to .8–1.2 for younger adults. The daily dose necessary to achieve lower blood levels may vary among older patients. As a general rule, starting lithium doses should be low (e.g., 150–450 mg/day), and dosage increments of 150–300 mg should be gradual.

The toxic profile of lithium in older persons differs in several important aspects from that of younger patients. Tremor and gastrointestinal upset occur in all age groups as side-effects. In older patients, however, the first, and often the most prominent, side-effects consist of a spectrum of neurotoxic symptoms. Subtle but progressive impairment of recent recall (anterograde amnesia), disorientation, aphasia, and irritability may appear as the first signs of excessive lithium dosage. This presents a double hazard: overdose and inaccurate interpretation of symptoms of cognitive impairment. Movement disorders are also early signs of toxicity, particularly irregular gait, decreased coordination, and dysarthria. Impaired consciousness may also develop at blood levels considered therapeutic in younger adults.

Reduced ability to clear lithium, increased receptor sensitivity, and heightened neurotoxicity suggest the use of lower lithium doses for older patients, in general. However, it is important to recognize that some older manic patients, particularly those with other psychiatric illness, sometimes require doses and blood levels equivalent to those needed by younger patients. Selecting the optimal therapeutic lithium dosage and blood level for any particular elderly patient, therefore, should be based on that patient's symptom profile and response to lithium, rather than on specific blood level.

VII. Treatment of Anxiety

When anxiety interferes with an older person's ability to cope with life or obtain pleasure, or when symptoms of anxiety become incapacitating, treatment is necessary. Treatment of the anxious older patient is usually limited to sympatomatic relief rather than to psychotherapeutic exploration of underlying psychic predispositions or causes. As a general principle, treatment should not be undertaken until symptoms have been thoroughly appraised. Physical illness, medications, or other nonpsychological causes of anxiety symptoms should be investigated, as well as coexisting depression.

A. Diagnostic Considerations

In older patients, symptoms of anxiety are not so clearly defined as in younger adults. Clinically significant anxiety symptoms commonly occur in states of depression and dementia, as well as secondary to physical illness or as a result of drug treatment.

In some cases, evaluation of anxiety in older persons reveals realistic needs and lack of resources that may suggest psychosocial intervention rather than pharmacotherapy. When anxiety is related to a clear precipitant, identification and clarification of this problem and discussion of alternative coping strategies may be sufficient treatment. If these approaches are ineffective, or if anxiety symptoms are incapacitating, interfere with function, or worsen other illness, antianxiety drugs may be an effective part of an overall treatment program. A decision to treat is often made for older patients who are in acute crisis (e.g., hospitalization, grief reaction, change in living circumstances) or for patients with long-standing characterological or personality disorders that have been responsive to antianxiety treatment.

Panic–phobic anxiety disorder does occur in older persons but is less prevalent than in younger adults and is often associated with physical illness and concomitant psychiatric disorder (Sheikh, 1990). There are no research studies or clinical reports describing the treatment of panic–phobic symptoms in older persons. Lacking specific guidelines for elderly patients, treatment approaches should follow those used for their younger counterparts. Drugs used for panic and phobic anxiety symptoms include high-potency benzodiazepines (alprazolam and clonazepam) and antidepressants. General recommendations regarding doses and guidelines for toxicity of these drugs are applicable for the treatment of panic and phobic anxiety symptoms.

Reviews of the pharmacologic treatment of anxiety in elders include those of Salzman (1990c), Hershey & Kim (1988), and Allen (1986).

B. Benzodiazepines

Among the most widely used drugs in the world, benzodiazepines are useful for the majority of elderly patients who require drugs as a treatment component for anxiety. They are used extensively in nursing homes to treat agitation and sleep disorders, as described by the clinical research of Pinsker & Suljaga-Petchel (1984) and Koepke, Gold, Linden, Lion, & Rickels (1982), Buck (1988), Beers et al. (1988), Beardsley et al., (1989). Several of these studies are critical of the basis for prescribing these (as well as other) psychotropic drugs for institutionalized elders. Objections include lack of documented mental health symptoms, concurrent use of different drug classes, insufficient monitoring, and seeming ignorance or indifference to possible harmful drug interactions.

Chronic benzodiazepine use is not unusual in older people. Daily use is common in older patients who are suffering from medical disorders, are in pain, or may be depressed. Chronic use may be inappropriate, however, and may lead to overuse and dependence. Clinical experience indicates that older patients are often reluctant to discontinue benzodiazepine treatment, even when the criteria for drug use are no longer present; physiological as well as psychological dependence leads to difficulty in relinquishing their use. Withdrawal reactions may include gastrointestinal upset, tremor, and agitation; seizures upon withdrawal have been reported but are unusual, occurring after abrupt cessation of very high dosages (APA Task Force, 1990).

Benzodiazepines are CNS sedatives. When prescribed for the older person together with other CNS sedatives (such as hypnotics, analgesics, alcohol, narcotics, and/or some antidepressants and neuroleptics), the combination is likely to produce confusion, memory loss, or disorientation.

1. Side-Effects

A very large and consistent literature documents the toxic effects of benzodiazepines in elderly patients (APA Task Force, 1990; Cook, Huggett, Graham-Pole, Savage, & James (1983); Ellinwood & Nikaido, 1987; Lucki, Rickels, & Gelber (1987); Pomara et al., (1985); Pomara, Deptula, Singh, & Monroy (1990). Four types of toxicity occur frequently in older persons at doses lower than in younger adults: sedation, ataxia, and falls, psychomotor slowing, and cognitive impairment (APA Task Force, 1990).

a. Sedation may be helpful at bedtime, but during the day it can impair function, and chronically sedated older people may become increasingly confused, belligerent, and agitated. Sedation also contributes to falls, psychomotor slowing, and some cognitive impairment.

b. Ataxia and falls as well as other signs of neuromuscular dyscoordination such as dysarthria and unsteadiness, obviously handicap older people, many of whom already have tremor or coordination difficulties arising from neurological disease. Evidence also points to increased risk and incidence of falls and consequent fractures associated with benzodiazepine use in the elderly (Hale, Stewart, & Marks, 1985; Rashi & Logan, 1986; Ray, Griffin, Schaffner, Baugh, & Melton, 1987).

c. Psychomotor slowing in the older patient is characterized by slowed reaction time, diminished accuracy in accomplishing motoric tasks, and impaired hand–eye coordination. Although only limited data document the toxic effect of benzodiazepines on driving skills in older persons, clinical experiences suggest that they may be more prone to benzodiazepine-impaired driving skills.

d. Cognitive impairment from benzodiazepine use is characterized by an anterograde amnesia, diminished short-term recall, increased forgetfulness, and decreased attention—all of which may resemble the early stages of a dementing illness. Some cognitively impaired older patients who take benzodiazepines for long periods may actually experience progressive benzodiazepine-induced cognitive toxicity, in addition to their neurologically induced cognitive dysfunction. Although the symptoms of organic brain disorders (such as Alzheimer's disease) are not reversible, benzodiazepine discontinuance may be associated with improved memory, reduced tension, and heightened concentration in these patients, as well as in persons with less or no cognitive impairment. For patients who are demented, it is possible to distinguish between two causes of symptom severity: that resulting from a dementing process and that resulting from the toxic effects of benzodiazepines (Salzman et al., in press).

2. Long Half-Life Benzodiazepines

This group of benzodiazepines undergoes complicated hepatic metabolism. Because these drugs have a long elimination half-life and, like heterocyclic antidepressants, produce active metabolites, their use can lead to build-up of potentially toxic substances. For these pharmacokinetic reasons, long half-life benzodiazepines (chlordiazepoxide, diazepam, chlorazepate, prazepam, halazepam, clonazepam, flurazepam) are not recommended for elderly patients.

3. Short Half-Life Benzodiazepines

This group of benzodiazepines (oxazepam, lorazepam, alprazolam, temazepam, triazolam) is preferred for older patients because the aging process does not interfere with their elimination from the body (Greenblatt & Shader, 1990). However, their use predisposes the older patient to a risk of discontinuance symptoms. As yet, no comparative data suggest that older patients, as a group, are more likely than young adults to develop these symptoms (APA Task Force, 1990). Clinical experience, however, suggests that some older patients are frightened by some of their withdrawal symptoms and consequently reluctant to discontinue their medication. This is especially true of benzodiazepine hypnotics, often used on a chronic, nightly basis for older nursing-home residents. When these drugs are discontinued, the rebound insomnia that commonly develops is so upset-

Table III

Antianxiety and Hypnotic Drugs

Generic name	Brand name	Usual geriatric dose range mg/day	Elimination half-life
Benzodiazepines (Short Half-life)			
Triazolam	Halcion	0.125–1	Very short
Oxazepam	Serax	10–60	Short
Temazepam	Restoril	15–60	Short
Lorazepam	Ativan	0.5–4	Short
Alprazolam	Xanax	0.25–2	Medium
Benzodiazepines (Long Half-life)			
Chlordiazepoxide	Librium	10–100	Long
Diazepam	Valium	2–30	Long
Clorazepate	Tranxene	3.75–15	Long
Halazepam	Paxipam	10–40	Long
Quazepam	Doral	7.5–15	Long
Flurazepam	Dalmane	15–60	Very Long
Clonazepam	Klonopin	0.125–0.5	Very Long
Barbiturates		Not recommended	
Antihistamines			
Diphenhydramine	Benedryl	25–100	Moderate
Chloral hydrate	Noctec	250–1000	Long

ting to most older people that they insist on returning to treatment with benzodiazepines despite toxic symptoms. Doses of short half-life benzodiazepines for older patients should be one third to one half the dosage given to younger adults.

C. Other Anxiolytic Drugs

Several classes of drugs other than benzodiazpines are also used to treat anxiety in older patients, although their use is less frequent and entails less-predictable response. These include buspirone, beta blockers, antidepressants, and neuroleptics. A recent report suggests that meprobamate, a potentially toxic anxiolytic, is still used by some elderly patients (Hale, May, Moore, & Stewart, 1988).

1. Buspirone

This nonbenzodiazepine anxiolytic produces unreliable antianxiety effects. Although research data suggest that it is as effective as benzodiazepines (Napoliello, 1986), limited clinical experience does not bear this out. Because clinical experience is relatively scant, recommendations for when it is indicated or contraindicated remain tentative. Case reports describing the use of buspirone for controlling severe agitation, disruptive behavior, and dementia differ; one report is positive (Colenda, 1988), another, negative (Strauss, 1988).

2. Beta Blockers

Although these compounds may substantially improve agitation and disruptive behavior in older patients, there have been no clinical trials using them in anxious elderly outpatients. The salutary effect of beta blockers in reducing autonomic symptoms associated with anxiety (e.g., sweating, tachycardia, palpitations) are well known in younger adults. However, research data, or even clinical reports, on their use in controlling these symptoms in anxious outpatients does not exist.

3. Antidepressants

Anecdotal reports suggest that antidepressants are effective in treating anxiety in young-adult outpatients, as well as in controlling panic disorder. Like beta blockers, however, neither research data nor published clinical experience on the use of either tricyclic antidepressants or MAOIs to treat anxiety in older people exists. Since anxiety and depression commonly coexist in older patients, antidepressants may have a special use in such mixed-symptom clinical pictures. However, no data suggest that antidepressants are especially useful for such patients, or more useful than single-drug antianxiety treatment with benzodiazepines. Furthermore, since the side-effects of antidepressants can be profound in older patients, the use of these drugs as routine antianxiety agents is not recommended.

D. Prescribing Guidelines for Anxiolytic Drugs for Older Patients

- Benzodiazepines and other drugs with antianxiety effects should be prescribed only when the patient's clinical condition warrants their use. Whenever possible, they should be used only for brief periods.
- Benzodiazepine toxicity is more frequent and more severe in older patients, regardless of the individual drug employed. They are more sensitive to sedation and dyscoordination effects as well as to effects of memory impairment, confusion, and disorientation.
- Long-term maintenance benzodiazepines and other anxiolytics should be limited to elderly patients who have demonstrated need for chronic treatment. In most cases, such patients have chronic physical or emotional illness.
- Chronic use of Benzodiazepines and other anxiolytics should be monitored frequently. These drugs should *not* be prescribed chronically for older patients when non-compliance or adverse drug interaction may interfere with their appropriate pharmacotherapeutic action.
- Short half-life benzodiazepines are the preferred psychotropic drug treatment for most older patients with anxiety.

E. New Research Directions

With the discovery of the anxiolytic properties of buspirone, future efforts will focus on other compounds of this azapyrone chemical class. Since these drugs affect serotonin receptors as part of their pharmacologic profile, other serotonergic drugs will be studied as potential anxiolytics for the elderly.

New research will also increase understanding of how neurotransmitters, receptors, and gene transmission contribute to anxiety and anxiety-related disorders such as panic and phobic anxiety. These advances, in turn, will facilitate the development of more specific anxiolytic drugs as well as other anxiety-reducing strategies that may affect older people.

VIII. Treatment of Sleep Disorders

Disordered sleep is not uncommon in older patients, due to normal age-related alteration in sleep patterns as well as to prevalent chronic pathologic conditions that interfere with sleep. These include respiratory distress (particularly sleep apnea), pain (especially from arthritis), drug toxicity, and depression. Before beginning a course of psychotropic drug use to treat sleep disturbance, a careful diagnostic evaluation of its etiology is mandatory.

A. Diagnostic Considerations

Complaints of disturbed sleep are most often described by older patients who awaken several times during the course of the night or in the early morning. When sleep is neither restful nor refreshing, daytime sleepiness takes the form of frequent daytime naps (to "make up" for sleep lost the night before), which, in turn, interfere with nighttime sleep—a cycle difficult to break. Strategies and regimens designed to prepare the body for sleep can sometimes lead to more restful, satisfying results. These include proper nutrition, daytime exercise, sleeping only in bed, going to sleep at the same time every night, and avoiding daytime naps.

Many psychotropic drugs (particularly sedative–hypnotics) and medications for physical illness (e.g., narcotics) have sedative properties that may interfere with normal sleep. Alcohol is also a well-known sleep disrupter; encouraging limits to or abstinence from alcohol may actually improve sleep, contrary to some long-held and deeply ingrained beliefs about its usefulness as a sedative. Stimulating drugs, such as some antidepressants, steroids, or thyroid hormone preparations, invariably interfere with sleep onset and duration. Pain and impaired respiration are medical conditions that frequently disrupt the sleep of older patients. Palliative treatment of such underlying physical disorders may help improve sleep.

Depression is usually associated with disturbed sleep, but early morning awakening may be a misleading symptom in older people, if an earlier rising hour represents age-related changes in the circadian cycle. Nonetheless, considering depression as a common cause of disturbed sleep in elderly persons is important, since vigorous antidepressant treatment may help improve sleep as well as depression.

B. Selection of Drug

Benzodiazepines are often used to treat the impaired sleep of elderly patients during brief hospitalization for medical or surgical treatment. Nonbenzodiazepine drugs are also sometimes used to treat sleep disturbances. Selection of a particular drug to alleviate sleep problems (like the selection of an antianxiety drug) is guided by the drug's pharmacokinetic properties, its side-effect profile, the patient's medical and emotional health, and the patient's history of prior sedative–hypnotic use. Reviews of psychotropic drugs to treat sleep disorders in older patients include those of Regestein (in press), Scharf & Jennings (1990), and Prinz, Vitiello, Raskind, & Thorpy (1990).

1. Benzodiazepines

Three benzodiazepines—flurazepam, temazepam, and triazolam—are used frequently for hypnotic purposes (Allen 1986; Gaillard, 1987; Regestein, in press). Flurazepam has an unusually long elimination half-life, which is further prolonged by the aging renal system's reduced capacity to clear active metabolites. This may produce unwanted daytime sedation in frail elders, particularly at higher doses. Temazepam has a short half-life but a slow onset of action. Triazolam, which has a very short half-life and no active metabolites, is an ideal benzodiazepine from the pharmacokinetic perspective. Unfortunately, its prolonged use may be associated with early-morning awakening (Kales, Soldatos, Bixler, & Kales, 1983), impaired memory, and strong drug dependence (APA Task Force, 1990). For these reasons, brief-duration use is recommended.

No current data support the therapeutic effectiveness of these drugs beyond 1 month, although surveys of nursing-home drug-prescription patterns indicate that long-term use is not unusual (Beardsley *et al.*, 1989; Beers *et al.*, 1988; Buck, 1988; Pinsker & Suljaga-Petchel, 1984;). Older residents of nursing homes themselves often believe that these drugs aid their sleep, and they are extremely reluctant to terminate their use. Preliminary data as well as clinical experience suggest that chronic use of benzodiazepine hypnotics may be associated with exacerbation of impaired cognitive function in older nursing-home residents, particularly those already suffering from mild and moderate dementia (Salzman *et al.*, 1990).

Clinicians therefore must weigh carefully the risks and benefits of the use of benzodiazepines as hypnotics on a regular basis. For some patients, long-term nightly use may be justified by chronic lack of sleep and the patient's perception of therapeutic efficacy. In patients with impaired cognition, disorientation, confusion, and socially inappropriate behavior, however, regular nightly use is not justified. For others, a good night's sleep may outweigh the risk of entailing some memory–cognitive loss.

2. Other Sedative Hypnotics

Other classes of psychotropic drugs are sometimes given to older patients to induce sleep. Sedating neuroleptics such as thioridazine in low doses or antidepressants with sedative side-effects such as trazodone and doxepin may be beneficial, particularly for the psychotic, demented, or disruptive older patient. Clinicians should keep in mind, however, that the use of these drugs is associated with the potential for anticholinergic, hypotensive, and cardiac side-effects. Barbiturates and nonbarbiturate hypnotics should not be given to older patients.

C. Prescribing Principles

The following guidelines are suggested for sleep disturbances:

- Whenever possible, avoid using drugs to induce sleep in older patients.
- If drug treatment of insomnia is deemed necessary, short half-life benzodiazepines are the preferred class of compounds in low doses.
- Brief or short-term use is preferable to long-term chronic nightly use.

IX. Treatment of Memory Loss and Cognitive Dysfunction _____

A. Diagnostic Considerations

Memory loss and cognitive decline are commonly associated with advanced age; virtually all people begin to experience forgetfulness in late middle age that gradually increases as age advances. Commonly manifest as forgetting names and recently acquired information (a book recently read or a movie seen), and inability to find the right word, this type of memory loss worries all who experience it. For most people, *age-associated memory impairment* does not signify pathologic CNS dysfunction. For others, however, initial forgetfulness progressively worsens to encompass significant decrements in all cognitive spheres—attention, orientation, ability to concentrate and to recognize people and objects, to speak coherently or comprehend spoken messages, as well as loss of short-term and long-term memory. Clinical overviews of the diagnosis and treatment of memory loss include those of Foster & Martin (1990), Crook, (1989), and Rosebush & Salzman (1988).

Just behind and sometimes in tandem with memory loss, behavior often deteriorates; extreme and irrational irritability and rage, agitation, psychotic thinking, extremely labile affect, and assaultiveness are frequent behavioral accompaniments of cognitive decline. This progressive deterioration of memory and other associated functions signifies presence of dementia, for which no clinically reliable treatments are currently available. Clinical assessment of functional performance (physical and psychological) in relation to cognitive decline is critical for sound diagnosis, prognosis, and treatment for older people, particularly when dementia is suspected or established (Reisberg, in press, Reisberg *et al.*, 1987).

In a recent assessment of clinically diagnosed demented patients in a U.S. community, over 10% of persons older than 65 years had "probable Alzheimer's disease" (Evans *et al.*, 1989). As the size of the elderly population increases, the prevalence of dementia will rise, as will the demand on clinicians, families, facilities, and society to deliver appropriate services.

B. Experimental Treatment Approaches

Numerous drugs and techniques have been studied; comprehensive reviews of the research described below include those of Tariot (in press), Crook, Johnson, & Larrabee (1990), and Gamzu & Gracon (1988). Early psychotropic drug-treatment strategies for dementia were based on theories of inadequate brain oxygenation or insufficient blood supply hyperbaric oxygen, anticoagulants, and other drugs that could presumably enhance the supply of brain nutrients (such as amino acid precursors and biogenic amine stimulants) were tried, but without success. The hypothesis that impaired cognition in dementia results from diminished CNS cellular metabolism led to tests of a large number of drugs that presumably enhanced metabolism, such as papaverine, procaine, cyclandelate, vincamine, isoxsuprine, cinnazerine, centrophenoxine. Although hydergine has been studied for more than 20 years and was once a widely prescribed drug in Europe and the United States for late-life memory loss, recent evidence shows only questionable efficacy (Thompson *et al.*, 1990).

A second treatment strategy focused on noötropics [from the Greek *noös* (mind) and *tropein* (toward)]. Thought to alter the genetic function of neuronal cells, these drugs (piracetam is one example) improve learned behavior somewhat in animals and invertebrates. In humans, however, therapeutic efficacy has been limited (Tariot, in press).

A third approach attempts to enhance the function of biogenic amines (norepinephrine, dopamine, serotonin). Although drugs such as clonidine, guanfacine, minaprine, L-tryptophan, bromocriptine, amantadine, memantine, and lysuride have been studied, each has had little meaningful efficacy (Tariot, in press). The modest beneficial effect of L-de-prenyl, a selective MAOI, in treating memory loss suggests a possible role for these drugs in treating the memory dysfunction of dementia (Tariot *et al.*, 1988).

One current research trend focuses on peptides—e.g., vasointestinal peptide, vas-opressin, and ACTH fragments. Many studies in this area indicate modest, unpredictable improvement with these substances, and exploration of their potential clinical utility continues.

An important and active area of current investigation for the psychotropic treatment of age-related memory and cognitive loss focuses on CNS acetylcholine neurotransmission. The central role of acetylcholine in memory function has been known for many years. Psychotropic drugs with anticholinergic properties (e.g., neuroleptics and heterocyclic antidepressants) reduce the efficiency of this neurotransmitter and markedly impair cog-nitive function in late life. The enzyme that transforms the dietary amino acid choline into the neurotransmitter acetylcholine diminishes during the course of the aging process. It is virtually absent from some parts of the brain in persons with Alzheimer's disease. These observations prompted development of cholinergic-enhancing strategies to treat memory loss. [History and documentation of this research focus are found in Bartus, Dean, Pontecorvo & Flicker, 1985; Coyle, Price, & DeLong, 1983; Davies & Wolozin, 1987; Tariot (in press), Whitehouse, 1987].

One such strategy attempts to increase acetylcholine precursors by increasing dietary intake of lecithin or phosphatidylcholine, but research has not yet yielded results that are reliable or sufficiently therapeutic (Little, Levy, Chuaqui-Kidd, & Hand, 1985). Attempts to inhibit the enzyme that metabolizes acetylcholine (acetylcholinesterase) have been somewhat more successful. Cholinesterase inhibitors such as physostigmine actually do increase cognitive function, although their effect is brief (Jenike, Albert, Heller, Gunther, & Goff, 1990; Stern, Sano, & Mayeux, 1988). The limited success of these studies prompted attempts to develop more long-lasting acetylcholine enhancers. Study results of cholinergic enhancers such as arecoline (Tariot *et al.*, 1988) and tetrahydroaminocrine (THA) (Kumar & Becker, 1989) have also supported the cholinergic-enhancing strategy, although the clinical utility of these approaches for age-associated memory impairment or for dementia remains questionable. Study of cholinergic precursors, some in combination with agents that enhance oxidative metabolism of neuronal tissue, will continue, and cholinergic substances such as acetyl-1-cannitine and long-acting physostigmine and re-lated cholinesterase inhibitors are likely to be the focus of future research efforts (Tariot, in press).

Future research to treat memory and cognitive disorders will build on the most promis-ing results of earlier work. Continued efforts will explore cholinergic peptides such as arginine vasopressin and ACTH fragments. Other peptides and hormones, such as melanocyte-stimulating hormone (MSH), growth hormone (GH), and endorphins are now being studied, as well as peptides such as the opiate antagonist melanocyte-inhibiting factor (MIF-1) and oxytocin. Studies are currently in progress of drugs that selectively enhance biogenic amines, such as the serotonin-reuptake inhibitor nicergoline and selec-tive MAOIs (cites). Drugs that affect neuronal-membrane function (e.g., phos-phatidylserine) or inhibit free radicals that destroy neurones, such as *N*-methyl-D-aspartate

(NMDA) receptor antagonists, *Gingko Biloba,* and nimodipine are also active areas of present and future inquiry. Finally, drugs that alter calcium channel function such as calcium channel blockers, or agents that block the build-up of calcium-activated "calpains" (proteins found in the brains of demented patients) have generated new research interest.

Memory function and other cognitive processes are complex, and attempts at single-treatment approaches to reverse dysfunction are probably too simplistic. At this stage of inquiry, research therefore aims at increased understanding of the CNS function implicated in impaired cognition. Effective therapeutic interventions will emerge when the knowledge base is broader, more specific, and capable of delineating the relationship among critical pathophysiological and neurochemical elements of cognitive processes.

X. Summary and Conclusions

Psychotropic drugs can benefit the older patient in acute emotional crisis or suffering from chronic recurrent symptoms of severe mental distress that cannot be alleviated solely by other interventions. Regardless of the symptoms being treated or the class of drug used, sound psychotropic treatment may be guided by the basic principles delineated in this chapter and summarized here.

- Careful review of the patient's current physical illness and medication regimen as part of the diagnostic process is mandatory when beginning treatment.
- The concomitant medication for physical illness that is almost inevitable for older patients may interact adversely with psychotropic drugs.
- Older patients are more likely to develop toxic effects from psychotropic drugs, even at doses and blood levels usually considered nontoxic in younger adults.
- The older patient's greater sensitivity to psychotropic drug effects, due to age-related CNS changes (pharmocodynamics), and the tendency of psychotropic drugs to exert greater effect for longer periods, due to age-related changes that alter drug disposition (pharmacokinetics), signify the need for lower starting doses and lower therapeutic and maintenance doses in order to avoid toxicity.
- Psychotropics should be used with caution, after other interventions prove ineffective.
- Close contact and frequent meetings with the older patient under treatment should be routine to assure optimal compliance and to monitor effects and reactions.

Despite the potential for mistreatment due to overdosing and the need to guard against it, it is important to emphasize that older patients suffering from emotional disorders are sometimes undermedicated for fear of producing toxicity. The geriatric psychopharmacology maxim, "Start low, go slow," is relevant and important, but most experienced clinicians would now add, "but don't quit." Underdosing and undertreating an older patient in distress may prolong symptoms and expose that person to side-effects without benefit of therapeutic response.

Supporting all treatment practice is the fact that older people, as a group, are the most heterogeneous in the population. Although principles of treatment for the "elderly" as a whole can be valid, sound clinical care requires that each patient be considered individually to account for unique symptom presentation, clinical picture, and medication response.

Some clinical emphases governing the clinician's rational use of psychotropic drugs outlined in this chapter become evident: choose drug treatment when all other treatment modes prove ineffective; be familiar with age-related changes intrinsic to psychotropic side-effects; appreciate the great diversity of the elderly population; and recognize the cautions necessary for safe psychotropic drug use when it is needed. Given what may appear to be considerable exceptions and proscriptions (particularly with regard to hazards and cautions), what, then, guides sound prescription?

First, alternatives to first-choice treatments are not appropriate in all circumstances and for all emotional disorders. For example, psychopharmacologic strategies for treating sleep disturbance and for alleviating the distress of the psychotic suicidally depressed elder will be vastly different, as will interventions for the chronically anxious person and the agitated person with moderate to severe dementia. Second, psychotropic treatment *can* aid emotionally disturbed older patients. And although therapeutic response cannot be assured, it is definitely aided and abetted by a comprehensive approach based on knowledge of each patient's physical and psychological status and informed by regular clinical monitoring. Third, knowledge of the age-related systemic, pharmacodynamic, and pharmacokinetic factors implicated in psychotropic drug effects can expand the clinician's means of enhancing therapeutic response and preventing adverse reactions. Fourth, use of lower doses is a proven means of implementing this knowledge. And, finally, the cautions, hazards, and dosages described here are recommendations based on our view of what is required currently to provide rational, attentive, compassionate psychotropic treatment. As our understanding of the complex of interrelated neurophysiological, neuropsychological, and neurochemical factors implicated in emotional disturbance and its treatment grows, these recommendations will both broaden and become more refined.

References

Abernethy, D. R. (In press). Psychotropic drugs and the aging process: Pharmacokinetics and pharmacodynamics. In C. Salzman (Ed.), *Clinical Geriatric Psychopharmacology*, 2nd ed. Baltimore, MD: Williams & Wilkins.

Alexopoulos, G. S. (In press). Treatment of depression. In C. Salzman (Ed.). *Clinical Geriatric Psychopharmacology*, 2nd ed. Baltimore, MD: Williams & Wilkins.

Alexopoulos, G. S., Young, R. C., Meyers, B. S., Abrams, R. C., & Shamoian, C. (1988). Late-onset depression. *Psychiatric Clinics of North America, 11*, 101–115.

Allen, R. M. (1986). Tranquilizers and sedative/hypnotics: Appropriate use in the elderly. *Geriatrics, 41*, 75–88.

American Psychiatric Association (1990). *Report of Task Force on Benzodiazepine Dependence, Toxicity, and Abuse*. Washington, DC: American Psychiatric Press.

American Psychiatric Association (1989). *Report of Task Force on Nursing Homes and the Mentally Ill Elderly*. Washington, DC: American Psychiatric Press.

Avorn, J. (1988). Medications and the elderly. In J. R. Rowe & R. W. Besdine (Eds.), *Geriatric Medicine* (pp. 114–121). Boston: Little, Brown.

Avorn, J., Dreyer, P., Connelly, K., & Soumerai, S. B. (1989). Use of psychoactive medication and the quality of care in rest homes: Findings and policy implications of a statewide study. *New England Journal of Medicine, 320*, 227–232.

Bartus, R. T., Dean, R. L., Beer, B. & Lippa, A. (1982). The cholinergic hypothesis of geriatric memory dysfunction. *Science, 217,* 408–417.

Bartus, R. T., Dean, R. L., Pontecorvo, M. J., & Flicker, C. (1985). The cholinergic hypothesis: A historical overview, current perspectives, and future directions. In D. Olton, E. Gamzu, & S. Corkin (Eds.), *Memory dysfunction: An integration of animal and human research from clinical and preclinical perspectives. Annals of the New York Academy of Sciences, 444,* 332–358.

Beardsley, R. S., Larson, D. B., Burns, B. J., Thompson, J. W., & Kamerow, D. B. (1989). Prescribing of psychotropics in elderly nursing-home patients. *Journal of the American Geriatrics Society, 37,* 327–330.

Beers, M., Avorn, J., Soumerai, S. B., Everitt, D. E., Sherman, D. S., & Salem, S. (1988). Psychoactive medication use in intermediate-care residents. *Journal of the American Medical Association* Nov 25, *260,* 20.

Black, J. L., Richelson, E., & Richardson, J. W. (1985). Antipsychotic agents: A clinical update. *Mayo Clinic Proceedings, 60,* 777–789.

Blazer, D., Williams, C. D. (1980). Epidemiology of dysphoria and depression in an elderly population. *American Journal of Psychiatry, 137,* 439–444.

Branconnier, R. J., & Cole, J. O. (1981). Effects of acute administration of trazodone and amitriptyline on cognition, cardiovascular function, and salivation in the normal geriatric subject. *Journal of Clinical Psychopharmacology, 1,* 82S–88S.

Branconnier, R. J., DeVitt, D. R., Cole, J. O., & Spera (1982). Amitriptyline selectively disrupts verbal recall from secondary memory of the normal aged. *Neurobiology of Aging, 3,* 55–59.

Brown, R. P., Sweeney, J., Loutsch, E., Kocsis, J., & Frances, A. (1984). Involutional melancholia revisited. *American Journal of Psychiatry, 141,* 24–28.

Buck, J. A. (1988). Psychotropic drug practice in nursing homes. *Journal of the American Geriatrics Society, 36,* 409–418.

Cohen, G. D. (1990). Anxiety and medical disorders. In C. Salzman & B. Lebowitz (Eds.), *Anxiety in the elderly* (pp. 47–62). New York: Springer.

Cohen-Mansfield, J., Marx, M. S., & Rosenthal, A. S. (1989). A description of agitation in a nursing home. *Journal of Gerontology, 44,* 77–84.

Cohen-Mansfield, J. (1986). Agitated behavior in the elderly: Preliminary results in the cognitively deteriorated. *Journal of the American Geriatrics Society, 34,* 722–727.

Colenda, C. C. (May 21, 1988). Buspirone in treatment of agitated demented patient. *Lancet,* ii, 1169.

Cook, P. J., Haggett, A., Graham-Pole, R., Savage, I. T., & James, I. M. (1983). Hypnotic accumulation and hangover in elderly patients: A controlled double-blind study of temazepam and nitrazepam. *British Medical Journal, 286,* 100–102.

Coyle, J., Price, D., & Delong, M. (1983). Alzheimer's disease: A disorder of cortical innervation. *Science, 219,* 1184–1190.

Creasey, H., & Rapoport, S. I. (1985). The aging human brain. *Annals of Neurology, 17,* 2–10.

Crook, T. (1988). Alzheimer's disease: New developments in treatment and symptom management research. *Psychopharmacology Bulletin, 21,* 31–38.

Crook, T. H. (1989). Diagnosis and treatment of normal and pathologic memory impairment in later life. *Seminars in Neurology, 9,* 20–30.

Crook, T. H., Johnson, B. A., & Larrabee, G. J. (1990). Evaluation of drugs in Alzheimer's disease and age-associated memory impairment. *Psychopharmacology Series (Berlin),* 37–55.

Curran, H. V., Allen, D., & Lader, M. (1987). The effects of single doses of alprazolam and lorazepam on memory and psychomotor performance in normal humans. *Journal of Psychopharmacology, 2,* 81–89.

Davies, P., & Wolozin, B. (1987). Recent advances in the neurochemistry of Alzheimer's disease. *Journal of Clinical Psychiatry, 48* (Suppl. 5), 23–30.

Devanand, D. P., Sackeim, H. A., & Mayeux, R. (1988). Psychosis, behavior disturbance, and the use of neuroleptics in dementia. *Journal of Comprehensive Psychiatry, 29*(4), 387–401.

Dupont, R. M., Cullum, C. M., & Jeste, D. V. (1988). Post-stroke depression and psychosis. *Psychiatric Clinics of North America, 11,* 133–150.

Ellinwood, E. H., & Nikaido, A. M. (1987). Perceptual–neuromotor pharmacodynamics of psychotropic drugs. In H. Y. Meltzer (Ed.), *Psychopharmacology: The third generation in progress* (pp. 1457–1466). New York: Raven Press.

Evans, D. A., Funkenstein, H. H., Albert, M. S., Scherr, P. A., Cook, N. R., Chown, M. J., Hebert, L. E., Hennekens, C. H., Taylor, J. O. (1989). Prevalence of Alzheimer's disease in a community population of older persons. *Journal of the American Medical Association, 262,* 2551–2556.

Feighner, J. P., Boyer, W. F., Meredith, C. H., et al. (1988). An overview of fluoxetine in geriatric depression. *British Journal of Psychiatry, 153* (Suppl. 3), 105–108.

Feighner, J. P., & Cohn, J. B. (1985). Double-blind comparative trials of fluoxetine and doxepin in geriatric patients with major depressive disorder. *Journal of Clinical Psychiatry, 46,* 20–25.

Folkman, S., Bernstein, L., & Lazarus, R. S. (1987). Stress processes and the misuse of drugs in older adults. *Psychology and Aging, 2,* 366–374.

Folstein, M. F., Maiberger, R., & McHugh, P. R. (1987). Mood disorder as a specific complication of stroke. *Journal of Neurosurgery and Psychiatry, 40,* 1018–1020.

Foster, J. R., & Martin, C. E. (1990). Dementia. In D. Bienenfeld (Ed.), *Verwoerdt's clinical geropsychiatry,* 3rd ed. (pp. 66–84). Baltimore, MD: Williams & Wilkins.

Friedel, R. O. (1978). Pharmacokinetics in the geropsychiatric patient. In M. A. Lipton, A. DiMascio, & K. F. Killian (Eds.), *Psychopharmacology: A generation of progress* (pp. 1499–1505). New York: Raven Press.

Gaillard, J. M. (1987). Place of benzodiazepines in the treatment of sleep disturbances. *Revue Medicale de la Suisse Romande, 107,* 717–720.

Gamzu, E. R., & Gracon, S. I. (1988). Drug improvement of cognition: Hope and reality. *Psychiatry & Psychobiology, 3,* 115–123.

Georgotas, A., Friedman, E., & McCarthy, M., (1983). Resistant geriatric depressions and therapeutic response to monoamine oxidase inhibitors. *Biological Psychiatry, 18,* 195–205.

Georgotas, A., Mann, J., & Friedman, E. (1981). Platelet monoamine oxidase inhibitors as a potential indicator of favorable response to MAOIs in geriatric depression. *Biological Psychiatry, 16,* 997–1001.

Georgotas, A., McCue, R. E., Hapworth, W., Friedman, Kim, Welkowitz, Chang, & Cooper (1986). Comparative efficacy and safety of MAOIs versus TCAs in treating depression in the elderly. *Biological Psychiatry, 21,* 1155–1166.

Gerner, R. H. (1984). Antidepressant selection in the elderly. *Psychosomatics, 25,* 528–535.

Gerner, R., Estabrook, W., Steuer, J., & Jarvik, L. (1980). Treatment of depression with trazodone, imipramine, and placebo: A double-blind study. *Journal of Clinical Psychiatry, 41,* 216–220.

Gerson, S. C., Plotkin, D. A., & Jarvik, L. F. (1988). Antidepressant drug studies, 1964–1966: Empirical evidence for aging patients. *Journal of Clinical Psychopharmacology, 8,* 311–322.

Glasser, M., Rabins, P. (1984). Mania in the elderly. *Age and Ageing, 13,* 210–213.

Glassman, A. H., Walsh, T., & Roose, S. P. (1982). Factors related to orthostatic hypotension associated with tricyclic antidepressants. *Journal of Clinical Psychiatry, 43,* 35–38.

Green, A. I., & Salzman, C. (1990). Clozapine: risks and benefits. *Hospital and Community Psychiatry, 41,* 379–380.

Greenblatt, D. J., Divoll, M., Harmatz, J. S., & McLaughlin, D. S., & Shader, R. I. (1981). Kinetics and clinical effects of flurazepam in young and elderly insomniacs. *Clinical Pharmacology and Therapeutics, 30,* 475–486.

Greenblatt, D. J., Sellers, E. M., & Koch-Weser, J. (1982). Importance of protein binding for the interpretation of serum or plasma drug concentrations. *Journal of Clinical Pharmacology, 22,* 259–263.

Greenblatt, D. J., & Shader, R. I. (1985). *Pharmacokinetics in clinical practice.* Philadelphia: Saunders.

Greenblatt, D. J., Abernethy, D. R., & Shader, R. I. (1986). Pharmacokinetic aspects of drug therapy in the elderly. *Therapeutic Drug Monitoring, 8,* 249–255.

Greenblatt, D. J., & Shader, R. I. (1990). Benzodiazepines in the elderly: Pharmacokinetics and drug sensitivity. In C. Salzman & B. Lebowitz (Eds.), *Anxiety in the elderly* (pp. 131–145). New York: Springer.

Greenwald, B. S., Marin, D. B., & Silverman, S. M. (1986). Serotoninergic treatment of screaming and banging in dementia. *Lancet, 20,* 1464–1465.

Gurwitz, J. H., Soumerai, S. B., & Avorn, J. (1990). Improving medication prescribing and utilization in the nursing home. *Journal of the American Geriatrics Society, 38,* 542–552.

Hale, W. E., May, F. E., Moore, M. T., & Stewart, R. B. (1988). Meprobamate use in the elderly. *Journal of the American Geriatrics Society, 36,* 1003–1005.

Helms, P. M. (1985). Efficacy of antipsychotics in the treatment of the behavioral complications of dementia: A review of the literature. *Journal of the American Geriatrics Society, 33,* 206–209.

Hershey, L. A., & Kim, K. Y. (1988). Diagnosis and treatment of anxiety in the elderly. *Rational Drug Therapy*, *22*, 3–6.

Holton, A., George, K. (1985). The use of lithium in severely demented patients with behavioral disturbance. *British Journal of Psychiatry*, *146*, 99–104.

Jarvik, L. (1981). Antidepressant therapy for the geriatric patient. *Journal of Clinical Psychopharmacology* (Suppl. 6), 55–61.

Jefferson, J. W., Greist, J. H., Ackerman, D. L., & Carroll, J. A. (1987). *Lithium encyclopedia for clinical practice*. Washington, DC: APPI.

Jenike, M. A. (1985c). The use of monoamine oxidase inhibitors in the treatment of elderly depressed patients. *Journal of the American Geriatrics Society*, *32*, 571–575.

Jenike, M. A., Albert, M., Heller, H., Gunther, A., & Goff, D. (1990). Oral psysostigmine treatment for patients with presenile and senile dementia of the Alzheimer-type: A double-blind, placebo-controlled trial. *Journal of Clinical Psychiatry*, *51*, 3–7.

Kalayam, B., & Shamoian, C. A. (in press). Treatment of depression: Diagnostic considerations. In C. Salzman (Ed.), *Clinical geriatric psychopharmacology*, 2nd ed. Baltimore, MD: Williams & Wilkins.

Kales, A., Soldatos, C. R., Bixler, E. D., & Kales, J. D. (1983). Early morning insomnia with rapidly eliminated benzodiazepines. *Science*, *220*, 95–97.

Koepke, H. H., Gold, R. L., Linden, M. E., Lion, J. R., & Rickels, K. (1982). Multicenter controlled study of oxazepam in anxious elderly outpatients. *Psychosomatics*, *23*, 641–645.

Kramer, M., & Schoen, L. S. (1984). Problems in the use of long-acting hypnotics in older patients. *Journal of Clinical Psychiatry*, *45*, 176–177.

Kumar, V., & Becker, R. (1989). Clinical pharmacology of tetrahydroaminoacridine: A possible therapeutic agent for Alzheimer's disease. *International Journal of Clinical Pharmacology, Therapy, and Toxicology*, *27*, 478–485.

Lamy, P. P. (1986). The elderly and drug interactions. *Journal of the American Geriatrics Society*, *34*, 586–692.

Lakshmanan, E. B., Mion, C. C., & Frengley, J. D. (1986). Effective low-dose tricyclic antidepressant treatment for depressed geriatric rehabilitation patients. *Journal of the American Geriatrics Society*, *34*, 421–426.

Larson, E. B., Kukull, W. A., Reifler, B. V., & Buchner, D. (1987). Adverse drug reactions associated with global cognitive impairment in elderly persons. *Annals of Internal Medicine*, *107* (2), 169–173.

Lazarus, L., L. W., Groves, L., Gierl, B., Pandey, G., Javaid, J. I., Lesser, J., Ha, Y. S., & Davis, J. (1986). Efficacy of phenelzine in geriatric depression. *Biological Psychiatry*, *21*, 699–701.

Lazarus, L. W., Newton, N., Cohler, B., Lesser, J., & Schweon, C. (1987). Frequency and presentation of depressive symptoms in patients with primary degenerative dementia. *American Journal of Psychiatry*, *144*, 41–45.

Leibovici, A., & Tariot, N. (1988). Carbamazepine treatment of agitation associated with dementia. *Journal of Geriatric Psychiatry and Neurology*, *1*, 110–112.

Liljequist, R., Linnoila, M., & Mattila, M. J. (1974). Effects of two weeks' treatment with chlorimipramine and nortriptyline, alone or in combination with alcohol, on learning and memory. *Psychopharmacology*, *39*, 181–186.

Liptzin, B. (In press). Treatment of mania. In *Clinical geriatric psychopharmacology*, 2nd ed. C. Salzman (Ed.). Baltimore, MD: Williams & Wilkins.

Liptzin, B., & Salzman, C. (1988). Psychiatric aspects of aging. In J. R. Rowe & R. W. Besdine (Eds.), *Geriatric medicine* (pp. 355–374). Boston: Little, Brown.

Little, A., Levy, R., Chuaqui-Kidd, C., & Hand, D. (1985). A double-blind, placebo-controlled trial of high-dose lecithin in Alzheimer's disease. *Journal of Neurology, Neurosurgery, and Psychiatry*, *48*, 736–742.

Lohr, J. B., & Bracha, H. S. (1988). Association of psychosis and movement disorders in the elderly. *Psychiatric Clinics of North America*, *11*, 61–81.

Lovett, W. C., Stokes, D. K., Taylor, L. B., Young, M. L., Free, S. M., & Phelan, D. G. (1987). Management of behavioral symptoms in disturbed elderly patients: Comparison of trifluoperazine and haloperidol. *Journal of Clinical Psychiatry*, *48*, 234–236.

Lucki, I., Rickels, K., & Gelber, A. (1986). Chronic use of benzodiazepines and psychomotor and cognitive test performance. *Psychopharmacology*, *88*, 426–433.

McAllister, T. W. (1983). Overview: Pseudodementia. *American Journal of Psychiatry*, *140*, 528.

Macdonald, J. B. (1985). The role of drugs in falls in the elderly. *Clinics in Geriatric Medicine, 1,* 621–636.

Mace, N. A., & Rabins, P. V. (1981). *The 36-hour day.* Baltimore, MD: Johns Hopkins Press.

Maletta, G. S. (1984). Use of antipsychotic medications. In *Annual Review of Gerontology and Geriatrics.* (pp. 175–220). New York: Springer.

Mattila, M. J., Liljequist, R., & Seppala, T. (1978). Effects of amitriptyline and mianserin on psychomotor skills and memory in man. *British Journal of Clinical Pharmacology, 5,* 53S–55S.

Moran, M. G., & Thompson, T. L., II. (1988). Changes in the aging brain: A review. *International Journal of Psychiatry in Medicine, 18,* 137–144.

Montamat, S. C., Cusack, B. J., & Bestal, R. E. (1989). Management of drug therapy in the elderly. *New England Journal of Medicine, 321,* 303–309.

Morgan, D. G., May, P. C., & Finch, C. E. (1987). Dopamine and serotonin systems in human and rodent brain: Effects of age and neurodegenerative disease. *Journal of the American Geriatrics Society, 35,* 334–345.

Morris, J. N., Hawes, C., Fries, B., Phillips, C. D., Mor, V., Katz, S., Murphy, K., Drugovich, M. L., & Friedlob, A. (1990). Designing the national Resident Assessment Instrument for nursing homes. *Gerontologist, 30,* 293–307.

Napoliello, M. J. (1986). An interim multicentre report on 677 anxious geriatric out-patients treated with buspirone. *British Journal of Clinical Practice, 40,* 71–73.

Nolan, L., & O'Malley, K. (1988). Prescribing for the elderly. Part II. Prescribing patterns: Differences due to age. *Journal of the American Geriatrics Society, 36,*(3), 245–254.

Peabody, C. A., Warner, D., Whiteford, H. A., Hollister, L. E. (1987). Neuroleptics and the elderly. *Journal of the American Geriatrics Society, 35,* 233–238.

Peabody, C. A., Whiteford, H. A., & Hollister, L. E. (1986). Antidepressants and the elderly. *Journal of the American Geriatrics Society, 34,* 869–874.

Phillipson, M., Moranville, J. T., Jeste, D. V., & Harris, M. J. (1990). Antipsychotics. *Clinics in Geriatric Medicine, 6,* 411–422.

Pinner, E., & Rich, C. L. (1988). Effects of trazodone on aggressive behavior in seven patients with organic mental disorders. *American Journal of Psychiatry, 145,* 1295–1296.

Pinsker, H., & Suljaga-Petchel, K. (1984). Use of benzodiazepines in primary-care geriatric patients. *Journal of the American Geriatrics Society, 32,* 595–598.

Pomara, N., Deptula, D., Singh, R. A., & Monroy, C. A. (1990). Cognitive toxicity of benzodiazepines in the elderly. In C. Salzman & B. Lebowitz (Eds.), *Anxiety in the Elderly* (pp. 175–196). New York: Springer.

Pomara, N., Stanley, B., Block, R., Berchon, R. Berchon R. C., Stanley, M., Greenblatt, D. J., Newton, R. E., & Gershon, S. (1985). Increased sensitivity of the elderly to the central depressant effects of diazepam. *Journal of Clinical Psychiatry, 46,* 185–187.

Prinz, P. N., Vitiello, M. V., Raskind, M. A., & Thorpy, M. J. (1996). Current concepts in geriatrics: Sleep disorders and aging. *New England Journal of Medicine, 323,* 520–526.

Rashi, S., & Logan, R. F. A. (1986). Role of drugs in fractures of the femoral neck. *British Journal of Medicine, 292,* 3.

Ray, W. A., Federspiel, C. F., & Schaffner, W. (1980). A study of antipsychotic drug use in nursing homes: Epidemiologic evidence suggesting misuse. *American Journal of Public Health, 70,* 485–491.

Ray, W. A., Griffin, M. R., Schaffner, W., Baugh, D. K., & Melton, L. J., III. (1987). Psychotropic drug use and the risk of hip fracture. *New England Journal of Medicine, 316,* 363–369.

Regestein, Q. (in press). Treaatment of sleep disorders. In C. Salzman (Ed.), *Clinical geriatric psychopharmacology,* 2nd ed. Baltimore, MD: Williams and Wilkins.

Reifler, B. V., Larson, Teri, L. & Poulson, M. (1986). Dementia of the Alzheimer's type and depression. Journal of the *American Geriatric Society, 34,* 855–859.

Reisberg, B., Borenstein, M. D., Saleb, S. P., Ferris, S. H., Franssen, E., Georgotas, A. (1987). Behavioral symptoms in Alzheimer's disease: Phenomenology and treatment. *Journal of Clinical Psychiatry, 48,* (Suppl.) 9–15.

Reisberg, B. (in press). Memory dysfunction and dementia: Diagnostic considerations. In C. Salzman (Ed.), *Clinical geriatric psychopharmacology* (2nd ed.) Baltimore, MD: Williams & Wilkins.

Reynolds, C. F., Kupfer, D. J., Hoch, C. C., Sewitch, D. E. (1985). Sleeping pills for the elderly: Are they ever justified? *Journal of Clinical Psychiatry, 46,* 9–12.

Risse, S. C., & Barnes, R. (1986). Pharmacologic treatment of agitation associated with dementia. *Journal of the American Geriatrics Society, 34,* 368–376.

Ritschel, W. A. (1988). *Gerontokinetics: The pharmacokinetics of drugs in the elderly.* Caldwell, NJ: Telford Press.

Robinson, R. G., & Price, T. R. (1982). Post-stroke depressive disorders: A follow-up study of 103 patients. *Stroke, 13,* 635–641.

Rockwell, E., Lam, R. W., & Zisook, S. (1988). Antidepressant drug studies in the elderly. *Psychiatric Clinics of North America, 11,* 215–233.

Rosebush, P. I., & Salzman, C. (1988). Memory disturbance and cognitive impairment in the elderly. In J. P. Tupin, R. I. Shader, & D. S. Harnett (Eds.), *Handbook of clinical psychopharmacology* (pp. 159–210). New York: Jason Aaronson.

Rovner, B. W., German, P. S., Brant, L. J., Clark, R., Burton, L., & Folstein, M. F. (1991). Depression and mortality in nursing homes. *Journal of the American Medical Association, 265*(8), 993–996.

Rovner, B., Kafonek, S., Filipp, L., Lucas, M. J., & Folstein, M. F. (1986). Prevalence of mental illness in a nursing home. *American Journal of Psychiatry, 143,* 1146–1149.

Rowe, J. R., & Besdine, R. W. (1982). Drug therapy. In J. R. Rowe and R. W. Besdine (Eds.), *Health and disease in old age.* (pp. 39–53). Boston: Little, Brown.

Salzman, C. (1982). A primer on geriatric psychopharmacology. *American Journal of Psychiatry, 139,* 67–74.

Salzman, C. (1984). Pharmacokinetics of psychotropic drugs and the aging process. In C. Salzman, Ed., *Clinical geriatric psychopharmacology* (pp. 32–48). New York: McGraw-Hill.

Salzman, C. (1985). Clinical use of antidepressant blood levels and the electrocardiogram. *New England Journal of Medicine, 313,* 512–513.

Salzman, C. (1986). Caution urged in using MAOIs with the elderly (letter to the editor). *American Journal of Psychiatry, 143,* 118–119.

Salzman, C. (1987a). Treatment of the depressed elderly patient. In H. J. Altman (Ed.), *Alzheimer's disease and dementia: Problems, prospects, and perspectives* (pp. 171–182). New York: Plenum Press.

Salzman, C. (1987b). Treatment of agitation in the elderly. In H. Y. Meltzer (Ed.), *Psychopharmacology: The third generation of progress* (pp. 1167–1176). New York: Raven Press.

Salzman, C. (1990a). Recent advances in geriatric psychopharmacology. In A. Tasman, S. M. Goldfinger, & Kaufman (Eds.), *Review of psychiatry* (pp. 279–292). Washington, DC: American Psychiatric Press.

Salzman, C. (1990b). Antidepressants. In P. F. Lamy (Ed.), *Clinical geriatric medicine* (pp. 399–410). Philadelphia: Saunders.

Salzman, C. (1990c). Practical considerations of the pharmacologic treatment of depression and anxiety in the elderly. *Journal of Clinical Psychiatry, 51,* (Suppl.), 40–43.

Salzman, C., Shader, R. I., & Pearlman, M. (1970). Psychopharmacology and the elderly. In R. I. Shader & A. DiMascio (Eds.), *Psychotropic drug side-effects* (pp. 261–279). Baltimore: Williams & Wilkins.

Salzman, C., Fisher, J., Nobel, K., & Wolfson, A. (in press), Cognitive improvement following benzodiazepine discontinuation in elderly nursing home residents: A single-blind study. *International Journal of Geriatric Psychiatry.*

Salzman, C. (in press). Treatment of anxiety. In C. Salzman (Ed.), *Clinical geriatric psychopharmacology,* 2nd ed. Baltimore, MD: Williams & Wilkins.

Salzman, C. (in press). Behavioral side-effects of benzodiazepines. In J. Lieberman & J. Kane (Eds.), *Adverse effects of psychotropic drugs* New York: Guilford Press.

Scharf, & Jennings, (1990). Sleep disorders. In D. Bienenfeld (Ed.), *Verwoerd's clinical geropsychiatry,* (pp. 178–194). Baltimore, MD: Williams & Wilkins.

Schmucker, D. L. (1984). Drug disposition in the elderly: A review of the critical factors. *Journal of the American Geriatrics Society, 32,* 144–149.

Schneider, L. S., Pollock, V. E., & Lyness, S. A. (1990). A metaanalysis of controlled trials of neuroleptic treatment in dementia. *Journal of the American Geriatrics Society, 38,* 553–563.

Severson, J. A. (1984). Neurotransmitter receptors and aging. *Journal of the American Geriatrics Society, 32,* 24–27.

Sheikh, J. I. (1990). Panic disorder. In C. Salzman & B. Lebowitz (Eds.), *Anxiety in the elderly* (pp. 251–266). New York: Springer.

Simpson, D. M., & Foster, D. (1986). Improvement in organically disturbed behavior with trazodone treatment. *Journal of Clinical Psychiatry, 47,* 191–193.

Small, G. W. (1988). Psychopharmacological treatment of elderly demented patients. *Journal of Clinical Psychiatry, 49* (Suppl), 8–13.

Spangnoli, A., Ostino, G., Borga, A., D'Ambrosio, R., Magiorotti, P., Todisco, F., Prattichizzo, W., Pia, L., & Corelli, M. (1989). Drug compliance and unreported drugs in the elderly. *Journal of the American Geriatrics Society, 37,* 617–624.

Spira, N., Dysken, M. W., Lazarus, L. W., Davis, J. M., & Salzman, C. (1984). Treatment of agitation and psychosis. In C. Salzman (Ed.), *Clinical geriatric psychopharmacology* (pp. 49–76). New York: McGraw-Hill.

Stern, Y., Sano, M., & Mayeux, R. (1988). Long-term administration of oral physostigmine in Alzheimer's disease. *Neurology, 38,* 1837–1841.

Stone, K. (1989). Mania in the elderly. *British Journal of Psychiatry, 155,* 220–229.

Strauss, A. (1988). Oral dyskinesia associated with buspirone use in an elderly woman. *Journal of Clinical Psychiatry, 49,* 322–323.

Sunderland, T. (in press). Neurotransmission in the aging central nervous system. In C. Salzman (Ed.), *Clinical geriatric psychopharmacology,* 2nd ed. Baltimore, MD: Williams & Wilkins.

Sunderland, T., Rubinow, D., Tariot, P. N., Cohen, R. M., Newhouse, P. A., Mellow, A. M., Mueller, E. A., & Murphy, D. L. (1987). CSF somatostatin in patients with Alzheimer's disease, older depressed patients, and age-matched control subjects. *American Journal of Psychiatry, 144,* 1313–1316.

Tamminga, C. A., & Gerlach, J. (1987). New neuroleptics and experimental antipsychotics in schizophrenia. In H. Y. Meltzer (Ed.), *Psychopharmacology: The third generation of progress* (pp. 1129–1140). New York: Raven Press.

Tariot, P. N. (in press). Neurobiology and treatment of dementia. In C. Salzman (Ed.), *Clinical geriatric psychopharmacology,* 2nd ed. Baltimore, MD: Williams & Wilkins.

Tariot, P. N., Sunderland, T., Cohen, R., Welkowitz, J., Newhouse, P. A., Murphy, D. L., & Weingartner, H. (1988). Multiple dose arecoline infusions in Alzheimer's disease. *Archives of General Psychiatry, 45,* 901–905.

Tariot, P. N., Sunderland, T., Cohen, R. M., Newhouse, P. A., Mueller, E. A., & Murphy, D. L. (1988). Tranylcyromine compared with L-deprenyl in Alzheimer's disease. *Journal of Clinical Psychopharmacology, 8*(1), 23–27.

Thompson, T. L., Filley, C. M., Mitchell, W. D., Culig, K. M., LoVerde, M., & Byyny, B. C. (1990). Lack of efficacy of hydergine in patients with Alzheimer's disease. *New England Journal of Medicine, 323,* 445–448.

Tingle, D. (1986). Trazodone in dementia. *Journal of Clinical Psychiatry,* (Letter to the Editor). *47,* 482.

Weiler, P. G., Mungo, D., & Bernick, C. (1988). Propranolol for the control of disruptive behavior in senile dementia. *Journal of Geriatric Psychiatry, 1,* 226–230.

Weintraub, M. (1990). Compliance in the elderly. *Clinics in Geriatric Medicine, 6,* 445–452.

Whitehouse, P. (1987). Neurotransmitter receptor alterations in Alzheimer's disease: A review. *Alzheimer Disease and Associated Disorders, 1,* 9–18.

Wragg, R. E., Jeste, D. V. (1988). Neuroleptics and alternative treatments. Management of behavioral symptoms and psychosis in Alzheimer's disease and related conditions. *Psychiatric Clinics of North America, 11,* 195–213.

Young, R. C., Alexopoulos, G. S., Shamoian, C. A., Dhar, & Kutt (1985). Plasma 10-hydroxynortriptyline and ECG changes in elderly depressed patients. *American Journal of Psychiatry, 142,* 866–868.

Yudofsky, S., Williams, D., & Gorman, J. (1981). Propranolol in the treatment of rage and violent behavior in patients with chronic brain syndromes. *American Journal of Psychiatry, 138,* 218–220.

Zimmer, J. G., Watson, N., & Treat, A. (1984). Behavior problems among patients in skilled nursing facilities. *American Journal of Public Health, 74,* 1118–1121.

Zisook, S. (1985). A clinical overview of monoamine oxidase inhibitors. *Psychosomatics, 26,* 240–246.

Environmental Intervention for Cognitively Impaired Older Persons

Victor Regnier and Jon Pynoos

I. Introduction
II. Twelve Environment–Behavior Principles
  A. Privacy
  B. Social Interaction
  C. Control, Choice, and Autonomy
  D. Orientation and Wayfinding
  E. Safety and Security
  F. Accessibility and Functioning
  G. Stimulation and Challenge
  H. Sensory Aspects
  I. Familiarity
  J. Aesthetics and Appearance
  K. Personalization
  L. Adaptability
III. Application of These Principles to Institutional Environments
  A. Privacy in One- and Two-Bed Rooms
  B. Corridors Designed for Sociability
  C. Decentralized Neighborhood Clusters
  D. Design That Supports Therapy
  E. Wayfinding and Orientation
  F. Outdoor-Space Treatments
  G. Family Orientation
  H. Environmental Intervention: Summary
IV. Home Settings: Strategies for Environmental Management
  A. Assessment
  B. Safety
  C. Accessibility and Functioning

Handbook of Mental Health and Aging, Second Edition

    D. Safety, Familiarity, and Stability
    E. Stimulation
    F. Privacy
    G. Social Interaction
  V. Future Directions
    References

I. Introduction

Research in aging and the environment ranges from theory-based behavioral science to applied work that identifies critical attributes of the environment for designers and policy makers. Behavioral science research primarily focuses on clarifying the relationships between characteristics of individuals and their environments. Applied design research, on the other hand, is oriented toward identifying critical aspects of the environment that can affect resident satisfaction and functional ability. The literature dealing with both applied and theoretical concerns is rich and varied. It has contributed to a clearer understanding of the relationship between individuals and their surrounding settings, as well as the impact of interventions, administrative policies, and the characteristics of support personnel.

Rather than reviewing the literature in theory-based research, this chapter focuses on identifying design responses for frail and cognitively impaired older persons in planned institutional settings and relatively unstructured home environments. Many of these design responses have been based on the perceived needs of the cognitively impaired, drawing on limited available experimental evidence or deductive assumptions. While it is becoming increasingly clear that the environment is important to the quality of life for cognitively impaired older persons, there is not yet enough research to assess the effectiveness of particular design features or environmental modifications.

Environmental design research literature is organized to conform to the information requirements of the design process or to provide guidance to practitioners and caregivers. Some analysts have chosen to organize information by room or type of space (AIA Foundation, 1985; Aranyi & Goldman, 1980; Calkins, 1988). This approach is popular because it can be used in the architectural programming process. Based on statements of desired behaviors within spaces, it frequently establishes design and management criteria for specific rooms.

Environmental information has also been organized in relation to the changing physiological or cognitive abilities of the older person. The most useful and widely recognized framework cited by design researchers is the competence-press model of Lawton and Nahemow (1973). In this model "adaptive behavior and positive affect are treated as outcomes of environmental demands that are commensurate with the bio-behavioral competence of the person," (Lawton, Altman & Wohlwill, 1984). The corollary to this model, the "environmental docility hypothesis," as described by Lawton *et al.* (1984), "holds that as competence decreases, behavior becomes increasingly determined by factors outside the person (i.e., the environment)." The simplicity of this model and its application to the range of housing types older people inhabit makes it a particularly powerful conceptual tool.

Conceptualizing the environment in terms of Lawton's model leads to interventions that maximize independence by treating the environment as a prosthesis. A variety of researchers have built on this work by developing psychological, physiological, and anthropometric criteria that are applied to original designs and design adaptations (Koncelik, 1976; Koncelik, 1982; Pynoos, Cohen & Lucas, 1989; Raschko, 1982; Valens, 1988). Such design guidelines attempt to "fit" the environment to the unique physiological and cognitive conditions an older person exhibits.

Concepts such as privacy and community can also be employed to structure design interventions. For example, in the publication *Low Rise Housing for Older People,* John Zeisel and his co-authors (Zeisel, Epp, & Demos, 1977) segment housing projects into six domains and 20 sub-domains. This type of approach starts with design concerns at the private scale of the unit and ends with broader "public" considerations of site-design and neighborhood relationship.

Design information can also be conceptualized as a component of planning and management (Chambliss, 1989; Lawton, 1975; NAHB, 1987; Parker, 1984). In this approach, the environment is assumed to be a tool that can be managed by staff and designed to meet the desires and needs of residents. Maintenance, neighborhood orientation, scheduled activities, and support services are integrated to form a management philosophy about housing environments.

Architectural case studies that review research findings are often an important vehicle for sharing project findings. Such case studies are used to illustrate behavioral responses to environmental situations. They are particularly effective in demonstrating how persistent activity patterns are expressed within a range of different physical environments. Hoglund (1985) uses European case studies to identify social and environmental attributes of buildings from other cultures; while Regnier (1985) and Howell (1980) develop guidelines from the consistent patterns of behavior uncovered through case study work.

Finally, guidelines are organized to conform to the process of design and development (CHAMP, 1987; Green, Fedewa, Johnstone, Jackson, & Deardorff, 1975; Welch, Parker & Zeisel, 1984). In this approach, design decisions at various stages of the development process are conceptualized as *choices* that specify potential directions for the housing form. These guidelines are often organized in a general-to-specific format that traces the project from initial feasibility to postoccupancy evaluation.

Although each of these approaches has its advantages and disadvantages, there is a need for a conceptual framework within which organized guidelines can be placed in relation to the needs of cognitively impaired older persons. Calkins (1988) does this by articulating five environmental and behavioral issues important in the design of nursing homes for confused residents. Cohen and his colleagues (Cohen et al., 1988) describe seven therapeutic goals that they believe relate to the design of Alzheimer's facilities. Similarly, Pynoos and Stacey (1985) specify seven therapeutic goals, Pynoos et al. (1989) identify nine therapeutic goals, and Lawton (1989) describes 11 goals considered applicable to environments for persons who have Alzheimer's disease. This chapter introduces 12 environmental and behavioral principles derived from design-based research that affect the behavior and quality of life of cognitively impaired older people in both purpose-built and conventional home environments.

II. Twelve Environment—Behavior Principles _____

A. Privacy

Provide opportunities for a place of seclusion from company or observation where one can be free from unauthorized intrusion. Privacy, such as having one's own room where one can be by oneself, provides a sense of self and separateness from others (Altman, 1977; Archea, 1977). Because of concerns over safety and the need for surveillance, many cognitively impaired older persons lose a great deal of privacy.

B. Social Interaction

Provide opportunities for social exchange and interaction. Social interaction can be therapeutic in that it allows older persons to make new friends, share problems, life experiences, ideas, and everyday events with others who also benefit from the exchange. Retirement housing, in particular, has been shown to encourage new friendship formation (Rosow, 1967) and result in increased life satisfaction and morale (Carp, 1987). Such opportunities are especially important for cognitively impaired older persons who may have difficulties in carrying on conversations.

C. Control, Choice, and Autonomy

Promote opportunities for residents to make choices and control events that influence outcomes. Older persons are more alienated, less satisfied, and more task dependent in settings that are highly restrictive. On the other hand, having real or perceived control and a sense of competency are enhancing characteristics (Langer & Rodin, 1976).

D. Orientation and Wayfinding

Foster a sense of orientation within the environment that reduces confusion and facilitates way finding. Feeling lost or disoriented within an environment is a frustrating and frightening experience that can affect one's sense of perceived competency and well-being. Large housing environments often rely on winding corridors, elevators, and anonymous double-loaded corridors that can exacerbate feelings of disorientation (Weisman, 1987). Older people who have experienced some memory loss especially need an environment that is easy to comprehend.

E. Safety and Security

Provide an environment that ensures each user will sustain no harm, injury, or undue risk. Older persons not only experience a high rate of home accidents, but also have more than twice the number of resulting deaths as other age groups (Pynoos, Cohen, Davis, & Bernhart, 1987). Loss of critical judgment and memory puts cognitively impaired persons at high risk of injuries and accidents in conventional settings.

F. Accessibility and Functioning

Consider manipulation and accessibility as the basic requirements for a functional environment. Older persons with cognitive impairments are also likely to experience physical problems in manipulating features in the environment (e.g., windows, doors, HVAC equipment, appliances) owing in part to chronic disabling diseases such as arthritis, or to controls that require complicated decision making. Problems with ambulation as well as limited reach capacity and muscle strength make it difficult to climb stairs, stoop, bend, sit, and stand (Steinfeld, 1987).

G. Stimulation and Challenge

Provide a stimulating environment that is safe but challenging. A stimulating environment keeps the older person active, alert, and aware and is especially important to combat boredom and passivity, which are common problems of persons with mobility and cognitive impairments.

H. Sensory Aspects

Changes in visual, auditory, olfactory senses should be accounted for in environments. Older people with age-related losses often experience problems with vision and hearing that can place them at a disadvantage in the environment (Hiatt, 1987). It appears that some physical incapacities, such as limited depth perception, are associated with cognitive diseases such as Alzheimer's. Environments that have high levels of sound or low lighting levels hinder safety, socialization, and manipulation of the environment.

I. Familiarity

Environments that use historical reference and solutions influenced by tradition can provide a sense of familiarity and continuity. Many cognitively impaired older persons experience problems with short-term memory but can recall images from the past. For some older people, moving from one housing environment to another can be a disconcerting process, especially when there is little continuity between these places (Hunt & Pastalen, 1987). Living in one's own home surrounded by personal objects and possessions or being allowed to bring them into a new setting can help maintain a familiar frame of reference. Newly built multiunit settings should also provide a familiar frame of reference in the way that they are laid out and used.

J. Aesthetics and Appearance

Design environments that appear attractive, provocative and non-institutional. The appearance of the environment sends a message to older persons, families, and friends about the physical and mental state of its residents. Housing environments that are institutional or dehumanized in appearance stigmatize residents (Hartman, Horovitz, & Herman, 1987). On the other hand, buildings that evoke residential images are likely to reflect more positively on their residents.

K. Personalization

Provide opportunities to make the environment personal and to mark it as the property of a single, unique individual. Self-expression or personalization reinforces an older person's sense of identity (Becker, 1977; Butterfield & Weidemann, 1987). It is also a way of demonstrating to others that a space is occupied by a particular individual with unique qualities, characteristics, and experiences. Personalization is a compelling intrinsic feature of living in one's own home.

L Adaptability

An adaptable or flexible environment can be made to fit changing personal characteristics. If older persons become cognitively impaired and/or physically frail, they often find that their environment no longer fits their capabilities. Consequently, some carry out activities in unsafe environments, give up some tasks, or move to another setting in spite of a strong preference to *age in place.* For a setting to meet the diminished capabilities of frail older persons, it must often include supportive features (e.g., ramps, grab bars, handrails) or have the capability to change over time (Pynoos *et al.,* 1987; Steinfield, 1987).

These twelve principles are particularly appropriate for cognitively impaired older persons living in settings that have a strong organizational or management component; a number of them are also valid in the home environment. Some of these principles are overlapping, and a few represent opposites. For example, social interaction and privacy can be viewed as two ends of a continuum. Safety–security and challenge can also represent opposing environmental characteristics. Although this list of principles may be incomplete, it provides a set of concepts on which to base design interventions and evaluation.

III. Application of These Principles to Institutional Environments ____

The following seven design responses have emerged from the design-behavior literature on purpose-built care settings for older persons. They represent ideas about physical environments currently being explored within nursing and assisted-living environments for older, frail, and confused residents.

A. Privacy in One- and Two-Bed Rooms

A long-standing controversy in the area of long-term care policy has been the need for privacy in the context of the patient room. This is often reflected in a debate over the one- versus two-bed rooms. The choice of placing one bed or two beds in a room and the configuration or layout of two beds within a single room involves issues of *privacy, control–autonomy,* and *personalization.*

The most interesting design work in this area has been that of Koncelik (1976, 1982). In his model designs for extended-care facilities, single rooms were specified. They contain provisions for privacy, personal storage, display, personalization, socialization, and personal hygiene. His designs stress control through the use of patient-accessible switches for lights, heating and cooling, entertainment (television and radio), and emergency call. Bed designs utilize a rolled, soft bolster for sitting, which invites family and friends to sit comfortably near the resident. This bed design supports dressing and grooming activities as well as safety. The bathroom modifications stress lateral storage, wheelchair accessibility, and fixture adaptations. For example, the design of integral handrails on both sides of the toilet add to its attractiveness and functionality.

The major choices available in nursing home room designs today are the conventional two-bed side-by-side arrangement, the toe-to-toe two-bed configuration, and the single-bed private room (Figure 1).

An excellent example of a single-bed room unit can be found in the new nursing facility for the Motion Picture Country House and Hospital in Woodland Hills, California. In this design, a window seat is combined with built-in storage cabinets and residentially trimmed furniture. An alcove credenza with storage space below is available for display items such as mementoes and photographs. Furthermore, access to the unit is through an entry alcove shared with three other units. On the outside, the building accommodates shared patio spaces. Each outdoor patio is accessible to and shared by four adjacent units. A trellis that hangs near the center of the terrace provides shade control. Thus each of the first floor units has access to an interior shared entry foyer and a shared exterior balcony.

The most common and efficient arrangement of two beds in a single room involves the side-by-side arrangement. This configuration has been criticized because it does not enhance options for privacy and can often create problems with territoriality. In most circumstances, the bed located closest to the entry door and bathroom "owns" this portion of the unit. Conversely, the bed near the exterior perimeter controls sunlight and natural ventilation. Such problems of territoriality have been difficult to overcome. Koncelik, however, has developed a system of furniture intended to resolve the issue of privacy and flexibility (Koncelik, 1982). He creates greater privacy with semi-full-height partitions

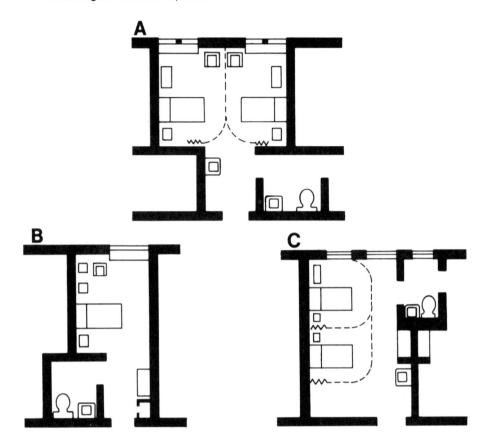

Figure 1   Three basic room configurations are commonly utilized in skilled nursing facilities today. (A) Two-bed room, toe-to-toe, (B) one-bed room, (C) two-bed room, side-by-side.

and a menu of additional features that can be added to the system. Koncelik's system has a module for coat storage, a corkboard for display, a drop-down writing desk, a book and display shelf, a cantilevered chest of drawers, and a lighting system mounted above the head of the bed (Figure 3).

The compromise between the private room and a side-by-side configuration is the *toe-to-toe* configuration. This configuration reduces the territorial problem caused by the side-by-side configuration, thereby enhancing privacy. Two-bed rooms organized in this way are slightly wider than the side-by-side configuration but are far more efficient than single room designs. Staff travel distances and access to nursing stations are also easier to resolve than in a single bed plan.

In the recently completed Joseph L. Morse Geriatric Center in West Palm Beach, Florida, a full-height partition offset to accommodate storage and desk space juts into the room, providing additional privacy and creating an alcove space that reinforces the feeling of separateness (Figure 4).

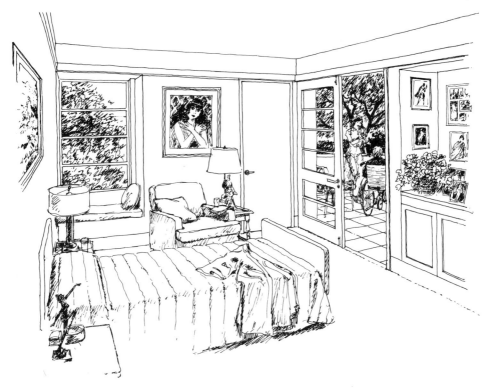

Figure 2 This private-room design by Bobrow-Thomas and Associates of Los Angeles for the Motion Picture and Television Fund Country House and Hospital opens onto a large shared balcony and contains a window seat, an alcove for storage and personalization, and space for a comfortable chair adjacent to the bed.

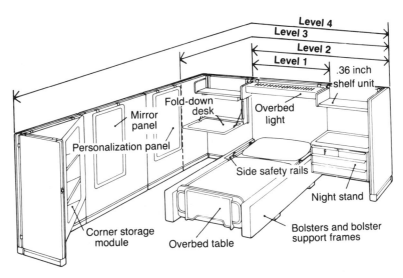

Figure 3 Koncelik's design for a furnishing system to be used in skilled nursing facilities utilizes four modules and a number of add-on features.

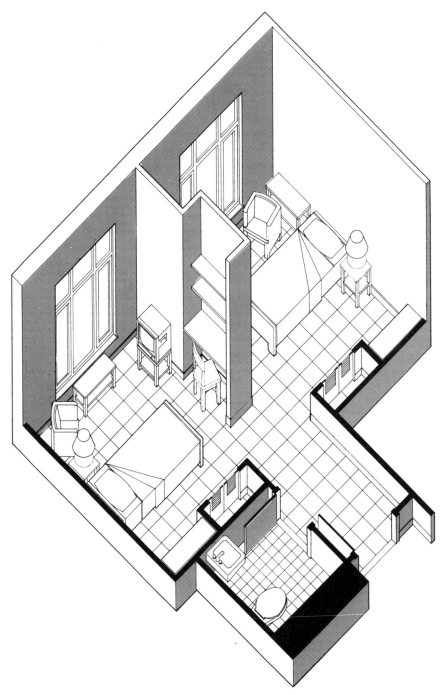

Figure 4   A semi-private toe-to-toe bed configuration provides privacy and independence. This design at the Joseph L. Morse Geriatric Center in West Palm Beach, Florida, is from the studio of Perkins, Geddis, Eastman of New York City.

Other creative approaches to the issue of privacy have involved the development of L-shaped rooms. One of the most interesting examples of this is the health center at the Glacier Hills retirement community in Ann Arbor, Michigan. In this design, the bathroom and entry space are situated between two rectangles juxtaposed at 90°. The room's shape accommodates the privacy and autonomy needs of two residents. An added benefit of this arrangement is flexibility. It can be transformed into a single-bed room with an adjoining living room. This provides autonomy for the two people sharing the room and allows the facility to cater to different personal needs (Figure 5).

B. Corridors Designed for Sociability

One typical institutional feature of a nursing home is the contiguous eight-foot-wide corridor that links resident rooms with therapy spaces, nurses' stations, and shared facilities. The contiguous nature of this pathway and its need to be separated from resident rooms and shared spaces by solid walls of fire-resistant construction, makes it a bleak and monotonous spatial extrusion. The corridor, however, is an active and vital conduit for guests, staff, materials, equipment, and general activity. As a result, residents see it as a

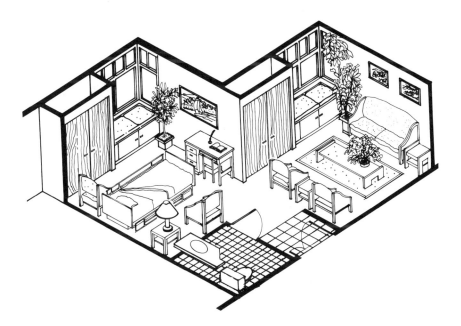

Figure 5 The L-shaped configuration designed for the Glacier Hills Nursing Center in Ann Arbor, Michigan, has the flexibility of accommodating two unrelated individuals in relatively private alcoves or, as the illustration demonstrates, a single person in a spacious one-bedroom with an adjacent living room. The design is from the Minneapolis studio of Ellerbe Becket, Inc.

metaphorical "street" where activity and interest abound. Corridors in long-term care settings are not designed to accommodate the vicarious interest of residents in viewing activity and movement. In most instances, corridors are designed simply to connect spaces. Rarely do they accommodate social opportunities.

Uniform lighting levels, an absence of variety in wall treatments, and monotonous material and color choices also add to its boredom. Creative corridor designs often deal with the potential of this space as a social environment. As a result the principles of *social interaction, appearance–aesthetics* and *orientation–wayfinding* hold the greatest opportunity for creative design exploration.

One of the simplest interventions is to widen the corridor to create alcoves adjacent to unit entries. This provides a visual break in the corridor configuration, and perceptually foreshortens corridor length. If wide enough, these alcoves can provide places where residents can rest as they move from one portion of the facility to another.

Personal expression at the unit edge is an idea best reflected in European models, where emphasis is placed on making the double-loaded corridor resemble an exterior design. For example, one English design for an assisted-living facility uses wood ceilings, a brick wall surface, a sisal mat in front of the door, a tile edge adjacent to the unit wall, a built-in seat, a display space, and a storage area to give the corridor wall a personal, individual appearance.

Small semiprivate sitting areas can also be developed between the unit portal and the corridor where an older resident can sit and view activity. This draws inspiration from the idea of the front porch, which creates a linkage between the privacy of the house and the public right-of-way of the street. European treatments of corridors frequently employ plant materials, natural light, wood and brick surfaces, and indirect lighting to add variety.

Facilities only one story in height can allow a designer to place skylights over the entry to each unit, creating a garden-like entry sequence. Built-in ledges throughout corridors can provide space for plants and areas where residents can sit when tired.

At the Motion Picture Country House and Hospital in Woodland Hills, California, the idea of a shared vestibule separated from the corridor by a 4-foot-high half wall provides a place for residents to sit, watch corridor activity and socialize. The change in spatial configuration also augments the typical eight-foot corridor width, adding variety and a sense of spatial hierarchy (Figure 6).

The Captain Eldrige Congregate House in Hyannis, Massachusetts, celebrates the notion of the *porch* arrangement in an alcove shared by two units. This porch, located inside the facility, overlooks a light-filled, two-story atrium. The indoor porch is outfitted with an operable double-hung window, a dutch door that can be opened on top or bottom, and a light that can be used by residents to signal their interest in socializing. This is all located within a space large enough for sitting or personalization. It is a flexible, ephemeral, permeable wall that allows connections to be made between the private unit and the semipublic realm of the facility.

Finally, the Lutheran Home in Arlington Heights, Illinois, uses dutch doors in the nursing unit. Residents can preserve privacy and connect to the corridor by opening the top portion of the door and leaving the bottom closed. Unfortunately, designs like this are discouraged because of over-restrictive fire codes that often require special, prohibitively expensive designs or require tedious and lengthy fire-rating tests.

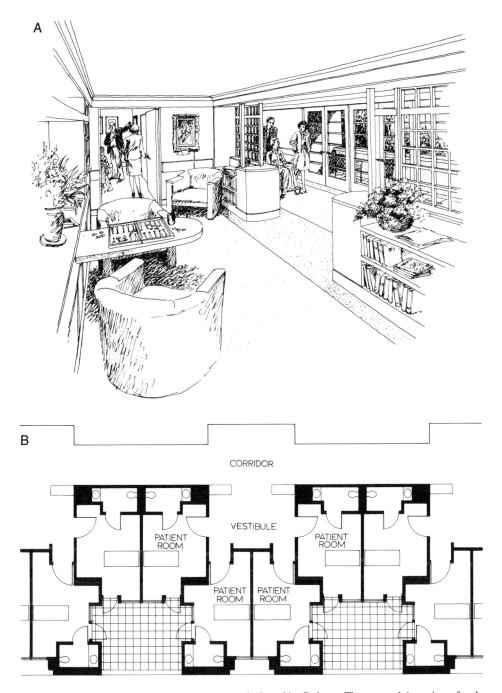

Figure 6 The corridor neighborhood concept designed by Bobrow-Thomas and Associates for the Motion Picture and Television Fund Country Home and Hospital in Woodland Hills, California, clusters four patient rooms around an interior vestibule. (A) layout design; (B) interior design.

C. Decentralized Neighborhood Clusters

Economy-of-scale efficiencies of staffing establish the size and bulk of many facilities. These often require 80–120 beds or units to optimize service production costs and regulatory requirements. The larger size and scale of these facilities often give them an institutional appearance. Unit layouts are frequently not organized to create smaller identifiable clusters or *neighborhoods* within a larger facility. Clustering units around program spaces where meals can be provided and therapy can take place is a very effective way to give a large institution a smaller-scale, neighborhood feeling. This organizational philosophy is very appropriate with severely impaired residents who have difficulties in ambulation or cognition. Clustering units around common areas can promote *social interaction,* provide better opportunities for *orientation and wayfinding,* while preserving *safety and security.* The result is a more intimate sense of scale, and a more attractive *aesthetic* appearance.

In this example (Figure 7), 12 beds are clustered around a decentralized nurse's station, a small lounge with outdoor access, and an area with tables where meals and therapy can be provided. This configuration makes it easy to move patients from their rooms to therapy and dinner activities while creating an intimate, residentially scaled, controllable environment.

In a Veterans Administration facility in Fresno, California, the end of a double-loaded corridor was widened and used for resident socializing. It was designed to accommodate several chairs and a table, thus increasing the sense of neighborhood. The perimeter of this lounge has skylights with indirect louvers, which allow the area to be daylighted from above.

Other projects, like the proposed Star Pavilion in Ontario, Canada, for Alzheimer's patients, break down the scale of the project into eight-bed bungalows. Each of these clusters is self-contained with its own individual dining and living room area. Thus dining, socializing, personal hygiene (including tub room), and service-support activities (clean or dirty laundry), are all decentralized in individual modules. The modules are linked by a continuous looped arcade that provides opportunities for wandering. This path overlooks an outdoor landscaped atrium (Figure 8).

D. Design That Supports Therapy

The placement, orientation, and relationship of therapy and dining spaces to resident rooms has also been used as the basis for conceptual design organization. Minimizing travel distance between a resident's room and common activity spaces has led to experimentation with plans that centralize these activities in one convenient location. These design schemes frequently increase *social interaction,* facilitate *orientation,* optimize *access* to activity spaces, and generally provide options for *stimulation.*

The classic application of this design idea is the Osmond plan at the Weiss Pavilion at the Philadelphia Geriatric Center. Here 25 resident rooms (40-bed capacity) are clustered around a 40 × 100 foot central space where physical therapy, meals, recreational activities, and craft activities are centered. A dining room is located at one end of the central

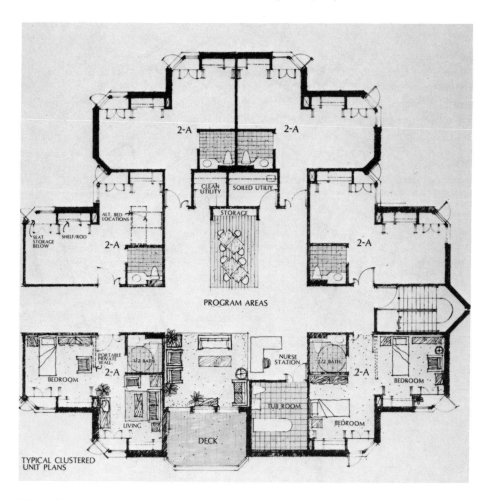

Figure 7   The Glacier Hills Nursing Center in Ann Arbor, Michigan, clusters eight flexible one or two bed rooms around a lounge and program space, thus accommodating a maximum of 48 beds on each floor in three distinct neighborhoods. The design was developed by Dale Tremain of the Minneapolis studio of Ellerbe Becket, Inc.

space, defined by a change in floor coloring and a screened partition. At the opposite end is a gazebo outfitted with physical therapy equipment. Also located at this end is a galley kitchen for activity of daily living training purposes. A nurses' station, located in the center of the large room, juts into the central space, providing visual access for observation. Some of these ideas have been further refined in the 24-unit Corinne Dolan Alzheimer's Center at Heather Hill in Chardon, Ohio. The center is designed as two *mirror-image* modules of 12 units and an enclosed activity room. Each set of units surrounds a triangular space. Within this large space is a fully equipped residential kitchen, a work space with counters, and a dining room. The peripheral pathway around the edge of this common space is used as an *ad hoc* wandering path by residents (Figure 9).

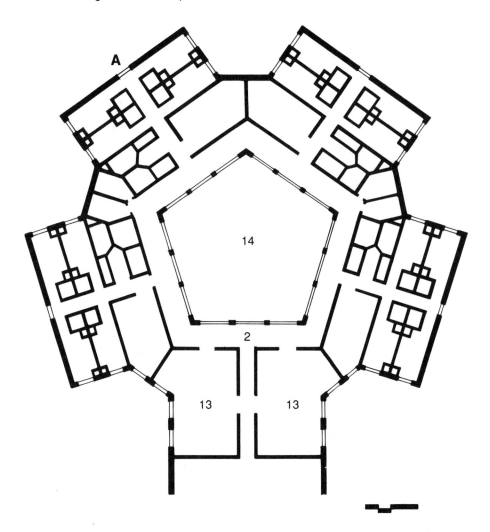

Figure 8   The Star Pavilion (A) planned for the Brotherhood Foundation in Scarborough, Ontario, uses a unique five-sided geometry to link 4 eight-bed bungalows around an outside, controlled-view patio. The architect is Siezenpiper Associates Inc. (From Cohen *et al.*, 1988). (B) Typical eight-bed bungalow plan.

These schemes typically minimize the distance between a resident's private room and communal activity space. Given the interest in engaging residents in a range of activities, plan configurations that require minimal staff outlays and make it easy for residents to *drop in* or *disengage* from activities are a major benefit.

E. Wayfinding and Orientation

Mentally impaired older persons are likely to need a strong sense of orientation to navigate a complex environment. Designs that facilitate *wayfinding and orientation* are also likely

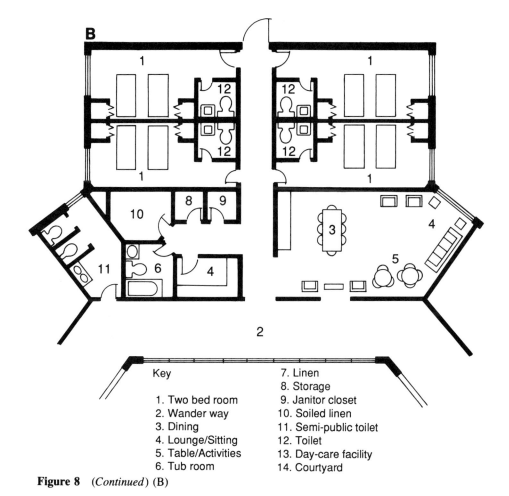

Figure 8 *(Continued)* (B)

Key

1. Two bed room
2. Wander way
3. Dining
4. Lounge/Sitting
5. Table/Activities
6. Tub room
7. Linen
8. Storage
9. Janitor closet
10. Soiled linen
11. Semi-public toilet
12. Toilet
13. Day-care facility
14. Courtyard

to increase residents' perceptions of *control and autonomy.*

One effective way to deal with the problem of wayfinding is to avoid a confusing building configuration. Projects that utilize symmetrical, round, or disorienting shapes for corridor configurations can create major problems in orientation. Maps and graphics can help by providing a mental image or pattern to guide users. Graphics are particularly useful in areas where reorientation is necessary (e.g., when a person exits an elevator on an upper floor or enters a building from the outside). Signs and graphics, however, are best used to clarify direction.

The most effective way to deal with orientation in a complex environment is architectural differentiation. In a study conducted by Weisman (1987), the vast majority of surveyed residents of an intermediate-care facility used elements of the environment such as plants, murals, doors, and artwork to orient themselves and find their way in a facility. Formal graphics intended for orientation purposes were cited far less often by residents. Weisman also cites the importance of *perceptual access* (Weisman, 1987). When it is

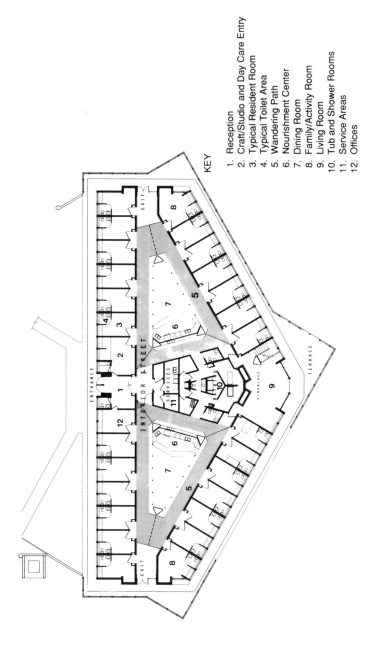

KEY

1. Reception
2. Craft/Studio and Day Care Entry
3. Typical Resident Room
4. Typical Toilet Area
5. Wandering Path
6. Nourishment Center
7. Dining Room
8. Family/Activity Room
9. Living Room
10. Tub and Shower Rooms
11. Service Areas
12. Offices

Figure 9 The Corinne Dolan Alzheimer Center at Heather Hill in Chardon, Ohio, consists of two identical wings used to test innovative environmental and programmatic ideas. The two-wing configuration allows for control group testing, unique in the area of environmental-design evaluation. The design is from Taliesen Associated Architects, Stephen M. Nemtin, design architect.

possible to see out of a facility or to view a centrally placed atrium or courtyard, wayfinding is enhanced.

F. Outdoor-Space Treatments

The use of courtyards, terraces, and balconies for controlled views, exercise, wandering, and retreat purposes is becoming more common. This not only aids in *orientation and wayfinding,* but also provides opportunities for *sensory stimulation,* and *aesthetic appreciation.*

Alzheimer's wandering gardens have become popular, because they provide restless patients with a positive feeling of release by allowing them to walk unencumbered. In the Alzheimer's unit at the Motion Picture Country House in Woodland Hills, California, an outdoor wandering garden has been created with several distinct microenvironments. Shaded and unprotected areas are located adjacent to a looped walkway, which moves from a wide, placid garden plaza near an aviary to a narrow, ramped pathway flanked by a turbulent stream. A range of nontoxic plant materials, several different seating choices, and open and protected rest areas, give the garden variety and complexity.

Sensory stimulation can also be an important attribute of outdoor spaces. A tiered, raised-bed design can allow residents in wheelchairs and walkers to have access to fragrant and/or pungent plant materials.

The idea of using the site context as an incentive for recreation and exercise activities is relatively unexplored. Although research in the area (Carstens, 1985; Regnier, 1985) illustrates its potential in independent housing, documentation of possibilities in care facilities is relatively meager.

One interesting application is a shared balcony designed for a new multistory nursing facility on the Douglass Gardens campus of the Miami Jewish Home. The architects selected an active balcony location near the elevator and nurses' station. Plant materials in a raised bed were used to buffer the balcony from interior spaces and an automatic sliding door was installed to facilitate movement of wheelchair-bound patients.

Courtyard spaces, because they are relatively self-contained, can provide the basis for water features, a gazebo, an active barbecue area, or a passive contemplation space. A courtyard can extend activities outside into a controlled area while efficiently utilizing the site.

G. Family Orientation

Involving family members in the lives of older residents is a goal of many facilities. The physical environment can play an important role here by establishing places within the facility where family members can socialize with residents outside their rooms. Family members may feel that an institution is a controlled, hospital-like environment where their presence is only tolerated and sometimes not encouraged. Transforming portions of the facility to *neutral territory* can make family members feel welcome.

Establishing a neutral, public zone adjacent to the front entry can allow family interactions to take place in a natural way. Alcoves for private conversations, and opportunities for reminiscence should also be pursued in common areas. Making a setting inviting to family members appeals to the principles of *social interaction, familiarity,* and *personalization.*

A creative approach to this concern has been pursued in the design of the Planetree unit in San Francisco, designed by Roselyn Lindheim. This project involved the redesign of a typical hospital ward into a more attractive environment for family members. The remodeled ward includes a lounge for family members and a small galley-type kitchen where snacks and other special meals can be prepared by family members for patients. It was originally designed to accommodate a range of special ethnic diets common to residents of this city, but the idea has utility for a range of different settings including long-term and assisted-care environments.

H. Environmental Interventions: Summary

The environment can become either a tool to support and focus ideas about therapy or a barrier to its implementation. Facilities that are managed well are often kept from pursuing their most effective work because negative aspects of the environment are antagonistic to therapeutic goals. Architects, management, and staff together must creatively respond by developing strategically designed environments that provide humane alternatives for the cognitively impaired.

IV. Home Settings: Strategies for Environmental Management _____

Institutional settings have captured the recent attention of designers in relation to housing older persons with cognitive problems such as Alzheimer's disease, but most cognitively impaired persons still reside in the home environment. The home setting has many advantages for cognitively impaired older persons. Because an older person is very likely to have lived in the home for a long period, strong attachments toward it have developed. The home itself represents a source of memories about events that occurred, such as family gatherings and the entertaining of friends. For an impaired older person who has short-term memory loss but still retains long-term memory, finding the way around the house may be much easier than trying to navigate a new environment. One's own home is also intrinsically personal. It reflects the taste and style of the older person in a way that is possible only to simulate in a planned environment. The home is a rich repository of items and belongings, including those stored in closets or attics, that can interest and involve the cognitively impaired older person. One's own home is also rooted in a neighborhood familiar to the older person. Persons in the neighborhood who may have known the older person before impairment occurred, understand their problems, and are supportive to the caregiver. Proximity may make it easier for such long-term friends to visit than if the cognitively impaired person moves to another setting.

While the home has many positive attributes, it also can be the source of frustration and danger for a cognitively impaired older person and his or her caregiver. Conventional homes and apartment units have been generally designed for active persons who function independently and have no cognitive impairments. Consequently, many aspects of the physical dwelling itself and the way it is used may need to be modified.

A. Assessment

Appropriate environment assessment is a key to maximizing the usefulness of the home environment for the well-being of cognitively impaired older persons (Pynoos *et al.*, 1989). The role of assessment is easiest to understand in relation to problem behavior such as outbursts, agitation, or confusion where the source of the behavior as well as the setting in which it occurred can be identified. Focusing on circumstances before and after a problem occurs may explain how behavior and symptoms develop or how they are connected to the environment. For example, was the environment changed? Were strange or unfamiliar sounds or shadows present in the room? Is a person's difficulty with vision or hearing contributing to the outburst? Is the activity too complex or confusing? Do problems occur in a particular part of the house? Environmental assessment is more difficult when inactivity or boredom exist. In such situations, trial and error may be required to introduce positive therapeutic environmental changes.

It should be noted that while some caregivers make modifications to home, others are unaware of the problems the environment presents and the potential positive impact of changes. Even those who recognize the relationship between behavior and the environment may be limited in terms of their ability to assess the environment and produce a range of appropriate adjustments. In addition, management of problem behavior can be highly variable, necessitating flexible responses from caregivers. For example, some Alzheimer's victims may wander during early parts of the illness, while others may never wander or do so only intermittently.

B. Safety

Diminished attention span and loss of critical judgment can make a conventional setting dangerous for a cognitively impaired person. To make the home safer, it may be necessary to simplify the environment by removing potentially dangerous hazards and objects such as sharp objects, poisonous materials, trailing wires or cords, loose mats, unsteady furniture, or weapons. Eliminating unnecessary items or reducing clutter may also make it easier for a cognitively impaired older person to get around without confusion. A clear path is especially important to older persons who have visual deficits and may have problems with depth perception.

C. Accessibility and Functioning

The aging process brings with it the likelihood of physical limitations that make it difficult to independently carry out tasks in the home without assistance. For example, chronic disabling diseases such as arthritis make it difficult to manipulate handles or knobs on windows, doors, heating, air conditioning, and appliances. Reduced reach capacity and muscle strength can affect bending, stooping, sitting, and standing. It often becomes troublesome to climb stairs, the most common complaint of older persons in relation to their homes. When these limitations are overlaid on mental impairments that affect judgment or motivation, older persons may find themselves underutilizing their homes, unnecessarily giving up activities, and becoming more dependent than they need be on assistance from others. Such excess disability or dependence may contribute to depression and further lack of motivation.

Modifications to the environment may help impaired persons perform many tasks and activities. Interventions in the area of accessibility and functioning require assessments of the older person's ability to perform activities in relation to environmental barriers. Ambulation, for example, may be hindered by changes in floor levels or grade changes between the front door and the street. Modifications such as ramps or handrails located appropriately and designed for good grasp control may assist older persons in climbing moderate grades. An older person may give up an activity such as bathing because he or she does not have the strength to get in and out of a tub safely. In such a situation non-skid strips on the bottom of a tub combined with grab bars or a transfer seat may provide an appropriate solution (Figure 10). Even if the impaired person cannot perform activities such as toileting or bathing independently, the addition of features such as grab bars make it easier and safer for the caregiver to provide assistance.

It is possible, of course, that an older, cognitively impaired person may give up activities such as bathing because of decreased interest in personal hygiene or increased fear. Resistance to bathing may come from embarrassment at having others involved in the task, fear of water, inability to remember how long it has been since last having bathed, depression, or simply the loss of desire. As in other areas, it is helpful to understand the causes of behavioral changes and look for simple physical modifications that help the older person carry out the task. For example, in cases where an older person values privacy in bathing or toileting, making physical changes such as those discussed above (e.g., grab bars) may assist him or her to independently carry out the activity without the direct assistance or surveillance of others. Checking water temperature and depth may reduce fears about scalding or drowning. Keeping a calendar of frequency of bathing may help an older person with memory problems recognize when the activity last occurred and when it is scheduled again. While removing or deactivating the lock on a bathroom door takes away a degree of privacy or control, it may reassure the impaired person that help is quickly available if needed. In other situations, such modifications may reduce the anxiety of the caregiver, who will then allow the cognitively impaired person to undertake the activity without assistance or surveillance.

D. Safety, Familiarity, and Stability

Home environmental modifications can be used to allow cognitively impaired persons to engage safely in activities that might otherwise be dangerous. For example, a common concern of caregivers is wandering outside the house. Rather than trying to eliminate wandering, it may be possible to enclose an area where this activity may take place or

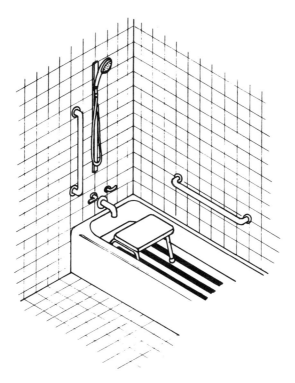

Figure 10 An older person's ability to continue using a bathtub can be enhanced through the installation of such features as a hand-held shower, grab bars, a bench-type seat, nonskid strips on the bottom, and lever-type control handles.

provide other forms of exercise, such as riding a stationary bicycle, which may reduce the need for wandering.

Appliances that cannot be used safely or are frustrating may need to be removed or modified. For example, taking the knobs off a stove may be necessary if the older person continues to forget to turn it off. In such cases, it may be possible to use devices that automatically turn off an appliance such as a tea kettle so that an older impaired person may continue to prepare hot drinks, soups, and other foods. To reduce frustration for those who may still try to use a device that has been *deactivated,* it may be useful to camouflage it. For example, some caregivers have installed complicated locks to keep older relatives from using a basement door. Because the impaired person has internalized the need to go to the basement for tasks such as doing the laundry, locks may only cause frustration. The door may be disguised by painting it to blend in with the wall or putting a poster over it (Figure 11). In such a case it might be better to move the activity to a place in the home where the impaired person can safely continue it.

While it may be necessary to simplify the environment, strategies that preserve a sense of familiarity and stability allow the home to retain its identity. This continues to provide

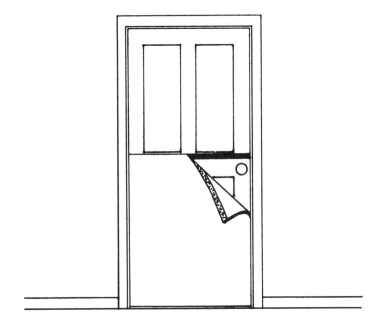

Figure 11 Sometimes "camoflaging" a door that leads to a dangerous area, such as a basement, can reduce the tendency of a confused older person to try to use it.

cues for orientation and activity. For example, modifying unsafe furniture and fixtures, rather than eliminating or replacing them, may allow older persons to keep familiar items that have sentimental value or provide comfort. Even slippery throw rugs can be secured with Velcro instead of being removed. Similarly, chairs can be made more supportive with the addition of cushions.

When the replacement or addition of items is necessary, it is important to take into account the impaired older person's ability to learn how to use new features. For example, a touchtone telephone may be easier for someone with arthritis to use, but more difficult for a cognitively impaired person familiar with a rotary telephone to operate. On the other hand, safety and security throughout the house can be enhanced with the installation of a number of *passive* items that do not require decisions by older confused persons. Such items include smoke detectors, lighting that goes on gradually as outside light levels diminish, grab bars, and railings. Bathtub and shower controls can be installed to keep water temperatures below the point at which a person could be scalded.

Stability and familiarity are important qualities of the home; therefore, changes should preserve a home-like atmosphere. Attractive, noninstitutional adjustments not only help the impaired person, but also reduce the reluctance a caregiver may have to make modifications. In addition, how a modification is introduced may make a difference. For example, involving the older person, when possible, in making choices about changes may increase the likelihood of a modification's being successful. In addition, singling out the most frustrating problem or starting with a minor change that the impaired person finds acceptable may work better than trying to solve everything at once.

E. Stimulation

While considerable attention has been paid to creating interesting activities for mentally impaired older persons, the ability of the environment to provide stimulation is often overlooked. Lawton's theory of environmental press suggests an environment should be safe but should also provide challenges appropriate to the abilities of the impaired person. Stimulation in the home setting may be enhanced by observing changes in daylight, daily weather and seasons through the addition of features such as window boxes, skylights, corner windows, and French doors. Greenhouses, aquariums, aviaries, vegetable gardens, and bird baths also help promote alertness and activity (Figure 12).

For those who experience memory problems, stimulation may be enhanced by displaying old photos or knickknacks that have special meanings associated with them but may not have been used in many years (Figure 13).

Older persons may be encouraged to take up activities such as sewing or handicrafts, which they may not have recently practiced. If a person feels bored or appears listless, moving him or her to another room or to a porch with enhanced views of street activity may promote interest.

One aspect of a stimulating environment is related to recognition and recall. While it may appear that the home environment is the most likely place for a cognitively impaired person to remember a room, it is still possible to lose the ability to differentiate rooms or to be able to get from one room to another. In such situations, it may prove helpful to

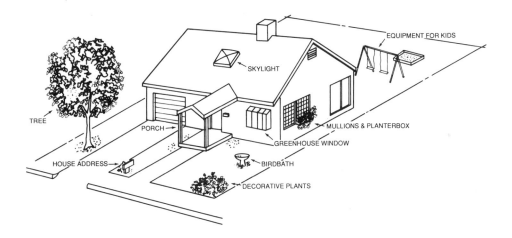

Figure 12 This diagram, adapted from the work of Robert Herman, AIA, San Francisco, shows a variety of features that can be added to a single-family house to provide stimulation and encourage interaction with neighbors and nature while, at the same time, indicating that a unique individual resides inside.

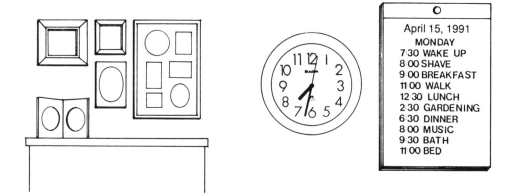

Figure 13   Special displays of old photos may provide a sense of familiarity and stimulation. In addition, large-faced, easy-to-read clocks and daily calendars may serve as reminders of scheduled activities.

reinforce recognition by placing a picture of a toilet on a bathroom door, putting up a sign pointing the way to the bathroom, or drawing a line on the floor leading to the bathroom. Even such a simple technique such as leaving the door open so an older person can see the toilet may help (Zgola, 1990).

Just as mentally impaired persons may suffer from a lack of stimulation, some aspects of the environment can be overstimulating and disorienting. For example, a room may be too noisy, causing agitation and distress. In such situations, the person may benefit from moving to a quieter area where soothing music is played. Shadows, particularly at sundown, may be disturbing to some impaired older persons. This type of anxiety may be ameliorated by adjusting the artificial light level in the house to become gradually brighter toward the end of the day. Some cognitively impaired older persons are confused by mirrors. Not recognizing themselves, they sometimes think that they have encountered another person and try to engage them in conversation. If the encounter with mirrors proves to be disturbing, it might be helpful to either remove or cover the mirrors.

F. Privacy

Privacy is important because it helps create a sense of self separate from others. In the home, it is usually provided by a bedroom or study where one can be alone. Sometimes, it is reinforced by rules, either stated or unstated, concerning when one can be disturbed. Older persons who suffer from cognitive impairments often lose privacy because of the need for surveillance and assistance from caregivers. The more surveillance can be reduced by modifying the environment for safety, or managed unobtrusively through devices such as intercoms, the more a sense of privacy can be preserved.

While the provision of privacy is important for the cognitively impaired person, it is of equal or greater importance for the caregiver. Persons with mental impairments may not respect the privacy of their caregivers, and open bedroom and bathroom doors without knocking or otherwise interrupt activities such as conversations. Sometimes persons with Alzheimer's disease follow their caregivers around the house. Caregiver privacy may be enhanced by isolating the living quarters of the impaired person or by limiting his or her access to certain areas occupied by other family members (Zgola, 1990). Locks can be installed on private rooms to prevent impaired persons from entering. Cognitively impaired persons may also sometimes lose or hide personal possessions. In some situations, it may be necessary to move items of value such as money, keys, and jewelry. When items such as keys have some intrinsic value or meaning to the impaired person, extra or "dummy" sets may be substituted.

G. Social Interaction

Cognitively impaired older persons living in their own homes are particularly susceptible to isolation that may contribute to depression. Social interaction may be enhanced by providing opportunities for interaction among these older persons, their neighbors, and visitors. Neighborhood connections can be created by adding a porch or bay windows. As Lawton (1989) has pointed out, a front porch, which can be secured if wandering is a problem, allows the person to sit where a conversation may occur with a neighbor or passerby, and, at the very least, provides the opportunity to observe pedestrians, children playing, and automobile traffic. Features such as flower boxes, outside mailboxes, personalized front doors, and play equipment for grandchildren or neighborhood children also can function as symbols of individuality and openness, encouraging neighborhood interaction.

V. Future Directions

Many of these proposed design interventions have been developed by analyzing institutional settings and modifications in the homes of mentally impaired older persons. The increasing number of reports in the literature suggest that designers, social-service practitioners (including mental health professionals), and family members are becoming more aware of the relationship between the environment and behavior of mentally impaired older persons.

Unfortunately, as Lawton (1989) has pointed out, because there is still a paucity of empirically validated design directives, the effectiveness of much of the current thinking and efforts to create more positive environments is still unsubstantiated. Hence, many of the interventions in the previous section were phrased as *may* rather than *will*. Because there is not yet a strong research base on which to predict the effect of the interventions on the lives of older persons, the extent to which one intervention will be more effective than another, and the degree to which a particular intervention will interact with others, are still unknown.

In purpose-built housing, our knowledge concerning the relationship between environment and behavior might be increased by following the method proposed by Zeisel (1981). In his approach, the building and its subcomponents become *hypotheses* and establish the research agenda. The best example in this regard is the Captain Eldridge Congregate House, which contains 20 design-behavior hypotheses that are stated as environmental intentions structured to support, protect, and connect residents. Facilities need to be developed that include provisions for testing hypotheses regarding the effect of the social and physical environment on the behavior and well-being of residents, staff, and visitors.

Ideally, such hypothesis testing would occur by varying different aspects of otherwise identical environments that house a randomized group of similar residents and then examining the outcomes. However, such research has been difficult to launch because of the complexity of buildings and their overall cost, the problems of obtaining verbal responses from many cognitively impaired residents, and the identification of comparable settings that differ only in a few dimensions. However, some experiments along this line are occurring at the Corinne Dolan Alzheimer's Center. The design of this facility—two mirror-image, 12-unit clusters—allows controlled interventions to be tested. One early finding of the research indicates that personal items located adjacent to each entry door have helped residents locate their dwelling units.

The great variation in home environments, caregiver coping skills, and the mental impairments of victims makes it much more difficult to obtain knowledge about how home modifications affect cognitively impaired older persons and their caregivers. It now seems wise to identify a wide range of modifications that caregivers and professionals can implement. In turn, observations from caregivers and social service professionals about what works will not only provide guidance about what to try but, as Lawton (1989) suggests, also will help formulate hypotheses for researchers to test in laboratory settings and planned environments.

References

AIA Foundation. (1985). *Design for aging: An architect's guide.* Washington, DC: AIA Press.

Altman, I. (1977). Privacy regulation: Culturally universal or culturally specific? *Journal of Social Issues, 33,* 66–87.

Aranyi, L., & Goldman, L. (1980). *Design of long-term care facilities.* New York: Van Nostrand Reinhold.

Archea, J. (1977). The place of architectural factors in behavioral theories of privacy. *Journal of Social Issues, 33,* 116–137.

Becker, F. D. (1977). *Housing messages* (Vol. 30. *Community development series*). Stroudsberg, PA: Dowden, Hutchinson, and Ross.

Butterfield, D., & Weidemann, S. (1987). Housing satisfaction of the elderly. In V. Regnier & J. Pynoos (Eds.), *Housing the aged: Design directives and policy considerations* (pp. 133–152). New York: Elsevier.

Calkins, M. (1988). *Design for dementia: Planning environments for the elderly and confused.* Owing Mills, MD: National Health Publishing.

Carstens, D. (1985). *Site planning and design for the elderly: Issues, guidelines, and alternatives.* New York: Van Nostrand Reinhold.

Carp, F. (1987). The impact of planned housing: A longitudinal study. In V. Regnier & J. Pynoos (Eds.), *Housing the aged: Design directives and policy considerations* (pp. 43–79). New York: Elsevier.

Chambliss, B. (1989). *Creating assisted living housing.* Denver: Colorado Association of Homes and Services for the Aging.

CHAMP. (1987). *Community guide to the development of congregate housing.* St. Paul, MN: Minnesota Board of Aging.

Cohen, U., & Weisman, G. (1991). *Holding on to home:* Designing environments for people with dementia. Baltimore, MD: Johns Hopkins University Press.

Cohen, U., Weisman, G., Ray, K., Steiner, V., Rand, J., & Toyne, R. (1988). *Environments for people with dementia: Design guide*. Milwaukee, WI: Center for Architecture and Urban Planning Research, University of Wisconsin-Milwaukee.

Green, I., Fedewa, B., Johnstone, C., Jackson, W., & Deardorff, H. (1975). *Housing for the elderly: The development and design process*. New York: Van Nostrand Reinhold.

Hartman, C., Horovitz, J., & Herman, R. (1987). Involving older persons in designing housing for the elderly. In V. Regnier, & J. Pynoos (Eds.), *Housing the aged: Design directives and policy considerations*. New York: Elsevier.

Hiatt, L. G. (1987). Designing for the vision and hearing impairments of the elderly. In V. Regnier & J. Pynoos (Eds.), *Housing the aged: Design directives and policy considerations*. New York: Elsevier.

Hoglund, D. (1985). *Housing for the elderly: Privacy and independence in environments for the aging*. New York: Van Nostrand Reinhold.

Howell, S. C. (1980). *Designing for the aging: Patterns of use*. Cambridge, MA: The MIT Press.

Hunt, M. E., & Pastalan, L. (1987). Easing relocation: An environmental learning process. In V. Regnier & J. Pynoos, (Eds.), *Housing the aged: Design directives and policy considerations*. New York: Elsevier.

Koncelik, J. (1976). *Designing the open nursing home*. Stroudsburg, PA: Dowden, Hutchinson and Ross.

Koncelik, J. (1982). Aging and the product environment. Stroudsburg, PA: Dowden, Hutchinson and Ross.

Langer, E., & Rodin, J. (1976). The effects of choice and enhanced personal responsibility for the aged. *Journal of Personality and Social Psychology, 34*, 191–198.

Lawton, M. P. (1975). *Planning and managing housing for the elderly*. New York: John Wiley and Sons.

Lawton, M. P. (1981). Sensory deprivation and the effect of the environment on management of the patient with senile dementia. In N. E. Miller and G. D. Cohen (Eds.), *Clinical aspects of Alzheimer's disease and senile dementia*. New York: Raven Press.

Lawton, M. P. (1979). Therapeutic environments for the aged. In D. Canter, & S. Canter (Eds.), *Designing for therapeutic environments: A review of research*. London: John Wiley and Sons.

Lawton, M. P. (1989). Environmental approaches to research and treatment of Alzheimer's disease. In E. Light & B. Lebowitz (Eds.), *Alzheimer's disease treatment and family stress*. Rockville, MD: National Institute of Mental Health.

Lawton, M. P., Altman, I., & Wohlwill, J. (1984). Dimensions of environment behavior research. In Altman, Lawton, & Wohlwill (Eds.), *Elderly people and the environment*. New York: Plenum Press.

NAHB. (1987). *Seniors and housing: A development and management handbook*. Washington, DC: National Association of Home Builders.

Parker, R. (1984). *Housing for the elderly: The handbook for managers*. Chicago: Institute of Real Estate Management.

Pynoos, J., Cohen, E., Davis, L. J., & Bernhardt, S. (1987). Home modifications: Improvements that extend independence. In V. Regnier & J. Pynoos (Eds.), *Housing the aged: Design directives and policy considerations*. New York: Elsevier.

Pynoos, J., Cohen, E., & Lucas, C. (1988). *The caring home booklet: Environmental coping strategies for Alzheimer's caregivers*. Los Angeles: Program in Policy and Services Research, Andrus Gerontology Center, University of Southern California.

Pynoos, J., Cohen, E., & Lucas, C. (1989). Environmental coping strategies for Alzheimer's caregivers. *American Journal of Alzheimer's Care and Related Disorders & Research. 4*, (8), 4–8.

Pynoos, J., & Stacey, C. (1985). Specialized facilities for senile dementia patients. In M. Gilhooly, S. Zarit, & J. Birren (Eds.), *The dementias: Policy and management*. Englewood Cliffs, NJ: Prentice Hall.

Raschko, B. (1982). *Housing interiors for the disabled and elderly*. New York: Van Nostrand Reinhold.

Regnier, V. (1985). *Behavioral and environmental aspects of outdoor space use in housing for the elderly*. Los Angeles: School of Architecture, Andrus Gerontology Center, University of Southern California.

Rosow, I. (1967). *Social integration of aged*. New York: Free Press.

Steinfield, E. (1987). Adapting housing for older disabled people. In V. Regnier & J. Pynoos (Eds.), *Housing the aged: Design directives and policy considerations*. New York: Elsevier.

Valens, M. (1988). Housing for Elderly People: A guide for Architects and Clients. New York: Van Nostrand.

Weisman, G. (1987). Improving way-finding and architectural legibility in housing for the elderly. In V. Regnier, & J. Pynoos (Eds.), *Housing the aged: Design directives and policy considerations*. New York: Elsevier.

Welch, P., Parker, V., & Zeisel, J. (1984). *Independence through interdependence*. Boston, Department of Older Affairs, Commonwealth of Massachusetts.

Zeisel, J., Epp, G., & Demos, S. (1977). *Low-rise housing for older people: Behavioral criteria for design* (HUD-483, September). Washington, DC: U.S. Government Printing Office.

Zeisel, J. (1981). *Inquiry by Design.* Monterey, CA: Brooks Cole Publishing.

Zgola, J. (1990). Alzheimer's disease and the home: Issues in environmental design. *American Journal of Alzheimer's Care and Related Disorders & Research. 5,* (3) 15–22.

Community and Home Care for Mentally Ill Older Adults

Linda K. George

I. Need for Mental Health Services: Heterogeneity of the Mentally Ill
II. Community-Based Mental Health Services
III. Mental Health–Service Use
    A. Treated Prevalence
    B. Predictors of Mental Health–Service Use
    C. Sector Choice for Treatment of Mental Health Problems
    D. Differences in the Content of Mental Health Treatment
    E. Service Use among Chronically Mentally Ill Older Adults
IV. Home Care of Mentally Ill Older Adults
    A. Consequences of Caregiver Burden
    B. Home Care for Chronically Mentally Ill Older Adults
V. The Interface between Community Care and Home Care
VI. Conclusions and Recommendations
    References

It is ironic that, at a time when there is more and better research about the causes of and effective treatments for psychiatric disorders, the mental health delivery system is underfunded and underutilized. During the past two decades, to choose an arbitrary but relevant time frame, progress has been achieved in psychiatric epidemiology and in research concerning the biological, psychological, and social antecedents of mental illness. There also has been progress in identifying effective treatments for psychiatric disorders. Older adults have profited from this knowledge and, indeed, it is primarily during the last two decades that significant progress has been made in identifying the similarities and differences in psychiatric disorders experienced in later life as compared with those experienced at earlier ages.

At the same time that knowledge about psychiatric disorders has grown, the mental health delivery system (a misnomer itself in that it implies a monolithic organization that does not exist) has been assaulted on multiple fronts. Third-party coverage for mental health treatments has eroded in the face of economic constraints and beliefs that mental health benefits often are overutilized. Community mental health centers (CMHCs) are berated for failing to serve the chronically mentally ill. Nursing homes have been identified as a major repository for chronically ill older adults, including the mentally ill. The homeless are certainly more visible and probably more numerous than previously—and a substantial proportion of the homeless are mentally ill. Just as older adults have profited from increased knowledge about psychiatric disorders, they have suffered from the erosion of mental health services.

This chapter addresses community and home care for mentally ill older adults. It begins with a brief review of epidemiologic data, which provide critical information about the need for mental health services among older adults. Major characteristics and limitations of community-based mental health services are described, as are patterns of and barriers to use. The importance of home care for mentally ill older persons is described, and it is argued that the interface between community and home care is particularly critical. Unless otherwise specified, *older adults* refers to persons age 65 and older. This is obviously an arbitrary cut-point; it was selected because it is compatible with the majority of previous research. In addition to providing a guide to what is to come, it also is prudent to note what is not covered in this chapter. First, although caregiving is described in the context of home care, a comprehensive review of the caregiving literature is not provided. Our focus is on mentally ill older adults rather than their caregivers. Second, examination of mental health services, though quite broad, does not include studies in which the efficacy of specific mental-health treatments (e.g., electroconvulsive therapy [ECT], reminiscence therapy) is evaluated.

I. Need for Mental Health Services: Heterogeneity of the Mentally Ill

One cannot understand patterns of community and home care for mental illness in later life without information about the degree to which older adults need mental health treatment and the kinds of psychiatric problems for which they need care. Epidemiologic literature is the primary and best source of such information. An earlier chapter in this volume provides detailed information about the epidemiology of mental disorders in later life (see Chapter 2). Here, epidemiologic data are reviewed briefly to set the stage for examining community and home care for mental disorders in later life.

The first lesson that epidemiology teaches is that the vast majority of older adults suffering from mental disorders are in the community, rather than in institutions (e.g., Blazer, 1989; George, Blazer, Winfield-Laird, Leaf, & Fischbach, 1988). The deinstitutionalization movement of the 1970s–1980s contributed to this trend, although it also resulted in the relocation of many older mental patients from state mental hospitals to nursing homes and other long-term care facilities (e.g., Aiken, 1990; Burns & Taube, 1990).

The best single measure of need for mental health treatment is the prevalence of psychiatric disorder. Recent epidemiologic data suggest that approximately 7–12% of older adults residing in the community have one or more psychiatric disorders—a figure somewhat lower than the 14–19% prevalence estimate for the adult population younger than age 65 (Burns & Taube, 1990; George *et al.*, 1988). These estimates also are somewhat lower than those from earlier studies (which often were in the 25–35% range). The more recent, lower estimates are more accurate than earlier estimates because of recent advances in case identification that assess criteria for psychiatric disorders beyond the presence of symptoms (e.g., severity of symptoms, concurrence of symptoms). As Burns and Taube (1990) note, more conservative prevalence estimates based on the most severe psychiatric problems are particularly important for mental health policy and planning when resources are scarce. Another advantage of more recent assessment tools is their focus on specific psychiatric disorders, whereas earlier tools frequently assessed global psychopathology (with no reference to specific diagnoses or syndromes). It is difficult to develop mental health policy or plan mental health programs without information about the prevalence of specific psychiatric disorders.

There is dissensus concerning the extent to which both the conventional diagnostic criteria of psychiatric practice (Diagnostic and Statistical Manual [DSM] III; American Psychiatric Association, 1980; DSM-III-R; American Psychiatric Association, 1987) and standard case-identification tools are *age-fair*. To the extent that there are specific psychiatric syndromes unique to later life and/or older adults express psychiatric disorders differently than do younger and middle-aged adults, both the criteria used to define psychiatric disorders and the tools used in case identification may be biased. For example, Blazer *et al.* note that the DSM-III criteria for schizophrenia may not be age-fair because the age of onset criterion precludes diagnosis of schizophrenia after age 44 (Blazer, George, & Hughes, 1988). Other data suggest that many older persons who report large numbers of psychiatric symptoms do not qualify for a diagnosis of psychiatric disorder (e.g., Blazer & Williams, 1980; Gurland, 1976). This pattern of high symptoms accompanied by low rates of disorder among older adults is not observed uniformly, however. Both Oxman *et al.* (Oxman, Barrett, Barrett, & Gerber, 1987) and Leaf *et al.* (1988) report that older adults have fewer symptoms of depression, on average, than younger adults, in addition to having lower rates of major depressive disorder. For our purposes, it is important to recognize that some older adults who do not qualify for a diagnosis of psychiatric disorder have substantial psychiatric symptoms and might profit from mental health treatment. Consequently, estimates of need based on the prevalence of full-blown psychiatric disorder may be conservative.

The population of community-dwelling older adults suffering from mental disorders is heterogeneous, and that variability has important implications for community and home care. One important source of variability is diagnosis. For our purposes, it is most useful to distinguish between organic mental disorders (i.e., dementias) and nonorganic mental disorders (affective and anxiety disorders are most common). Approximately 60% of the mental illness experienced by older adults is due to nonorganic psychiatric disorders, and the remaining 40% is due to organic mental disorders (e.g., George *et al.*, 1988). In contrast, nonorganic psychiatric disorders account for virtually all the psychiatric morbidity among younger adults (George *et al.*, 1988). This distinction is important for understanding patterns of community and home care among older adults in general and as compared to younger adults in particular. Affective and anxiety disorders, which are the majority of nonorganic psychiatric disorders experienced by both older and younger adults, are treatable and, though both disorders can be chronic and episodic, treatment is often effective. In contrast, although management to prevent excess disability is critical, there are no effective treatments for dementia.

Much of the available research concerning use of community-based mental health services focuses exclusively on nonorganic disorders. In these studies, a major component of the psychiatric morbidity experienced by older adults is neglected. Available research also demonstrates clearly that the distinction between organic and nonorganic mental disorders is critical because of stark differences in disease course, patterns of help-seeking, and treatment outcome. Consequently, the distinction between nonorganic and organic mental disorders will be maintained throughout this chapter.

An important subgroup of the mentally ill are persons with chronic mental illness [also referred to under current National Institute of Mental Health (NIMH) terminology as the severely and persistently mentally ill]. The chronically mentally ill are typically defined as persons with long histories of chronic and/or episodic mental illness, with constant or nearly constant residual disability (e.g., Aiken, 1990). NIMH and most public programs restrict definition of the chronically mentally ill to persons with specific diagnoses (primarily schizophrenia and schizophreniform disorder, recurrent major depression, and bipolar disorder) (Aiken, 1990). This definition excludes two major types of psychiatric disorders known to have chronic courses and to result in high levels of disability: substance-use disorders and organic mental disorders. Although substance-use disorders are relatively rare among older adults, organic mental disorders are very prevalent, as previously discussed.

Compared to other persons with psychiatric disorders, the chronically mentally ill tend to rely primarily on mental health services in the public sector (CMHCs and state hospitals), to live in poverty and receive public assistance for income and medical benefits, and to lack informal support networks (e.g., Gronfein, 1985; Mechanic, 1989; Okpaku, 1985). Consequently, chronically mentally ill older adults exhibit different patterns of community and home care than the broader population of older adults with psychiatric problems. Special attention will be paid to the chronically mentally ill throughout this chapter because they are severely mentally ill and because they account for a disproportionate share of public expenditures for mental health services. In these discussions, recall that persons with substance-use disorders and organic mental disorders have been excluded.

II. Community-Based Mental Health Services

Mental-health professionals and policy-makers have long believed that an ideal mix of community services would both provide effective treatment to the majority of the mentally ill and reduce the need for less desirable and more expensive inpatient care, especially long-term institutional placement (e.g., Maddox & Glass, 1989). Although there is no definitive description of the ideal mix of community services for the mentally ill, certain types of services are mentioned repeatedly in discussions of the continuum of care needed for community-based treatment of mentally ill older adults. The following list includes the services most frequently mentioned and is proposed by Burns and Taube (1990): evaluation–detection centers (including both specialty mental health settings and *gatekeepers* such as primary care physicians), outpatient treatment settings (which should include case management), day treatment and partial hospitalization settings, emergency- and crisis-intervention programs, home care to assist with activities of daily living (ADL), respite care for relief of informal caregivers, inpatient treatment to stabilize acute mental health problems, supervised housing (including assistance with ADL), and hospice (to be used primarily by late-stage dementia patients).

An adequate mix of community-based services for the mentally ill is thus very broad, including specialty mental health, general medical, and social services. Boundaries among mental health, medical, and social services are inherently amorphous because many services are relevant to both the physically and mentally ill. Moreover, providers of medical and social services should be qualified to develop and implement care plans that are responsive to the needs of the mentally ill.

To provide optimal community care for mentally ill older adults, more is needed than the simple availability of programs. Such programs work only to the extent that (1) mentally ill older adults are aware of and willing to make use of them, (2) referrals and coordination exist across programs and service providers, (3) eligibility criteria for service programs do not exclude segments of the population in need of services, and (4) potential service users have the means through private and/or public sources to pay for service use. Procedures such as outreach and case management evolved precisely because mere availability of programs does not ensure their appropriate use. Programs also are unlikely to survive in the long term unless third-party payors are convinced that investment in such services is both effective in terms of service-user outcomes and cost effective as compared to other options, including institutional care and/or reliance on nonreimbursed user fees.

The reality of community-based service systems is, of course, a far cry from ideal. Many communities do not have the range of services described above. Rural areas, for example, are especially unlikely to offer the mentally ill a continuum of care (e.g., Knesper, Wheeler, & Pagnucco, 1984; U.S. General Accounting Office, 1982). Services such as day treatment, respite care, and supervised housing are especially scarce in rural areas. Moreover, even when such services exist, they are unlikely to be able to effectively handle the total amount of community need. As described in more detail below, detection of mental illness remains a major problem among primary care physicians and other potential gatekeepers to the specialty mental health system (e.g., Waxman & Carner, 1984). And even when primary care physicians identify psychiatric disorder, they are unlikely to refer those patients for treatment in the specialty mental health sector (e.g., Waxman & Carner, 1984). Coordination of services remains a massive problem, and case management, though attractive in concept, has not yet proven to overcome this problem— nor is it available to most psychiatric patients. Eligibility criteria for service programs often exclude at least some of the persons who would be most likely to profit from service use. For example, many community programs exclude demented older adults. Publicly financed programs often can serve only low-income clients, leaving middle-income persons, who cannot afford the full cost of services out-of-pocket, without realistic access to services. Medicare benefits for specialty mental health services and related social services appropriate for the mentally ill are close to nonexistent (Goldman, Cohen, & Davis, 1985; Mumford & Siblinger, 1985). Medicaid will pay for a greater volume and range of services than will Medicare, but is available to only a small proportion of the older population and has a clear institutional bias. Moreover, Medicaid benefits vary widely across states, resulting in differential access to services.

Older adults with mental illnesses face a number of obstacles (less applicable to younger adults) to effective use of mental health services. First, some service programs categorically exclude services to demented persons (e.g., National Institute of Aging Task Force, 1980). Because dementia is strongly related to age, this problem disproportionately affects older adults. Second, older adults are more likely than younger adults to suffer from comorbid physical and mental illnesses (e.g., George, Landerman, Blazer, & Melville, 1989), increasing their risk of polypharmacy and side-effects due to drug interactions (e.g., Vestal, 1982). Thus, comorbidity complicates treatment and makes coordinated care especially important for mentally ill older persons. Third, evidence suggests that mental health providers have negative attitudes toward and are more reluctant to treat older patients (e.g., Gaitz, 1974; Gottleib, 1990). This factor can decrease outreach to older adults and create problems in access to mental health providers.

It is important to recognize that two service systems should be involved in providing community services to mentally ill older adults: the public mental health system (primarily CMHCs) and the aging services network. Available evidence, though scant and methodologically flawed (by very low response rates by CHMC administrators), suggests that formal relationships between CHMCs and Area Agencies on Aging (AAAs) are the exception rather than the rule. A survey of CHMC administrators indicated that 66% of the administrators reported an affiliation with their local AAAs, but only 25% had formal, contractual relationships (Lebowitz, Light, & Bailey, 1987; Light, Lebowitz, & Bailey, 1986). Not surprisingly, formal affiliation with the local AAA was associated with higher levels of investment in treating older adults. Those CMHCs with formal relationships to local AAAs provided a larger range of services to older adults, provided services to older adults in more settings, and provided mental health services to higher proportions of older adults (Lebowitz et al., 1987). One important component of developing a continuum of care for mentally ill older adults is input and consultation by mental health professionals to general service programs (e.g., home health care, supervised housing, hospice) (Burns & Taube, 1990). The research by Lebowitz and colleagues suggests that formal affiliation between mental health professionals and general aging programs increases the likelihood of such input.

Barriers to cooperation and coordination between CMHCs and AAAs reflect, in large measure, obstacles to coordination that characterize the service system more broadly: inadequate staff and other resources, lack of structural incentives for coordination, and lack of centralized control of the service system. In addition, mental health services are not a priority issue for many AAAs (Light et al., 1986). As discussed below, most mentally ill older adults seek help from primary care physicians. Consequently, increased cooperation between CMHCs and AAAs would solve only part of the fragmentation of community-based services for mentally ill older adults.

In summary, most older adults with mental illness confront a mix of community programs that is fragmented and may have sizeable gaps in the range of services available.

In addition, some programs may be unavailable because of exclusionary policies. It is likely that reimbursement will be inadequate for some services and nonexistent for others. As we turn to examination of patterns of service use by mentally ill older adults, we must keep in mind that those patterns reflect not only the help-seeking behavior of mentally ill older adults, but also the possibilities and obstacles that characterize and vary across local service delivery systems.

III. Mental Health Service Use

A. Treated Prevalence

When epidemiologists examine service use for physical and psychiatric disorders, they rely on the concepts of treated and untreated prevalence. Treated prevalence refers to the proportion of the population of persons with disease who are receiving care for that disease; untreated prevalence refers to the proportion of that same population who are not receiving care. Examining the treated prevalence of psychiatric disorders in later life provides an overview of mental health service use by older adults and a means of comparing service use by older adults with that of young and middle-aged adults.

Three recent studies provide estimates of treated and untreated mental illness among older adults. The first study, by Burns and Taube (1990), provides a national estimate for the noninstitutionalized elderly who exhibited psychiatric disorder during the past month. In addition to major nonorganic psychiatric disorders, the presence of severe cognitive impairment was included as a proxy for dementia. (Cognitive impairment is as close as epidemiologic researchers can come to identifying dementia in community studies. Both DSM-III and ADRDA (Alzheimer's Disease and Related Disorders Association) criteria for diagnosis of dementia require examination of clinical course and exclusion of other conditions based on extensive diagnostic tests—procedures that are not feasible in epidemiologic surveys.) Burns and Taube estimate a treated prevalence rate of 63% among older adults with psychiatric disorder. The second study, by George and colleagues (1988), examined the treated prevalence of psychiatric disorder in three community surveys (using identical methods of case identification and measurement of service use) for noninstitutionalized adults who exhibited psychiatric disorder in the past 6 months. Examination was restricted to nonorganic mental disorders and compared treated prevalence rates for adults aged 18–54 to those for adults aged 55 and older. Across the three communities, treated prevalence rates for adults aged 18–54 ranged from 38 to 58%; the range for adults aged 55 and older was 42 to 55%. Differences in treated prevalence across age groups were not statistically significant, suggesting that older adults were no more likely than their younger peers to lack treatment (although treated prevalence rates for all ages are lower than desirable). In addition, age was not a significant predictor of treatment *within* the samples of adults aged 55 and older. The third study focused exclusively on severe cognitive impairment and is a national estimate for adults aged 55 and older (George, Landerman, Blazer, & Anthony, 1991). Results indicated that 52% of persons 55 and older with severe cognitive impairment had received outpatient treatment in the past 6 months, and 31% had received inpatient treatment during the past year. Persons with severe cognitive impairment were less likely to have received outpatient treatment than were age peers without cognitive impairment, but were twice as likely to have received inpatient care.

These results provide an overview of the extent to which mentally ill older adults receive treatment for their psychiatric problems. But this broad view fails to adequately take into account at least three important distinctions: (1) differences for organic versus nonorganic mental disorder merit more detailed attention, (2) the distinction between help-seeking and volume of service use, and (3) the type of provider from whom mental health treatment is obtained. Moreover, treated prevalence rates by themselves do not provide information about the factors that predict service use.

First, with regard to the distinction between organic and nonorganic mental disorders, it is difficult to know how to interpret information about service use by persons with severe cognitive impairment. The data reported by George et al. (1991) indicate that severe cognitive impairment is associated with decreased outpatient care and increased inpatient care. Because there are no effective treatments for most dementias, it is not clear that decreased use of outpatient services by older adults with severe cognitive impairment represents problems in access to mental health services. Nonetheless, given the disability associated with dementia and the need for monitoring of secondary conditions, this pattern is of some concern. Moreover, the higher use of inpatient care suggests that hospitalization may substitute, in part, for outpatient service use among the severely cognitively impaired.

Treated prevalence rates provide cross-sectional "snapshots" of the extent to which ill persons receive medical care. Because they are cross-sectional, help-seeking and volume of care are confounded in treated prevalence rates. Help-seeking refers to receipt of any care and reflects the initiatives of mentally ill persons (and often their informal caregivers) to obtain care. Volume of health care, in contrast, reflects the joint decisions of patients and their physicians or other formal providers—indeed, volume of care often results primarily from the decisions of providers (e.g., the physician recommends treatment course, including number and schedule of visits). As described below, help-seeking and volume of care are characterized by different predictors, reinforcing the need to keep those two facets of health service use distinct.

Treated prevalence rates vary substantially depending on what kinds of providers are counted as relevant. In the three studies cited above, both specialty mental health providers (i.e., psychiatrists, clinical psychologists, psychiatric social workers) and general medical physicians were included as relevant sources of mental health treatment. This contrasts with many early studies in which only mental health professionals were viewed as appropriate sources of care. The decision to include general medical providers as relevant sources of treatment is a wise one, reflecting the fact that the majority of psychiatric disorders are identified and treated in the general medical sector (Regier, Goldberg, & Taube, 1978; Schurman, Kramer, & Mitchell, 1985). But this strategy also has two important implications. First, because of a more inclusive definition, treated prevalence rates are higher in recent than in earlier studies—this is largely, if not totally, a result of different methodologies rather than changes in access to and use of health services. Second, this issue reminds us that it is important to examine sector choice (i.e., the specialty mental health sector versus the general medical sector) and its implications for mental health treatment, an issue discussed further below.

Given the mix of services that are relevant to treatment of mental illness in the community, it would be helpful to know the proportion of persons with psychiatric disorder who obtain other services (e.g., home health care, day care). Unfortunately, available research does not provide such estimates.

B. Predictors of Mental Health Service Use

The major theory underpinning most studies of health service use was developed by Ronald Andersen and his colleagues at the University of Chicago (Aday & Andersen, 1975; Andersen, 1968; Andersen, Kravits, & Anderson, 1975). This simple, but highly useful, theory posits that health service use is a function of three generic classes of variables: predisposing characteristics, enabling factors, and need factors. Predisposing characteristics refer to social and attitudinal variables that predispose certain individuals to seek help from medical providers (e.g., sex, age, education, attitudes about the efficacy of medical treatment). Enabling factors refer to resources that facilitate health service use (e.g., income, health insurance, structural factors such as physician availability). Need factors are the signs and symptoms of disease and disability that can trigger the decision to seek health care. Andersen developed this theory to examine equity in access to health services. The theory has been used more broadly, however, to examine the multiple predictors of health service use.

Although the Andersen model has been applied primarily to health service use for physical illness, it also has proved useful for examining the predictors of service use for mental health problems. Those studies suggest that mental health treatment is viewed both by the public and by reimbursement programs as more discretionary than services for physical illnesses. As one would hope in an equitable health care system, need factors are the strongest predictors of service use for mental health problems (Kessler, Brow, & Broman, 1981; Kulka, Veroff, & Douvan, 1979; Leaf, Livingston, Tischler, Weissman, Holzer, & Meyers, 1985). Nonetheless, predisposing and enabling factors are stronger predictors of mental health service use than of general health service use. Lower income and education, being a member of a racial or ethnic minority, being male, and being old are all associated with lower likelihood of receiving mental health services in the presence of need for such services (Kessler et al., 1981; Kulka et al., 1979; Leaf et al., 1985). Note that although estimates of the treated prevalence of psychiatric disorders (reviewed earlier) do not suggest that older adults are less likely to receive mental health treatment than their younger peers, multivariate studies suggest that old age decreases the likelihood of treatment. This discrepancy appears to reflect the fact that treated prevalence rates do not take into account the multiple determinants of service use.

Another conceptual issue needs to be addressed with regard to the predictors of service use. As applied in previous research, the Andersen model has been used to predict both receipt of any service and volume of service use. But recent thinking suggests that these measures of service use need to be examined separately (George, 1986; Leaf et al., 1985). As noted earlier, the decision to seek or not seek treatment is largely in the hands of the individual. Thus, receipt of any care is a measure of help-seeking. In contrast, volume of service use is in large part the decision of the health care provider. A study by Leaf et al. (1985) clearly illustrates the importance of this distinction. Most dramatically, although need factors (subjective mental health status, DSM-III diagnoses, number of psychiatric symptoms, and functional status) were the strongest predictors of any care (i.e., help-seeking), they were not significant predictors of volume of care. Similarly, women were more likely to seek care in the presence of need, but sex was not a significant predictor of volume of care. Interestingly, age was the only significant predictor of both any care and volume of care. Both older (aged 65 and older) and younger (aged 18–24) adults were less likely to seek mental health treatment than adults aged 25–64 and, when treatment was obtained, received less care.

Although the Andersen model has dominated research on help-seeking for physical and mental illness, there are useful alternate theories of health-service use. Two major alternate theories are health-belief models (e.g., Kirscht, 1974; Rosenstock, 1974) and congruence models (e.g., Berkanovic & Telesky, 1982). These models focus on the beliefs, attitudes, and modes of symptom recognition and attribution that underpin decisions to seek health services. Research based on these theories adds a useful psychological and interpretive dimension to the social determinism of the Andersen model. In general, research results based on all three theoretical perspectives are consistent and additive, rather than discrepant (George, 1986; Krause, 1990). Of particular interest is the fact that the same subgroups that are identified as less likely to seek help in research based on the Andersen model (i.e., men, the old, racial and ethnic minorities) are identified in research based on health belief and/or congruence models to be less likely to recognize symptoms, attribute them to treatable illnesses, and view medical care as likely to be beneficial. The major difference between proponents of the Andersen model and advocates of health belief and congruence models is in recommendations for intervention. Investigators using the Andersen model focus attention on social structural factors such as reimbursement mechanisms and the supply of health providers. Those using health-belief and congruence models favor interventions targeted at individuals, especially health education.

C. Sector Choice for Treatment of Mental Health Problems

It is widely recognized that the general medical sector provides the majority of care to persons with psychiatric disorders (Regier *et al.*, 1978; Schurman *et al.* 1985). There is widespread concern that persons whose mental disorders are treated in the general medical sector receive lower quality care than that received by persons treated by mental health professionals. This concern is buttressed by substantial evidence that general medical providers (1) often fail to detect psychiatric disorder, (b) often fail to treat mental disorders when they are detected, and (3) often do not provide the most efficacious mental health treatments when they treat mental disorders (e.g., German *et al.*, 1987; Hankin & Oktay, 1979; Regier *et al.*, 1978). Inappropriate use of psychotropic medications by general medical providers is of particular concern, especially for older patients (e.g., Blazer, 1989; Vestal, 1982). There also is evidence that geriatricians, general medical providers are less likely to detect and appropriately treat like other mental disorders (Rapp & Davis, 1989; Waxman & Carner, 1984). Consequently, it is important to identify the predictors of sector choice.

There is considerable evidence that the majority of older adults seeking outpatient care for mental health problems are diagnosed and treated in the general medical sector. Using data from three community samples, George *et al.* (1988) found that older adults were twice as likely to receive mental health treatments from the general medical sector than from specialty mental health providers. Leaf *et al.* (1988) report similar distributions across general health and mental health sectors. Similarly, using data from the National Ambulatory Medical Care Surveys (NAMCS), Shurman *et al.* (1985) report that 80% of all older adults with primary or secondary psychiatric diagnoses were treated by non-psychiatrists. (The comparison here was psychiatrists versus nonpsychiatrist physicians—other mental health providers were not examined. In addition, the NAMCS excludes providers in public facilities such as CMHCs.) In contrast, however, Burns and Taube (1990) report that older adults treated for psychiatric disorders were about evenly split between general medical and mental health providers.

One of the primary reasons that the majority of psychiatric disorders are treated in the general medical sector is that primary care physicians typically do not refer patients with mental disorders to mental health professionals. Schurman *et al.* (1985), for example, report that nonpsychiatrist physicians refer only 5% of older patients with psychiatric disorders to mental health professionals, although it does appear that the most severely ill are most likely to be referred. Moreover, it appears that general medical providers are less likely to refer older than younger patients to mental health professionals. Goldstrom and colleagues documented that, even in a health center that included both general health and mental health providers, older patients with psychiatric disorders were less likely than younger patients to be referred to mental health specialists (Goldstrom *et al.*, 1987). Approximately 68% of younger patients with psychiatric disorders were referred to mental health professionals, as compared to 42% of older patients (note, however, that rates of referral for both age groups were relatively high, reflecting decreased referral barriers in that setting). Limited evidence also suggests that persons with low education and members of racial and ethnic minorities are less likely to be referred to mental health professionals than are the better educated and whites (e.g., Orleans, George, Houpt, & Brodie, 1985). As noted below, referral patterns have implications for the content of mental health treatment.

D. Differences in the Content of Mental Health Treatment

Available evidence strongly suggests that general medical providers treat psychiatric disorders differently than do mental health professionals. Because older adults are more likely than younger adults to obtain mental health services from general medical providers, these differences are important in understanding community care of mentally ill older adults.

It appears that both amount of time spent with patients and types of treatments used differ across general medical and mental health providers. Schurman *et al.* (1985) report that the average outpatient visit for treatment of a mental health problem is 19.6 min for general medical providers versus 44.3 min for mental health providers. This reflects the fact that general medical providers are much less likely than mental health professionals to provide psychotherapy. Psychotherapy is provided in 96% of visits to mental health providers, compared to 25% of mental health visits to general health providers (Schurman *et al.*, 1985). In contrast, general medical providers are far more likely than mental health providers to prescribe psychotropic drugs. Schurman *et al.* report that 78% of office visits for mental health problems among general medical providers include the prescription of psychotropic drugs, as compared to 25% of office visits to mental health providers. Studies restricted to older adults support this pattern. Burns and Taube (1990) estimate that older adults with psychiatric disorders treated in the general health care sector are four times more likely to receive psychotropic drugs as psychotherapy. Similarly, Larson *et al.* report that primary care physicians prescribe the majority of psychotropic drugs used by adults aged 55 and older, but record psychiatric diagnoses for only 34% of the older patients for whom they prescribe psychotropic drugs (Larson, Gardocki, Beardsley, Hidalgo, & Lyons, submitted). As Blazer (1989) notes, it is sobering to observe that older adults are the least likely to receive mental health treatment from mental health professionals, but are the most likely to receive psychotropic medications.

E. Service Use among Chronically Mentally Ill Older Adults

The chronically mentally ill represent the most severely disabled persons with psychiatric disorders. Consequently, it is ironic that there is almost no research concerning use of community services by chronically ill older adults. It is well established that CMHCs largely failed to provide community service and support for the chronically mentally ill. Many deinstitutionalized older mental patients are known to be in nursing homes, and some proportion are among the homeless. A recent study by Meeks and colleagues provides a profile of a small sample of deinstitutionalized chronically mentally ill older adults (Meeks *et al.*, 1990). Among the 65% of the sample living in the community, 59% were on psychotropic medications at the time of interview (60% of whom also were receiving other mental health treatments), but only 17% were seeing a mental health professional on a regular basis. Because this sample was recruited via use of CMHC records (thus excluding older adults who were placed in nursing homes at discharge and perhaps some who were homeless), it is likely that these results paint an overly rosy picture of mental health service use.

IV. Home Care of Mentally Ill Older Adults

The importance of home care for mentally ill older adults living in the community cannot be overstated. Indeed, were it not for the contributions made by family and friends, many mentally ill older adults who reside in the community would be in institutions. And, although informal sources of support cannot provide professional mental health services, home care is the primary source of assistance with the disabilities and functional impairments that typically accompany mental illness. The fact that home care is the bedrock of assistance for mentally ill older adults (indeed, for mentally ill adults of all ages) is widely acknowledged. It is surprising, therefore, that very little research addresses home care for the mentally ill. There is virtually no information about the number of mentally ill older adults who receive assistance from family and friends, the specific kinds of services provided by informal sources of support, or the impact of home care on the course and outcome of mental illness. Perhaps the best-documented fact is that lack of home care (either because caregivers are unavailable or because they are unwilling to continue to provide care) is one of the strongest predictors of institutionalization among the mentally ill elderly (e.g., Colerick & George 1986; George, 1984; Sommers, Baskin, Specht, & Shively, 1988). This is true for placement in both long-term psychiatric facilities and nursing homes.

Research on informal caregivers of impaired older adults has mushroomed during the past decade. Despite the tremendous growth of caregiving research, however, a number of issues remain unaddressed or inadequately studied. In particular, studies are lacking on the specific caregiving demands imposed by older persons with various illnesses and the impact of caregiving assistance on impaired older adults' level of functioning. For our purposes, it is relevant to note that much of the research base focuses on the family caregivers of demented older adults. A limitation of the research base is that no studies focus specifically on the caregivers of older persons with nonorganic psychiatric disorders. A large volume of research focuses on caregivers of *impaired* older adults, with impairment measured in terms of functional limitations rather than diagnosis. Unfortunately, it is not clear whether findings from such studies are applicable to the subset of family caregivers of older adults with mental illnesses other than dementia.

In this section, two issues will be reviewed: the consequences of caregiver burden, followed by a brief discussion of home care of the chronically mentally ill elderly.

A. Consequences of Caregiver Burden

There are now literally hundreds of studies demonstrating that the responsibilities of providing care to an impaired older adult often lead to demonstrable decrements in caregivers' well-being, as defined in multiple dimensions (i.e., financial status, physical health, and especially, social–leisure activities and mental health) (e.g., Chenoweth & Spencer, 1986; George & Gwyther, 1986; Zarit, Reever, & Bach-Peterson, 1980). This overall pattern of decreased well-being among family members is typically referred to as caregiver burden (Zarit *et al.,* 1980). Many of these studies are based on samples of caregivers serving older adults with organic mental disorders. None of these studies are based on samples of caregivers for older adults with nonorganic mental disorders, but it is reasonable to anticipate that those caregivers also are at risk of decreased well-being. It is possible, however, that providing care for a demented older adult is more burdensome than providing care to older adults with other impairments. Indeed, a limited research base supports this expectation (Houlihan, 1987; Scharlach, 1989).

One potential consequence of home care is increased risk of mental health problems among caregivers. Many caregivers are older adults—usually spouses of the care recipients, but sometimes children of the very old. Research suggests that a significant minority of family caregivers of demented older adults experience major depression (e.g., Cohen & Eisdorfer, 1989). An even larger proportion of caregivers experience psychiatric symptoms, albeit at levels below the thresholds for psychiatric diagnoses. Family caregivers also report high use of psychotropic medications (Clipp & George, 1990).

Another key concern is the extent to which caregiver burden affects the caregiver's ability to provide quality home care and the caregiver's willingness to provide home care for extended periods of time. A valid method of assessing quality of home care remains unavailable. Thus, there are no firm data indicating that caregiver burden reduces the quality of home care (though many investigators speculate that such is the case). There is evidence that caregiver burden is associated with increased propensity to institutionalize impaired older adults, and some of those studies are based on samples of family members caring for older adults with organic mental disorders (e.g., Colerick & George, 1986). The relationship between caregiver burden and institutional placement of impaired older adults is a major rationale for concern about the extent to which community-dwelling impaired older adults receive formal services as well as informal caregiving assistance. Investigators frequently speculate that timely use of formal community-based services can relieve caregiver burden sufficiently to prevent or delay institutional placement.

B. Home Care for Chronically Mentally Ill Older Adults

It is reasonable to expect home care to be at least as important for chronically mentally ill older adults as for other older people with psychiatric disorders. Unfortunately, research based on samples of chronically mentally ill older adults is very rare. The limited information available, however, supports the hypothesis that home care is critical to the ability of chronically ill older adults to remain in the community. Meeks *et al.* (1990) reported that home care from family members was the major factor distinguishing between deinstitutionalized chronically mentally ill older persons residing in the community and those residing in nursing homes. Similarly, Sommers and colleagues reported that lack of social support and degree of cognitive impairment were the strongest predictors of discharge from a state mental hospital to nursing homes rather than to community-based living arrangements (Sommers *et al.*, 1988). Indeed, some of the deinstitutionalized elderly in their study appeared to be in nursing homes only because of lack of social support—their physical and functional status did not suggest that nursing home placement was necessary because of need for medical care or supervision.

V. The Interface between Community Care and Home Care _____

Community care and home care are the foundations of the noninstitutional mental health care system. In addition to examining them separately, it also is important to examine the interface between community and home care. It is particularly important to know the extent to which home and community care work together to provide a continuum of mental health and related services to older adults with psychiatric disorders.

Two major hypotheses address the interface or links between community care and home care for older adults with mental disorders—indeed, for impaired older adults regardless of source of disability. The first hypothesis suggests that formal services typically are used as substitutes for informal services. Thus, the *substitution hypothesis* posits that formal services will be used primarily by persons without informal sources of support and/or by persons whose families cannot provide services (e.g., George, 1989; Noelker & Bass, 1989). In contrast, the *supplementation hypothesis* (also called the linking hypothesis) suggests that formal services are used to augment the contributions of caregivers (Noelker & Bass, 1989). A corollary of this hypothesis is that one of the contributions often made by family caregivers is helping to link impaired older adults to relevant formal agencies and programs (George, 1989). A more complex form of the supplementation hypothesis concerns *task differentiation.* According to this perspective, informal and formal services are used to accomplish distinct tasks, with formal and informal providers contributing the kinds of assistance each is best equipped to provide (e.g., Litwak, 1985).

Policy-makers prefer evidence favoring the supplementation hypothesis. If formal services are sought simply as a substitute for tasks formerly performed by family members, there is net gain in the cost of serving impaired older adults, presumably without comparable gain in the types and volume of services received by the older care recipients. As Greene (1983) points out, however, there are two kinds of substitution, with different implications. *Replacement services* represent true substitution in which there is no net gain for impaired older adults. *Respite services,* in contrast, may facilitate continued informal assistance and avert more costly institutional placement.

Though the issue of substitution versus supplementation is important, there are no studies of these competing hypotheses in the context of mental illness in later life. Research examining these hypotheses in the context of physical impairment has mixed results. With regard to use of physician services, both Krause (1988) and Cafferata (1987) report that older persons with strong support networks, especially those living with others, substitute informal support for use of outpatient medical care (though Cafferata notes that this pattern does not apply to hospitalization). Similarly, Soldo (1985) reports that impaired older persons receiving family care were less likely to use formal in-home services. But the supplementation hypothesis also receives support in previous research. In a longitudinal study of the introduction of community services for homebound older adults, Edelman and Hughes (1990) found no evidence of substitution. Instead, the formal services supplemented informal care, and the latter did not decrease over time. Similarly, Wan (1987) reported that size of the impaired elder's social network and availability of informal care was positively related to use of both social services and outpatient medical care. Noelker and Bass (1989) also found supplementation to be the dominant relationship between formal and informal services, although most of the caregivers in their study reported using no formal services. When used, formal services were supplementary, usually representing specialization of tasks between formal and informal providers. Tests of these competing hypotheses clearly merit further research, particularly with regard to older persons with psychiatric disorders. These conflicting results also suggest that attention might be fruitfully focused on determining the *conditions under which* substitution versus supplementation occurs, rather than continuing efforts to determine which hypothesis is "right."

One factor that may help to predict when substitution and supplementation are likely to occur is the distinction between strong and weak ties (Granovetter, 1973). Strong ties refer to primary relationships in which individuals are bound tightly and pervasively to others. Weak ties refer to less intimate and pervasive relationships, especially those developed in community organizations and other social groups. Granovetter documented the *strength of weak ties*—that the relatively formal and limited relationships that develop in community groups play an important role in providing individuals with access to information and services that may not be provided in more intimate relationships. One study suggests the strength of weak ties with regard to older persons' knowledge of community services. Chapleski (1989) found that weak ties were better predictors of service knowledge than strong ties. Specifically, non-kin relationships, memberships in clubs, ties with other service agencies, and moderate-size (as compared to large or small) kin networks were significant predictors of service knowledge. Obviously, knowledge of services has a far-from-perfect relationship with actual use of services (Chapleski, 1989; Greene & Monahan, 1987). In addition, though Chapleski studied 28 kinds of community services, the list did not include mental health services.

One of the problems in understanding use of community services for mental health problems is uncertainty about the process leading to service use and the persons involved in decisions about service use. For older persons with organic mental disorders, family caregivers are typically responsible for decisions about service use. For older persons with nonorganic mental disorders, decisions about service use are ambiguous and may reflect preferences of the mentally ill person, his or her family members or both. Additional research on the decision to use or not use formal services—and the types of services sought—is a priority issue for future research.

There is an implicit assumption in most literature that an effective interface between informal and formal service providers increases the quality of care received by impaired older adults. Though a number of studies suggest that receipt of informal and formal services typically results in a greater volume and variety of care, there is no concrete evidence that the quality of care is improved or that impaired older adults are better off as a consequence of receipt of care from both formal and informal providers. Another common assumption is that a proper balance of formal and informal care will help to delay or prevent institutionalization. There has been research on this issue, but the results are contradictory. Greene and Monahan (1987) found that caregivers' participation in support groups significantly decreased risk of institutionalization of the care recipients, controlling on other relevant factors. Similarly, Morris *et al.* found that case-managed home care offered at congregate housing sites decreased the rate of placement among older adults at high risk of institutionalization (Morris, Gutkin, Ruchlin, & Sherwood, 1987). On the other hand, Colerick and George (1986) found that receipt of formal services from community agencies was the strongest predictor of institutional placement of demented older adults over a 1-year interval, controlling on other factors. Clearly, many factors are involved in the decision to place an impaired older adult in a long-term care facility. Further research is needed to clarify the role that formal services play in institutionalization.

If integrated formal and informal services have benefits for impaired older adults and/or their family caregivers, efforts are needed to identify effective strategies for helping caregivers to obtain relevant community services in a timely manner. The fact that most caregivers of the impaired elderly, including older adults with organic mental disorders, are reluctant to use formal services is well documented (e.g., George, 1987; Noelker & Bass, 1989). But there also is evidence that caregivers of impaired older adults can be taught to make appropriate use of community services. For example, support groups and other programs can increase knowledge and awareness of relevant services (Chapleski, 1989; George & Gwyther, 1988). Similarly, an elegant experiment by Seltzer and colleagues suggests that informal caregivers can be taught to function as their relatives' case managers—and that such training results in increased use of appropriate community services without decreasing the contributions of informal service providers (Seltzer, Irvy, & Litchfield, 1987).

The interface between formal and informal care should be a priority area in future research. Such research has the potential to teach us a great deal about the benefits and limits of community care. The policy implications of such research are especially important. Although reimbursement of community services via Medicare and private health insurance has increased over the past decade, financial obstacles to use of community services remain formidable. Increased reimbursement for such services is unlikely in the absence of data documenting the benefits of such services for impaired older adults and their caregivers.

VI. Conclusions and Recommendations

Community and home care represent the majority of services received by mentally ill older adults. Most older adults with psychiatric disorders are in the community, yet only about half of them receive mental health services. The high untreated prevalence of psychiatric disorders among older adults has multiple antecedents, including problems of service availability and cost, fragmentation of services, and reluctance of mentally ill older adults and their caregivers to use mental health services. Most mentally ill older adults who seek care are treated by primary care physicians, raising concern about accurate identification and effective treatment of psychiatric disorders. Evidence about the interface of formal and informal services is scant, but it is clear that mental health policy and practice seldom take the contributions of mental patients' informal caregivers into account.

The need for additional research has been emphasized throughout this chapter. Three topics are especially attractive candidates for additional research about community and home care for older adults with psychiatric disorders. First, almost nothing is known about chronically mentally ill older adults. Information is needed about their numbers and characteristics, their use of community services, and the home care they receive. Second, more attention is needed to obtain comparable information about older adults with organic and nonorganic mental disorders. Although information about service use of older persons with nonorganic mental illnesses is relatively plentiful, we know very little about service use by demented older persons. Conversely, although we know quite a bit about home care of demented older adults, we know virtually nothing about the home care received by older adults with nonorganic psychiatric disorders. Third, and perhaps most important, we need to know more about the process and effects of help-seeking and service use among mentally ill older adults. Research is badly needed on the trajectories of care received by mentally ill older adults and the effects of different trajectories on outcomes. As compared to previous research, such studies would focus on distinctive patterns of care, selection factors that create different trajectories of care, and the long-term impact of patterns of mental health treatment.

Despite the need for more research, the current knowledge base permits selected policy recommendations. First, of particular concern is the large number of mentally ill older adults who receive no treatment. Programs are needed to identify these older persons and channel them into treatment. Given recent advances in knowledge about effective treatments for psychiatric disorders, untreated mental illness causes unwarranted suffering. Second, it is clear that community mental health services should be developed and delivered such that patterns of home care are taken into account. Third, mental health professionals must be willing and able to refer older patients and their families to other relevant service programs (e.g., day care, home health care, respite care). Effective mental health treatment includes services to compensate for the functional disabilities that accompany mental illness, as well as treatment of psychiatric disorders *per se*. Fourth and finally, though this is not a new recommendation, physicians and other providers in the general medical sector clearly would profit from additional training in the identification and treatment of mental disorders, as well as in the importance of referring the most seriously mentally ill to mental health specialists. There also is evidence that relatively inexpensive and simple procedures such as the use of psychiatric screening tools may be useful strategies for improving the identification and treatment of mentally ill older adults by primary care providers (e.g., German *et al.*, 1987).

The challenges of providing optimal community care to mentally ill older adults are substantial. Currently many mentally ill older adults are unable to take advantage of progress in the identification and treatment of psychiatric disorders. Forceful effort is needed to sustain progress in expanding knowledge about psychiatric disorders in later life and in using knowledge to inform mental health policy and practice.

Acknowledgments

Preparation of this chapter was supported by a grant from the National Institute of Mental Health (R01 MH43756).

References

Aday, L. A., Andersen, R. (1975). *Access to medical care*. Ann Arbor, MI: Health Administration Press.

Aiken, L. (1990). Chronic mental illness. In B. S. Fogel, A. Furino, & G. L. Gottleib (Eds.), *Mental health policy for older Americans: Protecting minds at risk* (pp. 239–256). Washington, DC: American Psychiatric Press.

American Psychiatric Association (1980). *Diagnostic and statistical manual of mental disorders, 3rd ed.* Washington, DC: American Psychiatric Association.

American Psychiatric Association (1987). *Diagnostic and statistical manual of mental disorders, 3rd ed., rev.* Washington, DC: American Psychiatric Association.

Andersen, R. (1968). *A behavioral model of families' use of health services*. Chicago: University of Chicago Center for Health Administration.

Andersen, R., Kravits, J., & Anderson, O. (1975). *Equity in health services*. Cambridge, MA: Ballinger.

Berkanovic, E., & Telesky, C. (1982). Social networks, beliefs, and the decision to seek medical care: An analysis of congruent and incongruent patterns. *Medical Care, 20*, 1018–1026.

Blazer, D. G. (1989). The epidemiology of psychiatric disorders in late life. In E. W. Busse & D. G. Blazer (Eds.), *Geriatric psychiatry* (pp. 235–262). Washington, DC: American Psychiatric Press.

Blazer, D. G., George, L. K., & Hughes, D. C. (1988). Schizophrenic symptoms in an elderly community population. In J. A. Brody & G. L. Maddox (Eds.), *Epidemiology and aging* (pp. 134–149). New York: Springer.

Blazer, D., & Williams, C. D. (1980). The epidemiology of dysphoria and depression in an elderly population. *American Journal of Psychiatry, 137*, 439–444.

Burns, B., & Taube, C. (1990). Mental health services in primary medical care and in nursing homes. In B. S. Fogel, A. Furino, & G. L. Gottleib (Eds.), *Mental health policy for older Americans: Protecting minds at risk* (pp. 63–84). Washington, DC: American Psychiatric Press.

Cafferata, G. L. (1987). Marital status, living arrangements, and the use of health services by elderly persons. *Journal of Gerontology, 42*, 613–618.

Chapleski, E. E. (1989). Determinants of knowledge of services to the elderly: Are strong ties enabling or inhibiting? *The Gerontologist, 29*, 539–545.

Chenoweth, B., & Spencer, B. (1986). Dementia: The experience of family caregivers. *The Gerontologist, 26*, 267–272.

Clipp, E. C., & George, L. K. (1990). Psychotropic drug use among caregivers of patients with dementia. *Journal of the American Geriatrics Society, 38*, 227–235.

Cohen, D., & Eisdorfer, C. (1989). Depression in family members caring for a relative with Alzheimer's disease. *Journal of the American Geriatrics Society, 36*, 385–389.

Colerick, E. J., & George, L. K. (1986). Predictors of institutionalization among caregivers of Alzheimer's patients. *Journal of the American Geriatrics Society, 34*, 493–498.

Edelman, P., & Hughes, S. (1990). The impact of community care on provision of informal care to homebound elderly persons. *Journal of Gerontology: Social Sciences, 45*, S74–S84.

Gaitz, C. M. (1974). Barriers to the delivery of psychiatric services to the elderly. *The Gerontologist, 14*, 210–214.

George, L. K. (1984). Institutionalized. In E. Palmore (Ed.), *Handbook on the aged in the United States* (pp. 339–354). Westport, CT: Greenwood Press.

George, L. K. (1986). *Psychological and social determinants of help-seeking.* (Position paper for Depression Awareness, Recognition, and Treatment Program). Rockville, MD: National Institute of Mental Health.

George, L. K. (1987). Easing caregiver burden: The role of informal and formal supports. In R. A. Ward & S. S. Tobin (Eds.), *Health in aging: Sociological issues and policy directions* (pp. 133–158). New York: Springer.

George, L. K. (1989). Social and economic factors. In E. W. Busse & D. G. Blazer (Eds.), *Geriatric psychiatry* (pp. 203–234). Washington, DC: American Psychiatric Press.

George, L. K., Blazer, D. G., Winfield-Laird, I., Leaf, P. J. & Fischbach, R. L. (1988). Psychiatric disorders and mental health service use in later life. In J. A. Brody & G. L. Maddox (Eds.), *Epidemiology and aging* (pp. 189–221). New York: Springer.

George, L. K., & Gwyther, L. P. (1986). Caregiver well-being: A multidimensional examination of family caregivers of demented adults. *The Gerontologist, 26*, 253–259.

George, L. K., & Gwyther, L. P. (1988). Support groups for caregivers of memory-impaired elderly: Easing caregiver burden. In L. A. Bond & B. M. Wagner (Eds.), *Families in transition: Primary prevention programs that work* (pp. 309–331). Beverly Hills, CA: Sage.

George, L. K., Landerman, R., Blazer, D. G., & Anthony, J. C. (1991). Cognitive impairment. In L. N. Robins & D. A. Regier (Eds.), *Psychiatric disorders in America.* (pp. 291–327). New York: Free Press.

George, L. K., Landerman, R., Blazer, D., & Melville, M. L. (1989). Concurrent morbidity between physical and mental illness. In L. L. Carstenson & J. Neale (Eds.), *Mechanisms of psychosocial influence on physical health, with special attention to the elderly* (pp. 9–22). New York: Plenum.

German, P. S., Shapiro, S., Skinner, E. A., Von Korff, M., Klein, L. E., Turner, R. W., Teitelbaum, M. S., Burke, J., & Burns, B. J. (1987). Detection and management of mental health problems of older patients by primary care providers. *Journal of the American Medical Association, 257*, 489–493.

Goldman, H. H., Cohen, G. D., & Davis, M. (1985). Economic grand rounds: Change in Medicare outpatient coverage for Alzheimer's disease and related disorders. *Hospital and Community Psychiatry, 36*, 909–942.

Goldstrom, I. D., Burns, B. J., Kessler, L. G., Feuerberg, M. A., Larson, D. B., Miller, N. E., & Cromer, W. J. (1987). Mental health services use by elderly adults in a primary care setting. *Journal of Gerontology, 42*, 147–153.

Gottleib, G. L. (1990). Market segmentation. In B. S. Fogel, A. Furino, & G. L. Gottleib (Eds.), *Mental health policy for older Americans: Protecting minds at risk* (pp. 135–156). Washington, DC: American Psychiatric Press.

Granovetter, M. (1973). The strength of weak ties. *American Journal of Sociology, 78,* 1360–1380.

Greene, V. L. (1983). Substitution between formally and informally provided care for the impaired elderly in the community. *Medical Care, 21,* 609–619.

Greene, V. L., & Monahan, D. J. 91987). The effect of a professionally guided caregiver support and education group on institutionalization of care receivers. *The Gerontologist, 27,* 716–721.

Gronfein, W. (1985). Incentives and intentions in mental health policy: A comparison of the Medicaid and community mental health programs. *Journal of Health and Social Behavior, 26,* 192–206.

Gurland, B. J. (1976). The comparative frequency of depression in various adult age groups. *Journal of Gerontology, 31,* 283–292.

Hankin, J., & Oktay, J. S. (1979). *Mental disorder and primary medical care: An analytical review of the literature* (DHEW Publication No. ADM-78-661). Washington, DC: U.S. Government Printing Office.

Houlihan, J. P. (1987). Families caring for frail and demented elderly: A review of selected findings. *Family Systems Medicine, 5,* 344–356.

Kessler, R. C., Brow, R. L., & Broman, C. L. (1981). Sex differences in psychiatric help-seeking: Evidence from four large-scale surveys. *Journal of Health and Social Behavior, 22,* 49–64.

Kirscht, J. P. (1974). The health-belief model and illness behavior. *Health Education Monographs, 2,* 387–408.

Knesper, D. J., Wheeler, J. R. C., & Pagnucco, D. J. (1984). Mental health services providers' distribution across counties in the United States. *American Psychologist, 39,* 1424–1434.

Krause, N. (1988). Stressful life events and physician utilization. *Journal of Gerontology: Social Sciences, 43,* S53–S61.

Krause, N. (1990). Illness behavior in late life. In R. H. Binstock & L. K. George (Eds.), *Handbook of aging and the social sciences* (3rd ed.) (pp. 227–244). New York: Academic Press.

Kulka, R. A., Veroff, J., & Douvan, E. (1979). Social class and the use of professional help for personal problems: 1957 and 1976. *Journal of Health and Social Behavior, 20,* 2–16.

Larson, D. B., Gardocki, G. J., Beardsley, R. S., Hidalgo, J., & Lyons, J. S. (submitted). *Psychotropics prescribed in the U.S. elderly in 1980 and 1981.*

Leaf, P. J., Berkman, C. S., Weissman, M. M., Holzer, C. E., Tischler, G. L., & Meyers, J. K. (1988). The epidemiology of late-life depression. In J. A. Brody & G. L. Maddox (Eds.), *Epidemiology and aging* (pp. 117–133). New York: Springer.

Leaf, P. J., Bruce, M. L., Tischler, G. L., Freeman, D. H., Weissman, M. M., & Meyers, J. K. (1989). Factors affecting the utilization of specialty and general medical mental health services. *Medical Care, 26,* 9–26.

Leaf, P. J., Livingston, M. M., Tischler, G. L., Weissman, M. M., Holzer, C. E., & Meyers, J. K. (1985). Contact with health professionals for the treatment of psychiatric and emotional problems. *Medical Care, 23,* 1322–1337.

Lebowitz, B. D., Light, E., & Bailey, F. (1987). Mental health center services for the elderly: The impact of coordination with area agencies on aging. *The Gerontologist, 27,* 699–702.

Light, E., Lebowitz, B. D., & Bailey, F. (1986). CMHCs and elderly services: An analysis of direct and indirect services and service delivery sites. *Community Mental Health Journal, 22,* 294–302.

Litwak, E. (1985). *Helping the elderly: The complementary role of informal networks and formal systems.* New York: Guilford Press.

Maddox, G. L., & Glass, T. A. (1989). The continuum of care: Movement toward the community. In E. W. Busse & D. G. Blazer (Eds.), *Geriatric psychiatry* (pp. 635–670). Washington, DC: American Psychiatric Press.

Mechanic, D. (1989). *Mental health and social policy* (3rd ed.). Englewood Cliffs, NJ: Prentice-Hall.

Meeks, S., Carstensen, L. L., Stafford, P. B., Brenner, L. L., Weathers, F., Welch, R., & Oltmanns, T. F. (1990). Mental health needs of the chronically mentally ill elderly. *Psychology and Aging, 5,* 163–171.

Morris, J. N., Gutkin, C. E., Ruchlin, H. S., & Sherwood, S. (1987). Housing and case-managed care programs and subsequent institutional utilization. *The Gerontologist, 27,* 788–796.

Mumford, E., & Siblinger, H. J. (1985). Economic discrimination against elderly psychiatric patients under Medicare. *Hospital and Community Psychiatry, 36,* 587–589.

National Institute on Aging Task Force. (1980). Senility reconsidered: Treatment possibilities for mental impairment in the elderly. *Journal of the American Medical Association, 244,* 259–263.

Noelker, L. S., & Bass, D. M. (1989). Home care for elderly persons: Linkages between formal and informal caregivers. *Journal of Gerontology: Social Sciences, 44,* S63–S70.

Okpaku, S. A. (1985). A profile of clients referred for psychiatric evaluation for Social Security Disability Income and Supplementary Security Income: Implications for Psychiatry. *American Journal of Psychiatry, 142*, 1037–1043.

Orleans, C. T., George, L. K., Houpt, J. L., & Brodie, H. K. H. (1985). How primary care physicians treat psychiatric disorders: A national survey of primary care physicians. *American Journal of Psychiatry, 142*, 52–57.

Oxman, T. E., Barrett, J. E., Barrett, J., & Gerber, P. (1987). Psychiatric symptoms in the elderly in a primary care practice. *General Hospital Psychiatry, 9*, 167–173.

Rapp, S. R., & Davis, K. M. (1989). Geriatric depression: Physicians' knowledge, perceptions, and diagnostic practices. *The Gerontologist, 29*, 252–257.

Regier, D. A., Goldberg, I. D., & Taube, C. A. (1978). The *de facto* U.S. mental health services system: A public health perspective. *Archives of General Psychiatry, 35*, 685–693.

Rosenstock, I. M. (1974). Historical origins of the health belief model. In M. Becker (Ed.), *The health-belief model and personal health behavior* (pp. 1–8). Thorofare, NJ: Slack.

Scharlach, A. E. (1989). A comparison of employed caregivers of cognitively and physically impaired elderly persons. *Research on Aging, 11*, 225–243.

Schurman, R. A., Kramer, P. D., & Mitchell, J. B. (1985). The hidden mental health network. *Archives of General Psychiatry, 42*, 89–94.

Seltzer, M. M., Ivry, J., & Litchfield, L. C. (1987). Family members as case managers: Partnership between the formal and informal support networks. *The Gerontologist, 27*, 722–728.

Soldo, B. (1985). In-home services for the dependent elderly. *Research on Aging, 7*, 281–304.

Sommers, I., Baskin, D., Specht, D., & Shiverly, M. (1988). Deinstitutionalization of the elderly mentally ill: Factors affecting discharge to alternative living arrangements. *The Gerontologist, 28*, 653–658.

U.S. General Accounting Office (1982). *The elderly remain in need of mental health services* (GAO/HRO Publication No. 82-1112). Washington, DC: U.S. Government Printing Office.

Vestal, R. F. (1982). Pharmacology and aging. *Journal of the American Geriatrics Society, 30*, 191–200.

Wan, T. H. (1987). Functionally disabled elderly: Health status, social support and use of health services. *Research on Aging, 9*, 61–78.

Waxman, H. M., & Carner, E. A. (1984). Physicians' recognition, diagnosis, and treatment of mental disorders in elderly medical patients. *The Gerontologist, 24*, 593–597.

Zarit, S., Reever, K., & Bach-Peterson, J. (1980). Relatives of the impaired elderly: Correlates of feelings of burden. *The Gerontologist, 20*, 649–655.

Mental Health and Aging: Hospital Care—A Nursing Perspective

May H. Wykle, Mary E. Segall, and Stephanie Nagley

I. Background
II. Admission of the Geriatric Mental Health Patient
III. Specific Behavior Problems in the Older Adult
   A. Depression
   B. Suicide
   C. Confusion and Wandering
   D. Anxiety and Somatization
   E. Paranoia and Hallucinations
   F. Physical Illness
IV. Formal Assessment
   A. Interdisciplinary Team Approach
   B. Plan of Care
V. Mental Health Interventions for Hospitalized Aged Persons
   A. Pharmacotherapy
   B. Electroconvulsive Therapy
   C. Discharge Planning
VI. Summary and Future Research Needs
   References

While community treatment of aged persons with psychiatric disorders is preferred, it may be necessary to hospitalize the older adult in a psychiatric setting. When elderly persons are admitted to a psychiatric hospital, specific age-sensitive care is required in order to provide the quality of service that will foster autonomy and self-esteem. This chapter will address hospital care for the older adult with mental health problems, reasons for admission to the hospital, specific behavior disorders in hospitalized older adults, assessment

Handbook of Mental Health and Aging, Second Edition
Copyright © 1992 by Academic Press, Inc. All rights of reproduction in any form reserved.

and care planning, the interdisciplinary team approach, mental health interventions, and discharge planning.

I. Background

Where are the mentally ill older persons? Data on the prevalence of mental disorders among elderly persons vary, but it is estimated that 15 to 25% of the aged older than 65 are purported to have mental health problems serious enough to require treatment (Blixen, 1989), yet fewer than 2% of persons seen in private psychiatric offices and only 4 to 6% of patients who receive community mental health services are older than 65. Prior to the 1960s, elderly persons with mental disorders who could no longer be maintained at home were placed in state hospitals and relegated to back wards, where care was primarily custodial. Then came the move to depopulate the state hospitals and return as many patients as possible to the community. By the mid-1960s, states restricted the admission of older persons to state mental hospitals (Berezin, Liptzin, & Saltzman, 1988). In the subsequent deinstitutionalization, many elderly patients with chronic mental illness were sent to nursing homes. Between 1969 and 1973 the percentage of elderly patients in state hospitals decreased by 40% (Whanger, 1980), while the percentage of aged persons with mental health problems in nursing homes increased anywhere from 19 to 40% (Spiro, 1982). Nursing homes were called *little state hospitals* or *backyard mental institutions* because the staff were unprepared to provide therapeutic psychiatric treatment (Collins, Stotsky, & Dominick, 1967). Nevertheless nursing homes became a primary source of care for aged persons with chronic mental illness, far exceeding the numbers in mental hospitals (Wykle, 1986). Although state and county mental hospitals still care for a small number of aged patients (Blixen, 1989), more than half of all nursing-home residents have psychiatric symptoms. Recent government legislation, the Omnibus Reconciliation Act (OBRA-87), is directed toward ensuring that patients in nursing homes receive formal psychiatric treatment services or are transferred to an appropriate care setting.

In all age groups a relatively small proportion of the population experiences problems with mental illness so severe that psychiatric hospitalization is necessary. In fact, one of the objectives of psychotherapeutic intervention is to thwart the need for hospitalization. Perhaps this underlies the lack of attention paid in the recent literature to inpatient psychiatric treatment of the older adult. Mental disorders account for fewer than 3% of acute care discharges of older adults, and individuals older than 65 years receive 7% of inpatient psychiatric services. Nevertheless, elderly persons are second only to those younger than 15 years with regard to first-listed diagnosis of mental disorders on discharge from inpatient psychiatric settings. Despite the small number of elderly persons who require inpatient psychiatric care, this group presents specific care issues that deserve the utmost attention. Planned acute hospital care can be very effective for the older psychiatric patient, particularly when certain therapies are best carried out in the institutional setting (Whanger & Myers, 1984). Research questions directed toward improving hospital care command high priority, given the expected rise in the number of older persons and the predicted increase in their mental health needs (Jarvik, 1982).

Ironically, elderly persons with psychiatric problems are commonly found on general hospital medical and surgical units. According to Lipowski (1983) 40 to 50% of older adults on medical–surgical units suffer from psychiatric disorders. The prevalence of depression in medically ill inpatients ranges from 12 to 45%, and depends largely on the way in which depression is measured (Koenig, Meador, Cohen, & Blazer, 1988; Magni *et al.*, 1985; Paykel, 1985). Thus older adults with mental health problems are found throughout the hospital and require an integrated team effort and collaboration to provide competent care.

Interest in the mental health of elderly persons over the past decade has been directed largely at those adults with dementia who reside either in the community or in nursing homes. In the past, attitudes and values of the hospital team toward the mental health care of aged persons has met with low enthusiasm. Older adults coming into the psychiatric hospital often present with physical illnesses for which they need attention. The aged person usually has three to four chronic illnesses, and the hospital stay for elderly patients in a psychiatric setting is generally longer than that of younger adults. In a retrospective study of aged cohorts discharged from an acute psychiatric hospital, elderly patients were found to have longer hospital stays and more physical problems than did younger patients (Nagley, Wykle, Nnewihe, & Collins, 1988). Aged persons in this study were treated differently by the hospital staff. Less-aggressive therapies were noted for those adults aged 65 and older, and older individuals required more hours of general nursing care. Not surprisingly, safety issues for older patients were mentioned more often in the aged patient records as were functional deficits. Many of the elderly patients were on multiple medications and had more cognitive deficits and sensory impairments than did the younger adults.

II. Admission of the Geriatric Mental Health Patient

Symptoms of depression, anxiety, dementia, and paranoia are the four most likely reasons for admission of an elderly person to an acute psychiatric setting. In a study of 152 elderly psychiatric inpatients, 63% were admitted for depression; 34%, for agitation; and 31%, for confusion (Nagley, Wykle, Nnewihe, & Collins 1988). Other reasons given for admission were delusional ideation and alcohol and drug abuse. The need for hospitalization is dependent on the severity of symptoms correlated with the capacity of the individual to accomplish the activities of daily living and to maintain a safe environment. Along with deficits in self-care, the individual may lack sufficient social support or have concomitant physical illness. According to Gurland and Cross (1983) problems with self-care, lack of social support, and physical illness are three common pathways to psychiatric mental health conditions.

Whanger (1980) reported that mental hospitals are again becoming treatment centers for older adults with psychiatric disorders, now that there is less pessimism regarding the older adult's response to therapy. Acute psychiatric hospitalization of elderly persons has brought about intense review and debate about whether elders should be treated on separate or specially designed psychiatric units or mixed with others. Examples of separate units include special units for dementia patients and geropsychiatric units.

The types of institutions in which elderly patients with psychiatric problems are commonly placed include general hospitals, psychiatric hospitals, nursing homes, and boarding care facilities. General hospitals may contain psychiatric units suitable for the treatment of acute mental illness and problems correctable within a brief period. Private mental hospitals may serve similar functions, with some providing longer periods of treatment. Public psychiatric hospitals care for many patients, both those with long-standing illness who have grown old in hospital settings and those whose psychiatric disturbance began late in life and have become chronic. Both skilled-care and intermediate-care nursing homes contain increasing numbers of psychiatric patients. Day hospitals and day-care centers, which are more widely available in Britain than in the United States, provide semi-institutional care for patients not requiring continuous care in a hospital. Day hospitals furnish diagnostic and minor treatment services and therapeutic, social, and recreational activities. Psychogeriatric day care may be included as an aspect of a psychiatric hospital, or may be separately managed. The psychiatric day hospital may ease the transition from hospital to community for some patients and provide a short-term alternative treatment for others; however, most participants have chronic psychiatric disabilities requiring long-term supportive care. This form of care is useful particularly for those with behavioral problems induced by organic brain impairment and for those with chronic or intermittent functional disorders (Busse & Blazer, 1980).

In old age, the separation of institutional and community life may become somewhat arbitrary. Institutional care is defined as 24-hr care in a setting regimented by rules and regulations, whereas community life is residence within a personal dwelling unit in the community. Gray areas such as board and care, foster care, and shared housing complexes for the aged are considered community residence. Older adults with mental health problems may be found in any of these care environments.

In sum, institutional care implies loss of some freedom owing to the rules or restrictions imposed on one's personal life space. Yet there are many levels of institutional care, with variations in services provided, personnel availability, payment mechanisms, and degrees of separation from community life. Institutional care for the elder with psychiatric problems may take place in an acute care hospital on a geropsychiatric unit, in an extended care facility, or in a residential and long-term care setting. Basic service goals for individuals in acute care include recovery and rehabilitation for maintaining functional activity. In the extended-care facility, those who are subacute or convalescing may continue rehabilitation, with teaching provided as a specific service to enable the patient's self-care and promote health. The major goal in residential and long-term care settings is to alleviate symptomatology and provide care and training in skills of daily living.

III. Specific Behavior Problems in the Older Adult _____

The major presenting psychiatric behaviors of elderly persons who are admitted to a psychiatric hospital occur in the following categories: depression, confusion, anxiety, and paranoia. This discussion briefly describes these disorders and specific hospital care.

A. Depression

Depression is the most frequent mental disorder reported in the elderly population. While depressive symptoms are common, diagnoses of clinical depression are less common because of the nature of depressive symptoms in the elderly person (Blazer & Williams, 1980; Katz, Curlik, & Lesher, 1988).

In older adults there is still a great deal to be understood about the coexistence of dementia, depression, and physical illness and how this mixture presents in assuring accurate diagnosis and treatment. In a study of 102 geriatric outpatients, Reifler, Raskind, and Kethley (1982) found that 23% of those with cognitive impairment were also depressed. Depression more often appeared in those with a mild degree of dementia. Elderly patients enter the care setting, including the acute-care psychiatric unit, often with complex physical and psychosocial needs, making accurate diagnosis troublesome and care delivery extremely challenging.

Depression, the most common cause of emotional disturbance in older adults, may have psychosocial or physiological etiology. Current research leaves little doubt that the neurophysiology is changed in depressed individuals, but physiological change cannot be embraced as the causative factor of depression any more than can struggles with psychosocial factors. In an effort to better understand the psychosocial factors at play in depressed elderly persons, Reed (1989) has conducted studies on the importance of developmental resources in depressed and nondepressed elderly. This work is based on lifespan development theory and incorporates the views of Peck (1968) and others who regard successful aging to be a result of the ability of individuals to transcend difficulties.

In these studies Reed has consistently demonstrated that the lack of developmental resources in elderly psychiatric inpatients was related to their depression. In 30 elderly inpatients with a diagnosis of primary major depression, 50% reported life development issues as the reason for hospitalization. These events were typical of what is found in older adulthood: problems related to relationships with children, concerns about physical health, and questions more existential in nature about life and death.

Another interesting finding from the work of Reed is that elderly persons who are not depressed use their developmental resources to challenge moments that could lead to depression. These are the times when mentally healthy older adults are able to transcend difficulties and engage in new behaviors and ways of thinking to move beyond issues. In the depressed elderly who were hospitalized, Reed found that once depression has set in, depression becomes the controlling factor, and the individual is unable to rally developmental resources.

Essentially, an explanation of depression based on the lack of appropriate developmental resources implies that many depressed older adults are using outdated resources to deal with life events. If developmental poverty is combined with neurophysiologic changes, there may be an increased risk for some elderly to develop depression. Several lines of research are open to much needed exploration: (1) the validity of developmental resources as a significant factor in the development of depression in older adults; (2) the factors that inhibit or enhance the use of appropriate developmental resources, and (3) approaches to the treatment of depression in elderly patients that increase their ability to use developmental resources effectively.

B. Suicide

Suicide remains a serious problem for depressed older adults (Osgood, 1985) and is among the 10 leading causes of death in the aged (Esberger & Hughes, 1989). Elderly persons who are considered at risk for suicide often require hospitalization. Butler (1978) believes that suicide in older adults is indeed preventable, hence the rationale for inpatient treatment. Although older people may be overtly suicidal, they do not always make overt suicidal threats. Their threats are often veiled, and staff should be cognizant of the behavior indicators for suicide in aged persons. Elderly white men in particular are successful in their suicide attempts. The suicide rate is highest in white males older than 85, especially those who are bereaved or suffering from a debilitating illness and physical pain. The potential for suicide is always considered when the elderly person is depressed (Gurland & Cross, 1983). Despite the import of indicators, suicide risk may go unrecognized by careproviders (Kermis, 1986). Staff often do not assess for a suicidal plan or are not aggressive in their assessment of the suicidal potential of hospitalized older adults.

A 93-year-old woman was admitted to an acute psychiatric ward from the intensive care unit following an overdose of sleeping pills. She was a pleasant-looking woman with white hair, somewhat obese, appearing younger than her age. She had recently moved north from Florida, where she had relocated with her husband some 20 years prior. He had recently died and her 65-year-old son brought her (against her wishes) to live with him and his wife. She did not like her daughter-in-law, saying, "She hates me like a poison," and felt "in the way" living in her son's home. Soon after her arrival, she saw a physician and asked him to prescribe sleeping pills, explaining that she was unable to sleep due to the change in location. She asked if he would just give her enough pills for a month until she was able to adjust to the move. She was given 30 tablets of Dalmane, which she took the next day while her son and daughter-in-law were at work. Fortunately, her son returned home early and found her. The staff on the psychiatric unit felt comfortable that she was no longer suicidal now that the son was aware of his mother's unhappiness. However, after a detailed assessment it was discovered that she was still very much suicidal and stated "I'll do it again."

Hospitalization may limit the opportunity for suicide but does not in itself reduce the suicidal ideation of the patient. The severely depressed hospitalized elderly patient needs support from the staff, continuous observation, and intensive therapy.

C. Confusion and Wandering

The incidence, prevalence, and consequences of confusion in hospitalized elderly persons is an area that needs further study; the softness of the data suggests the need for methodological consistency across studies. Available literature indicates that confusion was associated with 16 to 33% of the deaths of elderly persons admitted to general hospital care within a month of admission (Hodkinson, 1973; Seymour & Pringle, 1983). Simon and Cahan (1963) document the occurrence of 17% mortality of elderly patients within 1 month of admission to an acute psychiatric unit.

The geriatric patient is often admitted with or develops confusion during the hospital stay. The prevalence of confusion on admission for geriatric inpatients ranges from 10 to 40% for all types of facilities. Elderly patients admitted to inpatient medical–surgical settings have received the most attention with regard to confusion research. In one of the few studies conducted in an inpatient psychiatric setting, Simon and Cahan (1963) reported that 13% had confusion as a manifestation of dementia, and 33% had both acute psychotic symptoms and dementing processes. In a random sample of elderly psychiatric inpatients discharged from 1986 to 1987, Nagley et al., (1988) found that 31% had confusion listed as a reason for admission. No attempt was made in this study to differentiate whether the symptoms were acute, chronic, or both. The incidence of confusion during psychiatric hospitalization is less well known. For general medical units, the incidence of confusion ranges from 34 to 56% (Foreman, 1989; Gillick, Serrel, & Gillick, 1982).

Nurses, who provide the ongoing care of the hospitalized patient, use the term confusion to describe a constellation of behaviors that indicate impairments in cognition and behavior. Physicians, on the other hand, are more likely to use the term delirium, which is a transient global cognitive disorder of organic etiology (Lipowski, 1983). In either case, the patient will present with impairments in orientation, memory, abstract thinking, attention–concentration, and misinterpretations of the environment. Psychomotor behavior may range from hyper- to hypoactivity, and the sleep–wake cycle is disrupted, usually with greater lethargy occurring during the day and fragmented sleep at night.

As is so often the case in the care of the elderly, demonstrating a single cause for health problems is a difficult task. Confusion may stem from physiological alterations as well as psychosocial changes. Researchers generally agree that confusion is often the result of a number of coexisting factors (Foreman, 1986; Nagley, 1986; Wolanin & Holloway, 1980; Wolanin & Phillips, 1981). Small physiological shifts that would be inconsequential in younger patients take on dire consequences for elderly patients. The development of acute confusional states may be the result of such factors as fluid and electrolyte imbalance, hypo/hyperthermia, drug reactions, pain, fatigue, or sudden environmental changes as occur with hospitalization. Hospitalization and problems with mobility are two factors reported to be associated with the development of confusion in elderly patients (Roslaniec & Fitzpatrick, 1979; Williams et al., 1979). In addition, problems with elimination appear to be related to confusion in hospitalized elderly persons (Williams et al., 1985). Development or exacerbation of confusion is most likely in the oldest-old and inpatients who are physically frail. Patients with sensory deficits are at risk for the development of confusion as they are for the development of suspicious or paranoid behaviors.

Differentiating confusion from the symptoms of functional psychoses in elderly patients can be difficult because both disorders can present as cognitive impairment (Libow, 1973). Usually, however, careful consideration of pattern of onset, symptoms, and course of illness will lead to the correct diagnosis. Elderly patients with psychosis tend more toward bizarre hallucinations and illusions, whereas patients with acute confusion or delirium will experience hallucinations or illusions that seem more understandable. When the psychosis interferes with the stream of thought in addition to content (e.g., delusions and hallucinations) of thought, it is more likely to resemble confusion.

Wandering, often a manifestation of confusion, is the tendency to move about in what appears to be an aimless fashion. This clinical phenomenon is not well understood (Beck & Heacock, 1988), and may present in the elderly patient with dementia. Although initially regarded as aimless behavior, wandering is now thought to have distinguished forms. One form is goal-directed wandering, in that the person searches for someone or something and calls out repeatedly. The individual may display agitated behavior in a quasi-goal-oriented manner, indicating the need to accomplish a task or keep busy. Another wandering style is aimless in appearance, with the individual moving indiscriminately from one stimulus to the next.

A current explanation of wandering behavior is that the activity is a continuation of the individual's life-long pattern of coping with stress and reducing tension, or that it is agenda behavior (Beck & Heacock, 1988). The individual who has previously coped with stress by walking or engaging in a task such as cleaning (Snyder, Pyrek, & Smith, 1976) seems likely to be the one who wanders. In addition to an ingrained pattern of stress reduction, agenda behavior may represent the individual's need to recapture a sense of security and belonging by searching for situations that bring comfort.

One of the predominant concerns with regard to hospitalized elderly patients and related to the problem of wandering is the risk of falls. The elderly patient who wanders is most often confused, and the impaired cognitive functioning is a significant risk factor for falls (Steffl, 1984; Venglarik & Adams, 1985). In a study reviewed by Ebersole and Hess (1985), most falls occurred in the early evening hours, which may suggest that fatigue is a causative factor, as proposed by Venglarik and Adams (1985). Also indicated for causing falls are sedatives, tranquilizers, diuretics, and hypotensive agents (Kane, Oslander, & Abrass, 1989).

One remedy to this problem has been to restrain the patient to prevent falling. The use of restraints to maintain the safety of elderly patients, chemical or mechanical, is discouraged. While restraints may reassure the institutional caregiver, it is generally accepted that chemical and physical restraints increase the risk for cognitive impairment and further psychological if not physical deterioration (Wolanin & Phillips, 1981). At times, though, neuroleptics can be very effective when used to help the patients become more organized in their thinking or to reduce agitation so that the patients will be more accessible to intervention. Psychiatric hospitals where restraints are legally limited have the lowest percentage of restraint use with aged persons, less than 3% as compared to 20% in acute care settings (Bornstein, 1985; Frengley & Mion, 1986). Perhaps wandering is more tolerable in the psychiatric inpatient setting or in environments considered safe for the older adult to move about.

D. Anxiety and Somatization

Anxiety is subjectively expressed as worry and internalization of danger, a feeling of dread or panic, accompanied by a variety of psychophysiological symptoms (Herman, 1984). Anxiety diseases appearing in aged persons can be grouped in different ways, including (1) acute traumatic anxiety, (2) chronic neurotic anxiety, (3) obsessive-compulsiveness, and (4) phobias. In a random study of 728 community-dwelling elders, subjects rated nervousness as one of the top three symptoms across three different age cohorts (45–65 years, 65–75 years, and 75 years and older) and three different size communities (rural, midsize, and urban) (Haug, Wykle, & Namazi, 1989). This study underscores the prevalence of feelings of anxiousness among older adults. Anxiety in relation to loss of health, finances, friends, and family may lead to clinical symptoms of anxiety. As the level of anxiety increases, mental capacities become overworked, are paralyzed, and decompensate. Anxious behavior in the older adult that interferes with the activities of daily living and cannot be tolerated at home will lead to hospitalization; particularly if the anxiety is manifested as agitated behavior, with constant moaning, wringing of the hands, and continuous pacing. Caregivers will ask for help when the patient's behavior becomes uncooperative, demanding, and difficult to manage (Segall & Wykle, 1989). Aggressive behavior, both verbal and physical, is another symptomatic way of attempting to handle stress, a potentially maladaptive effort to overcome feelings of helplessness and powerlessness in the aged person. Anger in hospitalized older adults that is projected onto others or to self requires appropriate intervention to provide alternative approaches to restore a sense of autonomy and personal control. The hospital staff should make a conscious effort not to react negatively to the patient's hostility. Methods of intervening in aggressive behavior include anticipating the patient's demands. Helping the elderly person to express anger in socially acceptable ways prevents anger from building. It is important to support a sense of autonomy and give the elderly person an opportunity to participate in the planning of care. The capacity to tolerate stress in a hospital setting varies among older adults, particularly among those who are frail. Since anxiety is empathetically felt and communicated interpersonally, the hospital staff will need to address their own level of anxiety to reduce the spiraling effect of tension.

Somatization, verbalization of physical illness symptoms in response to emotional discomfort, and distress (Sakauye, 1986) can be considered a flight into illness in order to relieve anxiety. Somatization occurs in a number of psychiatric disorders and in aged persons who are distresssed. Many health professionals characterize such patients as hypochondriacs. Anxious elderly patients may attempt to legitimize their need for attention through such complaints. However difficult to manage, complaints of physical symptoms require careful assessment.

Other manifestations of anxiety, such as phobias and obsessive-compulsive behaviors, may warrant hospitalization of the older adult if the person becomes agitated, and the behavior interferes with activities of daily living (ADL) or becomes life threatening. In the acute stages of anxiety, intervention consists of support and environmental manipulation by the hospital staff.

E. Paranoia and Hallucinations

A small percentage of elderly persons are admitted to acute-care psychiatric hospitals with a diagnoses of paranoia. These patients are often suspicious and lack trust in others. They present with delusions of grandeur, jealousy, and persecution. Paranoia may or may not be accompanied by hallucinations.

A 74-year-old male was admitted to an acute psychiatric hospital with paranoid symptoms. He had gradually become more and more suspicious of his 72-year-old wife and was afraid of the children in the neighborhood. Often he would go out and yell at them. When he threatened to "shoot up" the neighborhood, the wife brought him to the hospital saying she no longer felt safe nor could she control his behavior. On admission he was threatening hospital staff, was unkempt, and was hearing voices. After several days of treatment with an antipsychotic medication, he improved markedly, and although his wife initially refused to have him home, he was discharged on medication, and no longer was delusional.

It is not unusual for elderly persons suffering from paranoia to accuse their spouses of infidelity. This behavior is not tolerated well by staff or family members, who have difficulty accepting the nonreality base of the jealousy toward the aged spouse. Often the older adult spouse who is being accused is devastated, and family members become angry and confront the absurdity of the accusation (Post, 1980). The delusional jealous spouse, however, if not treated, will grow more suspicious and resentful, harboring anger that may lead to abusive behavior toward the accused partner. Inpatient hospitalization may not only be necessary for treatment of the illness but may also be necessary to provide relief for the spouse. Other paranoid ideation includes accusations that others are taking their belongings or are "out to get them." These patients may believe that they are impoverished and cannot afford to stay in the hospital.

Although the older adult paranoid patients may prefer to be away from people, the isolation keeps them from reality. What is needed from the staff is understanding, encouragement, and social support to help the elderly person trust. The hospital environment can be protective for elderly paranoid patients while they are undergoing therapy. Interventions are directed toward counteracting the use of a self-validating autistic system. Occasionally paranoid reactions begin with some sensory impairment (e.g., hearing loss), and the inner world is used to replace sensory losses in the real world (Post, 1980). A physical assessment and measures to correct the impairment are essential parts of the treatment plan.

F. Physical Illness

Elderly patients are particularly demanding because of the vigilance that must be maintained with regard to their physical status and psychiatric needs. The physiological status of aged persons, especially the frail elderly, can be quickly thrown into a pathophysiological condition; therefore, basic physical needs require constant monitoring. Evidence of physiological imbalance frequently presents quietly and insidiously in frail older adults. The first indication of a physical problem is often the development or exacerbation of confusion.

As people grow older, the number of chronic illnesses compound and those adults older than 65 can have several chronic conditions. Therefore, it should be expected that elderly psychiatric inpatients will have a number of chronic physical illnesses. In a sample of 152 patients older than 65 discharged from an acute psychiatric setting during a 3-yr period, 86% claimed preexisting physical illness (Nagley et al., 1988). The largest portion of these illnesses were categorized as cardiovascular disease. This was significantly different from the middle-aged cohort used for comparison, in which were claimed few preexisting physical illnesses. Also significantly different from the younger cohort were the identified nursing problems for older inpatients, which dramatically indicated the need for basic physical care and extensive help with ADLs.

IV. Formal Assessment

Before instituting any therapies in the hospital setting, a comprehensive systematic multi-dimensional, functional, physical, social, and mental health assessment is done when the elderly person is admitted for hospital care. This assessment should be followed by an interdisciplinary team conference to evaluate the findings and determine a plan of care.

A. Interdisciplinary Team Approach

Interest in inpatient geriatric consultative teams recently has grown because of a greater appreciation of the difficulties that elderly persons experience with hospitalization and because prospective billing provides incentives for decreasing length of stay. A response to these changing needs is the inpatient geriatric consultative team (Miller *et al.*, 1988). These interdisciplinary teams consist of health care professionals seeking to maintain functional abilities in the hospitalized elderly person. A survey of 19 geriatric consultative teams was conducted by Winograd (Miller *et al.*, 1988) to understand how the typical inpatient geriatric consultative team functions. The most frequent major goal reported was the provision of geriatric assessments (80%) with discharge planning reported also as a major goal by 37%. Consultation as a review process for admission to a special geriatric ward was cited by one fifth of the respondents. Specific reasons cited for the consultation were: (1) placement and outpatient followup; (2) evaluation of reasons for the occurrence of problems, such as falls, incontinence, or decubitus ulcers; (3) evaluation of psychiatric problems; (4) help with ethical issues; and (5) assistance with decreasing length of stay.

B. Plan of Care

The plan of care follows the initial admission interview, health history, and assessment of the patient's psychosocial needs, mental and functional status, and environmental, family, and community resources. Interpretation of the data leads to the development of a comprehensive theory-based care plan that includes a list of problems and assets, goals, and plan of action including the patient, family, and interdisciplinary team. The plan of care includes interventions that will promote mental health, establish maintenance of function, promote communication, and provide safety and learning opportunities.

Implementation of the plan of care requires the expertise of the team to identify referral resources and establish the consistencies of approach to be used by staff. The plan of care is individualized, based on data and cultural variations that affect the health care of older adults, and requires continuous assessment for change, depending on the evaluation of outcomes (ANA, 1986).

V. Mental Health Interventions for Hospitalized Aged Persons _____

A number of concerns have been noted in the literature about the younger therapist and older client interaction (LeBray, 1984). Mental health professionals bring their own biases about the value of treating the psychogeriatric patient to the hospital setting. Some may believe that the situation of the aged is hopeless or that the elderly person would respond only minimally to treatment. Others argue that differences in the age of the therapist and the older adult speak to transference and counter-transference treatment issues. Therapists may have idealized feelings toward their older patients and look upon them as parents, or older patients may view young therapists as children. This relationship could be antagonistic to treatment. Such a situation calls for help from the interdisciplinary team, who can provide insight into the phenomenon. Treatment differentiation between the young and the old brings to bear ethical issues that also need to be examined within the interdisciplinary team. Most elderly persons respond to a more supportive form of therapy, which requires the therapist to be active, directive, and involved with the patient in a meaningful way. This interaction may go against the traditional thinking about therapy. However, since we know little about the developmental needs of those older than 65, the therapist has a rich opportunity to learn how older adults function and adapt to change during their hospitalization.

Recognizing the diversity in those persons older than 65, one would expect to see various degrees of response to mental health interventions. In the psychiatric field we are familiar with the so-called traditional therapies—individual, family, and group—and the somatic therapies, including psychotropic drugs and electroconvulsive therapy (ECT). Other forms of therapy utilized with elders include reminiscence groups, bereavement groups, guided imagery, exercise, remotivation, and reality-oriented groups, to name a few. Even with the traditional therapies, professional caregivers have historically been reluctant to utilize therapy with the older adult. Reasons for this attitude vary, ranging from the cost-effectiveness of treatment, the shortage of therapists with the expertise to work with the elderly, and the general attitudes, values, and beliefs of mental health professionals regarding the efficacy of treatment for the aged. Additionally, older adults themselves often possess negative attitudes and beliefs about mental illness, mental health professionals, and psychiatric hospitals that prevent them from seeking and accepting professional services. To a large degree, the current aged cohort has not held treatment for mental illness in high esteem.

Freud believed that by age 50, it was too late for classic psychotherapy or psychoanalysis. But we must remember that in Freud's time, the early 1900s, people were not living into the seventh, eighth, and ninth decade of life. Therefore, if the old of Freud's period had shorter life spans, there was some question as to whether or not to invest the time and energy in treatment. If analysis took seven years, at the end of that time a person over 50 was expected to be dead, and therapy would have been a waste. Today, however, a person depressed at 70 may live to be 90. So why live 20 years in misery, let alone face the deleterious effects that depression would have on the significant others, or the high cost, both in dollars and energy, to the individual?

Ebersole and Hess (1990) list 10 psychiatric interventions that can be utilized for the hospitalized older adult. These include brief psychotherapy, crises intervention, group work, family groups, confidants, peer counsels, reminiscence life review, and psychotropic drugs. Gatz, Popkin, Pino, and VandenBos (1985) provide a detailed overview of the interventions utilized with aged persons. They discuss studies that lend support to the efficacy of treatment for older persons. The authors conclude that across interventions, there are at least four common principles leading to change:

1. a sense of control, self-efficacy, and hope;
2. establishing a relationship with the helper;
3. providing or elucidating a sense of meaning; and
4. establishing constructive contingencies in the environment.

Recently there has been an increase in the number of positive research studies on the efficacy of various therapies with aged patients suffering from mental illness, thus providing a more optimistic view. Buckhart (1987) conducted a research synthesis of 41 controlled studies using meta-analysis techniques. She examined the type of treatment along with the subject response. Because elderly adults are seldom included in studies of traditional psychotherapy, a broader definition of therapy was used—any nondrug treatment nurses and others could provide and use in practice with a goal of relief of emotional distress and unacceptable behavior.

Six types of therapy were highlighted in the literature review: reality orientation, cognitive therapy, physical exercise, socialization, reminiscence, and interaction contact or touch. These types of therapy were examined for their differential effects on the mental health of elderly clients. Overall the subjects treated with any form of the six therapies tended to improve. Findings from the meta-analytic study supported the notion that elderly clients with mental health problems can benefit from treatment when compared to nontreatment controls. Further, the findings did not conclusively support superiority of any one treatment over another, or that a specific treatment was more beneficial for any mental health problem. Clearly there is a need for more study in this area.

Other studies have been conducted regarding individual therapies with a consensus that elders respond to treatment, especially if the mental health professional understands the aging process and the ways in which elders respond to mental illness differentially from younger adults. Ebersole and Hess (1990) nicely delineate differences in depressive symptoms across the life span, and most geropsychiatrists agree that depression in the elderly may present with strikingly different symptom manifestations.

A. Pharmacotherapy

Psychotropic drugs are commonly prescribed in the hospital setting, and their use is a major treatment modality for psychiatric patients. While these drugs are therapeutic for some major mental health disorders, they are to be approached with caution when treating the older adult. The staff must be aware of drug side-effects and how the age of the patient relates to the dosage, type, and frequency of administration. Aged persons can be very sensitive to psychotropic drugs owing to the physiological changes that occur from normal aging. Because of the increasing frequency of chronic illnesses among the aged, it is not unusual for these patients to have as many as four to five prescribed medications. Careful observation and monitoring of medication effects as well as symptom response are a most critical part of the aged person's psychiatric hospital care. Polypharmacy, altered pharmacologic response, and pharmacokinetic changes should be continuously evaluated.

Teaching the staff, patients, and families the appropriate use of medication is essential for the well-being of aged psychiatric patients and their aftercare. Pharmacotherapy is usually prescribed for patients along with other forms of geropsychiatric treatment. The relationship between the response to medications and response to the other therapies should be examined frequently. Mental health professionals need to be well informed about the medications that are prescribed for their clients.

B. Electroconvulsive Therapy

Older patients who have medication side-effects or respond poorly to medications and other therapies may be considered for electroconvulsive therapy. ECT has come under criticism for its use with hospitalized elderly psychiatric patients. It has been described in modern times as a safe, effective treatment for the elderly; yet some studies have shown that complications do increase with age, particularly in the old-old, those 75 and older (Burke, Rubin, Zorumski, & Wetzel, 1987). Therefore, in those situations in which ECT is used to treat older adults, special care and precautions are to be taken before, during, and after treatment. The elderly person using ECT requires intensive nursing care immediately following the procedure, and close observations between treatments. Current practice and guidelines for the use of ECT are much improved, so that ECT is considered as safe and effective for older persons as is other types of treatment (Calkins, Davis, & Ford, 1986).

C. Discharge Planning

The concept of the continuum of care is based on the recognition that elderly persons need different services at different stages in their hospitalization as health conditions and degree of illness change. The different health levels range from well elderly, whatever their chronological age, who need such services as recreation and legal aid, to the frail elderly who need 24-hr nursing care, to the severely ill who need medically oriented services. The varied individual needs and health conditions (often multiple illnesses) among the over 30 million elderly require many service options along a continuum (Maddox, 1987), and these options should be considered upon discharge.

Planning for the discharge of patients from acute-care hospitalization presents thorny problems for institutions, patients, and families. For older patients, the time immediately following hospitalization may be one of particular vulnerability. All participants—patients, institutional providers, and family—must cooperatively attempt to assess physical, emotional, and cognitive skills and weaknesses, and predict the likelihood of their change over time. Early assessment of the caregiver is critical in discharge planning. These analyses must be combined with (1) the patient's preferences, (2) the institution's evaluation measures designed to support the patient's caregiving potential, and (3) the financial realities. The process is most difficult, however, when the patient's mental capacity is diminished, and the patient indicates a clear and consistent preference that is opposed to the institution provider's recommendations for the patient's needs in the posthospital period (Harper, 1989).

In 1984 the Division of Legal and Ethical Issues in Health Care in the Department of Epidemiology and Social Medicine at Montefiore Medical Center and the Albert Einstein College of Medicine received a grant to add a lawyer to the interdisciplinary geriatric team in order to address the legal needs of hospitalized elderly patients. The premise of this project was that early legal intervention could assist in resolving some of these discharge-planning dilemmas by shifting the decision-making locus to a judge empowered to decide about complex situations and conflicting assertions of rights and duties (Dubler, 1987).

VI. Summary and Future Research Needs

In recent years there have been positive trends in geriatric mental health and a change in the treatment attitudes toward the hospitalized older adult. Hospitals have a major responsibility for providing and establishing high-quality mental and physical health care to older patients (Abrahams & Crooks, 1984). Research studies have demonstrated that older adults do respond positively to hospitalization and to a variety of therapeutic interventions. The future trend is to increase mental health promotion and to increase the utilization of community mental health services for the older adult. There remains a critical need to provide hospital care for those aged persons who require specialized inpatient psychiatric treatment. With the predicted increase in the older adult population, there is a mandate to provide better mental health services to improve the quality of life of aged persons. Further study of the developmental needs of elders and differential treatment of their mental health problems is imperative. The acute psychiatric hospital as a therapeutic environment of care also needs further study to determine the impact of the environmental press on both the physical and psychological well-being of the elderly person. Goldman (1984) states that we need to expand those medical, psychiatric, social, and economic programs in which we are already competent, and explore new ways to prevent and alleviate problems that interfere with well-being, develop adequate treatment resources, and contain costs.

References

Abrahams, J. P., & Crooks, V. J. (Eds.) (1984). *Geriatric mental health.* New York: Grune & Stratton.

American Nurses' Association. (1986). *Gerontological nursing curriculum.* Kansas City: American Nurses' Association.

APA Task Force on ECT. (1979). American Psychiatric Association. No. 14, Washington, DC.

Beck, C., & Heacock, P. (1988). Nursing and intervention for patients with Alzheimer's Disease. *Nursing Clinics of North America, 23*(1), 95–124.

Berezin, M. A., Liptzin, B., & Salzman, C. (1988). The elderly person. In A. M. Nicholi (Ed.), *The new Harvard guide to psychiatry.* (pp. 665–680). Cambridge, Massachusetts: Belnap Press of Harvard Univ. Press.

Blazer, D., & Williams, C. D. (1980). Epidemiology of dysphoria and depression in an elderly population. *American Journal of Psychiatry, 137*(4), 439–444.

Blixen, C. E. (1989). Aging and mental health care. *Journal of Gerontological Nursing, 14*(11), 11–15.

Bornstein, P. E. (1985). The use of restraints on a general psychiatric unit. *Journal of Clinical Psychiatry, 46,* 175–178.

Burke, W. J., Rubin, E. H., Zorumski, C. F., & Wetzel, R. D. (1987). The safety of ECT in geriatric psychiatry. *Journal of the American Geriatrics Society, 35,* 516–521.

Burkhart, C. (1987). The effect of therapy on the mental health of the elderly. *Research in Nursing and Health, 10,* 277–285.

Busse, E. W., & Blazer, D. G. (Eds.) (1980). *Handbook of geriatric psychiatry.* New York: Van Nostrand Reinhold.

Butler, R. N. (Ed.) (1978). *Overview on aging: Aging: The process and the people.* New York: Brunner/Hazel.

Calkins, E., Davis, P., & Ford, A. (1986). *The practices of geriatrics.* Philadelphia: Saunders.

Collins, J., Stotsky, B., & Dominick, J. (1967). Is the nursing home the mental hospital's back ward in the community? *Journal of the American Geriatrics Society,* 75–81.

Dubler, N. N. (1987, Summer). Introduction. *Generations, XI*(4), 6–8.

Ebersole, P. (1989). *Caring For the Psychogeriatric Client.* New York: Springer.

Ebersole, P., & Hess, P. (Eds.) (1990). *Toward healthy aging: Human needs and nursing response.* Baltimore: Mosby.

Esberger, K. K., & Hughes, S. T. (1989). *Nursing care of the aged.* Norwalk, CT: Appleton & Lange.

Foreman, M. D. (1989). Confusion in the hospitalized elderly: Incidence, onset and associated factors. *Research in Nursing and Health, 12*(1), 21–29.

Foreman, M. D. (1986). Acute confusional states in hospitalized elderly: A research dilemma. *Nursing Research, 35*(1), 34–38.

Frengley, J. D., & Mion, L. C. (1986). Incidence of physical restraints on acute general medical wards. *Journal of the American Geriatrics Society, 34,* 565–568.

Gatz, M., Popkin, S., Pino, C., VandenBos, G. R. (1985). Psychological interventions with older adults. In J. E. Birren, & K. W. Schaie (Eds.), *Handbook of the psychology of aging* (2nd ed.). (pp. 755–777). New York: Van Nostrand Reinhold.

Gillick, M. R., Serrel, N. A., & Gillick, L. S. (1982). Adverse consequences of hospitalization in the elderly. *Social Sciences in Medicine, 16*(10), 1033–1038.

Goldman, R. (1984). Forward. In J. P. Abrahams, & V. J. Crooks (Eds.), *Geriatric Mental Health* (pp. ix–xi). New York: Grune & Stratton.

Gurland, B., & Cross, P. S. (1983). Suicide among the elderly. In N. K. Aronson, R. Bennett, & B. J. Gurland (Eds.), *The acting-out elderly* (pp. 55–66). New York: Haworth.

Harper, H. (1989). Providing mental health services in the homes of the elderly. *Caring, 8*(6), 5–9, 52–53.

Haug, M., Wykle, M., & Namazi, K. (1989). Self-care among older adults. *Social Sciences and Medicine, 29,* No. 2, 171–183.

Herman, S. (1984). Anxiety disorders. In A. D. Whanger, & A. C. Myers (Eds.), *Mental health assessment and therapeutic intervention with older adults.* Rockville, Maryland: Aspen.

Hodkinson, H. M. (1973). Mental impairment in the elderly. *Journal of Royal College of Physicians, 7,* 305–317.

Jarvik, L. F. (1982). Aging and psychiatry. In *psychiatric clinics of North America* (pp. 5–9). Philadelphia: Saunders.

Kane, R. L., Ouslander, J. G., & Abrass, I. B. (1989). *Essentials of clinical geriatrics* (2nd ed.). New York: McGraw-Hill.

Katz, I. R., Curlik, S., & Lesher, E. L. (1988). Use of anti-depressants in the frail elderly. When, why, and how. *Clinical Geriatric Medicine. 4*(1), 203–222.

Kermis, M. D. (1986). *Mental health in late life: The adaptive process.* Boston: Jones and Bartlett.

Koenig, H. G., Meador, K. G., Cohen, H. J., & Blazer, D. G. (1988). Depression in elderly hospitalized patients with medical illness. *Archives of Internal Medicine. 148*(9), 1929–1936.

LeBray, P. (1984). Providing clinical geropsychology services in community settings. In J. P. Abrahams & V. J. Crooks (Eds.), *Geriatric mental health* (pp. 201–216). New York: Grune & Stratton.

Libow, L. S. (1973). Pseudo-senility: Acute and reversible organic brain syndromes. *Journal of American Geriatrics Society, 21,* 112–120.

Lipowski, Z. J. (1983). The need to integrate liaison psychiatry and geropsychiatry. *American Journal of Psychiatry, 140*(8), 1003–1005.

Maddox, G. (1987). *Encyclopedia of Aging* (pp. 145–147). New York: Springer.

Magni, G., Schifano, F., DeLeo, D., De Dominicis, G., Renecto, V., and Vianello, S. (1985). Evaluation of use patterns of psychotropic drugs in an Italian geriatric hospital. *Neuropsychobiology. 13*(1–2), 38–43.

Miller, R. L., Winograd, C., Frengley, D., Tsukuda, R., Katz, P., Barry, P., Shepherd, A., Cooney, L. (1988). Inpatient geriatric consultative teams. *Gerontology and Geriatrics Education, 8*(1/2), 35–52.

Nagley, S. J. (1986). Preventing confusion in your patients. *Journal of Gerontological Nursing, 12*(3), 27–31.

Nagley, S., Wykle, M., Nnewihe, A., & Collins, H. (1988). Age cohort comparison in an acute psychiatric setting. *The Gerontologist, 28,* 39A.

Osgood, N. (1985). *Suicide in the Elderly.* Rockville, MD: Aspen.

Paykel, E. S. (1985). The clinical interview for depression: Development, reliability, and validity. *Journal of Affective Disorders, 9*(1), 85–96.

Peck, R. (1968). Psychological developments in the second half of life. In B. L. Neugarten (Ed.), *Middle aging and aging* (pp. 88–92). Chicago: University of Chicago.

Post, F. (1980). Paranoid, schizophrenia-like and schizophrenia states in the aged. In J. E. Birren & R. B. Sloane (Eds.), *Handbook of mental health and aging* (pp. 591–615). Englewood Cliffs, NJ: Prentice-Hall.

Reed, P. G. (1989). Mental health of older adults. *Western Journal of Nursing Research, 11*(2), 143–157.

Reifler, B., Raskind, H., & Kethley, A. (1982). Psychiatric diagnoses among geriatric patients seen in an outreach program. *Journal of the American Geriatric Society, 30*(8), 530–533.

Roslaniec, A., & Fitzpatrick, J. J. (1979). Changes in mental status in older adults with four days of hospitalization. *Research in Nursing and Health, 2,* 177–187.

Sakauye, K. (1986). Interface of emotional and behavioral conditions with physical disorders in nursing homes. In M. S. Harper & B. D. Lebowitz, *Mental illness in nursing homes: Agenda for research.* Rockville, MD: National Institute of Mental Health.

Segall, M., & Wykle, M. (1988–89, Fall/Winter). The black family's experience with dementia. *The Journal of Applied Social Sciences, 13*(1), 170–191.

Seymour, D. G., & Pringle, R. (1983). Post-operative complications in the elderly surgical patient. *Gerontology, 29*(4), 262–270.

Simon, A., & Cahan, R. B. (1963). The acute brain syndrome in geriatric patients. In W. H. Mendel & L. J. Epstein (Eds.), *Acute psychotic reaction.* Psychiatric Research Reports of the American Psychiatric Association (No. 16, pp. 8–21). Washington, DC: APA.

Snyder, L. H., Pyrek, J., & Smith, K. C. (1976). Vision and mental function of the elderly. *The Gerontologist, 16*(6), 491–495.

Spiro, H. (1982). Reforming the state hospital in a centrified care system. *Hospital and Community Psychiatry, 33*(9), 722–727.

Steffl, B. (1984). *Handbook of Gerontological Nursing.* New York: Von Nostrand Reinhold.

Venglarik, J., & Adams, M. (1985). Which client is at high risk? *Journal of Gerontological Nursing, 11,* 28–30.

Whanger, A. D. (1980). Treatment within the institution. In E. Busse, & D. Blazer (Eds.), *Handbook of geriatric psychiatry.* New York: Van Nostrand Reinhold.

Whanger, A. D., & Myers, A. C. (1984). *Mental health assessment and therapeutic intervention with older adults.* Rockville, MD: Aspen.

Williams, M. A., Campbell, E. B., Raynor, W. J., Mucholt, M. A., Mlynarczk, S. M., & Crane, L. G. (1985). Predictors of acute confusional states in hospitalized elderly patients. *Research in Nursing and Health, 8,* 31–40.

Williams, M. A., Holloway, J. R., Winn, M. C., Wolanin, M. O., Lawler, M. L., Westlick, C. R., & Chin, M. R. (1979). Nursing confusional states in the elderly hip fracture patient. *Nursing Research, 28,* 25–35.

Wolanin, M. O., & Holloway, J. R. (1980). Relocation confusion: Intervention for prevention. In I. M. Burnside (Ed.), *Psychosocial care of the aged* (pp. 179–194). New York: McGraw-Hill.

Wolanin, M., & Phillips, L. (1981). *Confusion: Prevention and care.* St. Louis, MO: Mosby.

Wykle, M. H. (1986). *Mental health nursing: Research in nursing homes.* In M. S. Harper, & B. D. Lebowitz (Eds.), *Mental illness in nursing homes: Agenda for research* (pp. 325–347). Rockville, MD: National Institute of Mental Health.

Nursing Home Care

Benjamin Liptzin

I. Background
II. Epidemiology of Mental Disorders in Nursing Homes
   A. Prevalence of Problem Behaviors
   B. Mental Health Services in Nursing Homes
   C. Psychiatric Interventions in Nursing Homes: Assessment
   D. Pharmacologic Interventions
   E. Psychotherapeutic Approaches
   F. Behavioral and Environmental Interventions
III. Public Policy Issues
   References

I. Background

Nursing homes have developed as a major locus of health care for the elderly in the United States. Vladeck (1980) has reviewed the history of public policy with respect to the frail elderly and the development of nursing homes. Public facilities for the elderly were an outgrowth of the poorhouses and poor farms, which were operated by county governments. Private, nonprofit homes were founded by religious or ethnic organizations to provide decent living conditions for frail individuals who were widowed and unable to live alone. The Great Depression of the 1930s highlighted the needs of the millions of elderly Americans who were living in poverty. Social Security legislation was enacted to provide old age assistance that was noncontributory and means tested, and contributory pension benefits. The provision of minimal financial assistance made it possible for some frail elderly to afford institutional care and spurred the development of proprietary facilities. In the 1950s, Hill-Burton money from the federal government was extended from hospitals to nursing home construction. In addition to increasing the number of nursing home beds, nursing homes were also brought under a health care umbrella and away from the previous welfare image. This health care focus was confirmed with the passage of Medicare and Medicaid legislation in the mid-1960s. Medicare, which was universal, provided limited nursing home benefits for *extended care,* which was intended to help facilitate the transfer of patients out of expensive acute care hospitals. An afterthought at the time, but much more significant in the long run, was the expansion of federal contributions to state Medicaid programs for the poor and the inclusion of nursing home benefits in Medicaid. This guarantee of public funding for nursing home care led to a tremendous expansion in the number of nursing home beds over the next decade. In 1954, there were fewer than 300,000 nursing home beds in the United States. By 1963 that number was just over 500,000. With the availability of Medicaid funding, that number grew to 1.25 million beds by 1977 and to 1.5 million beds by 1989. Clearly, the large increase in the number of older persons, especially frail people older than 85, also contributed to the large increase in nursing home patients.

Before the enactment of Medicaid, many older persons who could not live independently or be managed by their families because of behavioral problems were admitted to and became long-term residents of state and county mental hospitals. From a peak of 558,922 residents of all ages in 1955 (28% aged 65+), the number of patients in state and county mental hospitals was gradually reduced to under 150,000 in 1989. Some of that decrease was accounted for by the philosophy of *deinstitutionalization,* which asserted that large mental hospitals were archaic warehouses and that community-based mental health facilities were more therapeutic. Another significant factor was the transfer of a large but unknown number of older residents to Medicaid-supported nursing homes and the diversion of many others, who formerly would have been admitted to public mental hospitals, to nursing homes. This strategy had the benefit for state and local governments of having the federal government pay approximately half the costs. This *transinstitutionalization* and diversion of patients has resulted in nursing homes now providing care for more mentally impaired older people than do public mental hospitals. Schmidt, Rheinhardt, Kane, and Olsen (1977), asserted that nursing homes had replaced the *back wards* of state hospitals. They complained that even though these facilities were *in the community,* patients received little therapeutic programming and deteriorated over time.

In summary, nursing homes have been transformed in the last 60 yr from a relatively small set of residential facilities for poor and frail older people to a large and expensive group of health care institutions, which provide the bulk of institutional care for mentally impaired older persons. The costs of this long-term institutional care have put enormous strains on state budgets and also exposed the glaring absence of long-term care benefits in public or private health insurance plans. The rest of this chapter will focus on the mental health problems and needs of older persons in nursing homes.

II. Epidemiology of Mental Disorders in Nursing Homes _____

Until recently, there was little systematic research on the prevalence of mental or behavioral disorders in nursing homes. Early studies found a high prevalence of psychiatric disorders and of behavioral problems. (Goldfarb, 1962; Miller & Elliott, 1976; Teeter, Garetz, Miller & Heiland, 1976) Often these problems were not noted in patient records or were stated in vague terms. Barnes and Raskind (1981) concluded that chart diagnoses for demented patients were inadequate, but that specific diagnoses could be assigned with careful examinations. They argued that specific diagnosis is important because it can lead to more accurate prognosis and management.

Using the diagnostic data available from the 1977 National Nursing Home Survey of the National Center for Health Statistics, Goldman, Feder, and Scanlon (1986) confirmed the high prevalence in nursing homes of patients with mental disorders and/or behavior problems. They concluded that of the 1.3 million nursing home residents in 1977, about 72,000 were classified as purely chronically mentally ill; 514,000, as purely chronically physically ill; 35,000, as having physical and mental diagnoses; and 561,000, as senile. These subpopulations differ in important ways and require different kinds of assistance.

Recent studies using careful epidemiologic methods have also demonstrated high rates of psychiatric disorder in nursing home residents. German, Shapiro, and Kramer (1986) reported that 37% of nursing home residents in East Baltimore had a diagnosable mental disorder, usually dementia. A high rate of clinically diagnosed depression (21%) was found by the same group in a later study, (Kafonek, Ettinger, Roca, Kittner, Taylor and German, 1989). Snowdon & Donnelly (1986) used the Geriatric Depression Scale (GDS) to screen for depression among residents of six nursing homes in Sydney, Australia, and found that of the 61% who could answer the questionnaire, more than one third were depressed. Studies using semistructured clinical interviews have also demonstrated a high prevalence of psychiatric disorders and behavioral problems in nursing home residents. (Chandler and Chandler, 1988; Merriam, Aronson, Gaston, Wey, Katz, 1988; Rovner, Kafonek, Filipp, Lucas, & Folstein, 1986).

In summary, a high proportion of nursing home residents have a diagnosable mental disorder. The majority have some form of dementia, which may require interventions even if the underlying disease is not reversible. Furthermore, a significant number have depression which is often treatable.

A. Prevalence of Problem Behaviors

In addition to studying the prevalence of specific psychiatric disorders, other investigators have tried to identify specific behavioral and emotional problems in nursing home residents, since these often require some management irrespective of diagnosis. Zimmer, Watson, and Treat (1984) found that 66% of nursing home patients had at least one significant behavioral problem such as verbal abuse, physical resistance to care, and physical aggressiveness. Jackson, Drugovich, Fretwell, Spector, Sternberg & Rosenstein, (1989) concluded that 26% of residents had engaged in some form of disruptive behavior within 2 weeks before assessment. Abusiveness (physical and verbal) and noisiness were identified as the most prevalent behavior types. Older residents and those with greater physical and cognitive impairments were more likely to exhibit behavior problems, but some cognitively intact residents exhibited disruptive behavior.

The general problem of *agitation* in nursing-home residents has been studied by Cohen-Mansfield and her colleagues and reported in a series of papers. Cohen-Mansfield and Billig (1986) presented a conceptual review of agitated behaviors in the elderly. Cohen-Mansfield, Marx, and Rosenthal (1989) provided a description of agitation in a nursing home setting. Cohen-Mansfield, Werner, and Marx (1989) showed that agitated behaviors were frequently observed in cognitively impaired residents. The most common agitated behaviors were strange noises, requests for attention, repetitious mannerisms, picking at things, strange movements, and pacing. Patterns of agitation were specific to each resident, and daytime agitation was positively associated with nighttime agitation. The same investigators (Cohen-Mansfield, Marx, & Werner, 1989) found no effect of a full moon on agitation in nursing-home residents.

The specific symptom of delusions was studied by Morriss, Rovner, Folstein, and German (1990) who found that 21% of 125 newly admitted nursing home patients had delusions. All delusional residents had cognitive impairment. A few had primary psychiatric disorders other than dementia (e.g., major depression, schizophrenia, or mania). The behavioral problems were often the reason for admission, and they persisted after admission. The staff of the nursing home infrequently identified and often inappropriately treated delusional patients. In another paper, Rovner, German, Broadhead, Morriss, Brant, Blaustein, and Folstein (1990) reported that 40% of demented patients had additional psychiatric symptoms, such as delusions or depression, and these patients were most likely to receive restraints or neuroleptics, and to require substantial nursing time.

A growing body of knowledge about nursing-home residents clearly indicates that large numbers have psychiatric and behavioral disorders that could benefit from careful mental health assessment and management. Currently, most such problems are inadequately documented and inappropriately managed.

B. Mental Health Services in Nursing Homes

Given the high prevalence of psychiatric and behavioral disorders in nursing home residents, it is important to review what mental health services are available to nursing-home residents and staff.

The Subcommittee on Long-Term Care of the Special Committee on Aging of the United States Senate cited many deficiencies in nursing-home care, including the lack of psychiatric care. This was particularly troublesome, given the trend noted earlier for patients to be transferred or diverted from public mental hospitals to nursing homes in the late 1960s. Glasscote, Beigel, and Butterfield (1976) concluded that most of the direct care in homes that had received patients from psychiatric facilities was provided by nursing aides with little or no training in how to care for frail old people. Medical care was minimal and provided largely by general practitioners who had no formal preparation for work with the elderly. Despite the presence of patients from psychiatric facilities, psychiatric consultation was rarely requested.

Another perspective on physician services in nursing homes was provided by Mitchell (1982). Using data from a national survey of 3,482 physicians in office-based practice, she found that only 28% had visited any nursing home during the previous week. Among psychiatrists in private practice, the figure was 11%. Mitchell concluded that large increases in reimbursement rates might be necessary to encourage more physicians to treat nursing home patients. In a follow-up study of physicians in Michigan, Mitchell (1986) found that in addition to concerns about reimbursement, physicians also complained that it took too much time, that they had few nursing-home patients in their practice, that they dislike the types of patients and conditions in nursing homes, that the nursing home had its own physicians, or that they were opposed to intrusive government regulations. Clearly the general problem of encouraging physicians (not just psychiatrists) to treat nursing-home patients requires more attention.

A number of model programs were developed and funded to provide mental health services to nursing-home residents, with a particular focus on patients transferred from public mental hospitals. These have been previously summarized (Borson, Liptzin, Nininger, & Rabins, 1989, pp. 15–22), and only a few will be described here. Stotsky (1967) developed a follow-up program for former mental hospital patients discharged to nursing homes with the focus on assistance to nursing-home staff rather than direct patient care. The intervention improved the chances of patients remaining in the home rather than being rehospitalized. Over time, however, the patients were found to have more symptoms, physical illness, and functional disability. In such programs, the psychiatric consultation is generally provided by salaried state employees or by staff hired through grants or contracts from state or federal agencies. Although most such programs were originally funded to provide specific follow-up to former mental hospital patients, some were able to broaden their scope to provide consultation to all nursing home residents in their service area. Unfortunately, many such programs have had to curtail services because of state and federal cutbacks in funding.

A different approach to providing psychiatric services in nursing homes is the development of a specialized psychiatric unit within a home. In a recent example of such a program, Gurian and Chanowitz (1987a) set up a demonstration unit in a proprietary nursing home. New staff were recruited and supplemented with a special psychosocial staff including a program director, a director of in-service training, a head psychiatric nurse, a psychiatric social worker, an occupational therapist, a psychiatrist, a group of case-managers, and a behavioral psychologist. Medical care was provided by a trained geriatric internist and trained nurse-practitioners. The program carefully screened referrals, and new admissions had an initial care plan developed with specific treatment goals. The focus was on decreasing antisocial behaviors and increasing functioning skills. Based on a careful evaluation, the authors concluded that the program had been successful in benefitting all patients and was cost-effective in preventing rehospitalization for most. Gurian and Chanowitz (1987b) also described the barriers and obstacles to the implementation of the program. Despite its demonstrated success, the program was discontinued for various reasons.

Another approach to providing psychiatric services in nursing homes involves regular visits by a psychiatrist. The visits usually include some direct services to patients (e.g., initial evaluations and followup visits) as well as consultation and training of nursing home staff. Tourigny-Rivard (Tourigny-Rivard & Drury, 1987) described her work with a 50-bed nursing home in rural Ontario, Canada. She visited monthly, and over a period of 18 months, evaluated 21 residents for symptoms such as *aggressive–uncooperative–agitated behavior* or *depressed appearance*. As might be expected, the initial referrals tended to be for more agitated patients, while over time, the staff became sensitized to the problems of more withdrawn patients. She also presented in-service programs on topics such as depression, death and dying, behavior therapy, and the use of psychotropic medications. While no attempt was made to collect systematic patient-outcome data, written comments from the nursing staff, nursing home physician, and administrators suggested that not only did specific patients improve but, in addition, there were improvements in staff attitudes toward psychiatric care, interdisciplinary relationships, staff confidence in their ability to handle emotionally disturbed residents, early detection of depression, and staff-initiated therapeutic programs for residents. A similar liaison model was described by Bienenfeld and Wheeler. (1989)

The above papers report the benefits of psychiatric consultation. Smyer, Cohn, and Brannon (1988) discussed consultation to nursing homes by nonphysician mental health professionals. Block, Boczkowski, Hansen, and Vanderbeck (1987) developed a consultation program that provided some basic knowledge of behavior therapy to nursing home aides, and training in the application of those techniques. Intervention programs for two of the most difficult residents were designed and implemented, leading to significant behavioral changes. Chartock, Nevins, Rzetelny, and Gilberto (1988) described their multidisciplinary program to assist nursing home staff to improve their understanding of the behavior of mentally impaired residents and to develop effective intervention skills. Evaluation data showed the program was effective in building knowledge and improving skills on the job.

Services of psychiatrists and other mental health professionals have been shown to be effective in nursing homes. Furthermore, these services are becoming more readily available.

C. Psychiatric Interventions in Nursing Homes: Assessment

In order to plan any interventions for the management of nursing home residents with psychiatric or behavioral problems, it is essential that a careful assessment be done. Nursing home residents often present with a complicated mixture of cognitive impairment, multiple physical problems, multiple medications, and behavioral symptoms that may be related to the above or to a primary psychiatric disorder. Information must be collected in all these areas in order to arrive at conclusions as to what is causing the problem and what interventions would be helpful.

A brief description of how to assess a geriatric patient will be given here. Other chapters in this handbook have provided more detail on different aspects of assessment (see Chapters 22 by Caine, 23 by La Rue, and 24 by Kemp). Since most referrals for psychiatric intervention in a nursing home are initiated by the direct-care staff, it is important to have them do their own assessment. In order to facilitate that process, it may be helpful to have the staff fill out the preconsultation form described previously (Liptzin, 1989). The form provides basic identifying information such as the patient's name, birthdate, marital status, admission date to the home, location admitted from, attending physician's name and telephone number, and nearest relative's name and phone number. Generally, the latter two should be told that a consultation has been requested so that there is no misunderstanding when the consultant calls for background information or initiates some form of intervention. Staff are asked to describe the resident's initial adjustment to the nursing home, since many problems stem from the initial adjustment period. The specific reason for the psychiatric consultation is requested along with the date of onset of the current problem and what was going on at the time the problem began. Past psychiatric history should be documented with records from other treating practitioners or facilities, something many nursing homes neglect to do. Medical diagnoses and current and past medications are listed, since they may be possible causes of the presenting problem or may complicate the treatment. A description is requested of the resident's mood, memory, and behavior, including appetite, sleep pattern, and tendency to wander, as well as the ability to carry out activities of daily living such as ambulation, feeding, toileting, and personal hygiene. Information about current involvement of family members or significant others is requested to provide clues to the current problem. Staff are asked to explain what they think is causing the current problem, including whether anything has happened in the last month to explain the current problem, or whether the problem has ever occurred before. The current treatment plan is described as well as what the staff would like or expect from the consultation. All of the above information is essential for a comprehensive assessment and helps the consultant determine how the staff understand the problem, and what types of intervention they are willing to entertain.

The information collected may suggest that the behavioral symptoms are a result of an underlying medical condition or medication side-effect rather than a primary psychiatric disorder. In such cases, there may be a more specific intervention than simply prescribing the psychotropic drug requested by the nursing home (Liptzin, 1989). For example, an 84-year-old nursing home resident was admitted to a psychiatric hospital because of *agitation,* which had developed over several days and become unmanageable. It was presumed that his underlying dementia was the cause and that he required sedating medication. However, on his admission physical examination, he was noted to have a fecal impaction. He was disimpacted, and his agitation disappeared. Careful attention to his bowel function prevented further recurrences. In another case, an 86-year-old woman was referred for evaluation of *paranoia* because she had barricaded herself in her room and was suspicious of her roommate. On history it was noted that the problem began after she was started on 60 milligrams of the steroid drug Prednisone. Her primary care physician agreed to taper and then discontinue the medication, and her paranoia disappeared. A final example illustrates the point that psychotropic medication is sometimes the cause of and not the solution to the presenting problem. An 85-year-old man was referred for *severe agitation* which had gotten acutely worse. He was severely demented and had been mildly agitated. As a result, his dose of thioridazine had been recently increased. It was after this increase that he became even more confused and agitated. In addition, he developed urinary retention, which required acute intervention. The thioridazine was stopped, and both his agitation and urinary problem improved.

A comprehensive assessment may lead to a variety of recommendations. In some cases the existing treatment approach may be adequate, and no further suggestions are necessary. In other cases, there may be suggestions for further medical work-up or treatment. Most often, some psychiatric intervention will be recommended. The next section discusses various interventions that are available and used in nursing homes.

D. Pharmacologic Interventions

1. Concerns about Psychotropic Drug Use in Nursing Homes

Medications can often be quite helpful in the treatment of nursing-home residents with psychiatric or behavioral problems. General principles of clinical geriatric psychopharmacology have been described in an earlier chapter of this handbook (see Chapter 26 by Salzman) There are special problems in drug prescribing for any older person because they are more sensitive to the side-effects of psychotropic drugs. Of all geriatric patients, nursing-home residents are the most challenging, because they tend to be older, more frail, and have multiple medical problems for which they take multiple medications, which can interact with psychotropic drugs. Given the side-effects and risks associated with psychotropic drug use in this population, the potential benefits need to be clear in order to justify their use.

Many studies have demonstrated that psychotropic drugs are frequently used in nursing home residents, and this has raised concerns about overmedication. For example, Schmidt, Rheinhardt, Kane & Olsen (1977) found that, over time, most patients received increased medication and became less active. They speculated that psychotropic medication was being used by the staff to achieve a more docile and compliant population, and that low activity levels were actually encouraged to maintain order in the nursing homes. The authors argued that nursing-home patients deteriorate because they receive little therapeutic intervention other than drugs to keep them quiet. In another study, Ray, Federspiel and Schaffner (1980) reported that a high proportion of nursing-home residents received antipsychotic drugs, often daily. Blazer, Federspiel, Ray and Schaffner (1983) expressed concerns about drug prescribing because of the high likelihood of anticholinergic side-effects from the psychotropic drugs prescribed to nursing-home residents. They suggested that a careful review of medications by an expert in psychopharmacology might reduce the morbidity of nursing-home residents.

Another large-scale study (Buck, 1988) demonstrated that of year-long residents, 60% received at least one psychotropic medication during the year. The author suggested that more detailed studies are needed of how decisions are made to prescribe psychotropic drugs to nursing-home residents. Utilizing data from the National Nursing Home Study Pretest, Burns and Kamerow (1988) showed a high prevalence of psychotropic drug prescriptions for a random group of nursing-home residents. Often there was no notation of a relevant symptom or diagnosis in the chart. The authors suggested a need for better and more careful documentation as well as better training for primary care physicians in the proper prescribing of psychotropic drugs. In a later paper, Beardsley, Larson, Burns, Thompson, and Kamerow (1989) reported that more than one fourth of the study patients had orders for more than one psychotropic medication. Nursing-home patients who received psychotropics had concurrent orders for an average of 3.3 nonpsychotropic medications, many of which could increase the possibility of drug interactions and potential side-effects.

Another study of medication use–misuse was done by Beers, Avorn, Soumerai, Everitt, Sherman and Salem (1988). More than half of all intermediate-care facility residents were receiving some psychoactive medication, and 26% were receiving antipsychotic medication. The authors concluded that the nursing-home population was exposed to high levels of psychotropic drug use, and that the drugs chosen were not optimal in terms of their side-effect profiles. In an accompanying editorial, Riesenberg (1988) echoed the authors' concerns, but cautioned that their study did not examine individual patients and could not determine whether the medication was warranted in each case. He did agree, however, that more careful use of psychotropic drugs in the institutionalized elderly could reduce the unwanted consequences of oversedation, orthostatic hypotension, and decreased cholinergic tone including mental deterioration, bowel and bladder dysfunction, and falls leading to hip fractures.

The concern about the effects of anticholinergic medications was borne out in a study by Rovner, David, Lucas-Blaustein, Conklin, Filipp, & Tune (1988). They found that patients with above the median anticholinergic blood levels had higher scores on the Psychogeriatric Dependency Rating Scales reflecting greater disability in dressing, personal hygiene, mobility, toileting, and urinary continence. The authors suggested that anticholinergic medications may cause excess disability in nursing-home patients and that a careful review of a patient's medication could help reduce this disability.

Avorn, Dreyer, Connelly and Soumerai (1989), in a study of 55 rest homes in Massachusetts, found that 55% of the residents were taking at least one psychoactive medication, with 39% receiving antipsychotic medication. In a more detailed study of residents in homes with high levels of antipsychotic drug use, they found half the residents had no evidence of participation by a physician in decisions about their mental health during the year of the study. Six percent of the residents had moderate or severe tardive dyskinesia, probably as a result of the medication. Most disturbing was that the staff had little understanding of the actions or side-effects of the psychoactive drugs they were dispensing to patients.

Concern about the prescription of neuroleptic drugs to institutionalized elderly is not limited to the United States. Nygaard, Bakke, and Breivik (1989) studied all residents in homes for aged people in Bergen, Norway, and found that 23% were receiving neuroleptic medication. There was increased use of neuroleptics with rising mental impairment, and decreased use with advanced age. Neuroleptic consumption was more frequent in persons representing a heavy workload, and in anxious, wandering, aggressive, restless, and incontinent residents. The authors argued that psychotropic medication may be used as a "substitute for human attention and stimulating surroundings (p. 173)."

In summary, many concerns have been expressed over the use of psychotropic medications in nursing homes because of the high potential for adverse effects, the limited involvement of physicians, and poor understanding by nursing staff of the risks and benefits of these medications. Although regulatory solutions have been suggested, educational approaches are more flexible and should be tried first.

2. Effectiveness of Psychotropic Medications

Given the concerns about psychotropic drug prescribing to nursing-home residents, it is remarkable that there are few, if any, controlled studies on the risks and benefits of medication use in this setting. This section will review available studies and present some previously published case examples (Borson *et al.*, 1989).

Barnes, Veith, Okimoto, Raskind, and Gumbrecht (1982) compared the therapeutic efficacy of thioridazine, loxapine, and a placebo in the treatment of behavioral disturbances in demented nursing-home residents. Each patient had at least three behavioral symptoms including irritability, hostility, agitation, anxiety, depressed mood, sleep disturbance, delusions, or hallucinations. Neuroleptic medications seemed to be effective for the specific behavioral problems of anxiety, excitement, emotional lability, and uncooperativeness. A few subjects benefitted greatly from drug treatment, but the majority of patients maintained on active medication were not rated markedly or even moderately improved at the end of the study. Furthermore, there was a prominent placebo effect. Patients treated with the active drugs experienced side-effects of sedation, extrapyramidal symptoms, and orthostatic hypotension, which may have limited their effectiveness. The authors recommended that social and environmental solutions be sought for these behavioral disturbances to avoid the use of medication, if possible.

Although much of the controversy about drug prescribing involves neuroleptic drugs, there are also questions about the proper use of antidepressant medications in this frail, older population. Even though several classes of antidepressants are available and effective for the treatment of serious depression and should not be withheld simply on the basis of the patient's age, many nursing-home residents do not tolerate the side effects of even the newer drugs (e.g., trazodone, fluoxetine, bupropion), which claim to have fewer side-effects. In such patients, electroconvulsive therapy (ECT) can be a safe and effective alternative, though it usually requires transfer to a hospital setting for the treatments. For example, an 87-year-old woman was admitted to a nursing home after falling at home and being hospitalized for a bruised hip. She became agitated and was quite disruptive because she constantly called out for help. When a staff member sat and talked with her, she would calm down, but as soon as she was left alone, she would start calling out again. Although it was clear that she was moderately demented, she was able to tell staff tearfully that she missed her home and her dog and wondered what had happened to him. She was unable to tolerate several antidepressants. A short course of ECT led to a dramatic improvement in her spirits. She stopped calling out and was able to enjoy visits from her family at a new nursing home near them. In cases of severe, psychotic or suicidal depression, ECT can be life saving.

The recognition and management of depression in demented patients is difficult. Rabins (1989) has reviewed the data on coexisting depression and dementia. In a study of outpatients, Reifler, Teri, Raskind, Veith, Barnes, White, and McLean (1989) compared imipramine to placebo in 61 patients with primary degenerative dementia of the Alzheimer's type who either met or did not meet DSM-III criteria for depression. After an 8-week trial, both groups improved significantly. The authors described their findings as positive since the patients improved, even though the specific antidepressant was not superior to placebo. They suggest that accurate detection can identify one area in which improvement may be possible against an otherwise poor prognosis. An example of the problem in recognition and of the benefit of treatment was an 82-year-old severely demented woman who was quite agitated and restless. The only evidence of depression was that she would occasionally walk by the nursing station, hold her head in her hands and say, "I feel so miserable." When asked what was bothering her, she was unable to describe her feelings or even remember that she had said anything. However, on a low dose of nortriptyline (10 mg b.i.d.) she was much less agitated, showed no more dysphoria, and could sit calmly in a chair in a group.

The treatment of elderly patients with bipolar disorder is also challenging. The *high* periods in such patients may be difficult to diagnose. Irritability, confusion, or paranoia may be present rather than the more typical elation, hyperactivity, grandiosity, and impulsiveness seen in younger patients who may spend excessively or become sexually indiscreet. In frail nursing-home residents there are also concerns about the narrow therapeutic range and the marked toxicity (e.g., confusion, tremors, ataxia) experienced at even low blood levels of lithium, the standard treatment for younger manic patients. However, Bushey, Rathey, and Bowers (1983) showed that used cautiously and monitored carefully, lithium could be quite effective in elderly bipolar nursing-home residents. A case example illustrates the effectiveness as well as the risks of lithium in such patients. A 78-year-old man with a long history of bipolar disorder and frequent episodes of mania as well as depression became unsteady on his feet and fell when his lithium level became too high. He was hospitalized for days in a comatose state and taken off lithium. He gradually woke up and stabilized medically and was transferred to a nursing home. He seemed slowed down, disinterested, and depressed until one morning when he woke up singing loudly and made crude sexual remarks to staff and other residents. He was placed back on lithium and became calmer and more appropriate. Since he was no longer depressed, he was motivated to return home to his wife where he remained for the last 7 yr of his life.

Although benzodiazepines are widely prescribed in nursing homes, this is usually for nighttime sedation and not for antianxiety effect. There are no nursing-home studies on the treatment of anxiety with either benzodiazepines or the newer antianxiety drug buspirone. Such studies should be done, since these drugs may be better tolerated than neuroleptics and may be as effective for anxiety or agitation.

Clearly, psychotropic medications are frequently used and can be extremely helpful for nursing-home residents. More education of nursing-home physicians and other staff as well as consultation with pharmacists and psychiatrists can help improve prescribing practices. More research is needed on the effectiveness of various psychotropic medications in frail, elderly nursing-home residents.

E. Psychotherapeutic Approaches

The use of psychotherapy in nursing homes has been rather limited to date. Mental health professionals who chose to work in nursing homes usually had only a limited amount of time and were asked to help with the management of many behavioral problems. This did not permit therapy sessions with individuals or groups on a regular basis. Until recent changes in Medicare, reimbursement for psychotherapy in nursing homes was quite limited. Beginning in 1990, there is no longer a limit on the number of psychotherapy sessions that will be reimbursed at 50% of the allowable fee. Although many patients are unable to pay the balance, it may be financially feasible for psychiatrists and psychologists whose services are covered to provide therapy in nursing homes. In contrast to earlier negative views about the suitability of psychotherapy for older persons, there is a growing recognition of its usefulness (see Chapter 25 by Newton and Lazarus, this volume).

Nursing-home residents without cognitive impairment can benefit as much as elderly patients in the community from the full range of psychotherapies. Psychotherapy with cognitively impaired residents is more controversial.

Goldfarb and Sheps (1954) described their psychotherapeutic work with cognitively impaired residents in a large home for the aged. Therapy consisted of 5- to 15-min sessions spaced far apart and structured to leave the patient with a sense of triumph or victory by having won an ally. This approach was designed to help manage the fear and rage that arose in the context of the resident's increasing helplessness and loss of physical, social, and economic resources. The goal was to encourage feelings of mastery in the resident. Based on their anecdotal experience, the authors suggested that such psychotherapy was helpful.

Several previously published case vignettes illustrate the value of brief focused psychotherapy sessions in cognitively impaired nursing-home residents (Borson et al., 1989, pp. 34–35). In both cases, daily sessions allowed the patients to work through the affect associated with their losses, accept the reality of their situation, develop a sense that the therapist was helpful and caring, and reestablish self-esteem.

In a controlled-outcome study of a brief psychotherapeutic intervention for withdrawn, apathetic, mostly bed- or chair-fast elderly patients, Power and McCarron (1975) used an interactive-contact approach emphasizing interpersonal stimulation. Physical touch, warmth, verbal and affective expressions of personal interest, and the sharing of simple nurturing tasks were designed as the therapeutic elements. After the 15 weeks of treatment and at followup, the treated group showed more improvement than did controls in their depression scores on the Brief Psychiatric Rating Scale.

In addition to individual psychotherapy, group therapies can also be very helpful in the nursing home and may be a more efficient use of a therapist's time. Herst and Moulton (1985) described several types of groups including a new resident's group, a confrontation group, a group formed to deal with issues of loss and grieving, and a life-review group. Group members discussed topics such as motivation to live, improvement of memory, social skills, and identity within the nursing-home setting.

A controlled study of group therapy in a nursing-home setting was carried out by Moran and Gatz (1987). They randomly assigned residents to either a task-oriented group to develop a welcoming project for newly admitted residents or an insight-oriented group that discussed issues of personal concern. These latter issues included how to get more privacy, have fun, help one's children, make friends and gain more control over personal space, diet, possessions, finances, visitors, noise, and roommates. Each group met once a week for twelve 75-min sessions. Before and after treatment, patients were assessed using rating scales for life satisfaction, psychosocial competence, trust, locus of control, and social desirability. The task group increased in internal locus of control and life satisfaction. The insight group increased in internal locus of control and in trust. Both groups improved more than controls assigned to a waiting list, but there were no clear differences between the two groups. Few patients dropped out, and many commented that they liked the groups.

In another randomized controlled study, Rattenbury and Stones (1989) compared the effects of reminiscence and current-topics group discussions on the psychological well-being of elderly nursing-home residents. Both interventions showed positive changes compared to a control group on measures of happiness–depression, activity, mood, and functional levels.

Despite the limited number of controlled studies to conclusively demonstrate the effectiveness of various approaches to psychotherapy in nursing homes, these interventions emphasize psychosocial interactions and should become more widely available.

F. Behavioral and Environmental Interventions

Given the high prevalence of behavioral disorders in nursing homes, a variety of behavioral and environmental interventions have been tried. Schwenk (1979) reviewed the literature on the effectiveness of Reality Orientation (RO), a set of techniques developed as a method of reducing confusion among institutionalized elderly. She concluded that serious methodological problems invalidated the results of most research on RO, but that the few adequate studies suggested that it sometimes helped reduce confusion but did not seem to increase autonomy or happiness. It is likely that any benefits are due to nonspecific rather than specific effects of the techniques used.

Physical restraint is a controversial behavioral technique, which is often used for cognitively impaired elderly to prevent wandering, falls, assaults on other residents, or disruption of medical treatment (e.g., pulling out catheters or intravenous lines). A recent review by Evans and Strumpf (1989) of available research questioned the benefits of this procedure and suggested the need to develop and test alternative measures. They pointed out that the problem is to balance autonomy, patient safety, and quality of life. Folmar and Wilson (1989) in a study of 112 nursing-home residents showed that low social performance puts a resident at risk of being restrained, but more frequently, the use of a restraint hampers a resident's performance of appropriate social behavior. Werner, Cohen-Mansfield, Braun, and Marx (1989) found that agitated nursing-home residents exhibited either the same amount or more agitated behaviors when they were restrained than when they were not restrained. They suggested that the act of restraining may itself contribute to manifestations of agitation. Furthermore, they questioned the effectiveness of restraints for preventing falls and described the adverse consequences of restraint use, including loss of dignity, muscle atrophy, osteoporosis, constipation, urinary retention, limb ischemia, and even death from strangulation. Powell, Mitchell-Pedersen, Fingerote, and Edmund (1989) demonstrated the feasibility of decreasing the use of both physical and chemical restraints in a geriatric population. From 1980 to 1986 the use of physical restraint fell dramatically, while the number of falls increased only slightly. Clearly, the risks and benefits of restraint use must be carefully considered, and alternatives tried whenever possible.

Wandering is a particular behavior that can be very troublesome in an unlocked nursing-home setting, but neither physical restraint nor chemical sedation is a good solution. Behavioral approaches to understanding and managing such behavior can often be helpful. Snyder, Rupprecht, Pyrek, Brekhus, and Moss (1978) identified three types of wandering behavior: (1) overtly goal-directed, searching behavior; (2) overtly goal-directed, industrious behavior, and (3) apparently nongoal-directed behavior. In addition, they suggested that three psychosocial factors may influence the tendency to wander: (1) lifelong patterns ot coping with stress; (2) previous work roles, and (3) a search for security. The authors recommended various approaches for dealing with the wandering behavior. Rehabilitation approaches included efforts to orient the person, to visit previous reference points in the community, to provide a vigorous schedule of physical and social activities, and to relieve anxiety. Compensatory approaches included the use of environmental cues such as signs, and environmental designs such as sheltered courtyards. The authors also worked closely with the staff to understand and chart the problem as well as to develop a consistent care plan for individual residents. When these care plans and other policy changes were implemented, the wandering subsided to a minimal level.

In a more recent paper, Rader (1987) described a specific, comprehensive program in a nursing home that resulted in a decrease in problem wandering, an increase in patient freedom and safety, and an increase in staff skill and comfort in handling wandering behaviors. Patients with potential wandering behavior were identified from the admission history or from observations during the first few days in the nursing home. These residents were given a special identification bracelet listing their name and a phone number to call if they were lost. All staff were alerted to the potential wandering behavior of the resident, and photographs identifying the resident were posted in the facility. A second intervention was the development of activities specifically designed for cognitively impaired residents. A program of music, exercise, and touching was designed and carried out in a small-group setting for an hour three times a week. It became clear that regular walks and other activities were an essential part of the care plan for these residents. The third approach was to teach staff more helpful ways to interact with cognitively impaired residents. Concrete, simple, and exact instructions were most effective. On a nonverbal level, staff were educated to use a gentle, calm tone of voice and physical stroking to quiet a confused person instead of getting angry and shouting, which increases agitation. Staff were encouraged, when possible, to accompany patients for short walks out of the facility, rather than forcing confused residents to stay inside. Attempts were made to understand the feelings and needs underlying the wandering behavior, such as a desire to go "home." The sense of being cared for and useful could be fostered by discussing the resident's family. A fourth approach established a specific set of procedures to use when a resident was thought to be missing from his unit. Over a 3-year period, the use of these approaches increased the safety of the residents at little extra time or cost. The staff experienced an increased sense of mastery and skill in dealing with confused residents. Fewer combative episodes and staff injuries were noted, and there was a decrease in the use of physical or chemical restraints.

The awareness of behavioral problems in cognitively impaired residents has also led in recent years to the development of *special care units* as one approach to the management of such patients (Maas, 1988). Rabins (1986) suggested that the advantages of such units include

1. staffing by persons specially trained to care for cognitively impaired residents;
2. a design that is physically safer and facilitates orientation;
3. reduction in behavioral problems with appropriate treatment;
4. concentration of the resources needed to care for these patients;

5. offering families the reassurance of specially designed surroundings and expert staff; and

6. sparing other residents the stress of living with severely cognitively impaired patients with behavioral problems.

Such units can also become valuable research and training resources for health care professionals. The potential disadvantages of such units include

1. the difficulty of attracting and retaining staff for a unit with such severely disturbed patients;

2. family resistance to having their relative placed on such a unit for fear it will precipitate a rapid decline, given the limited opportunity to interact with cognitively intact residents;

3. lower expectations for patients and less interest in identifying treatable problems; and

4. higher expense than routine nursing-home care.

Ohta and Ohta (1988) noted the wide variation in the developing special-care units. They identified the critical characteristics of such units with respect to philosophy, environmental design, and therapeutic approach. Philosophic differences include the definition of what makes a unit "special" for demented patients; is it these patients or the other nursing-home residents who are the primary beneficiaries; and is the focus on custodial or growth-promoting care? Environmental differences between programs include the size of the unit, type of room, architectural design, and space for wandering. Therapeutic approaches vary in terms of staff-to-patient ratios, consistency of staffing, staff training, patient admission and discharge criteria, and orientation ranging from custodial care to promotion of independent functioning. The authors suggest that given the heterogeneity of these special units, careful evaluation needs to be done to assess which program characteristics benefit which patients.

Several examples of such special programs or units have been described. McGrowder-Lin and Bhatt (1988) developed a "Wanderer's Lounge" program. From 3 to 5 PM daily, wandering residents were taken to a special room to participate in a program that included exercise, tossing a ball, refreshments, dancing, and a cool-down exercise. Positive changes were noted in each group member in target symptoms such as agitation or incontinence. Cleary, Clamon, Price, and Shullaw (1988) described a "Reduced Stimulation Unit" designed to reduce the level of stimulation and minimize reliance on memory. As a result of the program, weight loss was curtailed, patient agitation was diminished, restraint use was reduced, and wandering ceased to be a concern of staff or other patients. Family members were highly satisfied with the program and reported that patients were more calm and serene. Benson, Cameron, Humbach, Servino, and Gambert (1987) reported on 32 demented, elderly residents of a nursing home admitted to a specially designed dementia unit. There was an increased level of functioning in both mental and emotional status and basic functions of daily living at both 4- and 12-month follow-up evaluations. The improvement in scores was maintained despite an expectation that the dementia would progress. An example of specific design was the demonstration by Namazi, Rosner, and Calkins (1989) that exiting from a special unit could be reduced if the doorknob was concealed behind a cloth panel.

In contrast to the above enthusiasm for special care units, Holmes, Teresi, Weiner, Monaco, Ronch, and Vickers (1990) compared demented patients in such units to demented controls in the same four nursing homes and found no deleterious or beneficial effects associated with residence on a special unit. Similarly, Coleman, Barbaccia, and Croughan-Minihane (1990) reported that the hospitalization rate for demented patients was no lower and was possibly higher from a special-care unit compared to residents on a regular nursing-home unit. Clearly, more comprehensive evaluations are needed to determine the cost-benefit ratio and cost-effectiveness of such units.

III. Public Policy Issues

Nursing homes have received considerable attention from policy makers in the last few years as a result of the report "Improving the Quality of Care in Nursing Homes" published by the Institute of Medicine (1986). This led to enactment of new federal conditions of participation for long-term care facilities in the Medicare and Medicaid programs. The changes mandated by Public Law 100-203 include gradually phasing out the distinction between Skilled Nursing Facilities and Intermediate Care Facilities and establishing a single set of requirements for all nursing-home facilities. Among the new requirements are a physician visit every 60 days for all patients; at least a part-time medical director; a full-time social worker on staff for facilities with more than 120 beds; round-the-clock licensed nurses in all facilities with an RN on duty every day; qualified activities directors and dietitians in all facilities; mandatory training for all current and future nurse's aides; a comprehensive assessment of residents on admission, after any significant change in condition, and annually; a written plan of care that describes the medical, nursing, and psychosocial needs of the resident and how such needs will be met, initially prepared with the participation (to the extent practicable) of the resident or the resident's family or legal representative, by a team that includes the resident's attending physician and a registered professional nurse with responsibility for the resident, and is periodically reviewed and revised by such team after each assessment; a new emphasis on quality of life and resident's rights, including the right to participation in informed decisions about care and treatment, freedom from unnecessary chemical or physical restraints, physical or mental abuse, or involuntary seclusion, right to privacy, confidentiality, notification of legal rights and responsibilities, and of services available, and to freedom from involuntary transfer and/or discharge. The goal of all these new requirements is to "maintain the highest practicable physical, mental, and psychosocial well-being of each resident" (Nursing Home Reform Act, 1987).

While the above requirements are well intentioned, the draft regulations to implement them and the survey procedures to check for compliance are highly intrusive into clinical care. For example, the use of neuroleptics is severely restricted to certain clinical situations and their p.r.n. (as needed) use is discouraged. In addition, other than a requirement that states adjust their Medicaid rates to support the new requirements, there is no assurance that the additional funding needed to implement all the new requirements will be available.

One other major new provision grew out of concern that mentally ill patients were being "dumped" into nursing homes and were not receiving appropriate services. Preadmission screening is now required for all *mentally ill* and *mentally retarded* individuals to assure that they require the level of services provided by a nursing facility and do not require *active treatment* for their condition. Each mentally ill or mentally retarded resident of a nursing facility must also have an annual review to determine whether care in the nursing facility is still required or whether inpatient psychiatric services are needed. A resident is considered mentally ill if the individual "has a primary or secondary diagnosis of mental disorder [as defined in the Diagnostic and Statistical Manual of Mental Disorders, 3rd edition (DSM-III)] and does not have a primary diagnosis of dementia (including Alzheimer's disease or a related disorder)" (Nursing Home Reform Act, 1987). The determination as to who is mentally ill and whether they can be appropriately managed in a nursing home is to be made by "the state mental health authority (based on an independent physical and mental evaluation performed by a person or entity other than the state mental health authority." Many questions have been raised about the requirement for preadmission screening, and this has delayed the implementation. Although this requirement is intended to assure that mentally ill persons receive the appropriate services to meet their needs, they may be stigmatized and excluded from nursing facilities concerned about the risk they will not be paid. Furthermore, as this report has highlighted, most of the behavioral problems in nursing homes are a result of dementia, the one condition excluded from the preadmission screening and annual reviews. The discussion about these issues is ongoing, but the most sensible approach would seem to be to determine whether any applicant to a nursing facility needs the services provided there, rather than some lesser level of care, and then to assure that the appropriate care is provided.

One other area of public policy relevant to the provision of mental health services in nursing homes is the reimbursement for such services. As of January 1989, there is no longer an annual limit on benefits for outpatient *medical management* under Medicare, the national health insurance program that covers physician's services for most nursing-home residents. Such visits are, however, subject to 20% copayment, and that can limit the availability of such services. Furthermore, the reimbursement per visit is reduced somewhat if more than one patient is seen on the same day at the nursing home. Medicare patients can also receive unlimited psychotherapy benefits, but these are reimbursed with 50% copayment. Psychologists are also now eligible for Medicare reimbursement. With these changes in outpatient benefits, Medicare patients, including nursing-home residents, now have better coverage for outpatient psychiatric treatment than many younger, employed patients. Given the needs, it is hoped that an expansion in mental health services to nursing homes will result from these changes.

References

Avorn, J., Dreyer, P., Connelly, K., & Soumerai, S. B. (1989). Use of psychoactive medication and the quality of care in rest homes: Findings and policy implications of a statewide study. *New England Journal of Medicine, 320,* 227–232.

Barnes, R. F., & Raskind, M. A. (1981). DSM-III criteria and the clinical diagnosis of dementia: A nursing home study. *Journal of Gerontology, 36,* 20–27.

Barnes, R., Veith, R., Okimoto, J., Raskind, M., & Gumbrecht, G. (1982). Efficacy of antipsychotic medications in behaviorally disturbed dementia patients. *American Journal of Psychiatry, 139,* 1170–1174.

Beardsley, R. S., Larson, D. B., Burns, B. J., Thompson, J. W., & Kamerow, D. B. (1989). Prescribing of psychotropics in elderly nursing home patients. *Journal of the American Geriatrics Society, 37,* 327–330.

Beers, M., Avorn, J., Soumerai, S. B., Everitt, D., Sherman, D., & Salem, S. (1988). Psychoactive medication use in intermediate-care facility residents. *Journal of the American Medical Association, 260,* 3016–3020.

Benson, D. M., Cameron, D., Humbach, E., Servino, L., & Gambert, S. R. (1987). Establishment and impact of a dementia unit within the nursing home. *Journal of the American Geriatrics Society, 35,* 319–323.

Bienenfeld, D., & Wheeler, B. G. (1989). Psychiatric services to nursing homes: A liaison model. *Hospital and Community Psychiatry, 40,* 793–794.

Blazer, D. G., Federspiel, C. F., Ray, W. A., & Schaffner, W. (1983). The risk of anticholinergic toxicity in the elderly: A study of prescribing practices in two populations. *Journal of Gerontology, 38,* 31–35.

Block, C., Boczkowski, J. A., Hansen, N., & Vanderbeck, M. (1987). Nursing home consultation: Difficult residents and frustrated staff. *The Gerontologist, 27,* 443–446.

Borson, S., Liptzin, B., Nininger, J., & Rabins, P. V. (1989). *Nursing homes and the mentally ill elderly.* Washington, DC: American Psychiatric Association.

Buck, J. A. (1988). Psychotropic drug practice in nursing homes. *Journal of the American Geriatrics Society, 36,* 409–418.

Burns, B. J., & Kamerow, D. B. (1988). Psychotropic drug prescriptions for nursing home residents. *Journal of Family Practice, 26,* 155–160.

Bushey, M., Rathey, R., & Bowers, M. B. (1983). Lithium treatment in a very elderly nursing home population. *Comprehensive Psychiatry, 24,* 392–396.

Chandler, J. D., & Chandler, J. E. (1988). The prevalence of neuropsychiatric disorders in a nursing home population. *Journal of Geriatric Psychiatry and Neurology, 1,* 71–76.

Chartock, P., Nevins, A., Rzetelny, H., & Gilberto, P. (1988). A mental health training program in nursing homes. *The Gerontologist, 28,* 503–507.

Cleary, T. A., Clamon, C., Price, M., & Shullaw, G. (1988). A reduced stimulation unit: Effects on patients with Alzheimer's disease and related disorders. *The Gerontologist, 28,* 511–514.

Cohen-Mansfield, J., & Billig, N. (1986). Agitated behaviors in the elderly: I. A conceptual review. *Journal of the American Geriatrics Society, 34,* 711–721.

Cohen-Mansfield, J., Marx, M. S., & Rosenthal, A. S. (1989). A description of agitation in a nursing home. *Journal of Gerontology, 44:* M77–M84.

Cohen-Mansfield, J., Marx, M. S., & Werner, P. (1989). Full moon: Does it influence agitated nursing home residents? *Journal of Clinical Psychology, 45,* 611–614.

Cohen-Mansfield, J., Werner, P., & Marx, M. S. (1989). An observational study of agitation in agitated nursing home residents. *International Psychogeriatrics, 1,* 153–165.

Coleman, E. A., Barbaccia, J. C., Croughan-Minihane, M. S. (1990). Hospitalization rates in nursing home residents with dementia: A pilot study of the impact of a special care unit. *Journal of the American Geriatrics Society, 38,* 108–112.

Evans, L. K., & Strumpf, N. E. (1989). Tying down the elderly: A review of the literature on physical restraint. *Journal of the American Geriatrics Society, 36,* 65–74.

Folmar, S., & Wilson, H. (1989). Social behavior and physical restraints. *The Gerontologist, 29,* 650–653.

German, P. S., Shapiro, S., & Kramer, M. (1986). Nursing home study of the eastern Baltimore epidemiologic catchment area study. In M. S. Harper & B. D. Lebowitz (Eds.), *Nursing homes: Agenda for research* (pp. 27–40). Rockville, MD: National Institute of Mental Health.

Glasscote, R. M., Beigel, A., & Butterfield, A. (1976), *Old folks at homes.* Washington, DC: Joint Information Service of the American Psychiatric Association and the National Association for Mental Health.

Goldfarb, A. I. (1962). Prevalence of psychiatric disorders in metropolitan old age and nursing homes. *Journal of the American Geriatrics Society, 10,* 77–82.

Goldfarb, A. I., & Sheps, J. (1954). Psychotherapy and the aged: Brief therapy of interrelated psychological and somatic disorders. *Psychosomatic Medicine, 16,* 209–219.

Goldman, H. H., Feder, J., & Scanlon, W. (1986). Chronic mental patients in nursing homes: Reexamining data from the National Nursing Home Survey. *Hospital and Community Psychiatry, 37,* 269–272.

Gurian, B., & Chanowitz, B. (1987a). An empirical evaluation of a model geropsychiatric nursing home. *The Gerontologist, 27,* 766–772.

Gurian, B., & Chanowitz, B. (1987b). Barriers to implementation of a public/private model geropsychiatric nursing home. *The Gerontologist, 27,* 761–765.

Herst, L., & Moulton, P. (1985). Psychiatry in the nursing home. *Psychiatric Clinics of North America, 8,* 551–561.

Holmes, D., Teresi, J., Weiner, A., Monaco, C., Ronch, J., & Vickers, R. (1990). Impacts associated with special care units in long-term care facilities. *The Gerontologist, 30,* 178–183.

Institute of Medicine (1986). *Improving the quality of care in nursing homes.* Washington, DC: National Academy of Sciences.

Jackson, M. E., Drugovich, M. L., Fretwell, M. D., Spector, W. D., Sternberg, J., & Rosenstein, R. B. (1989). Prevalence and correlates of disruptive behavior in the nursing home. *Journal of Aging and Health, 1,* 349–369.

Kafonek, S., Ettinger, W. H., Roca, R., Kittner, S., Taylor, N., & German, P. S. (1989). Instruments for screening for depression and dementia in a long-term care facility. *Journal of the American Geriatrics Society, 37,* 29–34.

Liptzin, B. (1989). The nursing home resident as a psychiatric patient. In N. Billig & P. V. Rabins (Eds.), *Issues in geriatric psychiatry* (pp. 85–100). Basel, Switzerland: S. Karger.

Maas, M. (1988). Management of patients with Alzheimer's disease in long-term care facilities. *Nursing Clinics of North America, 23,* 57–68.

McGrowder-Lin, R., & Bhatt, A. (1988). A wanderer's lounge program for nursing home residents with Alzheimer's disease. *The Gerontologist, 28,* 607–609.

Merriam, A. E., Aronson, M. K., Gaston, P., Wey, S. L., & Katz, I. (1988). The psychiatric symptoms of Alzheimer's disease. *Journal of the American Geriatrics Society, 36,* 7–12.

Miller, M. B., & Elliott, D. F. (1976). Errors and omissions in diagnostic records on admission of patients to a nursing home. *Journal of the American Geriatrics Society, 24,* 108–116.

Mitchell, J. B. (1982). Physician visits to nursing homes. *The Gerontologist, 22,* 45–48.

Mitchell, J. B. (1986). Why won't physicians make nursing home visits? *The Gerontologist, 26,* 650–654.

Moran, J. A., & Gatz, M. (1987). Group therapies for nursing home adults: An evaluation of two treatment approaches. *The Gerontologist, 27,* 588–591.

Morriss, R. K., Rovner, B. W., Folstein, M. F., & German, P. S. (1990). Delusions in newly admitted residents of nursing homes. *American Journal of Psychiatry, 147,* 299–302.

Namazi, K. H., Rosner, T. T., & Calkins, M. P. (1989). Visual barriers to prevent ambulatory Alzheimer's patients from exiting through an emergency door. *The Gerontologist, 29,* 699–702.

Nursing Home Reform Act. (1987). Omnibus Budget Reconciliation Act of 1987. Public Law 100-203.

Nygaard, H. A., Bakke, K. J., & Breivik, K. (1989). Mental and physical capacity and consumption of neuroleptic drugs in residents of homes for aged people. *Acta Psychiatrica Scandinavica, 80,* 170–173.

Ohta, R. J., & Ohta, B. M. (1988). Special units for Alzheimer's disease patients: A critical look. *The Gerontologist, 28,* 803–808.

Powell, C., Mitchell-Pedersen, L., Fingerote, E., & Edmund, L. (1989). Freedom from restraint: Consequences of reducing physical restraints in the management of the elderly. *Canadian Medical Association Journal, 141,* 561–564.

Power, C. A., & McCarron, L. T. (1975). Treatment of depression in persons residing in homes for the aged. *The Gerontologist, 15,* 132–135.

Rabins, P. V. (1986). Establishing Alzheimer's disease units in nursing homes: Pros and cons. *Hospital and Community Psychiatry, 37,* 120–121.

Rabins, P. V. (1989). Coexisting depression and dementia. *Journal of Geriatric Psychiatry, 22,* 17–24.

Rabins, P. V., Rovner, B. W., Larson, D. B., Burns, B. J., Prescott, C., & Beardsley, R. S. (1987). The use of mental health measures in nursing home research. *Journal of the American Geriatrics Society, 35,* 431–434.

Rader, J. (1987). A comprehensive staff approach to problem wandering. *The Gerontologist, 27,* 756–760.

Rattenbury, C., & Stones, M. J. (1989). A controlled evaluation of reminiscence and current topics discussion groups in a nursing home context. *The Gerontologist, 29,* 768–771.

Ray, W. A., Federspiel, C. F., & Schaffner, W. (1980). A study of antipsychotic drug use in nursing homes: Epidemiologic evidence suggesting misuse. *American Journal of Public Health, 70,* 485–491.

Reifler, B. V., Teri, L., Raskind, M., Veith, R., Barnes, R., White, E., & McLean, P. (1989). Double-blind trial of imipramine in Alzheimer's disease patients with and without depression. *American Journal of Psychiatry, 146,* 45–49.

Riesenberg, D. (1988). Drugs in the institutionalized elderly: Time to get it right? *Journal of the American Medical Association, 260,* 3054.

Rovner, B. W., David, A., Lucas-Blaustein, M. J., Conklin, B., Filipp, L., & Tune, L. (1988). Self-care capacity and anticholinergic drug levels in nursing home patients. *American Journal of Psychiatry, 145,* 107–109.

Rovner, B. W., German, P. S., Broadhead, J., Morriss, R. K., Brant, L. J., Blaustein, J., & Folstein, M. F. (1990). The prevalence and management of dementia and other psychiatric disorders in nursing homes. *International Psychogeriatrics, 2,* 13–24.

Rovner, B. W., Kafonek, S., Filipp, L., Lucas, M. J., & Folstein, M. F. (1986). Prevalence of mental illness in a community nursing home. *American Journal of Psychiatry, 143,* 1446–1449.

Schmidt, L. J., Rheinhardt, A. M., Kane, R. L., & Olsen, D. M. (1977). The mentally ill in nursing homes: New back wards in the community. *Archives of General Psychiatry, 34,* 687–691.

Schwenk, M. A. (1979). Reality orientation for the institutionalized aged: Does it help? *The Gerontologist, 19,* 373–377.

Smyer, M. A., Cohn, M. D., & Brannon, D. (1988). *Mental health consultation in nursing homes.* New York: New York University Press.

Snowdon, J., & Donnelly, N. (1986). A study of depression in nursing homes. *Journal of Psychiatric Research, 20,* 327–333.

Snyder, L. H., Rupprecht, P., Pyrek, J., Brekhus, S., & Moss, T. (1978). Wandering. *The Gerontologist, 18,* 272–280.

Stotsky, B. A. (1967). A systematic study of therapeutic interventions in nursing homes. *Geriatric Psychology Monographs, 76,* 257–320.

Teeter, R. B., Garetz, F. K., Miller, W. R., & Heiland, W. F. (1976). Psychiatric disturbances of aged patients in skilled nursing homes. *American Journal of Psychiatry, 133,* 1430–1434.

Tourigny-Rivard, M. F., & Drury, M. (1987). The effects of monthly psychiatric consultation in a nursing home. *The Gerontologist, 27,* 363–366.

United States Senate, Subcommittee on Long-Term Care, Special Committee on Aging (1974). *Nursing home care in the US: Failure in public policy. Supporting Paper No. 1.* Washington, DC: U.S. Government Printing Office.

Vladeck, B. C. (1980). *Unloving care.* New York: Basic Books.

Weiss, I. K., Nagel, C. L., Aronson, M. K. (1986). Applicability of depression scales to the old person. *Journal of the American Geriatrics Society, 34,* 215–218.

Werner, P., Cohen-Mansfield, J., Braun, J., & Marx, M. S. (1989). Physical restraints and agitation in nursing home residents. *Journal of the American Geriatrics Society, 37,* 1122–1126.

Zimmer, J. G., Watson, N., & Treat, A. (1984). Behavioral problems among patients in skilled nursing facilities. *American Journal of Public Health, 74,* 1118–1121.

Forensic and Ethical Issues _____

Spencer Eth and Gregory B. Leong

I. Competency
    A. Competency in Civil Law
    B. Voluntary Informed Consent
    C. Competency in Criminal Law
II. Confidentiality
III. Boundary Issues
IV. Conclusion
    References

Forensic and ethical issues involving the aged encompass all of the ones that can be faced by any other adult; however, their frequency and complexity may be greater, reflecting age-dependent differences in the prevalence of important psychiatric and medical conditions that are the substrate for these legal and ethical concerns. Advancing age invariably results in a progressive loss of functional capacity of all biological systems. Further, old age is associated with an increasing likelihood of the specific degenerative changes within the central nervous system characteristic of dementia. Other body systems are also exposed to an accelerating risk of malfunction and disease, which can then directly, or indirectly through therapeutic intervention, give rise to organic mental syndromes. Finally, functional psychiatric disorders are well known to develop anew in later life (Jenike, 1985). The appearance of these mental and neuropsychiatric disturbances in the geriatric population plays a significant role in generating forensic and ethical concerns.

    This chapter will identify three critical themes that can clarify the legal and ethical analysis of the myriad problems found in a geriatric population at risk for mental, physical, and neuropsychiatric illnesses. The following clinical vignette serves to illustrate the themes of competency, consent, and confidentiality that will be explored in depth in the sections that follow (Veath, 1976). Mr. B is a 70-year-old Alzheimer's disease patient who has a history of cardiac arrhythmia. Mr. B has been confined to an intermediate-care facility because of his tendency to wander away from home and become lost. Mr. B's devoted wife of 50 years, who herself has grown quite frail, constantly laments her husband's deterioration, especially since he no longer consistently recognizes her during her daily visits with him. Although technically Mr. B is a voluntary patient in the facility, Mrs. B routinely provides consent for all medical procedures and treatments. One day, without her knowledge, Mr. B is transferred to a local hospital in order to replace the failing battery in his cardiac pacemaker. When notified of this action, Mrs. B expresses outrage and insists that nothing further be done to her husband. Mrs. B adamantly refuses permission for the minor surgery required to repair the pacemaker. As she explains: "What does he have to live for? Nothing! He has no memory, and he is slowly turning into a vegetable. I know he prefers death to that kind of miserable existence."

I. Competency

As suggested by the case of Mr. and Mrs. B, the concept of competency is central to any discussion of legal and ethical issues in the aged. Competency, or the lack of competency, play an important role in deciding whether older individuals, such as Mr. B, will be free to act in all of the ways that they have throughout their lives. For instance, deciding where to live, consenting to medical care, buying or selling assets, and writing a will all presuppose a person's competence. The loss of these capabilities, in a sense, results in a process of infantilization in which the senior citizen comes to rely increasingly on caretakers for life direction. It may, therefore, be useful to consider the emergence of competence at the other end of the life cycle.

Beginning at birth, American law grants a succession of rights and privileges to individuals as their chronological age advances. Federal and state regulations govern the precise age one may first vote, operate a motor vehicle, purchase alcohol, enter the armed forces, and practice medicine. In another context, the law determines a threshold age for exercising the right to a jury trial, for being found guilty of a crime, and for being subject to capital punishment. These age-dependent legal functions presume that a certain degree of cognitive maturation has accompanied chronological age. This generally occurs with the growth of a child according to accepted models of cognitive development (Piaget & Inhelder, 1969). Although the acquisition of relevant cognitive skills parallels to some extent the legal expectations of a juvenile (Billick, 1986), the age criteria for some older-adult activities appears driven by political processes rather than developmental capabilities. It is difficult to imagine the particular neuropsychological ability that first matures at 35 yr of age and only then qualifies a citizen to serve as President of the United States. Similarly, there does not appear to be a cognitive or functional marker of infirmity that defines 62 or 65 years as the appropriate age for entitlement to Social Security and Medicare benefits.

The principal legal concept that underlies the practice of forensic geropsychiatry in both the civil and criminal arenas is competency. In common parlance, competency refers to the capacity to understand the nature and consequences of an intended act. However, the actual legal usage of competency seems to defy precise definition, as it varies with the specific act that is being assessed, with the local statutes that set the criteria for that particular competency, and with the individual's functional ability and the context in which the act is to be carried out (Grisso, 1987). For legal purposes, adulthood routinely confers the status of competency for the full range of civil and criminal acts, unless there has been a formal adjudication of incompetency by the court.

The notion of *developmental competency,* or competency achieved through the acquisition of relevant cognitive skills (Billick, 1986), may serve as an analogy for the concept of *developmental incompetency,* which can arise when those cognitive skills are lost in the process of aging. While developmental competency carries the assurance of legal competency with the entrance into adulthood, developmental incompetency does not automatically render an individual incompetent at any age without a formal judicial hearing. Moreover, even if an individual is found incompetent to perform a certain act, that person is not necessarily incompetent for another.

A. Competency in Civil Law

Matters of civil law of interest to mental health practitioners may be divided into those actions that concern property and those that involve health care. In the property category, will-making, entering into a contract, and ability to manage finances cover the gamut of situations requiring an adult to be competent to participate in such acts. In the health care category, consent to medical treatment is the principal issue that involves both the competent and incompetent adult.

Competency to execute a will or testamentary capacity is probably the cardinal forensic issue encountered in the psychogeriatric population. In order to establish testamentary capacity, the following capabilities are typically required in all United States jurisdictions:

1. the individual knows that he or she is making a will;
2. the individual knows the nature and extent of his or her property;
3. the individual knows who are his or her natural heirs; and
4. the individual knows the effects of the manner in which his or her property will be disposed (Melton, Petrila, Poythress, & Slobogin, 1987).

Testamentary competency usually does not become an issue until after the author of the will, the testator, dies, and the validity of the will is challenged in Probate Court, often by a disinherited relative. Nonetheless, because many people are living longer with significant impairment in their cognitive functioning, wills could become increasingly susceptible to legal challenge (Redmond, 1987). The psychiatric evaluation of the testator could then be based only on a retrospective analysis of the mental state reconstructed from available historical data.

In assessing the contribution of mental disorder on testamentary capacity, only those aspects that directly affect the four criteria listed above are relevant for legal purposes. Mental disorder *per se* does not negate testamentary capacity. However, the judicial presumption of competency may be rebutted in court, especially in the presence of the disorientation of a delirium, the intellectual deterioration of a dementia, or the paranoid delusions of an organic or functional psychosis. In addition to impairment in one or more of the four essential criteria of a valid will, undue influence can also be used as a basis to nullify a will. Undue influence must have been exerted with sufficient force to overcome the free will of the testator and substitute the wishes of another person (Perr, 1981). Delusional thinking, which does not substitute the wishes of another person but replaces the will-maker's free choice with the product of psychosis, may also qualify as undue influence.

Closely related to testamentary capacity is the competency of an elderly person to enter into a legally binding contract, such as marital vows or a business agreement. A late-life wedding, especially when the elderly spouse has a considerable estate, can precipitate a dispute between the adult children and the new bride or groom. Likewise, when an elderly person purchases, or more likely sells an interest in a business or similar financial entity, his or her competency to enter into that contract can be contested by a concerned family member. The legal standard for competency to enter into a contract is similar to the standards for other legal competencies, and generally requires that the person know the nature and purpose of the contract, the probable consequences of the acts specified by the contract, and that the decision to enter into the contract is not the result of undue influence.

As in the case of testamentary capacity, the question of one's competency to contract turns on precisely how the mental disorder interferes with the proposed action. For example, a severely cognitively impaired individual will be unable to understand the many ramifications of a financial business transaction. Enforcement of that contract would thus demand a more stringent legal standard for competency than would hold for that same individual composing a will. Similarly, orientation in all spheres would seem to be necessary in order to wed, while this is not always an obligatory component for testamentary capacity. Challenges to marriages or business contracts can occur before the elderly person's death. Further, such challenges can be raised before the actual marriage or formal signing of a contract, and under these circumstances, an evaluation of mental status can be conducted while the individual in question is alive, rather than posthumously, as is the usual case in a disputed will.

What may arise more commonly than testamentary incapacity in persons suffering from declining mental health is a functional inability to manage appropriately the person's own finances. Such a person can have a proxy designated by the court to oversee the incompetent person's estate. Depending upon the particular state, the person so appointed is known as a conservator, probate guardian, or committee of the person. Procedures and legal standards for appointment of a substitute decision-maker vary by jurisdiction. From a clinical standpoint, competency in this area involves a cognitive as well as a functional ability to handle one's own finances. The mental functions that are often evaluated by the court include those basic to money matters, such as acquisition and conservation of resources, and those functions that organize the proper use of money to assure that basic independent life tasks are performed.

For states that have adopted the Uniform Probate Code, guardianship grants to a proxy decision-maker control over a person, while conservatorship grants a substitute decision-maker control over a person's property (Baker, 1986). Thus, guardians are empowered to offer medical consent and to select a suitable residence, including a nursing care facility, for their wards. In other states, the roles of the guardian and conservator may be reversed, but the essential functions of managing person and property are similar across jurisdictions. The courts generally look to family members or close friends as first choices to be appointed as surrogate decision-makers.

Cognitive impairment can progress beyond disabling a person from handling financial affairs to crippling one's ability to provide for the basic necessities of life. In many states there are mental health statutes governing situations in which an individual, as a result of mental disorders such as dementia or psychosis, cannot provide for or accept the offer of the basic necessities of life, such as food, clothing, and shelter. That individual can then be found *gravely disabled,* allowing for the court to appoint a guardian or conservator with specific delegated powers to remedy the individual's incapacities. Gravely disabled persons may be incapable of living by themselves or in the family home, dictating their admission to a locked facility. Mr. B, who was presented earlier in this chapter, could be deemed gravely disabled. Despite having a wife to care for him, Mr. B's penchant for wandering away from home, coupled with his lack of memory for the route back, placed him in continued peril.

In the context of a surrogate decision-maker's efforts to provide for the person's basic survival needs, there may arise a conflict between notions of individual autonomy and social paternalism. Though some elderly suffer from such severe cognitive impairment that the loss of independence and autonomy are inconsequential, most remain keenly aware of their dependent status. Unlike child development, in which increasing independence from parental control is achieved, the geriatric phase of the life cycle often heralds a unremitting reversal of autonomy. This issue is implicated in the demoralization experienced by the dependent elderly when first admitted to chronic care facilities, and may be an etiologic factor explaining the staggering morbidity and mortality suffered by this group.

A point of caution is indicated in discussing the problem of self-abuse or self-neglect in the aged. While cognitively impaired individuals not uncommonly perform these behaviors, such actions may also represent a method of suicide that is uniquely available to depressed, bedridden elderly. Health care providers should be alert to this form of *silent suicide,* which may be expressed through such acts as self-starvation or noncompliance with essential medical treatment (Simon, 1989). Psychiatrist Robert Simon (1989) surmises that the success rate of this method may approach 100%. Simon further argues that while some of these patients have nearly intact cognition, they are *affectively* incompetent to make health care decisions by virtue of their severe depression. By extension, professionals should be sensitive to the possibility that incompetence driven by affective disorders or pseudodementia (Wells, 1979) may be eroding the judgment and ability of many of the infirm elderly. If this is suspected, a formal psychiatric consultation may be helpful in resolving this question.

B. Voluntary Informed Consent

The issue of competency to consent to or refuse medical care is of utmost importance to patients, family members, and health care providers. Historically, physicians were afforded considerable latitude in discharging their duty to care for the sick (Jonsen, Siegler, & Winslade, 1986). Since physicians were asked to use their expertise to treat the patient, any infringement of their ability to act freely could negate their effectiveness and might result in harm. The desire, ability, and a request to help provides a powerful justification for the unlimited freedom to deliver medical care governed solely by the patient's condition. This model of beneficent medical paternalism flourished for millennia, only to be supplanted this century by case law that has irrevocably shattered the presumption that the physician is the final decision-maker. The glorious or perhaps inglorious tradition of medical paternalism, depending on one's views, has given way to a newer era of patients' rights (Katz, 1984).

In the landmark case of *Schloendorff v. Society of New York Hospital* (1914) (p. 126), New York state Justice Benjamin Cardozo opined:

> Every human being of adult years of sound mind has a right to determine what shall be done with his own body, and a surgeon who performs an operation without his patient's consent commits an assault for which he is liable in damages . . . this is true except in a case of an emergency where the patient is unconscious, and where it is necessary to operate before consent can be obtained.

More recently, a federal appellate court, in the case of *Canterbury v. Spence* (1972), mandated that the attending physician must disclose all information a reasonable patient would need to know in order to make an informed judgment about treatment. These decisions are but two of many court rulings that underscore the right of competent adult patients to all relevant information upon which to base a voluntary and informed choice whether to accept or refuse the recommended medical care in nonemergency situations. These then compose the three elements of a valid informed consent: information disclosure, competency, and voluntariness. Commentators have offered alternative conceptualizations of informed consent according to other organizing factors, such as communicating choices, understanding relevant information, appreciating the situation and its consequences, and manipulating information rationally (Appelbaum & Grisso, 1988). While such schema may be more clinically useful, they can be readily subsumed by the case law–derived components of informed consent suggested above.

In a valid informed consent, disclosure involves a process of explaining to the patient in the language of a layperson the following relevant elements: the nature and purpose of the proposed treatment, alternatives to that treatment, and the hoped-for benefits and possible risks of the proposed treatment and its alternatives, including the option of refusing treatment and allowing the disease process to progress naturally. Competency, in reference to a valid informed consent in medical situations, would depend on whether the patient retains the capacity to make a reasoned choice, even if the physician does not recommend the particular alternative selected by the patient. Voluntariness refers to a consent given without undue influence, such as that imposed by an implied threat of abandonment by the health care team or by a paranoid delusion involving the proposed treatment. Though the three elements of informed consent for medical treatment are listed separately, they are not necessarily mutually exclusive. In order to make a truly competent decision, the patient must have access to sufficient information (disclosure) and operate in an environment free of undue influence (voluntariness).

Closely following the emerging legal emphasis on information disclosure has been an evolution in the ethical standard of honesty in the doctor–patient relationship. As recently as a generation ago the policy of deception concerning catastrophic diagnoses was widely practiced. Compassionate physicians sincerely believed that it would be harmful to their patients to reveal the presence of a fatal illness. It is now generally accepted that lying is morally wrong and that physicians, regardless of motive, are not exempt from the duty to tell the truth (Bok, 1978). This view underscores the importance of the patient's standing as an autonomous moral agent. Further, there is empirical evidence confirming the supposition that patients wish to learn the truth no matter how painful it may be. For example, a survey of adult outpatients younger than 60 years found that virtually all would want to be informed of the diagnosis of Alzheimer's disease (Erde, Nadal, & Scholl, 1988).

The process of information sharing should respect individual patient needs. A delirious patient is rarely in a position to be confronted with complex cognitive material. Similarly, patients with dementia commonly present with characteristic fragility of their ego defenses. If suddenly challenged with an overwhelming cognitive task, a patient may respond with a catastrophic reaction of agitation and panic. Consequently, the discretionary withholding of information that would be immediately disturbing to an impaired patient is legally and ethically permissible under the rubric of therapeutic privilege. However, the physician retains an obligation to confide the necessary information as soon as possible within the limitations imposed by the patient's deficits (Overman & Stoudemire, 1988).

Every adult is presumed by law to be competent to offer voluntary informed consent. Not infrequently a patient will be referred for psychiatric consultation because of noncompliant or uncooperative behavior (Perl & Shelp, 1982). The idiosyncratic exercise of one's self-determination may or may not signify an underlying mental illness. If that patient is competent to consent, the choice of medical treatment is the exclusive right of the patient alone (Eth & Robb, 1986). However, many illnesses afflicting the elderly affect mentation and can render the patient less able to perform cognitive tasks. If an aged patient experiences difficulty comprehending the risks and benefits associated with treatment, the possibility of incompetence should be investigated. The physician is responsible for the rigorous, detailed assessment of the patient's mental status. The court is uniquely empowered to rule on whether that patient's cognitive and functional deficits necessitate the appointment of a substitute decision-maker. In most instances patients are deemed competent if they are capable of appreciating the elements of the consent process. Hence, they should be able to demonstrate an understanding of relevant information, a consideration of alternatives, and an ability to express their preference for or against treatment. Under this minimal standard some demented, psychotic, or severely depressed patients will be found competent to consent. From an ethical perspective, it has become clear that our society has placed an extraordinary value on individual liberty, daring to allow even patients with significant mental illness the right to choose the treatment option of their choice.

There are situations, especially in cases of permanent and severe cognitive dysfunction, in which geriatric patients lack the capacity to give informed consent. In *Superintendent of Belchertown State School v. Saikewicz* (1977), the Massachusetts Supreme Court ruled that the right to accept or reject medical treatment of a terminally ill, profoundly mentally retarded and incompetent 67-year-old patient residing in a state institution would be based on the substituted-judgement doctrine. However, since in fact since Saikewicz's retardation had resulted in lifelong incompetence, so that he had never previously expressed a preference on how to proceed if stricken with a terminal illness, his proxy consenter was forced to rely on an estimation of what would be in Saikewicz's best interests, rather than what he had indicated would be his preference in a comparable situation. The substituted judgement would attempt to formulate the exact decision that the incompetent person would have made if he or she were competent, by considering all of the positive and negative factors surrounding the alternative treatments according to the patient's own value system.

However, in these cases the court is the ultimate authority in rendering a substituted decision. The seminal precedent for this doctrine is the Karen Ann Quinlan case (*In re Quinlan*, 1976), in which the New Jersey Supreme Court granted this patient's father the authority to substitute his judgment, based on his unique relationship and insight, as to what his daughter would have wanted if she were competent under the actual circumstances.

Not all states consistently follow the doctrine of substituted judgement. For example, consider the celebrated New York case of *In re Eichner* (1981). Brother Fox was an 83-year-old Roman Catholic friar who had spoken of his desire never to be maintained by extraordinary means if stricken with a terminal illness. Unfortunately, he subsequently suffered a cardiac arrest during hernia surgery and lapsed into a persistent vegetative state requiring respiratory life support. The director of his religious order, Father Eichner, with the approval of Brother Fox's surviving relatives, asked to be appointed Brother Fox's guardian, in order to sanction the discontinuation of ventilatory assistance. The local district attorney opposed this request. Despite Brother Fox's death while on the respirator, the case worked its way through the New York court system, arriving at its highest court, the New York State Court of Appeals. The Court of Appeals held that the lower court had ruled properly in respecting Father Eicher's decision to terminate ventilatory assistance. But the court chose not to rely on the substituted-judgement doctrine, since there was clear and convincing evidence that Brother Fox had explicitly articulated his particular wish before becoming incompetent. Brother Fox's case illustrates the issue of an adult who, while competent, expressed his choice, and who later became incompetent as a result of illness. While precedents vary by state, the *Saikewicz* and *Eichner* cases demonstrate the dilemmas and complexities of law that can be encountered with geriatric persons who are incompetent to consent to their medical care.

Competent adults have the right not only to accept a proposed medical treatment in nonemergency situations, but also to decline permission, even if that decision ultimately leads to their death. Under these circumstances, treatment refusal confers a *de facto* right to die. However, the vicissitudes of medical illness are not such that a person will necessarily be competent at the time a decision to consent to medical treatment must be made. Thus, there needs to be a mechanism to ensure that competent patients who have preferences about their medical care will be permitted to control their destiny, even in the event of a terminal illness causing severe mental impairment. Since California's Natural Death Act of 1976, a total of 40 states have allowed the use of living wills (Baker, 1986). A living will is a written document prepared by a person while competent, which specifies the circumstances under which the declarant will permit the cessation of extraordinary treatment designed to prolong life, and thereby allow death in accordance with the natural progression of illness. The will must contain two signatures and can be revoked at any time (Baker, Perr, & Yesavage, 1986).

In 16 states with living-will laws, a separate statute provides for the creation of a durable power of attorney, which authorizes a named proxy to make health-care decisions in the case of an incapacitating illness (Regan, 1987). Although the option of designating an individual (attorney-in-fact) to assume responsibility for managing financial affairs is commonplace, the extension of this mechanism to medical decision making is by no means universal.

A durable power of attorney for health care, like a living will, allows for the possibility of future incompetency, but in addition, permits flexibility for situations that arise that are not specifically enumerated in the living will. This latitude maximizes the likelihood that the person's general wishes expressed while competent will be followed in case of future incapacity (Steinbrook & Lo, 1984). For example, the proxy nominated in the durable power of attorney document may refuse to permit the use of penicillin in the treatment of pneumonia for a comatose patient, even if there is record of instructions concerning the use of antibiotics.

With increasing numbers of geriatric patients entering psychiatric treatment, issues pertaining to terminal care have become inescapable and intensely controversial (Eth, 1990). Depending on a combination of medical factors, patients with advanced degenerative dementia and other catastrophic conditions may enter a terminal phase of their illness, during which time their level of function will have markedly deteriorated. Like Saikewicz and Brother Fox, many of these patients will have had guardians or other surrogate decision-makers appointed. However, the question of exactly what type of care is appropriate under these dire circumstances is being asked with great urgency (Bellacosa, 1990). Eventually, the painful decision must be faced about whether to initiate, continue, or withdraw the variety of life-support measures sustaining the patient (Wanzer et al., 1989). Hospital staffs quickly realize that their actions in initiating or withdrawing a life-sustaining treatment, such as mechanical ventilation, may become the proximate cause of death (Miles, Singer, & Siegler, 1989). The issue is especially difficult when the targeted treatment is the continued administration of fluid and nutritional support.

Until recently, a critical moral distinction was drawn between ordinary and extraordinary care (as illustrated by Father Eicher's opinion of artificial ventilation). Physicians and other health professionals were felt to be ethically obligated to deliver all ordinary forms of care to all patients. Extraordinary care, however, ought to be ordered only if there were a compelling reason to employ extreme measures. Over the last several years, our escalating technical sophistication has blurred the boundary between ordinary and extraordinary. For example, is hemodialysis, a procedure routinely performed at home, now to be considered ordinary, and therefore mandatory care for all terminally ill patients? The novel concept of proportionality, popularized by the President's Commission for the Study of Ethical Problems in Medicine (1983), has replaced the largely arbitrary and nonindividualized categories of ordinary and extraordinary care. Proportionate care can be defined as a treatment that has at least a reasonable likelihood of providing benefits that outweigh the burdens for that particular patient. In disproportionate care, the ratio of benefits to burdens is reversed. Thus, an ordinary-appearing treatment that briefly prolongs the life of a patient in agony is disproportionate care and ought to be avoided, while an extremely painful and intrusive procedure that is curative may be proportionate and highly desirable. Although introduced primarily by medical ethicists, this method of analysis has been embraced in several court decisions (e.g., *Barber v. Superior Court*, 1983).

The United States Supreme Court confronted the *right to die* issue for the first time in its 1989–1990 term (*Cruzan v. Director, Missouri Department of Health*, 1990). The case involved a request to discontinue gastrostomy feedings by the parents of a 32-year-old woman who had been in a persistent vegetative state for over 7 yr as a result of a motor vehicle accident. The Missouri high court held that there was insufficient evidence of the patient's own wishes about whether she would want the artificial feedings stopped, despite testimony by her family of her statements that she would never want to live as a "vegetable." The Supreme Court, in a five-to-four decision, ruled that nutrition and hydration are forms of medical treatment that can be refused by a competent patient in the same way as can any other care. However, a state may choose to require clear and convincing evidence of an incompetent patient's wishes about foregoing medical treatment before allowing a surrogate to terminate care. Therefore, in the absence of compelling evidence, the Court refused to grant Ms Cruzan's parents' request to discontinue feedings, although if such prior evidence were available for another comatose patient, artificial nutrition could be suspended.

An ethical consensus is forming around several policy positions in the care of elderly patients. Authority for all medical decisions rest exclusively with competent patients. For those patients who have been adjudicated incompetent to consent, their legal surrogate is entrusted with the right to make the relevant medical decisions for them. Consistent with local law, the surrogate should follow the patient's previously communicated instructions with regard to desirable forms of care (Lo, Rouse, & Dornbrand, 1990). Only in the absence of clear and convincing directives concerning the patient's preferences, the surrogate should choose a course consistent with the generally accepted interest in preserving life. In cases where further medical care imposes unacceptable burdens, as would be true for irreversibly comatose, terminally ill patients, then all such efforts may ethically cease. Disproportionate treatment of any type that confers no benefit, including fluid and nutritional support, would not be given. Hospital staff who hold dissenting religious or moral views may be replaced by other staff members comfortable with the agreed-upon-care plan.

A number of other issues remain outside the scope of moral consensus. Murphy (1988) has suggested that cardiopulmonary resuscitation (CPR) for severely demented patients in long-term care settings is never indicated. He contends that a substitute decision-maker's refusal to endorse a do-not-resuscitate (DNR) order in such cases may be motivated by guilt or misinformation. Accordingly, a physician ought to unilaterally withhold CPR since it is usually futile and always cruel to a patient who cannot comprehend its therapeutic intent. This argument is admittedly paternalistic and intensely controversial, as it explicitly conflicts with the rights of patients or their surrogates to expect and insist upon customary treatment efforts.

The practice of euthanasia, which has been exhorted as humane, remains both illegal and unethical in the United States. Active, voluntary euthanasia is the deliberate termination of a terminally ill patient's life at his or her own request. A number of medical institutions in Holland have developed procedures to enable physicians to participate in mercy killings in an acceptable and controllable manner (deWachter, 1989). The identical action openly perpetrated in an American hospital would surely result in prompt legal and professional sanctions (American College of Physicians, 1989). Nevertheless, patients' rights advocates, the Hemlock Society, and others continue to assert the desirability of permitting physicians to relieve a patient's suffering by granting an immediate, painless death. One medical commentator has woefully predicted that euthanasia programs in the United States are likely to appear in the near future (Sprung, 1990). However, the moral and legal objections to physician-assisted death seem to be well articulated and strongly held by most of the profession (Singer & Siegler, 1990).

C. Competency in Criminal Law

While the population of elderly adult criminals is certainly smaller than that of younger age groups, it is not altogether insignificant (Goldstein, 1987). If a geriatric criminal commits a crime while significantly mentally impaired, or later develops such an impairment, then the issue of mental competency in the criminal justice system could become a significant factor in the outcome of the legal proceedings.

The first occasion at which legal competency can arise in the criminal justice system involves the mental capacity to waive *Miranda* rights. These rights derive from the landmark U.S. Supreme Court decision, *Miranda v. Arizona* (1966), which required police officers to warn potential criminal defendants of their constitutional right against self-incrimination and their right to counsel before police interrogation. *Miranda* warnings also contain the caveat that should a defendant choose to speak to the police, those statements can be used as evidence in future legal proceedings. The waiver of these rights presumes that the act was voluntary, knowing, and intelligent. In essence, the forfeiture of *Miranda* rights parallels the informed-consent process permitting medical treatment. Thus, a certain minimal level of cognitive functioning is required in order for individuals competently to waive their rights.

Research has shown that minors have varying degrees of comprehension in executing a *Miranda* waiver (Ferguson & Douglas, 1970; Grisso, 1981). Moreover, case law has invalidated confessions obtained from minors whose competency to waive *Miranda* rights was considered faulty because of age (e.g., *In re Patrick W,* 1972) or mental retardation (e.g., *In re Roderick P,* 1979, 1980). A similar paradigm can be conceptualized for older adults. Those with impairment in cognitive function owing to dementia or other organic mental disorders could, in theory, be found incompetent to waive *Miranda* rights. This forensic issue would most likely be raised after the defendant had made legally damaging statements, if the question of competence had not been considered by the police at the time of the *Miranda* warning. In the absence of significant cognitive dysfunction, a *Miranda* waiver could permit the admission into evidence of an elderly suspect's confession, even if that confession was influenced by delusional beliefs or auditory hallucinations (*Colorado v. Connelly,* 1986).

The trial process for those accused of crimes begins with the first meeting with an attorney and does not conclude until the pronouncement of a sentence by the judge. The

Anglo-American legal tradition has shaped our belief that a defendant must be competent to stand trial throughout this period. Our present legal standard derives from the landmark U.S. Supreme Court case, *Dusky v. United States* (1960), which defines the criteria for competency to stand trial. In order to be found competent to stand trial, the defendant must demonstrate: (1) "sufficient present ability to consult with his lawyer with a reasonable degree of rational understanding," and (2) "a rational as well as factual understanding of the proceedings taken against him (p. 402).

Clinical evaluation of competency to stand trial has been well studied, with various investigators proposing the use of specific instruments to assess this competency (Grisso, 1987; McGarry, Lipsett, & Lelos, 1973). While the most frequent conditions associated with a legal finding of incompetency to stand trial are psychotic disorders, a severely cognitively impaired person could also meet at least one of the criteria necessary to qualify for incompetency to stand trial.

A finding of incompetency to stand trial does not dismiss the legal action against the defendant, but merely delays the courtroom proceedings until such time that the defendant's mental condition has improved and competency is restored. While most defendants with psychotic disorders can be effectively treated such that they regain competence, defendants suffering from mental conditions associated with permanent cognitive dysfunction are unlikely to improve to the extent that they can become competent to stand trial. Depending on the particular jurisdiction and the nature of the criminal charges, a defendant who will not be able to meet the standard in the foreseeable future may find the charges dismissed with or without accompanying civil commitment. In cases of minor crimes perpetrated by individuals who are unlikely to regain their competency in the foreseeable future, the U.S. Supreme Court (*Jackson v. Indiana,* 1972) has limited the incarceration of those defendants found incompetent to stand trial. In addition, several states have statutes setting specific time limits during which a defendant can be held as incompetent to stand trial.

Our legal definitions of who is capable of committing a crime derives from English common law (Platt & Diamond, 1966). With regard to age, all juveniles under 7 years were historically considered to lack the capacity to commit a crime, while criminal intent was possible under certain circumstances for minors between the ages of 7 and 14. Most states continue to follow English common law by providing young children an *infancy defense* of incompetency. For example, in California, minors under the age 14 are by law not capable of committing a crime, unless there is *clear proof* that they knew the wrongfulness of their behavior (*People v. Olsen,* 1984).

Another class of persons who are incapable of committing a crime are the insane. The District of Columbia and 47 states have established an insanity defense, based either on a variation of the *M'Naghten* rules (*Regina v. M'Naghten,* 1843) or on the American Law Institute (ALI) Model Penal Code rule (Callahan, Mayer, & Steadman, 1987). The *M'Naghten* prototype states that a defendant would have been legally insane if, at the time of the crime, he or she was incapable of knowing (understanding or appreciating) the nature and quality of the act or was incapable of distinguishing right from wrong. The ALI rule states that the defendant would have been legally insane if, at the time of the crime, he or she lacked substantial capacity to appreciate the criminality of the act, or to conform his or her behavior to the requirements of law. Putting aside a complex analysis of these insanity standards, both contain a wrongfulness clause by which a defendant can be found insane. Platt and Diamond (1966) have pointed out the similarity between the infancy defense for young children and the insanity defense used to negate criminal responsibility for older adolescents and adults. A critical component of the insanity defense involves the competency to commit a crime, or the capacity to comprehend that the act was wrong or illegal. Like young children, older adults who suffer from impairment in cognitive functioning may not have the requisite mental capacity to commit crimes, though they can have the physical ability to do so.

In many jurisdictions, laws providing for diminished capacity, diminished responsibility, or partial insanity can reduce the severity of the criminal charge if the defendant is convicted. For example, without proof that a person had the requisite mental state, a defendant who stood accused of homicide would be convicted of manslaughter instead of murder. Severely cognitively impaired individuals may qualify under these provisions. In addition, if a crime is committed while under the influence of medication-induced organicity, the perpetrator could be considered involuntarily intoxicated and thereby relieved of criminal responsibility on the basis of the insanity or unconsciousness defense. On the other hand, these defenses would be invalidated if the crime followed the knowing ingestion of alcohol or drugs, including prescription drugs, when the deleterious side-effects are understood. The increased vulnerability to the untoward effects of ingested substances, especially alcohol, with advancing age potentially raises the legal issue of voluntary intoxication in a variety of criminal cases.

The Supreme Court ruled in *Ford v. Wainwright* (1986) that convicts sentenced to capital punishment cannot be executed if they are mentally incompetent. Competency to be executed, though determined by state law, generally requires that an individual know the nature and consequences of the impending punishment, that is, the reason for the execution and its finality. In the *Ford* case, the prisoner first became incompetent when he developed a psychosis while incarcerated on death row. In contrast, the Supreme Court ruled that mental retardation *per se* was insufficient cause to commute a death sentence (*Penry v. Lynaugh,* 1989).

While execution is rare in adult prisoners, it is even less likely to occur in the geriatric population. In the penalty-phase hearing of a capital trial, the jurors are instructed to consider all mitigating as well as aggravating factors before imposing the death sentence (*Lockett v. Ohio,* 1978). In the case of an elderly defendant, advanced age itself could be construed as a mitigating factor, as well as the knowledge that the imposition of a long prison sentence accomplishes the same fatal outcome. There is, however, no upper age limit for execution, although a lower age limit of 16 years has been set (*Thompson v. Oklahoma,* 1988).

Competency to be a witness, or testimonial capacity, could arise in either the civil or criminal setting. The evaluation of this competency involves assessing the witness's reliability of memory, ability to perceive reality accurately, vulnerability to suggestion, and understanding of the obligation to testify truthfully (Melton, Petrila, Poythress, & Slobogin, 1987). Of particular relevance to the elderly witness is an evaluation of the reliability of memory, since disorders associated with aging are more likely to affect memory than the other three capacities. If a witness' fitness is challenged in court, the trial judge can conduct a qualification examination (voir dire) before that witness is permitted to testify.

II. Confidentiality

Confidentiality has stood the test of time as a fundamental covenant of medical practice; both the Hippocratic Oath and the current Principles of Medical Ethics (American Psychiatric Association, 1989) contain a pledge of silence regarding professional secrets. However, strict confidentiality is not an absolute value. Relevant patient information may be legally and ethically released at the patient's request, as necessary to protect life, or as required by law. Sharing information authorized by the patient presents no difficulties. Psychiatrists may also need to document certain confidential clinical data in order to institute civil commitment or conservatorship proceedings. In these instances, the decision to overrule a patient's insistence on secrecy is consistent with legal regulations and the desire to preserve life. In addition, all jurisdictions have enacted mandatory reporting laws to alert the authorities of potentially harmful conditions. For example, statutes commonly require health care providers to report patients suffering from any one of several communicable diseases to the local public health department. In the case of the elderly persons, there are two principal reportable conditions: elder abuse and the elderly person as a danger to society.

Akin to child abuse–reporting laws, many states have enacted statutes to protect the aged from abuse, which can assume many forms: passive or active neglect; verbal, emotional, or psychological abuse; physical abuse; material or financial misappropriation; and violation of rights (Kosberg, 1987). However, the problem is oftentimes invisible, as it occurs within the home and out of public view. Unlike child-abuse regulations, elder-abuse laws have been criticized as being imprecise, variable across jurisdictions, ineffective, and an infringement on personal liberty (Faulkner, 1982; Salend, Kane, Satz, & Pynoos, 1984).

Since the California Supreme Court decision of *Tarasoff v. Regents of the University of California* (1976), federal and state courts (Mills, Sullivan, & Eth, 1987) have adjudicated similar rules propounding the psychotherapist's legal duty to protect others when and if a patient has made a serious threat of physical harm toward an identifiable victim. In a situation of threatened violence toward others, the geriatric patient would be treated in an identical fashion as other adult patients. In a recent development, California has specifically mandated the reporting by physicians of diseases associated with dementia, including Alzheimer's disease and related disorders (§410, California Health and Safety Code; §§2500 and 2572, Title 17, California Code of Regulations). The purpose of this statute is the protection of motorists and pedestrians from a vehicle operator who may be impaired. In fact, several duty-to-protect cases involving psychiatric patients have arisen when third parties suffered injuries in automobile accidents (Felthous, 1990).

Perhaps the most common, though far less dramatic, are the conflicts over confidentiality arising in the context of involvement with the elderly patient's family. The wish to share clinical impressions with concerned relatives in order to facilitate treatment planning may clash with the patient's insistence that all clinical material remain private. Even in the first visit, the health care professional may wish to question family members in order to augment an incomplete or confusing history obtained from a cognitively impaired patient. In the case of a progressive dementia, the role of family support broadens as the patient becomes increasingly disabled. It is therefore advisable early in the treatment to obtain, while the patient is competent, written consent for release of information. Occasionally that permission is refused, as the incapacitated patients may insist on strict confidentiality as a way of gaining some control over their lives. This problem may be more likely in a situation in which adult children have assumed caretaking roles for their own parents. Interpretation of this dynamic may promote resolution of the conflict. If, however, the patient adamantly refuses to permit disclosure, the physician is effectively prevented from violating confidentiality until such time as the patient relents or a conservator is appointed by the court. Ultimately, appropriate medical information, such as the diagnosis of an hereditary disease, may be divulged to family members after the patient's death (American Psychiatric Association, 1987).

III. Boundary Issues

Despite numerous attempts at cost control, the total personal health care expenditures in the United States have continued to accelerate. Official forecasts predict that by the year 2000, this country will be devoting 15% of its entire production to health care (Aaron & Schwartz, 1990). Economic reality dictates that some form of rationing may be inevitable. Callahan (1990) in particular has criticized the explosion of expensive new medical technology and our expectation of unlimited scientific progress. In an era of budgetary controls, the use of new technology must be contained, even at the expense of potential life-extending benefits. Economists and ethicists have also decried the provision of excessive care to the dying, care that wastes finite resources and may actually harm rather than help fatally ill patients (Scitovsky & Capron, 1986).

Articles have appeared in the literature suggesting that physicians are already allocating scarce critical care resources according to such factors as bed availability and prognosis (Luce, 1990). What remains unresolved is the significance of age in determining the priority for scarce medical-care resources. Does the foreshortened life expectancy and diminished vigor of old age justify placing the elderly at the end of the waiting line for transplants, intensive care beds, and magnetic resonance imaging (MRI) scans? At least one commentator (Kilner, 1989) has argued that age *per se* is not an appropriate criterion; rather, medical factors independent of age should alone determine the patient's eligibility and priority for expensive and scarce specialized care. However, it has been abundantly clear that the elderly receive a disproportionately small share of the available mental health care services. While the average medical patient with a psychiatric diagnosis has a 40% chance of consulting a psychiatrist, the probability for an otherwise comparable elderly patient is only 3% (Schurman, Kramer, & Mitchell, 1985). Perhaps informal rationing of services to the aged is already occurring.

The importance of research in geriatric mental health cannot be overvalued. Without clinical investigation, progress in the understanding and treatment of psychiatric disorders will be stifled. Although there is no dispute over the need for research, there are many obstacles to its conduct in this patient population. For instance, as a function of cognitive deficits and old age, Alzheimer's disease victims, especially if they reside in long-term care facilities, are particularly vulnerable to exploitation by overzealous researchers. The best means of safeguarding the process of patient participation is through careful attention to the requirement of voluntary informed consent, which is generally recognized as a prerequisite for the inclusion of human subjects in biomedical research. Consent functions both to protect the unsuspecting patient from deceptive recruitment and to permit the willing patient to enter a study that promises little benefit and potential risk. Consequently, the consent process well serves the investigator and subject alike.

Informed consent for research, as for medical care, presupposes that the patient has the mental ability to comprehend the study procedures with their attendant risks and benefits. Incompetent patients lack the mental capacity to offer meaningful consent to treatment or research. However, it is these very patients, for example, those with pronounced Alzheimer's disease, who may be the most desirable subjects. Although the patient's surrogate can offer substitute consent for treatment, some constraints are placed on a surrogate's ability to expose another person to the research situation. The altruistic decision to sacrifice bodily integrity for the sake of others ought to be reserved for the individual in jeopardy (Eth & Mills, 1989). One approach to mitigating this limitation is to distinguish therapeutic from nontherapeutic research. According to this dichotomy, proxy decision-makers may freely approve those research projects in which there is the intent and reasonable probability of improving the health or well-being of the subject, such as an experimental drug protocol. Patients' representatives would be limited in their ability to consent to those nontherapeutic studies that carry only minimal risk. An innovative alternative to conventional surrogate-consent procedures has been proposed to facilitate research with patients suffering from progressive dementia (Schneiderman & Arras, 1985). Consent for future studies could be solicited from the patient in an early stage of illness while the patient was still competent. An argument could be made that the previously obtained consent would be binding later when the patient was no longer competent.

IV. Conclusion

This chapter's review of forensic and ethical issues may appear daunting at first glance. Many clinicians find these sorts of problems especially vexing, because they involve areas in the law and moral philosophy seemingly far removed from their usual medical and psychiatric concerns. However, taken together, these legal and ethical difficulties are seen to arise from a small number of manageable principles accessible to the professional reader. By identifying underlying themes of competency, consent, or confidentiality, a variety of common dilemmas can be framed and analyzed to suggest a reasonable resolution. In that vein, serious attention to the forensic and ethical domains will enhance clinical efficacy and personal satisfaction in working with this age group.

References

Aaron, H., & Schwartz, W. B. (1990). Rationing health care: The choice before us. *Science, 247*, 418–422.
American College of Physicians. (1989). Ethics manual. *Annals of Internal Medicine, 111*, 245–252, 327–335.

American Psychiatric Association. (1987). Guidelines on confidentiality. *American Journal of Psychiatry, 144,* 1522–1526.

American Psychiatric Association. (1989). Principles of Medical Ethics. Washington, DC: American Psychiatric Association.

Appelbaum, P. S., Grisso, T. (1988). Assessing patients' capacities to consent to treatment. *New England Journal of Medicine, 319,* 1635–1638; erratum 1989, 320, 748.

Baker, F. M. (1986). Legal issues affecting the older patient. *Hospital and Community Psychiatry, 37,* 1091–1093.

Baker, F. M., Perr, I. N., & Yesavage, J. A. (1986). *An overview of legal issues in geriatric psychiatry.* Washington, DC: American Psychiatric Association.

Barber v. Superior Court, 147 Cal. App. 3d 1006, 195 Cal. Rptr. 484 (1983).

Bellacosa, J. W. (1990). The fusion of medicine and law for *in extremis* health and medical decisions. *Bulletin of the American Academy of Psychiatry and the Law, 18,* 5–21.

Billick, S. B. (1986). Developmental competency. *Bulletin of the American Academy of Psychiatry and the Law, 14,* 301–309.

Bok, S. (1978). *Lying: Moral choice in public and private life.* New York: Pantheon.

Callahan, D. (1990). Rationing medical progress: The way to affordable health care. *New England Journal of Medicine, 322,* 1810–1813.

Callahan, L., Mayer, C., Steadman, H. J. (1987). Insanity defense reforms in the United States—post-Hinckley. *Mental and Physical Disability Law Reporter, 11,* 54–59.

Canterbury v. Spence, 464 F.2d 772 (D.C. Circuit 1972).

Colorado v. Connelly, 107 S.Ct. 515 (1986).

Cruzan v. Director, Missouri Department of Health, U.S. Supreme Court, No. 88-1503, (Decided June 25, 1990).

deWachter, M.A.M. (1989). Active euthanasia in the Netherlands. *Journal of the American Medical Association, 262,* 3316–3319.

Dusky v. United States, 362 U.S. 402 (1960).

Erde, E. L., Nadal, E. C., & Scholl, T. O. (1988). On truth telling and the diagnosis of Alzheimer's disease. *Journal of Family Practice, 26,* 401–403.

Eth, S. (1990). Psychiatric ethics: Entering the 1990s. *Hospital and Community Psychiatry, 41,* 384–386.

Eth, S., & Mills, M. J. (1989). Ethical issue (In organic mental syndromes). In T. B. Karasu (Ed.), *Treatments of psychiatric disorders* (pp. 994–1008). Washington, DC: American Psychiatric Association.

Eth, S., & Robb, J. W. (1986). Informed consent. In D. K. Kentsmith, S. A. Salladay, & P. A. Miya (Eds.), *Ethics in mental health practice* (pp. 83–110). Orlando, FL: Grune & Stratton.

Faulkner, L. R. (1982). Mandating the reporting of suspected cases of elder abuse: An inappropriate, ineffective and ageist response to the abuse of older adults. *Family Law Quarterly, 16,* 69–91.

Felthous, A. R. (1990). The duty to warn or protect to prevent automobile accidents. In R. I. Simon (Ed.), *American psychiatric press review of clinical psychiatry and the law,* (volume 1, pp. 221–238). Washington, DC: American Psychiatric Press.

Ferguson, B., & Douglas, A. C. (1970). A study of juvenile waiver. *San Diego Law Review, 7,* 39–54.

Ford v. Wainwright, 106 S.Ct. 2595 (1986).

Goldstein, R. L. (1987). *Non compos mentis:* The psychiatrist's role in guardianship and conservatorship proceedings involving the elderly. In R. Rosner & H. I. Schwartz (Eds.), *Geriatric psychiatry and the law* (pp. 269–278). New York: Plenum.

Grisso, T. (1981). *Juveniles' waiver of rights: Legal and psychological competency.* New York: Plenum.

Grisso, T. (1987). *Evaluating competencies.* New York: Plenum.

In re Eichner, 438 N.Y.S. 266 (1981).

In re Patrick W, 84 Cal.App.3d 520 (1978), vacated *California v. Patrick W,* 61 L.Ed.2d 870 (1979), on remand 104 Cal.App.3d 615 (1980), cert. denied 66 L.Ed.2d 824, (1981).

In re Quinlan, 70 N.J. 355 A.2d, cert. denied 429 U.S. 992, (1976).

In re Roderick P, 7 Cal.3d 801 (1972).

Jackson v. Indiana, 925 S.Ct. 1845, 32 L.Ed.2d 694 (1972).

Jenike, M. A. (1985). *Handbook of geriatric psychopharmacology.* Littleton, MA: PSG.

Jonsen, A. R., Siegler, M., & Winslade, W. J. (1986). *Clinical Ethics,* 2nd Ed. New York: Macmillan.

Katz, J. (1984). *The silent world of doctor and patient.* New York: Free Press.

Kilner, J. F. (1989). Age criteria in medicine: Are the medical justifications ethical? *Archives of Internal Medicine, 149,* 2343–2346.

Kosberg, J. I. (1987). Abuse of the elderly: an overview of the problem and solutions. In R. Rosner & H. I. Schwartz (Eds.) *Geriatric psychiatry and the law.* New York: Plenum.

Lo, B., Rouse, F., & Dornbrand, L. (1990). Family decision-making on trial: Who decides for incompetent patients? *New England Journal of Medicine, 322,* 1228–1232.

Lockett v. Ohio, 57 L.Ed.2d 870 (1978).

Luce, J.M. (1990). Ethical principles in critical care. *Journal of the American Medical Association, 263,* 696–700.

McGarry, A. L., Lipsett, P. D., & Lelos, D. (1973). Competency to stand trial and mental illness: Final report. (DHEW Publ. No. (HSM) 73-9105). Rockville, MD: National Institute of Mental Health.

Melton, G. B., Petrila, J., Poythress, N. G., & Slobogin, C. (1987). *Psychological evaluations for the courts.* New York: Guilford.

Miles, S. H., Singer, P. A., & Siegler, H. (1989). Conflicts between patients' wishes to forego treatment and the policies of health care facilities. *New England Journal of Medicine, 321,* 48–50.

Mills, M. J., Sullivan, G., Eth, S. (1987). Protecting third parties: A decade after *Tarasoff. American Journal of Psychiatry, 144,* 68–74.

Miranda v. Arizona, 384 U.S. 436, 1966.

Murphy, D. J. (1988). Do-not-resuscitate orders: Time for reappraisal in long-term-care institutions. *Journal of the American Medical Association, 260,* 2098–2101.

Overman, W., & Stoudermire, A. (1988). Guidelines for legal and financial counseling of Alzheimer's disease patients and their families. *American Journal of Psychiatry, 145,* 1495–1500.

People v. Olsen, 36 Cal.3d 638 (1984).

Perl, M., & Shelp, E. E. (1982). Psychiatric consultation masking moral dilemmas in medicine. *New England Journal of Medicine, 307,* 618–621.

Perr, I. N. (1981). Wills, testamentary capacity and undue influence. *Bulletin of the American Academy of Psychiatry and the Law, 9,* 15–22.

Penry v. Lynaugh, 109 S.Ct. 293Y (1989).

Piaget, J., & Inhelder, B. (1969). *The psychology of the child.* New York: Basic Books.

Platt, A., & Diamond, B. L. (1966). The origins of the "right and wrong" test of criminal responsibility and its subsequent development in the United States: An historical survey. *California Law Review, 54,* 1227–1258.

President's Commission for the Study of Ethical Problems in Medicine and Biomedical and Behavioral Research (1983). *Deciding to forego life-sustaining treatment.* Washington, DC: Government Printing Office.

Redmond, F. C. (1987). Testamentary capacity. *Bulletin of the American Academy of Psychiatry and the Law, 15,* 247–256.

Regan, J. J. (1987). Withholding life support from the elderly, or learning to live with high-tech death. In R. Rosner & H. I. Schwartz (Eds.), *Geriatric psychiatry and the law.* New York: Plenum.

Regina v. M'Naghten, 10 Cl.&F. 200, 8 Eng.Rep. 718 (1843).

Salend, E., Kane, R. A., Satz, M., & Pynoos, J. (1984). Elder-abuse reporting: Limitations of statutes. *Gerontologist, 24,* 61–69.

Schloendorff v. Society of New York Hospital, 211 N.Y. 125, 105 N.E. 92 (1914).

Schneiderman, L. J., & Arras, J. D. (1985). Counseling patients to counsel physicians on future care in the event of patient incompetence. *Annals of Internal Medicine, 102,* 648–693.

Schurman, R. A., Kramer, P. D., & Mitchell, J. B. (1985). The hidden mental health network. *Archives of General Psychiatry, 42,* 89–94.

Scitovsky, A. A., & Capron, A. M. (1986). Medical care at the end of life: The interaction of economics and ethics. *Annual Review of Public Health, 7,* 59–75.

Simon, R. I. (1989). Silent suicide in the elderly. *Bulletin of the American Academy of Psychiatry and the Law, 17,* 83–95.

Singer, P. A., & Siegler, M. (1990). Euthanasia—A critique. *New England Journal of Medicine, 322,* 1881–1883.

Sprung, C. L. (1990). Changing attitudes and practices in foregoing life-sustaining treatments. *Journal of the American Medical Association, 263,* 2211–2215.

Steinbrook, R., & Lo, B. (1984). Decision making for incompetent patients by designated proxy: California's new law. *New England Journal of Medicine, 310,* 1958–1601.

Superintendent of Belchertown State School v. Saikewicz, 370 N.E.2d (Mass 1977).

Tarasoff v. Regents of the University of California, 17 Cal.3d 425, 551 P.2d 334 (1976).

Thompson v. Oklahoma, 101 L.Ed.2d 702, 108 S.Ct. 2687 (1988).

Wanzer, S. H., Federman, D. D., Adelstein, S. J., Cassel, C. K., Cassem, E. H., Cranford, R. E., Hook, E. W., Lo, B., Moertel, C. G., Safar, P., Stone, A., & Von Eys, J. (1989). The physician's responsibility toward hopelessly ill patients. *New England Journal of Medicine, 320,* 844–849.

Wells, C. E. (1979). Pseudodementia. *American Journal of Psychiatry, 136,* 895–900.

Veatch, R. M. (1976). Death, dying, and the biological revolution. New Haven: Yale University Press.

Economic Issues and Geriatric Mental Health Care

Gary L. Gottlieb

I. Introduction
II. Economic and Health Policy Issues
III. The Medicare System
    A. Hospital Insurance (Part A)
    B. Supplemental Insurance (Part B)
IV. Medicaid
V. Private Insurance and Out-of-Pocket Expenditures
VI. Innovative Delivery Models: Cost Containment and Improved Access
VII. Conclusion
    References

I. Introduction

Financing mechanisms have influenced all aspects of psychiatric services for older adults (Goldman & Frank, 1990; Goldman, Taube & Jencks, 1987). Payment schemes and funding policy affect the selection of patient populations that are eligible for care, the organization and site of service delivery, provider discipline and behavior, and the process of care itself.

Government has driven the economy of geriatric mental health care. Older adults who were cared for in the almshouses and asylums of the nineteenth century helped to fuel the growth of the state hospital systems of the early and middle twentieth century as financial responsibility for the care of the seriously mentally ill was shifted from local to state government (Grob, 1983). The implementation of Medicare and Medicaid in the mid-1960s transferred substantial financial responsibility for the psychiatric care of the elderly from the states to the federal government. The indemnity design of these programs and the growth of private insurance stimulated the growth of private and general hospital psychiatric settings (Goldman *et al.*, 1987). At about the same time, deinstitutionalization in the context of poorly developed community resources and the federal and state support provided by Medicaid encouraged the use of nursing homes for the care of the chronically mentally ill older people (Goldman, Feder, & Scanlon, 1986). Additionally, limitations in reimbursement for outpatient specialty mental health services by Medicare and by other third parties have fortified the general health care sector as the dominant source of psychiatric services, particularly for the elderly (Regier, Goldberg, & Taube, 1978; Schurman, Kramer, & Mitchell, 1985). Prospective payment and nursing home reform, implemented in the 1980s, are now beginning to affect the nature of psychiatric care for older adults (English, Sharfstein, Scherl, Astrachan & Muszynski, 1986; Goldman *et al.*, 1987).

Providers and policymakers who seek to optimize the well-being of older Americans must understand the economic context of aging in late twentieth-century America. Similarly, a working knowledge of the structure of the geriatric mental health delivery system and the sources of payment for health and mental health services for the elderly is essential. This chapter highlights key financial and economic issues that affect the psychiatric care of older adults. The specific details regarding reimbursement of geropsychiatric services are provided and recent changes in third party payment schemes are described. Greater understanding of the terminology and subtleties of this system should help providers and consumers to cope with systematic barriers to the care of this exceptionally needy population.

II. Economic and Health Policy Issues

The size and diversity of the aging population are key determinants of the economic environment of geriatric mental health care. Just 30 years ago, about one of every eleven Americans was older than 65 years. Today, one in slightly more than eight Americans is older than 65. The U.S. Census Bureau (1987) anticipates that the elderly population will have grown by 23% to nearly 31 million during the 1980s. This growth is smaller than the landmark 28% growth experienced during the 1970s. The older population should grow by only about 10% in the 1990s and by 12% in the first decade of the next century, owing to relatively small Depression-era birth rates. This projected rate of expansion will yield approximately 39 million older Americans by 2010. Subsequently, the aging of the post–World War II baby-boom cohort will augment the older-than-65 population segment dramatically. By the year 2030, about 25% of the population, some 66 million people, will be in this age group.

The distribution of minorities among the elderly and sex differences in life expectancy have important economic consequences. Ethnic minorities account for a rapidly growing segment of the older population. In 1980, about 10% of persons older than 65 were nonwhite. However, about 15% of the elderly are projected to be from minority groups by the year 2025 (National Center for Health Statistics, 1987). Life expectancy at birth for whites exceeds that for African Americans by about 8%. However, at age 75, mortality rates for African Americans are lower than those for whites (National Center for Health Statistics, 1988). Very old African Americans are more likely to live at the poverty level and/or suffer from chronic illness than whites in the same age group (Soldo & Agree,

1988). The discrimination and underprivilege associated with minority status in the United States are exaggerated by the socioeconomic consequences of older age. Accrued social and financial resources are fixed and limited, barriers to health care services are more profound, and the need for nonhealth-related public services including housing, transportation, meals, and income maintenance is greater (Furino & Fogel, 1990; Markides & Mindel, 1987). Cultural differences may also affect the expression of illness and the ways in which minority individuals access the American health care system, designed for a predominantly white population (Hazzard, 1989).

There are approximately 1.5 women for every man older than 65, and about 2.5 women for every man older than 85 (U.S. Bureau of the Census, 1987). Traditional work roles and Social Security and pension provisions affect surviving women adversely. In general, continued earning potential from work and from pension income in late life is less for women than it is for men. Generally, older women have more limited financial assets. Inasmuch as they usually live longer than their spouses, they are more likely to become dependent on adult children and on the health care establishment to meet social and medical needs (Soldo & Agree, 1988).

There is extreme variability in the distribution of wealth and income among the elderly. The degree of this variability has confounded the development of rational social policy for older adults. The resulting political scenario has affected reimbursement and delivery of health and mental health services to the elderly.

Retirement is associated with a 30 to 50% reduction in income (Soldo & Agree, 1988). In 1986, almost 90% of men in their early 50s participated in the labor force, while only about 45% of men between the ages of 62 and 64 were still working (Schulz, 1988). After age 70, only about 10% of men and 4% of women are in the labor force. Elimination of a mandatory retirement age and the transformation of the American industry from domination by manufacturing to less physically demanding service and technology production may soon extend the working longevity of the population. In addition to the emotional and financial consequences of retirement, leaving the workforce may affect health insurance premium costs, the availability of specific insurance products and the possibility of participating in some health delivery systems [e.g., some health maintenance organizations (HMOs) and other managed systems].

The income reduction associated with retirement may affect standard of living adversely. Most older adults receive postretirement income from a combination of passive sources: Social Security benefits; public and/or private pensions; and income from savings or investments (Soldo & Agree, 1988). The magnitude of these earnings depends almost entirely on preretirement income. For many older individuals, these relatively fixed sources may be inadequate, and these people may suffer the consequences of poverty for the first time in their lives (Furino & Fogel, 1990). In 1986, one in eight people older than 65, or about 3.5 million Americans, had income below the poverty level. About 10% of the younger population were at that income level. Indigence increases with advanced age: about one fifth of people who live past the age of 85 have incomes at or below the poverty level. These rates are considerably more dramatic for women and for minorities. For example, 60% of African-American women older than 65 not living with their families had incomes below the poverty level in 1986 (Soldo & Agree, 1988).

Aging is not universally associated with poverty, however. More than 10% of households headed by an individual older than 65 have annual incomes over $40,000, and almost 13% of these households have net assets greater than $250,000 (Gottlieb, 1988).

This disparity in distribution of wealth and income has an important effect on social policy. Lawmakers frequently do not recognize the socioeconomic heterogeneity of the older population. Therefore, programs like Social Security and Medicare do not address completely the financial and health care needs of *all* older adults. Resulting gaps are filled in part by programs for the indigent, by private third-party insurance, and by out-of-pocket payments. These inequities are particularly important in mental health and in long-term care, where out-of-pocket payments compose a substantial component of costs to consumers (Gottlieb, 1988).

Continued growth in the number of older people increases demand for the products that elderly individuals are likely to consume. Inasmuch as many of the programs that benefit older adults are supported by contributions from the younger population, the growing ratio of older Americans to younger persons may affect society's ability to supply the goods, services, and payments that will be required to meet this expanding demand. There are currently about 19 Americans older than 65 per 100 people aged 18–64. This so-called dependency ratio is projected to double by 2050 (U.S. Bureau of the Census, 1987). Therefore, future policy initiatives must consider the potential need for the older generation to support a greater proportion of its own needs. Growth in the dependency ratio will influence future policy strategy substantially. It will also affect the labor market and national productivity. Therefore, medical and psychiatric interventions that promote the health and productivity of older workers will have social benefits that mirror individual improvements in function and quality of life (Hazzard, 1989; Furino & Fogel, 1990).

III. The Medicare System

Medicare is a social insurance program designed to provide medical care benefits for Americans older than 65. It was enacted in 1965 and initiated on July 1, 1966 under Title XVIII of the Social Security Act (Cutler & Fine, 1985; Gottlieb, 1988; US Senate Committee on Finance, 1978). The program was developed as a product of many years of debate regarding national health policy and in response to data derived from comprehensive evaluation of the needs of older adults provided by the Senate Select Committee on Aging. The program was expanded in 1972 to include younger disabled individuals and older adults who are not eligible for Social Security but who are willing to pay a monthly premium for coverage. Medicare coverage was extended in 1973 to provide medical coverage for individuals with end-stage renal disease. Currently, more than 32 million people are covered by Medicare. Ninety percent of these individuals are elderly (US Congress, Committee on Ways and Means, 1989).

Despite recent efforts to contain costs, expenditures for health care have grown remarkably and Medicare has made a substantial contribution to this expansion. In 1988, health care expenditures accounted for about 11% of the U.S. Gross National Product (GNP). Medicare outlays of close to $88 billion in 1988 accounted for approximately 7.6% of the federal budget and about 1.7% of the GNP [Physician Payment Review Commission (PPRC), 1989]. The inflation-adjusted average annual growth rate for Medicare expenditures per beneficiary was 5% during the 1970s and more than 5.5% for most of the 1980s (Long & Welch, 1988). Health care costs for the general population grew at rates of 3.6 and 4.3% over the same periods, respectively.

Specialty mental health services for older adults compose a miniscule fragment of total Medicare expenditures. Payments for treatment of psychiatric disorders total about 2.5% of Medicare spending. In contrast, between 7 and 18% of private insurers' reimbursements are for psychiatric services (Morrison, Janssen, & Motter, 1984). These data are more striking considering that more than 50% of all Medicare-covered psychiatric hospitalizations are for nonelderly disabled individuals (Goldman *et al.*, 1987). The relative underutilization of specialty mental health services by older Medicare beneficiaries may be attributed to the reinforcement of entrenched provider- and patient-induced barriers to care by economic disincentives and systematic stigmatization.

The Medicare benefit package is primarily designed to reimburse acute care services. Preventive services, long-term care, and dental services are excluded. Some services, including mental health care, are subject to limitations in coverage and substantial copayments. Therefore, under current conditions, Medicare covers only about 75% of hospital care for older adults, 2–3% of nursing home care, and about 58% of physician services, totaling slightly less than half of geriatric health care costs (PPRC, 1989; Waldo & Lazenby, 1984).

A. Hospital Insurance (Part A)

Through participation in the Social Security system, most Americans older than 65 are entitled to Part A coverage. The Part A Hospital Insurance (HI) Trust Fund is financed by Social Security payroll taxes paid by employers and employees.

Part A hospital coverage is limited to relatively brief inpatient stays, presumably for stabilization of acute conditions. Regulations describe coverage for *spells* of illness. A spell is defined as an inpatient episode that begins with hospital admission and ends with the close of the first period of 60 consecutive days after discharge. Therefore, a patient may be discharged and readmitted on several occasions during a given episode of illness and still be considered to be in the same spell, if 60 days have not elapsed between discharge and admission. For admission to general hospitals for nonpsychiatric and psychiatric diagnoses, there is no limit on the number of spells or *total lifetime* days covered. However, the maximum number of covered days during a single spell is 150 days.

There is no limit on the total number of hospitalizations or inpatient days covered for medical or surgical diagnoses or for psychiatric care in general hospitals. However, coverage for inpatient psychiatric care in facilities designated as free-standing psychiatric hospitals by the Health Care Financing Administration (HCFA) is limited to a total of 190 days during an individual's lifetime. Additionally, if an individual becomes Medicare eligible during the course of an episode of psychiatric hospitalization, Medicare may elect to cover less than the full 150 benefit days of that spell of illness. This provision is designed to restrict Part A psychiatric benefits to the active component of treatment and to prevent reimbursement for a person who may have been institutionalized for long periods of time.

Part A provides limited coverage for care in skilled nursing facilities (SNFs). However, services provided by domiciliary, personal care, and intermediate care facilities (ICFs) are not covered by Medicare. In order to be eligible for SNF benefits, an individual must have been hospitalized acutely for at least 3 consecutive days and nursing home admission must occur within 30 days of hospital discharge. HI covers up to 100 days of SNF care. Similarly, home health services are limited and must be related to acute and remediable conditions (American Psychiatric Association (APA) Office of Economic Affairs, 1986; Gottlieb, 1988; Waldo & Lazenby, 1984).

From 1966 until late 1983, Part A of Medicare paid for inpatient care through a retrospective cost-based reimbursement system. In an effort to prevent depletion of the Hospital Insurance Trust Fund by reducing hospital reimbursement costs, Congress and the Reagan administration enacted the Tax Equity and Fiscal Responsibility Act (TEFRA) of 1982. Emphasizing cost containment, TEFRA provided for limits on all inpatient operating costs and established target rates for cost increases. Financial incentives were designed to provide reduced hospital reimbursement if targets were not met and extra payments if limits were not exceeded. Reimbursement limits were adjusted to reflect patient mix, geographic location, and training costs. TEFRA mandated the development of legislation to replace cost-based reimbursement with a prospective payment system (PPS) (APA Office of Economic Affairs, 1986; English *et al.*, 1986; Frazier, Goldman & Taube, 1986; Scherl, English & Sharfstein, 1988).

Public Law 98–21 of the Social Security Amendments of 1983 established a PPS for Medicare. This PPS is based on a patient-discharge classification system that uses diagnosis-related groups (DRGs) to cluster patients who presumably require similar care. The DRG system groups patients into 23 major diagnostic categories and then assigns the discharge to one of 468 DRGs, derived from principal and secondary diagnoses, procedures rendered, and, to a lesser degree, age, sex, comorbidity, complications, and discharge status. Hospitals are paid a predetermined amount for each discharge according to the DRG that is assigned. Because this sum is independent of actual costs incurred, this payment mechanism is considered to be an incentive for efficient utilization of resources. If patients consume extraordinary resources or require prolonged inpatient care, they are classified as outliers. Medicare provides additional payments to the hospital for these patients at a rate considerably less than actual cost.

Fourteen of the DRGs apply to discharges for treatment of psychiatric disorders. Doubts concerning DRGs as accurate predictors of resource consumption for psychiatric disorders led to a temporary exemption from this payment method for free-standing psychiatric hospitals and for distinct psychiatric units in general hospitals. However, treatment of patients with primary psychiatric diagnoses in *scatter* beds on general medical and surgical units are reimbursed through the DRG system. In 1984, discharges from scatter beds accounted for about 46% of psychiatric cases reimbursed by Medicare (Goldman *et al.*, 1987).

Research evaluating the application of DRGs to psychiatric inpatient care has confirmed their inaccuracy in prediction of resource consumption. For all diagnoses, DRGs have been shown to account for only a limited proportion of the variation in individual lengths of stay (16–40%). They are considerably less accurate in predicting psychiatric utilization, generally accounting for less than 8% of the variance (English *et al.*, 1986;

Frank & Lave, 1985; Goldman, 1988). The American Psychiatric Association's comprehensive assessment of DRGs for psychiatry (English *et al.*, 1986) suggests that the similarity among patients within a given psychiatric DRG is extremely limited. Patients who require very brief hospitalizations are frequently clustered with individuals in need of much longer hospital stays. This assessment indicates that DRGs financially favor less severely ill patients and settings that provide short-term evaluation and limited treatment.

Free-standing psychiatric hospitals and exempted psychiatric units in general hospitals continue to be paid retrospectively by Medicare. However, these reimbursements were limited substantially by TEFRA. Medicare reimbursement for psychiatric inpatient treatment in these sites is capped at a ceiling rate established for each facility based on resource consumption during a base year (the first full fiscal year of operation after October 1, 1983). If the actual cost per case exceeds the target rate, the hospital must absorb the loss. If the cost is less than the TEFRA ceiling rate, the hospital may retain 50% of the difference up to 5% of the target rate.

The complex nature of psychiatric disorders in the elderly conflicts directly with these incentives. Incomplete evaluation of complicated patients in settings that are discouraged from employing expensive diagnostic technologies and treatment interventions may add unnecessary disability and ultimately generate substantially greater costs (Fogel, Gottlieb, & Furino, 1990a). Similarly, the high prevalence of medical disorders among older adults with psychiatric diagnoses renders DRGs and TEFRA caps inoperable. Patients with active medical diagnoses treated by psychiatric personnel in scatter beds and/or in exempt units have not been considered in research assessing these payment mechanisms. These comorbidities may add significantly to consumption of resources.

Several alternative strategies have been proposed to facilitate implementation of a PPS for psychiatry. While one method improves predictability of length of stay and other measures of resource consumption substantially, no system has been evaluated with adequately large data sets that are diverse enough to reflect the extremely differentiated nature of the mental health care delivery system (Goldman, 1988). Research in this area remains active, and improvements in policy in the near future are feasible.

B. Supplemental Medical Insurance (Part B)

Participation in the supplementary medical insurance (SMI) benefit program of Medicare Part B is voluntary. A monthly premium ($27.90 in 1989) is required for subscription. About 97% of Medicare Part A recipients purchase SMI benefits. The Part B Trust Fund is underwritten by general revenues from the federal treasury, trust fund interest, and subscriber premiums. The Part B premium is set by law at 25% of the average monthly benefit per enrollee. Premiums currently cover about one quarter of program expenditures (PPRC, 1989).

Physician services are paid by Medicare through a system called customary, prevailing, and reasonable (CPR). The payment rate, or reasonable allowed charge for a specific service is the lowest of the actual charge, a physician's usual charge for similar services (customary), the charge in the community for similar services provided by other physicians (prevailing) and the fiscal intermediary's (FI) usual reimbursement for comparable services to its policy holders under similar circumstances (PPRC, 1989; Gottlieb, 1988).

Part B benefits are subject to an annual deductible ($75 in 1990) and a copayment. For nonpsychiatric physician services and psychiatric inpatient services, the copayment equals 20% of reasonable charges. Coverage for medical and surgical visits is not limited by an annual number of visits or costs of resources consumed. However, when Part B psychiatric benefits were designed, mental illness was depicted as "lacking precise diagnostics and established treatment protocols expected to lead to specified outcomes within a defined period of time" (Cutler & Fine, 1985, p. 20). As a result, coverage for outpatient psychiatric treatment was limited severely. From the initiation of Medicare in 1966 through early 1988, total annual reasonable charges were set at $500, and the maximum annual Medicare reimbursement for outpatient psychiatric services was $312.50 or 62.5% of reasonable charges, whichever was lower. The 80% federal share, which was the maximum amount paid by Medicare to the psychiatrist or the patient, was $250 per year.

The Omnibus Budget Reconciliation Act of 1987 (OBRA-87) (Public Law 100-203) recognized, in part, the discrimination against services for mental disorders inherent in Part B. Coverage for outpatient psychiatric services was increased to $2,200 annually by 1989. However, the 50% copayment remained. Additionally, services for the medical management of psychiatric disorders were exempted from the $2,200 limit and are subject to the same 20% copayment as nonpsychiatric outpatient services. The Omnibus Budget Reconciliation Act of 1989 (OBRA-89; H.R.3299, Report 101–386) provided further improvement of the psychiatric outpatient benefit. Effective July 1, 1990, the annual dollar limit for outpatient mental health services was eliminated. However, the discriminatory 50% copayment and the Part A 190-day lifetime psychiatric hospital utilization limit were unaffected by the new law.

OBRA-89 was a watershed in its expansion of coverage for services provided by nonphysician providers. Until the enactment of this legislation, necessary services delivered by psychologists, social workers, therapists, nurses, and aides were reimbursable only under the *direct supervision* of a physician. Direct supervision is defined as immediate availability to provide assistance at the time of service. Exceptions to this rule included psychological testing and services provided by psychologists in some community mental health settings. The new law provided for direct reimbursement of psychologists in all settings. Direct reimbursement of clinical social worker services at the rate of 80% of the lesser of the actual charge or 75% of the amount paid to a psychologist is also provided. Social workers do not receive direct reimbursement when they provide services to an inpatient of a hospital or SNF as required for the facility's participation in Medicare Part A. OBRA-89 developed criteria regarding consultation with a physician for nonphysician providers. These criteria are vague and somewhat superficial. The provider must document that the patient has been informed of the desirability of consultation with the patient's primary care physician to consider potential medical conditions that may contribute to the patient's condition. Additionally, the provider must document written or verbal communication with the primary physician regarding the patient's treatment, unless the patient specifically refuses such contact. The law makes no provision for assessment or consultation with a psychiatrist. Reimbursement of services provided by psychiatric nurses and other therapists continues to require direct physician supervision (Conference Agreement—Mental Health Services, OBRA-89).

For the most part, direct patient treatment or evaluation is necessary in order to obtain Medicare reimbursement. Services rendered by telephone and patient contacts purely for the purpose of renewing a prescription that do not involve evaluation of patient status are not reimbursable. However, charges for obtaining treatment information from relatives or close associates of a patient who is unreliable or uncommunicative are allowable. Similarly, family counseling services are covered only when the purpose of counseling is to facilitate treatment of the identified patient.

At present, there are two procedures available for Medicare beneficiaries to receive benefits for provider services through Part B:

1. A provider may agree to *accept assignment* from SMI, thereby accepting the Medicare reasonable charge as payment in full. In this circumstance, the FI pays the approved amount less copayment and deductible to the provider directly. Coinsurance and deductible payments must be collected from the patient.
2. A provider may elect *not to accept assignment,* thereby not recognizing the Medicare-approved fee as payment in full. In this arrangement, in order to receive reimbursement at the CPR-determined level, the beneficiary must present an itemized bill from the provider to the FI. The patient receives reimbursement of 95% of the Medicare-approved fee less copayment and deductibles. The provider may bill the patient directly for the remaining balance. Providers who choose not to accept assignment still face limits in the fees that they may charge to Medicare recipients. The maximum allowable actual charge (MAAC) is based on a provider's profile of charges and adjustments made to the fee schedule for services rendered in the second quarter of 1984 or during the provider's first year of practice if it was subsequent to that time (PPRC, 1989). The MAAC is the highest fee that a nonparticipating provider may charge to a Medicare recipient. The nonparticipating physician must collect the entire fee directly from the patient.

OBRA–89 phases out MAAC limits and replaces them with new ceilings on balance billing, and it creates new incentives to accept assignment. Patients using nonparticipating providers will continue to be paid 95% of the Medicare-approved charge. In 1991, nonparticipating providers fees will be limited to the lesser of the physician's MAAC or 125% of the Medicare payment for nonparticipating providers. In 1992, this limit will fall to 120% of the payment for nonparticipating providers, and in 1993 and thereafter, the limit will be 115% of the Medicare payment amount for these providers. Additionally, since April 1, 1990, all providers are required to accept assignment from indigent Medicare beneficiaries who are also recipients of Medicaid. By 1992, acceptance of assignment will be required for care rendered to al Medicare recipients who are at or below the Federal poverty level (OBRA–89 Physician Payment Reform Summary Draft). Additionally, some states mandate all providers to accept assignment when treating Medicare beneficiaries.

Since the initiation of PPS for hospital services, the annual growth rate for costs of physicians' services has been more than twice the rate of growth for inpatient hospital services (Roper, 1988). The greatest contributors to this growth are rising prices for services and increases in the number of services consumed per beneficiary. Part B expenditures grew about 17% per year during the 1980s and they now account for about one third of Medicare expenditures (close to $35 billion in 1988) (PPRC, 1989). This growth has concerned policymakers and, in addition to the aforementioned expansion of coverage for mental health services, OBRA–89 stipulated the implementation of reform in methods of Medicare physician payment.

OBRA–89 provided for the development of expenditure targets or volume performance standards (VPS) to control growth in physician services. The Secretary of Health and Human Services is mandated to recommend to Congress an overall VPS growth rate before the beginning of each fiscal year. The VPS should be related to fee increases, growth in the size of the Medicare population, changes in service volume and intensity, and a volume performance factor ($-.5\%$ for FY 1990, -1% for FY 1991, -1.5% for FY 1992, and -2% thereafter). At the end of each year, the Secretary will compare actual growth in expenditures with the VPS and will use those data to determine the size of any fee adjustments (Psychiatric News, 1989; Physician Payment Review Commission, 1989).

OBRA–89 also provided for the development of a uniform Medicare fee schedule to replace the CPR payment system. The new fee schedule will be based on a resource based relative value scale (RBRVS), developed after extensive research led by Hsiao and his colleagues (1988) and input from the Physician Payment Review Commission (1989) and professional groups nationally. The RBRVS will be used to determine the relative values of about 7,000 different physician services. The relative value for each procedure will have three measurable components: the work it requires, practice expenses, and malpractice expenses. The proportions of each component will be based on a weighted average of specialty–specific practice expense and malpractice data. Approximately 60% of each fee will be adjusted for geographic variations in cost (Psychiatric News, 1989). The product of each relative value and a monetary conversion factor will determine the fee for each service.

The transition to the new fee schedule began in 1990 with reductions in payments for *overvalued procedures*. Existing fee schedules for anesthesia and radiology were adjusted to conform to the RBRVS fee schedule. The RBRVS fee schedule will be phased in gradually from 1992 to 1996 for most other specialties.

In an effort to correct for a system that financially reinforces the employment of costly technical procedures, the RBRVS emphasizes cognitive assessment, patient management and caring activities performed by providers (Hsiao, Braun, Kelly, & Becker, 1988). The work component of relative values is based primarily on the time, intensity, and stress associated with delivery of services. Case vignettes are assessed by provider panels in each specialty so that appropriate values can be assigned. Procedure codes from the Common Procedural Terminology (CPT-4) (American Medical Association, 1990) are employed to describe the procedure performed.

Preliminary efforts to apply the RBRVS to psychiatry have been seriously flawed. The vignettes designed originally were simplistic and unrepresentative of the broad spectrum of psychiatric practice. Measurements of clinical work performed and of practice costs were inconsistent, and efforts to develop work scenarios comparable to those encountered in other specialties considered the circumstances of psychiatric care poorly. Additionally, the CPT codes for psychiatry are extremely broad and, therefore, difficult to map onto the activities associated with specific vignettes (Fogel, 1990; Sharfstein, 1990). Therefore, Hsiao and his colleagues (1988) have reconvened a technical consulting group for RBRVS in psychiatry, and they are undertaking development of new vignettes and a new technical survey.

The first federal program requiring older adults to fund the increased medical needs of their own generation was the Catastrophic Coverage Act (CCA) of 1988. This legislation insured Medicare beneficiaries against some catastrophic health care costs. CCA required beneficiaries (predominantly individuals older than 65) to pay an additional premium to cover the costs of this coverage. Among other factors, the shifting of financial responsibility to potential recipients made CCA unacceptable politically, and this program was repealed in 1989.

IV. Medicaid

Medicaid is a social insurance program enacted by the federal government in 1965 to help to pay for medical care for indigent Americans by providing matching funds to the states. The Medicaid program requires states to provide minimum basic benefits in order to receive these matching funds. However, the program allows states to impose some restrictions on the types of services funded and the level of reimbursement for specific services. Therefore, Medicaid services for mental health care and for specific services for indigent older adults vary substantially among states. It is estimated that Medicaid pays for about 25% of all psychiatric care in the United States (English, Kritzler & Scherl, 1984; Gottlieb, 1988; Health Care Financing Administration, 1982).

Between 3 and 4 million individuals older than 65 receive Medicaid benefits each year. Older adults account for about 16% of all Medicaid beneficiaries, and the services they receive represent about 40% of program expenditures (Waldo & Lazenby, 1984). Most older Medicaid recipients are also Medicare subscribers. Many state Medicaid programs have Part B buy-in provisions. This strategy allows these states to reduce their risk for payment of physician services by paying Medicare SMI premiums on behalf of their older Medicaid recipients. Therefore, Medicaid is principally a coinsuror for many older adults. The program covers Medicare deductibles, copayments, uncovered physician services, and other services after Medicare benefits have been exhausted (Waldo & Lazenby, 1984). Fees for all Medicaid services are set by the states, and they are generally unrelated to prevailing or reasonable charges.

The flexible nature of the Medicaid program provides state governments with some discretionary power in the development of local benefits. Local needs often influence the nature of services offered. Numerous services that are not covered by Medicare may be available to indigent older adults. These include day-treatment programs (often longer term and broader than Medicare's hospital-based partial hospitals), home mental health services, and prescription drugs.

The Medicaid program is most important to older adults in its capacity as payor for long-term care services. Medicaid reimburses about 42% of all skilled and intermediate-level nursing-home utilization. Most states require that individuals spend down their assets below an established level before they become eligible for Medicaid benefits.

Medicare pays for only 2% of all long-term care costs. The balance of these expenses is borne out of pocket by patients and their families (Levit, Lazenby, Waldo, & Davidoff, 1985).

The nursing home may be the most important site for care of older adult psychiatric patients, particularly those with severe and chronic disorders like dementia, depression associated with medical illness and disability, and schizophrenia (Goldman *et al.*, 1986). Deinstitutionalization has transformed the nursing home into the last resort for care of many chronically psychiatrically ill younger and older adults. From the federal government's perspective, this process has shifted costs from the states (i.e., for state hospitals) to federally supported nursing-home beds paid for through Medicaid. In the nursing home reform provisions of OBRA–87, the federal government mandated preadmission psychiatric screening of nursing-home applicants. The legislation requires referral for *active psychiatric treatment* if it cannot be provided in the nursing home. These requirements could improve psychiatric care for disabled indigent older adults in nursing homes, while creating significant barriers to admission for others.

V. Private Insurance and Out-of-Pocket Expenditures _____

Out-of-pocket payments include health care costs that older adults must pay from personal or family income or from savings or loans. Out-of-pocket expenses include premiums for SMI and private *Medigap* policies, copayments, and deductibles for Medicare Parts A and B, charges imposed by providers who do not accept assignment that exceed Medicare-approved limits, and charges for uncovered services, including much of long-term care. In 1988, the average out-of-pocket health care cost per Medicare beneficiary excluding long-term care was almost $1,700. Long-term care costs affect about 5% of older adults and they average about $20,000 per year (PPRC, 1989; Moon, 1987). Overall, older adults spend about 15% of their income on medically related expenses. Older adults with psychiatric disorders may be affected disproportionately because copayments are higher, total psychiatric hospital days are limited, and the ability to continue to work to provide income may be more limited.

Seventy-one percent of older adults purchase private Medigap policies designed to cover deductibles and copayments in order to reduce risk related to out-of-pocket expenditures. Some of these policies also provide coverage for nursing care, physician's charges in excess of Medicare-approved charges, and prescription drug costs. Nursing home care not covered by Medicare is usually excluded from these policies. For outpatient psychiatric services, most Medigap policies reimburse only 12.5% of approved charges in addition to the 50% Medicare payment. This leaves a 37.5% copayment for the consumer, even if the provider accepts assignment (Gottlieb, 1988). The average Medigap premium is between $500 and $700 annually (PPRC, 1989). Therefore, poor Medicare beneficiaries without Medicaid, least able to afford the costs of major illness, are the least likely to have private supplemental insurance.

A small number of employed older adults and some retirees are required to retain company group private insurance as their primary coverage and use Medicare as a secondary insurer. These individuals are subject to the usual limitations on psychiatric benefits pervasive in insurance for younger adults.

In an attempt to promote managed care, TEFRA contains a provision that encourages the use of health maintenance organizations (HMOs) by elderly Medicare recipients (Iglehart, 1985). This allows qualified managed-care programs to contract directly with Medicare. Each month Medicare pays the contractor a premium equal to 95% of estimated fee for service costs to provide the complete Medicare benefit package to subscribers. The program allows HMOs to earn normal profit margins. However, cost savings above a predetermined rate must be used to provide extra services for elderly members.

The market for long-term care insurance has exploded over the past 5 years. This market has been poorly regulated, and prices and products vary remarkably. Policies frequently cover 2 or 3 years of care in a variety of facilities. Some policies also reimburse home-care services. Many of these policies exclude patients with psychiatric disorders, but they include coverage for patients with dementia. Premiums are often five times higher than those for Medigap policies, and deductibles and copayments are generally substantial.

VI. Innovative Delivery Models: Cost Containment and Improved Access

TEFRA initiated a series of broad steps to control the growth of American health care expenditures, particularly those for older adults. OBRA–89 reaffirmed this need by creating an agenda for further controlling the growth of individual provider-delivered services. During the 1980s and the early 1990s, government and the private marketplace have demanded a reduction in the cost of health care services. Because older adults are the dominant consumers of these services, they are the most likely to be affected by these changes. An emphasis on competitiveness in the marketplace, cost effectiveness, and cost containment, while creating some gaps in service delivery, especially for lower-income individuals, have also stimulated the development of innovative programs to improve access to care for older adults with mental illness within the constraints of fixed resources.

Public and private third parties have become preoccupied with cost containment and with risk management. Unfortunately, when these entities are unable to address these issues by improving efficiency and/or management, costs are often shifted to other payors, and risks may be shifted to providers or to insurance companies (Fogel, Furino, & Gottlieb, 1990b). The seeds of OBRA–87 emerged from the federal perception that state governments were shifting costs from state-run institutions to care for chronically mentally ill patients to Medicaid reimbursement, shared by the federal government, to fund inadequate care of these same individuals in nursing homes. While the nursing-home reform regulations of OBRA–87 had as their motivation reduction of this cost shifting, they also attempted to improve access to appropriate psychiatric services for older adults.

Similarly, the National Long-term Care Demonstration or Channeling Project was developed to provide assessment and appropriate care for community dwelling older adults at risk of institutionalization. In 12 states, the Department of Health and Human Services supported programs to substitute formal and informal community-based services for nursing-home care. While the principal motivation of this project was to reduce costs, this case management–based program also had as a major objective the improvement of quality of life for clients and informal caregivers and the use of the least restrictive alternative for the care of oftentimes indigent and always dependent older adults.

Two types of case management programs were instituted and evaluated from 1980 to 1985 in the Channeling Demonstration Project:

1. *Basic case management* tested the hypothesis that access was the major barrier for older adults to obtaining appropriate long-term care services. Each of the six sites testing basic case management received a fixed budget to be used only for payment for the case-management service itself.
2. The *financial-control case-management* model tested the hypothesis that inadequate public financing for community services was the cause of overutilization of nursing-home services. Clients were eligible for this project predicated on Medicaid eligibility for nursing-home admission and on evidence of disability in two or more of the basic activities of daily living (ADL), three severe impairments in the instrumental activities of daily living (IADL), or two severe IADL impairments plus one ADL impairment. Cognitive or behavioral impairments, presumably secondary to psychiatric disorders of functional or organic etiology, were considered to be equivalent to one severe impairment in IADL. Clients studied in this project had a mean age of 80 years and were more likely than the general older adult population to need postacute care after an acute episode of illness, were more likely to receive formal care from a community-care system, and were more likely to live alone.

Both case-management systems relied on five core functions: (1) a needs assessment to determine individual problems, available resources, and service needs; (2) planning of care to specify types and amount of care to be provided; (3) a management service to implement the plan; (4) a program to monitor services delivered; (5) reassessment to adjust care plans to changing needs (Phillips, Kemper, & Appelbaum, 1988).

The project was evaluated extensively. Compared to a simulated national population of age-matched individuals, clients in this program were considered to be very frail but not to be at a significantly higher risk of institutionalization. However, because they were often referred to the Channeling Project following an acute episode of care, they had a higher use of hospitals and other medical services. However, despite this level of frailty, only 13 to 14% of Channeling clients were in nursing homes after 1 year.

The expansion of case management and access to formal community services caused an incremental increase in costs. Total costs for basic case-management clients increased by 6%, while costs for financial-control case-management clients increased by 18% (Kemper, 1988). However, costs to individual clients were reduced by 7%, and assessments of quality of life for clients and their caregivers revealed significant improvement. Access to services improved; unmet needs were reduced; and satisfaction with care and service arrangements and life satisfaction improved in a number of domains (Robinson, 1990).

Another innovative model supported by HCFA to improve access to care and control and to costs is the *Social/Health Maintenance Organization* (S/HMO). In this managed system of health and long-term care, a single provider contracts to assume responsibility for a full range of health and support services in exchange for a fixed capitated premium. In a given service area, healthy *and* at-risk older adults are enrolled voluntarily to the system. Individuals must receive all covered services through S/HMO providers. Before enrollment and screening, applicants complete an extensive written form describing health status and functional ability. Impairments in function are related to physical mobility and to ADL. No specific information describing mental status or behavior is obtained. Individuals who have ADL impairments are placed on a waiting list to ensure a sufficient mix of healthy and impaired members in a given S/HMO. Because cognitive and behavioral problems are not included in this screen, it is conceivable that individuals with mental problems who do not suffer physical impairment might be accepted immediately. Psychiatric status and cognitive function are not assessed comprehensively until after individuals are accepted as members.

In the S/HMO model, case management is used extensively to control utilization of services and to improve access to needed care. Standard screens of cognitive function are employed regularly by case managers in order to identify individuals with impairment and to become aware of behavioral problems. Unfortunately, current S/HMO screens do not include assessments of mood or of behavioral discontrol (Robinson, 1990).

S/HMO models have done well in containing costs. Analysis of hospital use concluded that two S/HMO sites were at or very close to their capitation estimates, and two were substantially below their allocation. Researchers attribute reductions in hospital use to the efficacy of case management (Greenberg, Leutz, & Greenlick, 1988). S/HMOs report that the greatest impediment to providing mental health care is their inability to find psychiatrists to provide care to frail, older adults. The aforementioned limitations in screening for psychiatric problems and the absence of in-home services to assist with behavioral management limit the effectiveness of S/HMOs in caring for individuals with psychiatric disorders. Despite these limitations, this model may provide the framework for improved access to services for older adults.

Another model of capitated service delivery for at-risk older adults is the OnLok senior services program. This program, initiated in San Francisco in the early 1970s, has been replicated in four sites in other parts of the United States with support from foundations and the federal government. OnLok's services are geared to older adults who meet Medicaid eligibility standards for institutional care. Capitated costs of care are paid from income and from Medicaid. The monthly capitation rate is negotiated annually as full payment for all services.

OnLok depends entirely on a multidisciplinary team approach to care. This approach includes assessment, treatment planning, service delivery, and monitoring of care. Housing for community-dwelling individuals is provided through the Department of Housing and Urban Development's Section 202 grants program (Robinson, 1990). Mental health services are provided either through staff geriatric psychiatrists and other mental health specialists or through contracted services with outside providers. Through intensive case management and effective multidisciplinary teams and extensive community support, the OnLok programs have been successful in reducing overall social and health care expenditures, hospital days, and nursing-home days. There have been no systematic evaluations of mental health service utilization in OnLok programs (Robinson, 1990).

Older adults with more extensive resources have been able to purchase catastrophic long-term insurance from the private marketplace. Additionally, they have access to organized health care and living circumstances providing more comprehensive care through *life-care communities*. Life-care communities are owned by private for-profit and not-for-profit corporations and religious organizations. Life-care contracts generally require individuals to purchase a residential unit for a fixed entrance fee, typically ranging from $50,000 to $300,000, and they require a monthly service fee of anywhere from $400 to $3,000 per month. Life-care communities offer multiple levels of living and support. Independent apartments with available meal and activity services and access to medical care serve the largest segment of most communities. Additionally, personal care, intermediate care, and skilled nursing facilities may be available on site or by contract. These facilities provide social and health care security and long-term care insurance to middle class and wealthier consumers. Systematic assessment of mental health status and care for residents in these environments has not been undertaken (Robinson, 1990).

The emphasis on cost containment and the emergence of a competitive for-profit medical care establishment has stimulated the development of numerous products to reduce utilization of more costly and restrictive environments. Systematic assessment of the effects of in-home services, private agencies, and more innovative delivery systems on the mental health of the populations that they serve is eagerly awaited.

VII. Conclusion

The economic profiles and the health care needs of older adults are extensive, diverse, and they are complex. Despite extraordinary expenditures and recent policy improvements, enormous financial and organizational barriers to geriatric mental health care persist. Medicare policy has been the cornerstone of the organization and delivery of geriatric psychiatric services for nearly a quarter of a century. High copayments, service limitations, and poor reimbursement for services have reinforced discrimination and stigmatization of care for this rapidly growing population with established acute and chronic needs.

Recent legislation could begin to improve access to mental health services for older adults. New policies will open the door for a large group of providers to deliver services to the elderly. Additionally, the spirit of innovations in cost containment may reward the work inherent in the cognitive and caring activities of psychiatric providers. However, these steps are small and incremental, and they are superimposed on a fragmented system of care that has not reinforced quality or innovation. As this population grows in size, need, and influence, policymakers and mental health providers will be challenged to design a more comprehensive system that reduces systematic barriers to care.

Direct reimbursement of nonphysician specialty mental health providers may allow new models of service delivery for older adults to emerge. Collaborative and interdisciplinary programs that more aggressively address the need for greater access to preventive mental health services may now be developed. However, restrictions in fees for providers who care for older adults may reduce the incentive for practitioners to deliver services to geriatric patients. Similarly, restrictions on access to inpatient and ambulatory psychiatric settings by third parties may increase out-of-pocket expenditures and create greater barriers to badly needed mental health services.

Alternatively, the creative employment of capitated systems of care that include multiple levels of service delivery may improve overall quality of life and reduce utilization of acute and institutional services, while improving access to specialty mental health providers. Additionally, direct reimbursement of psychologists and social workers may enhance collaborative efforts with general medical practitioners. This may improve screening for psychiatric, behavioral, and cognitive disorders and facilitate appropriate referral and intervention.

References

American Medical Association. (1990). *Common Procedural Terminology* (4th ed.). Chicago, IL: Author.

American Psychiatric Association Office of Economic Affairs. (1986). *The coverage catalog* (pp. 403–420). Washington, DC: Author.

Cutler, J., & Fine, T. (1985). Federal health care financing of mental illness: A failure of public policy. In S. S. Sharfstein & A. Beigel (Eds.), *The new economics of psychiatric care* (pp. 17–37). Washington, DC: American Psychiatric Press.

English, J. T., Kritzler, Z. A., & Scherl, D. (1984). Historical trends in the financing of psychiatric services. *Psychiatric Annals, 14,* 321–331.

English, J. T., Sharfstein, S. S., Scherl, D. J., Astrachan, B., & Muszynski, I. L. (1986). Diagnosis-related groups and general hospital psychiatry: The APA study. *American Journal of Psychiatry, 143,* 131–139.

Fogel, B. S. (1990). Physician payment reform. In B. S. Fogel, A. Furino, & G. L. Gottlieb (Eds.), *Mental health policy for older Americans: Protecting minds at risk* (pp. 109–124). Washington, DC: American Psychiatric Press.

Fogel, B. S., Gottlieb, G. L., & Furino, A. (1990a). Minds at risk. In B. S. Fogel, A. Furino, & G. L. Gottlieb (Eds.). *Mental health policy for older Americans: Protecting minds at risk* (pp. 1–21). Washington, DC: American Psychiatric Press.

Fogel, B. S., Gottlieb, G. L., & Furino, A. (1990b): Present and future solutions. In B. S. Fogel, A. Furino, & G. L. Gottlieb (Eds.), *Mental health policy for older Americans: Protecting minds at risk* (pp. 257–277). Washington, DC: American Psychiatric Press.

Frank, R. G., & Lave, J. L. (1985). The psychiatric DRGs: Are they different? *Medical Care, 23,* 1148–1155.

Frazier, S. H., Goldman, H., & Taube, C. A. (1986). Psychiatry, Medicare and prospective payment (editorial). *American Journal of Psychiatry, 143,* 198–200.

Furino, A. F., & Fogel, B. S. (1990). The economic perspective. In B. S. Fogel, A. Furino, & G. L. Gottlieb (Eds.), *Mental health policy for older Americans: Protecting minds at risk* (pp. 23–36). Washington, DC: American Psychiatric Press.

Goldman, H. H. (1988). Overview of studies on psychiatric hospital care under a prospective payment system. In D. J. Scherl, J. T. English, & S. S. Sharfstein (Eds.), *Prospective payment in psychiatric care* (pp. 81–89). Washington, DC: American Psychiatric Association.

Goldman, H. H., Feder, J., & Scanlon, W. (1986). Chronic mental patients in nursing homes: Reexamining data from the national nursing home study. *Hospital and Community Psychiatry, 37,* 269–272.

Goldman, H. H., & Frank, R. G. (1990). Division of responsibility among payors. In B. S. Fogel, A. Furino, & G. L. Gottlieb (Eds.), *Mental health policy for older Americans: Protecting minds at risk* (pp. 85–95). Washington, DC: American Psychiatric Press.

Goldman, H. H., Taube, C. A., & Jencks, S. J. (1987). The organization of the psychiatric inpatient services system. *Medical Care, 25* (9 Suppl.), S6–S21.

Gottlieb, G. L. (1988). Financial issues affecting geriatric psychiatric care. In L. Lazarus (Ed.), Essentials of geriatric psychiatry (pp. 230–248). New York: Springer.

Greenberg, J., Leutz, W., Greenlick, M., Malone, J., Ervin, S., & Kodner, D. (1988). The social HMO demonstration: Early experience. *Health Affairs, 7,* 55–79.

Grob, G. N. (1983). *Mental illness and American society, 1875–1940.* Princeton: Princeton University Press.

Hazzard, W. R. (1989). Geriatric medicine: Life in the crucible of the struggle to contain health care costs. In J. D. McCue (Ed.), *The medical cost-containment crisis* (pp. 263–264). Ann Arbor, MI: Health Administration Press.

Health Care Financing Administration. (1982). *Medicare and Medicaid data book.* Washington, DC: Author.

Hsiao, W. C., Braun, P., Kelly, N. L., & Becker, E. R. (1988). Results, potential effects and implementation issues of the Resource-Based Relative Value Scale. *Journal of the American Medical Association, 260*(16), 2429–2438.

Iglehart, J. K. (1985). Health policy report: Medicare turns to HMOs. *New England Journal of Medicine, 312,* 132–136.

Kemper, P. (1988). Overview of the findings: The evaluation of the national long-term care demonstration. *Health Services Research, 23,* 161–174.

Levit, K. R., Lazenby, H., Waldo, D. R., & Davidoff, L. M. (1985). National health expenditures, 1984. *Health Care Financing Review,* 731–734.

Long, S. H., & Welch, W. P. (1988). Are we containing costs or pushing on a balloon? *Health Affairs, 7*(4), 113–117.

Markides, K. S., & Mindel, C. H. (1987). *Aging and ethnicity* (pp. 31–35). Newburg Park, CA: Sage.

Moon, M. (1987). The elderly's access to health care services: The crude and subtle impacts of Medicare changes. *Social Justice Research, 1*(3), 361–375.

Morrisson, L., Janssen, T., & Motter, L. (1984). *Evaluation of the Medicare mental health demonstration.* Silver Spring, MD: Macro Systems.

National Center for Health Statistics. (1987). *Health statistics in older persons; United States, 1986, vital and health statistics, series 3, no. 25* (DHSS Publication No. (PHS) 87-1409). Washington, DC. U.S. Government Printing Office.

National Center for Health Statistics. (1988). *Health, United States, 1987, Public Health Service* (DHHS Pub. No. PHS 88-1232). Washington, DC. U.S. Government Printing Office.

Phillips, B., Kemper, P., & Applebaum, R. (1988). The evaluation of the national long-term care demonstration, 4: case management under channeling. *Health Service Research, 23,* 67–82.

Physician Payment Review Commission. (1989). *Annual report to Congress* (pp. 7–28). Washington, DC. U.S. Government Printing Office.

Psychiatric News. (1989). New Medicare fee schedule gets Congressional approval. *Psychiatric News, 24*(24), 2, December 15.

Regier, D. A., Goldberg, I. D., & Taube, C. A. (1978). The *de facto* U.S. mental health services system. *Archives of General Psychiatry, 35,* 685–693.

Robinson, G. K. (1990). The psychiatric component of long-term care models. In B. S. Fogel, A. Furino, & G. L. Gottlieb (Eds.), *Mental health policy for older Americans: Protecting minds at risk* (pp. 157–177). Washington, DC: American Psychiatric Press.

Roper, W. L. (1988). *Statement before the Committee on Ways and Means.* Washington, DC. U.S. Congress, House of Representatives, September 29.

Scherl, D. J., English, J. T., & Sharfstein, S. S. (1988). Preface. In D. J. Scherl, J. T. English, & S. S. Sharfstein (Eds.), *Prospective payment of psychiatric care* (pp. xv–xxii). Washington, DC: American Psychiatric Association.

Schulz, J. (1988). *Economics of aging* (4th ed.) Dover, MA: Auburn House.

Schurman, R. A., Kramer, P. D., & Mitchell, J. B. (1985). The hidden mental health network. *Archives of General Psychiatry, 42,* 89–94.

Sharfstein, S. S. (1990). Payment for services: A provider's perspective. In B. S. Fogel, A. Furino, & G. L. Gottlieb (Eds.), *Mental health policy for older Americans: Protecting minds at risk* (pp. 97–107). Washington, D.C.: American Psychiatric Press.

Soldo, B. J., & Agree, E. M. (1988). America's elderly population. *Population Bulletin, 43*(3), 1–53 (September).

U.S. Bureau of the Census. (1987). *An aging world, International Population Reports, Series P-95, No. 78.* Washington, DC: U.S. Government Printing Office.

U.S. Congress, House of Representatives, Committee on Ways and Means. (1989). *Background material and data on programs within the jurisdiction of the Committee on Ways and Means.* Washington, DC: U.S. Government Printing Office.

U.S. Senate Committee on Finance. (1978). *Background material on health insurance.* Washington, DC: U.S. Government Printing Office.

Waldo, D. R., & Lazenby, H. C. (1984). Demographic characteristics and health care use by the aged in the United States: 1977–1984. *Health Care Financing Review, 6,* 1–29.

The Future

The Future of Mental Health and Aging

Gene D. Cohen

I. Historic Moment in the Field of Mental Health and Aging
   A. A Phenomenon of the Fourth Quarter of the Twentieth Century
   B. Lessons from Greek Mythology
II. Concepts Shaping the Direction of the Field
   A. Mental Illness in Later Life versus Normal Aging
   B. Modifying Mental Disorder in Later Life
   C. Modifying (Enhancing) Normal (Mentally Healthy) Aging
III. Research on Aging—Relevance to All Age Groups
   A. New Clues about Depression
   B. New Clues about Schizophrenia
IV. The Significance of Time and the Capacity to Change with Aging
   A. Age-Specific Strengths Influencing the Capacity to Effect Change
   B. The Influence of Time on Interpersonal Relationships in Later Life
V. Epidemiological Trends in Mental Health and Aging
   A. Alzheimer's Disease (AD)
   B. Depression
   C. Illicit Drug Abuse in Later Life
   D. The Mentally Healthy
   E. Special Older Population Groups
   F. Diverse Settings for Living and Care in Later Life
VI. The Mental Health–Physical Health Interface in Later Life
   A. Mental Health and Aging Interventions Influencing Somatic Recovery
   B. High Technology and Mental Health Services for Older Adults
VII. Public Policy and Social Values—Lessons from Anthropology
VIII. Selected Summary of Mental Health and Aging Trends toward the Future
IX. Conclusion
   References

I. Historic Moment in the Field of Mental Health and Aging ————

It is the historic moment in the field of mental health and aging. We are at remarkable time in the development of this field—a point from which a significant future should unfold in the treatment of mental disorders and the promotion of mental health in later life. There are many manifestations of what is historic about this period. Certainly the establishment of subspecialization in geriatric psychiatry stands out. Until 1978, in the history of the United States, there had been only one department of psychiatry offering specialized training in geriatric psychiatry. A decade later there were thirty. The dramatic growth in geropsychiatric training—a response to the burgeoning new knowledge base of mental health and aging and to major new demands to apply that knowledge—led the American Board of Psychiatry and Neurology to establish formal subspecialization in geriatric psychiatry as of 1991. Indeed, this historic growth of mental health and aging training programs and professional development has been an intertwining process throughout psychiatry, psychology, social work, and nursing. Comparable public policy changes have occurred at the same time, highlighted by the first major changes in Medicare reimbursement for outpatient mental health services for elderly patients since the inception of the Medicare Program a generation earlier. This look to the future builds on a related decade-earlier view. (Cohen, 1980).

A. Phenomenon of the Fourth Quarter of the Twentieth Century

To a large extent, the dramatic growth in the field of mental health and aging in the United States has been a phenomenon of the fourth quarter of the twentieth Century. It was not until 1975, for example, that the first federal center (in any country) for supporting studies of mental health and aging was established at the National Institute of Mental Health. It was also in 1975 that the National Institute on Aging became operational, under the direction of a geriatric psychiatrist. The Geriatric Research, Education, and Clinical Centers (GRECCs) of the Department of Veterans Affairs (VA) also started in 1975, and included an emphasis on mental health and aging. Shortly thereafter, the dramatic growth in mental health and aging training alluded to above occurred throughout psychiatry, psychology, social work, and nursing. Major new national and international professional societies and committees emerged, such as the American Association for Geriatric Psychiatry, Division 20 on Aging of the American Psychological Association, and the multidisciplinary International Psychogeriatric Association. Mental health and aging textbooks and journals (national and international) began to proliferate, the latter including *The Journal of Gerontological Social Work, Psychology and Aging,* and *International Psychogeriatrics.* Faculty development in mental health and aging moved into high gear, assisted by new categories of federal support, such as the Mental Health and Aging Academic Award for research teachers in nursing. The declaration of the 1990s as the "Decade of the Brain" by the U.S. Congress could easily have been referred to as the Decade of the *Aging* Brain because of the extraordinary research and public-policy focus on Alzheimer's disease. And the establishment of subspecialization in geriatric psychiatry—only the second formal subspeciality in the history of American psychiatry—catapulted the prestige of the mental health and aging field. All of this set an exciting stage for future developments (Cohen, 1989).

B. Lessons from Greek Mythology

Before looking further at the historic final 25 years of the twentieth century as a prelude to the future of mental health and aging, it is useful to look back some 25 centuries to the ancient Greek myth of Tithonos. Tithonos, a mere mortal, fell in love with Eos, the goddess of dawn. Eos, herself immortal and wanting to live forever with her lover, pleaded to almighty Zeus to bestow the immortality of the gods upon Tithonos. Zeus acquiesced, but while granting immortality, neglected to include eternal youth. As a result, Tithonos continued to grow older and older and more and more frail without dying. It is indeed extraordinary how this more than 25-century-old myth captures one of the great and growing concerns among researchers in gerontology today—that progress in extending average longevity not outpace progress in improving the quality of later life. In no area is this concern greater than from a mental health and aging perspective.

II. Concepts Shaping the Direction of the Field

There are many conceptual planes from which one can view the nature and direction of progress in the area of mental health and aging. One plane encompasses the continuum from basic to applied research; another spans biomedical and psychosocial areas of investigation; yet another plane contains studies ranging from a disease orientation to a focus on health promotion; still another moves from examinations of basic mechanisms of aging to age-associated problems of older adults. In all of these planes of scientific inquiry, ideas and new knowledge about mental health and aging are burgeoning.

Cutting across all of the above research planes are three evolving conceptual orientations that are generating important new hypotheses and directions for mental health and aging studies: (1) differentiating mental illness in later life from normal aging changes; (2) modifying mental disorder in later life; and (3) modifying (enhancing) normal (mentally healthy) aging. These orientations have resulted in historic departures in the ways changes associated with aging are viewed (Cohen, 1988).

A. Mental Illness in Later Life versus Normal Aging

Significant growth of gerontologic research on the processes of aging and geriatric research on the illnesses of later life has been, as previously described, largely a late twentieth century development. It was not until the mid-1970s that scientists and clinicians alike began with any depth to develop a more fundamental awareness that many of the negative mental changes experienced by older adults were, in fact, clinical manifestations of diseases rather than inevitable consequences of aging *per se*. Long-standing differences in how aging was perceived had blurred the distinction between clinical disorder and normal development in later life. This was the case in both art and science. Such differences can be seen in two famous views on old age from Shakespeare and Cicero.

In Act II, Scene 7 of Shakespeare's late sixteenth century play *As You Like It,* he wrote on old age as follows:

Last scene of all,
That ends this strange eventful history
In second childishness and mere oblivion,
Sans teeth, sans eyes, sans taste, sans everything.

On the other hand, Cicero, in his first century B.C. philosophical masterpiece, *De Senectute,* wrote on old age as follows (see Bartlett, 1955; p. 34):

Intelligence, and reflection, and judgment, reside in old men, and if there had been none of them, no states could exist at all

Both were seen as accurate reflections. How could the views both be accurate, while being opposite? The explanation is that Shakespeare was portraying illness in later life, while Cicero was describing normal aging. One of the best examples of this aging-versus-illness dichotomy is that of Alzheimer's disease. The disorder was formerly referred to as senility, a term that led the public to view dementia as an expected concomitant of advancing years. But in the mid-1970s, selective loss of central cholinergic neurons in Alzheimer's disease was discovered, and this led to the cholinergic hypothesis of the disorder and changed the way that cognitive impairment in later life was viewed (Davies and Mahoney, 1976).

Studies aimed at differentiating changes due to aging from those due to illness in later life continue to compose a major thrust of mental health and aging research today. At the same time, a new stream of investigation is gaining momentum—that aimed at modifying disorder in older adults.

B. Modifying Mental Disorder in Later Life

While conclusions that pervasive decline in later life was the norm with aging had interfered with the recognition of disorder in older adults, analogous conclusions that disease in elderly individuals could not be modified interfered with efforts to treat these patients. But new frontiers of investigation are revealing that even the most severe disorders in older patients may be modified (Cohen, 1990a). Consider, again, the case of Alzheimer's disease and pioneering research in this area.

In an important study, fibroblasts of skin cells of laboratory rats were genetically modified to secrete nerve growth factor (NGF) by infection with a retroviral vector (NGF promotes regeneration of damaged nerve cell processes such as axons and dendrites). The genetically modified skin cells were then implanted as autografts into the brains of rats that had received surgically induced lesions to the fimbria-fornix. Remarkably, the grafted cells survived and produced sufficient NGF to prevent the degeneration of cholinergic neurons that would have died without treatment. In addition, the protected cholinergic cells sprouted axons that projected in the direction of the cellular source of NGF (Rosenberg *et al.,* 1988). This suggests that a combination of gene transfer and intracerebral grafting may provide effective treatment for some disorders of the aging central nervous system historically viewed as causing untreatable mental impairment.

C. Modifying (Enhancing) Normal (Mentally Healthy) Aging

Theoretical and clinical advances are stalled owing to failure to distinguish disorder from normal aging changes and owing to failure to recognize the potential modifiability of later-life disorder once recognized. Progress in modifying normal aging changes has also been stalled. Because a characteristic is normal or typical does not inherently mean it cannot be enhanced. Concepts of health promotion are based on hypotheses of the potential enhancement of normal phenomena or capacities. Consider some enlightening research on speed of reaction, the slowing of which is a normal development with aging. The results of a 7-week study examining practice effects of videogame playing in persons 65 and older are interesting (Clark, Lanphear, & Riddick, 1987). Practice led to improvement in both speed and accuracy of response. Hence, behavioral intervention, i.e., mental processing practice exercises, led to performance increments, although normal aging is typically accompanied by decrements. Such findings have major ramifications for policy development and program planning aimed at enabling older adults to maintain independence for the maximal period.

1. Brain and Behavior Considerations with Aging

A focus on brain–behavior relationships in later life has opened yet another doorway toward enhancing normal aging. In the process, one of the biggest myths in the history of health science has been toppled—the myth that the brain is a static, nonresilient organ, especially with aging. But findings from brain research have provided new insights about the potential for brain plasticity (modifiability), including the plasticity of the normal aging brain (Cohen, 1988; Diamond, 1983). For example, experiments examining the impact of challenging and stimulating environments on the brains of rats revealed *thickened* and *heavier* cerebral cortex (the thinking part of the brain); greater activity of the enzyme acetylcholinesterase, which affects the metabolism of the neurotransmitter acetylcholine (viewed as being involved in memory and intellectual function); an increase in glial cells, which are believed to carry out a number of auxiliary metabolic functions to aid neurons (the primary cells of the cerebral cortex); and an increase in the number and projections of dendrites (projections from neurons that facilitate communication among these cells of higher intellectual activity). Moreover, all of these changes persisted in the aging brain. This research showed that behavioral stimulation influenced both neurochemistry and *neuroanatomy*. Behavior influenced brain structure and did not stop with aging. Those who have admonished "use it or lose it" in later life, referring to the brain aging analogously to muscle, have taken note of these findings and their logical ramifications for ongoing growth and development from a later life mental health perspective.

2. Normal Aging Means More Than the Mere Absence of Illness

Future studies are likely to reflect increased attention not only to modifying disorders in later life but to normal development as well. Increased attention will be paid to the fact that the opportunity for ongoing growth and development of the mind knows no endpoint in the life cycle—that this ongoing process is the ultimate manifestation of mentally healthy, normal aging (Cohen, 1988; McLeish, 1981). While the demographic explosion of older adults will mean larger numbers of mentally ill elderly individuals, there will be even greater numbers of mentally healthy elderly persons. Ever more educated and health-conscious new cohort groups of older adults will increasingly demonstrate the opportunity to age well, and at the same time will raise the shared sense of responsibility of society and science to intervene with those who age less well. Efforts will undoubtedly extend even beyond the goal of effecting healthy aging to the goal of achieving creative aging, as examples of ongoing creativity in later life become apparent—from Mahatma Ghandi to Grandma Moses (Cohen, 1988).

III. Research on Aging—Relevance to All Age Groups _____

The importance of research on aging for older adults is apparent. Less apparent, but equally important, is the potential value of research on aging for all age groups. Whenever any problem can be looked at through a different window, chances increase of seeing something previously overlooked. Attention to age offers a new window through which development and disorder across the life cycle may be viewed. Research on aging can provide a new piece to the puzzle about illness at any age (Cohen, 1979). In other words, a focus on aging or older adults in a given study might lead to new clues for younger subjects.

A. New Clues about Depression

A classic example of this concept can be found in the history of research on biogenic amine neurotransmitters and their theorized role in the etiology of depression. The biogenic amine hypothesis of mood disorder, simply stated, was that depression resulted from diminished levels of catecholeamines in the brain (Kaplan, Sadock, and Freedman, 1975). The efficacy of monoamine oxidase (MAO) inhibitors as antidepressants was viewed as supporting this hypothesis. MAO inhibitors act by inhibiting the action of the brain enzyme monamine oxidase, which breaks down the catecholeamine norepinephrine; norepinephrine has been found to be diminished in depression. According to the hypothesis, if the action of monoamine oxidase is inhibited (by the antidepressant), then norepinephrine can be elevated, and depression, alleviated. This seemed to be the case.

Studies on the aging brain found that monoamine oxidase levels increased with aging, while norepinephrine levels diminished (Salzman, 1984). According to the biogenic amine theory, then, one might expect to find the elderly as a whole becoming more and more depressed over time. This is not the case. In fact, there is evidence suggesting that primary depressions (depression in the absence of other disorders) may not be more prevalent in older persons than in younger adults (Blazer, 1990).

As research advanced on the relationship of biogenic amine imbalances and depression, new discoveries complicated the picture—among them certain changes in the aging brain (Veith & Raskind, 1988). If a reduction in norepinephrine levels coupled with an increase in monoamine oxidase activity in the aging brain does not result in a noticeable increase in the prevalence of depression, as would be expected by the biogenic amine depletion hypothesis, then more must be involved biochemically in the genesis of mood disorder. Research on elderly subjects suggested that further pieces to the puzzle of depression in general might be discovered through additional studies on older depressives. Such findings have given rise to newer theories, such as the *dysregulation hypothesis of depression,* which postulates disruption in mechanisms that regulate the activity rather than the level of neurotransmitters; the problem could be asynchrony in the interaction of two or more neurotransmitters (Siever & Davis, 1985).

B. New Clues about Schizophrenia

Views on schizophrenia have dramatically shifted, aided by findings from studies of the disorder in later life (Miller & Cohen, 1987). This applies both to those with late-onset schizophrenia and to those who have grown old with the disorder. Studying both of these groups can provide new pieces to the puzzle of schizophrenia regardless of age. For example, while the onset of schizophrenia is most common in young adults, why is it that certain people can go through so much of the life cycle before becoming symptomatic with the disorder? What is it about these older individuals that caused the onset of the illness to be postponed? New clues from studying elderly late-onset schizophrenics might translate into new interventions to postpone or prevent the earlier onset of the disorder in vulnerable younger persons.

Similarly, clues may be found about the disorder by studying those who age with it. For example, why is it that many early-onset schizophrenics display a *burnout* of their symptoms accompanied by better adjustment in later life (Bridge, Cannon, & Wyatt, 1978)? One theory has focused on the role of the neurotransmitter dopamine. The literature suggests that schizophrenic symptoms occur when the brain responds as if it has an excess of dopamine (Weiner, 1985). With aging, dopamine levels diminish. Findings from studies of aging lend further support to the dopamine hypothesis of schizophrenia. Based on the dopamine-excess view of the disorder, schizophrenics having a relatively high dopamine tone would—with the normal loss of dopaminergic tone with aging—gradually burn out, returning to normal mental and behavioral functioning. A related hypothesis, focused on the reduction in neurotransmitter levels of both dopamine and acetylcholine, has postulated that late-onset schizophrenia may represent a relative asynchrony between neurotransmitters; it postulates that greater loss of cholinergic than of dopaminergic tone leads to a relative excess in dopamine (Finch, 1985). Together, these studies of schizophrenia in later life add to the understanding of the disorder across the life cycle.

The future of mental health for all age groups will benefit from studies of aging and older adults because of additions to our basic understanding of health and illness from studying these phenomena in later life. In the process, the impact and prestige of the field of mental health and aging will continue to grow.

IV. The Significance of Time and the Capacity to Change with Aging

Much research, practice, and policy relevant to mental health and aging has been short-circuited because of misinformation about the significance of time and the capacity to change in later life. To be in one's seventh decade is too often seen as having little time left and little capacity to approach things differently. But paradox surrounds both time and change considerations with aging. This double paradox is delightfully captured in an observation by Somerset Maugham (see Sadavoy & Leszcz, 1987; p. 297):

> When I was young I was amazed at Plutarch's statement that the elder Cato began at the age of 80 to learn Greek. I am amazed no longer. Old age is ready to undertake tasks that youth shirked because they would take too long.

Life-expectancy data, of course, refer to average longevity from birth; by age 65, one is a survivor, with a new average longevity of increasing duration. Put in historical perspective, the time paradox becomes poignant. For example, in Rome, during the height of the Roman empire, average longevity from birth was only 22 years owing to death associated with childbirth, disease, famine, and war (Hendricks & Hendricks, 1977). Meanwhile, looking toward twenty-first century America, at age 65, average longevity approaches 20 years, with those older than 85 representing the fastest-growing part of the population. From a mental health and aging vantage point, be the issue psychotherapy or mental health promotion, there is typically ample time for most older adults to take action.

Moreover, research continues to add to our understanding about the capacity for growth in response to action in later life. As Poon (1987, p. 380) has pointed out, "when a number of variables associated with a learning task are taken into account, the chronological age of the learner has not been shown to provide a significant amount of influence on performance." Willis (1985, p. 843) reached a similar conclusion: "the research literature in adult developmental psychology demonstrates that older adults have a substantial learning potential and presents evidence of a special need for continuing educational opportunities in later life." The recognition of considerable longevity in the desire and ability to learn in later life should increasingly challenge the practices and policies of society in developing programs to promote mental health in older adults.

A. Age-Specific Strengths Influencing the Capacity to Effect Change

Because decrement in later life is expected, it is important to emphasize that many capacities continue independent of age. It is underappreciated that some strengths *emerge* in association with aging. Some changes that might be viewed as losses in earlier adulthood have been viewed as assets in older adults. Bertrand Russell (1960; p. 80) at age 87, in his characteristic style, gave an example of this point, recounting a conversation with friends who felt he might be concerned about his hair having turned white:

> They tell me that if only I took drugs my hair would turn black again. I'm not sure that I should like that because I find that the whiter my hair becomes the more ready people are to believe what I say.

Some abilities do indeed improve, and with increasingly well-educated and physically healthier older cohort groups, such late-life abilities will become more apparent. Some diverse examples:

- Vocabulary, an integral element aiding in the negotiation of one's environment, increases in the presence of a healthy, active later life (Granick & Patterson, 1971).
- The continued movement toward more and more specialization within contemporary societies will heighten attention to specific skills. A study of proofreaders found that, as a group, those older than 60 performed better than did younger workers (Clay, 1956).
- Areas of psychodynamic growth are also found in later life. Personal insight, a component of wisdom, is influenced by one's psychological resistance. Grotjahn (1955, p. 420) found that "resistance against unpleasant insight is frequently lessened in old age; demands of reality which in younger people are considered narcissistic threats may finally become acceptable." Indeed it was a 71-year-old (Sophocles) who, with insight, first wrote about Oedipus.

Given ongoing changes in the work force, the potential roles of older workers will undoubtedly increase and undergo significant redefinition. In this context, a greater appreciation of specific skills of older adults—which skills endure, which decline, which increase—present an important opportunity to creatively plan for the future workplace. The role of older persons as a national resource in this plan will become ever more apparent. An analogous situation applies to the roles of older adults in community services in which wisdom and accumulated life experience are rising in value. Knowledge derived from mental health and aging studies will expand our understanding of how to better preserve and utilize these assets of older adults.

B. The Influence of Time on Interpersonal Relationships in Later Life

In my own research on mentally healthy older adults (Cohen, 1990b), a number of the subjects have described interesting new phenomenologic opportunities as a factor of having more flexible time in later life. The interpersonal sphere of relationships with family, friends, and general acquaintances particularly stands out positively. Older persons relate that when they were younger and overwhelmed by demands from work and raising children, if a misunderstanding arose with another person, they often would not have the time to immediately clarify or resolve the conflict. As a result, the risk of tension mounted, or negative conclusions increased without adequate time to set things straight. Later life, with its altered demands, has provided them the opportunity to more immediately address misunderstandings and to allocate more time toward mending them. This is a good example of a positive aspect of mental health with aging to look forward to.

V. Epidemiological Trends in Mental Health and Aging _____

By 1990, there were more people older than 65 in the United States than the entire population of Canada that year—the equivalent of a nation of elderly within America. By 2050, it is projected that there will be more people older than 85 in the U.S. than the total 1990 population of Australia—the equivalent of a nation of the old-old within America. In the absence of curing or better controlling mental illness in later life, there will be some disturbing trends. The good news, though, is that the numbers of mentally healthy older adults will increase; mental *health* will continue to be the norm in later life. Controversy and debate surround the question as to whether older adults with serious illness will rise or fall as a *percentage* of the overall elderly population (Gilford, 1988). Still, the *numbers* with good mental health will rise. At the same time, the numbers with major illness will also be likely to rise, creating an ever-increasing challenge for society well into the twenty-first century. It is not just a matter of looking at demographic growth of the 65-and-older age group as a whole and determining the anticipated proportionate numbers with mental illness; there are some special considerations.

A. Alzheimer's Disease (AD)

This will be the greatest challenge. Already affecting approximately 4 million older adults at an estimated societal cost of $90 billion a year in 1990, in the absence of cure or control, the numbers and costs of this disorder by the middle of the twenty-first century will be staggering (Huang, Cartwright, & Hu, 1988; U.S. Congress Office of Technology Assessment, 1990). Because the risk is greatest in those 85 and older—the group that will grow fivefold from 1990 to 2050—there could be a tripling of those afflicted with AD. Worse, this could be accompanied by a related increase in the numbers of the *second patient*—family caregivers who succumb to depression under the enormous burdens they confront. The need for a massive assault from research and the launching of federally sponsored long-term care insurance has been strongly voiced by the congressionally appointed U.S. Department of Health and Human Services Advisory Panel on Alzheimer's Disease (1989).

B. Depression

Data on the prevalence of depression in later life vary (Blazer, 1990). It is important to consider one of the ways that depression is classified—primary versus secondary depressions (Klerman, 1982). Secondary depressions can occur as a consequence of physical illness or drug side-effect. Since the old-old are the group most at risk for physical illness and most in need of medication, the prevalence of secondary depressions in later life could rise significantly in the absence of research or treatment breakthroughs. This has broad ramifications for the need to escalate efforts to expand comprehensive services based on the bio–psycho–social model.

C. Illicit Drug Abuse in Later Life

Though illicit drug use in later life has been reported to be quite infrequent, cohort factors could change this—i.e., the experience of individuals growing up during the rise of the drug culture. When these individuals grow old, a higher percentage may carry with them lingering problems of substance abuse.

D. The Mentally Healthy

While the prevalence of other mental health problems in later life will also rise, in the absence of cure or control, owing to expanding demographics in the future, the mentally *healthy* will similarly become more apparent. With larger numbers of well-educated and physically healthy older persons in new aging cohorts, society will become more strongly challenged to develop mental health promotion programs for later life. Also, as a factor of changing cohorts, older adults will be more interested in seeking out mental health services when they are indicated. Action will increasingly be taken *by* older adults rather than *for* them.

E. Special Older Population Groups

Because the older age group is like a nation within a nation, it has all the diversity of any country. Accordingly, we need to focus policy, practice, research, and training efforts along special population group lines within the elderly population as a whole. Particular efforts need to be directed in the following areas.

1. Racial and Ethnic Minority Groups

By the middle of the twenty-first century there will be enormous shifts in the racial and ethnic profiles of older Americans. According to the 1980 Census, 8% of the elderly were black, 5% were Hispanic, and fewer than 2% were *other races* (Adler, Kitchen, & Irion, 1988). By 2050 it is projected that blacks will make up over 14% of the older population, with the Hispanic older population also growing at a faster rate than nonminority whites. Issues vary, of course, with minorities, and cultural and linguistic challenges apply more to some than others. But there are also cross-cutting issues common to most underserved population groups, one of these being the underdelivery of health services. This has even greater significance with older persons in the area of physical health–mental health interactions.

The greater frequency of general medical illness in minority groups adds to their multiple jeopardies from a mental health perspective, since major physical disorders are accompanied by a greater frequency of mental health symptoms and behavioral problems. Comparing blacks and whites older than 65, for example, one finds that blacks have over double the morbidity for hypertension (a major risk factor for multi-infarct dementia, influencing the prevalence of cognitive impairment in older blacks), over double the morbidity for diabetes; a 50% greater morbidity for diseases of the circulatory system, and a 50% greater morbidity for arthritis (Willis, 1989). The need to enhance comprehensive bio–psycho–social services becomes yet more apparent for the elderly as a whole.

2. Research on Minorities to Advance Mainstream Knowledge

Related to the earlier-discussed concept of research on aging, as a piece to the puzzle of understanding development and disorder independent of age, is the opportunity to advance knowledge in mainstream aging areas through studies of older racial and ethnic minority groups. Suicide offers a case in point. Suicide rates are higher among older

Anglo-whites than among older blacks, Hispanics, and Native Americans (Group for the Advancement of Psychiatry, Committee on Cultural Psychiatry, 1989). Through comparative studies of suicide among these different racial and ethnic groups, new understanding could emerge about risk factors and preventive interventions relevant to all older adults. Future research on minorities will provide the opportunity to better understand mental health and mental disorder not only in these special older population groups, but also in the elderly as a whole.

3. The Old-Old

As already alluded to, there will be a nation within a nation of old-old Americans by the middle of the twenty-first century. Everyone who will be in that age group then is alive today. While the field of aging is having increasing success in influencing general health and mental health practitioners to work with older patients, the impact has been more on the 65-to-80 age group. Attention to those aged 85 and older, the fastest-growing age group, is analogous to the lack of attention that used to be directed to those 65 and older in general. Some of the greatest changes in the field of aging will come from the growing focus on the old-old.

4. Older Women and Widows

Older women experience major challenges in several domains of special mental health relevance. They are particularly often widows, poorer than men, and much more likely to live alone. In 1930, 50% of the elderly population were women; by 1984, 60% were women. In 1980, women older than 85 outnumbered men that age by 2 to 1; by early in the twenty-first century, this ratio will be nearly 3 to 1. In 1984, 70% of men aged 75 and older were married, as compared to fewer than 25% of women in this age group. Apart from psychosocial ramifications, there are significant mental health service delivery problems related to the economic status and living situation of older women. These trends continue and need considerably greater planning and program development.

5. Older Adults Living Alone

As already alluded to, considerable numbers of older women live alone—41% of the noninstitutionalized in 1984. Many men also live alone, in numbers approaching 1 in 6. Dramatic shifts in family structure—e.g., fewer children, high divorce rates among caregiving children, geographical mobility of caregivers—complicate program planning based on the respective and interactive roles of informal and formal support systems. Here, too, much creative research and program planning are called for.

6. The Rural Elderly

It is estimated that approximately 1 in 4 older Americans lives in a rural area (Coward & Lee, 1985). Socioeconomic and services access issues are magnified on the average in this group in comparison to their urban counterparts. Meanwhile, a paucity of research from both mental illness and mental health vantage points exists on this special population group, which is another agenda item for the future.

F. Diverse Settings for Living and Care in Later Life

The growing diversity of settings for living and care for older adults is one of the most interesting changes in our midst, and one that creates innovative options for the future. As part of this changing process, a longstanding stereotype has taken a paradoxical twist. It used to be intimated—often in a patronizing manner—that one would be living like the elderly if attracted to high-density apartments with security personnel, recreation rooms, grounds and maintenance services, and resident managers to supervise the arrangements. Curiously, today, if a living arrangement were so described, who would you say lived there—elderly persons or yuppies? At one level this suggests that interesting new intergenerational living designs are more possible now and for the future than has long been the case, because of increasingly common goals for a desirable place to reside.

It is no longer a question of whether one should live at home or in a nursing home with advancing age. In addition to increasing choices, there is a growing continuum of arrangements based on an individual's level of dependency; these vary from highly individualized options scattered throughout the community to life-care facilities in one location. From a research perspective, there is an enormous need to study these different settings with the dual focus of understanding phenomenology pertaining to both mental-health promotion and mental-disorder intervention. Such knowledge is critical for mental health professionals to better advise people about the preferable living arrangement for them, what types of mental health programs might be planned for respective settings, and how mental health services might best be delivered. Such knowledge will also be of value for social-policy deliberations on what services should be covered by long-term care insurance. Additionally, this knowledge will be critical to foster another growing phenomenon in mental health and aging—the *home visit*. A brief clinical vignette illustrates the importance of in-depth understanding in this area of alternative settings for living and mental health care.

Case Example:

A consultation was requested on an 85-year-old woman, Mrs. R, who lived alone in an apartment building that provided the part-time services of a nurse, who was available in her office for purposes of supervising medication. The nurse did not make home visits. The consultation was requested because Mrs. R was becoming increasingly eccentric in her behavior, which the management felt was disturbing to other residents in the building. Other residents, however, had not complained to the family. Medication had been prescribed, but Mrs. R was reluctant and inconsistent about seeking the assistance of the nurse, whose supervision was needed for proper drug management.

Clinical assessment of Mrs. R at her apartment revealed some paranoid symptoms, which would be likely to respond very well to low dosages of neuroleptic medication and periodic supportive psychotherapy. But the impression was also that her setting was minimally tolerant of even mildly deviant behavior, resulting in a poor fit with little support and heightened tension for Mrs. R.

A recommendation was made to the family to have Mrs. R move to a similar setting that differed mainly in having a nurse available around the clock and who would make home visits as indicated. This more liberal service also suggested a higher tolerance level for problematic behavior at the alternative setting. Mrs. R did move, and the new arrangement was considerably better for her.

VI. The Mental Health–Physical Health Interface in Later Life _____

One of the characteristics that distinguishes older patients from younger ones is the greater likelihood of concurrent disorders, especially of mixed psychogenic and somatic origins. The influence of mental health on the course of overall health and the impact of mental health interventions on improving recovery from physical illness in later life are increasing—yet still greatly underrecognized—phenomena of major public health concern. This area will continue to loom as one of the most challenging and promising mental health and aging arenas well into the twenty-first century. Indeed, studies in this area offer us one of the greatest opportunities to understand interactions of biology and behavior to the benefit of all age groups. Table I offers some useful paradigms for examining different ways in which mental and physical health factors interact in elderly persons. They help frame ways that older patients can be approached clinically and ways that psychogeriatric research questions can be raised.

Since the prevalence of physical illness increases with aging—especially in the old-old—public health planning for the future needs to be much more cognizant of health and behavior relationships in later life than has been the case in the past. The growing body of research in this area since the early 1980s makes the case. Some examples follow.

Table I

Paradigms for Examining Relationships between Mental and Physical Health in Older Adults[a]

The impact of psychogenic stress that leads to physical health consequences
Example: Anxiety → gastrointestinal symptoms
The accurate diagnosis of gastrointestinal (GI) symptoms can be very difficult in the elderly, with research showing that as many as 5 of 9 older persons with GI trouble may experience psychogenic problems that lead to their physical discomfort.

The effect of physical disorder that leads to psychiatric disturbance
Example: Hearing loss → onset of delusions
More than 25% of the elderly have a hearing impairment; a sensory-deprivation phenomenon may lead to psychotic symptoms in certain vulnerable individuals; an increased frequency of hearing loss has also been identified in older adults with late-onset schizophrenia.

The interplay of coexisting physical and mental disorders
Example: Congestive heart failure + depression → further cardiac decline
Cardiac disorder and depression are two of the most common health problems of the elderly. A covert depression could bring about indirect suicidal behavior acted out by failure on the part of the patient to follow a proper schedule of medication; the resulting clinical picture could then be one of further deterioration in overall cardiac capacity.

The impact of psychosocial factors on the clinical course of physical health problems
Example: Diabetic with infected foot, living in isolation → increased risk of losing foot in absence of adequate social supports to help with proper medical management and followup
(More than two in five older women and nearly one in six older men live alone.)

---

[a]Adapted from Cohen (1985).

A. Mental Health and Aging Interventions Influencing Somatic Recovery

In a now classic study by Levitan and Kornfeld (1981), the investigators compared the clinical outcome of two groups of elderly patients surgically treated for fractured femurs. The *treatment* group of 24 patients aged 65 and older received mental health consultation during hospitalization, while the *control* group of 26 comparably aged subjects did not receive such consultation. The groups were matched as to reason for admission (broken hip), age, surgical intervention, hospital setting, and overall care—except for the mental health intervention. The treatment group revealed two major outcome differences from the control group. The treatment group had (1) a substantially shorter length of stay (30 versus 42 days, or a 29% reduction), and (2) a significantly improved clinical outcome (twice as many patients in the treatment group returned home rather than being discharged to a nursing home or other convalescent institution). A review of the literature a year later revealed 34 controlled studies of recovering surgical or heart attack patients with related results (Mumford, Schlesinger, & Glass, 1982).

How can one explain these results? There are both psychosocial and psychoimmunological explanations. Both consider the impact of depression and stress upon somatic recovery in older patients. The prevalence of depression is typically high in older adults hospitalized for physical health reasons. One study found that 24% of 406 elderly men seen for physical health problems in a primary health care setting complained of clinically significant symptoms of depression (Boorson *et al.*, 1986). Moreover, it is important to recognize the magnitude of dysfunction that depression alone can cause in comparison to major physical disorders. Results from the Medical Outcomes Study dramatically show that the impact of depressive symptoms can be equal to or more adverse than that of 8 major chronic medical conditions (Wells *et al.*, 1989). Of note was that depressive symptoms, with or without depressive disorder *per se,* resulted in poor functioning (e.g., impaired capacity to perform tasks and to carry out activities, and increased days in bed) comparable to or worse than those resulting from hypertension, diabetes, angina, advanced coronary artery disease, arthritis, back problems, lung problems, or gastrointestinal disorder.

The adverse impact of depression on hospital course can be understood psychosocially. Depression lowers motivation. The patient with depressive feelings is less motivated to aggressively participate in rehabilitative efforts and discharge planning, both of which can prolong hospitalization and make it more difficult to be discharged directly from hospital to home.

The adverse impact of depression on hospital course can also be understood psychoimmunologically. It appears that hospitalized older patients, more than younger ones, are at risk of experiencing compromised immunological functioning in response to depression and stress (Schleifer, Keller, Bond, Cohen, & Stein, 1989). Studies of depressed and severely stressed older caregivers of Alzheimer's patients report similar results, with negative immunological changes accompanied by an increased frequency of physical illness and increased utilization of general medical services (Kiecolt-Glaser & Glaser, 1989). A compromised immune system is less effective in helping with speedy repair of infected or damaged tissue.

Beyond the public health significance of mental health–physical health interactions is that of scientific opportunity. Since older adults are the group with the greatest frequency of concurrent mental health and general medical problems, they are the group most likely to show how behavior affects biology and how biology affects behavior. The opportunity to gain new insights into biology and behavior—and especially brain and behavior—through studies on older patients will not be lost on future investigators in general areas of science.

B. High Technology and Mental Health Services for Older Adults

High technology is all around us, but has made only a limited entry into mental health services for older adults. Its more noticeable use is in the area of diagnosis, as with sophisticated imaging [e.g., positron emission tomography or (PET)] techniques and new types of neuropsychological computerized assessment. But it is also headed toward care (Lieff, 1989; U.S. Congress Office of Technology Assessment, 1985).

- Computerized medicine boxes aid the patient in proper medication management. Computer programs will become more available for the practitioner to assist in drug management—e.g., software to evaluate potential adverse drug–drug interactions for patients taking psychotropics and other medications concurrently.
- Various computerized health-oriented alarms have already entered the home, such as those that signal cardiac arrhythmias. With new *smart house* technology—i.e., technology that allows houses to be wired for myriad computerized options—a range of creative electronic cues and crutches can assist the frail and cognitively impaired in the least-intrusive ways. For example, a sensor could be installed under the carpet by the bed, so that when an older person gets up at night, a light automatically goes on; a recording can also (analogous to a *fasten your seat belt* reminder) suggest that the person on antidepressants stand in place for a minute after getting out of bed, to reduce the risk of a drug-induced hypotensive reaction leading to a fall and potential hip fracture.
- In day-treatment programs for the cognitively impaired, discreet electronic devices are available for patients to wear around their ankles to signal a silent alarm should they wander out the door, thereby increasing individual freedom by reducing the need for restraints or excessive supervision.
- Two-way videos or video phones offer potential breakthroughs in improving the delivery of services to those who are home-bound or living in rural areas. A tremendous amount of information could be gathered by assessing the state of the patient's environment on the video, by seeing how nourished or hydrated patients appear, by examining their general appearance, by supervising the ingestion of medication, by evaluating for neuroleptic side-effects like tardive dyskinesia, and the like. Such systems could also be set up in day-treatment programs and nursing homes, thereby increasing the frequency of observation and interaction by mental health professionals not on the regular staff of such programs.
- Staff training and continuing education will also be assisted by more and more user-friendly computer educational programs.

The list will dramatically grow, creating all kinds of new opportunities for nonheroic high-technology mental health care practices and improved mental health services delivery.

Meanwhile, there is ample room for low-tech or no-tech innovations to enhance independence and social engagement (Morris, 1989). Consider those living alone. Numerous opportunities exist in our increasingly service-oriented society to initiate all kinds of imaginative socially oriented programs (both volunteer and entrepreneurial) to help mobilize frail and isolated individuals. Specially supervised clubs, providing adequate transportation for exercise, dinner, museum visits, theater, and travel, for example, can help transform many isolated and despondent existences. The combination of outreach and innovation will increase the number and impact of mental health–promotion programs in the future.

VII. Public Policy and Social Values—Lessons from Anthropology ___

At times, evolutionary perspectives influence views and values and, in turn, policies. Some argue that the dilemma of dealing with disability that creates a burden for the individual, family, and society alike is a historically new phenomenon—that our evolutionary ancestors were pragmatic in the *benign neglect* of disabled elders. It has been suggested that we can learn from such anthropological insights. But new findings about Neanderthals who inhabited the earth 100,000 years ago challenge such views of how early man and his society dealt with chronic disability. That these findings come from research on Neanderthals, who have been typically characterized as brutish, is all the more of note. It has now been found that Neanderthals

> were the first people who regularly buried their dead. . . . they regularly took care of their sick and aged. Most skeletons of older Neanderthals show signs of severe impairment, such as withered arms, healed but incapacitated broken bones, tooth loss, and severe osteoarthritis. Only care by young Neanderthals could have enabled such older folks to stay alive to the point of such incapacitation (Diamond, 1989; p. 55).

With an increase in contemporary debates about what resources should or should not go into the care of those at an advanced age, historical and anthropological perspectives add important new vantage points. Perhaps the area where this is most poignant from a mental health and aging perspective is in the area of Alzheimer's disease and related dementing disorders, the treatment and management of which is so much in the domain of mental health professionals. Such is logically the situation because the symptoms of *dementia* are *by definition* behavioral symptoms, and the best interventions to date for dementia include behavioral-management skills, psychotropic medications, and mental health support for the family. A mental health and aging knowledge base provides for state-of-the-art treatment for Alzheimer's disease today—treatment to alleviate symptoms and to maximize functioning at given points in the progression of the disorder (Group for the Advancement of Psychiatry, Committee on Aging, 1988). While recognition of the role of mental health interventions for Alzheimer's disease contributed to Medicare reform for improved outpatient mental health coverage, patients still lack long-term care insurance.

That the most affluent country in the world does not have an adequate and affordable long-term care insurance for the population as a whole is a growing public policy issue and social values concern. Important to note is that most Americans are not aware that they lack long-term care protection, the vast majority incorrectly thinking that Medicare provides such coverage (Williams & Katzman, 1988). Unfortunately, when it comes to chronic illness, most older Americans have *wrong-term* care insurance (acute-care coverage only). Meanwhile, intense study is underway to rectify this situation, with careful scrutiny of what long-term care services might be covered and what mechanisms might be utilized to finance them (Capitman, 1990). Because of the usually inseparable interplay of physical and mental health variables in those in need of long-term care, it will be critical to monitor the proper inclusion of mental health services in whatever long-term care package is eventually approved.

VIII. Selected Summary of Mental Health and Aging Trends toward the Future

Potential developments in the field of mental health and aging are pounding at the door. Selected likely developments are briefly summarized as follows.

(1) The ability to differentiate illness in older adults from aging changes *per se* will advance, moving from the level of manifest behavior to molecular biology, in understanding both mental health and mental disorder.
(2) Progress will continue in the ability of mental health professionals to modify clinical problems in later life.
   (A) *Major mental illness* (other than organic mental disorder) will better respond to
      (i) an improved state of the art in the use of behavioral and psychosocial interventions
      (ii) new pharmacologic agents with enhanced efficacy and fewer side effects
   (B) *Alzheimer's disease (AD)* and other organic mental disorders will become better managed through
      (i) the identification of diagnostic markers that will help in earlier and more accurate recognition of the disorder and in better predicting the duration of the disorder in individual cases
      (ii) further progress in treating comorbid problems causing excess disability, especially behavioral symptoms like agitation, wandering, depression, and delusions
      (iii) advances in understanding the underlying disease process of AD, which will lead to new somatic (e.g., pharmacologic) interventions that could postpone the onset of the disorder, slow its clinical course, and mitigate its symptoms
   (C) *General medical disorders* will become better managed through advances in the understanding of health-related behaviors such as
      (i) seeking appropriate diagnostic assessments (such as mammograms)
      (ii) improved exercise regimens

(iii) improved dietary habits

(iv) more informed participation in the treatment process

(D) *The risk of suicide,* which is greater in the elderly than in any other age group, will become better recognized and prevented in later life.

(3) The enhancement of psychological growth and creative capacity in later life will become a goal and outcome. This will come through

(A) *Progress in the development of health promotion techniques*

(B) *Age-specific creative patterns* becoming better recognized and understood, thereby spurring the development of more targeted approaches with older adults to tap into or release such potential

(4) New types of mental health interventions will emerge, particularly through the growth of knowledge of the interaction of mental health with overall health in later life and of brain–behavior relationships in older adults.

(A) *New classes of medications* for dealing with schizophrenia, depression, generalized anxiety, phobias, and alcohol abuse will come from improved understanding of brain–behavior relationships.

(B) *High-technology innovations*

(i) will permit greater patient and family capacity to manage cognitive impairment

(ii) will facilitate better access to mentally ill elders who are geographically isolated

(5) Increasing diversity in living and treatment settings will

(A) *create more options for individualized treatment*

(B) *require modifications in the clinical training experiences* of mental health professionals in order to optimally prepare them to deal with the problems and possibilities of providing interventions in such settings

(C) *lead to clinical practice moving to more natural locations* than the hospital and private office

(6) The growing numbers of older adults among ethnically and racially diverse populations will require modifications both in the training of mental health professionals and in the delivery of mental health services to more effectively deal with cultural variation among special population groups.

(7) Progress in research on aging will lead to increased average longevity that, on the one hand, will result in larger numbers of people who age well, with, on the other hand, larger numbers of ill persons at an advanced age—the latter being the most complex to treat. Treatment and care decisions for the latter group will create expanding ethical debates and dilemmas into which mental health professionals will be increasingly called.

(8) The field of mental health and aging will continue to grow.

IX. Conclusion

If the progress in the field of mental health and aging from 1975 to 1990 is any indication of what could follow in the next 15 years, the future should be comparably historic. The science has clearly moved into high gear. Old doubts about a unique knowledge base in this area have been done away with, replaced by the recognition of a critical new scientific literature that set the stage for subspecialization in geropsychiatry as well as Medicare reform for mental health coverage. The future should witness yet greater progress in understanding mental disorders in later life, in modifying these disorders, and in enhancing mental health for the vast majority of older adults.

Because a focus on aging affords new pathways to unanswered questions, the field will attract an increasing number of researchers from general areas within the broader scientific community. The opportunity, through research on aging, to gain new pieces to the puzzles of what causes mental disorder and what promotes mental health—independent of age—will create new horizons for academic careers in mental health and aging.

Meanwhile, on the service side, the field will be challenged by growing special population groups, significant changes within the family system, more diverse settings for living and care, and greater complexity in clinical manifestations of physical health–mental health interactions with extended average longevity.

The duration and meaning of time in later life will evolve, and the capacity for creative change with advancing age will become more apparent. This will be accompanied by greater acceptance and demand for mental health interventions. The interventions themselves will evolve, with greater innovation in human services and fundamentally new approaches via high technology. Conquering Alzheimer's disease and closing the gap between Tithonos' quantity and quality of life will be the field's greatest challenges.

References

Adler, M., Kitchen, S., & Irion, A. (1988). *Databook on the elderly 1987* (520–143/00027). Washington, DC: U.S. Government Printing Office.

Bartlett, J. (1955). *Familiar quotations* (p. 34). Boston: Little, Brown and Company.

Blazer, D. (1990). Epidemiology of late-life depression and dementia: A comparative study. In A. Tasman, S. M. Goldfinger, & C. A. Kaufman (Eds.), *Review of psychiatry* (Vol. 2, pp. 197–215). Washington, DC: American Psychiatric Press.

Boorson, S., Barnes, R. A., Kukull, W. A., Okimoto, J. T., Veith, R. C., Inui, T. S., Carter, W. & Raskind, M. A. (1986). Symptomatic depression in elderly medical outpatients. *Journal of the American Geriatrics Society, 34,* 341–347.

Bridge, T. P., Cannon, H. E., & Wyatt, R. J. (1978). Burned-out schizophrenia: Evidence for age effects on schizophrenic symptomatology. *Journal of Gerontology, 33,* 835–839.

Capitman, J. A. (1990). Policy and program options in community-oriented long-term care. In M. P. Lawton (Ed.), *Annual review of gerontology and geriatrics* (Vol. 9, pp. 357–388). New York: Springer.

Clark, J. E., Lanphear, A. K., & Riddick, C. C. (1987). The effects of videogame playing on the response selection processing of elderly adults. *Journal of Gerontology, 42,* 82–85.

Clay, H. M. (1956). A study of performance in relation to age at two printing works. *Journal of Gerontology, 11,* 417–424.

Cohen, G. D. (1979). Research on aging: A piece of the puzzle. *The Gerontologist, 19,* 503–508.

Cohen, G. D. (1980). Prospects for mental health and aging. In J. E. Birren & R. B. Sloane (Eds.), *Handbook of mental health and aging* (pp. 971–993). Englewood Cliffs, NJ: Prentice-Hall.

Cohen, G. D. (1985). Toward an interface of mental and physical health phenomena in geriatrics: Clinical findings and questions. In C. M. Gaitz & T. Samorajski (Eds.), *Aging 2000: Our health care destiny: Biomedical issues* (Vol. 1, pp. 283–299). New York: Springer-Verlag.

Cohen, G. D. (1988). *The brain in human aging.* New York: Springer.

Cohen, G. D. (1989). The movement toward subspecialty status for geriatric psychiatry in the United States. *International Psychogeriatrics, 1*(2), 201–205.

Cohen, G. D. (1990a). Biopsychiatry of Alzheimer's disease. In M. P. Lawton (Ed.), *Annual review of gerontology and geriatrics (Vol. 9*, pp. 216–231). New York: Springer.

Cohen, G. D. (1990b). Lessons from longitudinal studies of mentally ill and mentally healthy elderly: A 17-year perspective. In M. Bergener & S. I. Finkel (Eds.), *Clinical and scientific psychogeriatrics (Vol. 1*, pp. 135–148). New York: Springer.

Coward, R. T., & Lee, G. R. (Eds.). (1985). *The elderly in rural society: Every fourth elder.* New York: Springer.

Davies, P., & Mahoney, A. J. F. (1976). Selective loss of central cholinergic neurons in Alzheimer's disease. *Lancet, 2,* 1403.

Diamond, J. (1989). The great leap forward. *Discover, 10,* 50–60.

Diamond, M. C. (1983). The aging rat forebrain: Male–female left–right: Environment and lipofuscin. In D. Samuel, S. Algeri, S. Gershon, V. E. Grimm, & G. Toffan (Eds.). *Aging of the brain* (Vol. 22, pp. 93–98). New York: Raven Press.

Finch, C. E. (1985). A progress report on neurochemical and neuroendocrine regulation in normal and pathologic aging. In C. M. Gaitz & T. Samorajski (Eds.), *Aging 2000: Our health care destiny (Vol. 1*, pp. 79–90). New York: Springer-Verlag.

Gilford, D. M. (Ed.). (1988). *The aging population in the twenty-first century.* Washington, DC: National Academy Press.

Granick, S., & Patterson, R. D. (1971). *Human aging II: An eleven-year followup biomedical and behavioral study* (DHEW Publication No. (HSM) 71-9037). Washington, DC: U.S. Government Printing Office.

Grotjahn, M. (1955). Analytic psychotherapy with the elderly, I: The sociological background of aging in America. *Psychoanalytic review, 42,* 419–427.

Group for the Advancement of Psychiatry, Committee on Aging. (1988). *The psychiatric treatment of Alzheimer's disease.* New York: Bruner/Mazel.

Group for the Advancement of Psychiatry, Committee on Cultural Psychiatry. (1989). *Suicide and ethnicity in the United States.* New York: Bruner/Mazel.

Hendricks, J., & Hendricks, C. D. (1977). *Aging in mass society: Myths and realities.* Cambridge, Massachusetts: Winthrop Publishers, Inc.

Huang, L., Cartwright, W. S., & Hu, T. (1988). The economic cost of senile dementia in the United States. *Public Health Reports, 103,* 3–7.

Kaplan, H., Sadock, B., & Freedman, A. M. (1975). The brain in psychiatry. In A. M. Freedman, H. I. Kaplan, and B. J. Sadock (Eds.), *Comprehensive Textbook of Psychiatry II.* Baltimore, MD: Williams & Wilkins.

Kiecolt-Glaser, J. K., & Glaser, R. (1989). Caregiving, mental health, and immune function. In E. Light & B. D. Lebowitz (Eds.), *Alzheimer's disease treatment and family stress: Directions for research* (DHHS Publication No. (ADM)89-1569). Washington, DC: U.S. Government Printing Office.

Klerman, G. L. (1982). Depression and mania. In D. Oken & M. Lakovics (Eds.), *A clinical manual of psychiatry.* New York: Elsevier/North Holland.

Levitan, S. T., & Kornfeld, D. S. (1981). Clinical and cost benefits of liaison psychiatry. *American Journal of Psychiatry, 138,* 790–793.

Lieff, J. D. (1989). High technology and psychiatric care of the elderly. *International Psychogeriatrics, 1*(1), 87–101.

McLeish, J. A. B. (1981). The continuum of creativity. In P. W. Johnston (Ed.), *Perspectives on aging: Exploding the myth.* Cambridge, MA: Ballinger.

Miller, N. E., & Cohen, G. D. (1987). *Schizophrenia and aging.* New York: Guilford.

Morris, R. (1989). Challenges of aging in tomorrow's world: Will gerontology grow, stagnate, or change? *The Gerontologist, 29*(4), 494–501.

Mumford, E., Schlesinger, H. J., & Glass, G. V. (1982). The effects of psychological intervention on recovery from surgery and heart attacks: An analysis of the literature. *American Journal of Public Health, 72,* 141–151.

Poon, L. W. (1987). Learning. In G. L. Maddox (Ed.), *The encyclopedia of aging.* New York: Springer.

Rosenberg, M. B., Friedmann, T., Robertson, R. C., Tuszynski, M., Wolff, J. A., Breakefield, X. O., & Gage, F. H. (1988). Grafting genetically modified cells to the damaged brain: Restorative effects of NGF. *Science, 242,* 1575–1578.

Russell, B. (1960). *Bertrand Russell speaks his mind*. New York: Bard Books.

Sadavoy, J., & Leszcz, M. (1987). Treating the elderly with psychotherapy: The scope for change in later life (p. 297). New York: International Universities Press.

Salzman, C. (1984). Neurotransmission in the aging central nervous system. In C. Salzman (Ed.), *Clinical geriatric psychopharmacology*. New York: McGraw-Hill.

Schleifer, S. J., Keller, S. E., Bond, R. N., Cohen, J., & Stein, M. (1989). Major depressive disorder and immunity. *Archives of General Psychiatry, 46*, 81–87.

Siever, L. J., & Davis, K. L. (1985). Overview: Toward a dysregulation hypothesis of depression. *American Journal of Psychiatry, 142*, 1017–1031.

U.S. Congress, Office of Technology Assessment. (1985). *Technology and aging in America* (OTA-BA-264). Washington, DC: U.S. Government Printing Office.

U.S. Congress, Office of Technology Assessment. (1990). *Confused minds, burdened families* (OTA-BA-403). Washington, DC: U.S. Government Printing Office.

U.S. Department of Health and Human Services. (1989). *Report of the advisory panel on Alzheimer's disease* (DHHS Publication No. (ADM) 89-1644). Washington, DC: U.S. Government Printing Office.

Vieth, R.C., & Raskind, M.A. (1988). The neurobiology of aging: Does it predispose to depression? *Neurobiology of Aging, 9*, 101–117.

Weiner, H. (1985). Schizophrenia: Etiology. In H. I. Kaplan & B. J. Sadock (Eds.), *Comprehensive textbook of psychiatry/IV* (Vol. 1). Baltimore, MD: Williams & Wilkins.

Wells, K. B., Stewart, A., Hays, R. D., Burnam, M. A., Rogers, W., Daniels, M., Berry, S., Greenfield, S., & Ware, J. (1989). The functioning and well-being of depressed patients. *Journal of the American Medical Association, 262*, 914–919.

Williams, T. F., & Katzman, B. (1988). Public policy issues. In L. F. Jarvik & C. H. Winograd (Eds.), *Treatments for the Alzheimer patient* (pp. 147–154). New York: Springer.

Willis, D. P. (Ed.). (1989). *Health policies and black Americans*. New Brunswick, NJ: Transaction Publishers.

Willis, S. L. (1985). Toward an educational psychology of the older adult learner: Intellectual and cognitive bases. In J. E. Birren & K. W. Schaife (Eds.), *Handbook of the psychology of aging*. New York: Van Nostrand Reinhold.

Author Index _____

Aalto, U., 575, *581*
Abbott, M. H., 380, *402*
Abel, L. A., 254, *300*
Abelson, H. I., 537, *551*
Abernethy, D. R., 423–424, *427*, *428*, 729, 730, *756*, *758*
Abos, J., 495, *503*
Abou-Saleh, M. T., 500, *503*
Abrahams, J. P., 829, *829*
Abrahamsson, M., 262, *296*
Abram, H. S., 399, *400*
Abrams, R. C., 236, *246*, 381, 386, *400*, 530, 532, 537, 538, *545*, 738, *756*
Abramson, J. H., 542, *545*
Abrass, I. B., 822, *830*
Abusaura, L. C., 258, *300*
Ackerman, A. M., 330, *334*
Ackerman, D. L., 744, *759*
Ackerman, L. J., 589, *597*
Adam, M. J., 209, *227*
Adam, T., 186, *195*
Adams, A. J., 256, 264, *295*, *299*
Adams, C., 314, *335*
Adams, D. L., 358, *371*
Adams, F., 90, *96*
Adams, I., 177, *194*
Adams, K. M., 520, 527, *546*, *549*, 625, *639*
Adams, M., 822, *831*
Adams, R. D., 493, 497, *503*, *512*
Adams, W. L., 60, *66*, 522, *545*
Aday, L. A., 801, *810*
Adelstein, S. J., 861, *871*
Adey, M., 236, 244, *248*, 419, *431*
Adey, M. B., 15, *26*
Adey, V., 327, *337*, 617, *641*
Adinolfi, A. M., 177, *196*
Adlaf, E. M., 521, 523, 529, 530, *553*
Adler, F. H., 254, *295*

Adler, M., 903, *912*
Adler, W. H., 494–495, *507*
Adolfsson, R., 188, *194*, 486, *513*
Adreason, N. C., 47, *70*
Aflin-Slater, R. B., 540, *545*
Agid, Y., 488, *505*, 657, *668*
Agner, E., 540, *545*
Agranoff, B. W., 204, *224*
Agras, W. S., 414, *431*
Agree, E. M., 874–875
Aharon-Peretz, J., 624, *637*
Ahern, F. M., 436, *459*
Ahles, S., 393, *403*
AIA Foundation, 764, *790*
Aiello, G., 184, *197*
Aiken, L., 794, 796, *810*
Aitken, J. T., 158, *169*
Akerlund, B. M., 711, *713*
Akerlund, M., 486, *512*
Akiguchi, I., 159, *172*
Akiskal, H. S., 444, *457*
Alafuzoff, I., 188, *194*
Alagna, S. W., 539, *550*
Alair, A., 164, *172*
Alauddin, M., 484, *508*
Alavi, A., 205, *223*
Albert, M., 328, *337*, 754, *759*
Albert, M. L., 619, *637*, 656, *663*
Albert, M. S., 33, *68*, 201, 209, *224*, 237, *248*, 329, *331*, 391, *403*, 480, 482, 485, *505*, *507*, 644, 645, 646, *663*, *665*, 753, *758*
Alberts, M. J., 481, *511*
Aldrich, M. S., 204, *224*
Alexander, A. B., 420, *427*
Alexander, F., 524, *545*
Alexander, F. G., 672, *694*, 702, *713*
Alexander, G. E., 221, *223*

Alexander, J., 454, *461*
Alexopoulos, G., 381, *405*
Alexopoulos, G. S., *71*, 236, *246*, 381, 386,
    387, *400*, 448, 530, 532, 537, 538, *545*,
    730, 738, 742, *756*, *762*
Alexopoulous, G. S., 396, *407*
Allan, J. S., 576, *577*
Allen, M. J., 253, *295*
Allen, R. H., 485, 494, *504*, *508*
Allen, R. M., 746, 751, *756*
Allen, S. J., 182, *194*
Allison, Y., 184, *199*
Allman, J. M., 221, *224*
Alom, J., 495, *503*
Alpers, J. H., 422, *431*
Alpiner, J. G., 277, *295*
Alston, R. L., 152–153, *171*
Alterman, I., 56, *69*
Altman, I., 764, 766, *790*, *791*
Alvarez, S. L., 252–253, *304*
Alzheimer, A., 148, 156, 157, *169*
Amadio, L., 177, *194*
Amaducci, L., 214, *228*
Amaducci, L. A., 38, *66*
Ameblas, A., 383, *400*
American College of Physicians, 863, 867,
    868
American National Standards Institute, 268,
    295
American Nurses' Association, 825, *829*
American Psychiatric Association, 32, 57, *66*,
    326–327, *331*, 410, 412, *427*, 434, *457*,
    464, 465, 470, 473, 478, *503*, 517, 518,
    526, 530, *545*, 645, 656, *663*, 675, *694*,
    725, 746, 747, 748, 751, *756*, 795, *810*,
    866, 867, *869*
American Psychiatric Association Office of
    Economic Affairs, 878, 882, *889*
Amigo, E., 240, *247*, 687, 691, *696*
Ammann, W., 209, *227*
Amoore, J. E., 285, 286, *295*, *305*
Amoss, P. T., 84, *96*
Anaducci, L., 40, *72*
Anastasia, A., 348, *352*
Ancill, R. J., 533, *545*
Ancoli-Israel, S., 562, 564, 568, 571, 572,
    577, *578*
Anderasen, N. C., 391, *407*
Andersen, R., 801, *810*

Anderson, D. J., 589, *596*
Anderson, J. M., 153, *169*, *171*, 188, *196*
Anderson, J. R., 308, *331*
Anderson, O., 801, *810*
Anderson, V. E., 214, *226*
Anderson, W. F., 399, *402*
Anderson-Ray, S. M., 397, *407*
Andersson, H., 493, *513*
Anderton, B., 157, *172*
Andreasen, N. C., 47, *71*, 613, *637*
Andres, D., 312, *331*
Andres, R., 526, *554*
Angleitner, A., 358, *371*
Anglin, M. D., 536, 537, *545*
Angst, J., 384, *400*
Ankier, S. I., 393, *400*
Annab, L., 167, *173*
Anschutz, L., 318, *331*
Ansell, P. L., 253, *301*
Anthony, J., 523, 524, 526, *549*
Anthony, J. C., 28, 29, 32, 33, 35, 37, 39,
    40, 41, 43, 47, 48, 49, 52, 54, 56, 57,
    58, 59, 60, 62, 65, *66*, *67*, *68*, *69*, *70*,
    72, 410, 412, *430*, 531, 536, *551*, 618,
    637, 799, 800, *811*
Anthony, W., 675, 680, *694*
Anthony, W. A., 675, 676, *694*, *695*
Antonelli, A. R., 274, *295*
Apicella, A., 207, *228*
Appelbaum, P. S., 858, *869*
Appelbaum, S. L., 285, 287, 294, *297*
Appelt, G. D., 539, *545*
Applebaum, R., 886, *890*
Appleby, R. G., 280, *302*
Applegate, W., 682, *694*
Applegate, W. B., 530, *552*, 618, *637*
Apter, S., 221, *228*
Arai, Y., 177, *197*
Araki, F., 111, *117*
Aranyi, L., 764, *790*
Arato, M., 483, *506*
Arboleda-Florez, J., 440, *457*
Arbuckle, T. Y., 312, *331*
Archea, J., 766, *790*
Arenberg, D., 318, *336*, 356, *372*
Arendt, A., 180, *194*
Arendt, T., 180, *194*
Arey, L., 279, *295*
Arie, T., 530, 532, 542, *548*, *551*

Armanini, M., 500, *511*
Armbrecht, H. J., 526, *555*
Armstrong, D. M., 177, *196*, 487, *506*
Armstrong, H. F., 588, *596*
Arnold, L., 183, 189, *198*
Aronow, W. S., 541, *545*
Aronson, M., 191, *195*
Aronson, M. K., 14, *25*, 646, 652, *667*, 835, *851*
Aronson, S. M., 489, *509*
Arras, J. D., 868, *870*
Arregui, A., 184, *196*
Arvidson, K., 279, *295*
Asberg, K. H., 245, *246*
Ashcraft, M. H., 308, *331*
Asher, D. M., 496, *507*
Ashford, J. W., 215, *227*, 645, *666*, *668*
Ashikaga, T., 466, 467, 469, *474*
Ashton, H., 530, 532, 534, 535, *545*
Askinazi, C., 395, *400*
Astrachan, B., 874, 878, 879, *889*
Atack, J. R., 484, 487, 488, *504*, *505*, *509*
Atchley, R. C., 87, *96*, 364, 365, *372*, 704, *713*
Ather, S. A., 393, *400*
Atkinson, J., 258, *296*
Atkinson, J. H., 516, 523, 525, 528, *546*, *553*
Atkinson, J. W., 360, *372*
Atkinson, R. M., 516, 519, 520, 522, 524, 525, 526, 527, 528, 529, 537, *545*, *546*, *550*
Attneave, C., 110, *117*
Auchenbach, R., 382, *403*
Ausman, L. M., 524, *549*
Autio, L., 471, *474*
Auvinen, J., 575, *579*
Avery, D., 382, *400*
Avery, D. H., 560, 568, *581*
Avioli, L. V., 214, *223*
Avorn, J., 530, *546*, 728, 752, *757*, *758*, 840, 841, *849*, *950*
Axelrod, S., 290, 291, *295*
Azrin, N. H., 708, *716*

Baastrup, P., 384, *400*
Bacchetti, P., 495, *503*

Bach-Peterson, J., 805, *813*
Bachar, J. R., 381, 382, 398, 399, *401*
Bacher, Y., 486, *506*
Badash, D., 386, *402*
Baddeley, A., 317, *331*
Baddeley, A. D., 317, *337*
Bagley, C. R., 605, *638*
Bahrick, H. P., 331, *331*
Bail, G., 414, *431*
Bail, K., 260, *304*
Bailey, F., 17, *25*, 798, *812*
Bailey, P., 486, *506*
Bailey, R. B., 540, *546*
Baillie, M., 148, *169*
Baines, S., 710, 711, *713*
Bainton, B. R., 524, 525, *547*
Baird, P. A., 587, *596*
Baker, E. L., 38, *72*
Baker, F. M., 856, 860, 866, *869*
Bakke, K. J., 841, *851*
Baldessraini, R. J., 421, *427*
Baldinelli, L., 312, *336*
Baldridge, J. A., 523, *547*
Baldwin, R. C., 385, *401*
Baldy, R., 391, *403*
Ball, K., 260, 264, *295*, *296*
Ball, M. J., 188, *194*, 488, *503*
Ballard, P. A., 186, *196*
Balldin, J., 500, *503*
Ballenger, J. C., 417, 423, *427*
Baloh, R. W., 254, *305*
Balough, K., 280, *296*
Balter, M. B., 530, 531, 535, 538, *546*, *551*, *552*, *554*
Baltes, M. M., 363, *372*
Baltes, P. B., 330, *331*, 363, *372*
Bamford, K. A., 629, *638*
Ban, T. A., 424, *430*, 498, *510*
Banaji, M. R., 308, *331*
Banerjee, S. P., 184, *198*
Banford, D., 263, *296*
Bang, S., 328, *333*, 648, 652, *665*
Banks, P. G., 646, *663*
Bannister, R., 190, *194*
Baratz, R., 240, *248*
Barbano, H. E., 358, *372*, 437, 445, *457*
Barber v. Superior Court, 862, *869*
Barclay, G. H., 492, *506*
Bardolph, E. L., 151, *171*

Bareggi, S. R., 182, *194*, 564, *581*
Barker, W., 219, *224*, 624, *638*
Barker, W. W., 207, 211, *224*, 228
Barlow, D. H., 417, 422, *427*
Barlow, H. B., 258, *306*
Barnes, G. M., 523, 524, *546*
Barnes, R., 387, 394, *406*, 498, 499, 500, *503*, *510*, *512*, 733, 737, *761*, 842, *850*, *852*
Barnes, R. A., 907, *912*
Barnes, R. F., 384, 388, *404*, 500, *512*, 834, *849*
Barnes, R. H., 382, *401*
Baron, J.-C., 205, *227*, 228
Baron, M., 381, 382, *401*, 405
Barona, A., 651, *663*
Barr, A. N., 472, *474*
Barrat, J., 167, *173*
Barrett, J. E., 795, *813*
Barrett, P., 526, *554*
Barrett, T. R., 310, *331*
Barrett, V. W., 243, *247*
Barry, P., 825, *831*
Barry, S., 701, *717*
Bars, P., 282, 283, *296*
Barthel, D., 685, 689, *696*
Bartlett, J., 230, *246*, 896, *912*
Barton, R., 498, *504*
Bartoshuk, L. M., 282, 283, *296*
Bartus, R., 14, *24*, 617, *638*
Bartus, R. T., 180, *194*, 326, *332*, 732, 754, *757*
Barusch, A. S., 368, 369, *372*
Basen, M. M., 529, *546*
Baskin, D., 805, 806, *813*
Bass, D. M., 234, *246*, 807, 808, *812*
Bassey, J., 542, *548*
Basteris, L., 271, *303*
Bastida, E., 114, *115*
Bates, D., 691, *696*
Baugh, D. K., 747, *760*
Baum, B. J., 280, 282, 283, *306*
Baxter, C. F., 158, *172*
Baxter, L. R., 214, 220, 221, *223*, 226
Bayles, K. A., 649, 652–653, 657, *663*
Baylor, A. M., 346, 347, *352*
Beal, M. A., 164, *169*
Beal, M. F., 153, *169*, 486, 488, *503*, 508
Beamish, P., 42, *70*
Bean, P., 537, *546*

Beaney, R. P., 205, *227*
Beard, B. L., 260, *296*
Beard, C. M., 488, *510*
Beard, O. W., 523, *547*
Beardsley, R. S., 18, *23*, 530, *546*, 728, 746, 752, *757*, 804, *812*, 840, *850*
Beattie, B. L., 40, *68*, 209, *227*, 645, *668*
Beaumont, G., 394, *401*
Bebbington, P. E., 43, 46, 47, 48, *66*
Beck, A. T., 392, *401*, 417, 419, 422, *427*, 617, *637*, 709, *713*
Beck, C., 821, *829*
Beck, J., 126, *141*
Beck, R. W., 617, *637*
Becker, E. R., 882, 883, *890*
Becker, F. D., 768, *790*
Becker, J. T., 649, 650, 657, *665*, 666
Becker, M., 593, *597*
Becker, R., 754, *759*
Becker, R. E., 645, *668*
Beckham, K., 526, *548*, 710, *713*
Beckman, N., 278, *298*
Bednarski, P., 58, 60, *69*
Bednarski, P. B., 523, 524, 526, *549*
Beer, B., 180, *194*, 732, *757*
Beers, M., 530, *546*, 728, 752, *757*, 840, *850*
Begleiter, H., 516, *550*
Behan, D., 382, *407*
Behar, M., 539, *548*
Beigel, A., 836, *850*
Beiser, M., 110, *117*
Belal, A., 266, *296*
Belal, A., Jr., 266, *297*
Belbout, J., 481, *511*
Bell, A., 588, *596*
Bell, B., 260, *296*
Bell, J., 164, *169*
Bell, J. M., 486, *511*
Bell, P. A., 38, *67*
Bellacosa, J. W., 861, *869*
Bellchambers, M. J. G., 656, 657, *666*
Belle, S. H., 14, *26*, 649, *666*
Beller, S. A., 617, *640*
Bellini, F., 190, *195*
Belloc, N. B., 573, *577*
Benardo, L. S., 180, 190, *196*, 198
Benbow, S. M., 386, 396, *401*
Bengtson, V. L., 8, *25*, 103, *115*, 364, 365, *372*, *373*
Benjamin, Y. N., 713, *717*

Bennett, C., 261, *296*
Bennett, R., 448, *457*
Bennett-Levy, J., 313, *331*
Benson, D. F., 209, 210, 211, 215, 219, *223*, 227, 388, *405*, 447, *461*, 629, 632, 633, *638*, 645, 653, 656, *664*, *666*
Benson, D. M., 847, *850*
Benson, F., 653, *668*
Bentin, S., 205, *227*
Benton, A. L., 328, *331*, 646, 648, 653, *663*, 665
Benton, J. S., 182, *194*
Beran, B., 386, *402*
Berardi, A., 209, *223*
Berchon, R., 747, *760*
Berchon, R. C., 747, *760*
Berchou, R. C., 575, *580*
Berdzilovich, G. N., 491, *506*
Berent, S., 204, *224*
Beresford, T. P., 520, *546*
Berezin, M. A., 816, *829*
Berg, G., 214, 215, 216, 217, 222, *223*, *225*, 495, *504*, *513*, 645, *665*
Berg, G. W., 207, 213, *225*, *228*
Berg, L., 151, *170*, 646, 648, 651, 653, *663*, *666*, *669*
Berger, L. R., 495, *510*
Bergeron, C., 184, *198*
Berglund, M., 522, *552*
Bergman, H., 486, *506*
Bergman, K., 386, *404*
Bergman, M., 271, 274, 275, *296*, *303*
Bergmann, K., 31, *70*, 412, *427*, 473, *475*
Berkanovic, E., 802, *810*
Berkman, C., 239, *247*
Berkman, C. S., 680, 681, *694*, 795, 803, *812*
Berkman, L., 680, 681, *694*
Berkowitz, M. W., 442, *457*
Berkowitz, N., 240, *247*, 652, 667, 687, 691, *696*
Berkson, G., 590, *596*
Berlin, C. I., 275, *296*
Berman, J., 523, 525, 528, *553*
Berman, S. R., 13, *26*, 559, 561, 562, 564, 569, 571, 572, 576, *577*, *578*, *580*
Berney, S., 498, *510*
Bernhardt, S., 767, 768, *791*
Bernholz, C. D., 260, *296*
Bernick, C., 737, *762*

Bernstein, D. A., 422, *427*
Bernstein, L., 728, *758*
Bernstein, N., 328, *334*
Berrios, G. E., 471, 472, *473*
Berry, D. T. R., 562, *577*
Berry, J., 314, *335*
Berry, S., 907, *914*
Bertolucci, D., 520, *553*
Bertoni-Freddari, C., 177, *194*
Bertsch, J. D., 260, *299*
Besdine, R. W., 728, *761*
Besson, J. A. O., 624, 625, *638*, *639*
Bestal, R. E., 728, *760*
Bevan, J. A., 164, *170*
Beveer, W. C., 572, *577*
Bhatt, A., 847, *851*
Bhrolchain, M., 241, *246*
Bi Chiro, G., 495, *504*
Biaggioni, I., 539, *546*
Bialow, M., 388, *406*
Bielawska, C., 618, *638*
Bienenfeld, D., 838, *850*
Biesele, M., 84, *96*
Bigl, V., 180, *194*
Bigler, E. D., 151, *169*
Billick, S. B., 854, 855, *869*
Billig, N., 835, *850*
Billings, A. G., 239, 241, *246*
Binder, L. I., 483, *507*
Biorn-Henriksen, T., 386, *405*
Birch, D., 360, *372*
Bird, E., 184, *196*
Bird, E. D., 190, *197*, 493, *513*
Bird, H. R., 109, *115*
Bird, T. D., 182, 189, *194*, 480, *511*
Birkett, P., 688, 693, *695*
Birren, J. E., 4, 7, 10, *23*, 103, *115*, 208, *223*, 252, 262, 274, 292, *296*, *300*, 325, *337*, 340, 342, *352*, 365, *374*, 585, *596*
Bishop, E. R., 470, *474*
Bissette, G., 483, 486, *504*, *506*, *511*
Bixler, E. D., 751, *759*
Bixler, E. O., 564, 566, *579*
Bjork, E. L., 308, *331*
Bjork, J., 110, *117*
Bjork, R. A., 308, *331*
Black, B., 240, *247*, 687, 691, *696*
Black, F. W., 612, *641*
Black, J. L., 733, *757*
Blackman, D. K., 708, *716*

Blackstock, J., 618, *638*
Blackwell, B., 420, *431*
Blair, J., 651, *663*
Bland, R. C., 60, *69*
Blankfield, A., 64, *67*
Blass, J., 654, *668*
Blass, J. B., 618, *637*
Blass, J. P., 497, *504*
Blau, A., 646, 652, *667*
Blau, E., 654, *663*
Blaustein, J., 836, *852*
Blazeer, D., 798, *811*
Blazer, D., 14, *23*, 35, 37, 42, 58, 59, 62, 64, 65, *67*, *68*, 349, *352*, 380, 383, *401*, 438, 451, *457*, 470, *474*, 633, *637*, 681, *694*, 738, 739, *757*, 795, *811*, 819, *829*, 898, 902, *912*
Blazer, D. G., 28, 41, 42, 49, 51, 52, 54, 57, 58, *67*, *68*, 108, *115*, 380, 381, 382, 383, 384, 385, 386, 388, 389, 394, 397, 398, 399, *401*, *402*, *403*, *404*, *407*, 528, *546*, 617, *639*, 680, *694*, 794, 795, 799, 800, 802, 803, 804, *810*, *811*, 817, 818, *830*, 840, *850*
Blennow, K., 182, 189, *194*
Blessed, G., 30, 31, *67*, 154, 158, *173*, 180, *198*, 240, *246*, 484, 485, 487, 488, 490, *504*, *505*, *509*, *512*, 686, 691, *694*
Bleuler, E., 464, 466, 467, *474*
Bleuler, M., 185, *194*
Bliding, A., 420, *431*
Bliwise, D. L., 572, *577*
Bliwise, N. G., 572, *577*
Blixen, C. E., 816, *829*
Block, C., 838, *850*
Block, J., 135, *141*
Block, R., 575, *580*, 747, *760*
Blomstrand, C., 493, *513*
Bloom, F. E., 180, *198*
Bloom, S. R., 182, 183, 189, *195*
Blow, F. C., 520, *546*
Bloxham, C. A., 487, 488, *509*
Blum, L., 522, *546*
Blumenthal, J. A., 347, *352*
Blumenthal, M. D., 410, *427*
Blusewicz, M. J., 652, *666*
Boatman, R. A., 38, *68*
Boberg-Ans, J., 290, *296*
Bocca, E., 27, *296*
Boczkowski, J. A., 838, *850*

Bohman, M., 517, 524, *547*
Bokan, J. A., 571, *581*
Bolduc, P. L., 501, *511*
Boller, F., 488, *504*, 649, 656, *664*, *666*
Bolton, C. F., 289, 290, *296*
Bond, R. N., 907, *913*
Bondareff, W., 152, 154, *169*, *170*, 180, 188, *194*, *196*, 486, 491, *504*
Bonekat, J. W., 319, *332*
Bonett, D. G., 536, 537, *545*
Bongort, K., 360, *372*
Bonini, L., 182, *194*
Boone, D. R., 649, 652, *663*
Boone, K. B., 646, *664*
Boorson, S., 907, *912*
Booth, H., 622, *639*
Boothe, T., 207, *228*
Bootzin, R. R., 705, 708, *713*
Booze, L., 536, *550*
Booze, R. M., 190, *194*, 486, *504*
Borenstein, J., 497, *510*
Borenstein, M. D., 753, *760*
Borgatta, E. F., 523, *546*
Borgesen, S. E., 493, *512*
Borkovec, T. D., 422, *427*
Bornstein, P. E., 822, *830*
Bornstein, R. A., 659, *664*
Borrie, M. J., 523, 524, 526, *546*
Borson, S., 234, 239, 240, 245, *246*, *248*, 676, *697*, 837, 841, 844, *850*
Borst, M., 154, *169*
Bortin, L., 204, *228*
Borwein, B., 253, *301*
Bosse, R., 523, 541, *546*, *548*
Boston Collaborative Drug Surveillance Program, 423, *427*
Boszormenyi-Nagy, I., 713, *715*
Botwinick, J., 252, *296*, 328, *336*, 345, 346, 347, 349, *352*, 434, 436, *457*, 648, 653, *669*, 700, *713*
Bouchard, G. R., 522, 524, *548*, *549*
Bouchard, R., 486, *506*
Bouras, C., 191, *195*
Bousser, M.-G., 205, *227*, *228*
Boust, S. J., 617, *637*
Bowden, J. J., 422, *431*
Bowen, B., 219, 224, 624, *638*
Bowen, D. M., 182, 183, 188, *194*, *195*, *197*, 485, 486, *506*, *509*
Bowen, M., 7, *23*

Bowers, M. B., 843, *850*
Bowers, W., 454, *461*
Bowlby, J., 129, *141*
Bowman, M. J., 439, *457*
Boyd, J. H., 34, 35, 41, 49, 51, 57, 58, 60,
   71, 109, *116*, 410, 412, *430*, 531, 536,
   551
Boyko, R. B., 468, *474*
Boyton, R. M., 253, *303*
Bozza, G., 292, *303*
Braakman, R., 190, *196*
Bracco, L., 38, *66*
Bracha, H. S., 735, *759*
Braddick, O., 258, *296*
Braddock, D., 592, *597*
Bradford, D. C., 319, *332*
Bradley, R. M., 285, *296*
Bradley, W. G., 151, *171*
Brady, T. J., 623, 624, *639*
Braff, D., 329, *337*
Braffman, B. H., 491, *504*
Branch, L., 689, *694*
Branch, L. G., 604, 688, *694*
Branconnier, R. J., 661, *664*, 742, 743, *757*
Brandt, J., 652, *666*
Brandt, L. J., 268, *296*
Brane, G., 182, 189, *194*
Brannon, D., 838, *852*
Brant, L. J., 836, *852*
Brant-Zawadzki, M., 492, *505*, 624, *638*
Brauer, D., 701, *716*
Braun, J., 845, *852*
Braun, P., 882, 883, *890*
Brayden, J. E., 164, *170*
Breakefield, X. O., 896, *913*
Brecht, M. L., 536, 537, *545*
Breckenridge, J. N., 13, *24*
Breckenridge, J. S., 392, *407*, 709, *717*
Bredberg, G., 266, *296*
Breen, A., 328, *337*
Breen, A. R., 237, *248*, 660, *664*
Bregman, J. D., 590, *596*
Breier, A., 466, 467, 469, *474*
Breitbart, M., 496, *504*
Breitner, J., 468, *474*
Breitner, J. C. S., 40, *67*, 384, 387, 388,
   394, 397, *404*, 482, *504*
Breivik, K., 841, *851*
Brekhus, S., 845, *852*
Brendel, D. H., 559, *577*

Brennan, P. L., 525, *546*, *551*
Brenner, L. L., 804, 806, *812*
Brenner, R. P., 621, *637*
Breslau, L., 448, *457*
Breslow, N. E., 40, *67*
Brew, B., 495, *510*
Brewer, C., 497, *504*
Bridge, T. P., 89, *912*
Bridger, J. E., 158, *169*
Bridges-Webb, C., 530, *551*
Bridgewater, R., 523, *546*
Briest, J. C., 494, *508*
Brietner, J. C. S., 482, *508*
Brink, T., 327, *337*, 617, *641*
Brink, T. L., 15, *26*, 236, 244, *248*, 419, *431*
Brinkman, S. D., 150, *170*, 485, *504*
Brizzee, K. R., 253, 266, *302*
Broadbent, D., 323, *331*
Broadbent, D. E., 313, *331*
Broadhead, J., 836, *852*
Brock, M. A., 568, *577*
Broder, S., 495, *504*
Brodie, H. K. H., 803, *813*
Brodie, J., 205, *224*
Brody, A., 484, *509*
Brody, E., 369, *372*, 673, 676, 679, 686,
   690, 693, *694*, *696*
Brody, E. M., 618, *640*
Brody, H., 152, 154, 155, 159, *170*, *173*,
   176, 180, *194*, *199*, 266, *296*
Brody, J., 680, 681, *694*
Brody, J. A., 42, *73*, 496, *513*
Brodzinsky, D. M., 291, *300*
Broe, G. A., 39, *67*
Broman, C. L., 801, *812*
Bromley, D. B., 277, *296*, 410, *427*
Bromley, M. C., 713, *715*
Brook, P., 471, 472, *473*
Brook, P. B., 501, *509*
Brookbank, J., 341, 344 , 347, 348, *352*
Brookes, D. N., 590, *596*
Brooks, D. J., 205, *227*
Brooks, G. W., 466, 467, 469, *474*
Brooks, R., 209, 210, 212, *224*
Brooks, R. A., 211, 214, *224*
Broskowski, H., 525, 529, *548*
Brotherson, M. J., 593, *599*
Brouwers, P., 495, *513*
Brow, R. L., 801, *812*
Brower, K. J., 520, *546*

Browers, P., 650, *667*
Brown, A. L., 318, *331*
Brown, C. H., 29, 41, 59, *66, 70*
Brown, D. R., 52, 54, 56, *67*, 108, *115*
Brown, E., 537, *547*
Brown, G., 127, *141*, 419, *427*, 651, *670*
Brown, G. L., 396, *401*
Brown, G. W., 125, 127, *141*, 241, *246*
Brown, J. M., 388, *406*
Brown, L. L., 388, *401*
Brown, R., 381, 382, *401*
Brown, R. G., 487, *504*
Brown, R. P., 221, *228*, 498, *505*, 739, *757*
Brown, T., 237, 240, *247*
Brozek, J., 262, *296*
Bruce, M. L., 41, 42, 47, 48, *73*, 380, 384, *407*
Bruemmer, V., 191, *196*
Bruenberg, E., 438, *460*
Brugha, T. S., 619, *637*
Bruhn, P., 493, *512*
Bruininks, R. H., 589, *596*
Brummel-Smith, K., 109, *116*, 675, 692, *694, 695*
Brun, A., 149, 151, 156, *170*, 209, *223*, 491, *504*
Brunetti, A., 495, *504, 513*
Bruni, A., 214, *228*
Bruni, A. J., 40, *72*
Brust, J. C. M., 491, *504*, 656, 658, *664*
Bruton, C. J., 40, *67*
Bryant, G. O., 422, *431*
Buchner, D., 725, *759*
Buchsbaum, M. S., 207, *223*
Buchwald, N. A., 177, *196*
Buck, J. A., 728, 746, 752, *757*, 840, *850*
Buckingham, P., 205, *227*
Buckingham, T., 263, *296*
Bucknell, J. C., 611, *637*
Budinger, T. F., 209, 211, 214, 215, *225, 226*
Budzilovich, G. N., 189, *195*
Buell, S. J., 159, 161, 163, *170*
Bugiani, O., 191, *195*
Buhl-Auth, J., 110, *117*
Buhler, C., 120, *141*
Buie, D. H., 450, *459*
Bunney, W. E., 569, *578*
Buonanno, F. S., 623, 624, *639, 640*
Burg, A., 262, 263, *296*

Burghauser, R., 280, *306*
Burgio, K. L., 708, *713, 717*
Burke, D. M., 308, *331*
Burke, H., 687, 692, *694*
Burke, J., 802, 810, *811*
Burke, J. D., 34, 35, 41, 43, 49, 51, 56, 57, 58, 60, *67, 71*, 410, 412, *430*, 531, 536, *551*
Burke, J. O., 438, *460*
Burke, K. C., 43, 56, *67*
Burke, W. J., 396, *401*, 617, *637*
Burkhardt, C. R., 489, *504*
Burkhart, C., 827, 828, *830*
Burnam, A., 56, 58, 60, *69, 70*, 110, *115*, 536, *550*, 618, *638*
Burnam, M. A., 108, 109, 110, *115, 116, 117*, 907, *914*
Burns, B., 794, 795, 797, 798, 799, 804, *811*
Burns, B. J., 18, *23*, 530, *546*, 728, 746, 752, *757*, 802, 803, 810, *811*, 840, *850*
Burns, G. A., 481, *512*
Burns, M., 575, *577*
Burns, S., 657, *669*
Burres, M. J. K., 213, *228*
Burrows, G. D., 423, *427*
Burton, L. C., 18, *24*
Busby, W. J., 523, 524, 526, *546*
Buschke, H., 326, 328, *332, 333*, 646, 648, 651, 652, *664, 665*
Bushey, M., 843, *850*
Busse, E. W., 6, 11, *23, 26*, 362, *372*, 382, *401*, 410, *427*, 516, *546*, 818, *830*
Butler, F. K., 417, *430*
Butler, R., 132, *141*
Butler, R. M., 208, *223*
Butler, R. N., 107, 112, *115*, 204, *223*, 327, *332*, 410, *427*, 438, *457*, 700, 711, *713*, 820, *830*
Butterfield, A., 836, *850*
Butterfield, D., 768, *790*
Butters, N., 328, *336*, 526, *553*, 571, *577*, 652, *664*
Butzke, C., 691, *696*
Buysse, D. J., 559, 564, 566, 569, 572, *577*, *578*
Buzzelli, G., 292, *303*
Byme, D. G., 349, *352*
Byrd, M., 311, 312, *332*
Byrne, E. J., 489, *507*

Byrnes, V. A., 261, *296*
Byyny, B. C., 753, *762*
Bzowej, N., 184, *198*

Cadieux, D. W., 564, *579*
Cadieux, R. J., 566, *579*
Cadigan, D. A., 530, 535, *546*
Caey, P., 438, 439, *457*
Caffe, E. M., 498, *510*
Cafferata, G. L., 807, *811*
Cafferta, G. L., 593, *599*
Cahalan, D., 523, *546*
Cahan, R. B., 820, *831*
Cain, W. S., 284, 286, 287, 288, *303, 305*
Caine, E., 654, *664*
Caine, E. D., 14, *24*, 528, *547*, 604, 605,
    622, 629, 634, 635, *638, 639*
Cairl, R., 687, 692, *694*
Cajal, S., 486, *513*
Calden, G., 443, *457*
Calderini, G., 190, *195*
Caldwell, A. B., 566, *579*
Caldwell, J. H., 500, *512*
Calkins, E., 828, *830*
Calkins, M., 764, 765, *790*
Call, P., 496, *504*
Call, T. L., 586, 588, *597*
Callahan, D., 867, *869*
Callahan, J. J., 19, *24*
Callahan, L., 864, *869*
Callaway, R., 624, *639*
Callison, D. A., 588, *596*
Calloway, S. P., 391, *402*
Calne, D., 186, *195*
Calne, D. B., 209, *227*, 493, *507*
Caltagirone, C., 657, *665*
Camara, M., 271, *303*
Cambell, A. J., 523, 524, 526, *546*
Cameron, D., 847, *850*
Camp, C. J., 318, 330, *331, 332*
Campbell, D. W., 571, *578*
Campbell, E. B., 821, *831*
Campbell, F. W., 258, *296*
Campbell, J., 527, *550*
Campbell, K., 280, *303*
Campbell, K. B., 707, *716*
Campbell, M., 423, *431*

Campbell, M. J., 222, *227*
Campbell, S., 310, *334*
Campione, J. C., 318, *331*
Campisi, J., 167, *172*
Candy, J. M., 484, 487, 488, *504, 509*
Canino, G., 109, *115*
Canino, G. J., 60, *69*
Cannon, C. J., 340, *353*
Cannon, H. E., 899, *912*
Cannon, R. L., 588, *596*
Cannon, W. B., 417, *428*
Canterbury v. Spence, 858, *869*
Capel, W. C., 536, 537, *546, 547*
Capitani, E., 328, *332*
Capitman, J. A., 910, *912*
Caplan, B., 661, *664*
Capron, A. M., 867, *870*
Caraceni, T., 184, *197*
Cardoret, R. J., 47, *67*
Carella, F., 184, *197*
Carhardt, R., 272, *305*
Carkadon, M. A., 558, 561, 568, *577*
Carlsson, A., 40, *67*, 486, *513*
Carner, E. A., 797, 802, *813*
Carney, M., 396, *401*
Carni, E., 712, *715*
Carnicke, C. L. M., 389, *402*
Caro, J. P., 539, *547*
Carp, F., 766, *790*
Carpenter, T. A., 484, 488, *504, 505*
Carr, T., 624, *639*
Carrier, L., 486, *506*
Carroll, B. J., 236, *246*
Carroll, J. A., 744, *759*
Carrwel, P., 261, *305*
Carskadon, M. A., 566, 568, *577, 581*
Carson, R., 207, *228*
Carson, R. C., 355, *372*
Carson, R. E., 205, 218, 221, *225, 226*
Carstens, D., 781, *790*
Carstensen, L. L., 705, 706, 707, 709, *713*,
    804, 806, *812*
Carter, W., 239, *246*, 907, *912*
Cartwright, W. S., 902, *913*
Case, G. W., 535, *552*
Case, W. G., 422, *431*
Casella, V., 164, *172*
Casey, D. A., 445, *457*
Casey, P., 439, 440, *457, 461*

Casey, P. R., 438, 452, *457*
Cash, R., 488, *504*
Casperson, R. C., 252, *296*
Cassel, C. K., 861, *871*
Cassem, E. H., 861, *871*
Cassem, N. H., 395, *407*
Cassileth, B. R., 388, *401*
Castleden, C. M., 533, *547*
Cater, R., 111, *117*
Cath, S. H., 701, 702, *713*
Cattell, M., 90, *96*
Cattell, R. B., 436, 437, *457, 461*
Cauna, N., 289, *296*
Cavan, R. S., 399, *401*
Cavanaugh, J. C., 310, 313, 314, 316, 318, *332, 335*
Cavanaugh, S. V., 387, *401*
Cavanough, I. C., 357, *375*
Celesia, G. G., 472, *474*
Centers for Disease Control, 495, *504*
Ceorgotas, A., 497, *510*
Cerella, J., 260, *296*
Cermak, L. S., 314, *332*
Chahal, R., 41, 59, *66*
Chaisson, R. E., 495, *503*
Chakeres, D., 633, *639*
Chalke, H. D., 286, *297*
Chalkley, A. J., 417, 422, *428*
Chamberlain, W., 254, *297*
Chambliss, B., 765, *790*
CHAMP, 765, *790*
Chance, J., 687, 691, 692, *696*
Chance, J. M., 237, 240, *248*
Chancellor, A. H. B., 530, *551*
Chandler, J. D., 835, *850*
Chandler, J. E., 835, *850*
Chandra, S., 619, *639*
Chandra, V., 34, 38, *67, 70*
Chang, 743, *758*
Chang, J. Y., 207, 211, *224, 228*
Channing, M. A., 205, *224*
Chanowitz, B., 837, *851*
Chapleski, E. E., 808, 809, *811*
Chapman, W. P., 292, *297*
Chappell, N. L., 103, *117*, 359, *372*
Charbonneau, R., 486, *506*
Charness, N., 342, *352*
Charney, D. S., 381, *401*, 421, *428*
Charny, M., 542, *554*

Chartock, P., 838, *850*
Chase, G. A., 380, *402*, 467, 468, *475*, 500, *509*
Chase, N., 189, *195*, 491, *506*
Chase, T. H., 650, *667*
Chase, T. N., 209, 210, 211, 212, 214, 219, *223, 224, 227*
Chastain, R., 651, *663*
Chawluk, J. B., 205, *223*
Cheah, K.-C., 523, *547*
Chen, B., 186, *198*
Chen, C. H., 33, *70*
Chen, W., 347, *354*
Chenoweth, B., 805, *811*
Cherryman, G. R., 624, 625, *638*
Cherubin, C. E., 522, *551*
Chi, D., 151, *170*
Chi, M. T. H., 310, *332*
Chin, M. R., 821, *831*
Chiofolo, R., 692, *696*
Chmara, J., 399, *406*
Chown, M. J., 33, *68*, 201, 209, *224*, 480, 482, *505*, 753, *758*
Christensen, D. B., 538, 539, *552*
Christensen, J., 266, *304*
Christensen, K. J., 527, *555*, 653, *664*
Christenson, R., 470, *474*
Christians, B., 38, *68*
Christiansen, R. L., 284, *299*
Christie, J. E., 485, *505*
Christman, D. R., 205, 209, 210, 219, *224*
Christopher, F., 711, *713*
Christopherson, V. A., 524, 525, *547*
Christy, J. A., 656, *666*
Chuaqui-Kidd, C., 754, *759*
Chui, H., 680, *694*
Chui, H. C., 151, 152, *170, 171*, 180, *195*, 201, 209, *223*, 656, *664*
Chul, H. C., 488, *505*
Cimasoni, G., 284, *297*
Ciompi, L., 388, *401*, 466, 467, *474*
Cirignotta, F., 562, *579*
Cisin, I. H., 523, 537, 538, *546, 551, 552*
Clamon, C., 847, *850*
Clapp, L. E., 633, *639*, 656, 657, *666*
Clarfield, A. M., 486, *506*
Clark, A. W., 153–154, *173*, 485, *512*
Clark, C., 481, *511*
Clark, C. M., 207, 219, *223, 224*, 481, *509*

Clark, D. M., 417, 422, *428*
Clark, E., 647, *667*
Clark, E. O., 328, *334*, 651, 652, *666*
Clark, J. E., 897, *912*
Clark, T. B., 282, *304*
Clark, W. B., 59, *67*
Clark, W. C., 292, *297*
Clark, W. F., 103, *117*
Clarke, A. H., 415, *428*
Clarke, S., 169, *171*
Clarkson, A. D., 423, *431*
Clarkson-Smith, L., 312, *332*
Clay, H. M., 901, *912*
Clayton, P. J., 47, *71*, 130, *141*, 567, *577*
Clearly, T. A., 847, *850*
Cleary, P. D., 105, 112, *116*
Climo, J. J., 538, 539, *554*
Clipp, E. C., 805, *811*
Cloninger, C. R., 446, *457*, 517, 524, *547*, *552*
Clouston, T. S., 148, *170*
Coakley, J., 517, *550*
Coben, L. A., 651, *666*
Coburn, K. L., 645, *668*
Coburn, S., 575, *578*
Coccagna, G., 562, *579*
Coen-Cole, S., 654, *669*
Coffey, C. E., 14, *24*, 391–392, *401, 402*
Coffman, G. A., 445, *459*
Cogan, D. G., 253, *300*
Coghill, C. R., 153, *169*
Cohen, B., 467, 468, *475*
Cohen, B. F., 676, *694*
Cohen, C. I., 415, *428*
Cohen, D., 805, *811*
Cohen, D. J., 590, *596*
Cohen, E., 765, 767, 768, 783, *791*
Cohen, G., 14, *24*, 314, *332*, 368, *372*
Cohen, G. D., 10, 12, *24, 25*, 326, *332*, 677, 680, *694*, 798, *811*, 894, 895, 896, 897, 898, 899, 901, 906, *912, 913*
Cohen, H. J., 380, 384, 386, 388, 394, *404*, 617, *639*, 817, *830*
Cohen, J., 907, *913*
Cohen, L. D., 290, 291, *295*
Cohen, M. R., 676, *694*
Cohen, R., 484, *509*, 754, *762*
Cohen, R. M., 327, *332*, 386, *402*, 495, 500, *504, 512*, 654, *670*

Cohen, S., 106, *116*
Cohen, T., 284, *297*
Cohen, U., 765, *791*
Cohen-Mansfield, J., 14, *24*, 732, *757*, 835, 836, 845, *850, 852*
Cohler, B., 135, 137, *142*
Cohler, B. J., 77, *96*
Cohn, J. B., 393, *402*, 574, *578*, 743, *758*
Cohn, M. D., 838, *852*
Colarusso, C. A., 700, 703, 704, *713, 716*
Cole, J. O., 575, *581*, 742, 743, *757*
Cole, K. D., 313, *337*
Cole, M. G., 385, *402*
Colearo, C., 275, *296*
Coleman, P. D., 153, 154, 159, 161, 163, *170*, 177, *195*
Coleman, R. E., 347, *352*
Coleman, R. M., 564, *577*
Colenda, C. C., 738, 749, *757*
Colerick, E. J., 805, 806, 808, *811*
Collen, M. F., 292, 293, *306*
Colletti, P. M., 491, *504*
Collier, B., 486, *506*
Collins, G., 292, *297*
Collins, H., 817, 821, 824, *831*
Collins, J., 816, *830*
Colliver, J., 522, *547*
Colorado v. Connelly, 863, *869*
Colsher, P. L., 524, *547*
Colt, H. G., 540, *547*
Colton, J., 256, 265, *299*
Comalli, P., 324, *332*
Comar, M., 205, *228*
Comi, G., 564, *581*
Comis, R., 388, *403*
Committee on Personnel for Health Needs of the Elderly Through the Year 2020, 21, *24*
Comstock, G. W., 107, *115*, 397, *403*
Conklin, B., 539, *553*, 841, *852*
Conlon, P., 623, *638*
Conn, D. K., 456, *460*
Conneally, P. M., 40, *72*, 214, *228*
Connelly, K., 530, *546*, 841, *849*
Connelly, S., 324, *333*
Connolly, S. J., 564, *578*
Consolazione, A., 190, *195*
Constantinidis, J., 240, *246*, 493, *505*
Conwell, Y., 46, 48, *67*, 528, *547*, 634, *639*

Cook, B. L., 385, *402*
Cook, E., 110, 111, *116*
Cook, N. R., 33, *68*, 201, 209, *224*, 480, 482, *505*, 753, *758*
Cook, P. J., 533, *547*, 747, *757*
Cool, L., 104, *115*
Cooledge, N. J., 711, *714*
Coombs, D. W., 485, *506*
Cooney, L., 825, *831*
Cooper, A. F., 277, *297*, 468, *474*
Cooper, A. M., 451, *459*
Cooper, G., 205, *227*
Cooper, J. E., 109, *115*
Cooper, J. K., 529, 532, *552*
Cooper, K. L., 703, *713*
Cooper, P. F., 313, *331*
Cooper, T. B., 394, *403*, 574, *578*
Copeland, J., 232, *247*
Copeland, J. R. M., 38, 42, 46, *67*, 523, 530, 531, *553*, *554*
Coppen, A., 500, *503*
Corbin, K. B., 289, *297*
Corcoran, P., 677, *694*
Cordell, B., 483, *507*
Corenthal, C., 446, 451, 452, 454, *461*, *462*
Corkin, S., 322, 328, *333*, *335*, 653, *666*
Cornes, C., 574, *581*
Cornis, R., 47, *69*
Cornoni-Huntley, J., 358, *372*, 538, 539, *549*, 680, 681, *694*
Cornu, C., 261, *305*
Corsellis, A. N., 153, *171*
Corsellis, J. A. N., 40, *67*, 152–153, *171*, 182, 183, 189, *195*
Corso, J. F., 253, 266, 267, 268, 270, 271, 272, 274, 278, 279, 285, 288, *297*
Coryell, W., 396, *402*, 446, 451, 452, 454, *460*, *462*
Cosh, J. A., 290, *297*
Costa, P., 135, *142*
Costa, P. T., 436, 437, 445, *457*
Costa, P. T., Jr., 356, 358, *372*, 442, 445, *457*, *459*, 649, *664*
Cote, L., 388, *405*, 501, *508*, *511*
Cote, L. J., 501, *508*
Cotman, C. W., 180, 190, *195*, *196*, *197*, *198*, 483, *512*
Cotton, P. D., 585, *597*
Courtwright, D. T., 536, 537, *547*

Covi, L., 424, *429*
Coward, R. T., 904, *913*
Cowart, B. J., 282, 283, *306*
Cowen, P. J., 454, *459*
Cowgill, D., 84, *96*
Cox, C., 219, *227*, 634, *639*, 650, *667*
Cox, T. J., 536, *549*
Coyle, D. A., 388, *406*
Coyle, J., 754, *757*
Coyle, J. T., 485, *512*
Coyne, A. C., 258, *300*
Craig, T. J., 239, *246*
Craik, F. I. M., 310, 311, 312, 316, 322, *332*, 648, *664*
Crain, B. J., 486, *511*
Crambert, R. F., 263, *301*
Crane, L. G., 821, *831*
Cranford, R. E., 861, *871*
Crapper, D. R., 484, *505*
Crawford, J. R., 624, 625, *638*, *639*
Creasey, H., 39, *67*, 150, *172*, 207, *228*, 731, 732, *757*
Creasy, H., 151, *170*
Creese, I., 184, *196*
Cress, M., 391, *401*
Crider, D. M., 359, *375*
Crimmins, A., 312, *336*
Crockett, D. J., 645, *668*
Crockett, W. H., 364, *372*
Cromer, W. J., 803, *811*
Crook, T., 14, 15, *24*, *25*, *26*, 326, *332*, 345, *353*, 424, *428*, 617, *638*, 647, *664*, *667*
Crook, T. H., 647, 661, *666*, 753, *757*
Crooks, V. J., 829, *829*
Cross, A. J., 182, 183, 189, *195*
Cross, P., 33, 42, 46, 65, *68*, 243, *247*
Cross, P. A., 388, *401*
Cross, P. S., 31, *68*, 817, 820, *830*
Crossley, H. M., 523, *546*
Crow, T. J., 182, 183, 184, 189, *195*, *197*
Crowder, R. G., 308, *331*
Crowe, R. R., 417, *428*
Cruise, D. G., 349, *354*
Crusan, K., 527, *552*
Crutchfield, R. D., 108, *116*
Cruzan v. Director, Missouri Department of Health, 862, *869*
Crystal, H., 191, *195*, 328, *333*, 648, 652, *665*
Cubberley, L., 480, 498, 500, *507*, *511*

Cuellar, I., 113, *115*
Culig, K. M., 753, *762*
Cullum, M., 151, *169*
Cumming, E., 137, *142*
Cummings, E., 87, *96*
Cummings, J., 209, *223*
Cummings, J. L., 210, 211, 219, *223*, 388, *405*, 446, *460*, 471, *474*, 493, *505*, 624, 629, 632, 633, *637*, *638*, 653, 656, *664*, *668*
Cunningham, D. S., 482, *512*
Cunningham, W. R., 340, 341, 342, 344, 347, 348, 349, *352*
Cupp, C. J., 159, *170*
Cupples, L. A., 214, *224*
Curlik, S., 819, *830*
Curry, A. F., 468, *474*
Curtis, J. R., 520, *547*
Curtis, M., 487, 488, *509*
Curzon, G., 182, 188, *194*
Cusack, B. J., 728, *760*
Cutler, J., 876, 880, *889*
Cutler, N. R., 205, 207, 208, 209, 210, 211, 214, *224*, 645, *664*
Cutler, N. R. G., 150, *172*
Cutler, R. G., 148, *170*
Cutler, S. J., 314, *332*, 357, *372*
Cutting, J., 471, *474*
Cutting, J. C., 454, *459*
Czeisler, C. A., 560, 568, 576, *577*, *581*
Czirr, R., 446, *461*, 710, *717*
Czudek, C., 184, *198*

Dahl, R. E., 564, 572, *578*
Dal Toso, R., 190, *195*
Dalderup, L. M., 264, *297*
Dallosso, H., 530, 532, 542, *548*, *551*
Dalton, A. J., 493, *505*, 588, *597*
Daly, L. E., 541, *547*
Damas-Mora, J., 472, *474*
Damasie, A. R., 483, *507*
Damasio, A., 150, *170*
Damasio, A. R., 648, 653, *665*
Damasio, H., 150, *170*
D'Amato, C. J., 37, *71*, 191, *197*
D'Angelo, N., 526, *554*
Daniels, M., 907, *914*
Danziger, W., 151, *170*

Danziger, W. L., 328, *336*, 648, 651, 653, *666*, *669*
Darjes, R., 311, *337*
Darkins, A., 653, 656, *664*
Darnell, J. C., 538, *547*
Darrow, G., 120, 132, *142*
Darwin, C., 417, *428*
Darwish, A. K., 500, *505*
DaSilva, G., 702, *713*
Dastoor, D., 486, *506*
Dastur, D. K., 204, *223*
Davenport, L., 492, *505*, 624, *638*
David, A., 539, *553*, 841, *852*
Davidoff, L. M., 884, *890*
Davidson, A. N., 485, 486, *506*, *509*
Davidson, I. A., 38, 42, 46, 67, 523, 530, 531, *553*, *554*
Davidson, J., 389, *404*, 625, *639*
Davies, B., 395, *407*
Davies, G., 350, *352*
Davies, H. D., 500, *509*
Davies, P., 483, 485, *505*, *506*, *507*, 647, 652, *665*, 732, 754, *757*, 896, *913*
Davies, P. D., 281, *305*
Davies, R. K., 394, *402*
Davies, T., 500, *505*
Davis, B. M., 485, *508*
Davis, J., 743, *759*
Davis, J. M., 486, *504*
Davis, J. N., 190, *194*
Davis, K. L., 15, *26*, 328, *336*, 386, 387, 394, *403*, 482, 485, 486, *505*, *507*, *508*, 661, *669*, 899, *914*
Davis, K. M., 802, *813*
Davis, K. R., 623, 624, *639*
Davis, L. J., 525, 526, 527, 528, 529, *548*, *549*, 767, 768, *791*
Davis, M., 798, *811*
Davis, P., 828, *830*
Davis, P. B., 343, *353*
Davis, R. L., 700, 701, *715*
Davis, R. M., 541, 542, *548*
Davis, R. W., 525, *548*
Davison, A. N., 182, 183, 188, *194*, *195*, *197*
Davison, K., 605, *638*
Dawber, T. R., 256, 265, *299*
Dawes, L. R., 483, *513*
Dawson, G. W., 541, *547*
Dawson, P., 676, *694*

Day, N. E., 40, *67*
De Alarcon, R., 382, 389, *402*
de Beauvoir, S., 85, *96*
De Dominicis, G., 391, *404*
De Figueiredo, J. M., 484, *508*
de Jong, P. T. V. M., 262, *299*
De Leo, D., 391, *404*, 530, *547*, 817, *830*
De Leo, J. M., 150, *172*
De Leon, M. J., 240, *246*, 491, *506*
de Leon, M. J., 150, *170*, 189, *195*, 205,
    209, 210, 219, *224*, *227*, 240, *247*, 491,
    506, 654, *669*
De Met, E., 393, *403*
de Monasterio, F. M., 264, *300*
De Teresa, R., 153, *173*
de Waard, 262, *299*
Dean, L., 33, 42, 46, 65, *68*
Dean, R. L., 732, 754, *757*
Dean, R. L., III, 180, *194*
Dean, R. S., 655, *664*
Deardorff, H., 765, *791*
DeCarli, C. S., 219, *224*
Deckel, M. J., 562, *580*
Deely, P. J., 537, *547*
Defiore, C. H., 163, *170*
Deimling, G. T., 234, *246*
Deinard, S., 240, *247*
Deister, A., 467, 468, *474*
Deith, J., 314, *334*
DeKosky, S. T., 182, *195*
DeLabry, L. O., 522, 525, *548*, *549*
Delacourte, A., 165, 166, *172*
Delahunt, J., 422, *429*
Delanney, L. E., 191, *198*
D'Elia, L., 65, *667*
D'Elia, L. F., 328, *334*, 646, 651, 652, *664*,
    666
Delis, D. C., 647, 652, *664*, *666*, *668*
Della Court, M., 292, *303*
Delong, M., 754, *757*
DeLong, M. R., 221, *223*
DeLongis, A., 120, *142*
Dement, W. C., 558, 561, 566, 568, 569,
    572, *577*, *579*
Demming, J. A., 351, *353*
Demos, S., 765, *792*
Dennis, T., 488, *504*
Dent, D., 258, *303*
Deptula, D., 424, *430*, 747, *760*

Derenzo, S. E., 209, *225*
Derix, M. M. A., 660, *664*
Derogatis, L. R., 389, *402*, 419, *428*
Des Jarlais, D. C., 536, 537, *547*
DeSilva, H., 420, *431*
Desmond, D. P., 536, *550*
DeSouza, C., 527, *550*
DeSouza, E. B., 486, *505*
DeSouza, L. B., 488, *512*
Desrosiers, M. H., 202, 203, *228*
Dessonville, C., 13, *24*
Detels, R., 691, *696*
DeTeresa, R., 176, *198*
Detre, T. P., 394, *402*
Deustch, G., 221, *224*
Devanand, D. P., 221, *228*, 498, *505*, 733,
    757
Devaney, K. O., 253, *297*
DeVitt, D. R., 742, *757*
deWachter, M. A. M., 863, *869*
Dewey, M. E., 38, 42, 46, *67*, 523, 530,
    531, *553*, *554*
Dewhurst, J. R., 286, *297*
DeWit, H., 531, 535, *554*
Dhar, 730, 742, *762*
Dhillon, S., 562, *580*
Diamond, B. L., 864, 865, *870*
Diamond, J., 909, *913*
Diamond, M. C., 149, 152, 153, 159, *170*,
    897, *913*
DiChiro, G., 209, 210, 211, 212, 214, *224*
Dick, D. J., 487, 488, *509*
Dick, J. P. R., 618, *638*
Dickel, M. J., 566, *577*
Dickerson, M., 327, *332*
Dickerson, P. C., 705, *717*
Dickson, A. L., 646, *663*
Dickson, D., 191, *195*
Diebel, R., 657, *669*
Diener, E., 358, *372*
Difossey, A., 165, 166, *172*
Dillon, S., 438, 452, *457*
Dillon, W., 492, *505*, 624, *638*
Dilon, M. R., 485, *512*
DiMascio, A., 327, *336*
Dimsdale, J. E., 496, *512*
Dion, G., 680, *694*
Dirks, D., 272, *298*
Dirks, D. D., 274, *297*

Dismukes, K., 254, 265, *304*
Ditter, S. M., 488, *505*
Divoll, M., 423–424, *427*, *428*, 730, *758*
Dixon, R. A., 309, 310, 313, *332*, *334*
Djang, W. T., 14, *24*, 391–392, *401*
Doddi, S., 42, *429*
Dodson, M., 125, *142*
Dohrenwend, B. P., 105, *115*, 125, 128, *142*
Dohrenwend, B. S., 105, *115*, 125, 128, *142*
Dolan, L., 29, *70*
Dolan, R. J., 391, *402*, *403*
Dolcle, J. J., 705, *717*
Doliver, J. J., 261, *303*
Dolman, C. E., 153, *171*, 180, *197*
Dolman, C. L., 253, *297*
Dolphin, C., 469, *475*
Dominick, J., 816, *830*
Donaldson, G., 345, *353*
Donaldson, S., 689, *695*
Donley, J., 330, *334*
Donnelly, N., 835, *852*
Donovan, D. M., 516, *547*
Dorian, B., 448, 449, 450, 453, *460*
Dornbrand, L., 862, *870*
Dorpat, T. L., 399, *402*
Dorsa, D., 486, *510*
Dorsey, D., 214, *226*
Dorsey, D. A., 215, *227*, 645, *666*
Doty, R. L., 285, 286, 287, 294, *297*
Douglas, A. C., 863, *869*
Douvan, E., 801, *812*
Dowd, J., 103, *115*
Downing, R. W., 424, *429*
Doyle, J. T., 524, *549*
Doyle, M. C., 47, *67*
Drachman, D., 32, 40, *71*, *72*, 214, *228*,
    479, 481, *508*, *512*, 645, *667*
Drachman, D. A., 14, *26*
Drachman, D. B., 190, *197*
Drake, F., 388, *406*
Drance, S. M., 253, *297*
Drasdo, N., 263, *306*
Dravid, A., 177, *194*
Dresner, R., 328, *333*, 648, 652, *665*
Drew, L. R. H., 520, *547*
Drew, M. C., 191, *197*
Dreyer, P., 530, *546*, 841, *849*
Drinkwater, V., 534, *548*
Dritz, S., 495, *503*

Droller, H., 528, *547*
Drugovich, M. L., 835, *851*
Drury, M., 837, *852*
Dryman, A., 35, 43, 49, 52, 54, 56, 60, 62,
    68
Du Bois, B. C., 107, *115*
Du Boulay, G. H., 209, 219, *225*, 658, *665*
Duara, R., 205, 207, 208, 209, 210, 211,
    213, 214, 219, *224*, *226*, *228*, 624, *638*,
    645, 659, *664*, *667*, 687, 691, *696*
Dublin, W. B., 266, *297*
Dubno, J. R., 274, *297*
Dubois, B., 488, *505*, 657, *668*
Duchen, L. W., 493, *505*
Dudleston, K., 619, *638*
Duff, R. W., 524, *545*
Duffy, B., 32, 33, 35, 41, *68*
Duffy, F. H., 644, 645, *664*, *665*
Duffy, M., 713, *714*
Dufour, M., 522, *547*
Dufour, M. C., 520, *553*
Duke-Elder, W. L., 254, *297*
Duncan, W. C., 569, *578*
Duncan-Jones, P., 530, *551*
Dunham, R. G., 526, 529, *548*, *550*
Dunlop, J., 529, *548*
Duong, T., 164, 165, 166, *172*
Dupont, R. L., 423, *427*
Dupree, L. W., 525, 529, *548*, 679, *696*
Duquesnoy, N., 205, *228*
Durara, R., 240, *247*
Durham, N. C., 485, *511*
Dusky v. United States, 864, *869*
Dustman, R. E., 319, 329, *332*, *333*
Dyck, P. J., 289, 290, *296*
Dyrenfurth, I., 388, *405*, 501, *508*
Dysken, M. W., 500, *505*

Earl, N., 481, *511*
Easton, P., 31, *69*
Eaton, M. T., 388, *407*
Eaton, W. W., 35, 43, 49, 52, 54, 56, 60, 62,
    65, *67*, *68*, *70*, 107, 108, *115*, 349, *353*,
    468, *474*
Eberly, D. A., 679, *696*
Ebersole, P., 826, 827, *830*
Ebert, M. H., 344, *354*

Ebmeier, K. P., 624, 625, *638, 639*
Ebrahim, S., 530, 532, 542, *548, 551*
Eddy, J., 495, *504*
Edelman, P., 807, *811*
Edelstein, B. A., 705, *713*
Edelstein, H., 496, *505*
Edgerton, R., 586, *597*
Edmund, L., 845, *851*
Edwards, G., 536, *548*
Edwards, S., 327, *332*
Edwardson, J. A., 484, 488, *504, 505*
Egelhoff, C., 473, *475*
Ehlers, A., 421, *429*
Ehlers, C. L., 570, *579*
Ehlert, K., 710, 711 *713*
Ehmann, W. D., 484, *508*
Ehsani, A. A., 346, *354*
Eichling, J. O., 164, *172*
Eichorn, F., 279, *301*
Einstein, G. O., 317, *333*
Eisdorfer, C., 15, *26*, 240, *247*, 571, *580*,
    583, 585, *597*, 652, 659, *667*, 687, 691,
    696, 805, *811*
Eisenberg, R. L., 623, *640*
Ekerdt, D. J., 525, *548*
Ekholm, S., 622, *639*
Ekstrom, R. B., 351, *353*
El-Awar, M., 657, *665*
El-Mofty, A., 271, *303*
El Sobky, A., 500, *505*
Elam, C., 588, *596*
Eldridge, R., 484, *509*
Elias, J., 320, *337*
Elias, M. F., 346, *353*
Elias, P. K., 346, *353*
Ellinwood, E. H., 747, *757*
Elliot, D. F., 834, *851*
Elliott, D., 259, 264, *297, 306*
Elliott, D. B., 259, 262, *297*
Ellor, J., 397, *407*
Ellor, J. R., 538, *548*
Elsayed, M., 319, *333*
Embrey, J., 272, *298*
Embury, G. D., 533, *545*
Emery, C. F., 347, *352*
Emery, G., 392, *401*, 417, 422, *427*, 709,
    713, 714
Emery, O. B., 654, *666*
Emery, V. O. B., 14, *24*

Emmerich, M., 150, *170*
Endicott, J., 47, *70, 71*, 242, *246*, 387, *402*
Endo, S., 559, 566, *578, 580*
Engel, B. T., 708, *713, 717*
Engel, G. L., 604, 607, *638*
Engelhardt, J. L., 592, *597*
Engle-Friedman, M., 705, 708, *713*
Englehardt, H. T., Jr., 9, *24*
English, D. R., 494, *507*, 533, *550*
English, J. T., 874, 878, 879, 883, *889, 890*
English, R. J., 625, *639*
Englund, E., 149, *170*, 491, *504*
Ennis, J., 399, *406*
Epelbaum, J., 488, *505*
Epp, G., 765, *792*
Epstein, L. J., 528, *553*
Epstein, N., 419, *427*
Epstein, S., 365, *372*
Era, P., 290, *297*
Erbaugh, J., 617, *637*
Erde, E. L., 86, *859*
Erickson, R. P., 285, 288, *304*
Erikson, E., 79, 87, *96*, 132, *142*
Erikson, E. H., 120, *142*, 703, *714*
Erikson, H. E., 364, *372*
Erikson, J. M., 703, *714*
Erkinjuntti, T., 471, *474*, 492, *505*, 624, *638*,
    659, *665*
Erman, M., 496, *512*
Ermini, M., 177, *194*
Ernst, P., 386, *402*
Ervin, S., 887, *889*
Esberger, K. K., 819, *830*
Escher, M. C., 524, 525, *547*
Escobar, J. I., 108, 109, 110, *115, 116*, 618,
    638
Esiri, M. M., 182, 183, *194, 195*, 486, 489,
    506
Eslinger, P. J., 150, *170*, 648, 653, *665*
Esquirol, J. E. D., 611, *638*
Essen-Moller, E., 34, 37, *68*
Estabrook, W., 393, *403*, 574, *578*, 743, *758*
Esterson, F. D., 253, *303*
Eth, S., 859, 861, 866, 868, *869, 870*
Etholm, B., 266, *297*
Etienne, P., 486, 493, *513*
Ettinger, W. H., 384, *403*, 835, *851*
Ettlin, T. M., 621, *638*
Evans, C. C., 676, 680, *696*

Evans, D., 258, *298*
Evans, D. A., 33, *68*, 201, 209, *224*, 753, *758*
Evans, D. W., 258, *297*
Evans, H. M., 187, 188, *197*, 212, *227*
Evans, I. A., 480, 482, *505*
Evans, J. G., 37, 38. 40, 56, *68*
Evans, L. K., 572, *578*, 845, *850*
Evans, N. J. R., 212, *227*
Evarts, E., 168, *170*
Evenhuis, J. M., 585, 588, *597*
Everitt, D., 840, *850*
Everitt, D. E., 530, *546*, 728, 752, *757*
Eyde, D. R., 706, 713, *714*
Eyman, R. K., 586, 588, *597*
Ezrin-Waters, C., 180, *195*

Fabrega, H., 445, *459*
Factor, A., 592, *597*
Faek, A., 500, *505*
Fagg, G. E., 190, *195*
Fairbairn, A., 484, *504*
Fairbairn, A. F., 487, 488, 490, *509*
Fairbaum, A., 488, *505*
Falk, J. R., 383, 395, *407*
Fallen, H. J., 421, *429*
Farber, B., 593, *597*
Farber, J. F., 618, *638*
Farkas, M., 320, *333*
Farkas, T., 209, 210, *224*
Farneti, P., 562, *579*
Farolini, M., 495, *506*
Farr, R. K., 536, *550*
Farr, R. M., 539, *551*
Farrall, M., 481, *506*
Farrer, L. A., 214, *224*
Farrimond, T., 263, *298*
Farris, P. A., 386, *405*
Farrow, J. S., 482, *512*
Farrow, S., 542, *554*
Faulkner, D., 314, *332*
Faulkner, L. R., 866, *869*
Fauquette, A., 624, *640*
Fawcett, J., 399, *402*
Fay, M., 56, *69*
Featherstone, H. J., 494, *507*, 533, *550*
Fedder, D. O., 530, 535, *546*

Feder, J., 835, *850*, 874, 884, *889*
Federman, D. D., 861, *871*
Federspiel, C. F., 752, *760*, 840, *850*, *852*
Fedewa, B., 765, *791*
Fedio, P., 209, 210, 211, 212, 214, 219, *224*, *227*, 650, *667*
Fedoroff, J. P., 634, *640*
Feigenbaum, E., 711, *715*
Feighner, J. P., 393, *402*, 574, *578*, 743, *758*
Fein, G., 492, *505*, 624, *638*
Feinberg, I., 204, *227*, 572, *578*
Feinberg, T., 329, *333*
Feinson, M. C., 42, 64, *68*
Feld, S., 411, 412, *428*
Feldman, M. D., 539, *548*
Feldman, R. G., 40, *72*, 214, *228*, 481, *512*
Felten, D. L., 191, *196*
Felthous, A. R., 866, *869*
Fenner, M. E., 588, *597*
Fentem, P., 542, *548*
Fentem, P. H., 530, 532, *551*
Fenton, S., 399, *406*
Ferguson, B., 454, *461*, 619, *638*, 863, *869*
Ferguson, J., 485, *505*
Fernandez, F., 496, *507*
Ferrier, I. N., 182, 183, 189, *195*
Ferris, H., 150, *170*
Ferris, S., 14, *24*, 189, *195*, 345, *353*, 491, *506*, 617, *638*, 647, *664*
Ferris, S. H., 15, *24*, 205, 209, 210, 219, *224*, *227*, 240, 245, 246, 247, 248, 326, *332*, 497, *510*, 647, 654, *667*, *669*, 753, *760*
Fetting, J., 389, *402*
Feuerberg, M. A., 803, *811*
Fieschi, C., 38, *66*
Figiel, G. S., *4*, 14, 368, 391–392, *401*, *474*
Filipp, L., 539, *553*, 732, *761*, 835, 841, *852*
Fillenbaum, G., 15, *25*, 682, 687, 692, *695*
Fillenbaum, G. G., 108, *115*
Filley, C. M., 489, *504*, 659, *665*, 753, *762*
Filos, S., 237, 240, *248*, 687, 691, 692, *696*
Finch, C. E., 177, 179, 180, 181, 183, 186, 190, *195*, *196*, *197*, 483, *507*, 731, *760*, 899, *913*
Fine, T., 876, 880, *889*
Finger, T. E., 279, *298*
Fingerot, E., 845, *851*
Finlay-Jones, R., 49, *68*

Finlayson, R. E., 521, 525, 526, 527, 528, 529, 531, 535, 542, *548*, *549*
Finn, R. O., 495, *504*
Finney, J. W., 51, 525, *548*
Finset, A., 661, *669*
Fiore, M. C., 541, 542, *548*
Fischbach, R. L., 28, 41, 42, 49, 51, 52, 54, 57, 58, *68*
Fischer, C., 559, *578*
Fischer, R., 281, *299*
Fischer, S., 180, *194*
Fischer, W., 537, *552*
Fishburne, P. M., 537, *551*
Fishchel, M. A., 495, *513*
Fisher, J., 725, 752, *761*
Fisher, R. H., 647, 648, *669*
Fisher, R. S., 177, *196*
Fisher, S., 424, *429*, 483, *513*
Fisher, S. E., 41, 420, *430*
Fisk, A. D., 325, 330, *333*, *336*
Fisseni, H. J., 364, 365, *372*
Fitzgerald, D., 349, *352*
Fitzgerald, P., 313, *331*
Fitzpatrick, J. J., 821, *831*
Flanagan, T. J., 536, *550*
Fleiss, J., 242, *246*
Fleiss, J. L., 500, *506*, 686, 690, *695*
Flicker, C., 15, *24*, 651, 661, *665*, 754, *757*
Flood, D. C., 153, 154, 159, *170*
Flood, D. G., 163, *170*, 177, *195*
Florio, L. P., 41, 42, 47, 48, *73*, 380, 384, *407*
Flower, M. C., 525, 529, *549*
Foch, T. T., 344, *353*
Foelker, G. A., Jr., 15, *24*
Fogel, B. S., 875, 876, 879, 883, 885, *889*
Folkman, S., 120, *142*, 241, *247*, 365, 367, *373*, 525, *549*, 728, *758*
Folmar, S., 845, *850*
Folstein, M., 479, 501, *508*, *513*, 645, *667*
Folstein, M. F., 32, 33, 35, 40, 41, 49, *66*, *67*, *68*, *71*, 237, *247*, 345, 350, *353*, 380, *402*, 482, 500, *504*, *509*, 617, 618, *637*, *638*, 649, 653, *665*, 732, *761*, 835, 836, *851*, *852*
Folstein, M. R., 328, *333*
Folstein, S., 328, *333*
Folstein, S. E., 35, *68*, 237, *247*, 380, *402*, 617, *638*, 649, *665*

Fonagy, P., 532, 534, 535, *549*
Foncin, J.-F., 214, *228*
Fondacaro, M. R., 525, *551*
Fonein, J. F., 40, *72*
Fooken, I., 360, 361, *372*
Foos, P. W., 330, *333*
Force, F., 701, *717*
Ford, A., 675, 685, *695*, 828, *830*
Ford, C. V., 383, *406*
Ford, D., 542, *554*
Ford, D. E., 566, 567, *578*
Ford v. Wainwright, 865, *869*
Fordyce, W. E., 422, *428*
Foreman, M. D., 821, *830*
Forno, L. S., 184, 488, *506*
Forsling, M. L., 486, *512*
Forsythe, A., 618, *638*
Foster, D., 737, *762*
Foster, J. R., 753, *758*
Foster, N. L., 204, 209, 210, 211, 212, 214, 218, *224*, *225*, 650, *667*
Foster, T. E., 539, *550*
Fowler, J., 164, *172*
Fowler, J. S., 205, 209, 210, *224*
Fowler, L., 84, *96*
Fowler, N., 385, 389, 397, *401*, *403*
Fox, A. J., 491, *511–512*
Fox, G. A., 526, *554*
Fox, H., 491, *511–512*
Fox, P. T., 221, *224*, *228*
Foxall, M. J., 110, 111, *116*
Foy, A., 534, *548*
Foy, D., 685, *696*
Fozard, J. L., 254, 256, 257, 258, 259, 268, 272, 273, 274, 278, 280, 288, *296*, *298*, *303*, 316, *337*
Frackowiak, R. S. J., 202, 205, 209, 219, *224*, *225*, *227*
France, R. D., 389, *402*, *404*
Frances, A., 381, 382, *401*
Franceschi, M., 182, *194*
Francescki, M., 564, *581*
Francis, A., 739, *757*
Francis, P. T., 182, 183, *195*, 486, *506*
Frangione, B., 191, *195*
Frank, E., 570, 574, *579*, *581*
Frank, R. G., 873, *889*
Frankel, R., 701, 702, 703, 711, *715*
Franks, J. R., 278, *298*

Franssen, E., 219, 245, *248*, 497, *510*, 753, *760*
Frantz, A., 388, *405*, 501, *508*
Fratiglioni, L., 38, *66*
Frazier, S. H., 878, *889*
Fredericks, M. L. C., 264, *297*
Frederickson, H., 151, *170*
Frederickson, H. A., 150, *172*
Fredman, L., 386, *402*
Fredrickson, E., 47–48, *72*
Free, S. M., 736, *759*
Freed, D., 328, *333*
Freedman, A. M., 898, *913*
Freedman, J., 312, *337*
Freeman, D., 680, 681, *694*
Freeman, D. H., 541, *550*
Freeman, G. B., 191, *195*
Freeman-Browne, D., 40, *67*
Freiberg, U., 279, *296*
Freidenberg, D. O., 656, *666*
Freitag, W. Q., 576, *577*
Fremouw, W. J., 707, *713*
French, I. R., 484, *508*
French, J., 351, *353*
French, L. R., 38, *68*, *71*
Frengley, D., 825, *831*
Frengley, J. D., 740, *759*, 822, *830*
Fretwell, M. D., 835, *851*
Freud, S., 82, *96*, 129, *142*, 416, *428*, 699, *714*
Freund, G., 519, 520, 525, *548*
Friden, H., 188, *194*
Fridman, J., 31, *69*
Friedel, R. O., 729, *758*
Friedland, R. P., 209, 210, 211, 213, 214, 215, 216, 218, 221, 222, *225*, *226*, 645, 650, 652, *665*, *668*
Friedman, 743, *758*
Friedman, A. S., 327, *336*
Friedman, E., 743, *758*
Friedman, G. D., 292, 293, *306*, 524, *550*
Friedmann, T., 896, *913*
Fries, J., 686, 690, *695*
Frigerio, L., 191, *195*
Frisina, R. D., 266, 268, *298*
Fritch, W. W., 484, *508*
Fritz, R. B., 166, *172*
Frommelt, P., 214, *228*
Frommeti, P., 40, *72*

Frommlet, M., 571, *578*
Fruge, E., 14, 18, *24*, *25*
Fry, C., 78, *96*
Fry, J., 190, *196*
Fucci, D., 290, *302*
Fuchs, C. Z., 382, *403*
Fujikawa, D. G., 214, 215, *226*, *227*, 645, *666*
Fujimoro, M., 498, *510*
Fujiura, G. T., 592, *597*
Fukuda, H., 566, *580*
Fulcomer, M., 687, 692, *696*
Fuld, P., 191, *195*, 237, 240, *247*
Fuld, P. A., 492, *511*, 646, 647, 651, 652, 658, 659, *664*, *665*, *667*, *669*
Fulham, M. J., 495, *504*
Fuller, C., 84, 86, 90, *96*
Fullerton, A. G., 394, *402*
Fulling, K. H., 646, *669*
Fulton, J. P., 673, 677, *695*, *697*
Funkenstein, H., 201, 209, *224*, 480, 482, *505*
Funkenstein, H. H., 33, *68*, 753, *758*
Furad, F., 516, *549*
Furchtgott, E., 347, *353*
Furino, A., 879, 885, *889*
Furino, A. F., 875, 876, *889*
Furst, D. E., 540, *549*
Furtchgott, E., 286, *300*
Fyer, A. J., 421, *428*

Gabriel, E., 184, *198*
Gabrielli, W. F., 40, *71*
Gadjusek, D. C., 496, *507*
Gado, M., 151, *170*
Gado, M. H., 646, *669*
Gaeth, J., 272, *298*
Gafner, G., 712, *714*
Gage, F. H., 487, *506*, *510*, 896, *913*
Gahm, I. G., 575, *581*
Gainotti, G., 657, *665*
Gaitz, C. M., 411, 412, *428*, 798, *811*
Galatzer-Levy, R., 135, *142*
Gall, J., 439, *461*
Gallagher, D., 13, 15, *24*, *25*, *26*, 327, 328, 329, *335*, *337*, 392, *403*, *407*, 419, *431*, 446, *461*, 653, *668*, 699, 701, 707, 709, 710, *714*, *715*, *717*

Gallagher, D. E., 700, 701, 709, *714*
Gambert, S. R., 847, *850*
Gambetti, P., 488, *504*
Gammans, R. E., 424, *428*
Gamzu, E. R., 753, *758*
Gandolfo, C., 38, *66*
Ganley, S. P., 256, 265, *299*
Ganz, E., 209, *225*
Garber, H. J., 624, *639*
Garbin, A., 391, *404*
Gardillo, J. L., 501, *513*
Gardner, E. D., 289, *297*
Gardner, E. R., 538, *548*
Gardner-Keaton, H., 537, *551*
Gardocki, G. J., 804, *812*
Garetz, F. K., 834, *852*
Garner, W., 253, *298*
Garrett, N. J., 182, *198*
Garrett, T. J., 494, *508*
Garry, P. J., 60, *66*, 319, *333*, 522, *545*, 624, *639*
Garside, R. F., 420, *428*, *430*, 468, *474*
Gartner, A., 120, *142*
Garvey, A. J., 541, 542, *546*, *548*, 645, *665*
Garvey, P. M., 263, *304*
Garza, J., 592, *597*
Gaskell, P. C., 481, *509*, *511*
Gastaud, P., 261, *305*
Gaston, L., 710, *714*, *715*
Gaston, P., 14, *25*, 835, *851*
Gatz, C., 382, *402*
Gatz, M., 16, *24*, 363, *374*, 827, *830*, 844, *851*
Gauthier, L., 486, *506*
Gauthier, S., 486, 493, *506*, *513*
Gauvain, M., 15, *25*
Gay, J. R. A., 658, *668*
Gedye, A., 40, *68*
Geinisman, Y., 177, *195*
Geiwitz, J., 438, *460*
Gelber, A., 747, *760*
Geldard, F., 252, 272, 281, 289, *298*
Gelder, M. G., 51, *68*
Gelfand, D. E., 105, *115*
Geller, G., 520, *547*
Gemmel, H. G., 624, 625, *638*
Gemmell, H. G., 625, *639*
Gentes, C., 150, *170*
Gentes, C. I., 189, *195*, 205, *224*, 491, *506*

George, A. E., 189, *195*, 205, 209, 210, 219, *224*, *227*, 240, *246*, 491, *506*
George, A. F., 150, *170*
George, A. J., 47, *67*
George, C. F., 533, *547*
George, J. K., 14, *23*
George, K., 687, 692, *695*, 737, *759*
George, L., 356, 358, 365, *372*, *373*, *374*
George, L. K., 28, 34, 35, 37, 41, 42, 49, 51, 52, 54, 57, 58, 60, *68*, *71*, 108, *115*, 347, 349, *352*, 380, 383, 385, 397, *401*, *403*, 438, *457*, 794, 795, 798, 799, 800, 801, 802, 803, 805, 806, 807, 808, 809, *811*, *813*
Georgotas, A., 394, *403*, 574, *578*, 654, *669*, 743, 753, *758*, *760*
Gerber, C. J., 571, *580*
Gerber, I. E., 660, *666*
Gerber, P., 795, *813*
Gerdt, C., 654, *670*
Gerlach, J., 738, *762*
Germain, M., 486, *506*
German, P. S., 18, *24*, 384, *403*, 802, 810, *811*, 835, 836, *850*, *851*, *852*
Gerner, R., 393, *403*, 500, *511*, 743, *758*
Gerner, R. H., 220, 221, *223*
Gerner, T., 574, *578*
Gersch, B. J., 541, *549*
Gershon, S., 14, *24*, 240, *246*, 326, *332*, 345, *353*
Gerson, S., 388, *405*, 575, *580*
Gerson, S. C., 738, *758*
Gerteis, G., 40, *70*
Gescheider, G. A., 266, 268, *298*
Ghanbari, H. A., 483, *506*
Ghanim, A., 562, *580*
Gherardi, R., 495, *506*
Ghodse, A. H., 536, *548*
Giaccone, G., 191, *195*
Giambra, L. M., 330, *333*
Gibb, W. R. G., 489, *506*
Gibbon, M., 454, *461*, 609, *641*
Gibbs, H., 421, *429*
Gibbs, J. M., 205, *224*, 227
Giberson, R., 285, 286, 287, 294, *297*
Giblin, E. C., 564, 571, *581*
Gibson, G. E., 191, *195*, 497, *504*
Gibson, P. H., 177, 188, *195*, *196*
Gierl, B., 743, *759*

Gigy, L., 134, *142*, *143*
Gilbert, A. N., 287, *306*
Gilbert, J. G., 264, *298*
Gilberto, P., 838, *850*
Gilbertson, W. E., 538, *548*
Gilewski, M. J., 313, 314, *333*, *337*
Gilford, D. M., 902, *913*
Gilhome-Herbst, K., 277, *298*
Gilley, D. W., 186, *198*
Gillick, L. S., 821, *830*
Gillick, M. R., 821, *830*
Gillin, J. C., 344, *354*, 421, *431*, 569, *578*
Gillum, B., 357, *373*
Gillum, R., 357, *373*
Gilman, S., 204, *224*
Gilmore, M. M., 451, *459*
Ginsbert, M. D., 207, *228*
Ginsburg, A. P., 258, *297*, *298*
Giordano, J. A., 526, *548*, 710, *713*
Giovino, G., 541, *552*
Giovino, G. A., 541, 542, *548*
Girgis, G. N., 539, *550*
Girotti, F., 184, *197*
Gisell, J., 651, *670*
Gitman, L., 284, *297*
Gitting, N. S., 256, 259, *298*
Gittleman, B., 240, *247*, 687, 691, *696*
Giuli, C., 177, *194*
Giyanani, V. L., 623, *640*
Gjerris, F., 486, 493, *511*, *512*
Glanville, E. V., 281, *299*
Glanzer, M., 345, *354*
Glark, C. M., 219
Glaser, M., 383, *403*
Glaser, R., 19, *25*, 907, *913*
Glass, G. V., 907, *913*
Glass, L. E., 277, *298*
Glass, T. A., 796, *812*
Glasscote, R. M., 836, *850*
Glasser, M., 744, *758*
Glassman, A. H., 381, *403*, 500, *506*, 741, *758*
Glavin, Y., 445, *459*
Glen, A. I., 485, *505*
Glenner, G. G., 158, 165, *170*, 482, *506*
Gliklich, J. M., 421, *428*
Glucs, A., 263, *301*
Glynn, R. J., 522, 523, 524, 525, 541, *546*, *548*, *549*

Goate, A. M., 481, *506*
Goddard, D., 618, *641*
Godwin-Åusten, R. B., 489, *507*
Goetz, C. G., 186, *198*
Goetzinger, C. P., 272, *296*
Goff, D., 485, *507*, 754, *759*
Gold, D., 312, *331*
Gold, M. W., 152, *170*
Gold, R. L., 746, *759*
Goldberg, E. L., 397, *403*
Goldberg, I. D., 800, 802, *813*, 874, *890*
Goldberg, M., 319, *333*
Golden, C. J., 647, *665*
Golden, R., 33, 42, 46, 65, *68*, 617, *641*
Golden, R. R., 236, 244, *247*
Goldfarb, A. I., 237, *247*, 660, *666*, 834, 844, *850*
Golding, J. M., 54, 56, 57, *70*, 109, 110, *115*, *117*, 618, *638*
Goldman, A., 209, 210, *224*
Goldman, E., 523, *551*
Goldman, H., 878, *889*
Goldman, H. H., 798, *811*, 835, *850*, 873, 874, 877, 878, 879, *889*
Goldman, L., 764, *790*
Goldman, R., 829, *830*
Goldsmith, B. M., 536, 537, *547*
Goldsmith, J. M., 112, *115*
Goldstein, G., 647, *667*
Goldstein, R., 564, *579*
Goldstein, R. L., 863, *869*
Goldstrom, I. D., 803, *811*
Goli, V., 380, 386, 394, *404*
Goluboff, B., 204, *228*
Gomberg, E. L., 525, *548*
Gomberg, E. S. L., 59, 60, *68*
Gomez, F., 285, *301*
Gonatas, N. K., 157, *173*, 491, *504*
Gong, V., 327, 328, 329, *337*
Gonzales, J., 384, 388, 393, *404*
Gonze, M., 357, *373*
Goodell, H., 292, *298*, *304*
Goodgold, A., 491, *506*
Goodhardt, M. J., 182, 188, *194*
Goodin, D. T., 484, *508*
Gooding, W., 384, *406*
Goodman, A. G., 516, *549*
Goodman, B., 329, *333*
Goodman, J. D., 107, *115*

Goodman, L. S., 516, *549*
Goodman, S., 652, 654, *666*
Goodpaster, W. A., 439, 445, *461*
Goodwin, F. K., 569, *578*
Goodwin, J. S., 60, *66*, 319, *333*, 522, *545*
Gordon, A., 184, *199*
Gordon, C., 365, *372*
Gordon, E., 623, *639*
Gordon, J. R., 485, *504*
Gordon, M., 544, *551*
Gordon, M. M., 104, *115*
Gordon, M. N., 179, *197*
Gordon, P., 329, *333*
Gordon, T., 524, *549*
Gordon-Salant, S., 272, 273, 280, 288, *298*, *303*
Gorham, D. R., 617, *640*
Gorlin, R., 388, *406*
Gorman, J., 737, *762*
Gorman, J. M., 421, *428*
Gorsuch, R., 412, 419, *431*
Goss, J. R., 183, *196*
Gottfries, C. G., 182, 189, *194*, *196*, 486, *513*
Gottfries, I., 182, *196*
Gottleib, G. L., 798, *811*
Gottlieb, G. L., 876, 878, 879, 884, 885, *889*
Gottstein, U., 204, *225*
Goufries, C. G., 500, *503*
Gould, B., 256, *296*
Gould, R., 126, 134–135, *142*
Gouras, G., 219, *224*
Gove, W., 103, *115*
Gracon, S. I., 753, *758*
Grady, C. L., 150, *172*, 205, 207, 208, 209, 210, 211, 213, 214, 215, 216, 217, 218, 219, 221, 222, *223*, *224*, *225*, 226, 227, 645, *664*, *665*
Grady, J. G., 313, *332*
Graff-Radford, N., 150, *170*
Grafman, J., 495, *513*
Graham, I. M., 541, *547*
Graham, K., 522, 525, 527, 529, *549*
Graham-Pole, R., 533, *547*, 747, *757*
Grams, A. E., 314, *332*
Granger, C., 675, 685, 689, *695*
Granholm, E., 652, *664*
Granick, S., 901, *913*
Granovetter, M., 807, *812*
Grant, E., 343, *353*

Grant, I., 13, *24*, 527, *549*, 625, *639*, 652, 660, *664*, *665*
Grant, K., 660, *670*, 680, *697*
Graus, F., 495, *503*
Graves, A. B., 484, *506*
Graves, J. E., 347, *354*
Gray, B., 274, *305*
Gray, F., 495, *506*
Gray, J. W., 655, *664*
Gray, T. A., 388, *403*
Graybiel, A., 221, *225*
Grayson, D. A., 33, 42, *70*
Greden, F., 421, *431*
Greeley, A., 104, *115*
Green, A. I., 738, *758*
Green, I., 765, *791*
Green, M., 129, 130, *143*
Green, R., 712, 713, *714*
Green, R. L., 396, *401*
Greenberg, D., 184, *198*
Greenberg, J., 164, *172*, 593, *597*, 887, *889*
Greenberg, R., 381, *405*
Greenberg, R. L., 417, 422, *427*
Greenblatt, D. J., 423–424, *427*, *428*, 729, 730, 747, 748, *758*, *760*
Greenblatt, I. J., 575, *580*
Greenblatt, M., 396, *403*
Greene, H. A., 260, *298*
Greene, R., 712, 713, *714*
Greene, V. L., 110, *115*, 807, 808, *812*
Greenfield, J. P., 149, *170*
Greenfield, S., 907, *914*
Greenhouse, S. W., 208, *223*
Greenlick, M., 887, *889*
Greenough, P. G., 624, *639*
Greenough, W. T., 149, 152, *170*
Greenwald, B. S., 386, 387, 394, *403*, 485, *508*, 737, *758*
Greer, D., 685, 689, *695*
Grek, A., 680, *697*
Gresham, G., 689, *695*
Grey, B. A., 108, *116*
Gribben, K., 346, *353*
Griesinger, W., 611, *639*
Griest, J. H., 744, *759*
Griffin, B., 132, *142*, 703, *714*
Griffin, J. W., 190, *197*
Griffin, K., 500, *505*
Griffin, M. R., 540, *549*, 747, *760*
Griggs, D. S., 260, *296*

Grigor, R. R., 540, *549*
Grigson, B., 522, *547*
Grimes, A., 275, *298*
Grimes, A. M., 218, *225*
Grimshaw, L., 56, *68*
Grindle, J., 253, *301*
Grisold, W., 488, *507*
Grisso, T., 854, 858, 863, 864, *869*
Grob, G. N., 873, *889*
Grober, E., 326, 328, *332, 333*, 648, 652, 665
Grof, P., 384, *400*
Gronfein, W., 796, *812*
Gross, J. S., 494, *506*
Grosser, G. H., 396, *403*
Grossman, H. J., 584, *597*
Grossman, J. L., 316, *334*
Grotjahn, M., 701, 702, *714*, 901, *913*
Group for the Advancement of Psychiatry, 661, *665*
Group for the Advancement of Psychiatry, Committee on Aging, 909, *913*
Group for the Advancement of Psychiatry, Committee on Cultural Psychiatry, 904, *913*
Groves, L., 701, 702, 703, *715*, 743, *759*
Growden, J. H., 486, *508*
Growdon, J., 40, *72*, 214, *228*, 328, *333*
Growdon, J. H., 214, *224*, 487, *510*, 623, 624, 625, *639*, 653, *666*
Gruen, R., 120, *142*
Gruenberg, E. M., 28, 30, 32, 33, 35, 40, 41, 52, 59, *66, 68, 72*
Grundman, M., 617, *641*
Grunebaum, H., 137, *142*
Gruneberg, M. M., 318, *333*
Grunes, J., 132, *142*, 701, 702, 703, 711, *714, 715, 716*
Grzegorczyk, P. B., 280, *298*
Guider, R. L., 313, *337*
Guilford, J. P., 350, *353*
Guilleminault, C., 564, 575, *578*
Guiloff, R. J., 618, *638*
Gulaid, J. A., 541, *549*
Gulick, W. L., 266, 268, *298*
Gumbrecht, G., 498, 500, *503, 512*, 842, *850*
Gumbrecht, G. M., 500, *510*
Gummow, L., 329, *333*
Gunderson, J. G., 442, *460*
Gundke-Igbal, I., 157, *173*

Gunn, C. G., 166, 167, *171*
Gunther, A., 754, *759*
Gunther, J., 485, *507*
Gupta, B. K., 191, *196*
Gupta, M., 191, *196*
Gur, R. E., 205, *223*
Gurian, B., 837, *851*
Gurin, G., 411, 412, *428*
Gurland, B., 14, *24*, 31, 33, 42, 46, 65, *68*, 241, 242, *247*, 686, 688, 690, 693, *695*, 817, 820, *830*
Gurland, B. J., 15, *26*, 38, 42, 46, *67*, 109, *115*, 232, 234, 239, 243, 244, *247, 248*, 795, *812*
Gurling, H., 537, *553*
Gurney, C., 420, *428, 430*
Gurwitz, J. H., 728, *758*
Gusella, J. F., 40, *72*, 214, *228*
Gusella, J. I., 481, *512*
Gust, S. W., 540, *549*
Gustafson, L., 164, *171*, 209, *223*
Gustin, Q. L., 439, 445, *461*
Gutacker, P., 325, *337*
Guterman, A., 240, *247*, 652, 659, *667*, 687, 691, *696*
Guthrie, D., 177, *196*
Gutkin, C., 687, *697*
Gutkin, C. E., 808, *812*
Gutman, D., 75, 78, 85, 87, 94, *96, 97*
Gutmann, D., 9, *24*, 120, 132, 139, *142*, 703, *714*
Gutmann, D. L., 701, 702, 703, *713, 714, 715, 716*
Guttman, D., 521, 538, 542, *549*
Guy, D. W., 709, *714*
Guy, W., 498, *510*
Guze, B. H., 214, 220, 221, *223, 226*
Gwirtsman, H. E., 393, *403*
Gwyther, L. P., 805, 809, *811*
Gyldensted, C., 150, *171*

Ha, Y. S., 743, *759*
Haaland, K. Y., 624, *639*
Haan, E. A., 182, *194*
Haan, N., 366, *373*
Haas, A. P., 398, *403*
Hachinski, V., 646, *667*

Hachinski, V. C., 219, *225*, 491, 492, *506*, *511–512*, 658, 659, *665*
Haegerstrom-Portnoy, G., 264, *298*
Hagberg, J. M., 347, *354*
Hagborg, J. M., 346, *354*
Hagenlocker, K., 653, *666*
Haggett, A., 747, *757*
Hagnell, O., 28, 33, 34, 37, 38, 43, 46, 47, 62, *68*, *69*, *71*
Haigler, H. J., 483, *506*
Haines, J. L., 40, *72*, 214, *228*, 481, *509*, *512*
Hajdukovic, R. M., 573, *579*
Hakim, A. M., 488, *506*
Hakim, S., 493, *503*
Hakkinen, L., 253, *298*
Halaris, A., 393, *403*
Halberg, F., 573, *581*
Hale, W. E., 538, 539, *551*, 747, 749, *758*
Haley, W. E., 707, *714*
Halikas, J. A., 130, *141*, 567, *577*
Hall, F., 564, 572, *578*
Hall, F. T., 559, *577*
Hall, R. C. W., 520, 538, *546*, *548*
Hall, R. W. C., 423, *428*
Hall, T. C., 153, *171*
Hallett, C., 533, *547*
Halsey, H., 221, *224*
Halter, J. B., 486, *510*
Haltin, M., 493, *513*
Haman, K. L., 349, *352*
Hamer, J., 90, *97*
Hamer, R. M., 651, 654, *665*
Hamilton, J., 529, *548*
Hamilton, M., 236, *247*, 418, *428*, 617, *639*
Hamilton, S., 350, *352*
Hammarlund, E. R., 538, 539, *552*
Hammeke, T. A., 647, *665*
Hammen, C., 392, *406*
Hammen, C. L., 700, 701, 711, *716*
Hammer, M., 486, *511*
Hammond, K. M., 657, *665*
Hamsher, K. de S., 646, *663*
Hand, D., 754, *759*
Haney, C. A., 529, 538, *553*
Hankin, J., 802, *812*
Hanley, R., 499, *510*, 523, *552*
Hansen, C. C., 266, *298*

Hansen, D. B., 204, *223*
Hansen, L. A., 176, 177, *196*, *198*
Hansen, L. N., 153, *173*
Hansen, N., 838, *850*
Happersett, C., 107, *115*
Hapworth, W., 743, *758*
Harbaugh, R., 487, *510*
Harbaugh, R. E., 485, *506*
Harding, C. M., 466, 467, 469, *474*
Harding, J. S., 411, *429*
Harding, P. S., 59, *73*
Hardy, B., 395, *403*
Hardy, J. A., 481, *506*
Hardy, J. D., 292, *298*, *304*
Harker, J. O., 645, *669*
Harkins, S. W., 266, 267, 272, 292, 293, *298*, *302*, 329, *333*, 654, *665*
Harley, C., 347, *353*
Harman, M., 351, *353*
Harmar, A. J., 182, *197*
Harmatz, J., 423, *431*
Harmatz, J. S., 617, *641*, 730, *758*
Harp, S., 258, *298*
Harper, C., 497, *506*
Harper, M. S., 13, *24*
Harrah, C., 687, 691, 692, *696*
Harrah, C. H., 237, 240, *248*
Harrell, A. V., 537, *551*
Harrell, L. E., 624, *639*
Harrell, S., 84, *96*
Harrington, M. G., 496, *507*
Harrington, P., 536, *549*
Harris, H., 280, *298*
Harris, J. E., 316, *333*
Harris, M. J., 733, *760*
Harris, S., 363, *374*
Harris, T., 125, 127, *141*, 241, *246*
Harrop, R., 209, *227*, 493, *507*
Harrow, M., 394, *402*
Hart, R. P., 329, *333*, 347, 349, *353*, 651, 654, *665*
Hartford, J. T., 524, *549*
Hartley, A. A., 312, *332*
Hartley, J. T., 312, *333*
Hartman, B. K., 164, *171*, *172*
Hartman, C., 768, *791*
Hasher, L., 311, 324, *333*
Hasin, D., 47, *69*
Haskins, E., 327, 328, 329, *337*

Hassell, J., 483, *511*
Hastoe, T., 35, *69*
Hatazawa, J., 205, *227*
Hatziandreu, E., 541, *552*
Hatziandreu, E. J., 541, 542, *548*
Haug, H., 176, *196*
Haug, M., 822, *830*
Haugh, M., 157, *172*
Hauser, D. C., 486, *504*
Hauser, D. L., 491, *504*
Hausman, C. P., 318, *336*
Havasy, S., 711, *715*
Havasy-Galloway, S., 701, 702, 703, *715*
Havens, L. L., 607, *639*
Hawk, T. C., 214, *226*
Hawke, S. H., 526, *554*
Hawkes, J., 154, *171*, 486, *508*
Hawkins, J. E., Jr., 266, *299*
Hawkins, R. A., 210, 211, 212, 219, *223, 226*
Haxby, J. V., 151, *171*, 205, 207, 208, 209, 210, 211, 213, 214, 215, 216, 217, 218, 219, 221, 222, *223, 224, 225, 226, 227*, 645, *664, 665*
Hayashi, Y., 559, *578*
Haycox, J., 654, *668*
Hayman, A., 481, *511*
Haynes, A. R., 481, *506*
Haynes, C. S., 481, *509*
Hays, R. D., 907, *914*
Haywood, K. M., 254, *306*
Hazelwood, L., 708, *713*
Hazzard, W. R., 875, 876, *889*
Heacock, P., 821, 822, *829*
Health Care Financing Administration, 883, *889*
Healton, E. B., 494, *508*
Healy, M. J. R., 205, *227*
Heather, J. D., 202, 205, *225, 227*
Heaton, R. K., 659, 660, 661, *665*
Hebert, L. E., 201, 209, *224*, 480, 482, *505*, 753, *758*
Heckmann, T., 260, *299, 304*
Hedreen, J. C., 153–154, *178*, 472, *475*, 501, *513*
Hefti, F., 487, *510*
Heger, M., 659, *664*
Hegsted, D. M., 524, *549*
Heiden, J., 190, *196*

Heikkila, K., 562, *579*
Heikkinen, E., 290, *297*
Heiland, W. F., 834, *852*
Heilman, K., 319, *333*
Heinold, J. W., 542, *549*
Heinonen, O. P., 38, 39, 40, *72*
Heiring, J., 240, *247*
Held, K., 204, *225*
Helkala, E. L., 621, *641*
Helkala, E-L., 182, *198*
Heller, H., 485, *507*, 754, *759*
Heller, N., 572, *578*
Heller, T., 592, *597*
Helling, D. K., 538, 539, *549*
Helms, M. J., 34, *69*, 484, *507*
Helms, P. M., 385, *402*, 733, *759*
Helsing, K. J., 107, *115*
Helzer, J. C., 438, *460*
Helzer, J. E., 57, 58, 60, *66, 69*
Hemsi, L. K., 350, *353*
Henderson, A. S., 31, 32, 33, 38, 39, 40, 42, 60, *67, 69, 70*
Henderson, J. G., 494, *512*
Henderson, R. L., 263, *299*
Henderson, V. W., 151, *171*, 660, *666*
Hendin, H., 398, *403*
Hendler, J., 455, *459*
Hendricks, C. D., 900, *913*
Hendricks, J., 900, *913*
Hendrickson, A., 253, *306*
Hendrickson, D. E., 35o, 350, *352*
Hendrie, H., 618, *641*
Heninger, G. R., 421, *428*
Henkins, R. I., 284, *299*
Hennekens, C. H., 201, 209, *224*, 480, 482, *505*, 753, *758*
Henrichs, M., 389, *402*
Henry, N., 236, *247*
Henry, W., 87, *96*, 137, *142*
Hensel, H., 292, *299*
Herbert, L. E., 201, 209
Herbert, M. E., 467, *474*
Herbert, V., 539, *549*
Herfkens, R. F., 391–392, *401*
Herman, G. E., 272, *299*
Herman, G. F., 272, *306*
Herman, R., 768, *791*
Herman, S., 822, *830*
Hermann, C. K., 386, 387, 394, *403*

Hermanson, B., 541, *549*
Hermos, J. A., 522, 523, *548, 549*
Herold, S., 205, *227*
Herrmann, D. J., 313, 314, *333*
Herscovitch, P., 205, 218, 221, *225, 226*
Herscowitch, P., 417, *430*
Hershey, L. A., 624, *639*, 746, *759*
Herst, L., 844, *851*
Hertzog, C., 331, *334*, 340, 345, 346, *353, 354*
Hess, P., 826, 827, *830*
Hess, T. M., 330, *334*
Hesselink, J. R., 623, 624, *639*
Heston, L., 209, 210, 211, 214, *223, 224*, 645, *664*
Heston, L. L., 214, 215, *226*, 484, 493, *507, 512*
Heusman, R. H., 209, *225*
Hewitt, K. E., 588, *597*
Heyman, A., 15, *25*, 34, *69*, 108, *115*, 484, 485, *507, 511*
Heyman, A. L., 481, *509*
Hiatt, L. G., 767, *791*
Hichwa, R. H., 204, *224*
Hickey, N., 541, *547*
Hickey, W. F., 491, *504*
Hicks, S. P., 37, *71*, 191, *197*
Hidalgo, J., 804, *812*
Hier, D. B., 653, *666*
Hietanen, M., 656–657, *666*
Higbee, K. L., 314, *334*
Higgins, K. E., 264, *300*
Higgitt, A. C., 530, 531, 532, 534, 535, *549*
Hijdra, A., 660, *664*
Hilbert, N. M., 653, *666*
Hildebrand, H. P., 703, 704, *714*
Hill, B. K., 589, *596*
Hill, C., 654, *666*
Hill, C. D., 654, *669*
Hill, D., 654, *669*
Hill, M. A., 392, 393, *403, 406*, 446, *460*, 624, *637*, 653, 656, *664, 668*, 700, 711, *716*
Hill, R., 423, *432*
Hill, R. D., 649, 650, 651, 653, *669*
Himmelfarb, S., 349, *354*, 412, 420, *428*, 567, *580*
Himmelhoch, J. M., 382, *403*
Himwich, H., 588, *596*

Hinchcliffe, R., 250, 267, 271, *299*
Hingson, R., 523, *551*
Hinkle, P. E., 391, *402*
Hippius, H., 384, *400*
Hirano, A., 571, *578*
Hiris, E., 264, 280, *303*
Hirschfeld, R., 452, *460*
Hirschfield, M. A., 47, *70*
Hirschfield, R. M. A., 47, *71*
Hiscock, M., 539, *551*
Hobbs, W. J., 40, *72*, 214, *228*
Hoch, C. C., 13, *26*, 535, *552*, 559, 560, 561, 562, 564, 569, 571, 572, 573, 575, 576, *577, 578*, 580–581
Hoch, P., 396, *404*
Hodge, C. F., 152, *171*
Hodkinson, H. M., 820, *830*
Hoff, S. F., 190, *196*
Hoffman, E., 164, *172*
Hoffman, J. M., 214, *226*
Hofstetter, H. W., 253, 260, *299*
Hoglund, D., 765, *791*
Hokanson, J. E., 443, *457*
Holborn, P. J., 659, *666*
Holcomb, H. H., 207, *223*
Holford, T. R., 41, *73*
Holland, A. L., 649, *666*
Holland, J. C., 47, *69*, 388, *403*
Hollander, E., 56, *69*
Hollander, E. R., 486, *507*
Hollister, L. E., 732, 735, *760*
Holloszy, J. O., 346, *354*
Holloway, J. R., 821, *831*
Holman, H., 686, 690, *695*
Holman, L., 625, *639*
Holmes, L., 84, *97*
Holmes, M. M., 544, *551*
Holmes, V. F., 496, *507*
Holroyd, J., 594, *597*
Holton, A., 737, *759*
Holzer, C. E., 41, 42, 47, 48, *72, 73*, 386, 388, *405, 406*, 410, 412, *430*, 531, 536, *551*, 795, 801, 803, *812*
Holzer, C. E., III, 58, 60, *69*, 523, 524, 526, *549*
Homma, A., 386, *405*
Honigfeld, G., 469, *474*
Hook, E. W., 861, *871*
Horitz, B., 205, 221, *225*

Horn, J. L., 341, 345, *353*
Horner, J., 485, *511*
Hornykiewicz, O., 184, 190, *196*
Horovitz, J., 768, *791*
Horowitz, M., 277, *299*, 392, *403*, 704, 709, *714*
Horton, A., 40, *68*
Horvath, T. B., 485, *508*
Horvath, Z., 388, *403*
Horwitz, B., 204, 207, 210, 211, 213, 214, 215, 216, 217, 218, 221, 222, *225*, *226*, *228*
Horwitz, G. J., 163, *170*
Hossain, T. I., 484, *508*
Houck, P. R., 13, *26*, 561, 562, 564, 569, 571, 572, 576, *578*, *580*
Hough, R. L., 108, 109, 110, *115*, *116*, *117*
Houlihan, J. P., 805, *812*
Houpt, J. L., 389, *402*, 654, *669*, 803, *813*
Houston, M. J., 617, *637*
Howe, M. W., 708, *716*
Howell, N., 84, *96*
Howell, S. C., 765, *791*
Howell, T. H., 290, *299*
Howitz, B., 645, *665*
Hoxby, J. V., 151, *170*
Hoyer, W., 320, 321, 323, *333*, *334*, *335*
Hsiao, W. C., 882, 883, *890*
Hu, T., 902, *913*
Huand, O., 327, *337*
Huang, H. Y., 417, *430*
Huang, L., 902, *913*
Huang, P., 617, *641*
Huang, V., 15, *26*, 419, *431*
Hubbard, B. M., 153, *169*, *171*, 188, *196*
Huber, S. J., 633, *639*, 656, *666*
Hubert, L. E., 33, *68*
Huff, F. J., 14, *26*, 649, 653, *666*
Huffine, C. L., 525, *549*
Huggett, A., 533, *547*
Hughes, C. P., 151, *170*, 648, 651, 653, *666*, *669*
Hughes, D. C., 14, *23*, 108, *115*, 349, *352*, 380, 381, 382, 383, 385, 389, 397, *401*, *403*
Hughes, J. R., 540, *549*
Hughes, S., 807, *811*
Hughes, S. T., 819, *830*
Hughston, G. A., 711, *714*

Hulicka, I. M., 316, *334*
Hull, C. D., 177, *196*
Hull, C. L., 367, *373*
Hultsch, D. F., 309, 310, 313, 316, *332*, *334*
Humbach, E., 847, *850*
Hummert, M. L., 364, *372*
Hung, W. Y., 481, *509*
Hung, W-Y., 481, *511*
Hunt, A. L., 624, *639*
Hunt, M. E., 768, *791*
Hunt, W. C., 60, *66*, 522, *545*
Huntington, J. M., 262, *299*
Huppert, F. A., 33, *69*, 618, *641*
Hurley, B. F., 346, *354*
Hurley, J. R., 422, *429*
Hursch, C. J., 561, *581*
Hurst, L., 498, *504*
Hurst, N. C., 675, *695*
Hurt, R. D., 525, 526, 527, 528, 529, *548*, *549*
Hurtig, H. I., 205, *223*
Hurwitz, B. J., 485, *511*
Hurwitz, D., 240, *247*, 687, 691, *696*
Husain, M. M., 468, *474*
Hussian, R. A., 700, 701, 706, 711, *714*, *715*
Hutchins, G., 567, *580*
Hutchinson, J., 266, *304*
Hutton, J. T., 38, *68*, *71*, 254, 263, *299*, 484, *508*
Hwu, H. G., 60, *69*
Hyden, H., 155, *171*
Hyland, D. T., 330, *334*
Hyler, S. E., 455, *459*
Hyman, B. T., 483, *507*
Hymas, N., 467, *474*
Hynes, R., 264, *300*

Ibe, K., 539, *550*
Ichijo, M., 624, *639*
Ido, T., 164, *172*
Iglehart, J. K., 885, *890*
Ihara, K., 157, *171*
Iivanainen, M., 492, *505*
Ijspeert, J. K., 262, *299*
Iliff, L. D., 219, *225*, 492, *506*, 658, *665*
Imai, K., 619, *639*
Imber, S., 574, *581*

In re Eichner, 860, *869*
In re Patrick W, 863, *869*
In re Quinlan, 860, *869*
In re Roderick P, 863, *869*
Inciardi, J. A., 536, *552*
Ingham, C. A., 149, 152, *170*
Ingram, D. K., 179, *198*, *199*
Ingvar, D. H., 164, *171*, 205, 207, 208, 224
Inhelder, B., 854, *870*
Innocenti, G. M., 169, *171*
Insel, T. R., 56, *69*
Inui, T. S., 239, *246*, 907, *912*
Inzitari, E., 491, *511*
Iqbal, K., 157, *171*, 188, *194*, 484, *508*
Irion, A., 903, *912*
Irving, D., 154, *173*, 180, *198*, 490, *509*
Irwin, I., 186, 191, *196*, *198*
Ismail, A. H., 319, *333*
Iversen, L. L., 182, *198*
Iverson, I., 685, 689, *697*
Iverson, L. L., 183, 184, 189, *196*, *198*, 212, *228*, 486, *504*
Ivry, J., 809, *813*
Iwangoff, P., 182, 188, *194*

Jablensky, A., 31, *69*
Jackson, B., 675, 685, *695*
Jackson, C., 261, *305*
Jackson, G., 679, *696*
Jackson, J. S., 13, *24*
Jackson, M., 526, *554*
Jackson, M. E., 835, *851*
Jackson, R., 289, *299*
Jackson, S. W., 380, *403*
Jackson, W., 765, *791*
Jackson v. Indiana, 864, *869*
Jacobowitz, J., 355, *374*, 703, *715*
Jacobs, D., 572, *578*
Jacobs, S., 127, *142*
Jacobsen, J., 421, *429*
Jacobson, J. W., 585, 588, 589, *597*
Jacobson, S., 467, *474*
Jacoby, C. G., 391, *407*
Jacoby, R. J., 381–382, 391, *403*
Jacomb, P. A., 32, *69*
Jaffe, D. F., 624, *639*

Jaffe, J., 575, *577*
Jaffe, M., 675, 685, *695*
Jagenburg, R., 541, *551*
Jagoda, N., 279, *301*
Jagust, W. J., 213, 215, *226*, 652, 660, *668*
Jahoda, M., 9, *24*
Jajich, C. L., 541, *550*
Jamada, M., 209, *226*
James, I. M., 533, *547*, 747, *757*
James, L. A., 481, *506*
James, O. F. W., 523, 528, *546*, *555*
James, S. A., 386, *402*
Jamieson, C., 536, *550*
Jamieson, D. G., 205, *223*
Janicki, M. P., 583, 585, 586, 588, 589, *597*, 598
Janik, S. W., 529, *550*
Janis, I. L., 241, *247*, 369, *373*
Jankel, W. R., 472, *475*
Jansen, R., 495, *507*
Janssen, T., 877, *890*
Jaques, E., 132, *142*
Jarvik, L., 393, *403*, 410, *429*, 574, *578*, 743, *758*
Jarvik, L. F., 326, 328, *334*, 392, *406*, 645, 651, 652, 661, *666*, 700, 711, *716*, 738, *758*, 816, *830*
Jaspers, K., 30, *69*
Jassani, A., 709, *713*
Jatlow, P. L., 421, *428*
Javid, J. I., 743, *759*
Javoy-Agid, F., 488, *505*
Jayaram, G., 468, *475*
Jefferson, J. W., 744, *759*
Jellinger, K., 184, 188, *196*, *198*, 488, *507*
Jencks, S. J., 873, 874, 877, 878, *889*
Jenike, M. A., 391, *403*, 418, 420, 423, 424, *429*, 485, *507*, 519, *550*, 743, 754, *759*, 853, *869*
Jenkins, C. D., 420, *429*
Jenkins, R., 454, *459*
Jenner, F. A., 472, *474*
Jennett, B., 190, *196*
Jennings, J. R., 559, *577*
Jensen, B. A., 380, *402*
Jerger, J., 272, 273, 294, *299*
Jernigan, T. L., 527, *552*, 623, 624, *639*
Jerrom, G. W. A., 532, *552*
Jeste, D. V., 15, *24*, 732, 733, *760*, 762

Jimerson, D. C., 486, *510*
Joachim, C. L., 483, *507*
Joffe, R. T., 388, *403*
Joffee, F. R., 423, *428*
Johanson, C. E., 531, 535, *554*
John, E. R., 31, *69*
Johns, C. A., 485, *508*
Johnson, A. L., 182, *198*
Johnson, B. A., 753, *757*
Johnson, C. A., 264, *299*
Johnson, D. R., 711, *715*
Johnson, F. L., 110, 111, *116*
Johnson, H. A., 253, *297*
Johnson, J. A., 182, 183, 189, *195*
Johnson, K. A., 623, 624, 625, *639*
Johnson, R. C., 436, *459*
Johnson, R. E., 152, *170*
Johnson, S. A., 483, *507*
Johnson, T., 692, *696*
Johnsson, L. G., 266, *299*
Johnston, M. V., 487, *510*
Johnstone, C., 765, *791*
Jokela, J., 290, *297*
Jolkkonen, J., 182, *198*
Jolkkonin, J., 488, *507*
Jolley, D. J., 385, *401*
Jones, B., 261, *303*
Jones, B. E., 108, *116*
Jones, C. M., 292, *297*
Jones, G., 329, *334*
Jones, G. M. M., 541, *550*
Jones, H. E., 359, *373*
Jones, R., 677, *695*
Jones, S. R., 540, *546*
Jones, S. W., 280, *298*
Jones, T., 202, 205, 209, 219, *225, 227*
Jonsen, A. R., 857, *869*
Jordan, B. D., 632, *640*
Jordan, K., 438, *457*
Jorgensen, P., 470, *474*
Jorm, A. F., 32, 33, 39, *67, 69, 70,* 344, 345, 350, *353*
Joseph, J. A., 179, *198*
Josephm, H., 536, 537, *547*
Jost, G., 151, *170*
Joyner, R. E., 286, *299*
Joynt, R. J., 604, *638*
Judd, B. W., 492, *508,* 541, *553*
Jue, B. A., 537, *547*

Julian, C. E., 484, *509*
Jung, C., 120, 132, 134, *142*
Jung, C. G., 357, *373*
Juraska, J. M., 149, 152, *170*
Jyu, C. A., 539, *551*

Kafonek, S., 384, *403,* 732, *761,* 835, *851, 852*
Kahana, R. J., 702, *715*
Kahn, E., 559, *578*
Kahn, H. A., 256, 265, *299*
Kahn, J., 157, *172*
Kahn, M., 388, *406*
Kahn, R., 424, *429*
Kahn, R. L., 6, 16, 17, 19, *24,* 28, 72, 237, *247,* 593, *598,* 653, 660, *666*
Kahneman, D., 323, *334*
Kaiser, H., 590, *597*
Kakkai, T., 60, *70*
Kalab, M., 84, *97*
Kalayam, B., 381, 390, *405*
Kales, A., 559, 564, 566, *579,* 751, *759*
Kales, J. D., 559, *579,* 751, *759*
Kalinowsky, L., 396, *404*
Kalish, R. A., 114, *116,* 371, *373*
Kall, B. L., 110, *116*
Kalmus, H., 280, *298, 299*
Kalnin, A., 491, *506*
Kalnok, M., 356, 357, *373*
Kaltreider, N., 392, *403,* 709, *714*
Kamerow, D. B., 18, *23,* 530, *546,* 566, 567, *578,* 728, 746, 752, *757,* 840, *850*
Kameyama, M., 159, *172,* 210, *227*
Kaminsky, M., 711, *715*
Kamo, H., 209, *227,* 493, *507*
Kandel, E. R., 176, *196*
Kandler, K. S., 127, *142*
Kane, J., 469, *474*
Kane, J. M., 469, *474*
Kane, R. A., 681, 682, 684, 688, *695,* 866, *870*
Kane, R. H., 19, *24*
Kane, R. L., 681, 682, 684, 688, *695,* 822, *830,* 834, 840, *852*
Kania, J., 542, *550*
Kanjilal, G. C., 590, *596*
Kantor, J. S., 421, *429*

Kantor, S. J., 500, *506*
Kao, L. C., 186, *198*
Kaplan, A. R., 281, *299*
Kaplan, B. H., 386, *402*
Kaplan, H., 278, *299*, 898, *913*
Kaplan, M., 314, *335*
Kaplan, R. D., 451, *459*
Kaplan, W., 654, *669*
Kaplitz, S. E., 395, *404*
Kaprio, J., 186, *197*, 562, *579*
Karacan, I., 561, *581*
Karajgi, B., 422, *429*
Karamouz, N., 395, *400*
Karasu, T. B., 701, 712, *717*
Karis, C., 262, *301*
Karis, D., 331, *331*
Karlson, I., 182, 189, *194*
Karno, M., 34, 35, 41, 49, 51, 52, 54, 56,
    57, 58, 60, *67*, *70*, *71*, 109, 110, *115*,
    116, *117*, 380, 384, *407*, 618, *638*
Karno, R. L., 108, 109, *115*
Kasahara, Y., 33, *72*
Kase, C. S., 539, *550*
Kasl, S., 680, 681, *694*
Kastenbaum, R., 360, *373*
Kastrup, M., 439, 445, *459*
Kaszniak, A. W., 649, 652–653, *663*
Kathol, R. G., 422, *429*
Katon, W., 395, *404*
Katz, D., 484, *509*
Katz, I., 14, *25*
Katz, I. R., 384, *405*, 819, *830*
Katz, J., 858, *869*
Katz, P., 825, *831*
Katz, S., 234, 241, 242, *247*, 673, 675, 677,
    685, 689, *694*, *695*, *697*
Katzman, B., 910, *914*
Katzman, R., 13, *24*, 32, *71*, 237, 240, *247*,
    328, *334*, 479, 492, *508*, *511*, 645, 647,
    652, 658, *665*, *667*, *669*
Kaufman, E., 537, *547*
Kaufman, M. R., 702, *715*
Kaufman, S. R., 254, *300*
Kausler, D., 323, *334*
Kawas, C., 191, *195*
Kay, D. W. K., 31, 33, 40, 42, 60, *69*, *70*,
    386, *404*, 420, *429*, 468, *474*
Kay, W., 344, *354*
Kazniak, A. W., 15, *26*

Keefe, N. C., 656, *664*
Keegan, D. L., 539, *551*
Keenan, T., 480, *511*
Kehoe, L., 530, *551*
Kell, R. L., 271, *300*
Kellan, S. G., 29, *70*
Kelleher, E., 110, 111, *116*
Kelleher, M. J., 38, 42, 46, *67*
Keller, D. M., 687, 692, *694*
Keller, J. F., 713, *715*
Keller, M. B., 47, *70*
Keller, M. G., 47, *71*
Keller, S. E., *013*, 907
Kellet, J. M., 500, *503*
Kellett, J. M., 539, *552*
Kelly, C. D., 679, *696*
Kelly, G. A., 360, *373*
Kelly, M. J., 399, *406*
Kelly, N. L., 882, 883, *890*
Kelsey, T. G., 619, *639*
Kemp, B., 692, *695*
Kemp, B. J., 109, *116*
Kemp, W., 109, *116*
Kemper, P., 886, *890*
Kendell, R. E., 109, *115*
Kendig, N. E., 494–495, *507*
Kendrick, D. C., 649, *666*
Kennedy, C., 202, 203, *228*
Kennedy, J. S., 533, *545*
Kennie, D. V., 682, *695*
Kenshalo, D. R., 289, 290, 291, 292, *300*
Kentopp, E., 110, 111, *116*
Keohane, C., 495, *506*
Kermis, M. D., 820, *830*
Kernberg, O., 80, *97*, 132, *142*, 443, *459*,
    704, *715*
Kerr, T. A., 420, *428*, *430*
Kerridge, D. F., 660, *670*
Kerrige, D. F., 680, *697*
Kertesz, A., 624, 625, *639*
Keshaven, M. S., 500, *505*
Kessler, L. G., 29, 60, *70*, 107, *115*, 349,
    353, 803, *811*
Kessler, R., 207, *223*
Kessler, R. C., 105, 112, *116*, 801, *812*
Kessler, R. M., 205
Kethley, A., 521, 523, *552*, 819, *831*
Kethley, A. J., 538, 539, *552*
Ketonen, L., 492, *505*, 624, *638*

Kety, S. S., 202, 204, *223*, *226*
Keyl, P. M., 49, 52, 54, 65, *70*
Keys, A., 262, *296*
Khachaturian, Z. S., 487, *510*
Kidd, M., 157, *171*
Kido, D. K., 622, *639*
Kiecolt-Glaser, J., 19, *25*
Kiecolt-Glaser, J. K., 907, *913*
Kiely, M., 586, 587, 589, *598*
Kilburn, H., 108, *117*
Kilcourse, J., 419, *431*
Kilner, J. F., 867, *870*
Kiloh, L. G., 32, *70*, 328, *336*, 499, *507*, 653, *666*
Kilts, C. D., 486, *504*
Kim, C. B. Y., 263, *301*
Kim, J. H., 484, *508*
Kim, K. Y., 746, *759*
Kim, P. K. H., 536, *554*
Kim, Y., 656, *664*
Kimata, K., 483, *511*
Kimbrell, C. M., 286, *300*
King, D. A., 634, *639*
King, M. B., 525, 528, 530, 545, *550*, *553*
King, R. J., 414, *431*
Kini, M. M., 256, 265, *299*
Kinnamon, J. C., 279, *300*
Kinscherf, D. A., 446, *460*
Kinsel, V., 214, *225*
Kinsella, A., 469, *475*
Kirikae, I., 266, *300*
Kirkwood, T. B. L., 30, *70*
Kirscht, J. P., 802, *812*
Kirshner, H. S., 624, *641*
Kirshner, L. A., 702, *715*
Kishka, U., 621, *638*
Kissel, C., 486, *506*
Kissin, B., 516, *550*
Kitani, M., 541, *555*
Kitano, H. H., 111, *116*
Kitchell, M. A., 384, 388, *404*
Kitchen, S., 903, *912*
Kittner, S., 384, *403*, 835, *851*
Kitto, J., 240, *247*
Kivela, S. L., 42, 47, 48, *70*
Kivnick, H. Q., 703, *714*
Kiyak, A., 234, 240, 245, *248*
Kiyak, H. A., 676, *697*

Klasses, I., 369, *373*
Klatsky, A. L., 524, *550*
Klawans, H. L., 472, *475*
Kleban, M., 687, 692, *696*
Kleim, D., 323, *334*
Klein, D. C., 350, *354*
Klein, D. F., 417, 424, *429*
Klein, E., 120, 132, *142*
Klein, J. G., 437, 445, *460*
Klein, L. E., 802, 810, *811*
Klein-Schwartz, W., 536, *550*
Kleinbaum, D. G., 29, *70*, 386, *402*
Kleinhauz, M., 386, *402*
Kleinman, A., 113, *116*, 609, *639*
Kleinman, J. M., 291, *300*
Kleinman, J. S., 590, *598*
Klerman, G., 349, *353*, 419, *430*
Klerman, G. L., 46, 47, *70*, *71*, *73*, 234, *247*, 419, *429*, 635, *640*, 902, *913*
Klerman, L. V., 380, *405*
Klesges, R. C., 651, *666*
Kline, D. W., 253, 254, 258, 260, 262, 264, 265, *300*, *303*, *304*
Kline, G. E., 261, *305*
Kline, K., 676, *694*
Kling, A., 485, *512*
Klinger, A., 219, *224*
Klinowski, J., 484, *504*
Klotz, J., 382, *401*
Kluger, A., 209, 219, *227*
Knesper, D. J., 797, *812*
Kniepmann, K., 689, *694*
Knight, B., 701, *715*
Knight, R. T., 496, *505*
Knoblauch, K., 264, *300*
Knopman, D. S., 240, *247*, 609, *640*, 648, *666*
Knott, V. J., 349, *353*
Knox, L. A., 585, *597*
Kobari, M., 624, *639*
Kobasyashi, J., 659, *665*
Kobata, F. S., 106, 113, *116*
Kobayashi, H., 33, *72*
Kobayashi, S., 541, *555*
Koch-Weser, J., 730, *758*
Kochansky, G. E., 418–419, *429*
Kocsis, J., 381, 382, *401*, 739, *757*
Kodner, D., 887, *889*
Koegel, P., 536, *550*

Koenig, H. G., 380, 384, 386, 387, 388, 393, 394, 397, *404*, 617, *639*, 817, *830*
Koenigsberg, H. W., 451, *459*
Koepke, H. H., 746, *759*
Koepsell, T. D., 484, *506*
Kofoed, L., 542, *550*
Kofoed, L. L., 516, 519, 520, 524, 525, 526, 528, 529, 537, 538, *545*, *546*, *550*
Kohlmeyer, K., 33, *70*
Kohrs, M. B., 319, *335*
Kohut, H., 80, *97*, 704, *715*
Koi, M., 167, *173*
Kokmen, E., 34, *70*, *72*
Kolli, R., 422, *429*
Kolligian, J., Jr., 355, *374*
Koncelik, J., 765, 769, *791*
Kondo, J., 157, *171*
Konig, E., 253, 254, 271, *300*
Kopeikan, H., 500, *507*
Kopelman, M. D., 654, *666*
Koppel, C., 539, *550*
Koppel, H., 169, *171*
Koran, L. W., 619, *639*
Koresko, R. L., 572, *578*
Kornfeld, D. S., 907, *913*
Korsarek, E., 40, *68*
Korten, A. E., 33, 39, *67*, *70*
Kortman, K. E., 151, *171*
Korzun, A. H., 47, *69*, 388, *403*
Kosberg, J. I., 866, *870*
Koskenvuo, M., 186, *197*, 562, *579*
Koslowski, P. B., 166, *173*
Kosnik, W., 253, 254, *300*
Kosovsky, R., 386, *402*
Koss, B., 209, *225*
Koss, E., 210, 211, 213, 214, 215, 221, *225*, *226*, 652, *668*
Kothari, P., 211, *224*
Koziarz, B. J., 205. *224*
Kraemer, H. C., 619, *639*
Kraepelin, E., 383, *404*, 464, *474*
Kraft, P. G., 544, *551*
Krahn, D. D., 500, *505*
Kraines, R., 686, 690, *695*
Kraiuhin, C., 623, *639*
Kral, V. A., 654, *666*
Kramer, B. A., 395, *404*
Kramer, J. H., 647, 652, *664*, *666*
Kramer, J. J., 318, *331*

Kramer, M., 10, *25*, 29, 30, 34, 35, 41, 43, 49, 51, 52, 54, 56, 57, 58, 59, 60, 62, *66*, *68*, *70*, *71*, *72*, 410, 412, *430*, 531, *551*, 636, 835, *850*
Kramer, P. D., 800, 802, 803–804, *813*, 867, 870, 874, *890*
Kramer-Ginsberg, E., 386, 387, 394, *403*
Krause, N., 802, 807, *812*
Krauss, M. W., 585, 589, 590, 591, 592, 593, 594, *598*
Krauthammer, C., 635, *640*
Kravits, J., 801, *810*
Kricheff, I. I., 150, *170*, 210, *224*, 240, *246*
Krieger, M., 486, *506*
Kripke, D. F., 562, 564, 566, 568, 572, *577*, *579*
Krishnan, K. R. R., 389, 391, *402*, *404*, 468, *474*
Krishnan, S. S., 484, *505*
Kritzler, Z. A., 883, *889*
Kromer, L. F., 487, *507*
Kromer, L. J., 483, *507*
Kronauer, R. E., 576, *577*
Kronmal, R. A., 541, *549*
Krupka, L. R., 538, 539, *554*
Kruse, A., 363, 368, 369, *373*
Kryger, M. H., 558, 561, *579*
Ksiezak-Reding, H., 483, *507*
Kua, E. H., 59, *70*
Kubos, K. L., 47, *71*
Kudler, H. S., 394, *404*
Kuhar, M. J., 486, 488, *505*, *512*
Kuhl, D. E., 151, 164, *171*, *172*, 205, 207, 210, 211, 212, 214, 215, 219, *223*, *226*, 227, 645, *666*
Kuhlen, G. A., 360, *373*
Kukull, W. A., 239, *246*, 571, *581*, 725, *759*, 907, *912*
Kulka, R. A., 801, *812*
Kulys, R., 362, *373*
Kumar, A., 211, 214, *225*, 227
Kumar, V., 754, *759*
Kuo, W. H., 111, *116*
Kupfer, D. J., 13, *26*, 535, *552*, 559, 561, 562, 564, 569, 570, 571, 572, 573, 574, 576, *577*, *578*, *579*, *580–581*, *581*
Kupferer, S., 701, *717*
Kupper, L. L., 29, *70*
Kuramoto, R., 158, 166, *172*

Kuriansky, J., 686, 688, 690, *693*, 693, *695*
Kurland, L. T., 488, *510*
Kurnit, D. M., 481, *512*
Kurosaki, T., 687, 691, 692, *696*
Kurosaki, T. T., 237, 240, *248*
Kurz, D. J., 538, *548*
Kurze, T., 190, *196*
Kushnir, S., 486, *506*
Kuskowski, M., 500, *505*
Kusuda, M., 264, *300*
Kutcher, S. P., 395, *403*
Kutt, 730, 742, *762*
Kuwabara, T., 252, 253, *300*
Kuypers, J. A., 8, *25*, 364, *373*
Kvale, J. N., 384, 388, 397, *404*
Kvavilashvili, L., 317, *334*
Kwentus, J., 292, 293, *298*
Kwentus, J. A., 329, *333*, 347, 349, *353*, 651, 654, *665*
La Rue, A., 645, 651, 652, 654, 656, 658, 659, 661, *666*, *667*
Laakso, M., 182, *198*
Labell, J., 496, *512*
Labouvie-Vief, G., 310, 311, *334*
LaBudde, J. A., 424, *428*
Lachman, M. E., 363, *373*
Lader, M. H., 532, 534, 535, *549*
Laelber, C., 517, *550*
Laforet, G., 486, *504*
Lai, F., 481, *507*, 587, *598*
Lai, L. Y. C., 481, *506*
Laird, N. M., 522, 524, *548*
Laitman, L. B., 386, 387, 394, *403*
Lake, B., 438, *457*
Lake, R. C., 539, *550*
Lakin, K. C., 589, 592, *596*, *598*
Lakshamanan, E. B., 740, *759*
Lal, S., 486, 493, *513*
Lam, R. W., 15, *26*, 393, *406*, 738, *761*
Lammertsma, A., 205, *227*
Lamminsevu, U., 575, *579*
Lamontagne, A., 486, *506*
Lampe, T. H., 480, 486, 498, 500, *507*, *510*, *511*
Lamy, P. P., 539, 540, *550*, 726, *759*
Lancet editorial, 525, *550*
Landeman, R., 438, *457*
Landerman, R., 35, 37, *68*, 798, 799, 800, *811*

Landesman-Dwyer, S., 590, *598*
Landis, J. R., 191, *197*
Landis, R., 37, *71*
Landon, M., 489, *507*
Landsverk, J., 618, *638*
Landsverk, J. A., 110, *115*
Lane, M. H., 204, *223*, *227*
Langan, M. J., 284, *300*
Langer, E., 6, *26*, 766, *791*
Langinvainio, H., 562, *579*
Langsley, P. R., 702, *715*
Langston, J. W., 186, 191, *196*, *198*
Lanke, J., 33, 34, 37, 38, 43, 46, 47, 62, *69*, *71*
Lanphear, A. K., 897, *912*
Lansbury, C., 530, *551*
LaPierre, Y. D., 349, *353*
Larrabee, G. J., 15, *25*, 647, 661, *666*, *669*, 753, *757*
Larson, D. B., 18, *23*, 530, *546*, 728, 746, 752, *757*, 803, 804, *811*, *812*, 840, *850*
Larson, D. M., 437, 445, *457*
Larson, E., 386, *406*, 499, *510*
Larson, E. B., 14, *26*, 494, *507*, 533, *550*, 660, *664*, 725, *759*
Larson, E. V., 484, *506*
Larson, N. A., 491, *506*
Larson, S., 209, 210, 211, *224*
LaRue, A. D., 328, *334*
Lasker, B., 328, *334*
Lassek, A. M., 167, *171*
Lassen, N. A., 164, *171*, 204, *227*, 659, *665*
Lau, C., 491, *511–512*
Laulumaa, V., 488, *507*
Laux, L., 367, *373*
Lavelle, J., 112, *116*
Lavie, P., 564, *579*
Lavori, P. W., 47, *70*, *71*, 539, *551*
Lavy, S., 205, *227*
Lawler, M. L., 821, *831*
Lawrence, G. L., 660, *664*
Lawton, M., 687, 690, *696*
Lawton, M. P., 6, *25*, 384, *405*, 618, *640*, 673, 677, 679, *696*, 764, 765, 789, 790, *791*
Lawton, P., 679, 686, 690, 693, *696*
Lazaroff, A., 38, *67*
Lazarsfeld, P., 236, *247*
Lazarus, L. L. W., 743, *759*

Lazarus, L. W., 443, *459*, 701, 702, 703, 704, 711, *715*, *717*
Lazarus, R. S., 120, *142*, 241, *247*, 365, 367, *373*, 525, *549*, 728, *758*
Lazenby, H., 884, *890*
Lazenby, H. C., 877, 878, 883, *890*
Le Witt, P. A., 657, *669*
Leaf, P. J., 28, 41, 42, 47, 48, 49, 51, 52, 54, 57, 58, 60, *68*, *69*, 73, 380, 384, *407*, 410, 412, *430*, 523, 524, 526, 531, 536, *549*, *551*, 795, 801, 803, *812*
Leber, W. R., 526, *552*
Lebowitz, B., 437, 445, *457*
Lebowitz, B. D., 14, 17, *26*, 798, *812*
Lebowitz, M. R., 56, *69*
LeBray, P., 826, *830*
Lebrun-Grandie, P., 205, *227*, *228*
Lee, C. K., 60, *69*
Lee, D., 491, *511–512*
Lee, G. R., 904, *913*
Lee, J., 112, *116*
Lee, M. A., 421, *429*
Leenders, K. L., 205, *227*
Lees, A. J., 489, *506*
Legg, N. J., 209, 219, *225*
Lehman, H. E., 47, *70*
Lehr, U., 366, 368, 370, *373*, *375*
Leibovici, A., 737, *759*
Leibowitz, H. W., 256, 263, 265, *299*, *304*
Leid, J., 261, *305*
Leifer, D., 624, *640*
Leigh, S., 523, *546*
Leighton, A. H., 29, 46, 47, *71*, 411, *429*
Leighton, D. A., 252, *300*
Leighton, D. C., 411, *429*
Leirer, V., 327, *337*, 617, *641*
Leirer, V. O., 15, *26*, 419, *431*
Lekman, A., 182, 189, *194*
Lelkes, K., 280, *296*
Lelos, D., 864, *870*
Lemay, J. S., 539, *551*
LeMay, M., 622, *639*
Lemke, J. H., 538, 539, *549*
Lemke, S., 15, *25*
Lenders, M. B., 165, 166, *172*
Lenhardt, M. L., 266, 267, 272, *302*
Lennox, G., 489, *507*
Lenzi, G. L., 202, 205, 209, 219, *225*
Leon, L., 680, 681, *694*

Leon, R., 357, *373*
LeResche, L., 618, *637*
LeResche, L. R., 35, *66*
Lerner, W. D., 421, *429*
Lesher, E. L., 819, *830*
Less, A. J., 657, *667*
Lesser, J., 711, *715*
Leszcz, M., 700, 702, 711, *715*, *716*, 900, *914*
Leuba, G., 177, *196*
Leuchter, A., 645, *667*
Leung, J., 111, *117*
Leutz, W., 887, *889*
Leven, H. S., 150, *170*
Levensen, M. R., 455, *459*
Leventhal, H., 368, *374*
Leventhal, J., 617, 635, *640*
Leverenz, J., 488, *508*
Levi-Montalcini, R., 487, *508*
Levi-Strauss, C., 85, *97*
Levin, B. E., 617, *640*, 657, *667*
Levin, H. S., 646, 652, *667*
Levin, S., 279, *301*, 704, *715*
Levine, D. M., 520, *547*
Levine, M. S., 177, *196*
LeVine, R., 77, *97*
Levinson, D., 120, 132, *142*
Levinson, G. A., 704, *715*
Levinson, M., 120, 132, *142*
Levinson, P. K., 516, *551*
Levit, K. R., 884, *890*
Levitan, S. T., 907, *913*
Levitt, H., 278, *301*
Levy, J. K., 496, *507*
Levy, R., 350, *352*, 381–382, 391, *403*, 467, 468, *471*, *474*, 475, 754, *759*
Levy, S., 629, *638*
Levy-Bruhl, L., 84, *97*
Lewinsohn, P., 392, *404*
Lewinsohn, P. A., 700, 705, 707, *715*
Lewinsohn, P. M., 422, *429*, 707, *717*
Lewis, A., 470, *474*
Lewis, D. A., 222, *227*
Lewis, I. L., 410, *423*
Lewis, M. I., 327, *332*, 700, 711, *713*
Lewis, M. J., 415, *428*
Lewis, P. A., 542, *554*
Lewis, S., 523, *552*
Leys, D., 624, *640*

Lezak, M., 217, *227*
Lezak, M. D., 625, *640*, 651, *667*
L'Heureux, A., 488, *504*
Lhmermitte, F., 657, *668*
Li, D. K. B., 209, *227*
Li, G., 33, *70*
Li, S. R., 33, *70*
Liang, X., 186, *198*
Liban, C. B., 59, *72*
Liberman, M. A., 77, *96*
Liberman, R., 675, 676, 680, 685, *694, 696*
Libow, L. S., 494, *506*, 821, *830*
Lichstein, K. L., 423, *431*
Lieberman, L., 559, *578*
Lieberman, M. A., 122, 130, *143*, 241, *248*
Lieff, J. D., 908, *913*
Lieman, B., 317, *334*
Light, E., 14, 17, *25*, 798, *812*
Light, L. L., 308, *331*
Light, R. H., 646, *669*
Lilienfeld, A. M., 29, 40, *70*
Liljequist, R., 742, *759, 760*
Lin, N., 105, 106, *116*
Lincoln, J., 179, *196*
Lindboe, C. F., 153, *173*
Linden, M., 710, *715*
Linden, M. E., 746, *759*
Lindenbaum, J., 494, *508*
Lindesay, J., 385, 386, *405*
Lindgren, A. G. H., 492, *511*
Lindgvist, G., 493, *513*
Lindley, M. G., 282, *304*
Lindsay, R. D., 159, 163, *172*
Lindstrom, B., 155, *171*
Link, B., 47, *69*
Linn, B., 689, *696*
Linn, M., 689, *696*
Linn, M. W., 8, *25*
Linnoila, M., 56, *69*, 575, *579, 581*, 742, *759*
Linoli, G., 191, *195*
Linsk, N. L., 701, 708, *716*
Linton, M., 317, *334*
Lion, J. R., 746, *759*
Lipin, L. E., 489, *509*
Lipman, R. S., 424, *429*
Lipowski, Z. J., 329, *334*, 471, *474*, 816, 821, *830*
Lippa, A., 732, *757*

Lippa, A. S., 180, *194*
Lippert, G. P., 388, *403*
Lippi, A., 38, *66*
Lipsett, P. D., 864, *870*
Lipsey, J. R., 388, *406*, 634, *640*
Lipson, D. P., 538, 539, *549*
Lipton, M. A., 47, *70*
Liptzin, B., 744, *759*, 816, *829*, 838, 839, *851*
Lish, J. D., 234, *247*
Lishman, W. A., 447, *459*, 496, 497, *508*, 621, 632, 635, *640*
Liskow, B. I., 527, *550*
Liss, L., 285, *301*
Liston, E. H., 383, *406*, 656, 658, *667*
Lit, A., 260, *301*
Litchfield, L. C., 592, *598*, 809, *813*
Little, A., 754, *759*
Litwak, E., 807, *812*
Litzin, B., 837, 841, 844, *850*
Liu, W. T., 13, *24*
Liu, Z., 186, *198*
Livanainen, M., 624, *638*
Livera, P., 38, *66*
Livesley, W. J., 434, *459*
Livingston, M. M., 801, *812*
Livson, N., 134, 136, 137, *143*
Llabre, M. M., 617, *640*
Lo, B., 861, 862, *870, 871*
Lo, P., 188, *194*
Lo Verma, S., 209, *223*
LoCastro, J. S., 522, 523, 524, *548, 549*
Loch'h, C., 205, *227*
Locke, B. Z., 34, 35, 41, 43, 49, 51, 52, 54, 56, 57, 58, 60, 62, *68*, 108, *115, 171*, 358, *372*
Lockery, S. A., 106, 113, *116*, 525, 526, *551*
Lockett v. Ohio, 865, *870*
Locking, H., 399, *406*
Loeb, C., 658, *667*
Loeb, P., 709, *713*
Loewen, E. R., 316, *334*
Loewenstein, D., 219, *224*, 624, *638*, 687, 691, *696*
Loewenstein, D. A., 211, 240, *247*, 652, 659, *667*
Logan, R. F. A., 747, *760*
Logsdon, R. G., 659, *667*
Logue, P. E., 618, *638*

Lohr, J. B., 735, *759*
Lohr, W. D., 500, *509*
London, E., 189, *195*, 491, *506*
London, E. D., 179, *199*, 205, *224*
Long, G. M., 263, *301*
Long, S. H., 877, *890*
Longbrake, K., 659, *664*
Longley, W., 39, *67*
Loosen, P. T., 500, *508*
Lopez-Aqueres, W., 109, *116*
Loranger, A. W., 184, *196*, 454, *459*
Loring, D. W., 652, *667*
Lossinsky, A. S., 157, *173*
Lott, I. T., 587, *598*
Loutsch, E., 381, 382, *401*, 739, *757*
Love, D. W., 529, 532, *552*
LoVerde, M., 753, *762*
Lovett, W. C., 736, *759*
Lowe, J., 489, *507*
Lowe, J. I., 489, *507*
Lowe, S. S., 275, *296*
Lowenfeld, I. E., 252, *301*
Lowenson, R. B., 254, 263, *299*
Lowenstein, D., 207, *228*
Lowenthal, M. F., 470, *474*
Lowinson, J. H., 516, 536, *550*
Lubersky, M., 421, *431*
Lubin, R. A., 585, 586, 587, 588, 589, *598,*
    599
Lucas, C., 765, 783, *791*
Lucas, M. J., 234, *248*, 471, *475*, 558, *580,*
    732, *761*, 835, *852*
Lucas-Blaustein, M. J., 539, *553*, 841, *852*
Lucchelli, F., 328, *332*
Luce, J. M., 867, *870*
Luchins, D. J., 414, *429*
Lucki, I., 747, *760*
Lue, F., 564, *579*
Luft, A., 205, *227*
Lugaresi, E., 562, *579*
Lukianowicz, N., 456, *459*
Lum, O., 15, *26*, 327, *337*, 419, *431*, 617,
    641
Lundberg, A., 168, *171*
Lundquist, G., 384, *404*
Luria, A., 647, *667*
Lushene, R., 412, 419, *431*
Lusk, E. J., 388, *401*
Lutsky, N. S., 365, *373*

Lutze, M., 253, *303*
Lutzer, V. D., 592, *597*
Lyman, B. J., 260, 264, *304*
Lynch, G., 190, *197*
Lynch, P. E., 531, 532, 533, 534, *551*
Lyness, S. A., 733, *761*
Lyons, J. S., 804, *812*
Lyons, M., 455, *459*

Maas, M., 846, *851*
Macari-Hinson, M. M., 388, *406*
MacDonald, J., 384, *404*
Mace, N. A., 733, *760*
Mace, N. L., 234, *248*, 471, *475*, 558, *580*
MacEachron, A. E., 589, *597*
MacEwan, G. W., 533, *545*
Macfadyen, D., 28, *70*
MacGregor, R., 209, 210, *224*
Machizawa, S., 111, *117*
Machovski, L. V., 485, *512*
Mack, W., 151, *171*, 660, *666*
Mackay, A. V. P., 184, *196*
MacKenzie, S., 395, *403*
MacKenzie, T. B., 399, *404*
Mackenzie, T. B., 609, *640*
Macklin, D. B., 411, *429*
MacMillan, A. M., 411, *429*
MacMillan, D., 528, *550*
Macmillan, D., 473, *474*
MacVeigh, D., 259, *297*
Madden, D., 321, 322, *335*
Madden, D. J., 260, *298*, 320, *334*, 347, *352*
Maddox, G., 362, *372*, 828, *831*
Maddox, G. L., 796, *812*
Maddux, J. F., 536, *550*
Maffei, L., 258, *301*
Magaziner, J., 530, 535, *546*
Magni, G., 391, *404*, 817, *831*
Maguire, K., 395, *407*
Mahoney, A. J. F., 896, *913*
Mahoney, F., 685, 689, *696*
Mahoney, M. J., 422, *429*
Main, T. F., 450, *459*
Makinodan, T., 166, *171*
Makins, C., 282, *304*
Malatesta, C. Z., 356, 357, *373*
Malcolm, M. T., 523, *550*

Maletta, G. S., 733, *760*
Malin, H., 517, *550*
Maloff, D. R., 516, *551*
Malone, J., 887, *889*
Maloney, A. F. J., 184, *199*
Maloney, A. J. F., 485, *505*
Maltbie, A. A., 389, *402*
Maltese, A., 214, 215, *226, 227*, 645, *666*
Maltsberger, J. T., 450, *459*
Mamo, H., 205, *227*
Mandolini, A., 516, *551*
Manheimer, D. I., 530, 538, *546, 552*
Mann, A. H., 391, *402*, 454, *459*
Mann, D. A., 486, *508*
Mann, D. M., 179, *196*
Mann, D. M. A., 153, 154, *171*, 180, 187, 188, 189, 191, *196, 197*, 484, 485, *509, 513*
Mann, D. M. S., 154, *171*
Mann, J., 743, *758*
Mann, L., 369, *373*
Manning, R. G., 205, 207, 208, *224*
Mannlein, E. A., 110, 111, *116*
Manschreck, T. C., 624, *639*
Mansi, L., 209, 210, 212
Mant, A., 530, *551*
Mantobani, M., 562, *579*
Manton, K. G., 10, *25*, 398, 399, *401*, 438, *457*, 677, *696*
Manuelidis, E. E., 484, *508*
Manuelidis, L., 484, *508*
Mar, H., 483, *511*
Marcell, P. D., 494, *508*
Marcer, D., 533, *547*
March, S., 534, *548*
Marcopulos, B. A., 654, *667*
Marcusson, J. O., 179, *197*
Marcyniuk, B., 153, 154, *171*, 180, 187, 188, 189, *196, 197*
Margolin, R. A., 205, 207, 208, *223, 224*
Margolin, R. M., 645, *664*
Margraf, J., 421, *429*
Mariani, E., 564, *581*
Marin, D. B., 386, 387, 394, *403*, 737, *758*
Maritz, J. S., 64, *67*
Markesbery, W. R., 182, *195*, 484, *508*
Markides, K. S., 100, 104, 105, 110, 113, *116*, 875, *890*
Markley, R. P., 318, *318*

Markowitz, J. S., 234, *247*
Marks, 747, *758*
Marks, I. M., 52, *70*, 422, *429*
Marks, L. E., 281, 282, 283, 288, *296, 301, 305*
Marks, R. G., 538, 539, *551*
Markson, E. W., 103, *116*
Markush, R. E., 386, *405*
Marlatt, G. A., 516, *547*
Marmar, C. R., 710, *715*
Marmar, D. R., 710, *714*
Marmor, M. F., 253, *301*
Marmot, M. G., 524, *551*
Marneros, A., 467, 468, *474*
Marotta, R., 632, *640*
Marotta, R. F., 496, *504*
Marsden, C. D., 32, 33, *71*, 487, *504*, 618, *638*
Marsel-Mesulam, M., 240, *248*
Marsh, G. M., 485, *512*
Marshall, E., 490, *509*
Marshall, J., 209, 219, *225*, 253, *301*, 491, 492, *506*, 658, 659, *665*
Marshall, J. F., 191, *197*
Marshall, M., 110, *117*
Marskey, H., 491, *511–512*
Martello, J., 654, *670*
Martilla, R. J., 186, *197*
Martin, A., 650, *667*
Martin, C. E., 753, *758*
Martin, D. C., 560, 568, *581*
Martin, J. B., 153, *169*, 190, *197*, 486, *508*
Martin, J. C., 528, *551*
Martin, M., 317, 329, *334*
Martin, R. L., 40, *71*, 651, *666*
Martin, W., 186, *190*
Martin, W. R., 493, *507*
Martin, W. R. W., 209, *227*
Martin-Matthews, A., 103, *116*
Martron, K. I., 619, *639*
Marttila, R. J., 488, *508*
Martz, B. L., 538, *547*
Marx, M. S., 732, *757*, 835, 836, 845, *850, 852*
Masdeu, J., 191, *195*
Maskowitz, R., 675, 685, *695*
Mason, W., 564, 572, *577*
Mason, W. J., 562, 568, *577*
Massler, M., 288, *301*

Masson, H., 486, *506*
Massullo, C., 657, *665*
Mastrangelo, M., 564, *581*
Mastri, A. R., 214, *226*, 484, 493, *507, 512*
Masur, D., 191, *195*
Masur, D. M., 646, 652, *667*
Matarazzo, J. D., 651, *667*
Mathew, N. T., 658, *668*
Mathie, A. A., 485, *508*
Mathieson, I., 488, *506*
Mathis, C. A., 209, *225*
Matsumoto, A., 177, *197*
Matthews, C. G., 660, *665*
Mattila, M. J., 742, *759, 760*
Mattis, S., 328, *334*
Maule, A. J., 322, *336*
Maune, S., 590, *597*
Mauria, W. L., 567, *577*
Maurice, W. I., 130, *141*
Max, W., 15, *25*
May, F. E., 538, *551*, 639, 749, *758*
May, P. C., 179, 180, 181, *197*, 731, *760*
Mayer, C., 864, *869*
Mayer, M. J., 263, *301*
Mayer, R. J., 489, *507*
Mayeux, R., 388, *405*, 472, *475*, 485, 488,
    496, 498 *505*, 501, *508, 511, 512*, 617,
    635, *640*, 733, 754, *757, 762*
Mayo, S. C., 397, *405*
Mayol, R. F., 424, *428*
Mayse, E., 488, *505*
Mazure, C. M., 46, 48, *67*
Mazurek, M. F., 486, *508*
Mazza, D. L., 421, *429*
Mazziotta, J. C., 207, 214, 215, 220, 221,
    223, 226, 227, 645, *666*
Mazzuca, M., 165, 166, *172*
McAllister, I., 60, *70*
McAllister, T., 350, *353*
McAllister, T. W., 396, *406*, 654, *667*, 739,
    760
McAllister, V. L., 219, *225*, 492, *506*, 658,
    665
McAnulty, G., 644, 645, *664, 665*
McArthur, D., 594, *597*
McAvay, G., 567, 570, *581*
McCann, C., 689, *696*
McCann, U. D., 389, *404*
McCarley, T., 392, *406*, 700, 711, *716*

McCarron, L. T., 844, *851*
McCarthy, M., 647, *664, 667*
McCarthy, P., 278, *301*
McCarthy, P. D., 456, *459*
McCaudless, G. A., 275, *302*
McClearn, G., 344, *353*
McClearn, G. E., 436, *459*
McClellan, R. L., 623, *640*
McClelland, M., 384, *406*
McClintic, K. L., 646, *647*
McClure, D. J., 221, *227*
McConnell, F., 273, *303*
McCormick, A. Q., 253, *297*
McCrae, R., 135, *142*
McCrae, R. R., 356, 358, 365, *372, 373*,
    436, 437, 438, 442, 445, *457, 459*
McCue, M., 539, *551*, 647, *667*
McCue, R. E., 394, *403*, 574, *578*, 743, *758*
McCulloch, J. W., 456, *460*
McCusker, E., 39, *67*
McCusker, J., 522, *551*
McDaniel, M. A., 317, *333*
McDermott, J. R., 484, *508*
McDowd, J., 324, *334*
McDowd, J. M., 325, *337*
McDuff, T., 188, 189, *197*
McEvoy, J. P., 539, *551*
McEvoy, L. T., 58, 60, *69*
McFarland, R. A., 262, *301*
McGarry, A. L., 864, *870*
McGarvey, B., 15, *25*
McGee, N. D., 330, *333*
McGeer, E., 154, *171*
McGeer, E. G., 153, *171*, 179, 180, *197*,
    209, *227*, 493, *507*
McGeer, P. L., 153, 154, *171*, 179, 180, *197*,
    209, *227*, 493, *507*, 645, *668*
McGlashan, T. H., 439, 440, *459*
McGrath, C., 259, *301*
McGrowder-Lin, R., 847, *851*
McGuire, E. A., 526, *554*
McHugh, P. R., 35, *68*, 237, *247*, 328, *333*,
    345, 350, *353*, 617, *638*, 649, 653, *665*
McKee, B., 120, 132, *142*
McKee, D. C., 347, *352*
McKenna, P., 651, *668*
McKhann, G., 32, *71*, 479, *508*, 645, *667*
McKool, M., 90, *97*
McLaughlin, D. S., 730, *758*

McLean, P., 49, 387, 394, *406*, 500, *510*, *512*, 842, *852*
McLeish, J. A. B., 897, *913*
McNair, D., 424, *429*
McNair, D. M., 419, 420, *430*
McNeill, T., 483, *507*
McNicholas, W. T., 564, *579*
McNulty, T. F., 708, *717*
McWilliam, C., 523, 530, 531, *553*, *554*
McWilliams, J. R., 190, *197*
Meacham, J. A., 317, *334*
Meador, K. G., 384, 388, 394, *404*, 617, *639*, 817, *830*
Meares, R. A., 623, *639*
Mearrick, P., 534, *548*
Mechanic, D., 796, *812*
Meeks, S., 804, 806, *812*
Meerloo, J. A. M., 702, *716*
Mehl, L., 292, *297*
Mehler, M., 191, *195*
Mehraein, P., 163, *171*, 209, *226*
Mehren, B., 15, *25*
Mei-Tal, V., 381, 390, *405*
Meichenbaum, D., 422, *430*
Meier-Ruge, W., 182, 188, *194*
Meigs, J. W., 290, *303*
Meinhardt, K., 110, *117*
Meissner, W. W., 704, *716*
Melamed, E., 205, *227*
Melchior, C. L., 527, *553*
Mellinger, D. G., 530, 531, 535, *551*
Mellinger, G. D., 530, 531, 535, 538, *546*, *552*, *554*
Mellor, C. S., 464, *474*
Mellstrom, D., 541, *551*
Melton, G. B., 855, 865, *870*
Melton, L. J., III, 747, *760*
Meltzer, 469, *474*
Melville, M. L., 438, *457*, 798, *811*
Menaghan, E. G., 241, *248*
Menaloscino, F. J., 590, *598*
Mendels, J., 396, *405*
Mendelson, M., 617, *637*
Mendez, M., 653, 656, *664*
Mendez, M. F., 388, *405*
Mendlewicz, J., 48, *71*, 381, 382, *401*, *404*
Menninger, K. A., 277, *301*
Menustik, C. E., 526, 529, *554*
Merchant, A., 41, 59, *66*, 654, *668*

Meredith, W., 348, *354*
Meric, P., 205, *227*
Merriam, A. E., 14, *25*, 835, *851*
Merril, C. R., 496, *507*
Merrill, M., 544, *551*
Merz, G. S., 587, *599*
Messin, S., 564, *577*
Mesulam, M. M., 208, 217, *227*, 448, *459*
Mesulam, M.-Marcel, 169, *171*
Metter, E. J., 205, 207, 210, 212, 214, 215, 219, *226*, *227*, 644, 645, *666*, *667*, *669*
Meyer, B. J. F., 312, *336*
Meyer, J. S., 205, *227*, 347, *354*, 485, 492, *504*, *508*, 541, *553*, 624, *639*, 646, 658, *667*, *668*
Meyers, A. R., 523, *551*, 684, 688, *694*
Meyers, B. S., 48, *71*, 381, 390, *400*, *405*, 738, *756*
Meyers, C. E., 594, *598*
Meyers, J. K., 795, 801, 803, *812*
Mezey, R., 526, *554*
Mezzich, T. E., 445, *459*
Micelli, G., 657, *665*
Michels, R., 434, *460*
Midanik, L., 59, *67*
Middleton, R. S. W., 393, *400*, *405*
Miettinen, O. S., 29, 40, *71*
Miezin, F. M., 221, *224*
Milan, R., 190, *195*
Milberg, J., 495, *511*
Miles, L. E., 561, 566, 569, *577*, *579*
Miles, S. H., 537, *551*, 861, *870*
Millard, P. H., 385, *405*
Miller, A. K. C., 153, *171*
Miller, A. K. H., 152–153, *171*
Miller, B. E., 483, *506*
Miller, C., 157, *172*
Miller, D. C., 312, *336*
Miller, D. S., 388, *401*
Miller, E., 30, *71*, 649, *667*
Miller, F., 395, *405*, 531, 532, 533, 534, 535, *551*, *554*
Miller, F. D., 37, *71*, 191, *197*
Miller, I. J., Jr., 279, *301*
Miller, J., 189, *195*, 219, *224*, 491, *506*
Miller, J. D., 209, *227*, 537, *551*
Miller, J. H., 292, *296*
Miller, M. B., 834, *851*
Miller, N. E., 12, *25*, 803, *811*, 899, *913*

Miller, P., 329, *333*
Miller, P. L., 520, 523, 525, 528, *553*
Miller, P. S., 539, *551*
Miller, R. L., 260, *296*, 825, *831*
Miller, S. I., 526, 529, *554*
Miller, W. R., 350, *353, 354*, 834, *852*
Milligan, W. L., 347, *353*
Millodot, M., 290, *301*
Millon, T., 454, *460*
Mills, M. J., 866, 868, *869, 870*
Milne, J. S., 268, *301*
Milson, R., 308, *331*
Milton, R. C., 265, *299*
Mimpen, A. M., 272, 274, *302*
Minckler, J., 155, *172*
Mindel, C. H., 875, *890*
Minderhoud, J., 190, *196*
Miner, G. D., 484, *512*
Mink, I. T., 594, *598*
Minkoft, J. R., 500, *509*
Minstretta, C. M., 280, 290, *298, 305*
Mintun, M., 221, *228*
Mintz, J., 392, *406*, 700, 711, *716*
Mintzer, J., 659, *667*
Mion, C. C., 740, *759*
Mion, L. C., 822, *830*
Miranda v. Arizona, 863, *870*
Mirra, S. S., 488, *505*
Mirsen, T., 646, *667*
Mishkin, M., 218, 221, *225, 226, 228*
Misiak, H., 262, *301*
Mitchel-Pedersen, L., 845, *851*
Mitchell, A. L., 14, *26*
Mitchell, D. B., 648, *668*
Mitchell, J. B., 800, 802, 803–804, *813*, 836, *851*, 867, *870*, 874, *890*
Mitchell, M., 532, *552*
Mitchell, W. D., 753, *762*
Mitler, M. M., 573, *579*
Mitrushina, M., 647, 659, *668, 669*
Mittelman, D., 312, *336*
Miyakawa, T., 158, 166, *172*
Mizuno, N., 159, *172*
Mizutani, T., 488, *504*
Mjones, H., 472, *474*
Mlynarczk, S. M., 821, *831*
Moberg, D. D., 384, 388, 397, *404*
Moberg, P., 634, *641*
Mobley, W. C., 487, *510*

Mochizuki, Y., 279, *301*
Mock, J. E., 617, *637*
Modic, M. T., 624, *639*
Modlish, N. J. K., 592, *598*
Moeller, J. R., 221, *228*
Moertel, C. G., 861, *871*
Moffat, N., 661, *670*
Moffic, H. S., 388, *405*
Mohr, E., 219, *227*
Mohs, R. C., 15, *25*, 222, *228*, 328, *336*, 386, 387, 394, *403*, 482, 485, *505, 508*, 539, *551*, 661, *669*
Mohs, R. L., 486, *507*
Moldolsky, H., 564, *579*
Molgaard, C., 107, *115*
Molgaard, C. A., 109, *116*, 525, 526, *551*
Moline, M. L., 560, 568, *581*
Molleman, E., 369, *374*
Moller, M. B., 268, 270, 271, 273, 275, *301*
Mollica, R. F., 112, *116*
Molsa, P. K., 488, *508*
Moltzen, S., 619, *639*
Monahan, D. J., 110, *115*, 808, *812*
Mondini, S., 575, *578*
Monk, T. H., 559, 560, 575, *577, 580*
Monroy, C. A., 747, *760*
Monson, R. P., 29, 46, *71*
Montague, J., 50, *597*
Montamat, S. C., 728, *760*
Montgomery, R. J. V., 523, *546*
Monzingo, F., 279, *295*
Moon, M., 884, *890*
Moore, A. M., 205, 209, 210, 211, 214, *223, 224, 225*, 645, *664*
Moore, G. L., 399, *400*
Moore, M., 327, *335*, 653, *668*
Moore, M. T., 749, *758*
Moore, N. C., 277, *301*, 468, *474*
Moore, R. D., 520, *547*
Moos, B. S., 525, *551*
Moos, R., 105, 106, *116*
Moos, R. H., 15, *25*, 239, 241, *246*, 519, 525, *546, 548, 551*
Moran, J. A., 844, *851*
Moran, M. G., 731, *760*
Moranville, J. T., 733, *760*
Moretz, R. C., 157, *173*
Morgan, D. C., 183, *196*
Morgan, D. E., 274, *297*

Morgan, D. G., 177, 179, 180, 181, 183, 190, *195*, *197*, 731, *760*
Morgan, K., 530, 531, 532, 542, *548*, *551*
Morgenstern, H., 29, *70*
Mori, H., 483, *507*
Moriarty, K. M., 539, *550*
Morice, H. O., 709, *714*
Morin, C. M., 708, *716*
Morin, J., 486, *506*
Moriwaki, S., 114, *116*
Moriwaki, S. Y., 106, 113, *116*
Morr, 687, *697*
Morrell, R. W., 661, *668*
Morris, H. D., 150, *170*
Morris, J., 572, *580*
Morris, J. C., 15, *25*, 343, *353*, 646, *669*
Morris, J. N., 28, *71*, 380, *405*, 588, *599*, 808, *812*
Morris, P. E., 317, *334*
Morris, P. L. P., 634, *640*
Morris, R., 654, *669*, 909, *913*
Morris, V., 687, *697*
Morrison, J. D., 259, *301*
Morrison, J. H., 222, *227*
Morrison, T. R., 263, *301*
Morriss, R. K., 836, *851*, *852*
Morrisson, L., 877, *890*
Morrow, G. R., 389, *402*
Morrow, L., 656, *664*
Morse, R. M., 525, 526, 527, 528, 529, *548*, *549*
Mortel, K. F., 347, *354*, 492, *508*, 541, *553*, 646, *667*
Mortimer, J. A., 33, 37, 38, 38m *68*, *71*, 480, 484, 488, *505*, *508*
Morton, D. J., 107, 109, *115*, *116*
Morycz, R. K., 574, *581*
Moschitto, L. J., 423–424, *428*
Moscovitch, M., 312, 316, 317, *335*, *337*
Moses, H., 472, *475*
Moses, S., 279, *301*
Mosher, P., 699, *717*
Mosko, S., 566, *577*
Mosko, S. S., 562, *580*
Moskovitz, C., 472, *475*
Moskowitz, E., 689, *696*
Moskowitz, H., 424, *431*, 575, *577*
Moss, M., 687, 692, *696*
Moss, M. B., 644, *663*

Moss, R. J., 537, *551*
Moss, T., 845, *852*
Motoike, P., 392, *406*, 700, 711, *716*
Motte, J., 191, *197*
Motter, L., 877, *890*
Moulton, P., 844, *851*
Mountjoy, C. Q., 31, *71*, 182, 183, 187, 188, 189, *194*, *197*, *198*, 212, *227*, *228*, 486, *504*, 618, *641*
Mountjoy, C. Y., 152–153, *171*
Mouritzen Dam, A., 152, 153, *172*
Mucatel, M., 523, *551*
Mucholt, M. A., 821, *831*
Mueller, E. A., 56, *69*, 500, *512*
Mueller, G., 275, *298*
Mukherjee, S., 221, *228*
Mulcahy, R., 541, *547*
Mullan, J. T., 15, *25*, 241, *248*
Mullan, M. J., 481, *506*
Mullaney, J., 517, 524, *552*
Multhaup, K. S., 653, *664*
Mumford, E., 798, *812*, 907, *913*
Mungo, D., 737, *762*
Muniz, R. L., 571, *581*
Munk-Jorgensen, P., 470, *474*
Murphy, B. J., 263, *302*
Murphy, C., 280, 283, 284, 285, 286, 287, 288, *302*
Murphy, D. J., 862, *870*
Murphy, D. L., 56, *69*, 327, *332*, 386, *402*, 500, *512*, 569, *578*, 654, *670*, 754, *762*
Murphy, E., 13, *25*, 385, 386, 397, *405*
Murphy, E. A., 40, *67*
Murphy, J., 398, *405*
Murphy, J. B., 677, *697*
Murphy, J. M., 29, 46, 47, *71*
Murphy, S., 183, *197*
Murphy, S. M., 532, *551*
Murphy, S. T., 437, 445, *460*
Murray, G. B., 395, *407*
Murray, M. D., 538, *547*
Murray, R. M., 540, *551*
Murrel, S. A., 412, 420, *428*
Murrell, S. A., 349, *354*, 567, *580*
Mussen, P., 359, *374*
Muszynski, I. L., 874, 878, 879, *889*
Mycielska, K., 313, 325, *336*
Myerhoff, B., 104, *116*
Myers, A. C., 816, *831*

Myers, G. C., 10, *25*
Myers, J., 127, *142*
Myers, J. K., 34, 35, 41, 42, 49, 51, 57, 58, 59, 60, *69*, *73*, *171*, 410, 412, *430*, 523, 524, 526, 531, 536, *549*, *551*
Myers, R. H., 40, *72*, 190, *197*, 214, *224*, 228, 481, *512*
Myers, W. A., 445, *460*, 700, 702, *716*

Nabelek, A. K., 274, *302*
Nadal, E. C., 859, *869*
Naessen, R., 285, *302*
Nagai, T., 153, *171*, 180, *197*
Nagel, J. A., 254, 263, *299*
Nagel, J. S., 625, *639*
Nagley, S., 817, 821, 824, *831*
Nagley, S. J., 821, *831*
Nagoshi, C. T., 436, *459*
Naguib, M., 467, 468, *471*, *475*
NAHB, 765, *791*
Nahemow, L., 6, *25*
Nair, N. P., 486, 493, *513*
Nair, V., 486, *506*
Nakamura, S., 159, *172*
Nakaura, C. M., 525, 526, *551*
Namazi, K., 822, *830*
Nandy, K., 166, *172*
Napoliello, M. J., 424, *430*, 749, *760*
Naritomi, H., 205, *227*
National Academy of Sciences, 516, *552*
National Center for Health Statistics, 314, *335*, 874, *890*
National Institute for Occupational Safety and Health, 271, *302*
National Institute on Aging Task Force, 798, *812*
National Institutes of Health, 558, 560, 574, *580*
Navia, B. A., 495, *508*, 632, *640*
Nduaguba, M., 440–441, *460*
Neary, D., 182, 183, *194*, *195*, *197*, 485, 486, *506*, *509*
Nebes, R., 321, 333, *335*
Nebes, R. D., 571, *578*, 649, 657, *665*, *666*
Nee, L., 40, *72*, 214, *228*, 481, *512*
Nee, L. E., 484, *509*
Needels, D. L., 190, *197*
Neff, R. K., 47, *71*

Neider, J., 112, *117*
Neill, W., 324, *335*
Neirinck, L, 486, *506*
Neisser, U., 308, 313, *333*, *335*
Neito-Sampedro, M., 190, *197*
Nelson, E., 164, *172*
Nelson, H. E., 651, *668*
Nelson, J. C., 46, 48, *67*, 381, *401*
Nelson, J. P., 14, *26*
Nemerhoff, C. B., 486, *504*
Nemeroff, C. B., 391, *402*, 483, 486, *506*, *511*
Nemiroff, R. A., 700, 703, 704, *713*, *716*
Nerbonne, M., 266, *304*
Nerenz, D. R., 368, *374*
Nestadt, G., 41, 59, *66*, 654, *668*
Neufeld, R. R., 494, *506*
Neugarten, B., 137, *143*
Neugarten, B. L., 6, 11, *25*, 364, *374*
Neuman, A. C., 278, *302*
Neve, K. A., 191, *197*
Neve, R. L., 481, 483, *512*, *513*
Nevins, A., 838, *850*
New, P. F. J., 624, *639*
Newcomb, P. A., 541, 542, *548*
Newhouse, P. A., 500, *512*, 754, *762*
Newmans, S., 60, *69*
Newton, N., 701, 702, 703, *715*
Newton, N. A., 701, *716*
Newton, P., 13, *24*
Newton, R. E., 575, *580*, 747, *760*
Niaz, U., 35, *66*, 618, *637*
Nicholls, S., 272, *305*
Nickerson, R. S., 256, 265, *299*
Niederehe, G., 14, 15, 18, *24*, *25*, *26*, 327, *335*, 617, *640*, 653, 654, *666*, *668*
Nielsen, J., 37, 48, *71*, 386, *405*
Nielsen, P. E., 191, *195*
Nihira, K., 594, *598*
Nikaido, A. M., 747, *757*
Nininger, J., 837, 841, 844, *850*
Nishihara, K., 566, *580*
Nissen, M., 322, 328, *335*
Nissen, M. J., 328, *333*
Nnewihe, A., 817, 821, 824, *831*
Nobel, K., 725, 752, *761*
Nochlin, D., 480, 483, *511*
Noelker, L. S., 807, 808, *812*
Noh, S., 42, *72*, 239, *248*

Nolan, L., 726, 728, *760*
Nolen-Hoeksema, S., 327, *335*
Norberg, A., 709, *713*
Nordlund, D. J., 539, *553*
Nordstrom, G., 522, *552*
Nordstrom, S., 653, *664*
Norgen, R., 279, *302*
Norris, A. H., 526, *554*
Norris, F., 567, *580*
Norstad, N., 424, *430*
North, R., 659, *664*
Northern, B., 485, *509*
Novak, P., 204, *228*
Novotny, T. E., 541, 542, *548*
Nowlin, J. B., 420, *430*
Noyes, R., 452, *460*
Noyes, R., Jr., 451, 454, *460*
Nuessel, F. H., 364, *374*
Nutter, R. W., 349, *354*
Nyberg, P., 179, *197*
Nygaard, H. A., 841, *851*

Oakes, M., 30, *71*
Oakley, A. E., 484, 488, *504, 505*
Ober, A. B., 209, *225*
Ober, B., 215, *226*
Ober, B. A., 211, 213, 214, *225, 226*, 647,
  652, 654, *663, 664, 668*
Ober, H. A., 652, *666*
O'Brien, M. D., 658, *668*
O'Connor, D. W., 501, *509*
Oderda, G. M., 536, *550*
O'Donnell, B. F., 14, *26*
Oehlert, M. E., 648, *669*
Office of Technology Assessment, 328, *335*
Offord, K. P., 488, *510*
O'Gorman, T., 452, *460*
O'Hanlon, P., 319, *335*
Ohman, R., 34, 37, 38, *69*
Ohta, B. M., 847, *851*
Ohta, R. J., 847, *851*
Ohtani, K., 566, *580*
Ojesjo, L., 34, 37, 38, 43, 46, 47, 62, *69,
  71*
Okado, R., 177, *197*
Okazaki, H., 34, *72*, 489, *509*
Okimoto, J., 498, *503*, 842, *850*

Okimoto, J. T., 239, *246*, 384, 388, *404*,
  907, *912*
Okpaku, S. A., 796, *813*
Oktay, J. S., 802, *812*
Okudaira, N., 566, *580*
Okun, M. A., 356, 365, *373, 374*
Oldham, J. M., 454, *459*
Olivier, D. C., 29, 46, 47, *71*
Olsen, D. M., 834, 840, *852*
Olsho, L. W., 266, 267, 272, *302*
Olson, P. L., 261, 262, *302, 304*
Olson, P. R., 473, *475*
Olsson, J. E., 486, *512*
Olszewski, J., 149, *172*
Oltersdorf, T., 483, *509*
Oltmanns, T. F., 804, 806, *812*
Olzak, L. A., 258, *302*
Omalander, J. G., 423, *430*
O'Malley, K., 726, 728, *760*
Omenn, G. S., 541, *549*
O'Neill, P., 523, *552*
Onrot, J., 539, *546*
Opit, L. J., 423, *431*
Opjordsmoen, S., 470, *475*
Opler, M. E., 76, *97*
Ordy, J. M., 253, 266, *302*
Orlandi, M., 285, 288, *304*
Orleans, C. T., 803, *813*
Orr, N. K., 14, *26*
Orrell, M. W., 473, *475*
Orrison, W. W., 624, *639*
Ortega, S. T., 108, *116*
Orvaschel, H., 42, *73*, 410, 412, *430*, 531,
  536, *551*
Osborn, M. O., 280, *302*
Oseas, D., 324, *334*
Osgood, N., 819, *831*
Oshimura, M., 167, *173*
Osmond, I., 495, *503*
Oster, M., 47, 69, 388, *403*
Oster-Granite, M. L., 483, *513*
Osterweis, M., 129, 130, *143*
Ostfeld, A., 680, 681, *694*
Ostfeld, A. M., 541, *550*
Ostfield, A., 13, *24*
Ostrom, J. R., 538, 539, *552*
O'Sullivan, D. M., 214, *224*
O'Sulllivan, M., 679, *696*
Otto, W. C., 275, *302*

Ouellette, R., 234, *247*
Ouslander, J. G., 705, *716*, 822, *830*
Overall, J. E., 617, *640*
Overman, W., 859, *870*
Owaschel, H., 438, *460*
Owen, F., 184, *197*
Owen, M. J., 481, *506*
Owen, R., 184, *197*, 532, *551*
Owsley, C., 252–253, 258, 261, 264, *302*, *304*, *305*
Oxman, T. E., 795, *813*

Pachacek, T. F., 540, *549*
Paci, D., 177, *194*
Packan, D., 500, *511*
Paetau, A., 493, *512*
Pagan, D., 481, *512*
Pagnucco, D. J., 797, *812*
Pahkala, K., 42, 47, 48, *70*
Paisley, C. M., 588, *596*
Pakalnis, A., 633, *639*
Palin, A. N., 624, 625, *638*
Paljarvi, L., 182, *198*
Palmer, A. M., 182, 183, *194*, *195*, *197*, 486, *506*
Palmert, M. R., 483, *509*
Palo, J., 183, *197*, 471, *474*
Pals, J., 493, *513*
Pandey, G., 743, *759*
Panek, P. E., 436, 445, *461*
Pantano, P., 205, *228*
Panton, L. B., 347, *354*
Panzer, R., 622, *639*
Paolo, A. M., 648, *669*
Papanicolaou, A. C., 652, *667*
Papper, S., 423, *430*
Papsidero, J., 689, *694*
Parhad, I., 32, 33, 35, 41, *68*
Parhad, J. M., 153–154, *173*
Parham, I. A., 436, *460*
Paricak-Vance, M. A., 481, *511*
Parikh, R. M., 634, *640*
Parisi, J. E., 645, *664*
Parisi, S. A., 384, 387, 388, *406*
Park, D. C., 318, *335*, 661, *668*
Parker, G., 43, *71*
Parker, L., 564, 571, 572, *577*, *578*

Parker, R., 495, *511*, 765, *791*
Parkes, K. R., 313, *331*
Parkin, D., 399, *405*
Parks, H. J., 538, *552*
Parks, R. W., 645, *668*
Parmalee, P. A., 384, *405*
Parnetti, L., 182, 189, *194*
Parrott, J. M., 536, *554*
Parson, E. B., 108, *116*
Parsons, O. A., 526, *552*
Parsons, T., 8, *25*
Partanen, V. J., 621, *641*
Partinen, M., 562, *579*
Pascal, S., 207, 219, *224*, *228*, 624, *638*
Pascarelli, E. F., 536, 537, *552*
Pascualy, M., 634, *640*
Pascualy, R. A., 560, 568, *581*
Passafiume, D., 656, *664*
Pastalan, L., 768, *791*
Pate, B., 186, *196*
Pate, B. D., 209, *227*, 493, *507*
Patlak, C. S., 202, 203, *228*
Patronas, N., 218, *225*
Patronas, N. J., 209, 210, 211, 212, 214, *224*
Patten, P. C., 712, *716*
Patterson, D., 481, *512*
Patterson, R., 701, *716*
Patterson, R. D., 901, *913*
Patterson, R. L., 419, *430*, 673, 679, 680, *696*
Pattison, D., 590, *597*
Pauker, S., 467, 468, 469, *475*
Paul, E. A., 618, *638*
Paul, S. M., 419, *430*
Paul, T., 562, *580*
Paulson, G. W., 633, *639*, 656, *666*
Pavlov, I. P., 417, *430*
Paykel, E. S., 127, *143*, 241, *248*, 388, *405*, 817, *831*
Peabody, C. A., 500, *509*, 732, 735, 738, *760*
Peacock, E. J., 359, *374*
Pearce, B., 183, *197*
Pearce, J., 488, *509*
Pearlin, L. I., 15, *25*, 122, *143*, 241, *248*
Pearlman, M., 735, *761*
Pearlson, G., 46, 48, *71*, 634, *641*
Pearlson, G. D., 466, 467, 468, *475*, 500, *509*, 622, *640*

Pearson, J. C. G., 271, *300*
Pearson, J. L., 499, *509*
Peck, A., 237, 240, *247*, 492, *511*, 658, *669*
Peck, R., 819, *831*
Peddecord, K. M., 109, *116*, 525, 526, *551*
Pederzoli, M., 184, *197*
Pedone, D., 38, *66*
Peers, M. C., 165, 166, *172*
Pelham, A. O., 103, *117*
Pelton, S., 389, *404*
Pendleton, M. G., 661, *665*
Peng, M., 186, *198*
Penman, D., 389, *402*
Penner, L., 679, *696*
Pennybacker, M., 58, 59, 60, 62, 64, 65, *67*, 438, *457*
Penry v. Lynaugh, 865, *870*
Pentel, P., 539, *552*
People v. Olsen, 864, *870*
Peppers, L. G., 537, *546*
Perani, D., 205, *227*
Perel, J. M., 500, *506*, 574, *581*
Perez, F. I., 658, *668*
Pericak-Vance, M. A., 481, *509*
Perl, D., 484, *509*
Perl, M., 859, *870*
Perlin, S., 204, *223*
Perlmutter, M., 313, 314, *332*, *335*, 648, *668*
Perr, B., 500, *505*
Perr, I. N., 856, 866, *869*, *870*
Perrett, L., 497, *504*
Perrson, G., 42, *71*
Perry, E. K., 483, 484, 485, 487, 488, 490, *504*, *505*, *506*, *509*
Perry, G., 484, *509*
Perry, J. P., 443, *461*
Perry, M., 47, *69*, 388, *403*
Perry, R. H., 484, 485, 490, *504*, *509*
Perry, S., 632, *640*
Perry, S. W., 494, *509*
Person, D., 314, *335*
Persson, B., 149, *170*
Persson, G., 386, *405*
Peskin, H., 134, 136, 137, *143*
Peskind, E., 480, *511*
Peskind, E. R., 486, *510*
Peskund, E. R., 571, *580*
Pestonk, A., 190, *197*
Peters, N. L., 539, *552*

Peters, R. S., 8, *26*
Petersen, D. M., 536, *552*
Petersen, S. E., 221, *228*
Peterson, P. J., 473, *475*
Petit, H., 624, *640*
Petito, C. K., 495, *509*
Peto, J., 127, *141*
Petrie, W. M., 424, *430*, 498, *510*
Petrila, J., 855, 865, *870*
Petrosino, L., 290, *302*
Petry, S., 446, *460*
Pettigrew, K. D., 202, 203, *228*
Pfeffer, R., 687, 691, 692, *696*
Pfeffer, R. I., 237, *248*, 2240
Pfefferbaum, A., 527, *552*
Pfeiffer, E., 11, *23*, 367, *374*, 410, *427*, 687, 692, *694*, *696*
Pfohl, B., 454, *461*
Pfohl, B. M., 446, 451, 452, 454, *462*
Phelan, D. G., 736, *759*
Phelps, C. H., 487, *510*
Phelps, M., 164, *172*
Phelps, M. E., 205, 207, 210, 211, 214, 219, 220, 221, *223*, *226*, *227*
Phil, M., 219, *225*
Philip, A. E., 456, *460*
Philipose, V., 38, *67*
Phillips, B., 886, *890*
Phillips, B. A., 562, *577*
Phillips, L., 821, 822, *831*
Phillipson, E. A., 564, *579*
Phillipson, M., 733, *760*
Philpot, M. P., 541, *550*
Philpott, R., 47, *67*
Physician Payment Review Commission, 876, 877, 879, 881, 882, 884, *890*
Piacentini, S., 40, *72*, 214, *228*
Piaget, J., 854, *870*
Piasetsky, S., 389, *402*
Pichot, P., 382, *405*
Pickar, D., 327, *332*, 386, *402*
Pickett, H. G., 280, *302*
Pidcock, C., 38, *72*
Pierce, J., 541, *552*
Pierce, J. P., 541, 542, *548*
Piercy, F. P., 712, *716*
Pieri, C., 177, *194*
Pierotti, A. R., 182, *197*
Pignatiello, M. F., 330, *332*

Pillon, B., 657, *668*
Pinel, R., 611, *640*
Pinkston, E. M., 701, 708, *716*
Pinner, E., 737, *760*
Pino, C., 827, *830*
Pinsker, H., 530, *552*, 746, 752, *760*
Pitt, M. C., 254, *302*
Pitts, D. G., 255, 256, 259, *302*
Pitts, W. M., 439, 440, 445, *461*
Pizzo, P. A., 495, *504*
Plakun, E. M., 446, *460*
Plantinga, A., 284, 287, 288, *305*
Plasay, M. T., 646, *663*
Platt, A., 864, 865, *870*
Playmate, S. R., *507*, 550
Plein, J. B., 538, 539, *552*
Plester, D., 271, *303*
Plomp, R., 272, 274, *302*
Plopper, M., 109, *116*
Plotkin, D. A., 738, *758*
Ploye, P. M., 450, *460*
Plude, D. J., 320, 321, *335*
Plumb, C. S., 290, *303*
Plummer, M., 207, *227*
Podell, E. R., 494, *508*
Podgor, M., 264, *300*
Podlisny, M. B., 483, *509*
Podnieks, E., 357, *374*
Poirier, J., 495, *506*
Poiten, D., 481, *512*
Pokorny, A. D., 439, 445, *461*
Pokorny, J., 253, *303*
Poldinger, W., 384, *400*
Polinsky, J. L., 481, *512*
Polinsky, R., 214, *228*
Polinsky, R. J., 40, *72*
Polk, M., 624, *639*
Pollack, M., 660, *666*
Pollen, D., 40, *72*, 214, *228*
Pollitt, P. A., 501, *509*
Pollock, G., 132, *143*
Pollock, M., 237, *347*
Pollock, M. L., 347, *354*
Pollock, V. E., 733, *761*
Pomara, N., 388, *405*, 424, *430*, 575, *580*, 747, *760*
Pontecorvo, M. J., 754, *757*
Poon, L. W., 15, *26*, 177, *198*, 310, 316, 317, 318, *335*, *337*, 644, 661, *668*, 900, *913*

Popkin, M. K., 399, *404*
Popkin, S., 827, *830*
Popkin, S. J., 327, *335*, 653, *668*
Posner, M., 324, *335*
Posner, M. I., 221, *228*
Post, F., 277, *303*, 350, *352*, *353*, 383, 385, *406*, 414, *430*, 469, *475*, 499, *510*, 654, *668*, 824, *831*
Post, R. M., 350, *354*, 569, *578*, 654, *669*
Postman, L., 178, *198*
Potamianos, G., 539, *552*
Potter, J. F., 523, *546*, 590, *598*
Pottieger, A. E., 536, *552*
Poulsen, M., 386, *406*, 499, *510*
Poulter, M., 184, *197*
Poulton, J. L., 711, *716*
Powell, A. L., 653, *668*
Powell, C., 845, *851*
Powell, D. A., 347, *353*
Powell, G. F., 313, *331*
Power, C. A., 844, *851*
Power, K. G., 532, *552*
Poythress, N. G., 855, 865, *870*
Pozzilli, C., 209, 219, *225*
Prange, A. J., 41, *73*, 500, *508*
Prange, A. J., Jr., 494, *513*
Preen, O., 651, *663*
Prentice, R. L., 29, *71*
Present, P. A., 386, *405*
President's Commission for the Study of Ethical Problems in Medicine and Biomedical and Behavioral Research, 861, *870*
Press, G. A., 623, 624, *639*
Press, I., 90, *97*
Pressey, S. L., 351, *353*
Preston, C., 713, *717*
Preziosi, T. J., 501, *511*
Price, D., 32, *71*, 479, *508*, 645, *667*, 754, *757*
Price, D. D., 292, 293, *298*
Price, D. L., 153–154, *173*, 472, *475*, 486, 487, 488, *505*, *510*, *512*
Price, I. L., 485, *512*
Price, M., 847, *850*
Price, R. W., 495, *508*, *510*, 632, *640*
Price, T. R., 47, *71*, 388, *406*, 723, *761*
Price, T. R. P., 396, *406*
Pricep, L. S., 31, *69*
Prien, F., 498, *510*
Prifitra, A., 651, *667*

Pringle, R., 820, *831*
Prinz, P., 328, *337*, 559, 564, 571, *578*, *580*, *581*
Prinz, P. N., *26*, 113, 237, *247*, 560, 568, 571, *580*, *581*, 659, *667*
Pro, J. D., 188, *198*
Procacci, P., 292, *303*
Prohovnik, I., 221, *228*
Proud, G. O., 272, *298*
Proulx, G. B., 707, *716*
Prudic, J., 221, *228*
Prusoff, B., 419, *430*
Pruvo, J. P., 624, *640*
Pruyn, J., 369, *374*
Psychiatric News, 882, *890*
Pueschel, S. M., 568, 590, *598*
Pull, C., 382, *405*
Pulling, N. H., 261, *303*
Punch, J. L., 273, *303*
Purisch, A. D., 647, *665*, *668*
Pynoos, J., 765, 767, 768, 783, *791*, 866, *870*
Pyrek, J., 822, *831*, 845, *852*

Qu, Q-Y., 13, *24*
Quayhagen, M., 646, *669*
Quigg, J. M., 264, *299*
Quilliam, T. A., 289, *303*
Quinn, B. P., 530, *552*
Quirk, R. S., 539, *550*

Rabbitt, P., 319, *335*
Rabbitt, P. M., 321, *335*
Rabins, O. V., 234, *248*
Rabins, P., 46, 48, *71*, 383, *403*, 466, 467, *475*, 501, *510*, 634, *641*, 744, *758*
Rabins, P. V., 467, 468, 469, 471, *475*, 558, *580*, 635, *640*, 654, *668*, 837, 841, 844, 846, *850*
Rabkin, J. G., 125, 126, 127, *143*
Rachamin, B., 564, *579*
Rader, J., 846, *851*
Rae, D. S., 34, 35, 41, 43, 49, 51, 56, 57, 58, 60, *67*, *171*
Raffin, R. E., 422, *431*
Raffoul, P. R., 529, 532, *552*
Raghab, M., 498, *510*

Ragsdale, C. W., 221, *225*
Raichle, M. E., 164, *172*, 221, *224*, *228*, 417, *430*
Raiford, C. A., 278, *304*
Rajput, A. H., 488, *510*
Rall, T. W., 516, *549*
Rammohan, K., 633, *639*
Rampal, S., 209, 210, *224*
Ramsdell, D. A., 277, *303*
Ramsdell, J., 692, *695*
Rand, J., 765, *791*
Rao, K., 47, *71*
Rapaport, S. I., 211, 215, 216, 219, 221, 222, *226*, *227*
Rapaport, S. J., 150, *172*
Raphael, B., 129, *143*
Rapoport, S., 205, 207, 208, *224*, *225*
Rapoport, S. F., 151, *170*, *171*
Rapoport, S. I., 205, 207, 209, 210, 211, 214, 215, 216, 217, 218, 221, 222, *223*, *224*, *225*, *226*, *228*, 645, *664*, *665*, 731, 732, *757*
Rapp, S. R., 384, 387, 388, *406*, 802, *813*
Raschko, B., 765, *791*
Rashi, S., 747, *760*
Rasinski, K., 253, 254, *300*
Raskin, A., 15, *26*, 327, *336*, 617, *640*, 654, *668*
Raskin, M., 387, 394, *406*, 842, *852*
Raskind, C. C., 340, *353*
Raskind, H., 819, *831*
Raskind, M., 182, 189, *194*, 395, *404*, 487, 498, 499, 500, *503*, *510*, *512*, 521, *552*, 842, *850*, 907, *912*
Raskind, M. A., 239, *246*, 384, 388, *404*, 446, *461*, 480, 485, 486, 498, 499, 500, *507*, *509*, *510*, *511*, *512*, 571, *580*, 834, *849*, 898, *914*
Rasmussen, R., 527, *555*
Rasool, C. G., 493, *510*
Ratey, J. J., 421, *430*
Rathey, R., 843, *850*
Ratner, H. H., 312, *336*
Ratner, J., 486, *506*
Rattenbury, C., 844, *851*
Raval, J., 491, *504*
Ravens, J. R., 164, *172*
Ravid, R., 483, *506*
Ravindran, A. V., 47, *67*
Rawles, J. M., 254, *302*

Ray, K., 765, *791*
Ray, W. A., 540, *549*, 747, 752, *760*, 840, *850*, *852*
Raynor, W. J., 821, *831*
Reading, V. M., 263, *303*
Reason, J., 313, 325, *336*
Reasoner, J., 347, *352*
Rebok, G., 323, *334*
Rechsteiner, M., 489, *510*
Redfield, R., 80, *97*
Reding, M., 654, *668*
Redmond, D. E., 417, *430*
Redmond, F. C., 855, *870*
Reece, S., 111, *117*
Reed, B. R., 652, 660, *668*
Reed, J. E., 539, *550*
Reed, P. G., 819, *831*
Reed, R., 527, *549*
Reeder, T. M., 485, *506*
Reedy, M. N., 365, *372*
Reever, K., 805, *813*
Reeves, K., 110, *117*
Regan, J. J., 861, *870*
Regestein, Q., 751, *760*
Regestein, Q. R., 572, *580*
Regier, D. A., 43, 56, *67*, 108, 110, *115*, 438, *460*, 800, 802, *813*, 874, *890*
Regina v. M'Naghten, 864, *870*
Regnier, V., 765, 781, *791*
Reich, J., 440–441, 451, 452, 454, *460*
Reich, P., 399, *406*
Reich, T., 47, *70*, *71*, 396, *401*, 517, 524, *547*, *552*
Reid, A. A., 539, *550*
Reid, D. W., 647, 648, *669*
Reifer, B. B., 500, *512*
Reifler, B., 521, *552*, 819, *831*
Reifler, B. V., 14, *26*, 386, 387, 394, *406*, 484, 494, 499, *506*, *507*, *509*, *510*, 523, 533, *550*, *552*, 660, *664*, 842, *852*
Reifman, L., 437, 445, *460*
Reiger, D. A., 34, 35, 41, 49, 51, 57, 58, 60, *71*
Reiman, E. M., 417, *430*
Reinikainen, K. J., 182, *198*
Reinvang, I., 661, *669*
Reisberg, B., 15, *24*, 24, 205, 209, 210, *224*, *227*, 245, *246*, *248*, 497, *510*, 654, *669*, 753, *760*

Reisine, T. D., 184, *198*
Reiss, B. B., 501, *509*
Reiss, S., 590, *598*
Reitan, R. M., 648, *669*
Reith, M., 541, *550*
Reivich, M., 164, *172*, 202, 203, 205, *223*, 228
Reker, G. T., 359, *374*
Renfrew, J. W., 205, *224*
Rennels, M. L., 164, *172*
Renner, V. J., 4, 7, *23*, 103, *115*, 365, *374*
Resch, L., 180, *195*
Reske-Nielson, E., 266, *298*
Resnick, L., 495, *510*
Resnick, S. M., 205, *223*
Restifo, K., 562, 564, 571, *580–581*
Rey, A., 647, *669*
Rey, A. C., 350, *354*, 654, *669*
Reynaud, J., 271, *303*
Reynolds, C., 651, *663*
Reynolds, C. F., 13, *26*, 535, *552*, 559, 560, 561, 562, 564, 566, 569, 571, 572, 573, 574, 575, 576, *577*, *578*, *580*, *580–581*, 621, *637*
Reynolds, G., 486, *504*
Reynolds, G. P., 183, 184, 189, *198*, 212, *228*, 486, *504*
Reynolds, L., 528, *553*
Reynolds, M. A., 179, *199*
Rezek, D. L., 646, *669*
Rheinhardt, A. M., 834, 840, *852*
Rhoades, E., 110, *117*
Rhodes, C., 205, *227*
Rhyne, R., 60, *66*, 522, *545*
Rhyne, R. L., 624, *639*
Ricaurte, G. A., 191, *198*
Rice, D., 261, *303*
Rice, G. E., 312, *336*
Rice, J., 47, *70*, *71*
Rice, J. P., 517, 524, *552*
Rich, C. L., 737, *760*
Rich, J. A., 706, 713, *714*
Richard, J., 240, *246*, 493, *505*
Richards, B., 456, *460*
Richards, O. W., 261, *303*
Richardson, E. P., 624, *640*
Richardson, G. S., 568, 576, *577*, *581*
Richardson, J. S., 539, *551*
Richardson, J. W., 733, *757*

Richelson, E., 733, *757*
Richter, C., 280, *303*
Rickels, K., 422, 424, *429*, *431*, 535, *552*, 746, 747, *759*, *760*
Rickles, K., 424, *430*
Rickwood, D., 33, 42, *70*
Riddick, C. C., 897, *912*
Riddle, M. W., 347, *352*
Ridley, A., 289, *303*
Rieder, R. O., 455, *459*
Riederer, P., 184, *198*
Riege, W. H., 205, 207, 210, 212, 214, 215, 219, *226*, *227*, 645, *666*, *669*
Riegel, K. F., 358, *374*
Riekkinen, P., 488, *507*
Riekkinen, P. J., 182, *198*, 621, *641*
Ries, P. W., 267, *303*
Ries, R., 571, *578*
Riesenberg, D., 841, *852*
Riessman, F., 120, *142*
Rifkin, A., 422, *429*
Rifkin, B., 282, 283, *296*
Riley, J. N., 497, *511*
Rimer, B., 541, 542, *553*
Rinck, C., 527, *550*
Rinieris, P., 382, *406*
Rinne, J. O., 179, 180, *198*
Rinne, U. K., 186, *197*, 488, *508*
Rinot, Y., 205, *227*
Rios, D., 576, *577*
Ripeckyj, A., 701, 702, 703, *715*, *717*
Ripley, H. S., 399, *402*
Risberg, J., 220, *228*
Risse, S. C., 480, 486, 498, 500, *507*, *510*, *511*, 733, 737, *761*
Rissenberg, M., 345, *354*
Ritchie, I. M., 184, *199*
Ritchie, J. L., 500, *512*
Ritschel, W. A., 729, *761*
Ritzmann, R. F., 527, *553*
Rivera, V. M., 658, *668*
Robb, J. W., 859, *869*
Robbins, M. A., 346, *353*
Roberts, A. H., 126, *143*
Roberts, D. W., 485, *506*
Roberts, K., 530, *552*
Roberts, R., 113, *115*
Roberts, R. E., 110, *117*
Robertson, D., 519, 539, *546*, *553*

Robertson, E. A., 287, *304*
Robertson, L., 423, *431*
Robertson, R. C., 896, *913*
Robertson-Tchabo, E. A., 205, *224*, 318, *336*
Robey, R. R., 290, *302*
Robilliard, E., 292, *304*
Robiner, W. N., 609, *640*
Robins, L. N., 34, 35, 41, 49, 51, 52, 57, 58, 60, *67*, *69*, *71*, 438, *460*, 523, 524, 526, *549*
Robins, P. V., 733, *760*
Robinson, A., 420, *431*, 711, *715*
Robinson, D. W., 268, *303*
Robinson, G. K., 886, 887, 888, *890*
Robinson, P. K., 274, *302*
Robinson, R. G., 47, *71*, 388, *406*, 501, *511*, 634, 635, *640*, 723, *761*
Robitaille, Y., 493, *513*
Robson, J. G., 258, *306*
Roca, R., 384, *403*, 835, *851*
Rocca, W. A., 38, *66*
Roccaforte, W. H., 617, *637*
Rockwell, E., 15, *26*, 393, *406*, 738, *761*
Rodin, G. M., 399, *406*
Rodin, J., 6, *26*, 241, *247*, 363, 368, *374*, 567, 570, *581*, 766, *791*
Rodrigo, E. K., 530, *553*
Roenker, D. L., 260, *296*
Roessmann, U., 488, *504*
Rogers, H., 15, *25*
Rogers, J., 180, *198*
Rogers, J. C., 236, 240, 245, *248*, 673, 677, *696*
Rogers, J. G., 209, *227*
Rogers, K., 656, *664*
Rogers, R. L., 347, *354*, 492, *508*, 541, *553*, 646, *667*
Rogers, W., 907, *914*
Rogers, W. A., 325, *336*
Roman, G. C., 492, *511*
Romanoski, A., 41. 59, *66*
Romer, D., 590, *596*
Ron, M. A., 527, *553*
Ronda, J. M., 576, *577*
Ronge, H., 290, *303*
Ronningstam, E. F., 442, *460*
Room, R., 523, *553*
Roos, B. E., 182, *196*
Roose, S. P., 381, *403*, 741, *758*

Roper, W. L., 881, *890*
Roques, P., 481, *506*
Rorsman, B., 33, 34, 37, 38, 43, 46, 47, *69*, *71*
Rose, R. P., 414, *429*
Rose, T., 327, *337*, 585, *598*, 617, *641*
Rose, T. G., Jr., 619, *639*
Rose, T. L., 15, *26*, 318, *336*, 419, *431*
Rosebush, P. I., 753, *761*
Rosen, D. E., 271, *303*
Rosen, R., 392, *406*, 700, 711, *716*
Rosen, S. M., 205, *223*
Rosen, T. J., 14, *26*, 623, 624, 625, *639*
Rosen, W. G., 222, *228*, 328, *336*, 492, *511*, 658, 661, *669*
Rosenbaum, G., 651, *670*
Rosenbaum, J., 423, *430*
Rosenberg, G., 290, *303*
Rosenberg, G. A., 624, *639*
Rosenberg, L., 285, 286, 287, 294, *297*
Rosenberg, M. B., 896, *913*
Rosenbloom, M., 527, *552*
Rosenbloom, S., 150, *170*
Rosenblum, M., 495, *510*
Rosenstein, R., 501, *511*
Rosenstein, R. B., 835, *851*
Rosenstock, I. M., 802, *813*
Rosenthal, A. S., 732, *757*, 835, *850*
Roses, A. D., 481, *511*
Roslaniec, A., 821, *831*
Rosner, F., 522, *546*
Rosner, L., 491, *506*
Rosor, M., 184, *196*
Rosow, I., 8, *26*, 766, *791*
Ross, C. A., 500, 501, *509*, *513*
Rossor, M., 184, *198*
Rossor, M. N., 182, 183, 189, *198*, 212, *228*, 486, *504*
Rotem, Y., 279, *301*
Rotenberg, M., 528, *547*
Roth, G. S., 179, *198*
Roth, M., 30, 31, 32, 40, 42, 47, 48, 52, 54, *67*, *70*, *71*, *72*, 158, *173*, 182, 183, 187, 188, 189, *194*, *197*, *198*, 212, *227*, *228*, 240, *246*, 277, *303*, 417, 420, *428*, *430*, 466, 467, 468, *474*, *475*, 486, 490, 501, *504*, *509*, *512*, 618, *641*, 686, 691, *694*
Roth, T., 558, 561, *579*
Roth, W. T., 414, 421, *429*, *431*

Rothenbert, R., 495, *511*
Rotter, J. B., 363, *374*
Rourke, D., 651, *670*
Rouse, F., 862, *870*
Roussel, F., 262, *306*
Rovner, B., 732, *761*
Rovner, B. W., *53*, 500, *509*, 539, 738, *761*, 835, 836, 841, *851*, *852*
Rowe, J. R., 728, *761*
Rowe, J. W., 10, *26*, 28, 72, 593, *598*
Rowe, W., 90, *97*
Roy-Byrne, P., 421, *431*
Royall, O., 48, *72*
Ruberg, M., 488, *505*
Rubin, A. E., 564, *579*
Rubin, E. H., 446, *460*
Ruchlin, H. S., 808, *812*
Rudinger, G., 359, *374*
Ruff, R. M., 646, *669*
Ruhling, E. M., 319, *332*
Ruiz, P., 516, 536, *550*
Rundgren, A., 541, *551*
Rupprecht, P., 845, *852*
Rush, B., 611, *641*
Rush, J., 392, *401*
Rush, J. A., 709, *713*
Rushing, W. A., 108, *116*
Russakoff, L. M., 454, *459*
Russell, B., 900, *914*
Russell, D. E., 319, *332*
Russell, R. W., 492, *506*, 658, *665*
Russell, R. W. R., 219, *225*
Russo, J., 237, *248*, 328, *337*
Ruth, T., 186, *195*
Ruth, T. J., 209, *227*
Rutherford, G. W., 495, *503*
Rutherford, J. L., 396, *401*
Ryan, C., 526, *553*
Ryan, J. J., 648, *669*
Ryberg, S., 648, *666*
Rzetelny, H., 838, *850*

Sachdev, P., 624, *641*
Sachs, D. P. L., 541, 542, *553*
Sachs, H., 219, *224*
Sachs, H. J., 209, *227*
Sackeim, H. A., 221, *228*, 733, *757*

Sackellares, J. C., 204, *224*
Sackett, D. L., 40, 48, *72*
Sackett, G. P., 590, *598*
Sackheim, H. A., 498, *505*
Sacks, J. J., 541, *549*
Sacks, M., 531, 532, 533, 534, *551*
Sadavoy, J., 443, 448, 449, 450, 453, 456, *460*, 700, 702, 711, *715*, *716*, 900, *914*
Sadock, B., 898, *913*
Sadovnick, A. D., 587, *596*
Safai, B., 495, *513*
Safar, P., 861, *871*
Sahakian, B. J., 541, *550*
Sahakian, B. L., 473, *475*
Said, F. S., 253, *303*
Sainsbury, P., 399, *406*
St. Clair, D., 31, *72*
St. George-Hyslop, P., 40, *72*, 214, *228*, 481, *512*
Saint-Martin, M., 486, *506*
Sajadi, C., 440, *461*
Sakai, F., 205, *227*
Sakauye, K., 823, *831*
Sakurada, O., 202, 203, *228*
Sala, S., 328, *332*
Saleb, S. P., 753, *760*
Salem, S., 530, *546*, 728, 752, *757*, 840, *850*
Salend, E., 866, *870*
Salerno, J. A., 211, 219, *224*, *227*
Salkovskis, P. M., 417, 422, *428*
Sallis, J. F., 423, *431*
Salmon, D., 40, *72*, 214, *228*, 652, *664*
Salmon, D. P., 13, *24*, 328, *336*
Salob, S. P., 497, *510*
Salovey, P., 368, *374*
Salthouse, T. A., 311, *336*, 340, 342, *354*
Saltman, D., 530, *551*
Salzman, C., 14, *26*, 419, 421, 423, *430*, *431*, 498, *511*, 519, *553*, 575, *581*, 617, *641*, 725, 730, 733, 735, 736, 737, 738, 742, 743, 747, 752, 753, *758*, *761*, 816, *829*, 898, *914*
Samis, H. V., 687, 692, *694*
Samorajaski, T., 266, *303*
Samorajski, T., 524, *549*
Sample, P. A., 253, *303*
Sanchez, R., 576, *577*
Sandberg, B., 420, *431*
Sandler, A. M., 702, *716*

Sands, L. P., 348, *354*
Sanford, A. J., 322, *336*
Sanford, J. R. A., 558, *581*
Sangl, J., 593, *599*
Sano, M., 485, 501, *508*, *511*, *512*, 754, *762*
Santana, F., 109, *116*
Sapolsky, R., 500, *511*
Sargeant, W., 440, *460*
Sargent, F. I., 573, *581*
Sarna, S., 562, *579*
Sarwar, M., 150, *170*
Sashadri, T., 167, *172*
Saskin, P., 561, *581*
Sassin, J., 566, *577*
Sassin, J. F., 562, *580*
Sastre, J., 205, *227*
Sathananthan, G., 345, *353*
Sato, M., 483, *511*
Satti, M. H., 271, *303*
Sattin, R. W., 541, *549*
Satz, M., 866, *870*
Satz, P., 646, 647, 659, *664*, *668*, *669*
Saunders, F., 264, *300*
Saunders, P., 530, 531, *554*
Saunders, P. A., 523, *553*
Saunders, R. L., 485, *506*
Saunders, S. J., 525, 529, *549*
Saunders, W. B., 14, *24*, 391, *401*
Savage, D. G., 494, *508*
Savage, I. T., 533, *547*, 747, *757*
Savard, R. J., 350, *354*, 654, *669*
Sawa, G., 388, *403*
Sax, D. S., 190, *197*
Saxby, P., 710, 711, *713*
Sayre, C. I., 209, *227*
Sbordone, R. J., 647, *668*
Scanlon, W., 835, *850*, 874, 884, *889*
Schadé, J. P., 158, *172*
Schaffer, G., 316, 317, *335*
Schaffer, J. D., 498, *510*
Schaffner, W., 540, *549*, 747, 752, *760*, 840, *850*, 852
Schaie, J. P., 646, *669*
Schaie, K. W., 10, *23*, *26*, 311, 330, *336*, 342, 345, 346, *353*, *354*, 358, *374*, 436, 438, *460*, 587, *598*, 646, *669*
Schallert, T., 191, *198*
Schamoian, C. A., 381, 396, *407*
Schapira, K., 420, *428*

Schapiro, M., 645, *665*

Schapiro, M. B., 210, 211, 214, 215, 219, 221, *224, 225, 226, 227*

Scharf, 751, *761*

Scharlach, A. E., 805, *813*

Schecter, R., 237, 240, *247*

Scheff, S. W., 180, 182, 190, *195, 196, 198*

Scheibel, A. B., 159, 163, 164, 165, 166, 167, *172*

Scheibel, M. E., 159, 161, 163, 167, 168, *172*

Schell, D. A., 311, 312, *334, 336*

Schemper, T., 284, 286, *303*

Scherl, D., 883, *889*

Scherl, D. J., 874, 878, 879, 883, *889, 890*

Scherr, P. A., 33, *68*, 201, 209, *224*, 480, 482, *505*, 753, *758*

Schiebel, A. B., 253, *303*

Schiebel, M. E., 253, *303*

Schieber, F., 254, 255, 258, 262, 264, 272, 273, 280, 288, *300, 303*

Schifano, F., 391, *404*, 817, *831*

Schiffer, R. B., 629, *638*

Schiffman, S., 285, 288, *304*

Schiffman, S. S., 281, 282, 284, 288, *304*

Schimmel, H., 237, 240, *247*

Schlaepfer, T. B., 467, 468, *475*

Schlaepfer, W. W., 491, *504*

Schlageter, N. L., 207, 214, *226, 228*

Schlageter, S. L., 209, 210, 211, 215, *224, 225*

Schleifer, S. J., 388, *406*, 907, *914*

Schlesinger, H. J., 907, *913*

Schlesselman, J. J., 29, 40, *72*

Schlesser, M., 382, *407*

Schloendorff v. Society of New York Hospital, 858, *870*

Schluderman, E., 292, *304*

Schmaier, A. H., 482, *512*

Schmechel, D. R., 485, *511*

Schmidt, C. F., 202, *226*

Schmidt, L. J., 834, 840, *852*

Schmitt, F. A., 618, *638*

Schmitt, I., 485, *511*

Schmitz, R. E., 526, 529, *554*

Schmitz-Scherzer, R., 356, *374*

Schneck, M. K., 654, *669*

Schneck, S. A., 163, *172*

Schneider, C. L., 539, *553*

Schneider, E. L., 10, *26*

Schneider, L. S., 47–48, *72*, 733, *761*

Schneider, W., 362, 371, *374*

Schneiderman, L. J., 868, *870*

Schoenback, V. J., 386, *402*

Schoenberg, B., 34, *72*

Schoenberg, B. S., 34, 38, *67, 70*, 186, *198*

Schoenfeld, M., 190, *197*

Schoening, H., 685, 689, *697*

Schoenrock, S. A., 109, *116*

Scholl, T. O., 859, *869*

Schonefield, D., 287, *304*

Schonfeld, L., 525, 529, *548*

Schonfield, A. E. D., 308, *336*

Schor, C. M., 260, *299*

Schor, D., 260, *304*

Schow, R., 266, *304*

Schretlen, D., 646, *664*

Schrodt, C. J., 445, *457*

Schubert, D. S. P., 575, *581*

Schuckit, M. A., 516, 520, 523, 525, 528, 529, 536, 537, *545, 553*

Schuknecht, H., 266, *304*

Schuknecht, H. F., 266, *306*

Schulberg, H. C., 384, *406*

Schultz, N. R., 346, *353*, 438, *460*

Schulz, J., 875, *890*

Schulzer, M., 186, *195*

Schumacher, G. A., 292, *304*

Schuman, L. M., 38, *68, 71*, 484, *508*

Schupf, N., 585, 588, *599*

Schurman, R. A., 800, 802, 803–804, *813*, 867, *870*, 874, *890*

Schwab, J. J., 47, *72*, 386, 388, *405, 406*

Schwartz, J. H., 176, *196*

Schwartz, J. M., 220, *223*

Schwartz, M., 150, 151, *170, 172*, 205, *224*

Schweitzer, I., 395, *407*

Schweizer, E., 422, *431*

Schwenk, M. A., 845, *852*

Scialfa, C. T., 260, 263, 264, *304*

Scigliano, G., 184, *197*

Scitovsky, A. A., 867, *870*

Scjmale, A. M., 389, *402*

Scollo-Lavizzari, G., 621, *638*

Scott, J., 382, *402*, 411, 412, *428*

Scott, R., 33, 42, *70*, 191, *195*

Seab, J. P., 652, 660, *668*

Seals, D. R., 346, *354*

Sealy, A. P., 437, *461*
Seeman, M. V., 468, *475*
Seeman, P., 184, *198*
Segal, H., 702, *716*
Segal, J. H., 470, *475*
Segall, M., 823, *831*
Sehulster, J. R., 313, *336*
Seidler, F. J., 486, *511*
Seiler, W. O., 621, *638*
Seivewright, H., 439, 440, 442, *461*
Sekar, B. C., 624, *639*
Sekuler, R., 253, 254, 258, 260, 264, 265, *295*, *298*, *300*, *302*, *304*
Selesnick, S. T., 672, *694*
Seligman, H. P., 362, *374*
Seligman, M. E. P., 350, *354*, 426, *431*
Selin, C. E., 220, 221, *223*
Selkoe, D. J., 482, 483, 493, *507*, *509*, *510*, *511*, *512*
Sellers, E. M., 730, *758*
Seltzer, B., 38, *72*, 212, 213, *228*
Seltzer, M. M., 585, 586, 587, 589, 590, 591, 592, 593, 594, *598*, 809, *813*
Semla, T. P., 538, 539, *549*
Semple, S. J., 15, *25*
Seppala, T., 742, *760*
Serban, G., 127, *143*
Serduto, R. D., 265, *305*
Seretny, M. L., 655, *664*
Serrel, N. A., 821, *830*
Servino, L., 847, *850*
Sevensen, W. H., 443, *461*
Severson, J. A., 47–48, *72*, 731, *761*
Sewich, D. E., 535, *552*
Sewitch, D .E., 559, 561, 562, 564, 569, 571, 573, *580–581*
Seylaz, J., 205, *227*
Seymour, D. G., 820, *831*
Shadden, B. B., 278, *304*
Shader, R. I., 423–424, *427*, *428*, *431*, 617, *641*, 729, 730, 735, 748, *758*, *761*
Shafer, R., 573, *579*
Shafer, S., 126, *143*
Shaffra, A. M., 262, *306*
Shalat, S. L., 38, *72*
Shaman, P., 285, 286, 287, 294, *297*
Shamoian, C., 738, *756*
Shamoian, C. A., 236, *246*, 730, 742, *762*
Shanan, J., 77, *97*, 355, 365, 366, *374*

Shanas, E., 12, *26*
Shaper, A. G., 525, *553*
Shapira, J., 446, *460*
Shapira, K., 456, *461*
Shapiro, A. P., 540, *547*
Shapiro, H. B., 292, *296*
Shapiro, S., 35, 41, 43, 49, 52, 54, 56, 59, 60, 62, *66*, *68*, 802, 810, *811*, 835, *850*
Shapshak, P., 495, *510*
Sharfstein, S. S., 874, 878, 879, 883, *889*, *890*
Sharma, V. K., 523, 530, 531, *553*, *554*
Sharp, J. A., 254, *304*
Sharp, P. F., 624, 625, *638*, *639*
Sharpe, L., 688, 693, *695*
Sharpe, L. G., 164, *172*
Shaw, B., 392, *401*
Shaw, B. F., 709, *713*
Shaw, D. H., 569, *581*
Shaw, P., 473, *474*, 528, *550*
Shaw, R., 324, *336*
Shaw, S. M., 423, *431*
Shaw, T., 205, *227*, 485, *504*
Shazly, M., 500, *505*
Shea, J. P., 424, *428*
Shearer, H. W., 319, *332*
Sheehan, D. V., 424, *431*
Sheehan, M., 536, *548*
Sheehan, T., 84, *97*
Shefer, V. F., 152, *173*
Sheffield, B., 396, *401*
Sheikh, J. I., 410, 414, 419, 423, *431*, *432*
Shelley, C., 647, *667*
Shelp, E. E., 859, *870*
Shelp, F., 380, 386, 394, *404*
Shelton, A., 84, 86, *97*
Shen, Y. C., 33, *70*
Shenkin, H. A., 204, *228*
Shepherd, A., 825, *831*
Shepherd, M., 52, *72*
Sheps, J., 844, *850*
Shering, A., 485, *505*
Sherman, D., 840, *850*
Sherman, D. S., 530, *546*, 728, 752, *757*
Sherman, E. D., 292, *304*
Sherwin, I., 212, 213, *228*
Sherwood, S., 588, *599*, 687, *697*, 808, *812*
Shewchuk, R. M., 15, *24*
Shibayama, H., 33, *72*

Shifflett, P. A., 360, *374*
Shigeoka, J. S., 319, *332*
Shimamura, A. P., 328, *336*
Shinar, D., 264, *304*
Shindler, A. G., 653, *666*
Shinohara, M., 202, 203, *228*
Shiokawa, H., 280, 286, *304*
Shiverly, M., 805, 806, *813*
Shock, N. W., 259, *298*
Shopland, D., 541, *552*
Shoptaugh, C. F., 254, *306*
Shostak, M., 500, *506*
Shoulson, I., 629, 635, *638*
Shrout, P., 109, *115*
Shullaw, G., 847, *850*
Shulman, K., 395, *403*
Shulman, K. I., 383, *406*
Shuttleworth, E. C., 471, *475*, 633, *639*, 656, *666*
Siberfarb, P., 47, *69*, 388, *403*
Siblinger, H. J., 798, *812*
Siegel, D., 265, *305*
Siegel, J. S., 585, *599*
Siegelaub, A. B., 292, 293, *306*, 524, *550*
Siegler, H., 861, *870*
Siegler, I. C., 356, 363, *374*
Siegler, M., 857, 863, *869*, *870*
Siemsen, D., 258, 264, *302*
Siever, L. J., 899, *914*
Sigmon, A. H., 34, *69*, 484, *507*
Sigvardsson, S., 517, 524, *547*
Sikorski, L., 285, 286, 287, 294, *297*
Silberman, E., 350, *354*, 653, *669*
Silberman, E. K., 654, *669*
Silver, A., 710, *716*
Silver, R. L., 130, *143*
Silverberg, J. D., 395, *403*
Silverman, A. J., 382, *401*
Silverman, J., 382, *400*
Silverman, J. M., 482, *508*
Silverman, S. M., 737, *758*
Silverman, W. P., 585, 588, *599*
Silverskiold, P., 220, *228*
Silvestri, R., 575, *578*
Simchowitz, T., 148, 157, *173*
Simmons, L., 83, *97*
Simon, A., 442, *461*, 528, *553*, 820, *831*
Simon, R., 688, 693, *695*
Simon, R. I., 857, *870*

Simonson, E., 262, *299*
Simpson, D. M., 737, *762*
Simpson, J., 182, 184, *197*, *199*
Simpson, R. J., 532, *552*
Sims, N. R., 182, 183, *194*, *195*, *197*, 485, 486, *506*, *509*
Sims, P., 646, *667*
Sinall, R., 564, 572, *577*
Singer, H. S., 488, *512*
Singer, J., 355, *374*, 469, *474*
Singer, P. A., 861, 863, *870*
Singh, R., 424, *430*
Singh, R. A., 747, *760*
Sinnott, J. D., 317, *336*
Sipponen, J., 492, *505*, 624, *638*
Sitaram, N., 344, *354*
Sivak, M., 261, 262, *302*, *304*
Sjogren, H., 492, *511*
Sjogren, T., 492, *511*
Sjostrand, J., 262, *295*
Skaff, M. M., 15, *25*
Skalka, S. M., 254, *305*
Skelton-Robinson, M., 472, *474*
Skinner, E. A., 802, 810, *811*
Skorney, B., 529, *548*
Skurla, E., 236, 240, 245, *248*
Sladek, J. K., 191, *196*
Slager, U., 180, *196*, 488, *505*
Slater, E., 440, *460*
Slater, W. R., 388, *406*
Slatter, J., 385 , 386, *405*
Slauson, T. J., 64, 652, *663*
Slazer, U., 152, *170*
Sliders, W., 153, *169*
Sloane, M. E., 252–253, 258, 261, 264, *302*, *304*, *305*
Sloane, R. B., 47–48, *72*
Slobogin, C., 855, 865, *870*
Slotkin, T. A., 486, *511*
Sluss, T. K., 30, *72*
Small, G., 214, *226*
Small, G. W., 215, *227*, 645, *666*
Smallberg, S. A., 327, *332*, 344, *354*
Smallverg, A., 386, *402*
Smallwood, R. G., 560, 564, 568, 571, *581*
Smart, R. G., 59, *72*, 521, 523, 529, 530, *553*
Smiley, A., 424, *431*
Smiley, M., 384, 388, 393, *404*

Smirne, S., 182, *194*, 564, *581*
Smith, A. D.. 318, *335*
Smith, A. I., 484, *508*
Smith, A. M. R., 38, 42, 46, *67*
Smith, B., 680, *694*
Smith, B. L., 619, *637*
Smith, C. B., 188, *194*
Smith, C. C. T., 182, *194*
Smith, C. G., 285, *305*
Smith, C. H., 188, *198*
Smith, C. J., 490, *509*
Smith, D., 207, *228*
Smith, D. V., 279, *305*
Smith, E., 657, *667*
Smith, F. W., 624, 625, *638, 639*
Smith, I., 456, *460*
Smith, J. M., 469, *474*
Smith, J. S., 328, *336*
Smith, K. C., 822, *831*
Smith, R., 385, 386, *405*
Smith, R. B., 423–424, *428*
Smith, R. C., 485, *504*
Smith, R. E., 385, *402*
Smith, S. E., 281, *305*
Smith, V. C., 253, *303*
Smith, V. K., 424, *429*
Smolensky, M., 573, *581*
Smook, G., 347, *352*
Smyer, M., 687, 692, *695*
Smyer, M. A., 16, *24*, 838, *852*
Snow, A. D., 483, *511*
Snow, G., 648, *669*
Snow, W. G., 647, *669*
Snowden, J. S., 182, 183, *195*, 485, 486, *506, 509*
Snowdon, J., 473, *475*, 835, *852*
Snowdon, J. S., 182, *194*
Snyder, C., 324, *335*
Snyder, L. H., 822, *831*, 845, *852*
Snyder, S., 439, 440, 445, *461*
Snyder, S. H., 184, *196, 198*
Soave, P., 328, *332*
Sobe, A., 495, *506*
Sobol, A. M., 29, 46, 47, *71*
Soetaert, G., 624, *640*
Soffe, A. M., 204, *228*
Soininem, H., 621, *641*
Soininen, H., 38, 39, 40, *72*, 182, *198*, 488, *507*

Sokoloff, L., 164, *172*, 202, 203, 204, 205, 207, 208, *223, 224, 228*
Soldatos, C. R., 566, *579*, 751, *759*
Soldo, B., 807, *813*
Soldo, B. J., 874–875, *890*
Solomon, F., 129, 130, *143*
Solomon, K., 392, *406*
Som, P., 164, *172*
Sommers, I., 805, 806, *813*
Sonn, U., 245, *246*
Soper, H. V., 659, *669*
Sopolopski, J., 105, *117*
Sorbi, S., 40, *72*, 214, *228*
Sorensen, P. S., 486, *511*
Sorenson, S. B., 56, *70*
Soumerai, S. B., 530, *546*, 728, 752, 757, 758, 840, 841, *849, 850*
Soussaline, F., 205, *227*
Sox, C. H., 619, *639*
Sox, H. C., 619, *639*
Spacavento, L., 421, *429*
Spalding, E. M., 500, *503*
Spanton, S., 496, *508*
Spar, J., 500, *511*, 654, *666*
Spar, J. E., 328, *334*, 383, *406*, 645, 651, 652, *666, 667*
Spark, G. M., 711, *713*, 713, *716*
Spatz, E. L., 539, *550*
Spears, G. F. S., 523, 524, 526, *546*
Specht, D., 805, 806, *813*
Spector, A., 253, *298*
Spector, W. D., 677, *697*, 835, *851*
Speedie, L., 634, *641*
Speer, M. C., 481, *509*
Speilberger, C., 412, 419, *431*
Speilberger, C. D., 419, *430*
Speilman, A., 561, *581*
Spencer, B., 805, *811*
Spera, 742, *757*
Sperbeck, D. J., 706, *716*
Spieth, W., 346, *354*
Spiker, D. G., 559, 561, 562, 564, 571, *580, 580–581*
Spillane, J. A., 182, 188, *194*
Spinks, T., 205, *227*
Spinnler, H., 328, *332*
Spirduso, W. W., 346, 347, *352, 354*
Spiro, A., 437, *461*
Spiro, H., 816, *831*

Spirrison, C. L., 585, *597*
Spitz, P., 686, 690, *695*
Spitz, P. W., 540, *549*
Spitzer, A. R., 495, *513*
Spitzer, M. E., 281, *305*
Spitzer, R., 454, *461*
Spitzer, R. L., 242, *246*, 455, *459*, 609, *641*
Spokes, E., 184, *196, 198*
Spooner, J. W., 254, *305*
Spoor, A., 268, *305*
Spring, B., 539, *551*
Spring, W. D., Jr., 527, *555*
Sprung, C. L., 863, *871*
Squire, L. R., 328, *336*
Stabler, S. P., 494, *508*
Stack, J. A., 13, *26*, 561, 562, 564, 569, 571, 572, 576, *578, 580*
Stacy, C., 765, *791*
Stadian, E. M., 479, *508*
Stadlan, E. M., 32, *71*, 645, *667*
Staehelin, H. B., 621, *638*
Stafford, J. A., 34, *69*, 484, *507*
Stafford, J. L., 644, 645, *663*
Stafford, P. B., 804, 806, *812*
Stalgaitis, S., 423, *431*
Stamp, J. E., 179, *196*
Stanahan, S., 182, 189, *194*
Stanford, E. P., 107, 109, *115, 116*, 525, 526, *551*
Stangl, D., 446, 451, 452, 454, *461, 462*
Stanley, B., 575, *580*, 747, *760*
Stanley, M., 747, *760*
Staples, F., 109, *116*
Starcher, T., 495, *507*
Starkstein, S. E., 501, *511*, 634, 635, *640*
Starr, L. B., 47, *71*
Steadman, H. J., 864, *869*
Steele, C., 468, *475*, 501, *513*
Steele, V. G., 264, *306*
Steen, B., 541, *551*
Steer, R., 419, *427*
Steffl, B., 822, *831*
Stehr-Green, L., 495, *507*
Stein, M., 907, *914*
Steinberg, A., 111, *117*
Steinbrook, R., 861, *871*
Steiner, V., 765, *791*
Steiness, I., 290, *305*
Steinfield, E., 767, 768, *791*

Steingart, A., 491, *511–512*
Steinhouse, K., 399, *406*
Steinling, M., 624, *640*
Stella, A. G., 530, *547*
Stenback, A., 349, *354*
Stenchever, D., 523, *552*
Stengal, E., 399, *405*
Stephens, R. C., 529, 538, *553*
Stern, Y., 388, *405*, 485, 496, 501, *508, 511, 512*, 617, 635, *640*, 754, *762*
Sternberg, J., 835, *851*
Sternberg, R., 351, *354*
Steuer, J., 392, 393, *403, 406*, 743, *758*
Steuer, J. L., 700, 701, 711, *716*
Steven, J., 574, *578*
Stevens, J. C., 282, 284, 286, 287, 288, *305*
Stevens, S. S., 281, *305*
Stevenson, P. W., 273, *305*
Stewart, R. B., 747, *758*
Stewart, A., 618, *638*, 907, *914*
Stewart, C. K., 539, *546*
Stewart, D., 649, *664*
Stewart, G. D., 40, *72*, 214, *228*
Stewart, G. T., 536, 537, *547*
Stewart, M. A., 388, *406*
Stewart, M. S., 749, *758*
Stewart, R. B., 538, 539, *551*
Stiller, P., 688, 693, *695*
Stinson, F., 522, *547*
Stinson, F. S., 520, *553*
Stipec, M. R., 109, *115*
Stoesl, A. J., 209, *227*
Stoessel, A., 186, *196*
Stokes, D. K., 736, *759*
Stokes, E. J., 520, *547*
Stoller, E. P., 538, 539, *553*
Stolorow, R., 705, *716*
Stoltzman, R., 410, 412, *430*, 531, 536, *551*
Stone, A., 861, *871*
Stone, K., 635, *641*, 744, *762*
Stone, L. A., 292, *297*
Stone, R., 593, *599*
Stoneburner, R., 495, *511*
Stoner, S. B., 436, 445, *461*
Stones, M. J., 844, *851*
Storandt, M., 328, *336*, 346, 349, *352*, 648, 649, 650, 651, 653, *669*, 700, *716*
Stotsky, B., 816, *830*
Stotsky, B. A., 575, *581*, 837, *852*

Stoudemire, A., 654, *669*
Stoudermire A., 859, *870*
Strachan, R. W., 494, *512*
Strain, L. A., 103, *117*
Straker, M., 442, *461*
Strang, J., 537, *553*
Strassberg, D. S., 711, *716*
Strategy Council on Drug Abuse, 517, *554*
Strauss, A., 738, 749, *762*
Strauss, D., 392, *406*
Strauss, M., 652, *666*
Streib, G., 585, *599*
Streissguth, A. P., 528, *551*
Stricht, R., 274, *305*
Strick, P. L., 221, *223*
Strogatz, S. H., 576, *577*
Strouse, T. B., 388, *401*
Strout, P. E., 125, *142*
Strub, R. L., 612, *641*
Struble, R. G., 153–154, *173*, 485, *512*
Strumpf, N. E., 845, *850*
Studenski, S., 384, 388, *404*
Sturgeon, D. A., 439, *457*
Sturgis, E. T., 705, *717*
Sturgis, S. P., 261, *303*
Sturr, J. F., 261, *305*
Stuss, D. T., 447, *461*
Su, L., 388, *407*
Suddeth, J. A., 473, *475*
Sugar, J. A., 313, 314, 316, 317, *336, 337*
Sugiwara, O., 167, *173*
Suissa, S., 486, *506*
Suljaga-Petchel, K., 530, *552*, 746, 752, *760*
Sulkava, R., 488, 492, *505, 512*, 624, *638*
Sullivan, C., 523, *553*
Sullivan, C. F., 530, 531, *554*
Sullivan, D. C., 391–392, *401, 402*
Sullivan, G., 866, *870*
Sullivan, M. J., 419, *430*
Sullivan, P., 14, *26*
Sumi, S. M., 182, 188, 189, *194, 197, 198*, 480, 488, *508, 511*
Sumida, R. M., 220, 221, *223*
Summers, J. A., 593, *599*
Summers, W. K., 485, *512*
Sundaram, M., 205, 209, 210, 211, 214, 215, 216, 217, 222, *223, 224, 225*, 645, *665*
Sunderland, T., 218, *225*, 236, 240, 245, *248*, 484, 500, *509, 512*, 754, *762*

Sundet, K., 661, *669*
Sundquist, J., 486, *512*
Suominen, H., 290, *297*
Superintendent of Belchertown State School v. Saikewicz, 859, *871*
Surawicz, T. S., 541, 542, *548*
Surtees, P. G., 397, *407*
Susman, V. L., 454, *459*
Sussman, L., 52, 54, 56, 67, 108, *115*
Sutton, G. J., 268, *303*
Sutton, M. S., 585, *597*
Suzuki, J., 153, *171*, 180, *197*
Suzuki, J. S., 154, *171*, 179, *197*
Suzuki, S., 483, *511*
Svanborg, A., 541, *551*
Sved, S., 323, *334*
Svennerholm, L., 182, 189, *194*
Svingos, A., 263, *301*
Swanson, J. M., 311, 312, *332*
Swearer, J. M., 14, *26*
Sweeney, J., 381, 382, *401*, 739, *757*
Swenson, C., 535, *552*
Swenson, J. R., 496, *512*
Swift, C. G., 539, *554*
Swig, L., 495, *503*
Swinburne, H., 568, *581*
Sylvester, T. O., 254, *304*
Syme, S., 106, *115*
Symon, L., 219, *225*, 492, *506*, 658, *665*

Taborsky, G. J., 486, *510*
Tachiki, K., 485, *512*
Taeuber, C., 101, *117*
Tagliavini, F., 191, *195*
Tait, D., 589, *599*
Talland, G. A., 347, *354*
Talmor, N., 279, *301*
Tamminga, C. A., 738, *762*
Tang, Y. T., 575, *581*
Tanke, E., 419, *431*
Tanke, E. D., 423, *432*
Tannenhaus, M., 310, *334*
Tanner, C. M., 186, *198*
Tanridag, O., 624, *641*
Tanzi, R., 214, *228*
Tanzi, R. E., 40, *72*, 481, *512*
Tarasoff v. Regents of the University of Calfornia, 866, *871*

Tariot, N., 737, *759*

Tariot, P. N., 732, 753, 754, *762*

Tarlot, P. N., 500, *512*

Tarnowska-Dzidnszko, E., 163, *171*

Tarter, R. E., 497, *512*

Taska, L. S., 559, 561, 562, 564, 571, *580–581*

Taub, H. A., 261, *305*

Taube, C. A., 108, *115*, 800, 802, *813*, 873, 874, 877, 878, *889*, *890*

Tawakina, T., 492, *508*

Taylor, A. K., 325, *337*

Taylor, C., 536, *548*

Taylor, C. B., 414, *431*

Taylor, J. O., 201, 209, *224*, 480, 482, *505*, 753, *758*

Taylor, J. R., 329, *333*, 651, 654, *665*

Taylor, L. B., 736, *759*

Taylor, N., 384, *403*, 835, *851*

Taylor, P. J., 536, *554*

Taylor, R. L., 658, *668*

Taylor, W., 271, *300*

Teasdale, G., 190, *196*

Teeter, R. B., 834, *852*

Teitelbaum, M. S., 802, 810, *811*

Teleska, P., 650, *667*

Telesky, C., 802, *810*

Telles, C. A., 108, 109, *115*

Tenaglia, A. N., 388, *401*

Tenczer, J., 539, *550*

Tenney, Y. J., 317, *337*

Teravainen, H., 656–657, *666*

Teresi, J., 243, *247*

Teresi, J. A., 244, *247*

Teri, L., 14, *26*, 234, 240, 245, *248*, 386, 387, 394, *406*, 499, 500, *509*, *510*, *512*, 659, *667*, 676, *697*, 700, 705, *715*, 842, *852*

Termeer, J., 659, *664*

Terrence, L. R., 236, 244, *248*

Terry, R. D., 153, 157, *173*, 176, 177, *196*, *198*, 222, *227*, 492, *511*, 658, *669*

Terry, R. O., 647, 652, *665*

Tesar, G. E., 395, *407*

Tesfaye, Y., 486, *506*

Tetrud, J. W., 186, *196*

Thal, L. J., 617, *641*

Thase, M. E., 587, 588, *599*

Thoits, P. A., 127, *143*

Thomae, H., 356, 359, 360, 366, 367, *373*, *374*, *375*

Thomas, C. B., 484, *509*

Thomas, C. W., 536, *552*

Thomas, J., 467, 468, 469, *475*

Thomas, J. P., 258, *302*

Thomas, R., 191, *196*

Thomas, R. V., 495, *513*

Thomasen, A. M., 493, *512*

Thomlinson, B. E., 490, *512*

Thompson, J. W., 18, *23*, 530, *546*, 728, 746, 752, *757*, 840, *850*

Thompson, K. E., 484, *509*

Thompson, L., 419, *431*

Thompson, L. W., 13, 15, *24*, *25*, *26*, 313, 314, 327, 328, 329, *335*, *337*, 346, *352*, 392, *403*, *407*, 446, *461*, 653, *668*, 699, 700, 701, 707, 709, 710, *714*, *715*, *717*

Thompson, T. L., 753, *762*

Thompson, T. L., II, 731, *760*

Thompson v. Oklahoma, 865, *871*

Thornbury, J. M., 290, *305*

Thornton, J., 574, *581*

Thorpy, M., 561, *581*

Threatt, J., 166, *172*

Tibshirani, R. J., 35, *69*

Tierney, M. C., 647, 648, *669*

Tiller, J., 395, *407*

Tillman, T. W., 272, *305*

Timbers, D., 110, *115*

Timbers, D. M., 109, *116*

Timiras, P. S., 519, *554*

Timko, C., 363, *374*, 567, 570, *581*

Tingle, D., 737, *762*

Tinklenberg, J. R., 485, 500, *505*, *509*

Tiplady, B., 539, *554*

Tipper, S., 324, *337*

Tischler, G. L., 42, 58, 60, *69*, *73*, 380, 384, *407*, 410, 412, *430*, 523, 524, 526, 531, 536, *549*, *551*, 795, 801, 803, *812*

Tissot, R., 493, *505*

Tobin, J. D., 526, *554*

Tobin, S. S., 362, *373*, 397, *407*

Toffano, G., 190, *195*

Tohen, M., 680, *694*

Tolson, R. L., 526, 527, 529, *546*, *550*

Tombaugh, G., 500, *511*

Tomer, A., 340, 342, 347, 349, *352*, *354*

Tomiyasu, U., 159, 161, 163, 164, 165, 166, 167, 168, *172*
Tomlinson, A., 252, *300*
Tomlinson, B., 686, 691, *694*
Tomlinson, B. E., 30, 31, *67*, 154, 158, *175*, 180, 188, *196*, *198*, 240, *246*, 485, 490, *504*, *509*
Tomoeda, C. K., 649, 652, *663*
Toper, S., 179, *196*
Torii, S., 566, *580*
Torp, S., 153, *173*
Torpy, D., 588, *597*
Torvik, A., 153, *173*
Toth, R. F., 529, *550*
Tourigny-Rivard. M. F., 837, *852*
Tourtellotte, W. W., 184, *198*, 495, *510*
Toyne, R., 765, *791*
Trahan, D. E., 647, *669*
Trapp, G. A., 484, *512*
Treadway, C. A., 494, *513*
Treadway, C. R., 41, *73*
Treat, A., 835, *852*
Treat, N. J., 316, *337*
Tremaine, M., 279, *295*
Trent, A., 732, *762*
Trimble, M. R., 623, *638*
Trofatter, J. A., 481, *509*
Trojanowski, J. Q., 491, *504*
Tross, S., 47, *69*, 388, *403*
Troster, A. I., 651, *666*
Trotter, W. R., 280, *299*
Troughton, E., 451, 454, *460*
Truman, B., 495, *511*
Tsai, M., 385, *402*
Tsai, S. Y., 210, 211, 219, *223*
Tsuang, M. T., 469, *475*
Tsukuda, R., 825, *831*
Tsunematsu, T., 541, *555*
Tuck, R. R., 526, *554*
Tucker, C. M., 180, 187, 188, 189, 191, *196*
Tucker, G. J., 394, *402*
Tuke, D. H., 611, *637*
Tune, G. S., 568, *581*
Tune, L., 468, *475*, 539, *553*, 841, *852*
Tune, L. E., 467, 468, *475*
Tuokko, H., 40, *68*, 209, *227*, 645, *668*
Turetsky, B., 492, *505*, 624, *638*
Turkheimer, E., 151, *169*
Turnbull, A. P., 593, *599*

Turner, J. A., 526, 527, 529, *546*, *550*
Turner, R., 422, *429*
Turner, R. J., 28, 42, *72*, 239, *248*
Turner, R. W., 802, 810, *811*
Tuszynski, M., 896, *913*
Twelker, J. C., 264, *299*
Tym, E., 618, *641*
Tyrell, R. A., 263, *304*
Tyrer, P., 439, 440, 442, 454, *461*, 532, *551*

Uemura, E., 159, *170*, *173*
Uhde, T. W., 421, *431*
Uhlenberg, P., 101, *117*
Uhlenhuth, E. H., 530, 531, 535, *546*, *554*
Ulbrich, R. M., 107, *117*
Ulpian, C., 184, *198*
Ulrich, J., 191, *198*, *199*, 621, *638*
Ulrich, R. F., 569, *581*, 621, *637*
Underwood, B. J., 178, *198*
Underwood, S., 529, 538, *553*
Ungerleider, L. G., 218, 221, *225*, *226*, *228*
Upfold, L., 278, *305*
Urban, B. J., 389, *404*
Urquhart, A., 184, *199*
U.S. Bureau of the Census, 101, 102, 103, *117*, 874, 875, 876, *890*
U.S. Congress, House of Representatives, Committee on Ways and Means, 876, *890*
U.S. Congress, Office of Technology Assessment, 902, 908, *914*
U.S. Department of Health and Human Services, 100, *117*, 540, 541, 542, 543, *554*, 902, *914*
U.S. General Accounting Office, *813*, 897
U.S. Senate Committee on Finance, 876, *890*

Vachon, M. L. S., 130, *143*
Vaillancourt, D. R., 261, *303*
Vaillant, C. O., 437, *461*
Vaillant, G. E., 437, 443, *461*, 522, 536, *554*
Vale, W. W., 486, 488, *505*, *512*
Valenstein, E., 319, *333*
Valk, P., 492, *505*, 624, *638*
Valle, R., 13, *26*, 104, *117*
Van Allen, M., 648, 653, *665*

van Belle, G., 484, *506*
van den Berg, T. J. T. P., 262, *299*
van den Hoed, J., 561, *577*
Van Dyke, C., 492, *505*
Van Eerdewegh, P., 517, 524, *552*
Van Essen, D. C., 221, *224*
Van Gorp, W. G., 659, *669*
Van Hoesen, G. W., 483, *507*
van Knippenberg, A., 369, *374*
Van Natta, P., 397, *403*
Van Natta, P. A., 239, *246*
Van Nostrand, W. E., 482, *512*
Vandenberg, S. G., 436, *4459*
VandenBos, G. R., 827, *830*
Vanderbeck, M., 838, *850*
Vandermaas, M. P., 330, *334*
VanDerSpek, A. F. L., 204, *224*
Vanderzwaag, R., 530, *552*
VanDyke, C., 624, *638*
Vang, T. F., 112, *117*
VanKleuren, M. L., 481, *512*
vanMeeteren, A., 260, *305*
Varia, I., 391, *402*
Varon, S., 487, *506*
Vega, W., 110, *117*
Veith, R., 387, 394, *406*, 498, 499, 500, *503*,
    510, 842, *850*, *852*
Veith, R. C., 239, *246*, 384, 388, *404*, 446,
    461, 500, *512*, 634, *640*, 907, *912*
Vela-Bueno, A., 566, *579*
Vener, A. M., 538, 539, *554*
Venglarik, J., 822, *831*
Venn, R. D., 617, *641*
Venstrom, D., 286, *306*
Verbeeten, B. W. J., Jr., 660, *664*
Verdonik, F., 314, *335*
Verma, S., 618, *641*
Vernon, M., 689, *696*
Veroff, A. E., 622, *640*
Veroff, J., 411, 412, *428*, 801, *812*
Verrillo, R. T., 290, 291, *305*
Verrillo, V., 290 , 291, *305*
Verwoerdt, A., 382, *407*, 440, 442, 443, 445,
    461
Vestal, R. E., 526, 529, 541, *547*, *554*
Vestal, R. F., 798, 802, *813*
Vetter, N. J., 542, *554*
Vickio, C. J., 357, *375*
Victor, B. S., 421, *431*

Victor, M., 497, *512*
Vieth, R. C., 898, *914*
Vijayashankar, N., 154, 155, *173*, 180, *199*
Villa-Komaroff, L., 483, *513*
Viney, L. L., 241, *248*, 713, *717*
Vinoda, M. N., 456, *461*
Vitaliano, P., 328, *337*
Vitaliano, P. P., 237, *248*, 571, *580*, 660,
    664
Vitiello, M., 328, *337*
Vitiello, M. V., 13, *26*, 560, 564, 568, 571,
    578, *581*, 659, *667*
Viukari, M., 575, *579*, *581*
Vladeck, B. C., 833, *852*
Vogel-Sprott, M., 526, *554*
Vola, J. L., 261, *305*
Volicer, B. J., 526, *554*
Volicer, L., 526, *554*
Volkmar, F. R., 149, 152, *170*
Von Eys, J., 861, *871*
von Knorring, A.-L., 517, 524, *547*
Von Korff, M., 802, 810, *811*
Von Korff, M. R., 29, 35, 41, 59, 60, *66*, *70*
vonKorff, M. R., 618, *637*
Vonsattel, J. P., 190, *197*
Voorhoeve, P., 168, *171*
Vorhodt, A. W., 157, *173*
Vorstrup, S., 486, *511*
Voruganti, L. N. P., 523, 530, 531, *553*, *554*
Vos, J. J., 253, 260, *295*, *305*
Voss, K., 653, *664*
Voss, S., 284, 286, *303*
Vrabec, F., 253, *306*
Vroulis, G., 485, *504*
Vuorialho, M., 492, *505*, 624, *638*

Waddell, K. J., 536, 537, *547*
Waddington, J. L., 469, *475*
Wade, J. B., 654, *665*
Wagener, J. W., 272, *299*, *306*
Wagner, C., 689, *695*
Wagner, E., 211, *227*
Wagner, R., 351, *354*
Wainwright, W. W., 280, *306*
Waldo, D. R., 877, 878, 883, 884, *890*
Walker, A. P., 481, *511*
Walker, B., 544, *551*

Walker, C. A., 539, *547*
Walker, D. W., 497, *511*
Walker, M., 525, *553*
Walker, S. N., 543, *554*
Wallace, R. B., 524, 538, 539, *547, 549*
Waller, S. B., 179, *199*
Wallin, A., 182, 189, *194*
Walsh, D., 456, *459*
Walsh, D. A., 262, *306*, 384, 387, 388, *406*
Walsh, T., 741, *758*
Walsh-Sweeney, L., 318, *335*
Walter, D. O., 645, *667*
Wan, T. H., 807, *813*
Wand, E., 370, *375*
Wang, H.-S., 6, *26*
Wang, W., 186, *198*
Wang, Z., 13, *24*
Wannamethee, G., 525, *553*
Wanzer, S. H., 861, *871*
Ward, C. H., 617, *637*
Ward, R. A., 108, *117*
Ware, J., 907, *914*
Warheit, G., 110, *117*
Warheit, G. J., 47, 72, 107, *117*
Warick, Z. S., 288, *304*
Warner, D., 732, 735, *760*
Warren, E., 680, *697*
Warren, L. R., 272, *299, 306*
Wasson, W., 701, *717*
Waternavx, C., 680, *694*
Watkins, P. C., 40, *72*, 214, *228*, 481, *512*
Watson, A. B., 258, *306*
Watson, N., 732, *762*, 835, *852*
Watson, R., 319, *333*
Wattis, J. P., 528, *554*
Waugh, M., 526, *554*
Waxman, H. M., 797, 802, *813*
Waxman, R., 442, *457*
Wayne, G. J., 702, *717*
Weale, R., 252, 253, 264, *306*
Weale, R. A., 253, *303*
Weathers, F., 804, 806, *812*
Weaver, S., 310, *334*
Webb, W. B., 560, *581*
Weber, H., 367, *373*
Wechsler, D., 328, *337*, 616, *641*, 646, 647, *669*
Wechsler, H., 396, *403*
Weckowicz, T. E., 349, *354*

Weekers, R., 262, *306*
Wehr, T. A., 569, *578*
Weidemann, S., 768, *790*
Weiffenbach, J. M., 272, 273, 280, 282, 283, 288, *303, 306*
Weilburg, J. B., 624, *639*
Weiler, P. G., 737, *762*
Weinberg, G., 240, *247*, 687, 691, *696*
Weinberg, J., 701, 702, *717*
Weinberg, T., 484, *507*
Weinberger, D. R., 622, 623, *641*
Weinberger, M., 538, *547*
Weinberger, T., 34, *69*
Weiner, H., 645, *667*, 899, *914*
Weiner, R. D., 14, *24*, 391–392, *401, 402*
Weiner, W. J., 617, *640*
Weingartner, H., 205, 327, *332, 337*, 344, 350, *354*, 484, *509*, 653, 654, 657, *669*, 670, 754, *762*
Weingartner, H. W., 386, *402*
Weinreb, R. N., 253, *303*
Weintraub, M., 728, *762*
Weintraub, N. T., 494, *506*
Weintraub, R. J., 395, *400*
Weintraub, S., 240, *248*
Weis, P., 384, *400*
Weisman, G., 765, 766, 779, *791*
Weisman, K., 424, *430*
Weiss, H., 484, *509*
Weiss, K., 633, *639*
Weiss, M., 157, *173*
Weissman, M. M., 41, 42, 46, 47, 48, 49, 52, 58, 59, 60, *67, 68, 69, 73, 74*, 234, *247*, 380, 384, *407*, 410, 412, *430*, 438, *460*, 523, 524, 526, 531, 536, *549, 551*, 795, 801, 803, *812*
Weitzman, E. D., 560, 568, *581*
Welch, K., 481, *511*
Welch, P., 765, *791*
Welch, R., 804, 806, *812*
Welch, W. P., 877, *890*
Welkowitz, 743, *758*
Welkowitz, J., 754, *762*
Wells, C. E., 14, *26*, 343, *354*, 386, *407*, 419, *431*, 499, *512*, 653, 654, *670*, 857, *871*
Wells, D., 676, *694*
Wells, K. B., 110, *117*, 907, *914*
Wen, G. Y., 191, *199*

Werch, C. E., 60, 64, *73*, 522, 543, *554*
Werner, J. S., 264, *306*
Werner, M., 180, *194*
Werner, P., 836, 845, *850*, *852*
Wesner, R. B., 396, *407*
West, R., 314, *337*
West, R. L., 313, 316, *337*
Westbrook, M. T., 241, *248*
Wester, P., 179, *197*
Westermeyer, J., 112, *117*
Western Psychological Services, 647, *670*
Westervelt, F. B., 399, *400*
Westrick, M. L., 424, *428*
Wettstein, R. M., 387, *401*
Wetzel, R., 398, *405*
Wey, S.-L., 14, *25*
Whalley, L. J., 31, *72*
Whanger, A. D., 816, 817, *831*
Wheeler, B. G., 838, *850*
Wheeler, J. R. C., 797, *812*
Whitaker, D., 259, 262, 263, 264, *296*, *297*, *306*
Whitaker, L. S., 254, *306*
Whitbourne, S. K., 706, *716*
Whitcup, S., 395, *405*, 531, 532, 533, 534, *551*
Whitcup, S. M., 534, 535, *554*
White, C. L., 153–154, *173*
White, E., 387, 394, *406*, 484, 499, 500, *506*, *510*, *512*, 842, *852*
White, J., 214, *223*, *226*, 264, 280, *303*, 645, *664*
White, J. A., 493, *507*
White, J. F., 586, 588, *597*
White, P., 182, 188, *194*
White, R., 190, *197*
White-Campbell, M., 525, 529, *549*
Whiteford, H. A., 732, 735, 738, *760*
Whitehead, A., 350, *353*, 652, *670*
Whitehead, W. E., 420, *431*, 708, *713*, *717*
Whitehouse, P., 14, *24*, 326, *332*, 732, 754, *762*
Whitehouse, P. J., 153–154, *173*, 486, 488, 501, *505*, *512*, *513*, 656, *670*
Whitehouse, P.J., 485, *512*
Whitfield, J. R., 649, *664*
Whitlock, F. A., 456, *461*
Whitman, D., 651, *670*
Whitson, J. S., 483, *512*

Whitty, C. W. M., 616, *641*
Whybrow, P. C., 41, *73*, 494, *513*
Wiancko, D., 676, *694*
Wichman, A., 495, *513*
Wickramaraine, P. J., 47, *73*
Widaman, K. F., 588, *597*
Widerlov, E., 486, *504*
Widmer, R. B., 47, *67*
Wieland, R. G., 494, *513*
Wiens, A. N., 526, 529, *554*
Wiggli, U., 621, *638*
Wight, N., 483, *511*
Wikkelso, C., 493, *513*
Wikstrom, J., 183, *197*, 471, *474*
Wilbanks, W., 536, *554*
Wilcock, G. K., 182, 183, *194*, *195*, 486, *506*
Wilder, D., 693, *695*
Wilder, D. E., 232, 239, 243, *247*, *248*
Wilke, F., 687, 691, *696*
Wilkie, F., 240, *247*, 420, *430*, 652, 659, *667*
Wilkins, A. J., 317, *337*
Wilkinson, W. E., 34, *69*, 484, 485, *507*, *511*
Wilks, S., 148, *173*
Willenbring, M. L., 527, *555*
William, C. D., 738, 739, *757*
Williams, B. W., 660, *666*
Williams, C. D., 14, *23*, 42, 64, *67*, 349, 352, 451, *457*, 633, *637*, 795, *811*, 819, *829*
Williams, D., 571, *578*, 737, *762*
Williams, D. A., 113, *117*
Williams, D. E., 659, *667*
Williams, D. L., 275, *298*
Williams, G., 681, *694*
Williams, G. C., 30, *73*
Williams, J., 219, *227*, 501, *511*
Williams, J. B. W., 388, *405*, 454, 455, *459*, *461*, 501, *508*, 609, *641*
Williams, L. R., 487, *506*
Williams, M. A., 821, *831*
Williams, M. J., 264, 280, *303*
Williams, M. V., 274, *296*
Williams, P., 53, *553*
Williams, R., 420, *430*, 561, *581*
Williams, R. S., 191, *197*, 347, *352*, 481, *507*
Williams, T. F., 618, *637*, 910, *914*

Williamson, D. S., 712, *717*
Williamson, R., 481, *506*
Willis, D. P., 903, *914*
Willis, S. L., 342, *354*, 900, *914*
Willits, F. K., 359, *375*
Wilner, E., 496, *513*
Wilson, B. A., 661, *670*
Wilson, C. A., 680, *697*
Wilson, D., 278, *305*
Wilson, H., 845, *850*
Wilson, I. D., 30, *67*
Wilson, J., 33, 42, *70*
Wilson, J. R., 436, *459*
Wilson, L. A., 660, *670*
Wilson, R. S., 651, *670*
Wilson, T., 559, *579*
Wilson, W. H., 498, *510*
Wilson, W. P., 396, *401*
Winblad, B., 179, 188, *194*, *197*, 486, *513*
Winefield, H. R., 397, *407*
Wing, J. K., 619, *637*
Winick, C., 520, *555*
Winkelmann, R. K., 289, 290, *296*
Winkle, R. A., 564, *578*
Winlfield-Laird, I., 28, 41, 42, 49, 51, 52, 54, 57, 58, *68*
Winn, M. C., 821, *831*
Winocur, G., 312, *337*
Winograd, C., 680, *697*, 825, *831*
Winograd, C. H., 500, *509*, 660, 661, *666*, *670*
Winokur, A., 535, *552*
Winokur, G., 382, 383, 388, 396, *406*, *407*, 470, *475*
Winslade, W. J., 857, *869*
Winslow, L., 253, 254, *300*
Wirth, J. B., 467, 468, *475*
Wirth, L., 104, *117*
Wirtz, P. W., 537, *551*
Wise, R. J. S., 205, *227*
Wise, R. W., 526, *555*
Wisniewski, H., 157, 158, *171*, *173*
Wisniewski, H. M., 157, 166, *173*, 191, *199*, 484, *508*, 583, 587, *597*, *599*
Wisniewski, K. E., 191, *199*
Wisocki, P. A., 699, *717*
Witker, D. S., 483, *509*
Witney, P. M., 660, *670*, 680, *697*
Woelfel, M., 495, *511*

Wohlwill, J., 764, *791*
Wolanin, M., 821, 822, *831*
Wolanin, M. O., 821, *831*
Wold, D., 590, *597*
Wolf, A., 209, 219, *224*, *227*
Wolf, A. P., 164, *172*, 205, 209, 210, *224*, 240, *247*
Wolf, E., 260, 261, 262, *296*, *303*, *306*, 704, *715*
Wolf, G. L., 14, *26*
Wolf, P. A., 190, *197*
Wolf, R. S., 380, *405*
Wolfe, J., 652, *664*
Wolff, H. G., 292, *298*, *304*
Wolff, J. A., 896, *913*
Wolff, K., 710, *717*
Wolfson, A., 725, 752, *761*
Wolfson, L., 191, *195*
Wolinsky, M. A., 712, *717*
Wolozin, B., 732, 754, *757*
Wolozin, B. L., 483, *505*, *507*
Wong, C. W., 482, *506*
Wong, L., 256, *295*
Wong, L. S., 256, *295*
Wong, P. T. P., 359, *374*
Wong, S.-C., 13, *24*
Wood, J. S., 319, *332*
Wood, P. L., 486, 493, *513*
Wood, W. G., 526, *555*
Woodard, J. H. S., 488, *513*
Woodbury, M., 438, *457*
Woodhouse, K. W., 528, *555*
Woodrow, K. M., 292, 293, *306*
Woods, A. M., 274, *296*
Woods, S. W., 395, *407*
Woodward, J. A., 536, 537, *545*
Wooley, A., 590, *596*
Woolfolk, R. L., 708, *717*
Woolson, R. F., 469, *475*
World Health Organization, 31, 32, 57, *73*, 517, 518, *555*
Worthen, K., 126, *141*
Wortman, C. B., 130, *143*
Wragg, R. E., 732, 733, *762*
Wright, C. E., 263, *306*
Wright, J. L., 266, *306*
Wright, K., 349, *354*
Wright, L., 320, *337*
Wright, M., 310, *331*

Wyatt, R. J., 15, *24*, 569, *578*, 899, *912*
Wykle, M., 817, 821, 822, 823, 824, *830, 831*
Wykle, M. H., 816, *831*
Wyshak, G., 112, *116*
Wysocki, C. J., 287, *306*

Yaffe, L., 442, *457*
Yamado, M., 163, *171*
Yamagishi, M., 234, 240, 245, *248*, 676, *697*
Yamaguchi, F., 205, *227*
Yamaguchi, S., 541, *555*
Yamamoto, J., 111, *117*
Yamamura, H. I., 184, *198*
Yamaoka, L., 481, *511*
Yamaoka, L. H., 481, *509*
Yamashita, K., 541, *555*
Yang, L., 388, *407*
Yankaskas, B., 386, *402*
Yankner, B. A., 483, *513*
Yano, Y., 209, *225*
Yarchoan, R., 495, *504, 513*
Yarrow, M. R., 208, *223*
Yates, C. M., 182, 184, *197, 199*
Yates, M., 440–441, *460*
Yates, O., 153, 154, *171*
Yates, P. O., 154, *171*, 179, 180, 187, 188, 189, 191, *196, 197*, 484, 485, 486, *508, 509, 513*
Yates, W. R., 391, *407*
Yearick, E. S., 284, *300*
Yeh, E. K., 60, *69*
Yellowees, P. M., 422, *431*
Yen, M. S., 537, *547*
Yen, S. H., 483, *507*
Yeo, R. A., 624, *639*
Yesavage, J., 327, *337*, 500, *509*, 617, *641*
Yesavage, J. A., 15, *26*, 236, 244, *248*, 318, *336*, 419, 423, *431, 432*, 701, 712, *717*, 866, *869*
Yip, B., 111, 113, *117*
Ylinen, A., 488, *507*
Yoder, C., 654, *668*
Yonge, K. A., 349, *354*
Yoshii, F., 207, *228*
Youdelis, C., 253, *306*
Young, M. L., 736, *759*

Young, R. C., 236, *246*, 381, 383, 386, 395, 396, *400, 407*, 730, 738, 742, *756, 762*
Young, R. J., 319, *333*
Young, R. N., 708, *716*
Younkin, L. H., 483, *509*
Younkin, S. C., 483, *509*
Youssef, H. A., 469, *475*
Yu, E., 13, *24*
Yudofsky, S., 737, *762*

Zacks, R., 324, *333*
Zacks, R. T., 311, *333*
Zamel, N., 564, *579*
Zangaglia, O., 391, *404*
Zangwill, O. L., 616, *641*
Zaretsky, H., 709, *713*
Zarit, J. M., 14, *26*, 676, *697*
Zarit, S., 676, *697*, 805, *813*
Zarit, S. H., 14, *26*, 313, *337*, 653, *666*
Zarow, C., 152, *170*, 180, *196*
Zata, L., 492, *505*
Zatz, L., 624, *638*
Zec, R. F., 645, *668*
Zecca, L., 182, *194*
Zeidman, A., 525, 529, *549*
Zeisel, J., 765, 789, *791, 792*
Zeiss, A. M., 707, *717*
Zeldis, S. M., 421, *429*
Zelinski, E., 15, *25*
Zelinski, E. M., 313, 314, *333, 337*
Zemmers, R., 498, *511*
Zemuznikov, N., 571, *580*
Zepelin, H., 560, 568, *581*
Zgola, J., 788, 789, *792*
Zhang, M., 13, *24*
Zhao, Y. W., 33, *70*
Zigman, W. B., 585, 588, *599*
Zilhka, E., 219, *225*, 492, *506*, 658, *665*
Zimberg, S., 522, 529, *551, 555*
Zimmer, B., 13, *26*, 562, 564, 569, 571, 572, *580, 580–581*
Zimmer, J. G., 732, *762*, 835, *852*
Zimmerman, H. M., 571, *578*
Zimmerman, J. C., 560, 568, *581*
Zimmerman, M., 396, *402*, 446, 451, 452, 454, *461, 462*
Zimmerman, R. A., 491, *504*

Zimmerman, R. L., 484, *512*
Zinberg, N. W., 701, *717*
Zisook, S., 15, *26*, 329, *337*, 393, *406*, 738, 743, *761*, *762*
Zitrin, C. M., 421, *429*
Zivian, M. T., 311, *337*
Zonderman, A. B., 358, *372*, 437, 442, 445, *457*

Zorumski, C. F., 396, *401*
Zorzitto, M. L., 647, 648, *669*
Zubek, J. P., 292, *304*, 588, *596*
Zubenko, G. S., *26*, 114, 482, 491, *513*
Zucker, H. D., 388, *406*
Zung, W. W. K., 236, *248*
Zuo, C., 388, *407*
Zweig, R. M., 472, *475*, 488, 501, *512*, *513*

Subject Index

Acetycholine system
  aging changes in, 179–180
  Alzheimer's disease, in, 485–487
  cholinergic-enhancing strategies for memory
    loss, 754
  psychotropic drugs and, 731–732
Acquired immune deficiency syndrome
  (AIDS)
  dementia, 494–496, 631–632
  intravenous drug use and, 495, 537
  prevalence in elderly, 495
Activities of daily living (ADLs)
  assessment of, 684–693
  components of, 672–674
  hierarchial model of functional assessment
    and, 677–679
  long-term care eligibility and, 19–20, 886
Activity
  aging and, 356
Adaptation
  ethnic groups and, 106
  life crises and, 128–131
Addiction
  See Substance-use disorders
Adult life crises, 119–141
  adult-centered view of, 133–138
  cumulative vs. specific, 128–129
  definitions of, 120–121
  gender crisis at midlife, 135–136, 138, 703
  major crises, 368–371
  midlife crisis, 133–138
  models of, 124–125, 703
  psychiatric disorders and, 124–128
  relational investment and, 136–138
  spousal loss and, 129–131
  transformative, 131–138
  See also Life events

Affect
  aging and, 356, 357
  mental-status assessment of, 614
Affective disorders
  See Depression; Depressive disorders; Dys-
    thymia; Mania
African-Americans
  life expectancy of, 874
  population trends and, 100–102, 903
  poverty and, 874–875
  prevalence of mental disorders, in, 107–108
  racism and, 107
Age-associated memory impairment, 14, 326,
  751
Ageism, 134, 364
  mental health professionals and, 17, 701,
    826
  mental health services, in, 826
  See also Stereotypes
Age-related slowing, 149
  speech perception, and, 274, 276
  visual system, in, 262–264
Aging
  adjustment to, 364–371
  age-specific strengths, 900–901
  continuous developmental sequence, as,
    147, 169
  definition of, 103
  interpersonal relationships and, 901
  population trends, 22, 100–102, 874–876
  poverty and, 874–876
  secondary, 516
  statistical vs. deterministic models of, 293
  successful, 104, 113, 703, 897–898
  See also Brain aging; Intellectual aging;
    Neuronal aging; Normal aging; Senso-
    ry-perceptual aging

Agitation
  nursing home patients, in, 835–836, 839
  psychotropic treatment of, 732–738
Agoraphobia, 51–54, 413–414
Akathisia, 421, 735
Alcohol use, 524–525
Alcohol-use disorders, 390, 522–529
  age vs. cohort effects and, 522, 524
  clinical features, 527–528
  cognitive impairment and, 496–497, 525–
    526, 632, 633
  complications of, 527–528
  course, 528
  early vs. late-onset, 525
  epidemiology of, 522–524
  family patterns and, 526
  Korsakoff's syndrome, 344, 497, 632
  management/treatment, 529
  patterns of use and abuse, 524–527
  prevalence of, 522–524
Alcoholics Anonymous, 544
Alzheimer's disease, 478–487
  age of onset, 162–163, 182–183, 187–193,
    212–214
  aluminum and, 484
  amyloid and, 482–484
  cerebral metabolism and, 209–219
  clinical features, 479–480
  cognitive impairment in, 328–329, 245
  course, 189, 480
  CT measures and, 151
  diagnostic criteria, 32, 478–479
  Down syndrome and, 481, 587, 588, 595
  environmental toxins and, 484
  epidemiology of, 480, 902
  estimated risk of, 34
  family history and, 39–40, 214, 481–482
  gene-environment interaction model of, 38
  head trauma and, 38–40, 484
  interventions, 909
  neuropsychological testing, 328–329, 649–
    653
  pathophysiology, 149–151, 164–165, 182–
    183, 484–487
  personality changes in, 447–448, 479
  presenile vs. senile, 162–163
  prevalence, 33, 480
  risk factors, 37–41
  senescence theory and, 30–31, 38
  sleep disorders and, 564, 570–572
    societal cost of, 902
    treatment for, 896
    viral infection and, 38–40, 484
    See also Dementia; Differential diagnosis
Alzheimer's Disease Assessment Scale, 328,
    661
American Indians
  population trends and, 101
  prevalence of mental disorders in, 110–111
Analgesics
  prescription use and abuse, 535
Antidepressants, 739–744
  atypical, 737, 743–744
  cyclic, 393–394, 739–742
  frail elderly and, 842
  mixed anxiety–depression syndromes and,
    424, 749
  monoamine oxidase inhibitors (MAOIs),
    394–395, 742–743, 898
  treatment of insomnia with, 574–575
Antisocial personality
  burnout of traits with age, 440–441
Anxiety
  aging and, 356–357
  death, 357, 371
  definition of, 410
  depression and, 389
  hospitalization and, 822–823
  prevalence, 822
  psychopharmacologic treatment of, 745–750
  somatization and, 823
  See also Anxiety disorders
Anxiety disorders, 409–427
  assessment of, 418–419, 425
  classification of, 413–416
  epidemiology of, 411–413
  generalized anxiety disorder, 416
  medical illness and, 418, 420–422, 425
  mixed anxiety–depressive syndromes, 419–
    420, 424, 749
  models of, 416–417
  posttraumatic stress disorder, 415
  stress and, 126
  treatment, 422–425, 326
  See also Obsessive-compulsive disorder;
    Panic disorder; Phobias
Area Agencies on Aging (AAAs), 17, 798
Asian-Pacific Islanders
  population trends and, 101
  prevalence of mental disorders in, 111–112

Aspirin, 540
Assessment
 age-appropriate, 351, 795
 age-fair, 15
 psychiatric hospitalization and, 825
 psychiatric, in nursing homes, 838–839
 See also Functional assessment; Neuropsychiatric assessment; Neuropsychological assessment
Attention, 319–326
 definition of, 319
 depression, in, 327
 everyday, 325–326
 mental-status assessment of, 613
 selective, 319–325
Auditory aging, 265–278
 absolute sensitivity, 267–271
 auditory frequency analysis and discrimination, 271–272
 compensation for hearing loss, 277–278
 gender differences in, 270–271
 hearing aids, 277–278
 paranoid disorders and, 277
 phonemic regression, 272–274
 prevalence of hearing problems, 267
 relative contribution of noise and aging to,
  271
 social and psychological implications, 276–
  277
 sound localization, 272
 speech perception, 272–276
 structural changes, 265–266

Baltimore Longitudinal Study of Aging
 (BLSA)
 data on sensory-perceptual aging, 256–259,
  266, 268, 270, 280, 282
Barthel Index, 685, 689
Beck Depression Inventory, 617, 709
Behavioral interventions, 705–709
 nursing homes, in, 845–846
Benton Test of Visual Retention, 328
Benzodiazopines, 395, 423
 anxiety and, 746–747, 843
 side effects, 747
 treatment of anxiety with, 423–424
 treatment of depression with, 395
 treatment of insomnia with, 575–576, 751–
  752

Benzodiazopine-use disorders, 529–535
 assessment of, 534
 clinical features and complications, 532–
  533
 epidemiology of, 529–532
 management of, 534–535
 prevalence, 530–531
 prevention of, 535
 risk factors, 530–531
Bereavement, 103, 129–131, 904
 insomnia and, 566–567
Beta blockers, 424, 737, 749
Biogenic amine hypothesis, 14, 898
Bipolar disorder, 843
 See also Mania
Biopsychosocial perspective, 6, 604, 607, 902
Blessed Dementia Rating Scale, 240, 686, 691
Body monitoring, 6
Bonn Longitudinal Study on Aging (BOLSA)
 data, 356, 358, 359, 362, 363, 367, 368,
  370
Boston Naming Test, 651, 659
Brain aging, 147–169, 175–184
 behavior change and, 167–169
 accumulation of engrams and, 177–178
 age of onset in Alzheimer's disease and,
  187–193
 cerebral metabolism and, 204–209
 depression and, 47–48, 898–899
 gross changes, 149–151
 memory engrams and, 177–178
 microscopic changes, 151–163
 neurotransmitter systems and, 178–183
 plasticity of aging brain, 897
 schizophrenia, Parkinson's disease, and,
  184–187
 vascular changes, 163–167
 See also Neuronal aging
Brief Psychiatric Rating Scale, 439, 617
Brief Symptom Inventory, 709
Bupropion, 744

California Verbal Learning Test, 647, 648
Cambridge mental disorders of the elderly
 examination (CAMDEX), 618
Cardiovascular illness
 anxiety and, 421
 intellectual functioning and, 345–346

Caregivers
   behavioral interventions for cognitively im-
      paired, and, 708, 709
   caregiver burden, 805–806, 902
   coping strategies, 369–370
   developmental disability and, 592–594,
      596
   home care and, 804–806
   quality of life and, 234–235
Caregiving
   adult life crisis, as an, 121
   health/mental health implications of, 18–
      19, 64, 805
Case management
   elderly at risk of institutionalization and,
      885–886
Cattell 16 Personality Factor Inventory, 356
Center for Epidemiological Studies in Depression (CESD) Scale, 107, 111
Cerebral metabolism, 201–223
   age-related changes in, 204–209
   Alzheimer's disease in, 209–219
   cerebrovascular dementia, in, 219–220
   cognitive function and, 208–209, 214–219
   depression, in, 220–221
   measurement of, 202–204, 644
Chronically mentally ill, 796
   home care for, 806
   service use by, 804
Chronicity, 11–12
   effect on function, 680
   quality of life and, 238, 244
Circadian rhythms, 560–561
Clinical Dementia Rating, 240
Cognition
   capacity vs performance, 309
   cognition–emotion interactions, 360–371
   definition of, 308
   See also Attention; Intellectual functioning;
      Learning; Memory
Cognitive-behavioral interventions
   anxiety, for, 422–423
   depression, for, 709–710
   elderly and, 701
Cognitive Failures Questionnaire, 313
Cognitive impairment
   alcohol use and, 525–526, 633
   biological-deficiency hypothesis and, 193
   cerebral metabolism and, 201–208
   chronic benzodiazepine toxicity and, 533

functional impairment and, 240
   obsessive-compulsive disorder and, 56
   psychopharmacologic treatment of, 752–
      755
   severe, 34–37, 797–798
   ventricular enlargement and, 150–51
Cognitive theory
   anxiety and, 417
   personality, of, 360–317
Cohort-based analyses, 16
Cohort effects
   patterns of mental illness and, 12
   substance abuse and, 516–518
   use of services and, 16, 17
Color Aptitude Test, 264
Community mental health centers (CMHCs),
   17, 794, 798, 803
Community mental health services, 796–799
   ethnic minorities and, 112
   long-term care and, 20
Comorbidity, 10, 241, 680–681, 723–724,
   798, 824, 906
Competence-press model, 764–765
Competency, 854–866
   civil law, in, 855–857
   criminal law, in, 863–866
   definition of, 854–855
   testamentory capacity, 855–856
   voluntary informed consent, 857–863
Comprehensive Assessment and Referral Evaluation (CARE), 109, 688, 693
Computed tomography (CT), 150–151, 391,
   622–623, 644, 645
   diagnosis of multi-infarct dementia and,
      491–492
   guidelines for use, 623
Comrey Personality Scales, 436
Confidentiality, 866–867
Confusion
   hospitalized elderly, in, 820–821
   reality orientation and, 845
Consortium to Establish a Registry for Alzheimer's Disease (CERAD), 15
Continuous Visual Memory Test, 647
Controlled Learning and Cued Recall procedures, 648, 652
Coping, 106
   ethnic groups and, 106
   life crises, with, 365–371
   types of, 365–366

Countertransference
  elderly and, 701, 826
Creativity in later life, 898
Creutzfeldt-Jakob disease, 344, 496, 632
Culture, 75-96
  components of, 82-83
  cross-cultural field methods, 76-77
  defense mechanisms of, 81
  inner controls and, 81-82
  narcissism and, 80-81, 82-96 *passim*
  psychosocial role of, 78-80
  self-continuity and, 82
  traditional elders and, 83-88
  See also Deculturation
Cutaneous sensitivity, 288-292
  absolute touch sensitivity, 290
  haptic recognition, 291-292
  pain sensitivity, 292-293
  structural changes with age, 289
  temperature sensitivity, 292
  vibrotactile sensitivity, 290-291

Death anxiety, 357, 371
Deculturation, 88-96
  American values and, 92
  Druze and, 90-91
  gerophobia and, 93
  psychopathology and, 94-96
Deinstitutionalization, 794, 816, 834, 873-
  874, 884
Delayed Word Recall Test, 648
Delirium, 502-503, 626-629
  causes of, 627-628
  clinical features, 502, 627
  diagnostic criteria, 502
  differential diagnosis, 329
  EEG in detection of, 621, 626
  suspiciousness in, 471-472
  treatment, 502-503
Delusional disorder, 470
  diagnostic criteria, 465
  organic, 472-473
Delusions, 836
Dementia, 343-345, 629-633, 477-503
  alcohol and, 496-497, 633
  antipsychotic drugs and, 498
  attention in, 328-329
  behavioral problems in, 497-499

  causes of, 32, 630-633
  cerebrovascular, 219-220
  coexisting depression and, 386-387, 842
  cognitive functioning in, 327-330, 345-
    346
  cortical vs subcortical patterns, 630-631
  course, 478
  CT scans and, 151
  definition of, 32, 478, 629
  diagnosis of, 478
  epidemiology of, 32-41
  estimated risk, 34
  functional assessment of, 691-692
  Korsakoff's syndrome, 344, 497
  Lewy body disease, 489-490
  metabolic dementing disorders, 494, 632
  multiple sclerosis, 633
  neurosyphillis, 496
  normal-pressure hydrocephalus, 493-494,
    632
  prevalence of, 33, 343
  risk factors for, 37-41
  sleep disturbance in, 564, 570-572
  sundowning, 572
  suspiciousness in, 471-473
  See also Acquired immune deficiency syn-
    drome (AIDS); Alzheimer's disease;
    Creutzfeldt-Jakob disease; Differential
    diagnosis; Multi-infarct dementia; Par-
    kinson's disease; Pick's disease;
    Pseudodementia
Dementia syndrome of depression (DSD)
  See Pseudodementia
Dendrite systems, 158-163
Denial
  deculturation and, 95
  hearing loss and, 277
Dependency ratio, 876
Depression
  attentional processes in, 327
  biogenic amine hypothesis, 898
  brain aging and, 47-48, 898-899
  cerebral metabolism and, 220-221
  classification of, 348, 380-383
  cohort differences in risk of, 46-47
  course, 384
  developmental resources and, 819
  dysregulation hypothesis of, 899
  electroconvulsive therapy and, 394-395,
    828, 842

Depression (*cont.*)
  epidemiology, 41–48, 383–384
  estimated risk of, 42–46
  gender differences in, 46
  hearing loss and, 276–277
  hypothyroid-induced, 634
  intellectual functioning, 326–327, 349–351
  involutional melancholia, 46
  laboratory tests and, 390–391
  late-onset, 381–382
  life events and, 127–128, 367
  memory complaints, 501
  mortality rates and, 386
  neuropsychological findings, 327, 349–351, 654–655
  neuroradiological studies, 391
  Parkinson's disease and, 635
  personality disorders and, 451–452, 455–456
  poststroke, 634
  prevalence of, 41–42, 327, 349, 380, 383–384
  prognosis, 384–385
  psychopharmacologic treatment of, 393–395, 738–744
  psychotherapy for, 392–393, 709–710
  quality of life and, 233, 239
  risk factors, 46–48
  secondary, 634–635, 902
  sleep disturbances and, 564, 567, 569–570
  social support and, 396–397
  somatic recovery and, 907
  subcortical dementia and, 635
  treatment/management, 391–397, 709–710
  See also Anti-depressants; Differential diagnosis; Pseudodementia; Suicide
Depressive disorders
  diagnostic categories, 41, 380–381
  primary vs secondary, 634, 902
  See also Depression; Dysthymia; Mania
Developmental disability
  definition of, 584
Developmentally disabled elderly, 583–596
  cognitive abilities, 588
  definition of old age in, 584–585
  functional abilities, 588–589
  health and mental health status, 589–590
  family and informal supports, 592–594, 596

life expectancy, 586–587
population size, 585–586, 587
service sectors for, 590–592
Dexamethasone-Suppression Test (DST), 390–391, 500
Diagnostic Interview Schedule (DIS)
  data from ECA, 34–62, 111, 383–384, 566–567
Diagnostic-related groups (DRGs), 878–879
Differential diagnosis, 625–636, 649–660
  Alzheimer's disease vs. multi-infarct dementia, 658–660
  Alzheimer's disease vs. normal aging, 328–329, 649–653, 896
  Alzheimer's disease vs. Parkinson's disease, 656–658
  dementia vs. delirium, 329
  dementia vs. normal aging, 328–329, 649–653
  depression vs. delirium, 633
  depression vs. dementia, 329, 386–387, 499–501, 653–655, 819
  depression vs. other psychiatric disorders, 388–390
  mental illness vs. normal aging, 895–896
  primary and secondary depression, 387–388
  types of dementia, 328, 631, 656–660
Diogenes syndrome, 473, 528
Direct Assessment of Functional Status (DAFS), 687, 691
Disability
  quality of life and, 239–240
  See also Developmentally disabled elderly
Disengagement, 87, 136–137
Dopamine system
  aging changes in, 178–179, 184–187
  Parkinson's disease, in, 184–187
  personality disorders and, 446
  psychotropic drugs and, 731
  schizophrenia, in, 184–187, 899
Down syndrome
  Alzheimer's disease and, 481, 584, 587, 588, 595
  atypical aging in, 590, 596
  caregiving and, 593–594
  cognitive abilities and, 588
  life expectancy in, 586–587
  medical problems and, 589–590
  See also Developmentally disabled elderly

Drug use
   illegal, 536–539, 902
   See also Psychopharmacology; Substance
     use disorders
Durable power of attorney, 861
Dysthymia
   definition of, 381
   prevalence, 383

Elder abuse laws, 866
Elderly
   income, 875–876
   living alone, 904, 909
   rural, 904
Electroconvulsive therapy (ECT), 395–396,
   828, 842
Electroencephalogram (EEG), 620–621
Emotion
   age-related changes in affect, 356, 357
   aging and, 355–375
   cognition and, 360–371
Engrams, 177–178
Environmental docility hypothesis, 6, 764
Environmental interventions for cognitively
    impaired, 763–790
   home settings, in, 782–789
   hypothesis testing and, 789–790
   principles, 766–768
   See also Nursing home design
Epidemiological Catchment Area Program
    (ECA)
   data from, 34–62, 107–111, 383–384, 410,
    412–413, 438, 566–567
   description of, 34, 107
Epidemiological research
   causality and, 28–29
   diagnostic categories and, 31
   future directions, 63–65
   prevention and, 28–29
   risk factor research, 30–31
   strategies, 29, 63
Epidemiology, 28–65
   alcohol-use disorders, 522–524
   definition of, 28
   dementia, of, 32–41
   depressive disorders, of, 41–48
   mental disorders, of, in nursing homes,
    834–848

obsessive–compulsive disorder, of, 54–57
panic disorder, of, 48–51
personality disorders, of, 437–439
phobic disorders, of, 51–54
sedative-hypnotic drug use and problems,
   529–532
substance abuse disorders, of, 57–63, 516–
   521
trends in mental health and aging, 901–906
Error Proneness Questionnaire, 313
Ethnic groups
   community mental health and, 112
   ethnic minority women, 103, 114, 875
   melting pot theory, 104–105
   mental health services and, 112–114, 801,
    903
   minority status and, 104, 875
   physical illness in, 903
   population projections, 100–102, 874, 903
   prevalence of mental disorders in, 106–112
   psychosocial stress and, 105
   research on mental health and the aged and,
    13, 903–904
   social support and, 105–106
Ethnicity
   definition of, 104–105
Euthanasia, 862–863
Exercise
   memory and, 318–319
Extrapyramidial symptoms
   neuroleptics and, 734–735
Extraversion–introversion, 357–358, 437
Extreme group design, 330
Eyesenck Personality Inventory, 437

Falls, 822
Family
   role of, in therapy with ethnic populations,
    113
   See also Caregivers; Social support
Family therapy, 712–714
Farnsworth-Munsell 100-Hue test, 264
Fluoxetine, 743–744
Function
   definitions of, 762
   determinants of, 674–675
   effect of mental illness on, 679–681

Functional Activities Questionnaire (FAQ), 687, 691–692
Functional assessment, 671–694
  conceptual basis of, 672–679
  dementia patients, of, 691–692
  hierarchial model of, 677–679
  instruments, 684–693
  kinds of functional ability, 672–674
  principles of, 681–684
  See also Activities of Daily Living; Instrumental Activities of Daily Living
Functional Assessment Inventory (FAI), 687, 692

Gamma aminobutyric acid (GABA), 181
Gender, 103
Gender differences
  auditory aging, in, 270–271
  risk of depression, in, 46
  longevity, in, 101, 103
  risk of depression, in, 46
  risk of obsessive–compulsive disorder, in, 56–57
  sleep, in, 561
Gender trait reversal, 135–136, 138, 703
General Well-Being Schedule, 358
Generalized Additive Model (GAM), 35
Generalized anxiety disorder, 416
Generativity, 87, 132
Geriatric Depression Scale (GDS), 15, 327, 380, 617, 709
Geriatric psychiatry, 894
Geriatric Research, Education, and Clinical Centers (GRECCs), 894
Geriatric revolution, 10
Geriatrics
  training, 20–22
Gerontological revolution, 10
Global Assessment Scale (GAS), 242
Granovascular degeneration, 155–156
Group psychotherapy, 710–712
Guardianship, 856–857
Guilford-Zimmerman Temperament Scales, 356

Hachinski scale, 492
Hallucinations
  grief-related, 473

organic disease and, 472–473, 635
  paranoia and, 823–824
Halstead-Reitan Neuropsychological Battery, 346, 646
Hamilton Anxiety Rating Scale (HARS), 418–419
Hamilton Depression Rating Scale (HDRS), 617, 709
Health Assessment Questionnaire, 686, 690
Health maintenance organizations (HMOs), 885
Hearing loss
  See Auditory aging
Hidden Figures Test, 328
Hispanics, 241–242
  population trends and, 101–101, 903
  prevalence of mental disorders in, 108–110
Home care, 804–809
  community care and, 806–809
Home settings
  strategies for management in, 782–789
Home visits, 905
Hospital care
  See Psychiatric hospitalization
Huntington's disease, 190, 344
Hyperthyroidism
  anxiety and, 422
  dementia due to, 494
Hypochondriasis, 389
Hypothyroid-induced depression, 634

Incontinence
  behavioral treatment of, 707–708
Individual difference variables
  See Personality
Individual psychotherapy, 702–710
  behavioral interventions, 705–709
  empirical investigations, 709–710
  psychodynamic approaches, 702–705
Informed consent, 857–863, 868
Insomnia, 566–567
  treatment of, 707–708
Institutionalization
  personality disorders and, 448–451
  See also Nursing homes
Instrumental Activities of Daily Living (IADLs)
  assessment of, 684–693
  definition of, 673

hierarchial model of functional assessment and, 677–679
Instrumental Activities of Daily Living Scale, 618
Intellectual functioning, 339–351
  age-related decline, 341–342
  changes in structure of intelligence, 340–341
  dementia and, 343–345
  depression and, 348–351
  individual differences, 341–342
  physical health and, 345–348
Intelligence
  age-related changes in structure, 340–341
  methods of studying, 341
Interdisciplinary team approach, 825
Interpersonal relationships
  influence of time on, 901
Interventions
  behavioral, 705–709
  common principles of change, 827
  environmental, 763–790
  psychotherapeutic, 699–714
Iowa Dementia Battery, 648–649

Katz Index of ADL, 684, 685, 689
Kenny Self-Care Evaluation, 685, 689
Korsakoff's syndrome, 344, 497, 632

Learned helplessness, 350, 362, 426
Learning
  age-related differences in, 310–316
  definition of, 308–309
  longevity and learned behavior, 148
  potential in later life, 900
  See also Memory
Lewy body disease, 489–490
Life-care communities, 887–888
Life events, 119–141
  anxiety disorders and, 126
  chronological age and, 124
  consequences, 121–124
  daily hassles, 365–368
  depressive illnesses and, 127–128, 367
  family, 124
  mania and, 383
  marital, 123

modifiers, 122, 129
  occupational, 123
  personality disorders and, 441
  phobia and, 52, 126
  psychiatric disorders and, 124–128
  schizophrenia and, 126–127
  substance use disorders and, 519, 525
  See also Adult life crises
Life expectancy, 22, 900
  African-Americans, in, 874
Life review, 711
Life Satisfaction Index-Z Scale (LSI-Z), 110
Lipofuscin, 154–155
Lithium, 395, 737, 744–745, 843
Living wills, 860–661
Locus of control
  age-related changes in, 362–363
Longevity
  learned behavior and, 148
Long-term care, 19–20
  diversity of settings, 905
  insurance, 885, 909–910
Luria Nebraska Psychological Battery, 647

Magnetic resonance imaging (MRI), 151, 391, 623–624, 644
  diagnosis of multi-infarct dementia and, 491–492
Mania, 382–383, 635
  lithium treatment of, 395, 737, 744–745, 843
Marijuana
  prevalence of use in elderly, 537
Marital psychotherapy, 712
Mattis Dementia Rating Scale, 328–329
Medicaid, 873–874, 883–884
Medical ethics
  confidentiality, 866–867
  euthanasia, 862–863
  voluntary informed consent, 857–863
Medicare, 849, 873–874, 876–883
  hospital insurance, 877–879
  medigap policies and, 884–885
  supplemental medical insurance, 879–883
Medigap policies, 884–885
Memory, 308–319
  age-associated memory impairment (AAMI), 14, 326, 753
  age-related differences in, 310–316

Memory (*cont.*)
  capacity vs. performance, 309, 315–316
  cerebral metabolism and, 208–209
  definition of, 308–309
  environmental demand and, 311–312
  exercise and nutrition, 318–319
  everyday memory, 316–318
  lifestyle and, 312–313
  mental status assessment of, 615–617
  metamemory, 313–314
  mnemonics, 318
  model of, and aging, 309–310
  strategies, 315–316
Memory impairment
  age-associated, 14, 326, 751
  anticholinergic toxicity and, 742
  cholinergic-enhancing strategies and, 754
  dementia, in, 327–330, 344–345
  depression in, 326–327
  psychopharmacologic treatment of, 752–755
Memory Questionnaire, 313
Mental disorders
  adult life crises and, 124–128, 138–140
  age and, 10–11
  age invariance of, 15, 31
  age of onset and, 10–11
  biopsychosocial perspective, 6, 14, 604, 607, 902
  chronicity, 11–12
  cohorts and, 12
  diagnostic categories, 30–21
  effect of, on function, 679–681
  epidemiology of, 27–73?, 794–796
  insomnia and, 566
  modifying, in later life, 896
  organic vs nonorganic, 795–796
  prevalence, 795, 816–817
  prevalence of, in ethnic populations, 106–112
  prevalence of, in nursing homes, 834–835
  risk factors, 29, 30–31, 100
  See also individual disorders
Mental health
  culture and, 77–97
  defining elements, 7–9
  epidemiological trends in, 901–906
  norms, 7–8
  positive, 9, 339

  primary care and, 18
  relationship to physical health, 906–909
  trends in field of, 910–911
Mental health research and aging
  informed consent and, 868
  needs, 14–16
  progress in, 5–6
  trends in, 13–14
Mental health services
  ageism and, 826
  allocation of, to elderly, 867, 909
  barriers to, 17, 113, 700–701, 798–799, 826
  deinstitutionalization, 16, 794, 816, 834, 873–874, 884
  delivery models, 885–888
  developmental disability sectors, 590–592
  eligibility, 19–20, 797–798
  ethnic minorities and, 112–114, 801
  financing of, 873–889
  formal vs informal service use, 806–809
  general medical sector and, 18, 802–803
  help-seeking vs. volume of care, 800
  heterogeneity of mentally ill elderly and, 794–796
  home care, 804–806
  nursing homes, in, 836–838
  personnel needs, 20–21
  policy recommendations, 16–20, 810
  predictors of use, 801–802
  technology and, 908–909
  treated prevalence, 799–801
  underutilization of, by elderly, 17, 110, 700
  use of, by chronically medically ill, 804
  use of, by developmentally disabled elderly, 591–592
  See also Community mental health services; Psychiatric hospitalization
Mental hospitals
  See Psychiatric hospitalization
Mental retardation
  definition of, 584
  functional abilities and, 588–589
  life expectancy and, 586–587
  prevalence of, 585–586
  service use by persons with, 591
  See also Developmentally disabled elderly
Mental status assessment, 611–167
Mental status tests, 328

Metamemory, 313–314
  assessment instruments, 313
Metamemory in Adulthood Questionnaire, 313
Metamemory Questionnaire, 313
Methadone maintenance, 537
Michigan Alcoholism Screening Test (MAST),
  527
Middle age
  gender trait reversal in, 135–136, 138
Midlife crisis, 133–138
Millon Clinical Multiaxial Inventory (PAS)
Mini-Mental State Examination (MMSE), 35–
  36, 108, 111, 328–329, 617–618, 649,
  657–658, 659
Minnesota Multiphasic Personality Inventory
  (MMPI), 357, 440, 443
Multi-infarct dementia, 343–344, 490–492
  diagnostic criteria, 491
  differential diagnosis, 658–660
  estimated risk of, 34
  features, 343–344
  Hachinski scale, 492
  neuroimaging and, 491
  prevalence, 33, 343, 490
Multilevel Assessment Instrument (MAI), 687,
  692–693
Multiple sclerosis, 633

Narcissism, 80–81, 82–96 passim, 132
Narcissistic loss, 704–705
National Long-term Care Channeling Project,
  885–886
Neurofibrillary tangles, 156–157, 483–484
Neuroimaging, 621–625, 644–646
  depression and, 391
  diagnosis of dementia and, 491–493
  studies of brain aging, 149–151
Neuroleptics
  akathisia and, 421, 735
  behavioral disorders and, 733–736, 842
  institutionalized elderly and, 841, 848
  Parkinsonian and, 184, 469
  selection of, 736
  side effects, 734–736, 841
  treatment for schizophrenia with, 468–469
Neuronal aging
  Dendritic Systems, 158–163
  glial cells, 176–177

granovascular degeneration, 155–156
lipofuscins, 154–155
neurofibrillary tangles, 156–157, 483–484
neuronal loss, 152–154, 176–177
senile plaques, 157–158, 343, 482–483
structural and organizational changes, 154–
  158
Neuropeptides, 181, 486–487
Neuropsychiatric assessment, 603–637
  aims, 607–608
  biopsychosocial model, 604, 607
  case reasoning, 605–607
  clinical history, 608–611
  clinical laboratory assessment, 619–621
  final common behavioral pathways, 604–
    605, 636
  medical and neurological examination, 618–
    619
  mental-status assessment, 611–617
  neuroimaging and, 621–655
  neuropsychological testing and, 625
  standardized procedures, 617–618
  See also Differential diagnosis; Neuro-
    psychological assessment
Neuropsychological assessment, 643–633
  aims, 643
  neuroimaging research, 644–646
  old-age norms, 646–647
  testing, 625, 646–649
  treatment planning, in, 660–661
  See also Differential diagnosis; Neurop-
    sychiatric assessment
Neurosyphillis, 496
Neuroticism, 358, 438
Neurotropic factors
  Alzheimer's disease and, 487
Nocturnal myoclonus, 564–566
Noradrenergic system
  aging changes in, 180
  Alzheimer's disease, in, 486
  depression, in, 898–899
  Parkinson's disease, 488
  personality disorders and, 446
Normal aging
  differentiating from dementia, 328–329,
    649–655, 895–896
  enhancing, 897–898
  personality changes and, 445
Normal-pressure hydrocephalus, 493–494, 632

Norms
    abnormality and, 7–8
    old-age, 646–647
Nursing homes, 833–849
    assessment in, 838–839
    behavioral and environmental interventions,
        845–848
    history of, 833–834
    Medicare/Medicaid coverage and, 878,
        883–884
    mental health services in, 836–838
    pharmacologic interventions in, 840–843
    preadmission psychiatric screening, 849,
        884
    prevalence of problem behaviors in, 835–
        836
    prevalence of mental disorders in, 834–835
    psychotherapeutic approaches in, 843–845
    public policy issues, 848–849
    See also Nursing home design
Nursing home design
    centralization of activities, 776–778, 780
    corridors designed for sociability, 773–775
    decentralized cluster design, 776
    family orientation, 781–782
    outdoor space treatments, 781
    room configurations and privacy, 769–733
    special care units, 846–848
    wayfinding and orientation, 778–779

Object Memory Evaluation, 647, 659
Obsessive–Compulsive Disorder (OCD)
    cognitive decline and, 56
    definition of, 54
    epidemiology of, 54–57
Older Americans Resources Survey (OARS),
    110, 347, 687, 692
Old-old, 11, 585, 904
Olefactory aging, 285–288
    absolute olfactory sensitivity, 286
    compensating for losses in, 288
    structural changes, 285
    suprathreshold odor perception, 286–288
Omnibus Reconciliation Acts, 20, 816, 880–
    882, 884, 885
OnLok senior services program, 887
Operant learning, 706
Opioid dependence, 537

Orality
    deculturation and, 94
Organic hallucinoses, 472–473, 635
Over-the-counter (OTC) drugs, 538–549
    drug interactions, 727
    hypnotics, 538–539
    prevalence of use, 538
    stimulants, 539
    use and abuse, 538

Panic disorder, 413–414
    definition of, 48
    epidemiology of, 48–51
    quality of life and, 234
    treatment of, 746
Paranoia
    hospitalization for, 823–824
    See also Suspiciousness
Paranoid disorders
    hearing loss and, 277
    See also Delusional disorder
Paraphrenia, 466
Parenting
    adult children with developmental dis-
        abilities, 593–594
    parental imperative, 134–135
    transformative crisis, as a, 132
Parkinson's disease
    age of onset and, 190
    aging and, 184–187
    clinical features, 487
    dementia in, 487–490
    differential diagnosis, 656–658
    dopamine system and, 184–187, 190
    hallucinations in, 472
    neuropsychological testing, 656–658
    prevalence, 487–488
    relationship between depression and demen-
        tia in, 501–502
Performance Test of Activities of Daily Living
    (PADL), 686, 690
Personality
    adjusting to aging and, 364–371
    aging and, 355–371, 445–447
    cognitive theory and, 360–371
    culture and, 78–79
    definition of, 436
    extraversion-introversion, 357–358, 437,
        445

locus of control, 362–363
neuroticism, 358, 438
rigidity, 358
self-concept and, 364–365
stability of, 356–359, 435–437
stage theories, 436
time perspective, 360–362
traits, 434
Personality Assessment Schedule (PAS), 440,
454
Personality Diagnostic Questionnaire (PDQ),
441
Personality Disorder Examination, 454–455
Personality Disorder Questionnaire (PDQ),
454–455
Personality disorders, 433–457
assessment, 454–455
classification of, 435
definition of, 434
depression and, 451–452, 455–456
epidemiology of, 437–439
evolution of symptoms with age, 439–441
forced intimacy and, 449–451
institutionalization and, 448–449
life events and, 441
mature vs immature, 441
neurotransmitter function and, 446
organic factors in, 447–448
psychodynamic features, 443
residual and emergent, 445–447
suicide and, 456
symptom expression, 441–445
treatment, 452–453, 702
Philadelphia Geriatric Center Morale Scale,
380
Phobic disorders
definitions, 51
epidemiology of, 51–54
models of, 416–417
simple phobia, 414–415
social phobia, 414
stress and, 126
treatment of, 746
Phonemic regression, 272–274
Physical illness
impact on psychiatric symptoms, 723–724
psychiatric hospitalization and, 824
Physical Self-Maintenance Scale (PSMS), 686,
690
Pick's disease, 344, 492–493

Pittsburgh Sleep Quality Inventory, 569
Polypharmacy, 18, 726–727
Polysubstance-use disorders, 542–543
Positron emission tomography (PET), 151,
202–204, 493, 625, 644, 645, 908
Posttraumatic stress disorder, 415
Presbycusis, 267–271
Presbyopia, 253
Prescription drug-use disorders, 529–535
analgesics, 535
benzodiazopines, 529–535
Privacy
cognitively impaired and, 769–783, 788–
789
Prospective payment system (PPS), 878–
879
Pseudodementia, 14, 386–387, 419, 499,
633–634, 653–655
sleep disturbance and, 572–573
Psychiatric hospitalization, 815–829
assessment, 825
confusion in patients, 820–821
discharge planning, 828–829
interdisciplinary team approach, 825
interventions, 826–829
levels of care, 817–818
management of aggressive behavior, 823
reasons for admission, 817–818
restraints and, 822
Psychoanalytic model
anxiety, of, 416–417
Psychopharmacologic treatment, 721–756
adverse effects, 15
age-related changes in drug effect and,
729–732
anxiety, of, 423–425, 745–750
behavior disorders, of, 732–738
compliance problems, 728–729
complications in elderly, 723–729, 827–
828, 840
depression, of, 393–395, 738–744
disproportionate use with elderly, 804
drug interactions, 726–727
hospital settings, in, 827–828
mania, of, 744–745
nursing homes, in, 18, 529, 840–843
physical illness and, 723–724
prescribing patterns with elderly, 18, 529,
728
sleep disorders, of, 750–752

Psychotherapy
  behavioral interventions, 705–709, 845–846
  cognitive-behavioral, 392–393
  elderly and, 699–700, 826
  group, 710–712, 844
  individual, 702–710
  insight-oriented, 702
  marital, 712
  multigenerational family, 712–714
  nursing homes, in, 843–845
  principles of change, 827
  psychodynamic, 702–705
  supportive, 702
  therapeutic relationship, 700–702
PULSES, 685, 689

Quality of life, 229–246
  chronicity and, 238, 244
  definition of, 231
  diagnosis and, 232, 243
  domains, 232–239
  interaction among domains, 239–242, 245
  measurement, 237, 242, 244
  mental health problems and, 232
  subjective and objective, 234–236, 242–243
  time and, 237–239

Race
  definition of, 104
Rapid Disability Rating Scale (RDRS), 685, 689–690
Reality orientation, 710–711, 845
Reminiscence therapy, 711, 844
Restraints, 822, 845
Rey Auditory Verbal Learning Test, 647
Rigidity, 358
Right to die, 862

Sandoz Clinical Assessment Geriatric (SCAG) Scale, 617
Schedule for Affective Disorders and Schizophrenia (SADS), 709

Schizophrenia, 463–473
  aging and, 184–187, 899
  chronic with early onset, 469–470
  course, 464, 466
  definition of, 464
  diagnostic criteria, 464–466
  differential diagnosis, 388–389
  dopamine system and, 184–187, 899
  late-onset, 466–469, 899
  late-onset vs early-onset, 467–468
  risk factors for late-onset, 468
  stress and, 126–127
  treatment of, with neuroleptics, 468–469
Sedative-hypnotic drug use
  See Benzodiazepine-use disorders
Selective attention, 319–325
  data-driven vs memory-driven, 321–323
  facilitation-inhibition, 323–325
  Spatial Localization Hypothesis, 321
Selective Reminding Test, 646, 651
Self
  psychology of, 704–705
Self-concept, 364–365
Self-esteem
  elderly and, 704–705
Senescence, 10
Senescence theory, 30, 38
Senile dementia of the Alzheimer's type (SDAT)
  See Alzheimer's disease
Senile miosis, 252–253
Senile plaques, 157–158, 343, 482–483
Senile recluse syndrome, 473, 528
Sensory-perceptual aging, 251–295
  future research, 293–295
  peripheral vs central deficits, 293–294
  prevention, 295
  See also Auditory aging; Cutaneous sensitivity; Olefactory aging; Taste; Visual aging
Serotonin system
  aging changes in, 181
  personality disorders and, 446
Severe cognitive impairment, 34–37
  ECA definition and measurement, 34–35
  estimated risk of, 35–37
  treated prevalence, 797–798
Sex differences
  See Gender differences

Short Inventory of Memory Experiences, 313
Single photon emission-computed tomograph (SPECT), 625, 644, 645
Skilled nursing facilities
    See Nursing homes
Sleep
    age-dependent changes, 559–562, 571
    Circadian system, 560–561, 568
    EEG measures of, 559
    effects of drugs on, 751
    gender differences in, 561
    physiology of, 558–559
Sleep apnea, 389, 562–563
Sleep disorders, 557–576
    assessment, 573–574
    daytime sleepiness, 561, 567–568, 750–751
    dementia and, 570–572
    depression and, 389, 567, 569–570, 571
    insomnia, 566–567, 707–708
    mortality rates, 573
    nocturnal myoclonus, 564–566
    physical illness and, 569
    prevalence, 557–558
    pseudodementia and, 572–573
    sleep-disordered breathing, 389, 562–563
    snoring, 562
    treatment, 574–576, 707–708, 750–752
Smoking
    See Tobacco dependence
Smoking cessation, 541–542
Snoring, 562
Social/Health Maintenance Organizations (S/HMOs), 886–887
Social support
    definition of, 105–106
    depression and, 396–397
    ethnic groups, among, 105–106
    family, 18–19, 592–594, 712–714
Somatization, 823
Standardizes Assessment of Personality (SAP), 454
State-Trait Anxiety Inventory (STAI), 412, 419
Stereotypes
    mental health and aging, in, 4, 12
    See also Ageism
Stress
    coping with, 701

ethnic minorities and, 105–106
    locus of control and, 363
    personality disorders and, 339–445
    substance-use disorders and, 519, 525
    See also Adult life crises; Life events
Structured Clinical Interview for DSM-III-R Personality Disorder (SCID-II), 454–455
Structured Interview for DSM-III Personality Disorders (SID-P), 454–455
Subjective Memory Questionnaire, 313
Subjective well-being, 358–359
Substance dependence
    definition, 517
    diagnostic criteria, 518
Substance-use disorders, 515–545
    assessment of, 521
    benzodiazopine-use disorders, 529–535
    cohort and period effects and, 516–518
    definitions, 57, 516–517
    estimated risk, 60–62
    epidemiology of, 57–63, 516–521
    future case volume, 543
    illegal drug use, 536–537, 902
    management/treatment, 521–522
    opioid dependence, 536–537
    over-the-counter (OTC) drugs, 538–540
    polysubstance-use disorders, 542–543
    prescription drug-use disorders, 529–535
    prevalence, 58–60, 521
    prevention, 544–545
    risk factors, 62–63, 516–519, 520
    service planning, 543–544
    substance dependence, 517, 518
    tobacco dependence, 540–542
    under-recognition of, in later life, 519–520
    See also Alcohol-use disorders
Successful aging, 104, 113, 897–898
Suicide, 397–400, 819–820
    attempters vs completers, 456
    epidemiology of, 397–398
    management of suicidal patients, 399–400, 820
    personality disorder and, 456
    risk factors, 398–399, 820, 903–904
    silent, 857
Sundowning, 572
Suspiciousness, 470–472
    delirium, in, 471–472
    dementia, in, 471–472, 707

Suspiciousness (*cont.*)
  isolated, 470–471
  nonschizophrenic syndromes, in, 471

Tardive dyskinesia, 469, 735–736, 841
Taste, 278–284
  absolute taste sensitivity, 280–281
  flavor recognition, 284
  structural changes with age, 279–280
  suprathreshold taste perception, 281–284
Tax Equity and Fiscal Responsibility Act
    (TEFRA), 878–879, 885
Time perspective, 360–362
Tinnitis, 267
Tithonos
  myth of, 895
Tobacco dependence, 540–542
  health consequences, 540–541
  prevalence, 540
  smoking cessation, 541–542
Trazedone, 743
  treatment of agitation and, 737

Ventricular enlargement, 149–151
Visual aging, 252–265
  acuity, 255–257
  color sensitivity, 264
  contrast sensitivity, 257–259
  dynamic visual acuity, 262
  flicker sensitivity, 262–263
  motion sensitivity, 263–264
  oculomotor function, 254

psychophysical studies, 253–254
spatial resolution, 254–262
stereopsis, 259–260
structural changes, 252–253
temporal resolution, 262–264
visibility under adverse viewing conditions,
    260–262
visual pathologies, 265
visual search, 260

Wandering, 821–822, 845–846
  gardens, 781
  management of, 784–785, 822, 845–846,
    847
Washington University dementia battery, 648–
    649
Ways-of-Coping Questionnaire, 365
Wechsler Adult Intelligence Scale (WAIS),
    151, 341, 348, 349, 351, 356, 618, 647
Wechsler Memory Scale (WMS), 151, 328,
    646, 647
Widowhood, 103, 129–131, 904
Wills
  competency and, 855–856
Women, 103, 874, 904
  ethnic minority, 103, 114
  future time perspective of, 360–362

X-ray radiography, 622

Zung Depression Scale, 380